Contents in Brief

UNIT I OVERVIEW OF MATERNAL AND PEDIATRIC HEALTH CARE 1

1 The Nurse's Role in a Changing Maternal–Child Health Care Environment 3

2 Family-Centered and Community-Based Maternal and Pediatric Nursing 25

UNIT II FOUNDATIONS OF MATERNITY NURSING 43

3 Structure and Function of the Reproductive System 45

4 Special Issues of Women's Health Care and Reproduction 59

UNIT III PREGNANCY 97

5 Fetal Development 99

6 Maternal Adaptation During Pregnancy 117

7 Prenatal Care 135

UNIT IV LABOR AND BIRTH 165

8 The Labor Process 167

9 Pain Management During Labor and Birth 184

10 Nursing Care During Labor and Birth 202

11 Assisted Delivery and Cesarean Birth 238

UNIT V POSTPARTUM AND NEWBORN 259

12 The Postpartum Woman 261

13 Nursing Assessment of Newborn Transition 284

14 Nursing Care of the Normal Newborn 304

15 Newborn Nutrition 324

UNIT VI CHILDBEARING AT RISK 343

16 Pregnancy at Risk: Conditions That Complicate Pregnancy 345

17 Pregnancy at Risk: Pregnancy-Related Complications 381

18 Labor at Risk 409

19 Postpartum Woman at Risk 426

20 The Newborn at Risk: Gestational and Acquired Disorders 450

21 The Newborn at Risk: Congenital Disorders 478

UNIT VII HEALTH PROMOTION FOR NORMAL GROWTH AND DEVELOPMENT 515

22 Principles of Growth and Development 517

23 Growth and Development of the Infant: 28 Days to 1 Year 538

24 Growth and Development of the Toddler: 1 to 3 Years 557

25 Growth and Development of the Preschool Child: 3 to 6 Years 574

26 Growth and Development of the School-Aged Child: 6 to 10 Years 588

27 Growth and Development of the Adolescent: 11 to 18 Years 604

UNIT VIII FOUNDATIONS OF PEDIATRIC NURSING 621

28 Assessment of the Child (Data Collection) 623

29 Care of the Hospitalized Child 643

30 Procedures and Treatments 662

31 Medication Administration and Intravenous Therapy 680

UNIT IX SPECIAL CONCERNS OF PEDIATRIC NURSING 697

32 The Child With a Chronic Health Problem 699

33 Abuse in the Family 711

34 The Dying Child 722

UNIT X THE CHILD WITH A HEALTH DISORDER 741

35 The Child With a Sensory/Neurological Disorder 743

36 The Child With a Respiratory Disorder 775

37 The Child With a Cardiovascular/Hematologic Disorder 804

38 The Child With a Gastrointestinal/Endocrine Disorder 827

39 The Child With a Genitourinary Disorder 867

40 The Child With a Musculoskeletal Disorder 880

41 The Child With an Integumentary Disorder/Communicable Diseases 899

42 The Child With a Psychosocial Disorder 937

Appendix A: Standard and Transmission-Based Precautions 959
Appendix B: NANDA-Approved Nursing Diagnoses 961
Appendix C: The Joint Commission's "Do Not Use" Abbreviations, Acronyms, and Symbols 964
Appendix D: Good Sources of Essential Nutrients 965
Appendix E: Breast-feeding and Medication Use 966
Appendix F: Cervical Dilation Chart 968
Appendix G: Growth Charts 969
Appendix H: Pulse, Respiration, and Blood Pressure Values for Children 975
Appendix I: Temperature and Weight Conversion Charts 976
Appendix J: Recommended Childhood and Adolescent Immunization Schedules 979
Glossary 981
English-Spanish Glossary 996
References and Suggested Readings 1001
Index 1025

i

A-A-

Introductory Maternity & Pediatric Nursing

SECOND EDITION

N. Jayne Klossner, MSN, RNC
Director, Patient Care Improvement
Baptist Health System
San Antonio, Texas

Nancy T. Hatfield, MAE, BSN, RN
Former Program Director
Albuquerque Public Schools
Practical Nursing Program
Albuquerque, New Mexico

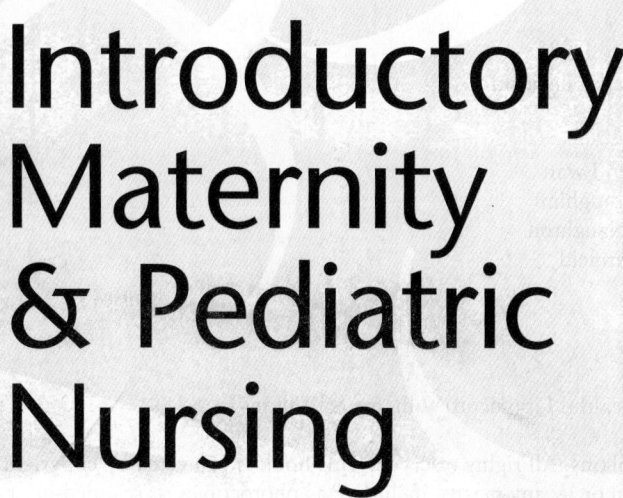 Wolters Kluwer | Lippincott Williams & Wilkins
Health
Philadelphia · Baltimore · New York · London
Buenos Aires · Hong Kong · Sydney · Tokyo

Executive Acquisitions Editor: Elizabeth Nieginski
Development Editor: Betsy Gentzler
Product Manager: Helene T. Caprari
Director of Nursing Production: Helen Ewan
Art Director, Design: Holly Reid McLaughlin
Art Director, Illustration: Brett MacNaughton
Manufacturing Coordinator: Karin Duffield
Production Services: Aptara

2nd Edition

9 8 7 6 5 4 3 2 1

Printed in China.

Library of Congress Cataloging-in-Publication Data
Klossner, N. Jayne.
   Introductory maternity & pediatric nursing / N. Jayne Klossner, Nancy T. Hatfield. — 2nd ed.
      p. ; cm.
   Includes bibliographical references and index.
   ISBN-13: 978-0-7817-8558-7 (hardback : alk. paper)
   ISBN-10: 0-7817-8558-8 (hardback : alk. paper) 1.   Maternity nursing. 2.   Pediatric nursing. I. Hatfield, Nancy T. II. Title.
III. Title: Introductory maternity and pediatric nursing.
   [DNLM: 1.   Maternal-Child Nursing—methods. 2.   Nursing Process. 3.   Pediatric Nursing—methods. WY 157.3 K66i 2010]
   RG951.K565 2010
   618.92'00231—dc22

                                                                                          2009022770

To Kevin
My husband, my partner, my friend—I love you with all my heart

To Katelyn, Joshua, and Jonathan
You are my heart. I love you always!

To Keri & Diane
You have made my sons happy, and you both are such wonderful mothers to my grandchildren. I couldn't have chosen better daughters-in-law had I tried.

Jayne

To John
My partner, my best friend; you are the light and love of my life!

To Mikayla and Jeff and Greg and Chelsea
You taught me about children, caring, and happiness and the joys of being a Mom!

To Sierra, Jaymin, Riley, and Hayley
Being your Nana has given me new understanding of the depth and meaning of love!

To Mom and Dad
Your unconditional love allowed me to be the child I was and the adult I am!

Nancy

Reviewers

Donna Alt, RN, MSN
Ivy Tech State College
Sellersburg, Indiana

Lisa Barrow
Nursing Professor
Kaskaskia College
Centralia, Illinois

Terry Bichsel, RN, BSN
Practical Nursing Coordinator,
Moberly Area Community College
Moberly, Missouri

Karen Brown, PhD
Associate Dean
Kirtland Community College
Roscommon, Michigan

Jacquelyn Bryant
Practical Nursing Instructor
Lanier Tech College
Oakwood, Georgia

Monica Cauley, RN, MSN, GCNS
Chair, Health Sciences
Lurleen B Wallace Community College
Opp, Alabama

Carol Lee Cherry, RN, MSN, CNE
Faculty, Nursing Program
Brown Mackie College,
Indianapolis, Indiana

Deirdre Conroy
License Practical Nursing
Cumberland County Technical
    Education Center
Bridgeton, New Jersey

Marsha Conroy, RN, MSN
Nurse Educator
Cuyahoga Community College
Cleveland, Ohio

Linda Crawford
Coastal Georgia Community College
Brunswick, Georgia

Annette Crew-Gooden
Trenholm State Technical College
Montgomery, Alabama

Susanne Cubberley, MSN, RN
Nurse Educator
Pinellas County Schools
Largo, Florida

Marian T. Doyle, RN, MSN, MS
Associate Professor, Nursing
Northampton Community College
Bethlehem, Pennsylvania

Yolanda P. Endaya, RNC, MSN, IBCLC
Assistant Patient Care Manager-
    Perinatal Services

Kansas City, Missouri
Adjunct Faculty- Practical Nursing
    Program
North Kansas City Missouri

Kimberly Friedmeyer, RN, MEd
Assistant Principal for Curriculum
Learey Technical Center
Tampa, Florida

Katherine Fukuyama, BSN, MEd
Department Head BSN Program
Vancouver Community College
Vancouver, British Columbia, Canada

Carol Gillis
Bucks County Community College
Newtown, Pennsylvania

Joanne Hartzell, RN, MS
Director of Tri County ROP Vocational
    Nursing Program
Director of Sutter Co. One Stop RN
    Refresher Program-Health Careers
Yuba City, California

Julie Hansen, MS, MA, RN
Faculty, Undergraduate Nursing &
    Nursing Accelerated Program
South Dakota State University
Brookings, South Dakota

Joyce Harper, RN, BSN
Vocational Nursing Instructor
Victoria College
Victoria, Texas

Charla K. Hollin, RN, BSN
Nursing Program Director
Rich Mountain Community College
Mena, Arkansas

Brenda J. Holmes, RN BS
Assistant Professor/ Adjunct Nursing
    Instructor
Practical Nursing Program
Brevard Community College
Cocoa, Florida

Susan C. Jewell, MS, RN
Nursing Department Chair
Ivy Tech Community College –
    Southern Indiana
Sellersburg, Indiana

Melissa Jones, RN, BSN
Practical Nurse Coordinator
Waynesville Practical Nursing School
Waynesville, Missouri

Mary Ann Kennedy, RNC, BSN, Master
    of Arts in teaching
Department Head of LPN Program
J.M. Wright Technical School
Stamford, Connecticut

Sharon Powell-Laney, RN, MSN
Coordinator of Practical Nursing
Jefferson County-DuBois A.V.T.S.
Reynoldsville, Pennsylvania

Donna Kuenstler, RN, MSN
Department Chair-Vocational Nursing
Sul Ross State University
Alpine, Texas

Lorraine Lowen
Nursing
Central New Mexico Community
    College
Albuquerque, New Mexico

Pamela Mahmoudi, RN, MS
Director of Tri Co. ROP Vocational
    Nursing Program-
Director of Sutter Co. One Stop RN
    Refresher Program-Health Careers
    Coordinator
Yuba City, California

Nadia Martindale
Vocational Nursing
Angelina College
Lufkin, Texas

Lori Moseley, RN, AAS, BS, MSN, CNE
Dean of Instruction for Health Sciences
Director of Nursing
Hill College
Hillsboro, Texas

Debbie Nolder
Division Chair, Associate
    Professor/Coordinator, PN
Maysville Community and Technical
    College
Maysville, Kentucky

Regina Okeowo, RN, MSN, MPH, CNE
Nurse Educator
Trenholm State Tech College
Montgomery, Alabama

Brenda Overton, RN, MSN
Assistant Professor, Nursing Program
Baltimore City Community College
Baltimore, Maryland

Raphael Pascua
College Director
Prime Career College
Vallejo, California

Rachel Poorman, RN, BSN
IOT LPN Online Instructor
Sinte Gleska University
Mission, South Dakota

Cheryl Puckett, OB-RNC, MSN
Associate Professor of Nursing
Bluegrass Community and Technical
    College
Danville, Kentucky

Rosemary Pullin, RN, BSN, CLNC
*Director of the Vocational Nursing
    Program*
Schreiner University
Kerrville, Texas

Lisa Richwine, RN, MSN, NP, CLNC
Faculty, Practical Nursing
Ivy Tech Community College
Anderson, Indiana

Ellie Riggs, RN, BSN, MS
Clinical Instructor
Wise County Career-Technical Center
Wise, Virginia

Sarah K. Roland, MSN, RN
ADN Instructor
Central Carolina Technical College
Sumter, South Carolina

Rebecca Romagna, RN, MSN
Nursing Instructor
Greater Altoona Career & Technology
    Center
Altoona, Pennsylvania

Marcia Scherer, RN, MS, PHN, LSN
Practical Nursing Instructor
Hennepin Technical College
Eden Prairie, Minnesota

Connie Scherger
Hennepin Technical College
Eden Prairie, Minnesota

Jacquie Scobie, RN, Master of Arts in
    Leadership and Training MA (LT)
Practical Nursing Program
College of New Caledonia
British Columbia, Canada

Lori Shortridge, RN, MScN
Faculty, Community and Health Studies
Kwantlen Polytechnic University
Surrey, British Columbia, Canada

Kristine Simoni
Anoka Technical College
Anoka, Minnesota

Mona D. Speak, RN, MSN, FNP-BC
Family Nurse Practitioner
Litton Family Medicine
Pennington Gap, Virginia

Dori Steers
Faculty, Practical Nursing Department
Rogue Community College
Medford, Oregon

Brigitte Thiele
*Coordinator of Practical Nursing
    Education*
Kennet Career and Technology Center
Kennett, Missouri

Sandra Thompson
Licensed Practical Nursing Staff
Mercer County Technical Education
    Center
Princeton, Wisconsin

Regina Torelli, MS, RN
LPN Instructor
Monmouth County Vocational School
    District
Neptune, New Jersey

Melissa Vander Stucken, BSN, RN
Vocational Nursing Instructor
Victoris College
Victoria, Texas

Jessica Webb
Lord Fairfax Community College
Middletown, Virginia

Dian Wright, BSN, AS, MBA, MSN
Department Chair
Ivy Tech Community College
Sellersburg, Indiana

Patti Yudelson, MSN, RN
Nurse Educator, Adult Practical
    Nursing Program
Western Suffolk BOCES
Huntington Station, New York

This second edition of *Introductory Maternity and Pediatric Nursing* reflects the underlying philosophy of love, caring, and support for the childbearing woman, the child, and the families of these individuals. The content has been developed according to the most current information available. In this text, we recognize that cultural sensitivity and awareness are important aspects of caring for the childbearing and child-rearing families. We also recognize that many children and pregnant women live in families other than traditional two-parent family homes and therefore refer to teaching and supporting the childbearing clients and family caregivers of children in all situations and family structures.

Maternal-child health care has seen a shift from the hospital setting into community and home settings. More responsibility has fallen on the family and family caregivers to care for the pregnant woman or ill child. We stress teaching the patient, the family, and the child, with an emphasis on prevention. The nursing process has been used as the foundation for presenting nursing care. Implementation information is presented in a narrative format to enable the discussion from which planning, goal setting, and evaluation can be put into action. The newest and most current NANDA terminology has been used for the possible nursing diagnoses for health care concerns.

Our goal in this text is to keep the readability of the text at a level with which the student can be comfortable. The second edition was carefully reviewed and edited to make what was a very readable text even more readable. In recognition of the limited time that the student has and the frustrations that can result from having to turn to a dictionary or glossary for words that are unfamiliar, we have attempted to identify all possible unfamiliar terms and define them within the text. This increases the reading ease for the student, decreasing the time necessary to complete the assigned reading and enhancing the understanding of the information. A full-color format, current photos, drawings, tables, and diagrams further aid the student in using this text. Hundreds of new drawings and photos are included in this second edition.

RECURRING FEATURES

In an effort to provide the instructor and student with a text that is informative, exciting, and easy to use, we have incorporated a number of special features throughout the text, many of which are included in each chapter.

Learning Objectives

Measurable student-oriented objectives are included at the beginning of each chapter. These help to guide the student in recognizing what is important and why, and they provide the instructor with guidance for evaluating the student's understanding of the information presented in the chapter.

Key Terms

A list of terms that may be unfamiliar to students and that are considered essential to the chapter's understanding is at the beginning of each chapter. The first appearance in the chapter of each of these terms is in boldface type, with the definition included in the text. All key terms can be found in a glossary at the end of the text.

Nursing Process

The nursing process serves as an organizing structure for the discussion of nursing care covered in the text. This feature provides the student with a foundation from which individualized nursing care plans can be developed. Each Nursing Process section includes the nurse's role in caring for the patient and family and also includes nursing assessment, relevant nursing diagnoses, outcome identification and planning, implementation, and evaluation of the goals and expected outcomes. Emphasis is placed on the importance of involving the family and family caregivers in the assessment process. In the Nursing Process sections, we have used current NANDA-approved nursing diagnoses. These are used to represent appropriate concerns for a particular condition, but we do not attempt to include all diagnoses that could be identified. The student will find the goals specific, measurable, and realistic and will be able to relate the goals to patient situations and care plan development. The expected outcomes and evaluation provide a goal for each nursing diagnosis and criteria to measure the successful accomplishment of that goal.

Nursing Care Plans

Throughout the text, Nursing Care Plans provide the student with a model to follow in using the information from the nursing process to develop specific nursing care plans. To make the care plans more meaningful, a scenario has been constructed for each one.

Nursing Procedures

Needed equipment and step-by-step instructions are included to help the students understand the procedures. These instructions can be easily used in a clinical setting to perform nursing procedures.

Family Teaching Tips

Information that the student can use in teaching the maternity patient, family caregivers, and children is presented in highlighted boxes ready for use.

Clinical Secrets

A recurring cartoon nurse provides brief clinical pearls. The student will find these valuable in caring for patients in clinical settings. Safety, nutrition, and pharmacology concerns, as well as other important issues to consider are highlighted.

Personal Glimpse With Learning Opportunity

Personal Glimpses, included in every chapter, present actual first-person narratives, unedited, just as the individual wrote them. Personal Glimpses offer the student a view of an experience an individual has had in a given situation and of that person's feelings about or during the incident. These narratives are presented to enhance the student's understanding and appreciation of the feelings of others. A Learning Opportunity at the end of each Personal Glimpse encourages students to think of how they might react or respond in the situation presented. These questions further enhance the student's critical thinking.

Cultural Snapshot

These boxes highlight issues and topics that may have cultural considerations. The student is encouraged to think about cultural differences and the importance of accepting the attitudes and beliefs of individuals from cultures other than his or her own.

Tables, Drawings, and Photographs

These important aspects of the text have been updated and developed in an effort to help the student visualize the content covered. Many color photographs in a variety of settings are included. The second edition also includes hundreds of new illustrations.

Key Points

Key Points listed at the end of each chapter help the student focus on important aspects of the chapter. The Key Points provide a quick review of essential content and address all Learning Objectives stated at the beginning of the chapter.

Internet Resources

At the end of each chapter, Web sites are included as resources for the student to gather information on certain conditions, diseases, and disorders. Web sites that offer support and information for families are listed as well.

LEARNING OPPORTUNITIES

In order to offer students opportunities to check their understanding of material they have read and studied, we have included many learning opportunities throughout the text.

Test Yourself

These questions interspersed throughout each chapter and are designed to test understanding and recall of the material presented. The student will quickly determine if a review of what he or she just read is needed.

Workbook

At the end of each chapter, the student will find a workbook section that includes:

- **NCLEX-Style Review Questions** are written to test the student's ability to apply the material from the chapter. These questions use the client-nurse format to encourage the student to critically think about patient situations as well as the nurse's response or action. Alternate format style questions have been included.
- **Study Activities** include interactive activities requiring the student to participate in the learning process. Important material from the chapter has been incorporated into this section to help the student review and synthesize the chapter content. The instructor will find many of the activities appropriate for individual or class assignments. Within the Study Activities, many chapters include an **Internet Activity** that helps the student explore the Internet. Each activity takes the student step by step into a site where he or she can access new and updated information as well as resources to share with patients and families. Some include fun activities to use with pediatric patients. These activities may require the use of Acrobat Reader, which can be downloaded free of charge.
- **Critical Thinking: What Would You Do?** questions present real-life situations and encourage the student to think about the chapter content in practical terms. These situations require the student to incorporate knowledge gained from the chapter and apply it to real-life problems. Questions provide the student with opportunities to problem solve, think critically, and discover his or her own ideas and feelings. The instructor also can use the questions as tools to stimulate class discussion. Dosage Calculations are found in the Workbook section of each pediatric chapter where diseases and disorders are covered. These questions offer the student practice in dosage calculations that can be directly applied in a clinical setting.

ORGANIZATION

The text is divided into 10 units to provide an orderly approach to the content. The first unit helps build a foundation for the student beginning the study of maternity and pediatric nursing. This unit introduces the student to caring for the childbearing woman and for children in various settings.

Maternity nursing content is covered in Units 2 through 6. Maternity topics that address the low-risk woman are covered first in Units 2 to 5. Unit 6 addresses issues related to at-risk pregnancy, childbirth, and newborn care. The instructor may choose to teach the normal content of pregnancy followed by the at-risk pregnancy chapters, if desired. However, the author designed the content so that normal considerations would be covered first followed by discussion of the at-risk woman, fetus, and neonate. This grouping ensures that all normal content is covered before any at-risk topics are addressed, which cuts down on the need for parenthetical content in the at-risk chapters. It also encourages the student to review the normal chapters when studying the at-risk content. This repetition of content is designed to help cement the student's understanding of the material. In Unit 6, the at-risk disorders are organized so that an explanation of the disorder is covered first followed by a discussion of medical treatment and nursing care.

Pediatric nursing content comprises Units 7 through 10. The basic approach to the study of caring for the child is organized within a unit discussing health promotion for normal growth and development for each age group. Subsequent units discuss foundational pediatric nursing topics as well as special concerns. Finally, the specific health problems seen in children are covered using a body systems approach. This approach, which is often used in nursing education curriculums, provides a user-friendly approach to the study of nursing care of children.

Unit 1, Overview of Maternal and Pediatric Health Care

Unit 1 introduces the student in Chapter 1 to a brief history of maternity and pediatric nursing, and discusses current trends in maternal-child health care and maternal-child health status issues and concerns. A brief discussion of the nursing process is also included. Chapter 2 follows with a discussion of the family, its structure, and family factors that influence childbearing and child rearing. The chapter introduces community-based health care and discusses the various settings in the community through which health care is provided for the maternity client and the child.

Unit 2, Foundations of Maternity Nursing

Unit 2 introduces the student in Chapter 3 to male and female reproductive anatomy, which is essential to the understanding of maternity nursing. The menstrual cycle and the sexual response cycle are also addressed. (Note: Pelvic anatomy is addressed in Chapter 8, and breast anatomy is addressed in Chapter 14.) Chapter 4 continues with a discussion of special reproductive issues to include family planning, elective termination of pregnancy, and issues of fertility.

Unit 3, Pregnancy

Unit 3 begins in Chapter 5 with a discussion of fetal development from fertilization through the fetal period. Chapter 6 introduces the student to diagnosis of pregnancy, physiologic and psychological adaptation of the woman during pregnancy; the chapter ends by outlining nutritional requirements of pregnancy. Chapter 7 covers the nurse's role in prenatal care and assessment of fetal well-being during pregnancy.

Unit 4, Labor and Birth

Unit 4 begins with a discussion of the labor process in Chapter 8. The four components of birth, the process of labor, and maternal and fetal adaptation to labor are covered. Female pelvic anatomy is discussed here. Chapter 9 introduces the student to concepts of pain management during labor and birth. The chapter begins with an overview of the characteristics and nature of labor pain as well as general principles of labor pain management. Nonpharmacologic and pharmacologic methods of pain management are reviewed. Chapter 10 covers the nurse's role during labor and birth to include assessment of the fetus through fetal monitoring and other methods. The nurse's role in each stage of labor is covered within the framework of the nursing process. The nurse-controlled delivery is also covered in this chapter. Chapter 11 discusses cesarean birth, version, cervical ripening procedures, induction and augmentation of labor, amnioinfusion, assisted delivery (including episiotomy, vacuum, and forceps delivery), and vaginal birth after cesarean.

Unit 5, Postpartum and Newborn

Unit 5 begins with a discussion of normal postpartum adaptation, nursing assessment, and nursing care in Chapter 12. Chapter 13 covers topics related to normal transition of the neonate to extrauterine life, general characteristics of the neonate, and the initial nursing assessment of the newborn. Chapter 14 presents the nurse's role in caring for the normal newborn and includes nursing care considerations in the stabilization and transition of the newborn, normal newborn care, assessment and facilitation of family interaction and adjustment, and discharge considerations. An emphasis is placed on teaching the new parents to care for their newborn. Chapter 15 delves into issues of infant nutrition. Breast-feeding and formula-feeding are presented, along with factors that affect a woman's selection of a feeding method, as well as advantages and disadvantages of each method. Physiology of breast-feeding, including breast anatomy, is covered here. The nurse's role in assisting the woman who is breast-feeding and the woman who is formula-feeding is also discussed.

Unit 6, Childbearing Atat Risk

Unit 6 begins with a focus on pregnancy at risk. Chapter 16 focuses on the pregnancy that is placed at risk by pre-existing and chronic medical conditions of the woman. This chapter covers the major medical conditions, such as diabetes and heart disease, as well as exposure to substances harmful to the fetus, threats from intimate partner violence, and age-related concerns on either end of the age spectrum. Chapter 17 introduces the student to the pregnancy that becomes at risk because of pregnancy-related complications and disorders.

Threats from hyperemesis, bleeding disorders of pregnancy, hypertensive disorders, and blood incompatibilities are presented. Chapter 18 covers topics associated with the at-risk labor, such as dysfunctional labor, preterm labor, postterm labor, placental abnormalities, and emergencies associated with labor and birth. Chapter 19 looks at the postpartum woman at risk. Postpartum hemorrhage, subinvolution, infection, thrombophlebitis, malattachment, grief reaction, and postpartum depression and psychosis are addressed. In Chapter 20, gestational concerns and acquired disorders of the newborn are discussed. Chapter 21 addresses congenital disorders of the newborn, including congenital malformations, inborn errors of metabolism, and chromosomal abnormalities.

Unit 7, Health Promotion for Normal Growth and Development

Unit 7 begins with Chapter 22, Principles of Growth and Development, which provides a foundation for discussion of growth and development in later chapters. The issues of children of divorce, latchkey children, runaway children, and homeless children and families are examined. Influences on and theories of growth and development are presented. The rest of this unit is organized by developmental stages, from infancy through adolescence. It includes aspects of normal growth and development.

Unit 8, Foundations of Pediatric Nursing

Unit 8 presents Chapter 28, which covers collecting subjective and objective data from the child and the family. The chapter also includes interviewing and obtaining a history, general physical assessments and exams, and assisting with diagnostic tests. Chapter 29 presents the pediatric unit, infection control in the pediatric setting, admission and discharge, the child undergoing surgery, pain management, the hospital play program, and safety in the hospital. Chapter 30 covers specific procedures for the pediatric patient as well as the role of the nurse in assisting with procedures and treatments. Chapter 31 includes dosage calculation, administration of medications by various routes, and intravenous therapy.

Unit 9, Special Concerns of Pediatric Nursing

Unit 9 begins with Chapter 32, which presents the concerns that face the family of a child with a chronic illness. The chapter discusses the impact on the family caring for a child with a chronic illness and the nurse's role in assisting and supporting these families. Chapter 33 explores the serious issue of child abuse in its many forms and addresses the problems of domestic violence and parental substance abuse and the impact that they have on the child. Chapter 34 concludes this unit with the dying child. Included in this chapter is a teaching aid to help the nurse perform a self-examination of personal attitudes about death and dying, as well as concrete guidelines to use when interacting with a grieving child or adult.

Unit 10, The Child With a Health Disorder

Unit 10 is structured according to a body systems approach as the basis for discussion of diseases and disorders seen in children. A brief review of basic anatomy and physiology of the body system discussed begins each chapter. Throughout the text, family-centered care is stressed. The nursing process and nursing care plans are integrated throughout this unit. Developmental enrichment and stimulation are stressed in the sections on nursing process. The basic premise of each child's self-worth is fundamental in all of the nursing care presented.

Appendices, Glossary, and References

Ten appendices are included at the back of the text and contain important information for the nursing student in maternity and pediatrics courses. Appendices include:

- Appendix A: Standard and Transmission-Based Precautions
- Appendix B: NANDA-Approved Nursing Diagnoses
- Appendix C: The Joint Commission's "Do Not Use" Abbreviations, Acronyms, and Symbols
- Appendix D: Good Sources of Essential Nutrients
- Appendix E: Breast-feeding and Medication Use
- Appendix F: Cervical Dilation Chart
- Appendix G: Growth Charts
- Appendix H: Pulse, Respiration, and Blood Pressure Values in Children
- Appendix I: Temperature and Weight Conversion Charts
- Appendix J: Recommended Childhood and Adolescent Immunization Schedules

The text concludes with a **Glossary** of key terms, an **English-Spanish Glossary** of maternity and pediatric phrases, and a listing of **References and Selected Readings**.

TEACHING/LEARNING PACKAGE
Resources for Instructors

Tools to assist you with teaching your course are available on the Instructor's Resource CD-ROM and on thePoint at http://thePoint.lww.com/KlossnerHatfield2e:

- The **Test Generator** lets you put together exclusive new tests from a bank containing over 1,200 questions, spanning the book's topics in both maternity and pediatrics, to help you in assessing your students' understanding of the material.
- An extensive collection of materials is provided for each book chapter:
  - **Pre-Lecture Quizzes** (and answers) are quick, knowledge-based assessments that allow you to check students' reading.
  - **PowerPoint Presentations** provide an easy way for you to integrate the textbook with your students' classroom experience, either via slide shows or handouts.

- **Guided Lecture Notes** walk you through the chapters, objective by objective, and provide you with corresponding PowerPoint slide numbers.
- **Discussion Topics** (and suggested answers) can be used as conversation starters or in online discussion boards.
- **Assignments** (and suggested answers) include group, written, clinical, and web assignments.
- **Case Studies** with related questions (and suggested answers) give students an opportunity to apply their knowledge to a client case similar to one they might encounter in practice.
- The **Image Bank** lets you use the photographs and illustrations from this textbook in your PowerPoint slides or as you see fit in your course.
- **Answers to Workbook Questions** from the book are provided.
- A sample **syllabus** provides guidance for structuring your maternity and pediatric nursing course.
- **Journal Articles** offer access to current research available in Lippincott Williams & Wilkins journals.

Resources for Students

Valuable learning tools for students are available on thePoint✴ at http://thePoint.lww.com/KlossnerHatfield2e. Many of these resources are also included on the free Student's Resource CD-ROM bound in the front of this textbook. Resources include:

- **NCLEX-style Review Questions** that correspond with each book chapter help students review important concepts and practice for the NCLEX.
- **Pediatric Dosage Calculation Problems** let students practice important calculation skills.
- **Watch & Learn Video Clips** demonstrate important concepts related to the developmental tasks of pregnancy, vaginal birth, cesarean delivery, breastfeeding, care of the hospitalized child, medication administration, and developmental considerations in caring for children. Icons appear in the text to direct students to relevant video clips.
- A **Spanish-English Audio Glossary** provides helpful terms and phrases for communicating with clients who speak Spanish.
- **Journal Articles** offer access to current research available in Lippincott Williams & Wilkins journals.

Contact your sales representative or visit www.LWW.com/Nursing for details and ordering information.

Acknowledgments

Many people were involved in the creation of this second edition of **Introductory Maternity and Pediatric Nursing.** We worked with some of these individuals on a frequent and ongoing basis, while others, we do not even know their names. With gratitude and appreciation we would like to express our thanks to all of the Lippincott Williams & Wilkins team whether they had a small or a large part in the process of publishing this textbook. We especially want to express our appreciation to:

Betsy Gentzler, Associate Development Editor, for her exceptional skill, expertise and precision in the ongoing revision of this text. Her ability to manage this project and her ideas and suggestions helped refine, strengthen, and improve the quality of this revision. Betsy, you are incredible!

Helene Caprari, Associate Development Editor and Product Manager, for stepping in to help complete the final aspects of the text, the ancillary materials, and getting the final project to production. Helene, we appreciate you!

Elizabeth Nieginski, Executive Acquisitions Editor, for her support behind the scenes managing the business aspects of the project.

Laura Scott, Senior Editorial Assistant, for her enthusiasm and help obtaining reviews and assisting with the many necessary administrative tasks.

Audrey Alt, Ancillary Editor, for her initial work planning the ancillary materials.

N. Jayne Klossner
Nancy J. Hatfield

Kevin, thank you from the bottom of the heart for all the support you have given me throughout this project. Thank you for making me laugh and helping me keep my sense of humor when it seemed the book would never be finished. Thank you, Frannie Rettig, for your faith in me that I could do this project when I first took it on. Thank you, Steve Angle for understanding when I had to miss choir rehearsals. Thanks to my boss, Jana Stonestreet, for allowing me to take PTO so I could finish this project. I couldn't have done it without all of you.

Jayne

My heartfelt thanks go to my husband, John, for his never-ending love, confidence, patience, and encouragement, and his sincere support of this project. His help with the everyday household responsibilities was invaluable in allowing me the time I needed to complete this text. I appreciate and thank my children Mikayla and Jeff, their spouses Greg and Chelsea, and my parents Edgar and Lucy Thomas for their love, phone calls, and positive words of encouragement-always just when I needed them. A special thanks to my grandchildren Sierra, Jaymin, Riley, and Hayley for reminding me how much I love children. My extended family and special friends offered support, listened to me, and gave me insight and advice-always affirming this project could be accomplished. Thank you all.

Nancy

Contents

UNIT I   OVERVIEW OF MATERNAL AND PEDIATRIC HEALTH CARE 1

1   The Nurse's Role in a Changing Maternal–Child Health Care Environment 3

Changing Concepts in Maternal–Child Health Care 4
  Development of Maternity Care 4
  Development of Pediatric Care 5
Current Trends in Maternal–Child Health Care 6
  Family-Centered Care 6
  Regionalized Care 6
  Advances in Research 8
  Bioethical Issues 8
  Demographic Trends 9
  Poverty 9
  Cost Containment 9
Payment for Health Services 12
  Private Insurance 12
  Federally Funded Sources 12
  Specialized Services 13
Maternal–Child Health Today 14
  Maternal–Infant Health Status 14
  Child and Adolescent Health Status 15
  Addressing Maternal–Child Health Status 17
The Nurse's Changing Role in Maternal–Child Health Care 18
Critical Thinking 20
The Nursing Process 21
  Assessment 21
  Nursing Diagnosis 21
  Outcome Identification and Planning 21
  Implementation 22
  Evaluation 22
Documentation 22

2   Family-Centered and Community-Based Maternal and Pediatric Nursing 25

The Family as a Social Unit 25
  Family Function 26
  Family Structure 27
  Family Factors That Influence Childbearing and Child Rearing 29
Health Care Shift: From Hospital to Community 31

Community-Based Nursing 31
Community Care Settings for the Maternity Client 32
Community Care Settings for the Child 33
Skills of the Community-Based Nurse 36
The Challenge of Community-Based Nursing 37
Rewards of Community-Based Nursing 38

UNIT II   FOUNDATIONS OF MATERNITY NURSING 43

3   Structure and Function of the Reproductive System 45

Male Reproductive System 45
  External Genitalia 45
  Internal Reproductive Organs 47
Female Reproductive System 49
  External Genitalia (Vulva) 49
  Internal Reproductive Organs 50
  Blood Supply for the Pelvic Organs 53
Regulation of Reproductive Function 53
  Puberty 53
  Menstrual Cycle 53
  Menopause 55
Sexual Response Cycle 55

4   Special Issues of Women's Health Care and Reproduction 59

WOMEN'S HEALTH ISSUES 59
Health Screening for Women 59
  Breast Cancer Screening 60
  Pelvic Examination and Pap Smear 61
  Vulvar Self-Examination 61
Common Disorders of the Female Reproductive Tract 63
  Menstrual Disturbances 63
  Infectious Disorders 66
  Disorders of the Uterus and Ovaries 67
  Pelvic Support Disorders 68
REPRODUCTIVE LIFE CYCLE ISSUES 70
Family Planning 70
  Planning Pregnancy 70
  Preventing Pregnancy 72
  Nursing Process for Assisting the Couple to Choose a Contraceptive Method 84

Induced Abortion 86
Infertility 87
  Causes of Infertility 87
  Initial Evaluation of Infertility 87
  Comprehensive Evaluation and
    Diagnostic Testing 89
  Management of Infertility 89
  Psychological Aspects of Infertility 91
  Nursing Care 91
Menopause 91
  Clinical Manifestations 91
  Treatment 92
  Nursing Care 92

UNIT III   PREGNANCY 97

5   Fetal Development 99

Cellular Processes 99
  Types of Cells 99
  Cellular Division 99
Stages of Fetal Development 101
  Pre-embryonic Stage 101
  Embryonic Stage 103
  Fetal Stage 104
Development of Supportive
Structures 104
  Fetal Membranes 104
  Amniotic Fluid 107
  Placenta 107
  Umbilical Cord 108
Fetal and Placental Circulation 109
  Fetal Circulation 109
  Placental Circulation 109
Special Considerations of Fetal
Development 111
  Teratogens and the Fetus 111
  Ectopic Pregnancy 112
  Multifetal Pregnancy 113

**6   Maternal Adaptation
During Pregnancy 117**

Signs of Pregnancy 117
  Presumptive (Possible) Signs 117
  Probable Signs 118
  Positive Signs 118
Physiologic Adaptation to Pregnancy 119
  Reproductive Changes 119
  Endocrine Changes 121
  Hematologic Changes 121
  Cardiovascular Changes 121
  Respiratory Changes 122
  Musculoskeletal Changes 122
  Gastrointestinal Changes 123
  Urinary Changes 123
  Integumentary Changes 123

Psychological Adaptation to
Pregnancy 123
  *First-Trimester Task: Accept
    the Pregnancy* 124
  *Second-Trimester Task: Accept
    the Baby* 124
  *Third-Trimester Task: Prepare
    for Parenthood* 125
Changing Nutritional Requirements of
Pregnancy 125
  *Energy Requirements and
    Weight Gain* 125
  Protein Requirements 126
  Mineral Requirements 127
  Vitamin Requirements 129
  Dietary Supplementation 130
  *Dietary Restrictions During
    Pregnancy* 130
  Special Nutritional Considerations 130

7   Prenatal Care 135

Assessment of Maternal
Well-Being During Pregnancy 135
  First Prenatal Visit 135
  Subsequent Prenatal Visits 139
Assessment of Fetal Well-Being
During Pregnancy 140
  Fetal Kick Counts 140
  Ultrasonography 140
  *Maternal Serum Alpha-fetoprotein
    Screening* 142
  *Triple-Marker (or Multiple-Marker)
    Screening* 142
  Amniocentesis 142
  Chorionic Villus Sampling 143
  *Percutaneous Umbilical Blood
    Sampling* 144
  Nonstress Test 144
  Vibroacoustic Stimulation 145
  Contraction Stress Test 145
  Biophysical Profile 145
The Nurse's Role in Prenatal Care 145
  *Nursing Process for Prenatal
    Care* 145

UNIT IV   LABOR AND BIRTH 165

8   The Labor Process 167

Four Essential Components of Labor 167
  Passageway 167
  Passenger 170
  Powers 172
  Psyche 174
The Process of Labor 174
  Onset of Labor 174

Mechanisms of a Spontaneous Vaginal
Delivery 176
Stages and Duration of Labor 176
Maternal and Fetal Adaptation
to Labor 179
Maternal Physiologic Adaptation 179
Maternal Psychological Adaptation 180
Fetal Adaptation to Labor 180

9 Pain Management During Labor
and Birth 184

The Pain of Labor and Childbirth 184
Uniqueness of Labor and Birth
Pain 184
Physiology and Characteristics of
Labor Pain 184
Factors Influencing Labor Pain 185
Pain Management Principles and
Techniques 185
Principles of Pain Relief During
Labor 185
Nonpharmacologic Interventions 186
Pharmacologic Interventions 191

10 Nursing Care During Labor and
Birth 202

The Nurse's Role During Admission 203
Immediate Assessments 203
Additional Assessments 205
Performing Routine Admission
Orders 208
The Nurse's Role: Ongoing Assessment of
Uterine Contractions and FHR 209
Monitoring Uterine Contractions 209
Monitoring FHR 211
The Nurse's Role During Each Stage
of Labor 217
Nursing Process During the First Stage
of Labor: Dilation 217
Latent Phase (Early Labor) 217
Active Phase (Active Labor) 220
Transition Phase 224
Nursing Process During the Second
Stage of Labor: Expulsion of the
Fetus 225
Nursing Process During the Third
Stage of Labor: Delivery of
Placenta 231
Nursing Process During the Fourth
Stage of Labor: Recovery 232

11 Assisted Delivery and Cesarean Birth 238

Induction of Labor 238
Indications 239
Contraindications 239

Labor Readiness 239
Cervical Ripening 240
Artificial Rupture of Membranes 241
Oxytocin Induction 241
Nursing Care 241
Assisted Delivery 241
Episiotomy 241
Vacuum-Assisted Delivery 242
Forceps-Assisted Delivery 243
Complications of Operative
Vaginal Delivery 244
Nursing Care 244
Cesarean Birth 244
Indications 244
Incidence 244
Risks 245
Maternal Complications 245
Fetal Complications 245
Incision Types 245
Steps of a Cesarean Delivery 247
Nursing Care 250
Vaginal Birth After Cesarean 254
Prerequisites 254
Contraindications 254
Risks and Benefits 254
Nursing Care 255

UNIT V POSTPARTUM AND NEWBORN 259

12 The Postpartum Woman 261

Maternal Adaptation During the
Postpartum Period 261
Physiologic Adaptation 261
Psychological Adaptation 265
The Nurse's Role in Postpartum Care 267
Nursing Process for the Early
Postpartum Period 267
Nursing Process for Postpartum Care
After Cesarean Birth 274
Nursing Process for Preparing the
Postpartum Woman for
Discharge 277

13 Nursing Assessment of Newborn
Transition 284

Physiologic Adaptation 284
Respiratory Adaptation 284
Cardiovascular Adaptation 285
Thermoregulatory Adaptation 286
Metabolic Adaptation 287
Hepatic Adaptation 287
Behavioral and Social Adaptation 288
Nursing Assessment of the Normal
Newborn 288
Initial Assessments at Birth 288

Continuing Assessments Throughout
Newborn Transition   288
Initial Admitting Assessment   289

14   Nursing Care of the Normal
Newborn   304

Newborn Stabilization and Transition   304
Nursing Process in Immediate
Stabilization and Transition of the
Newborn   304
General Newborn Care   309
Nursing Process in Providing Care to the
Normal Newborn   309
Discharge Preparation   314
Nursing Process in Preparing
the Newborn for Discharge   314

15   Newborn Nutrition   324

Selection of a Feeding Method   324
Factors That Influence Choice
of Method   324
Nursing Considerations   325
Breast-Feeding   325
Advantages and Disadvantages
of Breast-Feeding   326
Physiology of Breast-Feeding   327
Composition of Breast Milk   328
Nutritional Needs of the Breast-Feeding
Woman   329
Nursing Care of the Breast-Feeding
Woman   329
Formula-Feeding   335
Advantages and Disadvantages
of Formula-Feeding   335
Composition of Formula   336
Nursing Care of the
Formula-Feeding Woman   336

UNIT VI   CHILDBEARING AT RISK   343

16   Pregnancy at Risk: Conditions That
Complicate Pregnancy   345

Pregnancy Complicated by Medical
Conditions   346
DIABETES MELLITUS   346
Classification of Diabetes Mellitus   346
Treatment   347
Nursing Process for the
Pregnant Woman with DM   350
CARDIOVASCULAR DISEASE   352
Clinical Manifestations and
Diagnosis   353
Treatment   353
Nursing Care   354

ANEMIA   355
Iron-Deficiency Anemia   355
Sickle Cell Anemia   355
Nursing Care   356
ASTHMA   356
Clinical Manifestations and Diagnosis   356
Treatment   356
Nursing Care   357
EPILEPSY   357
Clinical Manifestations   358
Treatment   358
Nursing Care   359
INFECTIOUS DISEASES   359
TORCH   360
Sexually Transmitted Infections   364
Nursing Process for the Pregnant Woman
With an STI   368
Pregnancy Complicated by Intimate Partner
Violence   372
Clinical Manifestations and
Diagnosis   372
Treatment   373
Nursing Care   374
Pregnancy Complicated by
Age-Related Concerns   375
Adolescent Pregnancy   375
Pregnancy in Later Life   377

17   Pregnancy at Risk: Pregnancy-Related
Complications   381

Hyperemesis Gravidarum   381
Clinical Manifestations   382
Treatment   382
Nursing Care   382
Bleeding Disorders   383
Ectopic Pregnancy   383
Early Pregnancy Loss   384
Cervical Insufficiency   387
Gestational Trophoblastic Disease   387
Placenta Previa   389
Abruptio Placentae   390
Nursing Process for the Woman With a
Bleeding Disorder   392
Hypertensive Disorders in Pregnancy   394
Gestational Hypertension   394
Preeclampsia-Eclampsia   394
Chronic Hypertension and Preeclampsia
Superimposed on Chronic
Hypertension   403
Multiple Gestation   403
Clinical Manifestations   404
Treatment   404
Nursing Care   404
Blood Incompatibilities   404
Rh Incompatibility   404
ABO Incompatibility   405

18   Labor at Risk   409

Dysfunctional Labor (Dystocia)   409
  Complications   409
  *Clinical Manifestations and
    Diagnosis   409*
  Causes of Labor Dysfunction   410
  Treatment   410
  Nursing Care   411
Fetal Malpresentation   411
  Clinical Manifestations and Diagnosis   412
  Treatment   412
  Nursing Care   412
Premature Rupture of Membranes   413
  *Clinical Manifestations and
    Diagnosis   413*
  Treatment   413
  Nursing Care   413
Preterm Labor   414
  Clinical Manifestations and Diagnosis   414
  Treatment   415
  *Nursing Process for the Woman
    With Preterm Labor   415*
Postterm Pregnancy and Labor   417
  *Clinical Manifestations and
    Diagnosis   417*
  Treatment   418
  Nursing Care   418
Intrauterine Fetal Death   418
  Clinical Manifestations and Diagnosis   418
  Treatment   418
  Nursing Care   419
Emergencies Associated
With Labor and Birth   419
  Amniotic Fluid Embolism   419
  Shoulder Dystocia   420
  Umbilical Cord Prolapse   421
  Uterine Rupture   422
  *Placental and Umbilical Cord
    Abnormalities   422*

19   Postpartum Woman at Risk   426

Postpartum Hemorrhage   426
  Early Postpartum Hemorrhage   427
  *Nursing Process for the Woman with
    Early Postpartum Hemorrhage   428*
  Late Postpartum Hemorrhage   432
Postpartum Infection   432
  Endometritis   433
  Wound Infection   434
  Mastitis   436
  Urinary Tract Infection   437
Venous Thromboembolism   441
  Risk Factors   441
  Deep Vein Thrombosis   441
  Pulmonary Embolism   443

Postpartum Psychiatric Disorders   443
  Postpartum Depression   443
  Postpartum Psychosis   445
Special Postpartum Situations   445
  Grief in the Postpartal Period   445
  *Malattachment in the Postpartal
    Period   446*

**20   The Newborn at Risk: Gestational and
Acquired Disorders   450**

Variations in Size and Gestational
Age   451
  Gestational Age Assessment   451
  Neuromuscular Maturity   451
  Physical Maturity   451
  The Small-for-Gestational Age
    (Growth-Restricted)
    Newborn   451
  Contributing Factors   451
  Clinical Manifestations   453
  Complications   454
  Nursing Care   454
  The Large-for-Gestational Age
    Newborn   455
  Contributing Factors   455
  Potential Complications   455
  Nursing Care   455
  The Preterm Newborn   456
  Contributing Factors   456
  *Characteristics of the Preterm
    Newborn   456*
  Treatment of Complications   458
  *Nursing Process for the Preterm
    Newborn   459*
  The Postterm Newborn   466
  Contributing Factors   466
  *Characteristics of the Postterm
    Newborn   466*
  Potential Complications   466
  Treatment   467
  Nursing Care   467
Acquired Disorders   467
  Respiratory Disorders   467
  *Transient Tachypnea of the
    Newborn   467*
  Meconium Aspiration Syndrome   468
  Sudden Infant Death Syndrome   468
  Hemolytic Disease of the
    Newborn   469
  Causes   469
  Diagnosis   470
  Clinical Manifestations   470
  Treatment   470
  Nursing Care   471
  Newborn of a Diabetic Mother   471
  Clinical Manifestations   471

Nursing Care 472
NEWBORN OF A MOTHER WITH SUBSTANCE
    ABUSE 472
Fetal Alcohol Syndrome 472
Neonatal Substance Withdrawal 473
NEWBORN WITH A CONGENITALLY ACQUIRED
    INFECTION 473

21   The Newborn at Risk: Congenital
     Disorders 478

Congenital Malformations 479
CENTRAL NERVOUS SYSTEM DEFECTS 479
Spina Bifida 479
Nursing Process for the Newborn
    With Myelomeningocele 480
Hydrocephalus 482
Nursing Process for the
    Postoperative Newborn With
    Hydrocephalus 483
CARDIOVASCULAR SYSTEM DEFECTS: CONGENITAL
    HEART DISEASE 485
Development of the Heart 485
Common Types of Congenital
    Heart Defects 486
Risk Factors 489
Clinical Manifestations 489
Treatment and Nursing Care 489
GASTROINTESTINAL SYSTEM DEFECTS 491
Cleft Lip and Cleft Palate 491
Nursing Process for the Newborn
    With Cleft Lip and Cleft
    Palate 492
Esophageal Atresia and
    Tracheoesophageal Fistula 496
Imperforate Anus 498
Hernias 498
GENITOURINARY TRACT DEFECTS 500
Hypospadias and Epispadias 500
Exstrophy of the Bladder 500
Ambiguous Genitalia 500
SKELETAL SYSTEM DEFECTS 501
Congenital Talipes Equinovarus 501
Congenital Hip Dysplasia 502
Nursing Process for the Newborn
    in an Orthopedic Device or
    Cast 503
Inborn Errors of Metabolism 504
Phenylketonuria 506
Galactosemia 507
Congenital Hypothyroidism 507
Maple Syrup Urine Disease 508
Chromosomal Abnormalities 508
Down Syndrome 508
Turner Syndrome 509
Klinefelter Syndrome 510

UNIT VII   HEALTH PROMOTION FOR NORMAL
           GROWTH AND DEVELOPMENT 515

22   Principles of Growth and
     Development 517

Foundations of Growth and
Development 517
Patterns of Growth 518
Standards of Growth 518
Standards of Development 519
Influences on Growth and
Development 519
Genetics 519
Nutrition 520
Environment 522
Theories of Child Development 525
Sigmund Freud 525
Erik Erikson 527
Jean Piaget 529
Lawrence Kohlberg 530
Other Theorists 530
Developmental Considerations for
Communicating With Children and
Family Caregivers 531
Principles of Communication 531
Communicating With Infants 532
Communicating With Young
    Children 532
Communicating With School-Aged
    Children 533
Communicating With
    Adolescents 533
Communicating With
    Caregivers 533
The Nurse's Role Related to Growth and
Development 534

23   Growth and Development of the Infant:
     28 Days to 1 Year 538

Physical Development 538
Weight and Height 539
Head and Skull 539
Skeletal Growth and Maturation 539
Eruption of Deciduous Teeth 539
Circulatory System 540
Body Temperature and Respiratory
    Rate 540
Neuromuscular Development 540
Psychosocial Development 541
Nutrition 545
Addition of Solid Foods 546
Weaning the Infant 549
Women, Infants, and Children
    Food Program 549

Health Promotion and Maintenance   549
  Routine Checkups   549
  Immunizations   549
  Family Teaching   550
The Infant in the Health Care Facility   553

24   Growth and Development of the Toddler: 1 to 3 Years   557

Physical Development   558
Psychosocial Development   558
  Behavioral Characteristics   558
  Play   560
  Discipline   561
  Sharing With a New Baby   561
Nutrition   562
Health Promotion and Maintenance   563
  Routine Checkups   563
  Family Teaching   563
  Accident Prevention   567
The Toddler in the Health Care Facility   569
  Maintaining Routines   569
  Special Considerations   570

25   Growth and Development of the Preschool Child: 3 to 6 Years   574

Physical Development   575
  Growth Rate   575
  Dentition   575
  Visual Development   575
  Skeletal Growth   575
Psychosocial Development   576
  Language Development   576
  Development of Imagination   577
  Sexual Development   578
  Social Development   578
Nutrition   580
Health Promotion and Maintenance   581
  Routine Checkups   581
  Family Teaching   582
  Accident Prevention   583
  Infection Prevention   583
The Preschooler in the Health Care Facility   584

26   Growth and Development of the School-Aged Child: 6 to 10 Years   588

Physical Development   589
  Weight and Height   589
  Dentition   589
  Skeletal Growth   589
Psychosocial Development   590
  Development From Ages 6 to 7 Years   591

Development From Ages 7 to 10 Years   592
Nutrition   593
Health Promotion and Maintenance   594
  Routine Checkups   594
  Family Teaching   595
  Health Education   596
  Accident Prevention   598
The School-Aged Child in the Health Care Facility   598

27   Growth and Development of the Adolescent: 11 to 18 Years   604

Preadolescent Development   605
  Physical Development   605
  Preparation for Adolescence   606
Adolescent Development   606
  Physical Development   606
  Psychosocial Development   606
Nutrition   609
Health Promotion and Maintenance   610
  Routine Checkups   611
  Dental Checkups   611
  Family Teaching   612
  Health Education and Counseling   612
  Mental Health   616
  Accident Prevention   616
The Adolescent in the Health Care Facility   617

UNIT VIII   FOUNDATIONS OF PEDIATRIC NURSING   621

28   Assessment of the Child (Data Collection)   623

Collecting Subjective Data   623
  Conducting the Client Interview   623
  Obtaining a Client History   624
Collecting Objective Data   628
  Noting General Status   628
  Measuring Height and Weight   630
  Measuring Head Circumference   631
  Taking Vital Signs   631
  Conducting or Assisting with a Physical Examination   636
  Assisting With Common Diagnostic Tests   638

29   Care of the Hospitalized Child   643

The Pediatric Hospital Setting   644
  Early Childhood Education About Hospitals   644
  The Pediatric Unit Atmosphere   644

Pediatric Intensive Care Units 645
Safety 646
Infection Control 646
Importance of Caregiver Participation 647
Admission and Discharge Planning 649
Planned Admissions 649
Emergency Admissions 650
The Admission Interview 650
The Admission Physical
Examination 650
Discharge Planning 650
The Child Undergoing Surgery 651
Preoperative Care 651
Postoperative Care 653
The Hospital Play Program 655
The Hospital Play Environment 655
Therapeutic Play 656
Play Material 656

30 Procedures and Treatments 662
Nurse's Role in Preparation
and Follow-Up 662
Preparation for Procedures 662
Follow-up for Procedures 663
Performing Procedures
Related to Position 664
Using Restraints 664
Holding 665
Transporting 666
Positioning for Sleep 666
Performing Procedures Related to Elevated
Body Temperature 666
Control of Environmental Factors 667
Cooling Devices 667
Performing Procedures Related to Feeding
and Nutrition 667
Intake and Output Measurements 667
Gavage Feeding 667
Gastrostomy Feeding 667
Performing Procedures Related to
Respiration 670
Oxygen Administration 670
Nasal/Oral Suctioning 671
Tracheostomy Care 671
Performing Procedures Related to
Circulation 671
Heat Therapy 671
Cold Therapy 672
Performing Procedures Related to
Elimination 672
Enema Administration 672
Ostomy Care 672
Performing Procedures for Specimen
Collection 672
Nose and Throat Specimens 672
Urine Specimens 673
Stool Specimens 674

Assisting with Procedures Related to
Collection of Blood and Spinal Fluid 674
Blood Collection 674
Lumbar Puncture 675
Assisting with Procedures Related to
Diagnostic Tests and Studies 675

31 Medication Administration and
Intravenous Therapy 680
Medication Administration 680
Rights and Guidelines 680
Pediatric Dosage Calculation 681
Oral Administration 684
Ophthalmic, Otic, Nasal, and
Rectal Administration 685
Intramuscular Administration 686
Subcutaneous and Intradermal
Administration 687
Intravenous Administration 687
Intravenous Therapy 689
Fundamentals of Fluid and Electrolyte
Balance 689
IV Therapy Administration 691
Parenteral Nutrition Administration 692

UNIT IX   SPECIAL CONCERNS OF PEDIATRIC
NURSING 697

32 The Child With a Chronic Health
Problem 699
Causes of Chronic Illness in
Children 699
Effects of Chronic Illness on the
Family 699
Parents and Chronic Illness 700
The Child and Chronic Illness 701
Siblings and Chronic Illness 701
The Role of the Nurse 702
Nursing Process for the Family and the
Child With a Chronic Illness 702

33 Abuse in the Family 711
Child Abuse 711
Types of Child Abuse 712
Effects on the Child and Family 715
Nursing Process for the Child
Who is Abused 716
Domestic Violence in the Family 718
Effects on the Child and Family 718
Clinical Manifestations in the
Child 718
Parental Substance Abuse 718
Effects on the Child and Family 718
Clinical Manifestations in the
Child 718

34   The Dying Child 722

The Nurse's Reaction to Death and Dying 722
The Child's Understanding of Death 724
  Developmental Stage 724
  Experience With Death and Loss 725
  Awareness of Impending Death 726
The Family's Reaction to Dying and Death 728
  Family Caregivers' Reactions 728
  The Child's Reaction 729
  Siblings' Reactions 730
Settings for Care of the Dying Child 730
  Hospice Care 730
  Home Care 731
  Hospital Care 732
The Role of the Nurse 732
  Nursing Process for the Dying Child 732

UNIT X   THE CHILD WITH A HEALTH DISORDER 741

35   The Child With a Sensory/Neurological Disorder 743

Growth and Development of the Eyes, Ears, and Nervous System 743
  The Nervous System 743
  Sensory Organs 744
Vision Impairment 744
  Types of Vision Impairment 744
  Clinical Manifestations and Diagnosis 745
  Treatment and Education 747
  Nursing Care 747
Eye Conditions 747
  Cataracts 747
  Glaucoma 747
  Strabismus 747
  Eye Injury and Foreign Objects in the Eye 748
  Eye Infections 749
  Nursing Care for the Child Undergoing Eye Surgery 749
Hearing Impairment 749
  Types of Hearing Impairment 750
  Clinical Manifestations 750
  Diagnosis 750
  Treatment and Education 751
  Nursing Care 752
Otitis Media 752
  Clinical Manifestations 752
  Diagnosis 752
  Treatment and Nursing Care 752

Insertion of Foreign Bodies into the Ear or Nose 752
Reye Syndrome 753
  Clinical Manifestations 753
  Diagnosis 753
  Treatment 753
  Nursing Care 754
Acute or Nonrecurrent Seizures 754
  Clinical Manifestations and Diagnosis 754
  Treatment 755
  Nursing Process for the Child at Risk for Seizures 755
Seizure Disorders 756
  Clinical Manifestations 756
  Diagnosis 757
  Treatment 757
  Nursing Care 757
Haemophilus Influenzae Meningitis 759
  Clinical Manifestations 759
  Diagnosis 759
  Treatment 759
  Nursing Process for the Child With Meningitis 760
Cerebral Palsy 761
  Causes 761
  Prevention 762
  Clinical Manifestations and Types 762
  Diagnosis 762
  Treatment and Special Aids 762
  Nursing Care 763
Mental Retardation 764
  Causes 764
  Clinical Manifestations and Diagnosis 764
  Treatment and Education 765
  Nursing Process for the Child With Cognitive Impairment 765
Head Injuries 768
Drowning 769

36   The Child With a Respiratory Disorder 775

Growth and Development of the Respiratory System 775
Acute Nasopharyngitis (Common Cold) 776
  Clinical Manifestations 776
  Diagnosis 776
  Treatment and Nursing Care 776
Allergic Rhinitis (Hay Fever) 777
  Clinical Manifestations 777
  Treatment and Nursing Care 777
Tonsillitis and Adenoiditis 777
  Clinical Manifestations and Diagnosis 777

Treatment and Nursing Care 777
Nursing Process for the Child Having a
  Tonsillectomy 778
Croup Syndromes 779
  SPASMODIC LARYNGITIS 779
  Clinical Manifestations and
    Diagnosis 779
  Treatment and Nursing Care 779
  ACUTE LARYNGOTRACHEOBRONCHITIS 780
  Clinical Manifestations and
    Diagnosis 780
  Treatment and Nursing Care 780
  EPIGLOTTITIS 780
  Clinical Manifestations and
    Diagnosis 780
  Treatment and Nursing Care 780
Acute Bronchiolitis/Respiratory Syncytial
Virus Infection 781
  Clinical Manifestations 781
  Diagnosis 781
  Treatment and Nursing Care 781
Asthma 781
  Clinical Manifestations 782
  Diagnosis 782
  Treatment 782
  Nursing Process for the Child With
    Asthma 785
Bacterial Pneumonia 788
  Clinical Manifestations 788
  Diagnosis 788
  Treatment 788
  Nursing Process for the Child With
    Pneumonia 788
Cystic Fibrosis 793
  Clinical Manifestations 793
  Diagnosis 794
  Treatment 794
  Nursing Process for the Child With Cystic
    Fibrosis 795
Pulmonary Tuberculosis 799
  Clinical Manifestations 799
  Diagnosis 799
  Treatment 800
  Prevention 800

37   The Child With a Cardiovascular/
     Hematologic Disorder 804

Growth and Development of the
Cardiovascular and Hematologic
Systems 804
Differences Between the Child's and
Adult's Cardiovascular and Hematologic
Systems 805
Congestive Heart Failure 805
  Clinical Manifestations 805
  Diagnosis 806

Treatment 806
Nursing Process for the Child With
  Congestive Heart Failure 806
Rheumatic Fever 807
  Clinical Manifestations 807
  Diagnosis 808
  Treatment 808
  Prevention 809
  Nursing Process for the Child With
    Rheumatic Fever 809
Kawasaki Disease 811
  Clinical Manifestations 811
  Diagnosis 811
  Treatment and Nursing Care 812
Iron Deficiency Anemia 812
  Clinical Manifestations 812
  Diagnosis 812
  Treatment and Nursing Care 812
Sickle Cell Disease 813
  Clinical Manifestations 813
  Diagnosis 814
  Treatment 814
  Nursing Process for the Child With
    Sickle Cell Crisis 814
Thalassemia 815
  Clinical Manifestations 816
  Treatment and Nursing Care 816
Hemophilia 816
  Mechanism of Clot Formation 816
  Common Types of Hemophilia 816
  Clinical Manifestations 817
  Diagnosis 817
  Treatment 817
  Nursing Process for the Child With
    Hemophilia 817
Idiopathic Thrombocytopenic
Purpura 820
  Clinical Manifestations and
    Diagnosis 820
  Treatment and Nursing Care 820
Acute Leukemia 820
  Pathophysiology 820
  Clinical Manifestations 820
  Diagnosis 820
  Treatment 820
  Nursing Process for the Child With
    Leukemia 821

38   The Child With a Gastrointestinal/
     Endocrine Disorder 827

Growth and Development of the
Gastrointestinal and Endocrine
Systems 828
  Gastrointestinal System 828
  Endocrine System and
    Hormonal Function 828

Gastrointestinal Disorders   829
  MALNUTRITION AND NUTRITIONAL
    PROBLEMS   829
  Protein Malnutrition   829
  Vitamin Deficiency Diseases   829
  Mineral Insufficiencies   830
  Food Allergies   830
  Nursing Process for the Child With
    Malnutrition and Nutritional
    Problems   831
  CELIAC SYNDROME   832
  Clinical Manifestations   833
  Diagnosis   833
  Treatment   833
  Nursing Care   833
  GASTROESOPHAGEAL REFLUX   834
  Clinical Manifestations   834
  Diagnosis and Treatment   834
  Nursing Care   834
  COLIC   834
  Clinical Manifestations and
    Diagnosis   834
  Treatment and Nursing Care   835
  DIARRHEA AND GASTROENTERITIS   835
  Clinical Manifestations   835
  Diagnosis   836
  Treatment   836
  Nursing Process for the Child With
    Diarrhea and Gastroenteritis   836
  PYLORIC STENOSIS   839
  Clinical Manifestations   839
  Diagnosis   839
  Treatment   839
  Nursing Process for the Child With
    Pyloric Stenosis   839
  CONGENITAL AGANGLIONIC
    MEGACOLON   842
  Clinical Manifestations   842
  Diagnosis   842
  Treatment   842
  Nursing Process for the Child Undergoing
    Surgery for Congenital Aganglionic
    Megacolon   843
  INTUSSUSCEPTION   845
  Clinical Manifestations   845
  Diagnosis   845
  Treatment and Nursing Care   845
  APPENDICITIS   846
  Clinical Manifestations   846
  Treatment   846
  Nursing Process for the Child With
    Appendicitis   846
  INTESTINAL PARASITES   848
  Enterobiasis (Pinworm Infection)   848
  Roundworms   848
  Hookworms   848
  Giardiasis   849

  INGESTION OF TOXIC SUBSTANCES   849
  Emergency Treatment   850
  Treatment Steps in Order of
    Importance   850
  LEAD POISONING (PLUMBISM)   850
  Sources of Chronic Lead
    Poisoning   850
  Clinical Manifestations   852
  Diagnosis   852
  Treatment and Nursing Care   852
  Prognosis   852
  INGESTION OF FOREIGN OBJECTS   853
  Treatment and Nursing Care   853
Endocrine Disorders   854
  TYPE 1 DIABETES MELLITUS   854
  Pathogenesis   854
  Clinical Manifestations   855
  Diagnosis   855
  Treatment   855
  Nursing Process for the Child With
    Type 1 Diabetes Mellitus   857
  TYPE 2 DIABETES MELLITUS   862
  Clinical Manifestations and
    Diagnosis   862
  Treatment   863
  Nursing Care   863

**39   The Child With a Genitourinary
Disorder**   867

**Growth and Development of the
Genitourinary System**   867
Urinary Tract Infections   868
  Clinical Manifestations   868
  Diagnosis   868
  Treatment   868
  Nursing Process for the Child With a
    Urinary Tract Infection   869
Enuresis   870
Acute Glomerulonephritis   870
  Clinical Manifestations   870
  Treatment   871
  Nursing Care   872
Nephrotic Syndrome   872
  Clinical Manifestations   872
  Diagnosis   872
  Treatment   872
  Nursing Process for the Child With
    Nephrotic Syndrome   873
Wilms' Tumor (Nephroblastoma)   875
Hydrocele   875
Cryptorchidism   875
Menstrual Disorders   875
  PREMENSTRUAL SYNDROME   876
  DYSMENORRHEA   876
  AMENORRHEA   876
Vaginitis   877

40   The Child With a Musculoskeletal Disorder   880

Growth and Development of the Musculoskeletal System   880
Fractures   881
　Treatment and Nursing Care   881
Osteomyelitis   888
　Clinical Manifestations and Diagnosis   888
　Treatment   888
　Nursing Care   888
Muscular Dystrophy   888
　Clinical Manifestations and Diagnosis   888
　Treatment and Nursing Care   888
Legg-Calvé-Perthes Disease (Coxa Plana)   890
　Clinical Manifestations and Diagnosis   890
　Treatment and Nursing Care   890
Osteosarcoma   890
　Clinical Manifestations and Diagnosis   890
　Treatment and Nursing Care   890
Ewing's Sarcoma   891
　Clinical Manifestations and Diagnosis   891
　Treatment and Nursing Care   891
Juvenile Rheumatoid Arthritis   891
　Clinical Manifestations   891
　Treatment and Nursing Care   891
Scoliosis   892
　Diagnosis   892
　Treatment   892
　Nursing Process for the Child With Scoliosis Requiring a Brace   894

41   The Child With an Integumentary Disorder/Communicable Diseases   899

Growth and Development of the Integumentary and Immune System   899
Integumentary Disorders   900
　SEBORRHEIC DERMATITIS   900
　MILIARIA RUBRA   900
　Clinical Manifestations   900
　Treatment and Nursing Care   900
　DIAPER RASH   900
　Clinical Manifestations   900
　Treatment and Nursing Care   901
　CANDIDIASIS   901
　Clinical Manifestations   901
　Treatment and Nursing Care   901
　IMPETIGO   902
　Treatment   902
　Nursing Care   902

ACNE VULGARIS   902
　Clinical Manifestations   902
　Treatment and Nursing Care   903
Fungal Infections   903
　TINEA CAPITIS (RINGWORM OF THE SCALP)   903
　Clinical Manifestations   903
　Treatment and Nursing Care   903
　TINEA CORPORIS (RINGWORM OF THE BODY)   903
　TINEA PEDIS   903
　TINEA CRURIS   904
Parasitic Infections   904
　PEDICULOSIS   904
　Clinical Manifestations   904
　Treatment and Nursing Care   904
　SCABIES   905
　Clinical Manifestations   905
　Treatment and Nursing Care   905
Allergic Disorders   905
　ATOPIC DERMATITIS (INFANTILE ECZEMA)   906
　Clinical Manifestations   906
　Diagnosis   906
　Treatment   906
　Nursing Process for the Child With Infantile Eczema   907
　SKIN ALLERGIES   908
　Clinical Manifestations   908
　Treatment   908
　PLANT ALLERGIES   908
　Clinical Manifestations   909
　Treatment   909
Bites   909
　ANIMAL BITES   909
　SPIDER BITES   909
　TICK BITES   909
　SNAKE BITES   910
　INSECT STINGS OR BITES   910
Burns   910
　Types of Burns   910
　Emergency Treatment   912
　Treatment of Moderate to Severe Burns: First Phase—48 to 72 Hours   913
　Complications   915
　Long-term Care   916
　Nursing Process for the Child With a Burn   916
Sexually Transmitted Infections   921
　GONORRHEA   921
　CHLAMYDIAL INFECTION   921
　GENITAL HERPES   921
　SYPHILIS   921
　Clinical Manifestations   921
　Treatment   923
　ACQUIRED IMMUNODEFICIENCY SYNDROME   923
　Clinical Manifestations and Treatment   924

Nursing Process for the Child With
     AIDS   924
Infectious Mononucleosis   927
     Clinical Manifestations   927
     Diagnosis   927
     Treatment and Nursing Care   928
Communicable Diseases of Childhood   928
     Prevention   933
     Nursing Care   933

42   The Child With a Psychosocial
Disorder   937

Autism   937
     Clinical Manifestations   937
     Diagnosis   938
     Treatment   938
     Nursing Care   938
Attention Deficit Hyperactivity
Disorder   939
     Clinical Manifestations   939
     Diagnosis   939
     Treatment and Nursing Care   939
Enuresis and Encopresis   940
School Phobia   940
     Clinical Manifestations   940
     Treatment and Nursing Care   940
Suicide   940
     Clinical Manifestations   940
     Treatment and Nursing Care   941
Substance Abuse   941
     Prevention and Treatment   942
     ALCOHOL ABUSE   943
     TOBACCO ABUSE   944
     MARIJUANA ABUSE   944
     COCAINE ABUSE   944
     NARCOTIC ABUSE   945
     OTHER ABUSED DRUGS   945
Nonorganic Failure to Thrive   945
     Clinical Manifestations   946
     Diagnosis   946
     Treatment   946

Nursing Process for the Child With
     Nonorganic Failure to Thrive   946
Eating Disorders   948
     ANOREXIA NERVOSA   948
     Characteristics   948
     Clinical Manifestations and
          Diagnosis   948
     Treatment and Nursing Care   948
     BULIMIA NERVOSA   949
     Clinical Manifestations and
          Diagnosis   949
     Treatment   950
     Nursing Process for the Child With
          Anorexia Nervosa or
          Bulimia Nervosa   949
Obesity   955
     Clinical Manifestations and
          Diagnosis   955
     Treatment   955

Appendix A: Standard and Transmission-Based
     Precautions   959
Appendix B: NANDA-Approved Nursing
     Diagnoses   961
Appendix C: The Joint Commission's "Do Not Use"
     List of Abbreviations, Acronyms, and Symbols   964
Appendix D: Good Sources of Essential Nutrients   965
Appendix E: Breast-feeding and Medication Use   966
Appendix F: Cervical Dilation Chart   968
Appendix G: Growth Charts   969
Appendix H: Pulse, Respiration, and Blood Pressure
     Values for Children   975
Appendix I: Temperature and Weight Conversion
     Charts   976
Appendix J: Recommended Childhood and Adolescent
     Immunization Schedules   979
Glossary   981
English-Spanish Glossary   996
References and Suggested Readings   1001
Index   1025

OVERVIEW OF MATERNAL AND PEDIATRIC HEALTH CARE

1 The Nurse's Role in a Changing Maternal–Child Health Care Environment

KEY TERMS

actual nursing diagnoses
capitation
case management
critical pathways
dependent nursing actions
independent nursing actions
infant mortality rate
interdependent nursing actions
maternal mortality rate
morbidity
nursing process
objective data
outcomes
prospective payment system
puerperal fever
risk nursing diagnoses
subjective data
utilization review
wellness nursing diagnoses

LEARNING OBJECTIVES

On completion of this chapter, you should be able to:

1. Discuss factors influencing the development of maternity and pediatric care in the United States.
2. Describe how current trends in maternal–child care have affected the delivery of care to mothers, infants, and children in the United States.
3. Name three ways that nurses contribute to cost containment in the United States.
4. Describe sources of payment for health services for pregnant women and children.
5. Discuss maternal–child health status in the United States.
6. Discuss two possible reasons the United States ranks low compared with other developed countries in terms of infant mortality rate.
7. Discuss major objectives of *Healthy People 2010* as they relate to maternal and pediatric nursing.
8. List new roles of nurses providing maternal and pediatric nursing care.
9. Discuss how nurses use critical thinking skills in maternal and pediatric nursing.
10. List the five steps of the nursing process.
11. Explain the importance of complete and accurate documentation.

AS A NURSE preparing to care for today and tomorrow's childbearing and child-rearing families, you face vastly different responsibilities and challenges than did the maternal and pediatric nurse of even a decade ago. Nurses and other health professionals are becoming increasingly concerned with much more than the care of at-risk pregnancies and sick children. Health teaching, preventing illness, and promoting optimal (most desirable or satisfactory) physical, developmental, and emotional health have become a significant part of contemporary nursing.

Scientific and technological advances have reduced the incidence of communicable disease and helped to control metabolic disorders such as diabetes. As a result, health care practitioners increasingly provide health care outside the hospital. Patients now receive health care in the home, at schools and clinics, and from their primary care provider. Prenatal diagnosis of birth defects, transfusions, other treatments for the unborn fetus, and improved life-support systems for premature infants are but a few examples of the rapid progress in child care.

Controversy continues to rage about choices in family planning. In January 1973, a Supreme Court decision declared abortion legal anywhere in the United States. Since that time, various groups have tried to convince Congress to pass legislation that would make all abortions illegal, or at least restrict a woman's access to abortion services. In the 1990s, bitter debate between "pro-life" and "pro-choice" groups raged. This debate seems likely to continue for many years.

Tremendous sociologic changes have affected attitudes toward, and concepts in, maternal–child health. American society is largely suburban, with a population of highly mobile persons and families. The women's movement has focused new attention on the needs of families

3

in which the mother works outside the home. Escalating divorce rates, changes in attitudes toward sexual roles, and general acceptance of unmarried mothers have increased the number of single-parent families. Many people have come to regard health care as a right, not a privilege, and expect to receive fair value for their investment. In addition, the demand for financial responsibility in health care has contributed to shortened hospital stays and alternative methods of health care delivery.

The reduction in the incidence of communicable and infectious diseases has made it possible to devote more attention to such critical problems as preterm birth, congenital anomalies, child abuse, learning and behavior disorders, developmental disabilities, and chronic illness. Research in these areas continues; as these findings become available, nurses will be among the practitioners who will help translate this research into improved health care for pregnant women, children, and families.

However, in order to translate relevant medical research into nursing practice, you must understand the predictable but variable phases of pregnancy and of a child's growth and development. It is also necessary to be understanding of and sensitive to the importance of family interactions.

CHANGING CONCEPTS IN MATERNAL–CHILD HEALTH CARE

Maternity care has changed dramatically throughout the years as attitudes and opinions have altered. Historically, maternity care was a function of lay midwives, and most births occurred in the home setting. As knowledge increased about birth interventions and physicians developed methods of infection prevention, the family physician became the provider of choice for prenatal care, and hospitals, instead of homes, became the accepted place to give birth.

In today's society, as the health care consumer has become more knowledgeable, two different trends have emerged. On one hand, as lawsuits have become more common with large judgments leveled against practitioners, maternity care has become increasingly specialized. Obstetricians often provide routine prenatal and delivery care. Frequently a maternal-fetal medicine specialist, a physician who specializes in the care of women with high-risk pregnancies, follows the at-risk client. Neonatologists provide expert specialized care to at-risk newborns. On the other hand, the consumer movement has promoted the view that birth is a natural process in which little intervention is required. Therefore, some women choose midwives to provide maternity care, and some elect to deliver at home or in birthing centers, which provide a home-like atmosphere.

Child health care has evolved from a sideline of internal medicine to a specialty that focuses on the child and the child's family in health and illness through all phases of development. Technologic advances account for many changes in the last 50 years, but sociologic changes, particularly society's view of the child and the child's needs, have been just as important. The development of, and current trends in, maternal and child health care are discussed briefly in the following sections.

Development of Maternity Care

In colonial times, most births occurred at home. The lay midwife, who had no formal education, attended the woman throughout labor and birth. Women of the community shared experience and knowledge about childbirth. Childbirth was truly a woman's affair.

As physicians became educated in the practice of midwifery and began to use instruments such as forceps, to which the midwives had no access, physicians began to replace lay midwives as the attendant at deliveries. Few women became physicians because of the cultural pressures for a woman to fulfill the roles of housewife and mother.

Physicians began to rely increasingly on interventions to assist the natural process of labor and hasten delivery. Lay midwives mainly provided support and encouragement to a woman during her labor and relied on nature to take its course. Therefore, as more physicians began to attend deliveries, labor came to be viewed as an illness, or at the very least, a dangerous condition that required the skillful intervention of a physician. Two major developments greatly influenced the way maternity care was practiced in the United States—acceptance of the germ theory and development of anesthesia to decrease the pain of childbirth.

Acceptance of the Germ Theory

Before scientists knew the principles of infection transmission, it was common for a woman to develop **puerperal fever**, an illness marked by high fever caused by infection of the reproductive tract after the birth of a child. Puerperal fever was often fatal. Although rates of infection and mortality (deaths) were much higher in hospitals, women who delivered at home also were susceptible to puerperal fever.

In the late 1700s, Alexander Gordon, a Scottish physician, was the first to recognize that puerperal fever was an infection transmitted to patients by physicians and nurses as they moved between treating patients with puerperal fever and attending births or caring for women who had already delivered. The work of two other men, Oliver Wendell Holmes and Ignaz Philip Semmelweis, confirmed Gordon's infection theory, and the development of interventions to stop the transmission of puerperal fever began.

In 1842, Oliver Wendell Holmes, the famous American poet, physician, and professor of anatomy and physiology at Harvard University, wrote an essay on puerperal fever based on conclusions he made after observing physicians in clinical practice. He strongly advocated that a physician who performed autopsies on individuals who died of infection[1] should not attend women during childbirth. Ignaz Philip Semmelweis (1818–1865), a German-Hungarian physician, made similar observations in his practice. He noticed a dramatic difference in rates of puerperal fever between two maternity wards, one in which medical students practiced, the other run by midwives. The death rate in the ward attended by medical students was two to three times higher than that of the ward in which the midwives delivered. Semmelweis noticed that the only difference between the two wards was that the medical students would dissect cadavers and then go immediately to the maternity ward to examine patients. The midwives, of course, did not dissect cadavers. Then a physician friend of Semmelweis died from a cut he sustained while examining a woman who died of puerperal fever. These observations convinced Semmelweis that the infection spread by the hands of the physicians. He began requiring medical students to wash their hands in a chlorinated lime solution between examinations. Immediately, the mortality rate fell from approximately 18% to 1%, equivalent to the death rate in the midwives' ward.

The medical community largely ignored Holmes' advice and Semmelweis' work. Efforts to prevent the spread of infection did not begin in earnest until Louis Pasteur, a French chemist and microbiologist, proved that microorganisms cause infection. Joseph Lister, a British surgeon, embraced Pasteur's theory. Lister used carbolic acid as an antiseptic during surgery and greatly improved the survival rates of his surgical patients. His research and persistence led to general acceptance of the germ theory by physicians in Europe and the United States. As physicians began to use antiseptic techniques during the childbirth process, maternal mortality rates fell.

Easing the Pain of Childbirth

The development and use of anesthesia during childbirth was the change that most influenced wealthy and middle-class women to begin delivering their children in hospitals, rather than at home. In the 1920s and 1930s, a method called "twilight sleep" greatly increased the number of women who chose to deliver in hospitals. Physicians administered morphine and scopolamine at the beginning of labor to induce twilight sleep. Morphine eased the pain of labor and scopolamine, an amnesiac, induced a hypnotic-like state that caused the woman to be unable to recall the pain of labor. This development allowed women to enjoy painless childbirth and gave the physician more control over the birth process. Therefore, the public came to view the hospital as the safest and most humane place in which to deliver a baby.

---

[1] He specified puerperal fever, erysipelas, and peritonitis as types of infection that could be transmitted and cause puerperal fever in a woman who had just delivered.

Development of Pediatric Care

Pediatrics is a relatively new medical specialty, developing only in the mid-1800s. In colonial times, epidemics were common, and many children died in infancy or childhood. In some cases, disease wiped out entire families. Sometimes, white society deliberately exposed Native American children to new and fatal diseases; other times transmission of these diseases was unwitting. Medicine men then cared for these children, who often died. Children of slaves received only the care their slave owner cared to provide.

Families were large to compensate for the children who did not live to adulthood. Society viewed children as additional hands to help with the family farm chores. Sick children often were cared for by the adults in the family or by a neighbor with a reputation of being able to care for the sick.

The first children's hospital opened in Philadelphia in 1855. Until that point in Western civilization, children were not valued, except as contributors to family income. Physicians treated hospitalized children as small adults. Often, children shared the same hospital bed with an adult. Unfortunately, early institutions for children were notorious for their unsanitary conditions, neglect, and lack of proper infant nutrition. Well into the 19th century, mortality rates were commonly 50% to 100% among institutionalized children in asylums or hospitals.

Many view Arthur Jacobi, a Prussian-born physician, as the father of pediatrics. Under his direction, several New York hospitals opened pediatric units. He helped found the American Pediatric Society in 1888. During the early 1900s, intractable diarrhea was a primary cause of death in children's institutions. Initiation of the simple practices of boiling milk and isolating children with septic conditions lowered the incidence of diarrhea. This practice of pasteurizing milk was instrumental in decreasing the rate of death in children.

After World War I, a period of strict asepsis began. Institutions provided individual cubicles for babies and strictly forbade nurses to pick up the children, except when necessary. Nurses draped clean sheets over the crib sides, leaving infants with nothing to do but stare at the ceiling. These practices did not consider the now recognized importance of toys in a child's environment; besides, prevailing thought was that such objects could transmit infection. Parents could only visit for half an hour or perhaps 1 hour each week, and institutional rules forbade them to pick up their children under penalty of having their visiting privileges revoked.

Despite these precautions, high infant mortality rates continued. One of the first people to suspect the cause was Joseph Brennaman, a physician at Children's Memorial Hospital in Chicago. In 1932, he suggested that the infants suffered from a lack of stimulation; other concerned child specialists became interested. In the 1940s, Ren Spitz published the results of studies showing that deprivation of maternal care caused a state of dazed stupor in an infant. He believed this condition could become irreversible if the child remained separated from the mother. He termed this state "anaclitic depression." Spitz also coined the term *hospitalism,* which he defined as "a vitiated condition of the body due to long confinement in the hospital" (*vitiated* means feeble or weak). Later, the term came to be used almost entirely to denote the harmful effects of institutional care on infants. Another physician, Bakwin, found that infants hospitalized for a long time actually developed physical symptoms that he attributed to a lack of emotional stimulation and a lack of feeding satisfaction.

Working under the auspices of the World Health Organization, John Bowlby of London thoroughly explored the subject of maternal deprivation. His 1951 study, which received worldwide attention, revealed the negative results of the separation of child and mother due to hospitalization. Bowlby's work, together with that of associate John Robertson, led to a re-evaluation and liberalization of hospital visiting policies for children.

In the 1970s and 1980s, Marshall Klaus and John Kennell, physicians at Rainbow Babies and Children's Hospital in Cleveland, carried out important studies on the effect of the separation of newborns and parents. They established that early separation may have long-term effects on family relationships and that offering the new family an opportunity to be together at birth and for a significant period after birth may provide benefits that last well into early childhood (Fig. 1-1). These findings also have helped to modify hospital policies. Hospital regulations changed slowly, but they gradually began to reflect the needs of children and their families. Isolation practices have been relaxed for children who do not have infectious diseases; children are encouraged to ambulate as early as possible and to visit the playroom, where they can be with other children. Nurses at all levels who work with children are prepared to understand, value, and use play as a therapeutic tool in the daily care of children.

■ Figure 1-1 The mother, father, and infant son soon after birth. (Photo by Joe Mitchell.)

Table 1-1 highlights selected milestones in maternal-child health care development.

CURRENT TRENDS IN MATERNAL–CHILD HEALTH CARE
Family-Centered Care

Society began to view childbirth as a safe and natural process as maternal and infant mortality rates began to fall. Women questioned the need for intense intervention in every birth. Also in question were the effects that medications and anesthesia had on the fetus. Many women began to insist on natural childbirth methods that allowed nature to take its course with minimal medical involvement. Some women voiced the desire for increased control over decisions about the timing and extent of interventions during labor and birth.

These efforts throughout the 1970s, 1980s, and 1990s led to family-centered maternity care, which eventually became the norm for American hospitals. Physicians and other health care practitioners began to respect the rights of women to participate in planning the type of care given during labor and birth. Husbands were at first allowed, and then encouraged, to participate in the birth process. Hospitals allowed siblings greater access to their mother and the new baby. Birthing rooms and later labor, delivery, and recovery rooms (LDR) replaced the old assembly-line system of moving from a labor room, to a delivery room, to a recovery room. In many hospitals, mothers and newborns remain together and receive care from one nurse. This type of postpartum care takes the place of the older model, in which a nursery nurse cared for the baby in the nursery and a postpartum nurse took care of the mother.

Family-centered pediatric nursing is a new and broadened concept in the health care system of the United States. It is no longer acceptable to treat children merely as clinical cases with attention given exclusively to their medical problems. Instead, health care practitioners must recognize that children belong to a family, a community, and a particular way of life or culture and that these factors influence the child's health (Fig. 1-2). A philosophy that separates children from their backgrounds leads to care that meets their needs only in a superficial manner, if at all. Even if nursing takes place entirely inside hospital walls, family-centered care pays attention to each child's unique emotional, developmental, social, and scholastic needs, as well as physical ones. Family-centered nursing care also strives to help family members alleviate their fears and anxieties and to cope, function normally, and understand the child's condition and their role in the healing process (see Chapter 2).

Regionalized Care

During the past several decades, there has been a definite trend toward centralization and regionalization of maternity and pediatric services. Providing high-quality medical care for the at-risk patient necessitates transporting the

Table 1-1 ▊ SELECTED MILESTONES IN MATERNAL–CHILD HEALTH IN THE UNITED STATES

Time Period	Accomplishments
1800s	• Development of smallpox vaccination led to eventual eradication of smallpox. • Public school movement laid the foundation for free education for all children in the United States. • Society for prevention of cruelty to children established. • Pediatrics recognized as a special branch of medicine. • Establishment of children's hospitals in most large cities by the mid-1890s.
1900–1909	• National child labor committee formed that laid the foundation for strong state and federal child labor laws.
1910–1919	• Pasteurization recognized as best way to ensure safe milk for infants and general population. • Establishment of The Children's Bureau to investigate and report on child health issues and resolve problems through legislation and the political process. • National birth registry established. Vital statistics record keeping highlighted causes of high mortality rates and stimulated change to improve.
1920–1929	• Adoption by Congress of the Maternity and Infancy Care Act (better known as the Sheppard Towner Act) funded many child and adult health programs. • Child Health Day established to focus national attention on the unique health needs of children.
1930–1939	• Milk fortified with vitamin D leads to the eventual eradication of rickets. • Discovery of vitamin K leads to the prevention of hemorrhagic disease in newborns. • Title V of the Social Security act became law, providing programs for maternity, infant, and child care. It is the longest-standing public health legislation in American history and continues to work to improve the health of women and children. • March of Dimes-initiated research defeated polio. March of Dimes continues to work to prevent birth defects, prematurity, and infant mortality.
1940–1949	• Children's Bureau active in the establishment of the United Nations International Children's Emergency Fund (UNICEF). • Centers for Disease Control (CDC) established. The CDC is now globally recognized as a leading force in public health expertise.
1950–1959	• American College of Obstetrics & Gynecology (ACOG) formed. • Polio vaccine developed.
1960–1969	• Phenylketonuria (PKU) screening test routinely administered to infants. Prevents many cases of mental retardation. • Birth control pills approved for use. The pill allowed women control over their childbearing. • The National Institute of Child Health and Human Development (NICHD) established to conduct and support research and training for maternal and child health issues. • All states developed child abuse reporting laws. • Measles and rubella vaccines licensed. • Head Start program established to help children who live in poverty get a "head start" on learning, social development, and health care. • Medicaid (Title XIX) established to provide health insurance coverage to low-income women and children. • Migrant Health Program established to provide prenatal and infant care services to migrants, seasonal farm workers, and their families.
1970–1979	• Developmental Disabilities Service Act passed. Initiated a multifaceted mandate to organize services for individuals with developmental disabilities. • Special Supplemental Food Program for Women, Infants, and Children (WIC) created. • Supplemental Security Income Disabled Children's Program (SSI/DCP) provided cash payments to the families of low-income children with disabilities.
1980–1989	• Child Safety Seats laws passed. • Institute of Medicine (IOM) issued a report: Preventing Low Birth Weight that focused national attention on this important issue. • The United Nations ratified the "Rights of Children" charter.
1990–1999	• The Individuals with Disabilities Education Act (IDEA) provides money to help pay for special education for children with disabilities from birth to age 21. • Healthy Start Program initiated to reduce infant mortality. • Healthy Child Care America campaign implemented. • The State Children's Health Insurance Program (SCHIP) Title XXI added to Social Security Act.
The new millennium	• Children's obesity epidemic recognized. • No Child Left Behind Act signed into law. • Two new vaccines approved: rotavirus and cervical cancer.

Source: MCH Timeline: History, Legacy and Resources for Education and Practice. Funded by the Maternal and Child Health Bureau, Health Resources and Services Administration, US Department of Health and Human Services. Retrieved January 17, 2007, from http://mchb.hrsa.gov/timeline.

External factors
Physical variables
Biological variables
Social variables
Cultural variables

Internal factors
Personal characteristics
Physiological processes
Growth and development
Behavior/Temperament

■ **Figure 1-2** Internal and external factors that influence the health and illness patterns of the child.

pregnant woman or the child to medical teaching centers with the best resources for diagnosis and treatment. To contribute to economic responsibility by avoiding duplication of services and equipment, the most intricate and expensive services and the most highly specialized personnel are available in the centralized location: maternal-fetal medicine specialists, neonatologists, pediatric neurologists, adolescent allergy specialists, pediatric oncologists, nurse play therapists, child psychiatrists, neonatal and pediatric nurse practitioners, and clinical nurse specialists. In these large regional centers are geneticists, at-risk antenatal units, neonatal intensive care units, computed tomography scanners, burn care units, and other highly specialized equipment and units.

Regionalized care often takes the maternity, neonatal, and pediatric patient far from home. Family caregivers must travel a longer distance to visit than if the patient were at a local suburban hospital. Family-centered care becomes even more important under these circumstances. Measures are taken to keep the hospitalization as brief as possible and the family close and directly involved in the patient's care. For the child in particular, separation from the family is traumatic and may actually retard recovery. Many of these regionalized centers (tertiary care hospitals) have accommodations where families may stay during the hospitalization of the pregnant woman, the neonate, or the child.

Advances in Research

Huge technological and scientific advances emerged at the same time the movement for family-centered care was gaining momentum. It became possible to save premature and low-birth-weight infants who previously would not have survived. Researchers perfected diagnostic techniques. Surgical techniques to intervene on the fetus while in utero have been developed. New research and techniques make it possible to detect and treat children born with congenital problems and disorders almost immediately after birth. Pediatric specialists and specialty units add to the ability to treat childhood disorders sooner, thus decreasing the effect of the concern on the child and family. These are only a few examples of the research advances.

Questions that influence maternity care are guiding many biomedical research projects today. Two areas of intense scientific inquiry are the prediction and prevention of preterm labor and the causes, prevention, and treatment of preeclampsia, a condition exclusively found in pregnancy marked by high blood pressure, edema, and loss of protein in the urine. Progress in the prevention and/or treatment of these disorders would decrease maternal and infant mortality rates significantly.

Gene therapy currently treats certain immune disorders. Scientists are studying ways to prevent and treat genetic disorders with gene therapy, which will likely be possible in the near future. Many animal, human, and stem cell studies are underway to better understand and treat a variety of obstetric disorders. Researchers and practitioners have made much progress in understanding and treating infertility. Other examples of current studies include the identification of genes that are responsible for the unique characteristics of Down's syndrome and therapies to treat intrauterine growth retardation (IUGR), a condition in which the fetus fails to gain sufficient weight.

Bioethical Issues

An ethical issue is one in which there is no one "right" solution that applies to all instances of the issue. Ethical decision making is a complex process that should involve many groups of individuals with varying experiences and perspectives. Recent scientific and medical advances have raised bioethical issues that did not exist in times past. Examples of bioethical issues that are present in our world today include the Human Genome Project (HGP), prenatal genetic testing, surrogate motherhood, and rationing of health care.

The HGP began in 1990 with the purpose of studying all of the human genes and how they function. Although completed in 2003, analyses of the data will continue for years to come. New concepts and ideas regarding many aspects of health and disease emerge as research continues. Identification of gene mutations in people who may be carriers of genetic disorders or who may be at risk for developing inherited disorders later in life has been a big part of the research findings in the project. Genetic testing and counseling is one area greatly affected by the HGP. Another focus of the HGP is to detect predisposition to certain diseases that do not become evident until adulthood. The ability to study the human gene and factors related to the inheritance of disease and disorders has an impact on the future health of all individuals.

Today it is possible to know many things about a child before the child is born. Ultrasound can reveal the gender of the fetus and certain abnormalities early in pregnancy. Amniocentesis and chorionic villus sampling show the entire genetic code of the fetus. In this way, diagnosis of many chromosomal abnormalities can occur during the first trimester. This knowledge allows the parents to make decisions about continuing the pregnancy or preparing to cope with a child who has a genetic disorder. Some parents want to know everything possible before the child is born, whereas others do not wish to interfere with the natural order of things and decline any type of prenatal testing.

Many ethical questions surround prenatal testing. Is it right to end a pregnancy because a child has a mild genetic abnormality? Will we become a society in which parents can choose or reject an unborn child based on his or her genetic code? Is it right to bring a child into the world with a severe defect, which may cause him and his caregivers untold pain and suffering? Is it okay to make life and death decisions based on quality of life? Or is any form of life sacred regardless of the quality? Because of technology that makes prenatal diagnosis possible, these and other ethical questions abound.

Surrogacy is an arrangement whereby a woman or a couple who is infertile contract with a fertile woman to carry a child. The fetus may result from in vitro fertilization techniques; then the embryos created from such techniques are implanted in the surrogate woman's womb. At other times, the surrogate mother becomes pregnant by artificial insemination with the sperm of the man or with the sperm of an unknown donor. Surrogate motherhood is a situation fraught with ethical dilemmas. Questions that surround this issue include the following: Who has the right to make decisions about the pregnancy? Who is legally obligated for the unborn child? What if one or the other of the parties changes their minds before the end of the pregnancy? What happens if the infant is born with a genetic disorder that leaves him physically or mentally disabled?

Did you know?

Many professional organizations have developed guiding principles for making certain ethical decisions. For example, the American Academy of Pediatrics (AAP) recommends that the rules surrounding adoption be used to guide decision making in surrogacy cases. This principle helps safeguard the rights of the child in this unusual situation.

A phenomenon that some have referred to as "rationing of health care" is on the rise. On the one hand, there have been enormous advances in knowledge, technology, and the ability to intervene to change outcomes. Some conditions that were untreatable in the past can now be treated and even cured. On the other hand, individuals who live in poverty are less likely to have access to these treatments and cures. Ethical questions that arise in this situation include the following. To which services should all citizens have access regardless of ability to pay? What services are appropriate to exclude if the consumer cannot afford payment?

Demographic Trends

Several demographic trends are influencing the delivery of maternal–child health care in the United States. The aging of society and the tendency of American families to have fewer children have caused a shift in focus from the needs of women and children to those of older adults. This trend along with budget deficits has shifted fund allocation away from health care programs and research that enhance the health care of women and children.

The growing percentage of minority populations in relation to white, non-Hispanic populations in the United States will continue to affect health care. Nurses and other health care providers need to provide culturally appropriate care. Practitioners must assess the use of nontraditional methods of healing and over-the-counter herbal remedies and integrate these methods into the plan of care. More and more nurses must accommodate the unique needs of these populations.

Poverty

One social issue that greatly influences maternity and pediatric care is the problem of poverty. Unfortunately, poverty rates are rising in this country, with a disproportionate number of women and children affected (DeLashmutt, 2007). A woman who lives in poverty is less likely to have access to adequate prenatal care. Poverty also has a negative impact on the ability of a woman and her children to be adequately nourished and sheltered. A woman who lives in poverty is at risk for substance abuse and exposure to diseases such as tuberculosis, human immunodeficiency virus/acquired immunodeficiency syndrome (HIV/AIDS), and other sexually transmitted infections. Each of these factors increases the chance of adverse outcomes for childbearing women and their children.

Cost Containment

Cost containment refers to strategies developed to reduce inefficiencies in the health care system. Inefficiencies can occur in the way consumers use health care. For example, taking a child to the emergency department (ED) for treatment of a cold is inappropriate use. It would be more efficient to treat the child's cold at a clinic.

Inefficiencies also can relate to the setting in which health care is given. For example, in the past, physicians admitted all surgical patients to the hospital the night, or sometimes even several days, before the scheduled procedure. This practice demonstrates an inefficient use of the hospital setting. Preparation of the patient for surgery takes place more efficiently on an outpatient basis without reducing quality.

Inefficiencies also can exist in the production of health services. For example, a neonatal intensive care unit (NICU) is a highly specialized, costly unit to operate. If every hospital in a large city were to operate a NICU, this would be an inefficient production of health services. It is more cost effective to have one large NICU for the entire region.

Cost Containment Strategies

Health care costs continue to increase at a rate out of proportion to the cost of living. This situation has challenged local, state, and federal governments; insurance payers; and providers and consumers of health care to cope with skyrocketing costs while maintaining quality of care. Some major strategies to help control costs include prospective payment systems, managed care, capitation, cost sharing, cost shifting, and alternative delivery systems.

Prospective Payment Systems

A **prospective payment system** predetermines rates paid to the health care provider to care for patients with certain classifications of diseases. The insurer pays these rates regardless of the costs that the health care provider actually incurs. This system tends to encourage efficient production and use of resources. The government first developed prospective payment systems in an attempt to control Medicare costs. These systems include diagnosis-related groups (DRGs) for inpatient billing; ambulatory payment classifications (APCs); and home health, inpatient rehabilitation facility, and skilled nursing facility prospective payment systems.

Managed Care

Managed care is a system that integrates management and coordination of care with financing in an attempt to improve cost effectiveness, use, quality, and outcomes. Managed care evolved from the old "fee-for-service" type of health insurance, in which insurers paid providers of care the amount they billed to provide a service. Under managed care plans, both the provider of service and the consumer have responsibilities to help control costs. Discussion of the main types of managed care plans— health maintenance organizations (HMOs), preferred provider organizations (PPOs), and point-of-service (POS) plans—takes place in the section "Payment for Health Services."

Capitation

Capitation is one method managed care plans use to reduce costs. The insurer negotiates a fixed amount per person for the health care provider to provide services for enrollees. The health care provider is obligated to provide care for the negotiated amount, regardless of the actual number or nature of the services provided.

Cost Sharing and Cost Shifting

Cost sharing refers to the costs that the patient incurs when using his or her health insurance plan. Examples of cost sharing are co-payments and deductibles. When costs go up, health insurance plans often increase the amount of deductibles and co-payments before they raise the price of the insurance premium. Cost shifting is a strategy in which the cost of providing uncompensated care for uninsured individuals passes to people who are insured. Often, cost shifting results in higher premiums, co-pays, and deductibles.

Alternative Delivery Systems

Another way to control costs is to provide alternative delivery systems. Many hospitals found that it is cost efficient to send a patient home earlier and provide follow-up care using a home health agency. Skilled and intermediate nursing and rehabilitation facilities and hospice programs are other examples of alternative delivery systems.

Nursing Contribution to Cost Containment

Specific cost-containment strategies that nurses have been instrumental in implementing include health promotion, case management, and critical care paths. Nurses are the primary providers of **utilization review**, which is a systematic evaluation of services delivered by a health care provider to determine appropriateness and quality of care, as well as medical necessity of the services provided.

Nurses have long advocated health promotion activities as a valuable way to maintain quality of life and control health care costs. Health promotion involves helping people to make lifestyle changes to move them to a higher level of wellness. Health promotion includes all aspects of health: physical, mental, emotional, social, and spiritual. Many nurses and nursing organizations lobby for increased spending on health promotion and illness prevention activities. For example, nurses may testify at a public hearing that it is more cost effective to provide comprehensive prenatal care for low-income women than to pay high "back end" costs of highly specialized care in a NICU for a preterm baby. Nurses also may lobby for low-cost programs to provide periodic screening examinations in schools. The argument in this example is that it is cheaper to screen for illness and provide early treatment than to provide care when a disease is well advanced and harder to treat.

Although nurses are not the only licensed professionals qualified to provide case management, many case managers

Table 1-2 ▌ CRITICAL PATH FOR SCHOOL-AGER WITH LONG-LEG CAST AFTER FRACTURE

	Day One	Day Two
Diagnostic Tests	CBC X-ray left leg.	
Assessments	Establish baseline neurovascular status, then neurovascular checks every 2 hours. Inspect cast. Assess head, chest, and abdomen for other injuries. Assess skin integrity.	Perform neurovascular checks every 4 hours. Teach family to perform neurovascular checks. Inspect cast. Teach family cast inspection. Assess skin integrity. Teach family skin integrity assessment.
Diet	Diet as tolerated.	Diet as tolerated. Provide instruction on adding foods rich in protein.
Activity	Elevate leg when lying or sitting. Start nonweight-bearing crutch walking. Initiate safety precautions.	Elevate leg when lying or sitting. Assess ability to use nonweight-bearing crutch walking for discharge. Maintain safety precautions.
Medications	Tylenol with codeine for pain as ordered.	Tylenol with codeine for pain as ordered. Tylenol for pain as ordered.
Psychosocial	Assess developmental status. Promote self-care (bathing, dressing, grooming, etc.). Provide diversional activities. Assist in continuing school work. Teach safety.	Provide instruction on diversional activities for home. Instruct family on how to promote self-care. Reinforce safety teaching.
Discharge Planning	Teach cast care. Teach crutch walking. Arrange for home tutoring.	Provide written instructions and obtain feedback on cast care. Provide written instructions and obtain feedback on crutch walking. Provide written instructions for home tutoring. Include family and child in teaching. Arrange for follow-up appointment.

A critical pathway is an abbreviated form of a care plan used by the entire multidisciplinary team. It provides outcome-based guidelines for goal achievement within a designated length of stay.

are nurses. **Case management** involves monitoring and coordinating care for individuals who need high-cost or extensive health care services. An at-risk pregnant woman with diabetes is a good candidate for case management because she requires frequent monitoring of blood sugars and coordination of several health care providers.

Concerns about cost containment, quality improvement, and managed care have led many facilities to develop a system of standard guidelines, termed **critical pathways**. Critical pathways are standard care plans used to organize and monitor the care provided. They include all aspects of care, such as diagnostic tests, consultations, treatments, activities, procedures, teaching, and discharge planning. Other names for critical pathways are caremaps, collaborative care plans, case management plans, clinical paths, and multidisciplinary plans. To ensure success, the critical pathways must be a collaborative effort of all disciplines involved, and all members of the health team must follow them.

The nursing process is part of the underlying framework of critical pathways. Nursing diagnoses and intermediate and discharge outcomes are necessary to avoid fragmenting care. Documentation of nursing interventions and outcomes is essential to the overall process. Understanding the nursing process thoroughly is essential to achieve accountability when providing care in a setting in which critical pathways are used (Table 1-2).

Test Yourself

✔ Name two major developments that contributed to the modernization of maternity care in the United States.

✔ The work of which pediatric reformer led to the liberalization of hospital visiting policies for pediatric patients in the 1950s?

✔ Define "prospective payment system."

PAYMENT FOR HEALTH SERVICES

Health care insurance often facilitates access to and use of health care services. Typically, families with health care insurance are more likely to have a primary care provider and to participate in appropriate preventive care (*Healthy People 2010*, 2001). Statistics provided by *Healthy People 2010* and supported by the midcourse review (2006) show that more than 44 million people in the United States do not have health insurance. Of this number, 11 million are children.

Most employers provide some form of medical insurance for employees and their families; or families may elect to purchase their own insurance apart from an employer. In either situation, this type of insurance is called private insurance. For those who are uninsured, the federal and state governments provide means to access health care services. In addition, specialized services, often funded by local, state, or federal governments or administered by private organizations, are available.

Private Insurance

Individuals and families can obtain private insurance through work benefits, or through individual means. The policyholder pays a monthly fee for the insurance coverage. The policyholder is responsible for paying the preset co-payment for any health services needed. Before the onset of managed care, medical services traditionally were paid for on a fee-for-service basis. Physicians billed for their services, and insurance providers paid whatever was charged. However, with technological advances and skyrocketing costs, managed care was born in an effort to contain costs and make health care affordable. Managed care insurance plans include HMOs and PPOs (Box 1-1).

Some insurance companies provide physicians fixed amounts to provide health care to individuals, regardless of the actual costs involved. This system discourages physicians from ordering costly laboratory and diagnostic tests or from giving treatments of questionable therapeutic benefit. It has also encouraged physicians to see more patients, which decreases the amount of time available to individual patients.

Managed care has had multiple effects on individual consumers of health care. Consumers pay higher premiums with higher deductibles and co-payment amounts. At the same time, they have fewer choices. The consumer may choose from a limited number of providers that belong to an HMO or who are "in network" if the insurance plan is set up as a PPO. Review panels chosen by the HMO or PPO have the right to review and decline services deemed unnecessary. Usually the consumer cannot appeal these decisions. This situation has led to a consumer movement for the right to sue these companies when decisions negatively affect the individual's health.

This is not to say that all of the effects have been negative. Managed care has provoked the health care industry to be more cost conscious and fiscally temperate. Health care providers are less likely to order expensive tests and procedures unless there is an unmistakable benefit. However, health care costs, particularly pharmaceutical costs, have continued to increase out of proportion to other costs of living.

> ### Box 1-1   ■   COMPARISON OF MANAGED CARE PLANS
>
> **Health Maintenance Organizations (HMOs)**
> With an HMO, the insurer
> - contracts with selected health care providers and facilities to provide health care services to its policyholders.
> - pays a fixed amount of money in advance to the provider or facility.
>
> The insured person (policyholder)
> - chooses health care providers and facilities from the approved provider list for their HMO.
> - pays flat fees associated with particular services.
> - usually cannot visit a specialist without preapproval from the insurer.
>
> **Preferred Provider Organizations (PPOs)**
> With a PPO, the insurer
> - also contracts with selected health care providers and facilities to provide health care services to policyholders.
> - does not prepay the provider or facility.
> - closely evaluates providers and facilities for unnecessary services.
> - may deny claims.
>
> The policyholder
> - has more choices for service providers when they choose a PPO versus an HMO.
> - may choose to access services from a provider that is not on the preferred provider list, although this may increase the policyholder's out-of-pocket expense for services rendered.

Federally Funded Sources

Medicaid

Medicaid was founded in 1965 under Title XIX of the Social Security Act. This federal program supplies block grants to states to provide health care for individuals who have low incomes and meet other eligibility criteria. Under broad federal guidelines, each state develops and administers its own Medicaid program; therefore, eligibility requirements and application processes vary from state to state. Pregnant women and children who meet the income guidelines qualify for this program (Centers for Medicare & Medicaid Services, 2005).

Although Medicaid has helped address the problem of access to health care for some childbearing women and some children, the process for applying is often complex and confusing. Many women and children who qualify do not benefit from the program. Concerned citizen groups in many states are working to modify the application process and find ways to assist eligible individuals to apply for and receive Medicaid.

State Child Health Insurance Program

Many families make too much money to qualify for Medicaid; however, health insurance is not available or affordable to them. Because of this problem, many pregnant women and children do not get adequate health care, particularly preventive care, such as prenatal care, well-child visits, and immunizations. In response to this need, the federal government instituted another block grant program to states under Title XXI of the Social Security Act. The State Child Health Insurance Program, also known by its acronym "SCHIP" or simply "CHIP," was enacted in 1997 as part of the Balanced Budget Act.

SCHIP provides health insurance to newborns and children in low-income families who do not otherwise qualify for Medicaid and are uninsured. Sliding scales based on total family income determine premiums and co-payment amounts. Emphasis is on preventive care and health promotion in addition to treatment for illness and disease. One of the requirements for states to participate in SCHIP is that each state must develop an outreach program to inform and enroll eligible families and children.

Special Supplemental Nutrition Program for Women, Infants, and Children

One federally funded program that continues to successfully meet its goal to enhance nutritional status for women and children is the Special Supplemental Nutrition Program for Women, Infants, and Children (WIC). WIC began serving low-income, nutritionally at-risk pregnant, breast-feeding, and postpartum women and their children (as old as 5 years) in 1974. The Food and Nutrition Service administers this grant program, which distributes monies to state agencies to provide benefits to eligible citizens.

Local health departments, hospitals, and clinics in all 50 states provide WIC services. Women and children must first meet income eligibility requirements, and then a trained health professional (such as a nurse, social worker, or physician) screens for nutritional risk factors based on federal guidelines (Fig. 1-3). Nutritional risk factors are categorized as medically based risk and diet-based risk. Examples of medical risk factors include conditions such as young maternal age, anemia, poor pregnancy outcomes, and being underweight. Diet-based risk includes diets with deficiencies in any of the major food groups, vitamins, or minerals. Because there are not unlimited funds available, at-risk women are screened according to predetermined categories of priority.

The WIC program is one of the federal government's success stories. Eligible women and their children receive food vouchers to redeem at participating grocery stores. The vouchers allow the woman to purchase foods that

■ **Figure 1-3** A trained registered nurse screens a pregnant woman and child at a WIC clinic. If the woman meets income and nutritional eligibility requirements, she may receive vouchers to purchase nutritious foods.

are high in at least one of the following nutrients: protein, iron, calcium, and vitamins A and C. Fortified cereals, milk, eggs, cheese, peanut butter, and legumes are examples of eligible foods. Although breast-feeding is encouraged, if a participant chooses to bottle-feed, the WIC program provides formula assistance up to 6 months of age (FNS/USDA, 2006).

Specialized Services

Other institutions and organizations are available across the United States to provide health care services to children for special conditions, regardless of the family's ability to pay. Two examples are the Shriners Hospital for Children and Easter Seals Early Childhood Intervention (ECI) program. The Shriners Hospital provides a wide variety of services at no charge to children with orthopedic disorders, burns, spinal cord injuries, and cleft lip and palate. Services provided to children include evaluation by specialists, diagnostic testing, surgical management, and provision of prostheses and other orthopedic devices for correction. There are no eligibility requirements, financial or otherwise, to qualify for Shriners services.

The Early Childhood Intervention (ECI) program, sponsored by Easter Seals, is available for the child with disabilities or developmental delays. This program can provide needed services for all children until the age of

Here's how you can help!

Provide the patient and family with a list of available community health care resources. This information can be of great help, especially if the family needs financial assistance to afford adequate medical treatment.

3 years, free of charge to any family. The services provided include evaluation and weekly therapy for rehabilitation. A therapist also can go to the patient's home to provide needed therapy. A referral from the health care provider is all that is required to qualify for this type of assistance.

MATERNAL–CHILD HEALTH TODAY

The Centers for Disease Control and Prevention (CDC) and the National Centers for Health Statistics track measures of our nation's health. Birth and death rates, life expectancy, and morbidity rates are examples of health statistics. The statistics of particular interest to the maternity and pediatric nurse include maternal, infant, and child mortality rates. In addition to tracking statistics, the CDC develops and supports programs and interventions to improve maternal/child health.

Maternal–Infant Health Status

Mortality (death) rates are statistics recorded as the ratio of deaths in a given category to the number of individuals in that category of the population. The CDC reports all mortality rates relating to the fetus, neonate, and infant as the number of deaths for every 1,000 live births. Reporting of maternal deaths is per 100,000 live births because these deaths, fortunately, are uncommon. Box 1-2 defines selected terms used in vital statistics.

The **infant mortality rate** is the number of deaths during the first 12 months of life per 1,000 live births. The **maternal mortality rate** refers to the number of maternal deaths per 100,000 live births caused by a pregnancy-related complication that occurs during pregnancy or during the 42 days after pregnancy. Maternal mortality rate provides a measure of the likelihood that a pregnant woman will die from maternal causes. Box 1-3 lists the leading causes of infant and maternal deaths.

Both infant and maternal mortality rates have fallen dramatically since the early 1900s. At that time, for every 1,000 live births, approximately 100 infants died before they reached their first birthday. In 1940, that number had dropped to a little less than 50 deaths per 1,000 live births—a decline greater than 50%! Between 1940 and 2005, the rate steadily decreased to 6.87 deaths per 1,000 live births (Fig. 1-4). Maternal mortality rates at the turn of the century were from 600 to 900 deaths per 100,000 live births and decreased to 12.1 deaths per 100,000 live births by 2003 (Fig. 1-5).

Notwithstanding these remarkable advances, much work remains. The United States lags behind 21 other

---

Box 1-2 ▌ SELECTED VITAL STATISTIC DEFINITIONS

Birth rate: The number of live births per 1,000 population (in a calendar year).

Fetal death: The intrauterine death of a fetus before delivery.

Fetal mortality rate: Most states define fetal mortality as the number of fetal deaths of 20 weeks or more gestation for every 1,000 live births.

Neonatal mortality rate: The number of infant deaths during the first 28 days of life for every 1,000 live births.

Infant death: Death of a live-born child before his or her first birthday (includes neonatal death).

Infant mortality rate: The number of infant deaths per 1,000 live births within a calendar year (includes neonatal mortality rate).

Maternal mortality rate: The number of maternal deaths per 100,000 live births caused by a pregnancy-related complication that occurs during pregnancy or during the 42 days after pregnancy.

Source: The National Center for Health Statistics. NCHS Definitions. Retrieved October 17, 2007, from http://www.cdc.gov/nchs/datawh/nchsdefs/list.htm.

Box 1-3 ▌ LEADING CAUSES OF INFANT AND MATERNAL MORTALITY IN THE UNITED STATES

Infant Mortality

The three leading causes of infant death for the year 2004 (the latest year for which data are available; 2005 preliminary data are very similar) listed in descending order:

1. Congenital malformations, deformations, and chromosomal abnormalities (20.1%)
2. Disorders related to short gestation and low birth weight (16.6%)
3. Sudden infant death syndrome (SIDS) (8.0%)*

Maternal Mortality

The three leading causes of pregnancy-related death for the years 1991 to 1999 (the latest decade for which long-term comparative data are available) listed in descending order:

1. Embolism (20%)
2. Hemorrhage (17%)
3. Pregnancy-related hypertension (16%)[†]

*Source: Miniño, A. M., Heron, M., Murphy, S. L., & Kochanek, K. D. (2007). Deaths: Final data for 2004. *National Center for Health Statistics.* Retrieved January 13, 2007, from http://www.cdc.gov/nchs/products/pubs/pubd/hestats/finaldeaths04/finaldeaths04.htm.

[†]Source: Centers for Disease Control. (2003). Pregnancy-related mortality surveillance, United States, 1991–1999. *MMWR surveillance summaries.* Retrieved January 13, 2007, from http://www.cdc.gov/mmwr/preview/mmwrhtml/ss5202a1.htm.

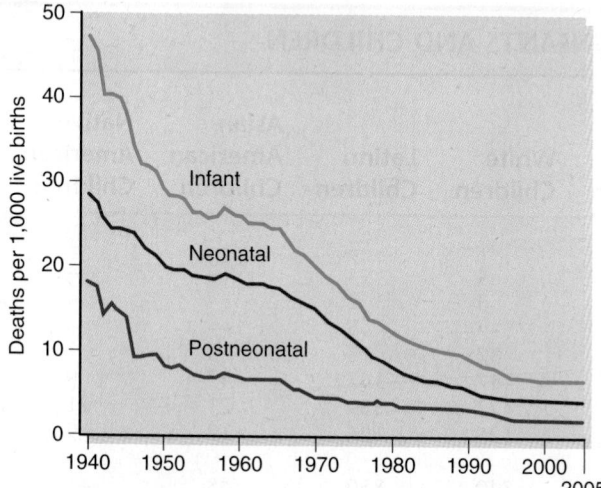

NOTE: Rates are infant (under 1 year), neonatal (under 28 days), and postneonatal (28 days–11 months) deaths per 1,000 live births in specified group.
SOURCE: CDC, NCHS, National Vital Statistics System, Mortality.

■ Figure 1-4 United States infant mortality rate by year (1940–2005). (From Kung, H. C., Hoyert, D. L., Xu, J. Q., & Murphy, S. L. [2008]. Deaths: Final data for 2005. National Vital Statistics Reports, 56[10]. Hyattsville, MD: National Center for Health Statistics. Retrieved September 20, 2008, from http://www.cdc.gov/nchs/data/nvsr/nvsr56/nvsr56_10.pdf)

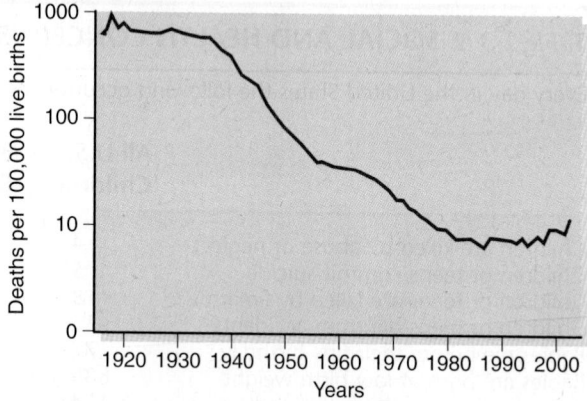

NOTE: Prior to 1933, data for birth-registration states only.

■ Figure 1-5 United States maternal mortality rate by year (1915–2003). (From Hoyert, D. L. [2007]. Maternal mortality and related concepts. National Center for Health Statistics. Vital Health Stat, 3[33]. Retrieved September 20, 2008, from http://www.cdc.gov/nchs/data/series/sr_03/sr03_033.pdf)

industrialized nations in maternal mortality statistics. Since 1982, the maternal mortality rate has hovered between 7 and 8 deaths per 100,000 live births. The *Healthy People 2000* goal[2] of 3.3 maternal deaths per 100,000 live births set in 1987 is still unrealized. In 2004, the latest year for which data are available, the maternal mortality rate was 13.1 (Miniño et al., 2007).

In addition, there is racial disparity in maternal mortality rates. In 2003, the maternal mortality rate for black women was 3.5 times the rate for white women (Hoyert et al., 2006). A black woman is almost twice as likely as a white woman to experience a pregnancy complication and is four times more likely to die of a complication of pregnancy. If the United States could eliminate the disparity, the overall rate would fall considerably (CDC, 2005).

The United States also lags behind many other industrialized nations with regard to infant mortality. The U.S. infant mortality rate for 2003 was 6.75; more than twice that of Japan, the country with the lowest reported rate of 3.3 (The World Factbook, 2007). Many factors may be associated with high infant mortality rates and poor health. Low birth weight and late or nonexistent prenatal care are main factors in the poor rankings in infant mortality. Other major factors that compromise infants' health include congenital anomalies, sudden infant death syndrome, respiratory distress syndrome, and in-

creasing rates of HIV. Low birth weight and other causes of infant death and chronic illness are often linked to maternal factors, such as lack of prenatal care, smoking, use of alcohol and illicit drugs, pregnancy before age 18 or after age 40, poor nutrition, lower socioeconomic status, lower educational levels, and environmental hazards.

Both infant and maternal mortality rates are much higher among nonwhite populations; studies repeatedly attribute high mortality rates to lack of adequate prenatal care and an increased birth rate among the high-risk group of adolescent girls and young women 15 to 19 years of age. The lack of adequate financial resources, insurance, and education regarding birth control and health care in general contributes to this situation.

Child and Adolescent Health Status

In the first half of the 20th century, many children died during or after childbirth or in early childhood because of disease, infections, or injuries. Technological and socioeconomic changes have influenced both the health problems today's children face and the health care they receive. Communicable diseases of childhood and their complications are no longer a serious threat to the health of children. As the 21st century begins, health problems for children focus much more on social concerns (Table 1-3). A summary of these issues follows; more in depth coverage of specific issues occurs throughout the text.

Infectious diseases such as polio, diphtheria, scarlet fever, measles, and whooping cough once posed the greatest threat to children. However, today, the largest risk to all children and adolescents is unintentional injury, frequently the result of motor vehicle accidents. Other unintentional injuries include drowning, falls, poisonings, and fires. Families, communities, and government agencies minimize the risks of injury-related death through protection and safety measures.

---

[2]*Healthy People 2000* were national health goals set in 1987. For further information on the *Healthy People* initiative see the Web site: http://www.health.gov/healthypeople/

Table 1-3 ■ **SOCIAL AND HEALTH CONCERNS FOR INFANTS AND CHILDREN**

Every day in the United States the following occurrences take place:

	All U.S. Children	Black Children	White Children	Latino Children	Asian American Children	Native American Children
Children are killed by abuse or neglect	4	—	—	—	—	—
Children or teens commit suicide	5	—	4	—	—	—
Children or teens are killed by firearms	8	3	3	2	—	—
Children or teens die from accidents	35	—	—	5	—	—
Babies die before their first birthday	77	22	37	13	3	1
Babies are born at low birth weight	888	219	447	167	47	9
Babies are born to teenage mothers	1,154	284	477	359	21	21
Babies are born to mothers who received late or no prenatal care	367	92	125	126	19	9
Babies are born into poverty	2,447	723	749	850	45	41
Children are arrested for drug abuse	380	103	270	—	3	3
Children are arrested for violent crimes	181	83	94	—	2	2
Students drop out of high school each school day	2,756	506	1,345	856	11	—

Source: Children's Defense Fund, 2005
Note: not all totals equal 100%.

Morbidity refers to the number of persons afflicted with the same disease condition per a certain number of population. Morbidity rates among children often are associated with environmental and socioeconomic issues. According to the American Academy of Pediatrics (AAP), the increasing complexity in the environment seems to have created new morbidities that greatly affect the child's psychosocial development. These include:

- School problems, including learning disabilities and attention difficulties
- Child and adolescent mood and anxiety disorders
- Adolescent suicide and homicide, which is increasing alarmingly
- Firearms in home
- School violence
- Drug and alcohol abuse
- HIV and AIDS
- Effects of media on violence, obesity, and sexual activity

Historically, disease conditions affecting children were very different from those affecting adults. Today, an increasing number of health conditions that used to be seen only in adults are occurring in children. For example, hyperlipidemia and hypercholesterolemia are appearing more frequently in children. Statistics reveal an increase in the number of children older than 12 years of age identified with hypertension (elevated blood pressure). Obesity is another major health concern in children. According to the National Health and Nutrition Examination Survey (NHANES), from 2003 to 2004, 17% of children and adolescents between the ages of 2 and 19 years were overweight or obese. In addition, children are now included in the statistics for patients experiencing depression. For example, major depressive disorder occurs in approximately 1% to 3% of children, and dysthymic disorder (chronic depression with no clearly defined well periods) occurs in 1% of children and 8% of adolescents.

Developmental problems related to socioeconomic factors are on the rise, including mental retardation, learning disorders, emotional and behavioral problems, and speech and vision impairments. Lead poisoning appears to be a major threat to the child's developmental well-being. Although strict laws have minimized the amount of lead in gas, air, food, and industrial emissions, many children live and play in substandard housing areas where exposure to chipped lead-based paint, dust, and soil often occurs.

Other prevalent factors that affect children's health include respiratory illness, violence toward children in the form of child abuse and neglect, homicide, suicide, cigarette smoking, alcohol and illicit drug use, risky sexual behavior, obesity, and lack of exercise.

Establishment of healthy living habits takes place in early childhood. Many schools educate students about the hazards of tobacco, drugs, and the importance of exercise, nutrition, and safe sex. Many also provide immunization and screening programs. However, there is still a need for improvements and increases in the number of educational and support programs available to children, families, and communities. The program goals should be to alleviate many child health problems and provide children with adequate tools to make healthy living choices well into adulthood.

Addressing Maternal–Child Health Status

The United States has successfully improved the health of women and their children in many areas. Examples include the Newborn Hearing Screening program to reduce preventable complications of early hearing loss. Another success is the 50% reduction in cases of sudden infant death syndrome (SIDS) after initiation of the Back to Sleep campaign. The Breast-Feeding Friendly Workplace initiative has increased the proportion of women who breast-feed for at least 6 months (Brush et al., 2005). Immunization against infectious diseases is one of the most significant public health achievements of the 20th century. The CDC sponsors National Immunization Awareness Month (NIAM), with the goal of increasing awareness about immunizations across the life span and to promote the benefits of immunization.

Still, much work remains. Box 1-4 lists the Centers for Disease Control (CDC) recommendations of ways to continue to decrease maternal and infant mortality. National initiatives to reduce infant and child mortality include The National Maternal and Child Health Bureau (MCHB) Center for Child Death Review, The National Fetal and Infant Mortality Review (NFIMR) Program, the Pregnancy Risk Assessment Monitoring System (PRAMS), and *Healthy People 2010*.

The National MCHB Center for Child Death Review

The National MCHB Center for Child Death Review (CDR) is a national resource center funded by the U.S. Department of Health and Human Services. The center aims to better understand how and why children die in order to prevent other deaths and improve the health and safety of children. The center offers a wide range of services to state and local CDR teams including technical assistance, training, and support; resources and tools; a national CDR reporting system; coordination with other review teams; collaboration with other child health, safety, and protection programs and organizations; and promotion of CDR to national organizations (CDC, 2006).

Box 1-4 ▌ OPPORTUNITIES TO REDUCE MATERNAL AND INFANT MORTALITY

Prevention measures to reduce maternal and infant mortality and to promote the health of all childbearing-aged women and their newborns should start before conception and continue through the postpartum period. Some of these prevention measures include the following:

Before Conception
- Screen women for health risks and pre-existing chronic conditions, such as diabetes, hypertension, and sexually transmitted diseases.
- Counsel women about contraception and provide access to effective family planning services (to prevent unintended pregnancies and unnecessary abortions).
- Counsel women about the benefits of good nutrition; encourage women especially to consume adequate amounts of folic acid supplements (to prevent neural tube defects) and iron.
- Advise women to avoid alcohol, tobacco, and illicit drugs.
- Advise women about the value of regular physical exercise.

During Pregnancy
- Provide women with early access to high-quality care throughout pregnancy, labor, and delivery. Such care includes risk-appropriate care, treatment for complications, and the use of antenatal corticosteroids when appropriate.

- Monitor and, when appropriate, treat pre-existing chronic conditions.
- Screen for and, when appropriate, treat reproductive tract infections including bacterial vaginosis, group B streptococcus infections, and human immunodeficiency virus.
- Vaccinate women against influenza, if appropriate.
- Continue counseling against use of tobacco, alcohol, and illicit drugs.
- Continue counseling about nutrition and physical exercise.
- Educate women about the early signs of pregnancy-related problems.

During Postpartum Period
- Vaccinate newborns at age-appropriate times.
- Provide information about well-baby care and benefits of breast-feeding.
- Warn parents about exposing infants to second-hand smoke.
- Counsel parents about placing infants to sleep on their backs.
- Educate parents about how to protect their infants from exposure to infectious diseases and harmful substances.

From Centers for Disease Control. (1999). Healthier mothers and babies. *MMWR: Morbidity and Mortality Weekly Report, 48*(38), 849–856. Retrieved October 17, 2007, from http://www.cdc.gov/mmwr/PDF/wk/mm4838.pdf

The National Fetal and Infant Mortality Review (NFIMR) Program

The NFIMR Program is a collaborative effort between the MCHB and the American College of Obstetricians and Gynecologists (ACOG) that addresses fetal and infant mortality issues. The purpose of the program is similar to that of the Center for CDR, to better understand the causes of fetal and infant mortality so that implementation of prevention measures can occur. The program includes a resource center that provides information and advice about implementing NFIMR methods (CDC, 2006).

Pregnancy Risk Assessment Monitoring System (PRAMS)

The CDC initiated PRAMS in 1987 because infant mortality rates were no longer declining as rapidly as they had in prior years. In addition, the incidence of low birth weight infants had changed little in the previous 20 years. The goal of the PRAMS project is to improve the health of mothers and infants by reducing adverse outcomes such as low birth weight, infant mortality and morbidity, and maternal morbidity. PRAMS provides state-specific data for planning and assessing health programs and for describing maternal experiences that may contribute to maternal and infant health (CDC, 2006). Research indicates that maternal behaviors during pregnancy may influence infant birth weight and mortality rates. Issues that PRAMS has addressed include HIV counseling for pregnant women, physical violence during pregnancy, nutritional intake of folic acid by women of childbearing age, postpartum depression, and unintended pregnancy.

Healthy People 2010

In 1990, a national consortium of more than 300 organizations developed a set of objectives for the year 2000, *Healthy People 2000*. Prevention of illness, or health promotion, was the underlying goal of these objectives. States were encouraged to set their own objectives. Priority areas specifically affecting children were identified. The initiative has continued, and *Healthy People 2010* outlines two basic goals for health promotion and disease prevention (*Healthy People 2010*, 2001):

1. Increase quality and years of healthy life
2. Eliminate health disparities

These goals are broken down into focus areas and attainment objectives. Many of the focus areas and objectives directly relate to pregnant women and children and their health care (Box 1-5). Nurses caring for pregnant women and children use these objectives as underlying guidelines in planning care.

Looking toward the future, the Healthy People program is already seeking input from communities across the nation to develop *Healthy People 2020*. Assessments of major risks to health and wellness, changing public health priorities, and emerging technologies related to health awareness and prevention will be used to develop the goals, objectives, and action plan for *Healthy People 2020*.

Test Yourself

✔ Name the number one cause of maternal mortality in the United States.

✔ Name one health care milestone related to women or children for each decade of the twentieth century.

✔ What are the two basic goals for health promotion and disease prevention outlined by *Healthy People 2010*?

THE NURSE'S CHANGING ROLE IN MATERNAL–CHILD HEALTH CARE

The image of nursing has changed, and the horizons and responsibilities have broadened tremendously in recent years. The primary thrust of health care is toward prevention. In addition to the treatment of disease and physical problems, modern maternal–child care addresses prenatal care, growth and development, and anticipatory guidance on maturational and common health problems. Teaching also is an important aspect of caring for the childbearing and child-rearing family. Nurses educate clients on a variety of topics, from follow-up of immunizations to other, more traditional aspects of health.

As a nurse at any level, you are legally accountable for your actions and assume new responsibilities and accountability with every advance in education. Practicing in maternity and pediatric settings at any level requires keeping up to date with education and information on how to help patients and where to direct families for help when they need additional resources. When functioning as a teacher, adviser, and resource person, it is important to provide information and advice that is correct, pertinent, and useful to the person in need.

Advanced practice nurses, in particular the certified nurse midwife (CNM) and nurse practitioners—family, neonatal, and pediatric—have taken a significant place in caring for childbearing and child-rearing families. The family nurse practitioner (FNP) provides primary care for women and their families. When pregnancy occurs, the FNP usually refers the woman to a CNM or obstetrician for prenatal care. The neonatal nurse practitioner (NNP) specializes in the care of the neonate. Hospital NICUs and neonatologists employ NNPs to provide care for premature and other sick newborns. The pediatric nurse practitioner (PNP) specializes in primary care of the child. Some of these nurses specialize in school nursing or oncology, among other areas. In addition, the clinical nurse

Box 1-5 ■ HEALTHY PEOPLE 2010: FOCUS AREAS RELATED TO CHILDBEARING WOMEN AND CHILDREN

Focus Area: Access to Quality Health Services
Goal: Improve access to comprehensive, high-quality health care services.
  Persons with health insurance
  Single toll-free number for poison control centers
  Special needs for children
  Early (starting in the first trimester) and consistent prenatal care
Focus Area: Educational and Community-Based Programs
Goal: Increase the quality, availability, and effectiveness of education and community-based programs designed to prevent disease and improve health and quality of life.
  School health education
  School nurse-to-student ratio
  Community health promotion programs
  Patient and family education
  Culturally appropriate and linguistically competent community health promotion programs
Focus Area: Environmental Health
Goal: Promote health for all through a healthy environment.
  Safe drinking water
  Elevated blood lead levels in children
  School policies to protect against environmental hazards
  Toxic pollutants
Focus Area: Family Planning
Goal: Improve pregnancy planning and spacing and prevent unintended pregnancy.
  Adolescent pregnancy
  Abstinence before age 15 and among adolescents aged 15 to 17 years
  Birth spacing
  Contraceptive use
  Male involvement in pregnancy prevention
  Pregnancy prevention and sexually transmitted disease (STD) protection
  Insurance coverage for contraceptive supplies and services
  Problems in becoming pregnant and maintaining a pregnancy
Focus Area: HIV
Goal: Prevent HIV infection and its related illness and death.
  Condom use
  Screening for STDs and immunization for hepatitis B
  Perinatally acquired HIV infection
Focus Area: Immunization and Infectious Diseases
Goal: Prevent disease, disability, and death from infectious disease, including vaccine-preventable diseases.
  Hepatitis B and bacterial meningitis in infants and young children
  Antibiotics prescribed for ear infections
  Vaccination coverage and strategies
Focus Area: Injury and Violence Prevention
Goal: Reduce injuries, disabilities, and deaths due to unintentional injuries and violence.
  Child fatality review
  Deaths from firearms, poisoning, suffocation, motor vehicle crashes

  Child restraints
  Drownings
  Maltreatment and maltreatment fatalities of children
Focus Area: Maternal, Infant, and Child Health
Goal: Improve the health and well-being of women, infants, children, and families.
  Fetal, infant, child, adolescent deaths
  Maternal deaths and illnesses
  Prenatal and obstetric care
  Low–birth-weight and very low–birth-weight, preterm births
  Developmental disabilities and neural tube defects
  Prenatal substance exposure
  Fetal alcohol syndrome
  Breast-feeding
  Newborn screening
Focus Area: Nutrition and Overweight
Goal: Promote health and reduce chronic disease associated with diet and weight.
  Overweight or obesity in children and adolescents
  Iron deficiency in young children and in females of childbearing age
  Anemia in low-income pregnant females
  Iron deficiency in pregnant females
Focus Area: Physical Fitness and Activity
Goal: Improve health, fitness, and quality of life through daily physical activity.
  Physical activity in children and adolescents
Focus Area: Sexually Transmitted Diseases
Goal: Promote responsible sexual behaviors, increase access to quality services to prevent STDs and their complications.
  Responsible adolescent sexual behavior
  STD complications affecting females
  STD complications affecting the fetus and newborn
  Screening of pregnant women
Focus Area: Substance Abuse
Goal: Reduce substance abuse to protect the health, safety, and quality of life for all, especially children.
  Adverse consequences of substance use and abuse
  Substance use and abuse
Focus Area: Tobacco Use
Goal: Reduce illness, disability, and death related to tobacco use and exposure to secondhand smoke.
  Adolescent tobacco use, age, and initiation of tobacco use
  Smoking cessation by adolescents
  Exposure to tobacco smoke at home among children
Focus Area: Vision and Hearing
Goal: Improve the visual and hearing health of the nation.
  Vision screening for children
  Impairment in children and adolescents
  Newborn hearing screening, evaluation, and intervention
  Otitis media
  Noise-induced hearing loss in children

Adapted from National Center for Health Statistics. (2001). *Healthy people 2010.* Hyattsville, MD, Author.

specialist (CNS) is a nurse with advanced education, prepared to provide care at any stage of illness or wellness. Both the registered nurse (RN) and the licensed practical or vocational nurse (LPN/LVN) often work in the pediatric clinic setting or as a nurse on an acute pediatric unit.

As a nurse, you may care for children and their families in a variety of settings. Some of these settings include schools, homes, and ambulatory settings. In schools, nurses have become much more than Band-Aid dispensers: they monitor well children, including their immunizations and their growth and development. School nurses are often present or are consultants in classroom health education programs and often serve on committees that evaluate children with educational and social adjustment problems. For children with long-term or chronic illnesses, home care nurses can help provide care in the home. This home care often occurs in collaboration with other health care professionals. Pediatric nurses play an important role in ambulatory care settings; these settings help avoid separating the child from the family and provide a less costly means of administering health care to children. In addition, nurses contribute to health care research that will help lead to more improvements in the care of children and their families.

Health teaching is one of the most important aspects of promoting wellness. Such teaching for children and families may be concerned with safety, nutrition, health habits, immunizations, dental care, healthy development, and discipline. As a nurse, you may often be in a position to do incidental teaching, as well as more organized formal teaching. Some examples of possible teaching opportunities include those in a hospital work environment, such as helping the child and family understand a diagnosis or proposed treatment, understanding medications, and providing teaching materials to children and families. In the community, you can be an advocate for healthy living practices and policies or can serve as a volunteer in community organizations to promote healthy growth and development and anticipatory guidance. You can become involved with schools to offer knowledge and expertise in wellness practices. You can also serve as a role model to others in practicing good health habits. Use every opportunity to contribute to and encourage healthy living practices.

This text identifies teaching opportunities and supplies teaching suggestions throughout. However, during any teaching be alert to the abilities of the pregnant woman or child and family to understand the material. By using methods of feedback, questions and answers, and demonstrations when appropriate, confirm that the patient and family understand the information. This also gives you the opportunity to reinforce any areas of weak knowledge. With experience, all nurses can become very competent teachers.

A Personal Glimpse

My Grandpa's eyes gave me my first vision of nursing. A licensed practical nurse, he filled my head with hospital stories and my belly with chocolate milk. He saw people hurt by pain and fear, and he made them feel better. I wasn't much bigger than the children he saw, but I knew I wanted to make them feel better too. So I went to nursing school in the same hospital where I shared chocolate milk with Grandpa.

My pediatric nursing career started at graduation 25 years ago. Back then, the community pediatric unit was always filled to capacity. Outpatient and critical care services for children were minimal, so disorders ranged from the mild to the severe. Newborns through teens were treated for everything from mild diarrhea to significant trauma. But two things remained constant regardless of age or diagnosis: the pain and the fear.

Soon, helping sick children feel better was no longer enough. I realized early in my career that the best way to help was to prevent children from getting sick in the first place. So I went back to school, through baccalaureate and masters' degrees, to become a pediatric nurse practitioner (PNP). Seventeen years later, I still practice as a PNP in a rural community.

Changes in health care have put more emphasis on the various nonhospital settings, where most children receive care. Healthy children are less likely to become ill and more likely to become healthy adults. Prevention and health promotion are essential. They should be part of the care of all children (and adults!), including those who are hospitalized. I always take the time to teach the importance of immunizations, proper nutrition, growth, and development. A little goes a long way, and there is tremendous satisfaction in knowing that I've helped to ease pain and fear before they have a chance to get started.

Mary

Learning Opportunity: What are the challenges for the nurse caring for the child in a community health setting? Describe the priorities of the pediatric nurse in health

CRITICAL THINKING

In all nursing roles in maternal–child health care, it is important to use clinical judgment and purposeful thought and reasoning to make decisions; doing so leads to positive outcomes for the patient. This process is critical thinking. Collect data and use skills and knowledge to make a conscious plan to care for the patient and family. As you carry out the plan, continue to evaluate the care of the patient, keeping the desired outcomes always in mind. By using critical thinking, you can be more proficient and effective at meeting the needs of the patient. Critical thinking involves a systematic process used while following the nursing process.

THE NURSING PROCESS

The **nursing process** is a proven form of problem solving based on the scientific method. The nursing process consists of five components:

- Assessment
- Nursing diagnosis
- Outcome identification and planning
- Implementation
- Evaluation

Based on the data collected during the assessment, nurses determine nursing diagnoses, plan and implement nursing care, and evaluate the results. The process does not end here but continues through reassessment, establishment of new diagnoses, additional plans, implementation, and evaluation. The goal is to identify and deal with all the patient's nursing problems (Fig. 1-6).

Assessment

Nursing assessment is a skill that is practiced and perfected through study and experience. The practical-vocational nurse collects data and contributes to the child's assessment. It is important to be skilled in understanding the concepts of verbal and nonverbal communication; concepts of growth and development; anatomy, physiology, and pathophysiology; and the influence of cultural heritage and family social structure. Data collected during assessment of the pregnant woman or child and family form the basis of all nursing care for the patient.

Assessment and data collection begin with the admission interview and physical examination. During this phase, a relationship of trust begins to build between you and the family. This relationship forms more quickly when you are sensitive to the family's cultural background. Careful listening and recording of **subjective data** (data spoken by the child or family) and careful observation and recording of **objective data** (data you can observe) are essential to obtaining a complete picture.

Nursing Diagnosis

The process of determining a nursing diagnosis begins with analysis of information (data) gathered during the assessment. Along with the registered nurse or other health care professional, the practical-vocational nurse participates in the development of a nursing diagnosis based on actual or potential health problems that fall within the range of nursing practice. These diagnoses are not medical diagnoses; rather, nursing diagnoses describe the patient's response to a disease process, condition, or situation. Nursing diagnoses change as the patient's responses change; therefore, diagnoses are in a continual state of re-evaluation and modification.

There are three classifications of nursing diagnoses: actual, risk, and wellness diagnoses. **Actual nursing diagnoses** identify existing health problems. For example, a child who has asthma may have an actual diagnosis stated as *Ineffective Airway Clearance related to increased mucus production as evidenced by dyspnea and wheezing.* This statement identifies a health problem the child actually has (ineffective airway clearance), the factor that contributes to its cause (increased mucous production), and the signs and symptoms. This is an actual nursing diagnosis because of the presence of signs and symptoms and the child's inability to clear the airway effectively.

Risk nursing diagnoses identify health problems to which the patient is especially vulnerable. These identify patients at high risk for a particular problem. An example of a risk nursing diagnosis is *Risk for Injury related to uncontrolled muscular activity secondary to seizure.*

Wellness nursing diagnoses identify the potential of a person, family, or community to move from one level of wellness to a higher level. For example, a wellness diagnosis for a family adapting well to the birth of a second child might be *Readiness for Enhanced Family Coping.*

The North American Nursing Diagnosis Association (NANDA) first published an approved list of nursing diagnoses in 1973; since then, NANDA has revised and expanded the list periodically. The revision and development of nursing diagnoses continues to keep them current and useful in describing what nurses contribute to health care.

Outcome Identification and Planning

To plan nursing care for the patient, data must be collected (assessment) and analyzed (nursing diagnosis) and outcomes identified in cooperation with the child and family caregiver. These **outcomes** (goals) should be specific, stated in measurable terms, and include a time

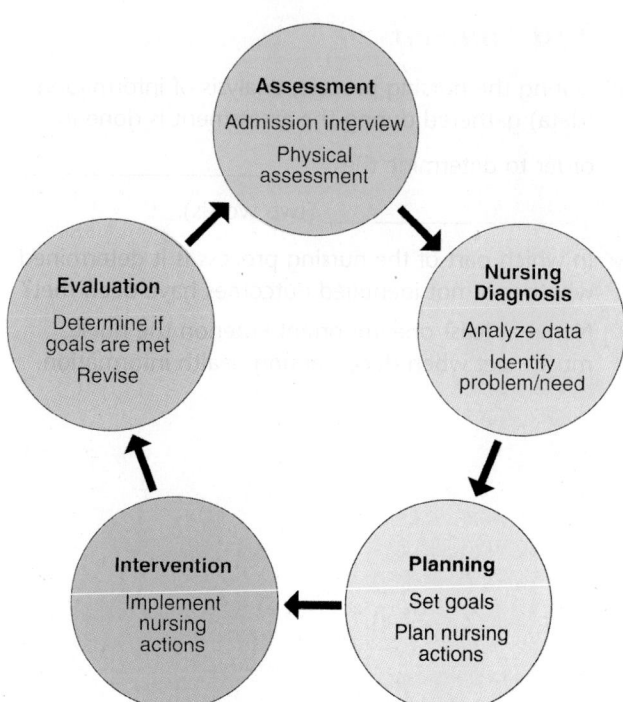

■ **Figure 1-6** Diagram of the Nursing Process.

frame. For example, a short-term expected outcome for a child with asthma could be "The child will demonstrate use of metered-dose inhaler within 2 days." The goal must be realistic, patient-focused, and attainable. Although the RN may identify a number of possible diagnoses and outcomes, he or she must review them, rank them by urgency, and select those that require immediate attention.

After selecting the first goals to accomplish, the RN must propose nursing interventions to achieve them. This is the planning aspect of the nursing process. These nursing interventions may be based on clinical experience, knowledge of the health problem, standards of care, standard care plans, or other resources. Interventions must be discussed with the patient and family to determine if they are practical and workable. Interventions are modified to fit the individual patient. If standardized care plans are used, they must be individualized to reflect the patient's age and developmental level; cognitive level; and family, economic, and cultural influences. Expected outcomes are set with specific measurable criteria and time lines.

Implementation

Implementation is the process of putting the nursing care plan into action. The actions may be independent, dependent, or interdependent. **Independent nursing actions** are actions that may be performed based on the nurse's own clinical judgment, for example, initiating protective skin care for an area that might break down. **Dependent nursing actions**, such as administering analgesics for pain, are actions that the nurse performs as a result of a physician's order. **Interdependent nursing actions** are actions that the nurse must accomplish in conjunction with other health team members, such as meal planning with the dietary therapist and teaching breathing exercises with the respiratory therapist.

Evaluation

Evaluation is a vital part of the nursing process. The practical nurse participates with other members of the health care team in the patient's evaluation. Evaluation measures the success or failure of the nursing plan of care. Success is determined by whether the patient has met identified outcomes. The criteria of the nursing outcomes determine if the interventions were effective. Like assessment, evaluation is an ongoing process. If the goals have not been met in the specified time, or if implementation is unsuccessful, the nurse may need to reassess and revise a particular intervention. Possibly the outcome criterion is unrealistic and needs to be discarded or adjusted. It is important to assess the patient and family to determine progress adequately. Both objective data (measurable) and subjective data (based on responses from the patient and family) are used in the evaluation.

DOCUMENTATION

One of the most important parts of nursing care is recording information about the patient on the permanent record. This record, the patient's chart, is a legal document and must be accurate and complete. Nursing care provided and responses to care are included. In maternity and pediatric settings, documentation is extremely important because records can be used in legal situations many years after the fact. These records include nurses' observations and findings, and they help explain and justify the actions taken.

You may complete various forms of documentation, including admission assessments, nurse's or progress notes, graphic sheets, checklists, medication records, and discharge teaching or summaries. Many health care settings use computerized or bedside documentation records. Whatever the system or form used, chart concise, factual information. Everything written must be legible and clear and include the date and time. Document nursing actions, such as medication administration, as soon as possible after the intervention to ensure the action is communicated, especially in the care of childbearing women and children.

Test Yourself

✔ During the nursing process, analysis of information (data) gathered during the assessment is done in order to determine the _____ _____ (two words).

✔ In which part of the nursing process is it determined whether or not identified outcomes have been met?

✔ Name at least one important criterion the nurse must meet when documenting health information.

Key Points

➤ Two major developments that changed maternity care in the United States were acceptance of the germ theory that led to decreased deaths from infection and the development of obstetric anesthesia to ease the pain of childbirth.

➤ Many changes have taken place in the care of children in the past century. Until the early part of the 20th century, society viewed children as miniature adults and expected them to behave that way.

➤ The concept of family-centered care developed in conjunction with the consumer movement that led childbirth to be viewed as a safe and natural process. Family-centered pediatric care recognizes that children should receive care within the context of their families and cultural norms.

➤ Regionalization of care contributes to economic responsibility by avoiding duplication of services and expensive equipment.

➤ Ethical dilemmas are by definition difficult to decide and involve complex choices and conflicts. Ethical decision making requires careful consideration and input from a variety of sources.

➤ Recent advances in research have led to new ethical dilemmas that must be addressed by health care providers. Examples include the Human Genome Project, prenatal genetic testing, surrogate motherhood, and rationing of health care.

➤ The increase in the number of older Americans, the tendency for American families to limit the number of children, and budget deficiencies have influenced a shift in focus away from programs for childbearing women and their infants.

➤ Poverty and the "rationing of health care" are social issues that have a negative impact on the health of childbearing women and children and increase the chance that complications will occur.

➤ Rising health care costs and shrinking budgets have led to attempts to reform health care. Managed care has become the norm of American health care. Attempts to contain health care costs have led to the development of prospective payment systems (such as HMOs and PPOs) and capitation. Nurses have been especially helpful with the cost-containment strategies of utilization review, critical pathways, and case management.

➤ Payment for health services for pregnant women and children may be provided through private insurance; federally funded programs such as Medicaid, SCHIP, or WIC; and specialized programs that offer services to children with special conditions.

➤ One way in which the health status of a nation is measured is through morbidity (illness) and mortality (death) rates. Measures particularly useful to maternity and pediatric health include maternal and pediatric mortality rates.

➤ The three leading causes of infant mortality are congenital disorders, prematurity and low birth weight, and sudden infant death syndrome. The three leading causes of maternal mortality are embolism, hemorrhage, and pregnancy-related hypertension.

➤ Although its infant mortality rate is improving, the United States still remains behind most other industrialized countries. Low birth weight and lack of or inadequate prenatal care are two major causes of this problem.

➤ Technologic and socioeconomic changes have influenced child health status. Many previous health concerns, such as communicable diseases of childhood have been eliminated. Health problems for children today focus more on social concerns.

➤ *Healthy People 2010* set goals for health care with a focus on health promotion and prevention of illness as the nation approaches the year 2010.

➤ The role of the nurse has changed to include the responsibilities of teacher, adviser, resource person, and researcher, as well as caregiver.

➤ Critical-thinking skills must be used to take data collected and use it to develop a plan to meet the desired outcomes for the maternity and pediatric patient.

➤ The nursing process is essential in the problem-solving process necessary to plan nursing care. The five steps of the nursing process include assessment, nursing diagnosis, outcome identification and planning, implementation, and evaluation.

➤ Accurate and timely documentation is essential for providing a legal record of care given. This is particularly important to the maternity and pediatric nurse because legal action can occur many years after an event.

INTERNET RESOURCES

Forum on Child and Family Statistics
www.childstats.gov
U.S. Department of Health and Human Services
www.dhhs.gov
USDA Food and Nutrition Service
www.fns.usda.gov/wic

Healthy People 2010
www.health.gov/healthypeople
Human Genome Project Information
www.ornl.gov/sci/techresources/Human_Genome/home.shtml
Shriners Hospitals for Children
http://shrinershq.org/Hospitals/Main

Workbook

■ NCLEX-STYLE REVIEW QUESTIONS

1. Preventing and treating infections during childbirth have reduced maternal and infant mortality rates. Of the following, which scientific advancement has done the *most* to improve neonatal mortality statistics?

    a. Control of puerperal fever
    b. Use of anesthesia during labor
    c. Enforcement of strict rules in hospitals
    d. Treatment advances for preterm infants

2. The nursing process is a scientific method and proven form of which process?

    a. Cost containment
    b. Problem solving
    c. Oral communication
    d. Health teaching

3. The nurse collects data and begins to develop a trust relationship with the patient in which step of the nursing process?

    a. Assessment
    b. Planning
    c. Implementation
    d. Evaluation

4. The nurse carries out nursing care for the patient in which step of the nursing process?

    a. Assessment
    b. Planning
    c. Implementation
    d. Evaluation

5. In caring for patients, a health care team often uses critical pathways. Which of the following are reasons critical pathways are used? (*Select all that apply.*) The critical pathway

    a. decreases cost for the patient and hospital.
    b. helps to establish a trusting relationship with patients.
    c. is followed by all members of the health team.
    d. provides organization for the care of the patient.
    e. includes all treatments and procedures.

■ STUDY ACTIVITIES

1. Choose the three social issues you think have the highest impact on health care concerns of children (use Table 1-3). Using these issues, complete the following table.

	How Does This Issue Affect Children's Health Care?	What Is the Nurse's Role in Dealing With This Issue?
Social issue		
Social issue		
Social issue		

2. Go to the following Internet site: http://web.health.gov/healthypeople/. At "Healthy People—Leading Health Indicators," click on "What are the Leading Health Indicators?"

    a. Make a list of the leading health indicators.
    b. Hit the back arrow and return to "Leading Health Indicators." Click on "Resources for Action." What is a resource site you could share with a family caregiver regarding health care access?
    c. What is a resource site you could share with someone needing information on injury or violence?

3. Discuss how children were cared for in institutions in the 19th and early 20th centuries. Describe the hospital care of infants and children in the period immediately after World War I.

■ CRITICAL THINKING: WHAT WOULD YOU DO?

1. A new mother tells you that her husband makes a few dollars an hour over the minimum wage, so her new baby is not eligible for Medicaid. She sighs and wonders aloud how she is going to pay for the medical bills. What would you say to the new mother? Does she have any options? If so, what are they?

2. Describe sociologic changes that have affected child health concepts and attitudes.

3. While working, you overhear an older nurse complaining about family caregivers "being underfoot so much and interfering with patient care." Describe how you would defend open visiting for family caregivers to this person.

2 Family-Centered and Community-Based Maternal and Pediatric Nursing

KEY TERMS

blended family
case management
client advocacy
cohabitation family
communal family
community-based nursing
couplet care
cultural competency
extended family
nuclear family
primary prevention
secondary prevention
single-parent family
socialization
stepfamily
tertiary prevention

LEARNING OBJECTIVES

On completion of this chapter, you should be able to:

1. Identify the primary purpose of the family in society.
2. Discuss the functions of the family.
3. Discuss the types of family structure.
4. List factors that have contributed to the growing number of single-parent families.
5. Describe how family size and sibling order affect children.
6. Explain the trend for families to spend less time together.
7. Identify the focus of community-based health care.
8. Describe advantages of community-based health care for the pregnant woman, child, and family.
9. Differentiate between primary, secondary, and tertiary prevention and give one example of each.
10. Discuss community care settings for the maternity and pediatric client.
11. List the skills needed by a community health nurse.
12. Explain the information a nurse needs to successfully teach a group of individuals.
13. Describe how child advocacy helps children in community-based health care.
14. Discuss challenges, issues, and rewards of community-based nursing.

EACH PERSON is a member of a family and a member of many social groups, such as church, school, and work. Families and social groups together make up the fabric of the larger society. It is within the context of the family and the community that an individual presents him- or herself to receive health care. When caring for maternity and pediatric patients, it is critical for you to recognize the context of the patient's needs within the patient's family and community.

THE FAMILY AS A SOCIAL UNIT

The arrival of a baby changes forever the primary social unit—a family—in which all members influence and are influenced by each other. Each subsequent child joining that family continues to reshape the individual members

and the family unit. In addition, the community affects family members as individuals and as a family unit.

Nursing care of women and children demands a solid understanding of normal patterns of growth and development—physical, psychological, social, and intellectual (cognitive)—and an awareness of the many factors that influence those patterns. It also demands an appreciation for the uniqueness of each individual and each family. For nursing care to be complete and as effective as possible, you must consider the identified patient as a member of a family and a larger community.

Throughout history, family structure has evolved in response to ongoing social and economic changes. Today's families may only faintly resemble the nuclear families of 30 or 40 years ago, in which the father worked outside the home and the mother cared for the children. In an estimated 60% to 70% of today's families with school-aged children, only one parent lives at home. More than 50% of American women with a child younger than 1 year of age work outside the home. Changes such as these place bigger demands on parents and have contributed to the growing demands on public institutions to fill the gaps. "Blended" families or step-families have created other major changes in family structure and interactions within the family. Divorce, abandonment, and delayed childbearing are all contributing factors.

Family Function

The family is civilization's oldest and most basic social unit. The family's primary purpose is to ensure survival of the unit and its individual members and to continue society and its knowledge, customs, values, and beliefs. It establishes a primary connection with a group responsible for a person until that person becomes independent.

Although family structure varies among different cultures, its functions are similar. The family serves two functions in relation to society: to reproduce and to socialize offspring. For each family member, the family functions to provide sustenance and support in the five areas of wholeness: physical, emotional, intellectual, social, and spiritual.

Physical Sustenance

The family is responsible for meeting each member's basic needs for food, clothing, shelter, and protection from harm, including illness. The family determines which needs have priority and chooses the resources used to meet those needs. Sometimes families need help obtaining the proper resources. For instance, a community program might partially fulfill a pregnant woman's nutritional needs. Some families need help learning to set priorities. For example, very young parents may benefit from parenting classes to learn to set priorities for infant and child care.

Traditionally, division of labor between the mother and the father was very clear. The mother provided total care for the children, and the father provided the resources to make care possible. These attitudes have changed so that in a two-parent family, each parent has an opportunity to share in the joys and trials of child care and other aspects of family living. In the **single-parent family**, one person must assume all these responsibilities.

> **Don't be quick to judge!**
> It is easy to forget how many responsibilities a single parent has. You may be able to help by finding a Big Brother or Big Sister program in your community, in which an older teen or young adult "adopts" a child and provides special social opportunities for him. For instance, the Big Brother may take the child to a ball game.

Emotional Support

The process of parental attachment to a child begins before birth and continues throughout life. Encouragement of early interaction between the new parents, and the newborn enhances this process.

Research studies continue to support the importance of early parent–child relationships to emotional adjustment in later life. Research supports that healthy parent–child attachment relates significantly to two variables: sensitivity of the parent in responding to the child's signals and the amount and nature of interaction (O'Gorman, 2006). A difference of only a few hours of interaction per day may constitute a critical period in the emotional bond between parent and child. Although specific results of these studies are controversial, there is general agreement that young children are highly sensitive to psychological influences, which may have long-range positive or negative effects.

Within the family, children learn who they are and how their behavior affects other family members. Children observe and imitate the behavior of family members. They quickly learn which behaviors the parents reward and which behaviors bring punishment. Participation in a family is a child's primary rehearsal for parenthood. How parents treat the child has a powerful influence on how the child will treat future children. Studies show that abused children often grow up to abuse their own children.

Intellectual Stimulation

Many experts suggest that parents read to their unborn children and play music to provide early stimulation. It is unknown when the fetus can actually hear, but it is clear that the newborn recognizes and finds comfort in his or her parents' voices.

The need for intellectual development continues throughout life. The small infant needs to have input through his five senses to develop optimally. Many parents buy brightly colored toys and play frequently with their infants to facilitate this stimulation. Talking and reading to the infant and small child is another way parents fulfill this function.

Socialization

Within the family, a child learns the rules of the society and culture in which the family lives: its language, values, ethics, and acceptable behaviors. The family accomplishes this process, called **socialization**, by training, education, and role modeling. The family teaches children acceptable ways of meeting physical needs, such as eating and elimination, and certain skills, such as dressing oneself. The family educates children about relationships with other people inside and outside the family. Children learn what their society permits and approves and what it forbids.

Each family determines how to accomplish goals based on its principles and values. Family patterns of communication, methods of conflict resolution, coping strategies, and disciplinary methods develop over time and contribute to a family's sense of order.

Spirituality

Spirituality addresses meaning in life. Each family bases its values and principles in large part on its spiritual foundation. Although religion is one way that a family may express spirituality, religion is not the only way to define spirituality. Cultivating in children an appreciation for the arts (literature, music, theater, dance, and visual art) gives them the basis from which to begin their own spiritual journey.

Family Structure

Various traditional and nontraditional family structures exist. The traditional structures that occur in many cultures are the nuclear family and the extended family. Nontraditional variations include the single-parent family, the communal family, the stepfamily, and the gay or lesbian family. The adoptive family can be either a traditional or a nontraditional structure.

Nuclear Family

The **nuclear family** is composed of a man, a woman, and their children (either biological or adopted) who share a common household (Fig. 2-1). This was once the typical American family structure; now, fewer than one third of families in the United States fit this pattern. In many cases, patterns of living show a move away from life-long marriage and the nuclear family toward serial dissolution and formation of partnerships, either by cohabitation or by remarriage (Pacey, 2005). The nuclear family is a more mobile and independent unit than an extended family, but it is often part of a network of related nuclear families within close geographic proximity.

■ **Figure 2-1** The nuclear family is an important and prominent type of family structure in American society.

Extended Family

Typical of agricultural societies, the **extended family** consists of one or more nuclear families plus other relatives, often crossing generations to include grandparents, aunts, uncles, and cousins. The needs of individual members are subordinate to the needs of the group, and the family considers children an economic asset. Grandparents aid in child rearing, and children learn respect for their elders by observing their parents' behavior toward the older generation.

Here's an important tip.

In some cultures, the extended family plays an important role in everyday life. It may be challenging, but when the extended family comes to visit the new mother and newborn, work with them to accommodate their needs.

A Personal Glimpse

Living with both my mother and grandmother definitely has its advantages. Even though I had a male figure around me while I was growing up, it wasn't really the same as having a father who would always be there. I lived with my aunt and her family along with my mother and my grandmother. I had my uncle or cousin to turn to if I needed advice that my mother or my grandmother couldn't give me. However, my uncle wasn't always around, neither was my cousin, so a lot of my questions were left unanswered. Questions that I didn't think anybody else other than a man could answer. I learned a lot of things on my own, whether it was by experience or by asking somebody else.

Things are different now. It's only my mother, my grandmother, and myself. As I grow older, I'm finding that I can open up to the both of them a lot more. There is no reason to keep secrets. I can tell them anything and they understand. Actually they are a lot more understanding than I thought they would be about certain things. Every day I'm realizing that I can tell them anything.

People often ask me what it is like not knowing about my father. They ask me if I'm curious about my father. And I say, "Of course I'm curious. Who wouldn't be?" I also tell them that love is a lot stronger than curiosity. I love and care about my mother and grandmother more than anything in this world. No one father could ever give me as much love and devotion as the two of them give me. And I wouldn't give that up for anything.

Juan, age 15 years

Learning Opportunity: Where would you direct this mother in your community to go to find opportunities for her son to interact with male adults who could be positive role models for him? What are the reasons it would be important for this child to have appropriate adult male role models? If someone other than the biological parent has raised a child, what are some of the reasons these individuals seek their biological parents?

Single-Parent Family

Rising divorce rates, the women's movement, increasing acceptance of children born out of wedlock, and changes in adoption laws reflecting a more liberal attitude toward adoption have combined to produce a growing number of single-parent families. The percentage of single-parent households increased from 19.5% in 1980 to 28.2% in 2004, and women head most of these households (United States Bureau of Census, 2007). Although this family situation places a heavy burden on the parent, no conclusive evidence is available to show its effects on children. At some time in their lives, more than 50% of children in the United States may be part of a single-parent family.

Communal Family

During the early 1960s, increasing numbers of young adults began to challenge the values and traditions of the American social system. One result of that challenge was the establishing of communal groups and collectives, or a **communal family.** This alternative structure occurs in many settings and may favor either a primitive or a modern lifestyle. Members of a communal family share responsibility for homemaking and child rearing; all children are the collective responsibility of adult members. Not actually a new family structure, the communal family is a variation of the extended family. The number of communal family units has decreased in recent years.

Gay or Lesbian Family

In the gay or lesbian family, two people of the same sex live together, bound by a formal or informal commitment, with or without children. Children may be the result of a prior heterosexual mating or a product of the foster-child system, adoption, artificial insemination, or surrogacy. Although these families often face complex issues, including discrimination, studies of such families show that membership in this type of family does not harm children (Patterson, 1996; Downs & James, 2006).

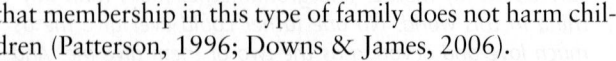

Did you know?
The children of a gay or lesbian family are no more likely to become homosexual than are children of heterosexual families.

Stepfamily or Blended Family

The **stepfamily** consists of a custodial parent and children and a new spouse. As the divorce rate has climbed, the number of stepfamilies has increased. If both partners in the marriage bring children from a previous marriage into the household, the family is usually termed a **blended family.** The stress that remarriage of the custodial parent places on a child seems to depend in part on the child's age. Initially there is an increase in the number of problems in children of all ages. However, younger children apparently can form an attachment to the new parent and accept that person in the parenting role better than can adolescents. Adolescents, already engaged in searching for identity and exploring their own sexuality, may view the presence of a nonbiological parent as an intrusion. When each partner brings children from a former marriage into the family, the incidence of problems increases. Second marriages often produce children of that union, which contributes to the adjustment problems of the family members. However, remarriage may provide the stability of a two-parent family, which may offer additional resources for the child. Each family is unique and has its own set of challenges and advantages (Pacey, 2005).

Cohabitation Family

In the nuclear family, the parents are married; in the **cohabitation family,** couples live together but are not married. The children in this family may be children of earlier unions, or they may be a result of this union. These families may be long lasting, and the cohabitating couple may eventually marry, but sometimes such families are less stable because the relationships may be temporary. In any family situation with frequent changes in the adult relationships, children may feel a sense of insecurity.

Adoptive Family

The adoptive family falls into a category of its own, whether the family structure is traditional or nontraditional. The parents, child, and siblings in the adoptive family all have challenges that differ from other family structures. A variety of methods of adoption are available, including the use of agencies, international sources, and private adoptions. Paperwork, interviews, home visits, long periods of waiting, and often large sums of money all contribute to the potential stress and anxiety a family who decides to adopt a child goes through. Sometimes, adopted children have health, developmental, or emotional concerns. Many have been in a series of foster homes or have come from abusive situations. The family who adopts a child of another culture may have to deal with the prejudices of friends and family. These factors add to the challenges the adoptive family faces.

Some research shows that "open adoption," in which the identity of the birth and adoptive parents is not kept a secret, is less traumatic for the birth mother, child, and adoptive family. The adoptive parents must work out legal issues in advance to decrease the painful situations that can occur if a birth mother changes her mind about giving up her child for adoption.

A complete physical examination of the newly adopted child is indicated soon after the adoption. The practitioner obtains basic information regarding the child's health, growth, and development, and then discusses any problems or concerns with the adoptive family. The feelings of the parents as well as the siblings need to be explored and support given. Throughout childhood and into adulthood, adopted children often continue to have questions and need emotional support from health care personnel.

Family Factors That Influence Childbearing and Child Rearing

Family Size

The number of children in the family has a significant impact on family interactions. The smaller the family, the more time there is for individual attention to each child. Children in small families, particularly only children, often spend more time with adults and, therefore, relate better with adults than with peers. Only children tend to have more advanced language development and intellectual achievement.

Understandably, a large family emphasizes the group more than the child. Less time is available for parental attention to each child. There is greater interdependence among these children and less dependence on the parents (Fig. 2-2).

Sibling Order and Gender

Whether a child is the firstborn, a middle child, or the youngest also makes a difference in the child's relationships and behavior. Firstborn children command a great deal of attention from parents and grandparents. The parents' inexperience, anxieties, and uncertainties also affect firstborn children. Often the parents' expectations for the oldest child are greater than for subsequent children. Generally, firstborn children are greater achievers than their siblings are.

With second and subsequent children, parents tend to be more relaxed and permissive. These children are likely to be more relaxed and are slower to develop language skills. They often identify more with peers than with parents.

Gender identity in relation to siblings also affects a child's development. Girls raised with older brothers tend to have more male-associated interests than do girls raised with older sisters. Boys raised with older brothers tend to be more aggressive than boys raised with older sisters.

Parental Behavior

Many factors have contributed to the change in the traditional mother-at-home, father-at-work image of the American family (Fig. 2-3). Sixty-five percent of American mothers of children younger than age 18 years work outside the home. Some mothers work because they are the family's only source of income, others because the family's economic status demands a second income, and still others because the woman's career is highly valued. More than half of all children between the ages of 3 and

■ Figure 2-2 Children from large families learn to care for one another. Many older children are expected to help with homework and prepare after-school snacks. (Photo by Joe Mitchell.)

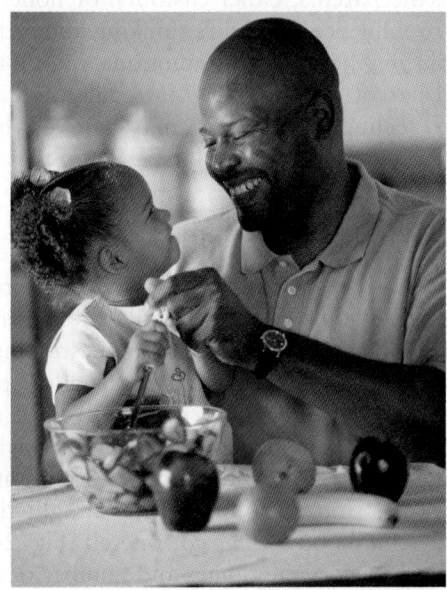

■ Figure 2-3 In some American families, traditional roles are being reversed. The father cares for the children while the mother is at work.

5 years spend part of their day being cared for by someone other than their parents.

Many factors contribute to the trend for families to spend less time together. Both parents may work; the children participate in many school activities; family members watch television, rather than talking together at mealtime, or eat fast food or individual meals without sitting down together as a family; and there is an emphasis on the acquisition of material goods, rather than the development of relationships. All these factors contribute to a breakdown in family communication, and they are typical of many families. Their impact on today's children, the parents of tomorrow, is unknown.

Divorce

From 1970 to 1990, the number of divorces increased every year. Although there has been a slight decrease in this number in recent years, more than 1 million children younger than age 18 years have been involved in a divorce each year. Although these children are obviously affected, it is difficult to determine the exact extent of the damage. Children whose lives were seriously disrupted before a divorce may feel relieved, at least initially, when the situation is resolved. Others who were unaware of parental conflict and felt that their lives were happy may feel frightened and abandoned. All these emotions depend on the children involved, their ages, and the kind of care and relationships they experience with their parents after the divorce.

Children may go through many emotions when a divorce occurs. Feelings of grief, anger, rejection, and self-worthlessness are common. These emotions may follow the children for years, even into adulthood, even though children may understand the reason for the divorce. In addition, the parents, either custodial or noncustodial, may try to influence the child's thinking about the other parent, placing the child in an emotional trap. If the noncustodial parent does not keep in regular contact with the child, feelings of rejection may be overwhelming. The child often desperately wants a sign of that parent's continuing love.

Culture

Each person is the product of a family, a culture, and a community. In some cultures, family life is gentle and permissive; other cultures demand unquestioning obedience of children and expect children to endure pain and hardship stoically. The child may be from a cultural group that places a high value on children, in which relatives and friends give children lots of attention, or the child may be from a group that has taught the child from early childhood to fend for oneself (Fig. 2-4).

Culture influences the timing and number of children desired by the childbearing family. Values and beliefs about birth control, abortion, and sexual practices influence the choices individuals and couples make about childbearing.

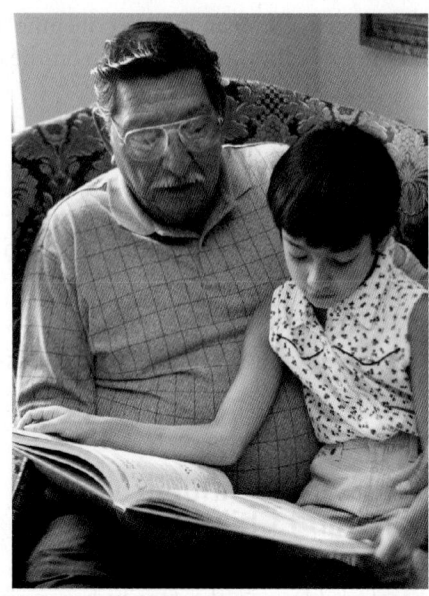

■ **Figure 2-4** Many cultural preferences are seen in families. In some cultures, extended family members such as grandparents participate in raising children. (Photo by Joe Mitchell.)

Culture also determines the family's health beliefs and practices. Respect for a person's cultural heritage and individuality is an essential part of nursing care. To plan culturally appropriate and acceptable care, it is important to understand the health practices and lifestyle of families from various cultures. Rather than memorizing a list of generalized facts regarding different cultures, it is more useful to develop **cultural competency**, the capacity to work effectively with people by integrating the elements of their culture into nursing care (Schim, Doorenbos, & Borse, 2006; Sealey, Burnett, & Johnson, 2006). To develop cultural competency, you must first understand cultural influences on your life. These influences include surface cultural influences (e.g., language, food, clothing), as well as hidden cultural influences (e.g., communication styles, beliefs, attitudes, values, perceptions). Only after recognizing these influences on your own life is it possible to recognize and accept the different attitudes, behaviors, and values of another person's culture.

Integrating cultural attitudes toward food, cleanliness, respect, and freedom in nursing care are of utmost importance. Be especially sensitive to the fears of the child who is separated from his or her own culture for the first time and finds the food, language, people, and surroundings of the health care facility totally alien. Cultural competency promotes cooperation from the child and family, and minimizes frustration. These factors are essential in restoring health so that the child may once again be a functioning part of the family and the community, whatever the cultural background.

Test Yourself

✔ Name one way that family size affects a child's development.

✔ What are two factors that contribute to American families spending less time together?

✔ Define cultural competency.

HEALTH CARE SHIFT: FROM HOSPITAL TO COMMUNITY

In the last century, health care has gone through a number of changes. The sophisticated health care currently available is extremely expensive and has strained health care funding to a point where other health care approaches have become necessary. This need for change has led to the emergence of community-based health care and an emphasis on wellness and preventive health care.

The shift to community-based health care has influenced normal and at-risk maternity care. Many women with limited resources choose to obtain prenatal care from local health department clinics. A pregnant woman who develops complications can sometimes receive care at home with the assistance of a nurse case manager who helps to coordinate her care. This allows the woman to receive high-quality care at a lower cost than if she were to require hospitalization. Community-based programs such as Women, Infants, and Children (WIC) provide nutritional screening and assistance for the low-income pregnant woman and her small children.

The shift to community-based health care also has been a positive factor in children's care. The health care community no longer views the child simply as a person with an illness, but rather as a child who is a member of a family from a certain community with deep-seated cultural values, social customs, and preferences. Learning about the child's community and using that knowledge improves the level of care the child receives. In the community, the child can also receive preventive care and wellness teaching not previously available unless one was ill in the hospital setting.

Community-Based Nursing

Community-based nursing focuses on prevention and is directed toward persons and families within a community. The goals are to help persons meet their health care needs and to maintain continuity of care as they move through the various health care settings available to them.

The role of the nurse who works in the community is different from that of the hospital nurse. Generally, the nurse in the community focuses on **primary prevention**, health-promoting activities that help prevent the development of illness or injury. This level of prevention includes teaching regarding safety, diet, rest, exercise, and disease prevention through immunizations and empha-

sizes the nursing role of teacher and client advocate. Examples of primary prevention are a school nurse giving a drug education program to a fourth-grade class, and a nurse in a maternity clinic giving teaching tips on proper nutrition during pregnancy.

In some community settings, the nurse's role focuses on **secondary prevention**, health-screening activities that aid in early diagnosis and encourage prompt treatment before long-term negative effects arise. Such settings are clinics, home care nursing, and schools. The nurse participates in screening measures such as height, weight, hearing, and vision. During child assessments and follow-up, the nurse compiles a health history and collects data, including vital signs, blood work, and other diagnostic tests as ordered by the health care practitioner. One example of secondary prevention is when the school nurse identifies a child with pediculosis (head lice). The school nurse contacts the child's family caregivers and provides instructions on the care of the child and other family members to eliminate the infestation. Another example of secondary prevention is a community clinic nurse's identification of a pregnant adolescent who is gaining insufficient weight and is possibly anemic. The nurse works with the family caregiver to review the family's dietary habits and nutritional state. This would help determine if the problem is limited to the pregnant adolescent or if other family members are also malnourished and if there is lack of knowledge or inadequate means. After finding these answers, the nurse can help the family caregiver provide better nutrition for the family and focus on nutritional issues unique to the pregnant adolescent.

Tertiary prevention, health-promoting activities that focus on rehabilitation and teaching to prevent further injury or illness, occurs in special settings. For example, community-based health care interventions might help the at-risk infant or child through special intervention programs, group homes, or selected outpatient settings focusing on rehabilitation, such as an orthopedic clinic. A young rural family with a child who has spina bifida and who needs urinary catheterization several times a day is another example of tertiary prevention. The family brings the child regularly to a specialized clinic at a major medical center. The family has no insurance, and the cost of catheters is such that the family caregivers feel they can no longer afford them. The nurse helps the family explore additional resources for financial help, such as an organization that will help fund their trips to the clinic for regular appointments. The nurse also finds a source to cover the costs of catheters and other incidental expenses.

Such a broad selection of settings and roles places nurses in a remarkable situation. An advantage of community-based health care is that pregnant women and children receive care in settings familiar to them—homes, schools, or community centers. In the community setting, the child's caregivers can more freely make choices; for instance, they may be more able to follow a child's medication regimen at home, rather than in the hospital, because the family may view the hospital as a strange territory. Although involved in direct care, the nurse in the community spends a great part of his or her time as a communicator, teacher, administrator, and manager.

Community Care Settings for the Maternity Client

Prenatal and Postpartum Home Health Care

Nurses often made home visits in the early days of public health nursing. Through the years, the setting for health care gradually shifted to clinics and offices. Recently, in an effort to meet the challenges of cost-containment and poor access to care, some organizations and researchers have reinstituted home visits by nurses.

Current evidence shows that at-risk mothers and infants experience better health outcomes when nurses go to the home for visits throughout pregnancy and the first year of the child's life. Positive results include increase in positive maternal–infant interaction, decreases in substance abuse and pregnancy rates, longer time between pregnancies, lower incidence of child abuse and neglect, as well as improvements in economic status (Gardner & Deatrick, 2006; Jack, DiCenso, & Lohfeld, 2005). One recent study demonstrates that home nurse visits during the postpartum period can be very helpful to decrease return to smoking after pregnancy (Groner et al., 2005).

Settings for Birth

Cultural beliefs, political beliefs, and personal preferences guide the mother's choice of a birth setting. For example, on the United States western frontier during the mid- and late-1800s, women gave birth in their homes, attended by female family members or female neighbors. These women cared for the older children, helped with chores, and stayed with the new mother during the early postpartum period, when possible. Today, in most parts of the world, the choices of birth settings are primarily home, birthing centers, and hospitals (Fig. 2-5).

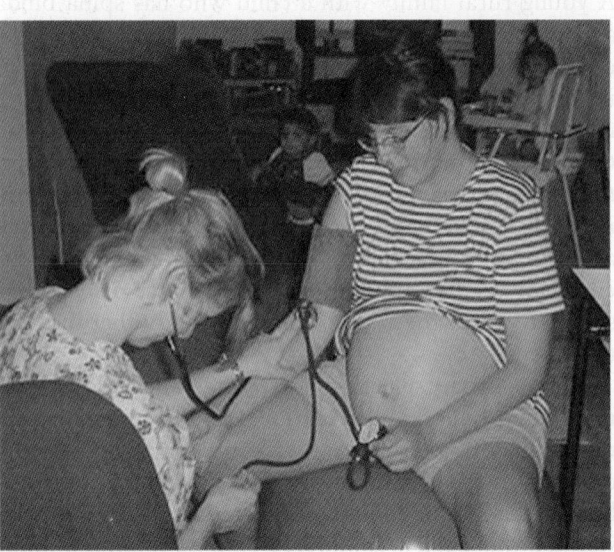

■ Figure 2-5 There are many different settings in which a woman can choose to give birth. These decisions are influenced by preferences regarding methods of pain control and general beliefs about how a birth should be managed. **(A)** Hospital LDRP. **(B)** Birthing center. **(C)** Home setting. (Photos A and C by Joe Mitchell. Photo B by Gus Freedman.)

Home

In the early 20th century, home births were the norm before the availability of anesthesia and pain medication in the hospital setting. Today, home births occur rarely. A woman may choose to deliver at home for a variety of reasons. She may desire a more comfortable setting or more control over birthing conditions and positions. In addition, a woman may prefer to give birth at home so that she can take care of her healthy newborn, rather than experiencing periods of separation while her baby is cared for in a hospital nursery.

Midwives usually attend births at home; physicians rarely do. Some are lay midwives, often trained through apprenticeships with experienced lay midwives. Others are formally trained certified nurse midwives (CNMs) who practice independently in home settings and clinics with physician backup for consultation and referral. Laws in individual states regulate the practice of midwifery.

There is debate over the safety of giving birth at home. In particular, the American College of Obstetricians and Gynecologists continues to oppose home birth. However, a recent large study (Johnson & Daviss, 2005) found that women who deliver at home with a CNM experience fewer medical interventions than women who deliver in hospitals and the neonatal and maternal mortality rates are similar.

Birthing Centers

Since the early 1980s, birthing centers have increased in popularity and availability in some areas of the United States. The environment is usually comfortable with furnishings and lighting designed to make the laboring woman and her family feel welcome. There often are family areas (e.g., kitchens and sitting rooms) and bathrooms with showers and/or whirlpool tubs. Birthing centers employ a variety of health care professionals, including registered nurses (RNs), CNMs, licensed practical or vocational nurses (LPNs/LVNs), and doulas (specialized birth attendants). Medical interventions occur rarely, so physicians are seldom present. However, birthing centers often are affiliated with a variety of obstetricians and pediatricians as consultants.

Midwives at birthing centers screen prospective patients and only accept low-risk women as patients. Most birthing centers have medical equipment such as intravenous lines, fluids, oxygen, newborn resuscitation equipment, infant warmers, and local anesthesia for repair of tears or infrequently performed episiotomies. Mild narcotics are available, as is oxytocin for control of postpartum bleeding. If a laboring woman decides she wants an epidural anesthesia, or if she presents with complications that put her or her baby at risk, the midwife arranges for transport to a hospital. The latest Cochrane Review (Hodnett et al., 2005) concludes that home-like birth settings are associated with increased maternal satisfaction and fewer medical interventions.

Hospitals

Americans accepted childbirth in a hospital setting as the norm by the 1920s. By 1950, the vast majority of births in the United States took place in hospitals. Today, 99% of births in the United States are in hospitals, with 92% attended by medical doctors (MDs). Doctors of osteopathic medicine (DOs) and midwives attend most of the other 8% of births in U.S. hospitals.

Until the 1970s, giving birth in a hospital required the woman to endure uncomfortable procedures (e.g., enemas, shaving); to labor, deliver, and recover in separate rooms; and to be separated from her newborn until several hours after birth. In the mid-1970s, patients began to be more consumer-oriented. They began to "shop around" for family-centered maternity care, which included more time with their babies and less time moving from room to room. Hospital administrators and physicians began to listen to consumer needs, and hospital policies began to change. As a result, the trend in many hospitals is to promote family-centered maternity care in more home-like settings. Most hospitals today offer combination labor-delivery-recovery rooms (LDRs). The rooms are larger to accommodate family support and to allow health care professionals enough room to attend the birth. In addition, LDRs are aesthetically appealing, with home-like furnishings, wallpaper, softer lighting, and showers in the bathrooms.

Some hospitals have initiated combination labor-delivery-recovery-postpartum rooms (LDRPs). This arrangement further reduces the number of locations to which a woman is moved during her hospital stay. **Couplet care**, another concept that some hospitals have embraced, places the healthy mother in the same room with her newborn as long as there is no medical indication for separation. One nurse is responsible for the care of both. This practice encourages early bonding and provides time for new parents to learn to care for their newborns before discharge. Parents learn to recognize their newborns' cues and, therefore, are better prepared to care for their newborns at home.

Test Yourself
- ✔ Define primary prevention.
- ✔ Give one example of tertiary prevention.
- ✔ List three childbirth settings.

Community Care Settings for the Child

Care for a child occurs in a wide variety of community settings. Some settings provide primarily wellness care, whereas others provide specialized care for children with a particular diagnosis or condition. These include outpatient settings, home care, schools, camps, community centers, parishes, intervention programs, and group homes.

Outpatient Settings

There are a variety of outpatient settings for children. As the health care delivery system continues to move into the community, more settings will emerge. Outpatient settings are organized according to who offers the services and who pays for them. Public (tax-supported) outpatient clinics may be an extension of a hospital's services, or a regional, county, or city health department may be the sponsor. Private (based on fees charged) clinics are owned and operated by corporations or individuals and operate for a profit. A third system is the growing network of health maintenance organizations (HMOs). Some HMO plans charge a small co-payment for each visit. However, under the HMO system, the family is not free to choose the specialty care the child may receive. The child's primary care provider determines what, if any, specialized care the child needs and who will administer that care (see Chapter 1).

Community needs dictate clinic services. Examples include a well-baby clinic offered by the county health department, an orthopedic clinic offered by a regional children's hospital, or a pediatric clinic of an HMO. Infants, children, and caregivers use the clinics for education, anticipatory guidance, immunizations, diagnosis, treatment, and rehabilitation.

A Personal Glimpse

The clinic is where you go when you're on the public access card and cannot afford real insurance. You hardly see the same doctor twice. A lot are interns working out their internship.

My baby was about 2 months old when he developed a bumpy rash on the crown of this head. I took him to the clinic because it was spreading and I didn't know what it could be. A doctor who I could hardly understand was on duty. This was the same doctor that told me I had chickenpox when I was pregnant (I didn't). He looked at the rash and looked at me very strange, then said, "This looks similar to a rash connected to HIV." He requested a test for AIDS! You cannot know the thoughts that go through your head. How? Where? Who? Why? Then, I remembered that I had been tested when I first found out I was pregnant and it was negative. Since Jack, the baby's father, and I had not been with anyone else, I knew there must be another reason for this rash.

That doctor never took a sample to test or asked another doctor to come in and look at the rash. I took little Tommy home and started to use an ointment I'd heard about on his head every day for about a month. The rash went away, and I've changed clinics since—like they're not all really the same. You get what you pay for.

Michelle

Learning Opportunity: What feelings do you think this mother might have been experiencing in this situation? What specific things could the nurse do to be of support and help to this mother?

A specialty clinic focuses on one aspect of an infant or child's well-being, for instance dentistry, oncology, sickle cell anemia, or human immunodeficiency virus/acquired immunodeficiency syndrome (HIV/AIDS). Some health department clinics specialize in at-risk infants born to drug-addicted mothers, children of parents with a history of child abuse, or low-birth-weight infants. Nurses in these clinics devote much of their efforts to parental education and guidance, as well as follow-up services for the child.

Home Health Care

Infants, children, and their families make up a significant proportion of the home health care population. Shortened acute care stays have contributed to the increasing number of children cared for by home nurses. Children are often more comfortable in familiar home surroundings (Fig. 2-6). Children and infants can be successfully treated for many conditions at home, where they and their caregivers are more comfortable, and they can receive the love and attention of family members. The child's caregivers feel more confident about performing treatments and procedures when they have the guidance of the home nurse. Common conditions for which an infant or child may receive home care services include:

- Phototherapy for elevated bilirubin levels
- Intravenous antibiotic therapy for systemic infections
- Postoperative care
- Chronic conditions, such as asthma, sickle cell anemia, cystic fibrosis, HIV/AIDS, and leukemia and other cancers
- Respirator (ventilator) dependence
- Reconstructive or corrective surgery for congenital malformations
- Corrective orthopedic surgery

Other home health care team members may include a physical therapist, speech therapist, occupational therapist, home schooling teacher, home health aide, primary health care provider (physician or nurse practitioner),

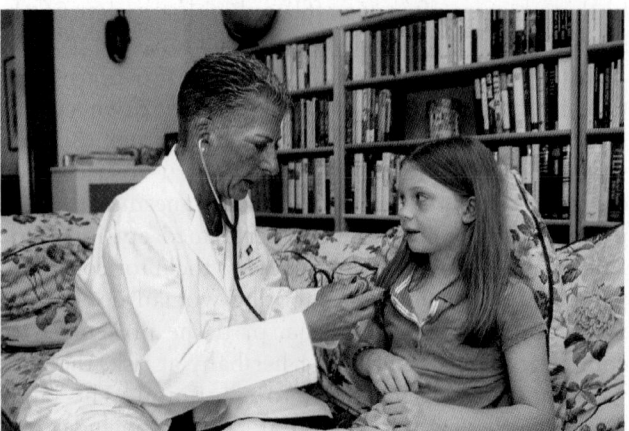

■ Figure 2-6 During a visit by the nurse, the child is comforted by the familiar surroundings of her home.

and social worker. Members of the team vary with the child's health needs.

Schools and Camps

Schools and camps have been sites for provision of health care for many years, but the role of health care professionals in these settings has expanded (Fig. 2-7). The school nurse may be responsible for classroom teaching, health screenings, immunizations, first aid for injured children, care of ill children, administering medication, assisting with sports physicals, and identifying children with problems and recommending programs for them. Classroom teaching geared for each grade level can cover personal hygiene, sex education, substance abuse, safety, and emotional health.

Many mainstreamed children have chronic health problems that need daily supervision or care; for example, a child with spina bifida who needs to be catheterized several times each day or a diabetic child who needs to perform glucose monitoring and administer insulin during school hours. The school maintains health records on each child. Some schools have clinics that provide routine dental care, physicals, screening for vision, hearing, scoliosis, tuberculosis, and follow-up on immunizations. Children learn to know the school nurse over a number of years and usually establish a comfortable, friendly relationship that often aids the nurse in helping the child solve his or her health problems.

The camp nurse knows the child for a much briefer time, but many camp nurses establish warm relationships with the children in their care. Camp nurses provide first aid for campers and staff, maintain health records, teach first aid and cardiopulmonary resuscita-

tion (CPR), offer relevant health education, maintain an infirmary for ill campers, and dispense tender loving care to homesick children.

At camps for children with special needs, the campers' health care needs determine the type of nursing care required. For example, at a camp for diabetic children, the nurse may teach self-administration of insulin and the many aspects of diabetic care. Other camps may cater to children with developmental delays, physical challenges, or chronic illness such as asthma or cystic fibrosis. Others have specific purposes, such as weight control or behavior management. In each of these settings, the nurse provides basic health care with individualized health teaching, based on the camp population. Each type of camp brings its own challenges and rewards; the benefits to the children and their families are often exceptional.

Community Centers, Parishes, and Intervention Programs

Community centers and parishes provide care relevant to a particular community. Parish centers may sponsor outreach programs in a church, synagogue, or other religious setting. These centers design services to meet community needs. For example, in areas with many homeless persons, centers may provide basic health care and nutrition. These centers may also provide food, clothing, money, or other resources. Other centers may provide childcare classes for new mothers or young families.

Some communities offer walk-in or residential clinics for special purposes, such as teen pregnancy, alcohol and drug abuse, nutritional guidance, and family violence. Other specialized clinics offer programs on HIV/AIDS, cancer, and mental health; provide maternal and well-baby care; and offer day care services for children or the elderly.

In many communities, volunteer service organizations such as the Lions Club, Rotary Club, Shriners, or Kiwanis provide care. Some of these organizations have specific goals. For example, the Shriners sponsor clinics for children with orthopedic problems.

In any community center, there are people who can benefit from the services of health care professionals. Often, the health services focus on education and other primary prevention practices. Nurses help design safety, exercise, and nutrition programs; provide basic immunization services; conduct parenting classes; organize crisis intervention programs for youth and teens; and help organize health fairs. The health care staff may be paid or may work on a volunteer basis, or there may be a combination of paid and volunteer staff.

These programs can provide many services to smaller groups of infants and children with special needs. Federal or state funds may support such intervention programs offered through the school district or private associations for developmentally delayed, physically challenged, or emotionally disturbed children. The interventions are often multidisciplinary, consisting of a team

■ Figure 2-7 The school nurse cares for a young boy who injured his knee. In addition to first aid, the school nurse's duties include counseling, health education, and health promotion.

of professionals who work together to meet the multiple needs of the child.

Professional teams may consist of a teacher, psychologist, neurologist, physical therapist, social worker, physician, and nurse. The most important team members are the family caregivers and the child, and it is essential to include them in planning meetings and program intervention development. The nurse's role as a team member involves interpreting diagnoses or medical orders to other team members and the family, teaching the family how to provide care for a medically fragile child, and effectively integrating the family into intervention programs.

Residential Programs

Residential programs, often called group homes, provide services for a number of health needs. Those geared primarily toward children include chemical dependency treatment centers and homes for children with mental or emotional health needs, pregnant adolescents, and abused children. These homes vary in size and setup according to the children's needs.

Depending on the number of children a home serves, a nurse may contract to provide specific services. The nurse may work for the local health department or for a corporation that owns several group homes. For example, in a home with six children with minimal disabilities, the nurse may visit every 2 weeks to meet with and educate the staff, update health records, and provide immunizations. This may be all the health care service the home requires to maintain its group home license.

Homes that serve many children or that serve children with very complex needs may need to have nurses 24 hours a day. Often, licensing standards require this complete coverage in addition to meeting the health care needs of the children. Some homes hire a multidisciplinary team of health care practitioners that may include nurses; medical social workers; psychologists; physical, speech, or occupational therapists; special education teachers; home health aides or attendants; and physicians. Not all the team members provide services to group homes on a full-time basis.

Skills of the Community-Based Nurse

The nursing process serves as the foundation of nursing care in the community, just as it does in a health care facility. Communication with the patient and family is essential. Teaching is a fundamental part of community-based care because of the emphasis on health promotion and preventive health care. Case management is necessary to coordinate care and monitor case progress through the health care system.

The Nursing Process

The focus of the community-based nurse is the patient within the context of the family. The initial family assessment interview provides information about how various family members affect the pregnant woman or the child and his or her condition. Noticing cues in the environment provides additional information. Upon completion of data collection and assessment, the RN and health care team focus on identifying the nursing diagnoses based on the family's strengths, weaknesses, and needs. Family interaction and cooperation leads to collaborative goal setting and proposed interventions. The ongoing nursing process requires that the nurse evaluate these interventions as the cycle continues.

Communication

Positive, effective communication is fundamental to the nursing process and the care of childbearing and child-rearing families in the community. Establishing rapport with the patient and the family, understanding and appropriately responding to cultural practices, and being sensitive to the needs of the patient and family all require good communication skills. (See Chapter 22 for further discussion of communicating with children and family caregivers.)

Teaching

Teaching and health education are key components of community-based nursing care. Health care often involves teaching families, small groups of children, family caregivers, members of extended families, and large groups of children, on various topics that focus on primary prevention (Fig. 2-8).

> **Here's an idea.**
> When teaching a group with which you are unfamiliar, ask the group leader for demographic information to help develop an appropriate teaching plan.

To teach a group successfully, it is important to know the needs of the target population and have the appropriate teaching skills,

■ **Figure 2-8** The nurse takes the opportunity to provide patient education regarding normal growth and development to these mothers attending a mom and baby class with their infants.

strategies, and resources. Important information about the group includes age, educational level, ethnic and gender mix, language barriers, and any previous teaching the group has had on the subject. Knowledge of growth and developmental principles will help to identify the appropriate level of information, learning activities, and average attention span. Additional information includes any available teaching resources, group size, seating arrangements, and other advantages or restrictions of the environment. For instance:

- Are the chairs movable for small-group discussions?
- Is there a videocassette recorder or DVD player available to show a video?
- Can the children go outside?
- Will a lot of noise disturb others in the building?
- Will the classroom teacher or teacher's aide attend?

A successful group teaching experience relies on a prepared nurse educator.

Case Management

Case management, a systematic process that ensures that a client's multiple health and service needs are met, may be a formal or an informal process. In formalized case management, the agency or insurer who pays for the health care services predetermines the contact with the client. In other settings, the nurse may determine the needed follow-up and either provide the services, or assist with referrals to obtain services.

In formalized case management, the insurer pays for nursing services. Care plans and protocols clearly outline the case manager's role, and the insurer determines limits to service. In community agencies where nursing services are part of the overall service (for instance, schools or group homes), the intensity of follow-up is determined by the agency's philosophy, available resources, and the nurse's perception of the role and her individual skills.

Client Advocacy

Client advocacy is speaking or acting on behalf of clients to help them gain greater independence and to make the health care delivery system more responsive and relevant to their needs. The nurse working in a community setting may often develop a long-standing relationship with childbearing and child-rearing families because of the continuous nature of client contact in an outpatient, school, or other setting. This type of relationship may allow the nurse to discover broader health and welfare issues. Examples of interventions include:

- Teaching a family about the services for which the pregnant woman or child is eligible.
- Assisting the family to apply for Medicaid or other forms of health care reimbursement.
- Identifying inexpensive or free transportation services to medical appointments.

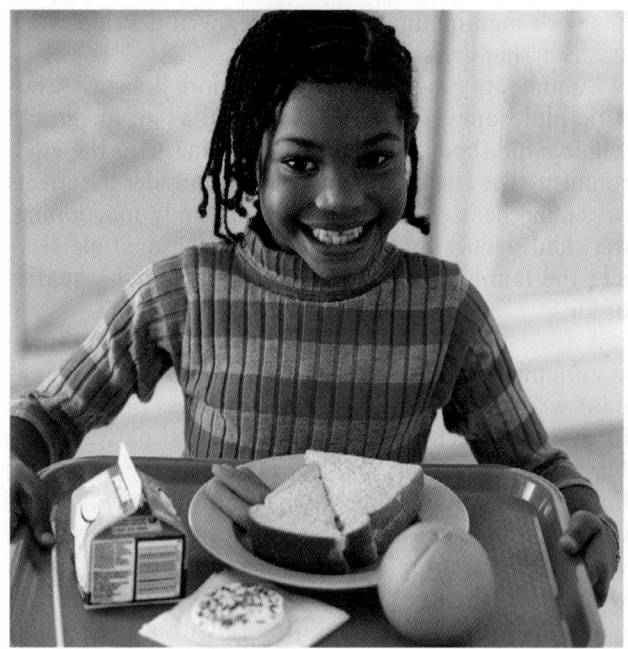

■ **Figure 2-9** A nurse advocate can help the child enter a school lunch program so that nutritional needs are met.

- Making telephone calls to establish eligibility for and to acquire special equipment needed by a physically challenged child.

Examples of client advocacy are limitless and include health and social welfare services that intertwine in ways that families cannot manage alone. One example is assistance with referrals and acquisition of needed resources. As a member of a health care team, the nurse assists with the referral process. This process focuses on the childbearing or child-rearing family obtaining the appropriate services and resources. Improving the childbearing or child-rearing family's health or quality of life is the goal of interventions. It is important to be knowledgeable about community resources, contact persons, details of appropriate applications, and other required documentation (Fig. 2-9).

The Challenge of Community-Based Nursing

There are differences between caring for childbearing and child-rearing families in a hospital or clinic and caring for them in community settings. Community-based work requires a different set of skills.

Unique Aspects of Community-Based Nursing

Community-based nursing practice is autonomous. The community nurse must be self-reliant to be successful. There may not be many other health care practitioners with whom to consult; those available may be physically distant. Providing childbearing and child-rearing families with high-quality care requires well-developed assessment and decision-making skills.

Community practice tends to be more holistic. A holistic philosophy views the individual as an integrated whole mind, body, and spirit interacting with the environment. The community nurse must consider the effects of the mother's or child's health on family functioning, the child's educational progress, and the multiple services the family and child need to improve the quality of life.

A final difference is the focus on wellness. Some community settings have a population of at-risk pregnant women and children with an illness or diagnosis in common, such as diabetes or cerebral palsy. Working with these groups involves managing the disease or limitations with a wellness focus. For instance, the focus might be on teaching a group of pregnant women with diabetes about diabetic diets. Another example would be showing how the child with cerebral palsy can be included comfortably within the regular classroom.

In most areas where the community nurse works, the focus is on wellness. Women and children are well but may be going through growth and developmental crises. The nurse intervenes to ease the transition from one developmental stage to another. The nurse provides anticipatory guidance to family caregivers and emphasizes preventive health practices. Teaching health-promotion practices to pregnant women and children is another activity of primary importance.

Issues Facing Pregnant Women, Children, and Families

Nurses who work in the community encounter the complex issues facing childbearing and child-rearing families. Caring for pregnant women, children, and families within their own environments allows the nurse to better understand their unique needs.

Poverty is a major issue that affects all aspects of recovery and responses to care. For many families, a lack of resources hinders compliance and takes its toll on the health of all family members. Services and resources may be inaccessible because of cost, location, or lack of transportation. Sometimes, family caregivers see such services as unnecessary. Poverty, lack of information, questionable decisions about priorities, and ineffective coping skills affect the health of pregnant women, children, and families in significant ways. Nurses frequently encounter the results of this lack of resources in emergency departments, neonatal intensive care units (NICUs), and in acute care beds of children's units.

The community nurse must explore these issues with the family caregivers. When a pregnant woman delays prenatal care, what issues surround this behavior? When a family does not follow up with an orthopedic appointment for a new cast application on the legs of a 6-month-old infant, what factors influenced their decision? When a family caregiver saves half of the antibiotic suspension for another child in the family with similar symptoms, what motivates this decision? When a single parent keeps a physically disabled and developmentally delayed 9-year-old son at home in one room of the apartment, what types of caregiving services and information might afford benefit?

Test Yourself

✔ Name two conditions for which a child or infant could receive home health care.

✔ Define client advocacy.

✔ Name three unique aspects of community-based nursing.

Rewards of Community-Based Nursing

The nurse in community-based settings sees the client over time. This allows the nurse to have a broader understanding of the context within which the individual and family lives. The clinic nurse may see the same family for different problems over a period of many years. The camp or school nurse watches children grow and gets to know siblings and families over time. A group-home nurse works intensely with a group of developmentally disabled children and learns to know each one and rejoice in their small triumphs. A nurse in a home for pregnant teens works with a young mother throughout her pregnancy and takes pleasure in the birth of a healthy baby.

For the community nurse, rewards come slowly and in different ways. A school nurse may diligently work over several months with a child and family and a community service organization to obtain a pair of glasses for the child. This nurse may feel rewarded when the child no longer comes into the school nurse's office with headaches and is doing better in class work. The camp nurse may help a homesick camper design a way to stay in touch with his or her parents and may encourage the camper to participate in camp activities. This nurse may also find reward when the camper returns each season. The nurse in a group home for teenage foster children with behavioral problems may help the teens develop a theater group that presents plays about safe sex and responsible teen dating to other group homes, high school classes, or community service organizations. This nurse may find reward after a year of work with the teens when they write the scripts, build the sets independently, and declare that they enjoy the theater group more than any other activity in the residence. This nurse may also find a deeper reward when he or she realizes that because of the theater group, there are fewer behavioral problems and the teens' self-esteem is high.

Community nurses work in many ways to prevent unnecessary hospitalization. Examples of health problems that the community nurse seeks to prevent include injuries to a child not appropriately secured in a car seat, severe burns to the face of a toddler from grabbing a tablecloth and spilling a cup of coffee, a near-drowning in a backyard pool, an infant who fails to thrive because the parents do not know that infants need specific amounts of formula, or a pregnant teen who contracts HIV because she does not practice safe sex.

The community nurse helps families develop the skills and knowledge they need to make decisions that affect their lives and those of other family members. In this way, families can learn and practice preventive health care. With a focus on wellness, the community nurse provides a service that eventually improves the health of the entire community.

Key Points

- The family is the basic social unit. It provides for survival and teaches the knowledge, customs, values, and beliefs of the family's culture.
- The basic functions of the family are to reproduce and to socialize children to function within the larger society. To meet the needs of individual members, the family also functions to provide support in the five areas of wholeness: physical, emotional, intellectual, social, and spiritual.
- The nuclear family and the extended family are the two types of traditional family structures that exist in most cultures. The single-parent family, communal family, gay or lesbian family, and cohabitation family are four examples of nontraditional family structures.
- Mobility, changing attitudes about children born out of wedlock, divorce, women working outside the home, and changes in adoption laws all have contributed to an increase in single-parent families.
- Family size affects the child's development. Children from small families receive more individual attention and tend to relate better to adults. Children from large families develop interdependency skills.
- Birth order also influences development. First-born children tend to be high achievers. Subsequent children are often more relaxed and are slower to develop language skills.
- Families tend to spend less time together than in the past for many reasons—both parents may work, the children participate in many school activities, families often do not eat together, and there is an emphasis on acquisition of material goods, rather than the development of relationships.
- Community-based health care focuses on wellness and prevention and on helping persons and families meet their health care needs.
- Community-based health care is advantageous for the pregnant woman, child, and family because it allows the individual to receive care within the context of the community and culture. Identifying and meeting needs within the community may also allow for less costly care than that provided in a hospital setting.
- Primary prevention focuses on preventing illness and injury. An example is a nurse in a maternity clinic giving teaching tips on proper nutrition during pregnancy.
- Secondary prevention involves health screening activities that aid in early diagnosis and encourage prompt treatment before long-term negative effects occur. An example is a school nurse who identifies a child with head lice, then contacts the family caregivers with instructions on how to rid the child and family members of infestation.
- Tertiary prevention involves health-promoting activities that focus on rehabilitation and teaching to prevent additional injury or illness. An example is a child with spina bifida who requires frequent catheterizations and trips to a specialized clinic. The nurse assists the family to find resources so that proper care and medical monitoring can continue to prevent the development of additional problems.
- Prenatal and postpartum home health care can help decrease the cost of care as well as increase access to care, especially for at-risk populations. Settings for birth include the home, birthing centers, and hospitals.
- Community-based care for pediatric clients occurs in outpatient settings and through home health care. Children's health care needs may be addressed and met in school and in specialized camp settings. Many communities have centers and programs that children and families can access for health care services.
- The community-based nurse uses the nursing process to plan and provide care to families and groups, communicates effectively, teaches individuals

and groups, performs case management, and practices client advocacy.

➤ An effective community nurse educator must identify and assess the target population by determining the age, educational level, ethnic and gender mix, language barriers, and any previous teaching the group may have had. The nurse must assess each audience and gear the teaching appropriately using appropriate materials.

➤ The community nurse functions as a child advocate by taking actions to improve the child's health or quality of life. One example of child advocacy is a nurse assisting with the referral process to help the child and family obtain the services and resources needed to maintain health.

➤ Community-based nursing provides the nurse an opportunity to function autonomously in a holistic, wellness focused environment. Issues of poverty, lack of information, questionable decisions about priorities, and ineffective coping skills must be explored with families. Seeing positive outcomes and improved health status, often over a period of time, is rewarding for the community-based nurse.

INTERNET RESOURCES

Cultural Competence:
　www.air.org/cecp/cultural.
Minority Health:
　www.omhrc.gov/omhhome.htm.
Minority Health and Health Disparities:
　www.cdc.gov/omhd/default.htm

Discovery Health:
　www.health.discovery.com
Kids Health:
　www.kidshealth.org/kid
KinderStart:
　www.kinderstart.com

Workbook

■ NCLEX-STYLE REVIEW QUESTIONS

1. In working with families, the nurse recognizes that different family structures exist. Which of the following examples best describes a blended family? A family in which

    a. the adult members share in homemaking as well as in child rearing.
    b. both partners in the marriage bring children from a previous marriage into the household.
    c. grandparents live in the same house with the grandchildren and their parents.
    d. partners of the same sex share a household and raise children together.

2. One role of the nurse in a community-based setting focuses on primary prevention. An example of primary prevention would be

    a. screening children for vision in a preschool.
    b. teaching bicycle safety in an after-school program.
    c. identifying head lice in a child in elementary school.
    d. exploring financial help for a client in a home setting.

3. One role of the nurse in a community-based setting focuses on secondary prevention. An example of secondary prevention would be

    a. screening children for vision in a preschool.
    b. teaching about nutrition in an after-school program.
    c. recommending a group home setting for an adolescent.
    d. administering immunizations to infants in a clinic.

4. One role of the nurse in a community-based setting focuses on tertiary prevention. An example of tertiary prevention would be

    a. testing children for hearing loss in a preschool.
    b. teaching bicycle safety in an after-school program.
    c. administering immunizations to infants in a clinic.
    d. exploring financial help for a client in a home setting.

5. A mother of a child being cared for in a home setting makes the following statements. Which statement *best* illustrates one of the positive aspects of home health care?

    a. "My family gets to visit once a week when my child is in the hospital."
    b. "I can do my child's care since you taught the procedure to me."
    c. "Our insurance pays for us to go to the well-child clinic."
    d. "The neighbor's child likes being in the group home."

6. When a nurse is doing teaching in a community-based setting, it is *most* important for the nurse to

    a. ask questions about the histories of those present.
    b. use posters that everyone in the group can read.
    c. tell the participants about the nurse's background.
    d. know the needs of the audience.

■ STUDY ACTIVITIES

1. Survey your community to discover the community-based health care providers available. Use the information you found to complete the following table.

Community-Based Health Care Providers	How Are They Funded?	What Types of Health Care for Children Do They Provide?

2. Using the information you obtained above, evaluate your community's health care services by answering the following:

    a. Does your community have adequate health care services for childbearing and child-rearing families?
    b. Are funding concerns an issue for your community? In what ways?
    c. What other services do you think are needed to care for the childbearing and child-rearing families in your community?

3. Select a community-based setting and outline the services that a nurse in that setting should ideally provide. Include the resources needed to provide the services.

4. Go to the following Internet site: http://www.culturediversity.org. At "Transcultural Nursing," click on "Cultural Competency."

    a. What is the definition of cultural competence?
    b. What are the five essential elements necessary for an organization to become culturally competent?
    c. What are the four major challenges to attaining cultural competency?

5. Go to the following Internet site: http://www. lehman.cuny.edu/faculty/jfleitas/bandaides/. At "Bandaides & Blackboards," click on "Kids." Go to "Lots of Stories" and click on the star.

   a. In working with school-age children, what are some of the stories in this site you would encourage the children to read?

   b. List the topics and diseases included in the stories that you could share with school-age children.

■ CRITICAL THINKING: WHAT WOULD YOU DO?

Apply your knowledge of the family and the nurse's role in the community to the following situations.

1. Nine-year-old Shawn has become withdrawn, his school grades have fallen, and he complains of having headaches and stomachaches since his parents' divorce 3 months ago. He lives with his mother during the week and visits his father, who lives with a girlfriend, on weekends.

   a. What concerns do you think Shawn's parents would have about his changes in behavior and his physical complaints?

   b. What advice would you offer Shawn's parents regarding these concerns?

   c. What could these parents do to help Shawn better adjust to the divorce?

2. You are making a home visit to the Andrews family because their newborn needs home phototherapy treatment for 3 to 5 days. You find 6-year-old Samantha ill with bronchitis. Both parents smoke. Outline a teaching plan for these caregivers regarding the health of their family.

3. Mrs. Perez, a second-grade teacher, asks you to teach a unit on personal hygiene to her class.

   a. Identify the information you will need from Mrs. Perez.

   b. Describe how you will present the lesson to these children.

UNIT II

FOUNDATIONS OF MATERNITY NURSING

3

Structure and Function of the Reproductive System

KEY TERMS

climacteric
corpus luteum
endometrium
epididymis
gametes
menarche
menstruation
mons pubis
myometrium
ovulation
prepuce
seminiferous tubules
spermatogenesis
vas deferens
vestibule
vulva

LEARNING OBJECTIVES

On completion of this chapter, you should be able to:

1. Explain two major functions of the reproductive system.
2. Label an anatomic drawing of the female and male reproductive systems, including external genitalia and internal anatomy.
3. Discuss major functions of each reproductive structure, gland, and organ.
4. Trace the path of sperm through the male reproductive system, from the site of formation to ejaculation from the body.
5. Describe the process of semen production.
6. Compare hormonal regulation of male reproductive function with that of the female.
7. Illustrate the inter-relationships of the ovarian and uterine cycles and the overall menstrual cycle.
8. Describe and compare the male and female sexual response cycles.

THE OBSTETRIC nurse counsels prospective parents before and throughout pregnancy and childbirth. This responsibility requires a working knowledge of reproductive anatomy and physiology and the menstrual cycle. This knowledge guides the selection of appropriate interventions for the childbearing woman and her family.

The main purpose of the male and female reproductive systems is to produce offspring. Male testes produce and female ovaries contain **gametes** or sex cells, spermatozoa (sperm) in the male and ova (eggs) in the female. Each gamete contains one half of the genetic material needed to produce a human baby. However, some of the structures in the reproductive tract serve dual purposes. Most often, these alternate functions have to do with urinary elimination because the urinary and reproductive systems are closely connected.

You will notice that most structures in the reproductive tract are paired (e. g., testes, ovaries, labia majora, labia minora) and that male and female reproductive systems are complementary; for example, male testes and female ovaries; male scrotum and female labia majora; and male glans penis and female clitoris. It is important to know that the pituitary gland governs reproductive hormone production and function (Fig. 3-1).

MALE REPRODUCTIVE SYSTEM

Sometimes, people do not fully appreciate the man's contribution to childbirth because of the focus on the pregnant woman and her growing fetus. However, the father's role is crucial to this process. His genetic material not only determines the sex of the unborn child, but also influences numerous other inherited traits. The male reproductive anatomy consists of external and internal reproductive organs. The purpose of the male reproductive tract is to allow for sexual intimacy and reproduction of offspring and to provide a conduit for urinary elimination.

External Genitalia

The man's external reproductive organs, the external genitalia, consist of the penis and scrotum (Fig. 3-2).

Penis

The penis serves a dual role as the male organ of reproduction and as the external organ of urinary elimination. The penis is composed of a bulbous head, the glans penis or glans, and a shaft. The glans is the most sensitive area on the penis because it contains the greatest concentration of nerve endings. This part of the penis is analogous

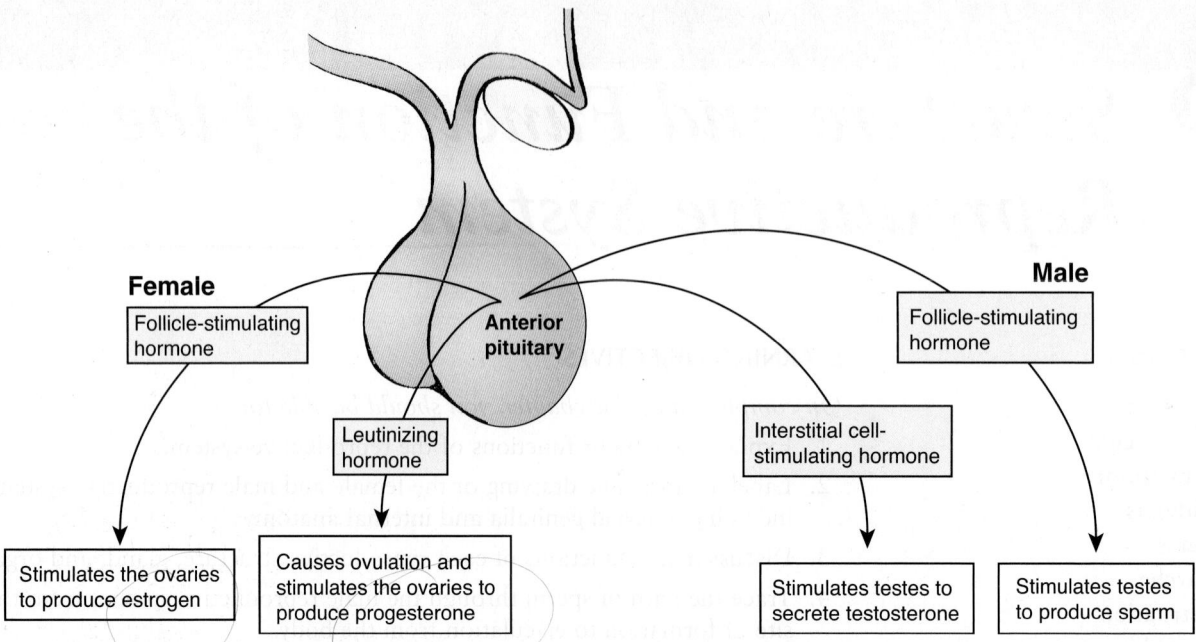

■ Figure 3-1 Hormones of the anterior pituitary stimulate the reproductive system in the male and the female.

to the clitoris in the female. At birth, a layer of tissue, the **prepuce** or foreskin, covers the glans.

Three columns of erectile tissue compose the shaft of the penis (Fig. 3-3): the paired cavernous bodies (corpus cavernosa) and the spongy body (corpus spongiosum). The cavernous bodies are parallel, and the spongy body lies atop them in the midline. The spongy body is cradled in the channel formed at the junction of the cavernous

Make a note of this.

The prepuce is removed in the surgical procedure called circumcision. If the parents choose to do this optional procedure, it is usually done within the first few days of life. Although adult males can undergo circumcision (usually for medical reasons), this procedure is not often done in adulthood.

bodies. A thick sheath called the tunica albuginea encases each column. Two layers of fascia encircle all three columns along the length of the shaft. The fascia gives the penis support, allowing it to become a firm structure during sexual stimulation.

The erectile tissue is well supplied with blood vessels and nerves. When the penis is stimulated sexually, parasympathetic nerves cause the veins in the shaft to dilate. The sinuses within the erectile tissue fill up with blood causing an erection. The erect penis is capable of penetrating the female vagina during sexual intercourse. If the erect penis is stimulated to ejaculation within the vagina, it deposits sperm in the female reproductive tract.

The urethra passes through the shaft of the penis within the spongy body. It functions to eliminate urine from the bladder and to transport semen to the woman's vagina during ejaculation.

Scrotum

The scrotum is an external sac that houses the testes in two internal compartments. The main functions of the scrotum are to protect the testes from trauma and to regulate the temperature within the testes, a process that is extremely important to the production of healthy male gametes. The ideal temperature within the scrotum is approximately 96°F, just slightly lower than normal body temperature. The skin of the scrotum is greatly pigmented and folded into furrows called rugae. When either the environmental or the body temperature is hot, the cremaster muscle within the scrotal sac remains relaxed so that the testes dangle down, away from the warmth of the body. If the temperature is cold, the

Scrotum ———

——— Penis shaft

——— Glans penis

■ Figure 3-2 Male external genitalia. (Photo by B. Proud.)

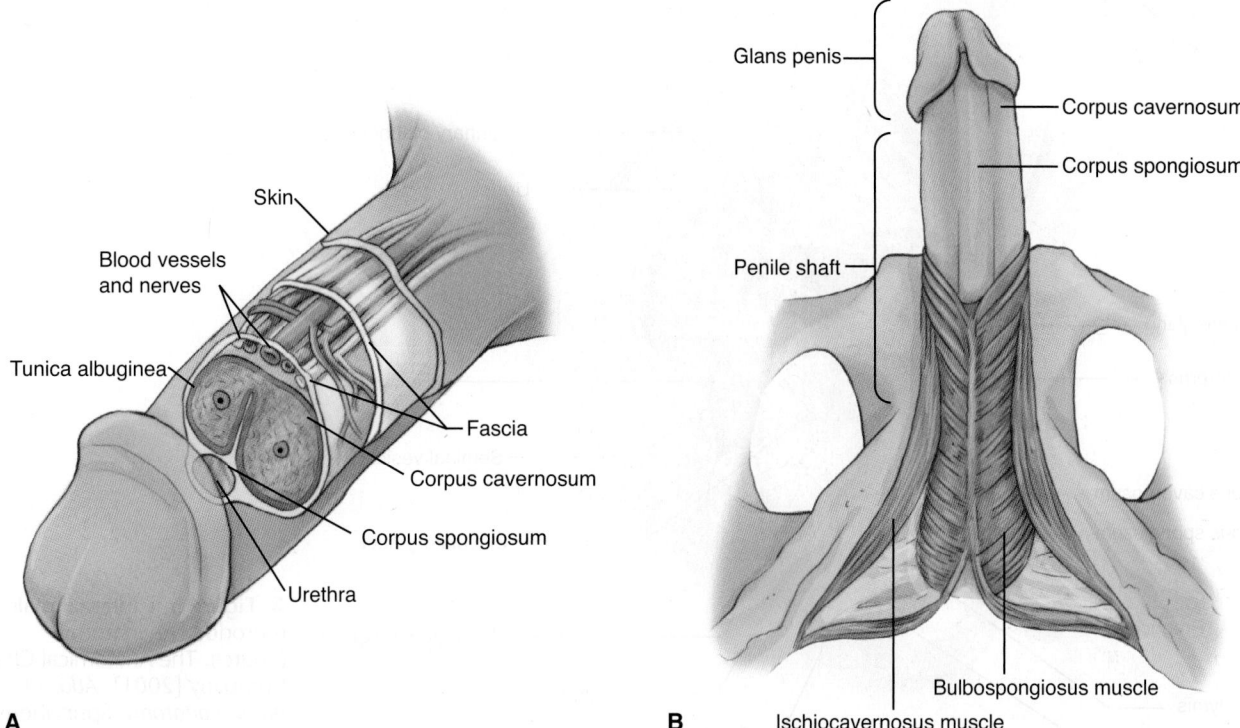

■ **Figure 3-3** Internal structure of the penis. **(A)** Notice the three columns of erectile tissue; these are well supplied with blood and nerve tissue. The cavernous bodies (corpus cavernosa) contain sinuses that fill with blood during an erection. The urethra traverses the shaft encased within the spongy body (corpus spongiosum). **(B)** This view of the ventral aspect shows how the spongy body lies in relation to the cavernous bodies. Notice how the root of the penis is anchored to the pelvis by the tough connective tissue and muscle.

cremaster muscle contracts, pulling the scrotum in toward the man's body, thereby increasing the temperature in the testicles.

Internal Reproductive Organs

Male internal reproductive organs include the testes and a system of glands and ducts that are involved in the formation of nutrient plasma and the transport of semen out of the man's body (Fig. 3-4).

Testes

The testes are two oval organs, one within each scrotal sac (Fig. 3-5). The testes serve two important functions: production of male sex hormones, androgens, and formation and maturation of spermatozoa. Each testis is about 4 cm long by 2.5 cm wide and is divided into lobes. The lobes contain **seminiferous tubules,** tiny coils of tissue in which **spermatogenesis,** production of sperm, occurs. Interstitial cells surround the seminiferous tubules and produce the androgen testosterone, which is necessary for the maturation of sperm. A system of tiny tubes called the rete testis lead from the seminiferous tubules to the **epididymis,** an intricate network of coiled ducts on the posterior portion of each testis that is approximately 6 m (20 ft) in length. It is here that sperm mature. Table 3-1 provides a summary of the hormones that influence male reproduction.

Many physicians recommend that men (ages 15 years and older) perform testicular self-examination (TSE) monthly to detect early changes associated with testicular cancer. Refer to Chapter 27 for how to perform TSE.

Ductal System

The **vas deferens** is the muscular tube in which sperm begin their journey out of the man's body. It connects the epididymis with the ejaculatory duct. The vas deferens is sheathed in the spermatic cord, which also contains the blood vessels, nerves, and lymphatics that serve the testes. The left spermatic cord is usually longer than the right so that the left testis hangs lower than the right.

The spermatic cord (and vas deferens contained within it) leads into the abdominal cavity through the inguinal canal, arches over the urinary bladder, and then

This is an important teaching tip.

Sperm production is most efficient when the temperature within the testes is slightly lower than core body temperature. Constrictive clothing (e. g., tight jeans) holds scrotal contents close to the body. The resultant transfer of heat can reduce sperm production and possibly lead to male infertility.

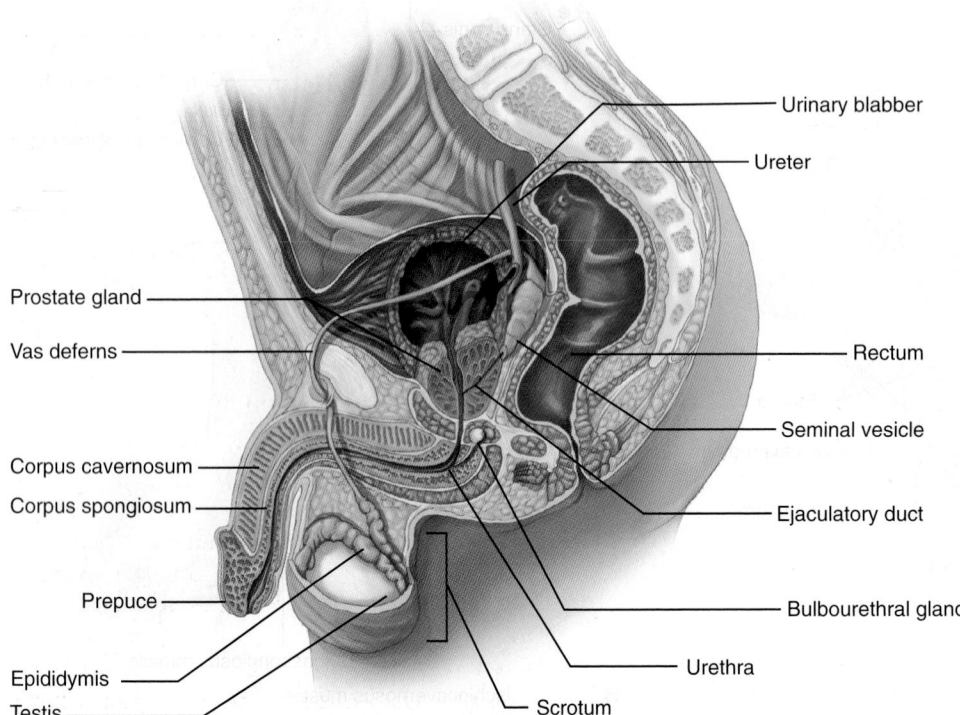

■ **Figure 3-4** Internal male reproductive anatomy. (Source: The Anatomical Chart Company [2001]. *Atlas of human anatomy.* Springhouse, PA: Springhouse.)

curves downward on the posterior side of the bladder. It is at this point that the vas deferens joins with the ejaculatory duct. The paired ejaculatory ducts then connect with the single urethra, which transports the sperm out of the man's penis during ejaculation.

Accessory Glands and Semen

The seminal vesicles are paired glands that empty an alkaline, fructose-rich fluid into the ejaculatory ducts during ejaculation. The prostate is a muscular gland that surrounds the first part of the urethra as it exits the urinary bladder. It is approximately the size of a chestnut. The prostate secretes alkaline prostatic fluid when the gland contracts during ejaculation. The bulbourethral (Cowper's) glands secrete an alkaline fluid that coats the last part of the urethra during ejaculation.

The alkaline fluids secreted by these glands are nutrient plasmas with several key functions, including:

■ Enhancement of sperm motility (i.e., ability to move)
■ Nourishment of sperm (i.e., provides a ready source of energy with the simple sugar fructose)
■ Protection of sperm (i.e., sperm are maintained in an alkaline environment to protect them from the acidic environment of the vagina)

The alkaline fluids and sperm combination is a thick, whitish secretion termed semen or seminal fluid. An average human ejaculate has a volume of 1 to 5 mL and contains several hundred million sperm. Table 3-2 describes (in order) the journey of sperm from formation in the seminiferous tubules to the path out of the body via the urethra.

■ **Figure 3-5** Internal structure of a testis.

Table 3-1 ▌ HORMONAL CONTROL OF MALE REPRODUCTIVE FUNCTIONS

Hormone	Source	Reproductive Functions
Follicle-stimulating hormone	Anterior pituitary	• Stimulates production of sperm in the seminiferous tubules
Interstitial cell-stimulating hormone[1]	Anterior pituitary	• Stimulates the interstitial cells to secrete testosterone
Testosterone	Interstitial cells	• Assists sperm to mature • Influences the development of secondary sex characteristics (facial and pubic hair growth, deepening of the voice, growth of the penis)

[1]Homologous to luteinizing hormone in the female.

Test Yourself

✔ What is the general term that refers to male and female sex cells?

✔ Name two important functions of the testes.

✔ Trace a sperm through the male reproductive tract to outside of the body beginning at the seminiferous tubules. Name all the ducts and glands along the way.

FEMALE REPRODUCTIVE SYSTEM

The female reproductive tract consists of external genitalia, or **vulva,** and internal reproductive organs. The purpose of the female reproductive tract is to allow for sexual intimacy and fulfillment and to produce children through the processes of conception, pregnancy, and childbirth. Each part of the female reproductive tract contributes in some way to these purposes.

The bony pelvis and mammary glands are also part of the female reproductive system. Chapter 8 describes the bony pelvis, and Chapter 14 discusses breast anatomy in conjunction with infant nutrition and lactation. Chapter 27 explains how to do a self-breast examination, an important procedure to detect breast cancer in the early stages.

External Genitalia (Vulva)

The external genitalia consist of the mons pubis, labia majora and minora, clitoris, vestibule, and perineum. Figure 3-6 illustrates these structures.

Mons Pubis

The **mons pubis,** or mons, is a rounded fatty pad located atop the symphysis pubis. Coarse pubic hair and skin cover the mons. The function of the mons is to protect the pelvic bones during sexual intercourse.

Labia

The labia majora (singular: labium majus) are paired fatty tissue folds that extend anteriorly from the mons pubis and then join posteriorly to the true perineum. Labia majora are covered with pubic hair, are vascular, and contain oil and sweat glands. Inside the labia majora

Table 3-2 ▌ A SPERM'S JOURNEY THROUGH THE MALE REPRODUCTIVE TRACT

Event	Site
Formation of sperm	Seminiferous tubules (paired)
Maturation of sperm	Epididymis (paired)
Path into the abdominal cavity	Vas deferens (paired)
Connecting duct between vas deferens and urethra	Ejaculatory duct (paired)
Path out of the man's body	Urethra (single)

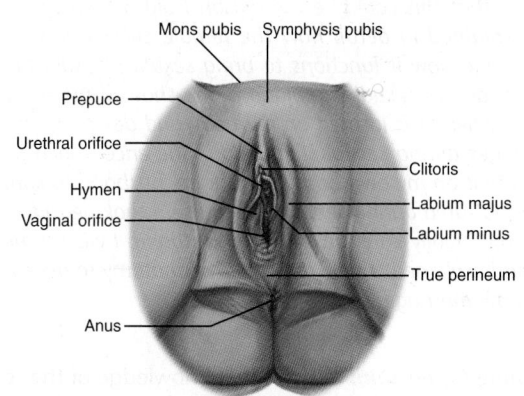

■ Figure 3-6 Female external genitalia.

are the labia minora (singular: labium minus), paired erectile tissue folds that extend anteriorly from the clitoris and then join posteriorly to the fourchette, a tissue fold that is formed where the labia minora meet posteriorly. The labia minora are thinner than the labia majora, are hairless, contain oil glands, and are sensitive to stimulation.

Clitoris

The clitoris is a hooded body composed of erectile tissue located at the apex of the labia minora. The clitoris, similar to the glans penis, is highly sensitive and allows the woman to experience sexual pleasure and orgasm during sexual stimulation. The prepuce is the hooded structure over the clitoris.

Vestibule

The vestibule is the area between the labia minora. The urethral meatus (opening to the urethra), paraurethral (Skene's) glands, vaginal opening or introitus, and Bartholin glands are located within the vestibule. The

paraurethral and Bartholin glands are each paired glands whose secretions moisten the delicate vaginal mucosa and raise the pH of vaginal fluid during sexual intercourse to enhance sperm motility.

The hymen is an avascular fold of tissue located around or partially around the introitus. It varies in shape from woman to woman and throughout an individual woman's reproductive life span. In the past, people believed that an intact hymen was evidence of female virginity. However, activities other than sexual intercourse, such as heavy physical exertion or the use of tampons, can tear the hymen, so the appearance of this tissue is not a reliable method of determining virginity.

Perineum

The true perineum is a band of fibrous, muscular tissue that extends from the posterior portion of the labia majora to the anus. Several sets of superficial and deep muscle groups meet at the perineum to provide support for pelvic structures. The perineum and muscles of the pelvic floor are capable of great expansion during childbirth to allow for delivery of the fetus. These structures are also subject to the stresses and trauma of childbirth. The delivery attendant sometimes cuts an episiotomy into the perineum. Uncontrolled tearing and lacerations can also occur. The woman may experience stress incontinence or prolapse of pelvic organs later in life if lacerations are not repaired properly or if they do not heal appropriately.

> **Be careful!**
>
> It is easy to confuse the clitoris with the urethral meatus. When preparing to insert a urinary catheter, carefully locate the urethral meatus between the labia minora below the clitoris. If you touch the sensitive tissue of the clitoris with the catheter, you may cause the woman pain.

Internal Reproductive Organs

The internal reproductive organs include the vagina, uterus, fallopian tubes, and ovaries. Figure 3-7 illustrates the internal reproductive structures.

Vagina

The vagina, or birth canal, is a muscular tube that leads from the vulva to the uterus. From the opening within the vestibule, it slopes up and backward to the cervix. Because the walls of the vagina extend beyond the uterine cervix, the cervix dips into the vagina and forms fornices, which are archlike structures or pockets. The posterior fornix is largest because the posterior vaginal wall is longer than the anterior wall (approximately 9 and 7 cm long, respectively). Because of its location and size, the posterior fornix provides the physician ready access to the peritoneal cavity for certain invasive procedures.

A Personal Glimpse

For the first 12 years of my marriage, I never experienced an orgasm. My husband and I married very young, just out of high school. In the early years of marriage, sex was okay but never great for me. Then, after three kids and no sleep, I really did not enjoy sex. I began to think there was something wrong with me. Why couldn't I enjoy sex when everyone else seemed to enjoy it? I began to speak confidentially with my nurse practitioner at my obstetrician's office. She had delivered two of my kids and I trusted her completely. I explained my concerns to her. She said that this is a very normal concern and that I was right to come see her. She said she would perform a physical examination to rule out any physical reasons for my lack of interest in, and enjoyment of, sex. A few days after the examination, we sat in her office and talked. She told me that I was in great physical shape, my lab work looked fine, and my reproductive tract was healthy. She asked what kind of stimulation my husband provided before intercourse. I said none. She explained that this could be the reason I did not enjoy sex. She explained in detail how the female clitoris was designed and how it functions to bring sexual pleasure and orgasm during sexual stimulation. She showed me drawings of where it is located on my body and described how it changes during sexual stimulation. She encouraged me to locate it on my own body and ask my husband to stimulate that area during sexual intercourse. I took her advice and now I really enjoy sex with my husband. I wish someone had explained female reproductive anatomy to me earlier in my marriage.

Donna

Learning Opportunity: How does knowledge of the reproductive tract help nurses take care of women who desire greater sexual satisfaction?

Ureter
Ovary
Fallopian tube
Urinary bladder
Symphysis pubis
Urethra
Clitoris
Rectum
Uterus
Cervix
Vagina

■ **Figure 3-7** Internal female reproductive anatomy. (Source: The Anatomical Chart Company [2001]. *Atlas of human anatomy.* Springhouse, PA: Springhouse.)

The vagina serves several important functions. The inner folds, or rugae, allow the vagina to stretch during birth to accommodate a full-term infant. In addition, normally, the vagina maintains an acidic pH of 4 to 5, which protects the vagina from infection. The vagina receives the penis during sexual intercourse and serves as the exit point for menstrual flow.

This is a good patient teaching point.
The acidic environment of the vagina is protective. Any change that alters the pH multiplies the risk for irritation and infection. Douches, tampons, or sanitary pads that contain deodorant, and antibiotic therapy are examples of substances that can alter the pH of the vagina.

Uterus

The uterus, or womb, is a hollow, pear-shaped, muscular structure located within the pelvic cavity between the bladder and the rectum. In the nonpregnant woman, the uterus is approximately 7.5 cm long by 5.0 cm wide (at the widest portion) and weighs approximately 40 g. The uterus normally tips forward and rests just above the urinary bladder (see Fig. 3-7). The functions of the uterus are to prepare for pregnancy each month, protect and nourish the growing child when pregnancy occurs, and to aid in childbirth. The uterus (Fig. 3-8) is divided into four sections:

■ cervix
■ uterine isthmus
■ corpus
■ fundus

The cervix is a tubular structure that connects the vagina and uterus. The outer os (opening) dips into the vagina, and the inner os opens into the uterine isthmus, the lower portion of the uterus. The cervix normally has a tiny slit that allows sperm to enter and the menstrual flow to exit. During childbirth, the cervix must be thin and open fully so that the baby can be born. The ciliated epithelium that lines the inner walls of the cervix produces mucus that lubricates the vaginal canal and protects the uterus from ascending infectious agents.

The uterine isthmus is a narrow neck portion or corridor that connects the cervix to the main body of the uterus. During pregnancy and childbirth, the uterine isthmus is referred to as the lower uterine segment. This is the thinnest portion of the uterus and does not participate in the muscular contractions of labor. Because the tissue is so thin, the lower uterine segment is the area that is most likely to rupture during childbirth.

The corpus is the main body of the uterus, and the fundus is the topmost section. The walls of the corpus and fundus have three layers. The perimetrium is the tough outer layer of connective tissue that supports the uterus. The middle layer is the **myometrium,** a muscular layer that is responsible for the contractions of labor. The muscle fibers of the myometrium wrap around the uterus in three directions: obliquely, laterally, and longitudinally. This muscle configuration allows for tremendous expulsive force during labor and birth. The **endometrium** is the vascular mucosal inner layer. This tissue changes under hormonal influence every month in preparation for possible conception and pregnancy.

Four paired ligaments provide support and hold the uterus in position (see Fig. 3-8). These ligaments anchor

Fundus of uterus

Fallopian tube

Corpus of
the uterus

Uterus
Perimetrium

Myometrium

Endometrium

Abdominal opening
of fallopian tube

Internal os of cervix

External os of cervix

Vagina

Cervix

Rugae

Bartholin's gland

Ovary

Ovarian ligament

Artery and vein

Broad ligament

Uterine isthmus

Round ligament

■ **Figure 3-8** Anterior view of the female reproductive tract. The right fallopian tube and ovary, uterus, and vagina are shown in a cross-sectional view to demonstrate the internal structure of these organs.

the uterus at the base (cervical region), leaving the upper portion (corpus) free in the pelvic cavity. The *broad ligament* is a sheet of peritoneum that attaches the lower sides of the uterus to the sidewalls of the pelvis. The right and left *cardinal ligaments* anchor the walls of the cervix and vagina to the lateral pelvic walls. The *round ligaments* are paired fibromuscular bands that tip the uterus forward and hold it in an anteflexed position. They extend from the anterior/lateral portions of the uterus to the labia majora. The round ligaments are homologous to the spermatic cord in the male. The *uterosacral ligaments* anchor the lower posterior portion of the uterus to the sacrum.

Fallopian Tubes

The paired fallopian tubes (also known as oviducts) are tiny, muscular corridors that arise from the superior surface of the uterus near the fundus and extend laterally on either side toward the ovaries. They are 8 to 14 cm in length. Each fallopian tube has three sections. The isthmus, which means a neck or narrow section, is the medial one third of the tube that connects to the uterus. The ampulla is the middle portion of the tube. The infundibulum is the outer portion that opens into the lower abdominal cavity. At the outer edges of the infundibulum are fimbriae, fingerlike projections that undulate gently over the ovaries.

The tubes have a critical role in conception. When the ovary releases an egg, the undulating movements of the fimbriae attract the egg toward the fallopian tube. Once the egg is within the tube, muscular contractions and

beating of tiny cilia propel it toward the uterus. If sperm are present, fertilization of the egg is possible. Fertilization most frequently occurs in the ampulla section of the tube. The tubes secrete lipids and glycogen to provide nourishment to the fertilized egg as it makes its way to the uterus. The functions of the fallopian tubes are to provide a site for fertilization, a passageway, and a nourishing, warm environment for the fertilized egg to travel to the uterus.

Ovaries

The ovaries, two sex glands homologous to the male testes, are located on either side of the uterus. They are similar to almonds in size and shape. The broad and ovarian ligaments provide support to the ovaries. The functions of the ovaries are to produce the female hormones estrogen and progesterone, which are responsible for female secondary sex characteristics; to store ova and help them mature; and to regulate the menstrual cycle in response to anterior pituitary hormones (see discussion in the Menstrual Cycle section).

Every female is born with all the ova (eggs) that she will ever have. Typically, females are born with approximately 2 million eggs, many of which will deteriorate during childhood. The ovaries normally re-

You do the math.

If one ovum matures every month during the childbearing years (from age 12 through 50), a woman would only use 456 ova. Because on average a baby girl is born with 2 million immature ova, there are significantly more available than will ever be used.

lease the remaining ova at a rate of one per month until the woman's reproductive years are over.

Blood Supply for the Pelvic Organs

The pelvic organs have a rich blood supply (Fig. 3-9). The internal iliac artery arises from the common iliac artery and supplies the pelvic organs, gluteal region, hip, and medial thigh. The vaginal and uterine arteries, both of which arise from the anterior division of the internal iliac artery, supply the vagina and uterus, respectively. The ovarian artery, which supplies the ovaries and oviducts, branches directly from the abdominal aorta. The internal pudendal artery is the primary blood supply to the perineum. This artery branches from the anterior division of the internal iliac artery and supplies the anus, superficial and deep perineal muscles, clitoris, and posterior aspect of the labia majora.

Several major veins drain the tissues of the pelvic organs. The ovarian vein, which drains the ovary, the distal part of the fallopian tube, and ureter, intersects directly with the inferior vena cava on the right and on the left connects with the left renal vein. The uterine and vaginal venous plexuses drain the uterus, fallopian tubes, and vagina. A plexus is a network of veins that forms multiple tributaries. These plexuses connect with the uterine and vaginal veins to drain into the internal iliac vein. The external and internal pudendal veins allow deoxygenated blood from the perineal region to flow into the femoral, great saphenous, and internal iliac veins.

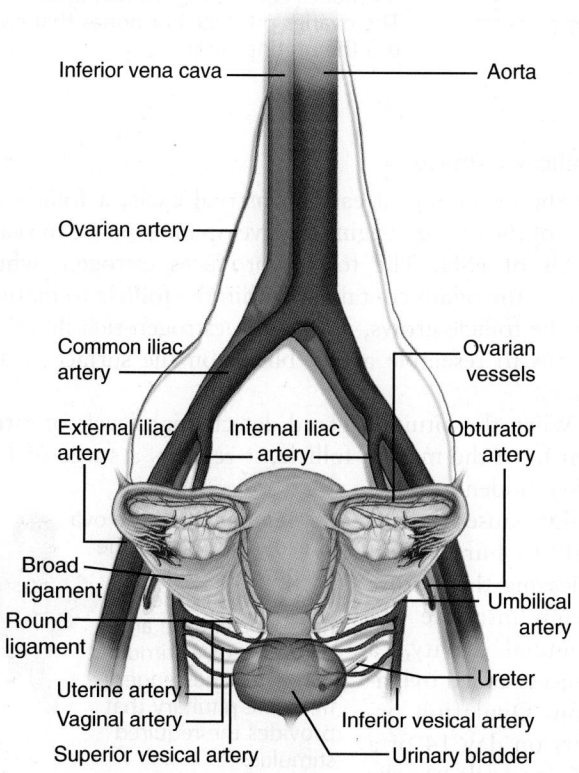

Inferior vena cava ——— ——— Aorta

Ovarian artery ———

Common iliac artery ———

Ovarian vessels

External iliac artery ———

Internal iliac artery ———

Obturator artery

Broad ligament ———

Round ligament ———

Umbilical artery

Uterine artery ———

Vaginal artery ———

Ureter

Superior vesical artery ———

Inferior vesical artery

Urinary bladder

■ **Figure 3-9** Pelvic blood supply.

REGULATION OF REPRODUCTIVE FUNCTION
Puberty

Puberty is the time of life in which the individual becomes capable of sexual reproduction. Puberty occurs on average between the ages of 10 and 14 years. This phase is marked by maturation of the reproductive organs and development of secondary sex characteristics, external physical evidence of sexual maturity. Secondary sex characteristics include female breast development, growth of pubic and axillary hair, growth of external genitals (labia and penis), appearance of facial hair, and deepening of the voice in the male.

The changes associated with puberty happen in response to hypothalamic and pituitary hormones. Secondary sex characteristics develop in an orderly sequence, although the timing may be varied between individuals. Breast budding in the female is usually the first physical sign noted and occurs between the ages of 10 and 12 years, on average. Appearance of pubic hair usually occurs just before **menarche**, the first menstrual period. Menarche occurs most frequently between the ages of 12 and 14 years.

Menstrual Cycle

The menstrual cycle, or the female reproductive cycle, refers to the recurring changes that take place in a woman's reproductive tract associated with menstruation and the events that surround menstruation. **Menstruation**, the casting away of blood, tissue, and debris from the uterus as the inner lining sheds, is variable in amount and duration. On average, flow lasts 4 to 6 days, with a total blood loss of 25 to 60 mL. Although this loss is seemingly negligible, with time it can contribute to low iron stores and anemia.

The menstrual cycle encompasses the events that transpire in the woman's reproductive organs between the beginnings of two menstrual periods. Hormones from the ovaries and the pituitary gland regulate these cyclical changes. The average cycle lasts 28 days, approximately one month; however, there are great variations between women, and an individual woman's cycle

> **Don't get lost in the details!**
>
> When you understand the menstrual cycle, you will then be able to understand the process of conception, and you will be better prepared to counsel families on how to prevent pregnancy or how to increase the probability that pregnancy will occur.

— Controlled by hypothalamus

— Anterior pituitary

FSH   LH   — LH peak triggers ovulation

Maturing follicle

Degenerating corpus luteum

Corpus luteum

Ovulation

Day 1–5   Day 6–14   Day 15–26   Days 27 and 28

Ovarian hormones

Estrogen   Progesterone

Glands
Arteries
Veins

Thickness of endometrial lining during the menstrual cycle

Uterine phases	Menstrual	Proliferative	Secretory	Isch-emic	Men-strual
Ovarian phases	Follicular		Luteal		

Days   1   5   14   26   28

■ **Figure 3-10** A 28-day (average) menstrual cycle. The anterior pituitary hormones control the ovarian cycle. The ovaries produce hormones that control the uterine cycle.

may vary in duration from cycle to cycle. For ease of understanding, the following discussion of the menstrual cycle is based on the average 28-day cycle.

There are two main components of the menstrual cycle: the ovarian cycle and the uterine cycle. Although each cycle is discussed separately below, it is important to remember that both cycles work together simultaneously to produce the menstrual cycle (Fig. 3-10). Changes in cervical mucus take place during the course of the menstrual cycle; these changes are also discussed.

Ovarian Cycle

Cyclical changes in the ovaries occur in response to two anterior pituitary hormones: follicle-stimulating hormone (FSH) and luteinizing hormone (LH). There are two phases of the ovarian cycle, each named for the hormone that has the most control over that particular phase. The follicular phase, controlled by FSH, encompasses days 1 to 14 of a 28-day cycle. LH controls the luteal phase, which includes days 15 to 28.

Follicular Phase

At the beginning of each menstrual cycle, a follicle on one of the ovaries begins to develop in response to rising levels of FSH. The follicle produces estrogen, which causes the ovum contained within the follicle to mature. As the follicle grows, it fills with estrogen-rich fluid and begins to resemble a tiny blister on the surface of the ovary.

When the pituitary gland detects high levels of estrogen from the mature follicle, it releases a surge of LH. This sudden increase in LH causes the follicle to burst open, releasing the mature ovum into the abdominal cavity, a process called **ovulation**. Ovulation occurs on day 14 of a 28-day cycle. As the

Remember, all of the ova already exist within the ovaries in an immature state. In order to ripen, or mature, an ovum needs a stimulus. FSH is the messenger from the pituitary that provides the required stimulus.

ovum floats along the surface of the ovary, the gentle beating of the fimbriae draws it toward the fallopian tube.

Luteal Phase

After ovulation, LH levels remain elevated and cause the remnants of the follicle to develop into a yellow body called the **corpus luteum**. In addition to producing estrogen, the corpus luteum secretes a hormone called progesterone. If fertilization does not take place, the corpus luteum begins to degenerate, and estrogen and progesterone levels fall. This process leads back to day 1 of the cycle, and the follicular phase begins anew.

Test Yourself

✔ Which hormone is responsible for ovulation?

✔ What is the main purpose of FSH?

✔ What structure produces progesterone?

Uterine Cycle

The uterine cycle refers to the changes that occur in the inner lining of the uterus. These changes happen in response to the ovarian hormones estrogen and progesterone. There are four phases to this cycle: menstrual, proliferative, secretory, and ischemic.

Menstrual Phase

The onset of menstruation signals day 1 of the menstrual cycle. During the menstrual phase of the uterine cycle, the uterine lining is shed because of low levels of progesterone and estrogen. At the same time, a follicle begins to develop and starts producing estrogen. The menstrual phase ends when the menstrual period stops on approximately day 5 of the cycle.

Proliferative Phase

When estrogen levels are high enough, the endometrium begins to regenerate. Estrogen stimulates blood vessels to develop. The blood vessels in turn bring nutrients and oxygen to the uterine lining, which begins to grow and become thicker. The proliferative phase ends with ovulation on day 14.

Secretory Phase

After ovulation, the corpus luteum begins to produce progesterone. This hormone causes the uterine lining to become rich in nutrients in preparation for pregnancy. Estrogen levels also remain high to maintain the lining. If pregnancy does not transpire, the corpus luteum gradually degenerates, and the woman enters the ischemic phase of the menstrual cycle.

Ischemic Phase

On days 27 and 28, estrogen and progesterone levels fall because the corpus luteum is no longer producing them. Without these hormones to maintain the blood vessel network, the uterine lining becomes ischemic. When the lining starts to slough, the woman has come full cycle and is once again at day 1 of the menstrual cycle.

Test Yourself

✔ What is the main function of estrogen during the menstrual cycle?

✔ Which hormone is active only during the secretory phase of the uterine cycle?

✔ What happens to the uterine lining during the ischemic phase?

✔ What causes the ischemic phase to occur?

Cervical Mucus Changes

Changes in cervical mucus take place over the course of the menstrual cycle. Some women use these characteristics to help determine when ovulation is likely to happen. During the menstrual phase, the cervix does not produce mucus. Gradually, as hormonal changes transpire and the proliferative phase begins, the cervix begins to produce a tacky, crumbly type of mucus that is yellow or white. As the time of ovulation draws near, the mucus becomes progressively clear and thin with lubricating properties; the mucus resembles raw egg white. At the peak of fertility (i.e., during ovulation), the mucus has a distensible, stretchable quality called spinnbarkheit (see Chapter 4 for further discussion of cervical mucus changes that indicate ovulation). After ovulation, the mucus again becomes scanty, thick, and opaque.

Menopause

Menopause refers to the time in a woman's life when reproductive capability ends. Gradually the ovaries cease to function, and hormone levels fall. The woman begins to experience irregular menstrual cycles until they finally end. The time during which these changes gradually take place is called the **climacteric**. The average age at which menopause occurs is between 47 and 55 years.

SEXUAL RESPONSE CYCLE

Sexuality is part of our human nature. Nature has provided us with the capacity to give and receive pleasure through the process of sexual stimulation. Therefore, a discussion of reproduction would be incomplete without mention of the physiology of sexual response.

There are two underlying physiologic responses to sexual stimulation in both men and women: vasocongestion and myotonia (muscular tension). These two processes are fundamental to almost all physiologic responses that take place during sexual arousal.

Vasocongestion occurs in the pelvic organs during sexual excitement because the arteries dilate, allowing inflow of blood that is greater than venous capacity to drain the area. The result is widespread congestion of the pelvic tissues. Vasocongestion leads to erection of the penis and clitoris, vaginal lubrication, and engorgement of the labia and testicles. Other tissue, such as the nipples and earlobes, may also be affected.

Myotonia is present throughout the body during sexual arousal and orgasm. It is evident in voluntary and involuntary contractions. Facial grimacing, spasmodic contractions of the hands and feet, and the involuntary muscular contractions during orgasm are the most notable examples of myotonia.

There are four phases of the sexual response: excitement, plateau, orgasm, and resolution. These phases occur in both sexes and follow the same general patterns, regardless of the method of sexual stimulation.

During the excitement phase, the woman's clitoris engorges and enlarges, the labia majora separate, and the labia minora increase in size. The uterus increases in size and begins to elevate. For the man, excitement leads to erection of the penis, thickening of the scrotal sac, and testicular elevation. In both sexes, increases in heart rate, blood pressure, and respirations mark the onset of the excitement phase. Some individuals experience a "sex flush," a reddening of the skin on the chest and neck.

Duration of the excitement phase is from several minutes to several hours.

No set event marks the beginning of the plateau phase. Vasocongestion and myotonia continue, and the heart rate and blood pressure remain elevated. For the female, the outer third of the vagina engorges, the clitoris retracts behind its hood, and the labia minora deepen in color. The uterus is fully elevated in the pelvic cavity. The head of the penis in the male engorges further, and the testes remain engorged and elevated. The plateau phase is typically a few seconds to several minutes in duration.

A series of muscular contractions marks orgasm, the climax of sexual response. The clitoris remains retracted behind the hood, and the outer third of the vagina, rectal sphincter, and uterus undergo rhythmic contractions. The male experiences contractions of the urethra, base of the penis, and rectal muscles, as well as emission and expulsion of semen.

During resolution, the muscles gradually relax, and there is a reversal of vasocongestion. The heart rate, blood pressure, and breathing return to normal. The clitoris descends, and the labia and internal organs return to their prearousal positions and color. The male loses his erection, the testes descend, and the scrotum thins.

Key Points

➤ Two major functions of the reproductive system are to produce offspring and to provide the experience of pleasure through physical intimacy.

➤ The testes and ovaries are responsible for the production of sex cells, or gametes.

➤ Male external genitalia include the penis and scrotum. The penis serves to eliminate urine from the bladder and functions to deposit sperm in the female reproductive tract for the purposes of reproduction. The scrotum regulates the temperature and protects the testes from trauma.

➤ The testes and ductal system compose the man's internal reproductive tract. Spermatogenesis occurs in the testes, and the ductal system serves as the exit route for sperm from the man's body.

➤ Sperm are formed in the seminiferous tubules and mature in the epididymis. During ejaculation, sperm travel from the epididymis through the paired vas deferens and ejaculatory ducts to the urethra and out of the body.

➤ Sperm need an alkaline environment and an energy source to be motile. The seminal vesicles (paired), prostate gland, and the bulbourethral glands (paired) contribute alkaline secretions to semen. The seminal vesicles also contribute fructose, an energy source for sperm.

➤ Testosterone, FSH, and interstitial cell-stimulating hormone (ICSH) are the male hormones responsible for production of sperm and the development of secondary sex characteristics.

➤ The female external genitalia, or vulva, includes the mons pubis, labia majora, labia minora, clitoris, urethral meatus, vaginal opening, and Bartholin glands. The vestibule is the area within the boundaries of the labia minora and includes the urethral meatus, vaginal opening, and Bartholin glands.

➤ The vagina is an internal reproductive organ that functions as the female organ for sexual intercourse, exit point for the menstrual flow, and as the birth canal. Rugae, or folds, allow for stretching during the birth process.

➤ The main divisions of the uterus are the cervix, isthmus, corpus, and fundus. The walls of the uterus have three layers: perimetrium (protective cover), myometrium (muscle), and endometrium (lining).

➤ The fallopian tubes lead from the uterus toward the ovaries. The isthmus is the narrow portion near the uterus. The ampulla is the middle portion, and the infundibulum is the outer portion close to the ovaries. Fimbriae on the infundibulum make wave-like motions over the ovary to guide the released ovum toward the fallopian tube.

- The ovaries are homologous to the male testes. The ovarian hormones, estrogen and progesterone, play a major role in the menstrual cycle and in the development of secondary sex characteristics in the female.
- The menstrual cycle begins with day 1, the start of menstrual flow. The cycle encompasses the ovarian cycle and the uterine cycle. FSH and LH from the pituitary govern the ovarian cycle, and estrogen and progesterone from the ovaries guide the uterine cycle.
- The sexual response cycle is divided into four phases: excitement, plateau, orgasm, and resolution. Vasocongestion and myotonia are the primary physiologic processes that contribute to sexual response in both the male and female.

INTERNET RESOURCES

Male
www.healthac.org/male.html
www.nlm.nih.gov/medlineplus/malereproductivesystem.html

Female
www.healthac.org/female.html
www.nlm.nih.gov/medlineplus/femalereproductivesystem.html

Menstrual Cycle
en.wikipedia.org/wiki/Menstrual_cycle
www.4woman.gov/faq/menstru.htm
www.fwhc.org/health/moon.htm

Workbook

■ NCLEX-STYLE REVIEW QUESTIONS

1. You are teaching a male client about the male reproductive system. You ask him which gland provides the sugar that gives the sperm energy to move. Which answer indicates that he correctly understands your teaching?

   a. Bartholin gland
   b. Bulbourethral gland
   c. Epididymis
   d. Seminal vesicles

2. The vagina is a hostile environment for sperm. What characteristic of semen protects sperm from the vaginal environment?

   a. Acidic fluid
   b. Alkaline fluid
   c. Presence of testosterone
   d. Secretions from seminiferous tubules

3. You are preparing to perform a urinary catheterization on a female client. In which location will you expect to find the urinary meatus?

   a. Above the clitoris
   b. Below the vaginal opening
   c. On the true perineum
   d. Within the vestibule

4. You are caring for a woman in labor. The doctor is concerned that the uterus might rupture. Which part of the uterus requires the closest assessment because it is the thinnest part of the uterus?

   a. Corpus
   b. Fundus
   c. Inner cervical os
   d. Lower uterine segment

5. Which ovarian hormone regulates the proliferative phase of the uterine cycle?

   a. FSH
   b. LH
   c. Estrogen
   d. Progesterone

■ STUDY ACTIVITIES

1. In each row of the table, you will find either a male or a female reproductive organ listed. In the column that is missing information, fill in the name of the homologous reproductive organ.

Male Reproductive Organ	Female Reproductive Organ
Glans penis	
	Round ligaments
	Ovaries
Foreskin or prepuce	

2. In your clinical group, have a discussion as to why it is important for a nurse to understand the menstrual cycle.

■ CRITICAL THINKING: WHAT WOULD YOU DO?

Apply your knowledge of reproductive anatomy and physiology to the following situation.

1. Doug and Nancy, a young married couple, ages 26 and 22 years, respectively, have not been using any contraception for the past year, but Nancy has not become pregnant. Doug is a rancher and dresses in cowboy gear, including tight jeans. He works in a hot, humid environment for 10 to 12 hours almost every day.

   a. Using your knowledge about male reproductive anatomy, what is one possible reason pregnancy has not occurred?
   b. What advice might be helpful for Doug to increase the likelihood that pregnancy will occur?

2. Nancy complains of frequent vaginal infections. During an office interview, Nancy tells you that she douches at least once per week.

   a. What other questions should you ask regarding Nancy's hygiene habits?
   b. What advice might be helpful for Nancy to decrease her risk for vaginal infections?

4

Special Issues of Women's Health Care and Reproduction

KEY TERMS

abstinence
amenorrhea
coitus interruptus
dysmenorrhea
dyspareunia
elective abortion
endometriosis
gestational surrogate
induced abortion
infertility
menorrhagia
metrorrhagia
perimenopause
postcoital test
spinnbarkeit
therapeutic abortion

LEARNING OBJECTIVES

On completion of this chapter, you should be able to:

1. Describe health-screening recommendations for women.
2. Differentiate between dysmenorrhea and premenstrual syndrome (PMS).
3. Explain the clinical manifestations, treatment, and nursing care for endometriosis.
4. Discuss risk factors for pelvic inflammatory disease (PID).
5. Explain causes and risk factors for pelvic support disorders.
6. Discuss the significance of family planning.
7. Compare and contrast methods of contraception.
8. Explain advantages and disadvantages for each method of contraception.
9. List possible causes for fertility problems.
10. Identify diagnostic testing used related to fertility problems.
11. Discuss treatment options available for fertility problems.
12. Discuss the psychosocial effects of fertility problems.
13. Identify major considerations for the perimenopausal and postmenopausal woman.

THIS CHAPTER examines issues related to women's health and reproduction. Women's health issues include preventive health care, menstrual disorders, pelvic infections, disorders of the uterus and ovaries, and pelvic support disorders. Issues related to the reproductive life cycle include family planning and contraception, elective termination of pregnancy, infertility, and menopause. Friends and family members may turn to you, the nurse, as a resource for questions about women's health issues, becoming pregnant, contraception, or infertility. Therefore, the nurse's role in women's health and reproductive life cycle issues is also discussed.

Several *Healthy People 2010* goals relate to the topics in this chapter. Selected goals include:

- Reduce breast and cervical cancer death rates.
- Increase the number of females who comply with screening recommendations, specifically pap tests and mammography.
- Increase the proportion of intended pregnancies.
- Promote responsible sexual behaviors, strengthen community capacity, and increase access to quality services to prevent sexually transmitted infections (STIs) and their complications.
- Reduce the proportion of adults aged 50 years and older with osteoporosis.

WOMEN'S HEALTH ISSUES

Women's health issues encompass a broad variety of topics. Current research is highlighting the unique needs of women in relation to medical–surgical conditions, such as diabetes, heart disease, and stroke. Although these topics are critical to the overall health of women, this chapter focuses on conditions that occur universally, or near universally, in women.

HEALTH SCREENING FOR WOMEN

Health promotion is a broad concept that involves educating and assisting individuals to make behavior and lifestyle modifications for the prevention or early detection and treatment of disease. Because nurses are trusted health care professionals, individuals and families often turn to them for information and advice on health-related matters. As a result, health promotion for women is an area in which nurses can have great influence.

Health screening is a component of a comprehensive health promotion plan. Screening tests do not diagnose disease. Instead, a positive result indicates the need for more thorough testing. The following discussion encompasses screening procedures that promote the early detection of disorders that are unique to, or occur commonly in, women.

Breast Cancer Screening

Breast cancer is the most frequently diagnosed malignancy in women and ranks second (behind lung cancer) among cancer deaths in women. Each year in the United States, there are more than 200,000 new cases diagnosed and more than 40,000 deaths caused by breast cancer. Detection of breast cancer before axillary node involvement increases the chance for survival (American Cancer Society [ACS], 2005). Therefore, the American Cancer Society (ACS) recommends a three-pronged approach to screening for early identification of breast cancer: breast self-awareness, clinical breast examination, and mammography (ACS, 2006). Educate women regarding the importance of each screening test and how to perform breast self-examination (BSE), as indicated.

Breast self-awareness may involve BSE. BSE is a self-scheduled, systematic approach the woman uses to check her breasts. In the past, monthly BSE was recommended. The ACS now presents BSE as optional because current research indicates that performing BSE does not decrease mortality associated with breast cancer. However, the ACS recommends that each woman know how her breasts normally look and feel, and if she finds changes, she should immediately report them to a physician (ACS, 2006). (Refer to Chapter 27 for instructions on how to perform BSE.)

Clinical breast examination involves inspection and palpation of the breasts by a practitioner. The ACS recommends that a woman in her 20s and 30s should have a clinical breast examination at least every 3 years. When the woman reaches 40 years of age, she should schedule a yearly clinical breast examination.

At 40 years of age, the woman should begin having a yearly mammogram. Mammography is a screening tool that uses very–low-dose x-ray for examination of breast tissue. Mammography is useful in the early detection of cancer because it can detect a breast tumor or abnormality 2 years before the woman or the primary care provider can palpate it. For this procedure, the breast is placed on a platform and compressed firmly between the platform and a plastic paddle (Fig. 4-1). Routine views

A

B

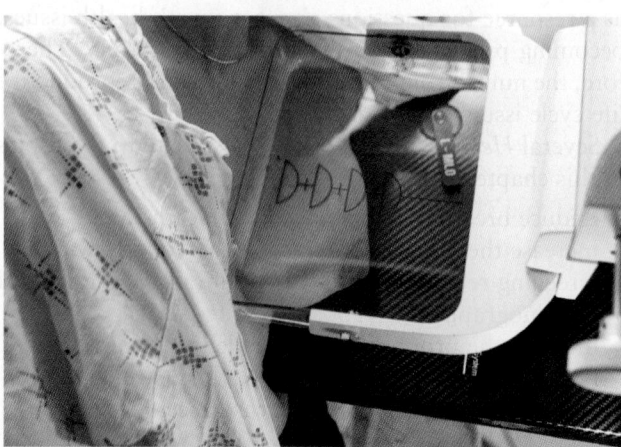

C

■ Figure 4-1 Mammography. **(A)** Mammography equipment. **(B)** A top-to-bottom view of the breast. **(C)** A side view of the breast.

include a top-to-bottom and a side view. The compression can be uncomfortable for some women. The most common recommendation is to schedule the examination for the week after the menstrual period, when the breasts are less tender, to minimize discomfort.

Pelvic Examination and Pap Smear

Every woman should have a yearly physical examination. A pelvic examination should be part of the total physical examination. A pelvic examination detects changes associated with certain gynecologic conditions such as infection, inflammation, pelvic pain, cancer, and other disorders. The Papanicolaou test (Pap smear) is one part of the pelvic examination.

The pelvic examination begins with the woman in lithotomy position. The practitioner palpates and examines the appearances of the structures of the vulva. Then, the practitioner inserts a speculum to examine the walls of the vagina and the cervix. When the cervix is clearly visible, the practitioner swabs the cervix to obtain cell samples for the Pap smear and secretions to culture for pelvic infection. A bimanual examination follows the speculum examination. The practitioner inserts two lubricated fingers into the vagina with one hand and uses the other hand to palpate uterine and ovarian structures through the abdominal wall. Frequently, a rectal examination to test for fecal occult blood and/or to palpate the rectovaginal wall completes the examination. See Nursing Procedure 4-1 for guidance in assisting the practitioner to collect a Pap smear.

The Pap smear is an important screening tool for cervical cancer. In fact, the incidence of cervical cancer has decreased by 70% between 1950 and 1970, with another 40% decrease since 1970. These decreases relate to the routine performance of Pap smears because of early detection and prompt treatment of precancerous changes (National Cancer Institute, 2006). The American Cancer Society's current (2006) guidelines recommend that the woman obtain the initial Pap smear approximately 3 years after she first has sexual intercourse, or by 21 years of age, whichever comes first. Subsequent Pap smears should occur annually in women younger than 30 years of age. Healthy women aged 30 years and older may require a Pap smear only every 2 to 3 years. The woman's primary care provider may advise the woman who has the human immunodeficiency virus (HIV) or is otherwise immunocompromised, and the woman who has other risk factors for cervical cancer to continue to have annual Pap smears (ACS, 2006). The American College of Obstetricians and Gynecologists (ACOG) continues to recommend annual pelvic examinations for all women, even when a Pap smear is not required (ACOG, 2004).

Vulvar Self-Examination

Some primary care practitioners recommend that women older than 18 years (and those younger who

---

Nursing Procedure 4-1
ASSISTING WITH COLLECTION OF A PAP SMEAR

EQUIPMENT

Examination table with stirrups or foot pedals
Drapes
Sterile gloves for the examiner
Speculum
Swab for the Pap test
Glass slide
Fixative
Sterile lubricant (water-soluble)

PROCEDURE

1. Explain procedure to the patient (Fig. A).
2. Instruct the patient to empty her bladder.*
3. Wash hands thoroughly.
4. Assemble equipment, maintaining sterility, as indicated (Fig. B).
5. Position patient on stirrups or foot pedals so that her knees fall outward.

A

B

(continues on page 62)

Nursing Procedure 4-1

ASSISTING WITH COLLECTION OF A PAP SMEAR *(continued)*

C

D

E

F

G

H

6. Drape the patient with a sheet or other draping for privacy, covering the abdomen but leaving the perineal area exposed.
7. Open packages as needed.
8. Encourage the patient to relax.
9. Provide support to the patient as the practitioner obtains a sample by spreading the labia (Fig. C); inserting the speculum (Fig. D); inserting the cytobrush (Fig. E) and swabbing the endocervix; and inserting the plastic spatula (Fig. F) and swabbing the cervix.

10. Transfer specimen to container (Fig. G) or slide. If a slide is used, spray fixative on the slide.
11. Wash hands thoroughly.
12. Label specimen according to facility policy.
13. Rinse reusable instruments and dispose of waste appropriately (Fig. H).
14. Wash hands thoroughly.

Note: A full bladder interferes with the pelvic examination and causes discomfort for the woman.

are sexually active) should perform a monthly self-examination of the external genitalia. As with BSE, the major value of the monthly vulvar self-examination is that the woman will become familiar with her own normal anatomy. Using a hand mirror and an adequate light source, the woman should inspect her vulva for any lesions, growths, reddened areas, unusual discharge, or changes in skin color. She should also take note of any changes in sensation, such as itching or pain. Caution the woman that although most changes are not cancerous, she should report all changes to her primary care practitioner for evaluation.

COMMON DISORDERS OF THE FEMALE REPRODUCTIVE TRACT

There are several commonly occurring female reproductive tract disorders. Many involve disorders of menstruation. Others are related to or caused by infections or decreased support of the pelvic floor.

Menstrual Disturbances

Disturbances of the menstrual cycle include increased or decreased frequency; absent, excessive, or irregular bleeding; and pain. Nursing intervention depends on the cause and treatment of the disorder, but may include providing information about recommended treatments or prescribed medications, caring for the woman before and after a procedure, and providing emotional support and reassurance.

Amenorrhea

Amenorrhea refers to the absence of menstruation. A 16-year-old girl who is developing normally and yet does not experience menarche (the first menstrual period) has *primary amenorrhea. Secondary amenorrhea* is the cessation of menstrual periods after they have occurred previously (Chandran, 2006).

The presence of regular menstrual periods is a sign of health. Regular menses signal that the pituitary and ovarian connection are working together properly and that appropriate amounts of sex hormones are present.

Because pregnancy is the most common cause of amenorrhea in women of reproductive age, a pregnancy test is often the first test performed when a woman presents with this symptom. Once the practitioner rules out pregnancy as a cause, the next step is a thorough review of systems.

Endocrine symptoms, such as hot flashes, night sweats, and vaginal dryness, associated with amenorrhea often indicate ovarian dysfunction. Many factors can cause the ovaries to stop working prematurely. These include history of radiation therapy or chemotherapy to treat cancer and unknown causes. Systemic symptoms may indicate disorders of the hypothalamus and pituitary. Factors that can interfere with normal hypothalamic function include excessive exercise; endocrine disorders, such as hyper- or hypothyroidism; human immunodeficiency virus/acquired immunodeficiency syndrome (HIV/AIDS); malnutrition; and major psychiatric disorders.

If there are no associated endocrine symptoms, the problem may be in the outflow tract. The ovaries may be functioning normally, but if adhesions have scarred the endometrium (Asherman syndrome), it will not respond to ovarian stimulation. Imperforate hymen or underdevelopment of the lower reproductive tract does not allow the menstrual flow to escape.

A thorough assessment by physical examination, history taking, and laboratory testing to identify the underlying cause and direct medical intervention. The underlying cause guides subsequent treatment.

Atypical Uterine Bleeding

There are several types of atypical (abnormal) uterine bleeding. Heavy or prolonged bleeding, **menorrhagia,** is the most common menstrual complaint and can lead to anemia if left untreated. **Metrorrhagia** refers to menstrual bleeding that is normal in amount but occurs at irregular intervals between menstrual periods. Metrorrhagia that occurs with hormonal contraceptives is called breakthrough bleeding. This type of bleeding frequently decreases over time.

Many of the factors that contribute to amenorrhea can also cause menorrhagia, including ovarian dysfunction. A thorough history and physical can rule out systemic causes. Other uterine conditions, such as polyps and fibroids, can cause menorrhagia. If there are no readily apparent causative factors, the practitioner may initiate a trial of oral progestin therapy. If this therapy does not work, the practitioner might insert an intrauterine device that releases progestin into the uterine cavity. The advantage of this therapy is that systemic hormone levels remain low because the hormones discharge directly into the uterine cavity. If traditional measures do not work, another therapy option is endometrial ablation, removal of the uterine lining (Vega, 2006). Hysterectomy, surgical removal of the uterus, remains a treatment alternative when other measures fail.

> **This is worth noting.**
> Pregnancy is the most common cause of abnormal bleeding during the reproductive years. Bear in mind that any woman of childbearing age who presents with atypical or irregular bleeding may be pregnant.

Dysmenorrhea

Dysmenorrhea is painful or difficult menses. Primary dysmenorrhea refers to painful menstrual periods that are not associated with a disease process. Secondary dysmenorrhea is painful menses secondary to pelvic pathology. This discussion focuses on primary dysmenorrhea, which is the more common of the two conditions. Discussion of secondary dysmenorrhea occurs in conjunction with the associated disease process.

Primary dysmenorrhea results from the action of prostaglandins on the uterus during ovulatory cycles. Prostaglandins contribute to dysmenorrhea in two ways.

> **Don't get confused.**
> Primary dysmenorrhea is not the same thing as premenstrual syndrome (PMS). A woman can have both conditions, but they are separate entities.

They cause the uterus to contract, which leads to painful cramping, and they decrease blood flow to the myometrium, which contributes to lactic acid buildup and additional pain.

Primary dysmenorrhea affects as many as 50% of women during their childbearing years. It occurs at a higher rate in younger women who have not borne children. As age and parity increase, the incidence of primary dysmenorrhea decreases. Risk factors that increase the severity of symptoms include earlier age at menarche, long and/or heavy menstrual flow, smoking, and a family history of the condition (Calis et al., 2006).

Clinical Manifestations

Primary dysmenorrhea typically begins within 6 months to 2 years after menarche. Major symptoms consist of severe intermittent cramping in association with constant pain in the lower abdomen, which may radiate to the lower back or upper thighs. General malaise, fatigue, dizziness, nausea and vomiting, diarrhea, and headache frequently accompany the spasmodic cramping. Symptoms usually begin shortly before or with the onset of menstrual flow.

The practitioner must rule out secondary dysmenorrhea before initiating treatment. The first step is to do a thorough history and physical and a pelvic examination, along with a variety of diagnostic procedures, to identify any underlying causes. If a causative factor exists, treatment begins to cure the underlying condition or control its symptoms. When there is no identified secondary cause, the practitioner diagnoses primary dysmenorrhea.

Treatment

The most effective treatments to date have been nonsteroidal anti-inflammatory drugs (NSAIDs) and oral contraceptives (birth control pills), given alone or in combination. NSAIDs, such as ibuprofen, naproxen, and meclofenamate, reduce symptoms by lowering prostaglandin levels and intrauterine pressure. NSAIDs are most effective when taken around the clock, as soon as menstrual flow begins. They are less effective when taken on an as-needed basis. Gastrointestinal distress is the most common side effect (Calis et al., 2006).

Oral contraceptives relieve symptoms by inhibiting ovulation, which thins the endometrial lining and decreases prostaglandin production. Sometimes the practitioner prescribes NSAIDs together with oral contraceptives to obtain adequate symptom control.

One promising new therapy for patients who do not respond to NSAIDs or oral contraceptives is the selective estrogen-receptor modulator (SERM) tamoxifen (Pierzynski et al., 2006). Alternative therapies that sometimes decrease dysmenorrhea include relaxation and massage, yoga, acupuncture, and herbal or homeopathic remedies.

Nursing Care

Nursing care of the woman with primary dysmenorrhea involves education about the condition and its treatment and interventions to relieve pain. Explain medication actions, common side effects, measures to reduce side effects, and timing of administration. Reassure the woman that sometimes medication changes occur several times before the best therapy for her symptoms is determined. Reinforce that she should take her NSAIDs on a schedule, rather than waiting until the pain begins or becomes severe.

Several nonpharmacologic interventions can help relieve the pain associated with dysmenorrhea. Heat can be soothing. Suggest the use of hot baths or heating pads. Sometimes changing positions can be helpful. Some women report relief when they assume a knee-chest position. Pain is usually less severe when the woman is in good general health. Encourage adequate exercise, diet, rest, and hygiene. Discourage smoking. Reassure the woman that the pain has a physiologic, not emotional, cause (Edmundson et al., 2006).

> ### Test Yourself
> ✔ Define amenorrhea.
> ✔ What is the medical term for irregular menstrual flow?
> ✔ What is the difference between primary and secondary dysmenorrhea?

Premenstrual Syndrome

Winer and Rapkin (2006) estimate that about 20% to 40% of all women experience PMS. PMS entails physical and behavioral symptoms that occur cyclically during the last half of the menstrual cycle.

Although the exact causes of PMS remain unknown, research shows that PMS symptoms are very complex and do not arise from one single causal factor. In fact, PMS results from the interplay between the central nervous system, the endocrine system, and other factors, such as genetics.

Premenstrual dysphoric disorder (PMDD) is a more severe form of PMS. PMDD includes all of the physical symptoms of PMS with additional and more debilitating emotional symptoms. Approximately 3% to 8% of menstruating women experience PMDD (Rapkin, 2006).

Clinical Manifestations

Most women experience some discomfort just before the menstrual period, most commonly breast tenderness, food cravings, and pelvic heaviness or bloating. The key factors that distinguish these normal discomforts from PMS are the cyclical nature and interference with normal functioning that occur with PMS.

PMS presents with a wide variety of symptoms, which may be physical, behavioral, or both. The symptoms can be highly distressing for the woman and her family. In making a diagnosis of PMS, the crucial component is the cyclical nature of the symptoms. ACOG lists four physical symptoms and six affective or behavioral symptoms used for diagnosis (Box 4-1).

Diagnostic criteria include:

- At least one characteristic physical and one characteristic behavioral sign or symptom (see Box 4-1) must occur during the last half of the menstrual cycle.
- The woman should be asymptomatic before ovulation, and there must be at least 7 symptom-free days in each cycle.
- Symptoms reported must be severe enough to affect relationships, work, and daily lifestyle.
- Diagnosis must be made based on symptoms that are charted as they occur, rather than depending on recall. PMS diaries are useful for this purpose (Pradhan & Lim, 2006).

Typically, the severity of symptoms progresses over time. In the early stages of PMS, women describe symptoms beginning a few days before their period that stop when bleeding begins. With time, symptoms begin to appear 1 to 2 weeks before the onset of menses. Some women describe a cluster of symptoms occurring at the time of ovulation, followed by a symptom-free week, then a recurrence of symptoms a week before menses. PMS does not equate with dysmenorrhea. Many women with symptoms of PMS do not have pain with menses.

Treatment

Pregnancy and menopause are the only true cures for PMS. Treatment aims to alleviate specific signs and symptoms. Some studies show that supplementation with vitamin B_6, calcium, and magnesium are beneficial. Certain diuretics can reduce bloating. NSAIDs can relieve PMS symptoms. Clomipramine (Anafranil) and naproxen sodium (Anaprox) are particularly beneficial. Antianxiety or antidepressant medications and stress-reduction techniques may also provide benefit. New research shows that cognitive behavioral therapy, which is short-term, structured therapy that focuses on the influence of thinking patterns on behavioral choices, is very effective in reducing symptoms of PMS. Hormonal suppression of ovulation or surgical removal of the ovaries is reserved for severe cases of PMS.

PMDD responds to treatments similar to those used for PMS. In addition, low-dose antidepressant therapy during the last half of the cycle has been effective in treating the severe mood swings and other emotional problems that interfere with work productivity and social relationships (Rapkin, 2006).

Nursing Care

Assist the woman to find ways to decrease stress. A healthy lifestyle contributes to a general sense of well-being. Encourage regular exercise, even when she is experiencing symptoms. Research shows that exercise can decrease symptom severity. Encourage reduction or elimination of caffeine and alcohol. Explain that limiting salt intake may decrease symptoms of bloating. Family Teaching Tips: Relief Measures for PMS describes additional relief measures.

Endometriosis

Endometriosis is a painful reproductive and immunologic disorder in which tissue implants resembling endometrium grow outside of the uterus. The tissue implants respond to cyclic hormonal changes in a manner similar to that of endometrial tissue, causing menstrual-like internal bleeding that leads to inflammation, scarring, and adhesions in the pelvic and abdominal cavities (Lynch, 2006). The condition occurs in 5% to 10% of women and is a leading cause of infertility and chronic pelvic pain (Aeby & Hiraoka, 2006).

Clinical Manifestations

Some women with advanced endometriosis are essentially asymptomatic and are unaware of the disease until the condition presents during abdominal or pelvic surgery. Other women may experience debilitating, almost continuous pelvic pain, with only minimal abnormal tissue growth. The woman typically experiences the most pronounced symptoms right before the onset of the menstrual period (Mounsey, Wilgus, & Slawson, 2006).

Cyclic pelvic pain that occurs in conjunction with menses is a classic symptom, as is menorrhagia. The pain and bleeding can involve the bladder, leading to hematuria, or can affect the bowel, leading to blood in the stools and painful defecation. Chronic pelvic pain, dysmenorrhea, and **dyspareunia**, painful intercourse, are other common symptoms. Although endometriosis appears to play a role in infertility for some women, others experience no apparent difficulty with conception.

Family Teaching Tips

RELIEF MEASURES FOR PMS

DIET

- Reduce (or eliminate) caffeine intake (including coffee, tea, colas, and chocolate).
- Avoid simple sugars (as in candy, cakes, cookies).
- Reduce salt intake (pickles, fast foods, chips).
- Eat a diet rich in complex carbohydrates and low in fat, particularly in the 2 weeks before the menstrual period.
- Use the following nutritional supplements (Pradhan & Lim, 2006):
  - 1,200 mg of calcium per day in divided doses
  - 200–400 mg of magnesium per day
  - 6 grams of L-Tryptophan per day from ovulation to menses
  - Vitex agnus-castus, or chasteberry, extract
- Eat six small meals per day (to stabilize blood glucose levels).

EXERCISE

- Do aerobic exercise, such as walking or jogging, several times each week.

STRESS MANAGEMENT

- Note your pattern of PMS symptoms and alter your schedule to minimize stressors when symptoms are most severe.
- Use interventions such as relaxation techniques, massage, and warm baths.
- Consider cognitive-behavioral therapy, a short-term, structured psychotherapeutic approach that focuses on the interplay of your current thinking patterns with behavior choices.

SLEEP AND REST

- Maintain a regular sleep schedule.
- Drink a glass of warm milk before bedtime.
- Schedule exercise for early morning or early afternoon.
- Give yourself a quiet time to relax just before going to bed.

Endometriosis is difficult to diagnose due to the varied symptoms. In addition, the practitioner can easily attribute the symptoms to other conditions. Physical examination reveals pelvic tenderness, particularly during menses. Laparoscopy is the primary diagnostic tool for endometriosis because the surgeon can directly visualize the characteristic endometrial lesions and take biopsy samples. Disadvantages include that laparoscopy is an invasive surgical technique.

Treatment

Treatment decisions depend on the severity of symptoms and/or disease, desire for fertility, and the woman's treatment goals. The woman with mild pain may respond well to NSAIDs and oral contraceptives (Falcone, 2005). Medical therapy for severe symptoms aims to suppress ovulation and induce an artificial menopause, which in turn results in suppression of abnormal tissue and relief of pain. These treatment options include using mifepristone (RU-486); gonadotropin-releasing hormone (GnRH) agonists, such as goserelin and leuprolide; or danazol, a synthetic steroid analog (androgen) that inhibits luteinizing hormone (LH) and follicle-stimulating hormone (FSH). Side effects include symptoms associated with menopause, such as labile emotions, hot flashes, and vaginal dryness.

Surgical intervention can be conservative (reproductive function is maintained), semi-conservative (destroys reproductive function, but maintains ovarian function), or radical, which involves removal of the uterus and ovaries. The goal of conservative surgery is to destroy the abnormal tissue while preserving reproductive ability. The surgeon uses laser or diathermy techniques to ablate (destroy) the lesions (Huntington & Gilmour, 2005).

Nursing Care

Chronic pain is a common nursing diagnosis for the woman with endometriosis (Huntington & Gilmour, 2005). Evaluate the character and severity of pain. Assist the woman to find ways to cope with and decrease pain. Biofeedback, acupuncture, and physical therapy are examples of alternative pain management options (Falcone, 2005). Encourage the use of analgesics, as ordered.

Provide emotional support. Frequently the woman has suffered years of pain before the practitioner makes a diagnosis. Allow the woman to ventilate. She may particularly have this need if the endometriosis is causing infertility problems. Encourage the woman to ask questions. Assist the woman and her family to make treatment decisions by providing information regarding the advantages, disadvantages, possible risks, and likely outcomes of each treatment option.

Infectious Disorders

Infections of the reproductive tract can cause permanent damage, such as infertility and chronic pelvic pain. Sexually transmitted organisms cause many of these infections. Chapters 16 and 40 discuss STIs. This section covers toxic shock syndrome (TSS) and pelvic inflammatory disease (PID).

Toxic Shock Syndrome

TSS is a rare illness typically caused by an exotoxin produced by the bacteria *Staphylococcus aureus*, although infection with streptococcus pyogenes can also cause TSS. TSS was first recognized in 1978; authorities quickly noticed that the majority of cases occurred in women who were using certain types of high-absorbency tampons. Shortly thereafter, manufacturers made changes to the composition and absorbency of tampons, and TSS cases declined dramatically. However, women who use tampons, diaphragms, or contraceptive sponges are still at risk for the illness. In fact, there are reports of increased incidence of TSS in recent years (Kelley, 2005).

TSS starts suddenly with a high fever (>102°F), nausea, vomiting, abdominal pain, a rapid drop in blood pressure, watery diarrhea, headache, sore throat, and muscle aches. Within 24 hours, a sunburnlike rash develops. The skin, particularly on the palms and soles, may peel approximately 1 to 2 weeks later. Treatment requires hospitalization, often in an intensive care setting, intravenous fluids, and antibiotics.

Nurses can be helpful in the prevention of TSS. Teach the woman who uses tampons to wash her hands thoroughly before and after inserting or removing tampons. She should use the lowest absorbency that will handle her menstrual flow, change tampons frequently (at least every 2 to 3 hours) or alternate tampons with sanitary napkins, and never use more than one tampon at once. Between periods, tampons should be stored away from heat and moisture to help prevent bacterial growth. The woman should frequently remove and clean any vaginal device (e.g., a diaphragm or vaginal sponge) that she is using.

Pelvic Inflammatory Disease

PID is a broad term used to refer to inflammation of any portion of a woman's reproductive tract, such as uterus, fallopian tubes, or ovaries. PID occurs most commonly in association with untreated STIs, in particular gonorrhea and Chlamydia (Workowski & Berman, 2006). Untreated PID can lead to scarring, ectopic (tubal) pregnancy, and chronic pelvic pain. Peritonitis and sepsis are other life-threatening complications. Each year in the United States, approximately 1 million women will have an acute episode of PID, and 20% of these will require hospitalization (Hill & Lockrow, 2005). Rates are highest for adolescent girls who have multiple sexual partners and do not use condoms.

Clinical Manifestations

Major symptoms include lower abdominal pain and abnormal vaginal discharge. Other symptoms include chills, fever, vomiting, dyspareunia, menorrhagia, dysmenorrhea, fatigue, loss of appetite, backache, and painful or frequent urination. Some women are asymptomatic but can still experience permanent damage.

Diagnosis is made by a complete history and physical to include a pelvic examination. Generally, specimens are collected and cultured for STIs. Other tests that may be ordered include ultrasound, endometrial biopsy, or laparoscopy.

Treatment

Frequently it is impossible to identify the causative organism, so current guidelines suggest that practitioners prescribe at least two wide-spectrum antibiotics. Sometimes two courses of antibiotics are necessary. Treatment can occur on an outpatient basis in approximately 75% of cases of PID. Occasionally hospitalization is required for intravenous antibiotic therapy. Sex partners of the woman with PID must also receive antibiotic treatment, even if they do not have symptoms.

Nursing Care

Patient teaching is an important nursing function for the woman with PID. Discuss the transmission, treatment, and prevention of infection. Encourage the woman to take all of her antibiotics, even after she starts to feel better. Explain the use of any prescribed pain medications. Explain the importance of treatment of her partner to prevent reinfection. Instruct the woman to avoid sexual intercourse until she finishes the full course of antibiotics and her partner is treated. Because douching can force bacteria into the reproductive tract, it is contraindicated (Cottrell, 2006).

Instruct the woman on ways to prevent STIs and PID in the future because the more frequently she experiences these infections, the more likely the infection will lead to scarring and infertility (Hill & Lockrow, 2005). The best way to prevent PID is to avoid sexual intercourse or to remain in a monogamous relationship—in which both partners are sexually faithful to the other. The next best way is for the woman's partner to use latex condoms for every act of sexual intercourse. Diaphragms and other barrier methods afford some protection but are not as reliable as condoms.

Disorders of the Uterus and Ovaries
Cervical Polyps

Cervical polyps are benign tumors that hang on a stemlike pedicle and protrude through the cervical os. Cervical polyps are associated with infection and chronic inflammation. Postcoital (after intercourse) bleeding, metrorrhagia, menorrhagia, and leukorrhea (white or yellow vaginal discharge) are associated symptoms. The practitioner can visualize cervical polyps during a speculum examination of the cervix and may remove them during the procedure. Tissue is sent to pathology for microscopic examination. The practitioner usually prescribes prophylactic antibiotics after removal of the polyps.

Uterine Fibroids

Uterine leiomyomata, or fibroids, the common name, are benign estrogen-responsive tumors of the uterine wall that often regress with menopause. Fibroids occur in 20% to 50% of women over the age of 30 and are much more common in black women than in white women (Thomason, 2005). Many are asymptomatic; however, the tumors can enlarge and cause pelvic pressure, pain, and menstrual irregularities. They can be particularly problematic during pregnancy. Diagnosis is made via bimanual pelvic exam; transvaginal or abdominal ultrasound; sonohysterography, injection of contrast media into the uterus with transvaginal ultrasound; or hysteroscopy, insertion of a scope through the cervical canal into the uterine cavity (Griffin & Wilder, 2005).

Therapy depends on the symptoms and whether or not the woman wishes to retain fertility. The presence of uterine fibroids is the most common reason cited for hysterectomy and may be the treatment of choice if the woman does not want a future pregnancy. A less radical procedure, myomectomy (removal of the fibroid), is the traditional option for the woman who wishes to maintain fertility. The surgeon sometimes chooses laparoscopy to remove multiple fibroids. Laparoscopy can preserve fertility in some patients.

A newer procedure, uterine artery embolization, uses a technique similar to heart catheterization to introduce a catheter into the uterine artery and then inject a substance that flows to the arteries supplying the fibroids and blocks them. The fibroids shrink after the procedure because of decreased blood supply. Women have successfully carried pregnancies after uterine artery embolization, but researchers recommend more studies (Cockey, 2005). The newest treatment option is noninvasive magnetic resonance imaging-guided focused ultrasound. This treatment preserves the uterus, but researchers do not recommend the procedure for the woman who desires to become pregnant (Hesley et al., 2006).

Pharmacologic options are also available. Hormonal regulation with GnRH agonists can shrink fibroids. Treatment with mifepristone can also be effective. The newest drug available is asoprisnil, which specifically targets the uterine vessels (Doskoch, Faherty, & Gibb, 2005).

Ovarian Cysts

Two types of functional ovarian cysts can develop: follicular and luteal. The type is dependent on when in the menstrual cycle the cyst develops. Most ovarian cysts develop during the childbearing years; however, cysts are possible at any time in the female life cycle (Helm, 2005).

Ovarian cysts are usually benign but can lead to complications, such as hemorrhage (which can be life threatening), ovarian torsion (twisting), inflammation, rupture, necrosis, and bacterial infection leading to septic shock. Pelvic adhesions, infertility, and chronic pelvic pain syndrome are chronic complications that can occur.

The diagnostic challenge is to distinguish between benign cysts and malignancy. Transvaginal and abdominal ultrasound done simultaneously is the most effective method for diagnosing an ovarian cyst. Laparoscopy allows for diagnosis and removal of cysts, although many cysts do not require surgical intervention and will resolve spontaneously. Some practitioners adopt a "wait and see" approach, which normally results in regression

of the cyst. The mainstay of medical therapy is oral contraceptives, which regulate the menstrual cycle and may cause regression of a cyst or prevention of additional cyst formation.

Pelvic Support Disorders

Three types of support hold the pelvic organs in place: endopelvic fascia, ligaments, and paired muscle groups of the pelvic floor. These support structures function like a hammock to support the urethra, bladder, small intestine, rectum, uterus, and vagina. Problems occur when support structures relax or weaken, allowing the organs to drop down or protrude through the vaginal wall.

The names of pelvic support disorders correspond to the affected organs:

- Cystocele occurs when the bladder bulges into the front wall of the vagina.
- Rectocele occurs when the rectum protrudes into the back wall of the vagina.
- Enterocele occurs when the small intestine and peritoneum jut downward between the uterus and rectum.
- Uterine prolapse occurs when the uterus drops down into the vagina.

Figure 4-2 illustrates pelvic support disorders.

The most common causes of pelvic support disorders are pregnancy, vaginal birth, and aging. Some medical experts think cesarean birth may be protective against pelvic support disorders, although this theory is controversial. Women with a history of multiple vaginal births are at the highest risk for pelvic support disorders. Other causes include obesity, chronic coughing, frequent straining during bowel movements, heavy lifting, hysterectomy, nerve disorders, injuries, and tumors (Harvard Women's Health Watch, 2005).

Clinical Manifestations

Pelvic support disorders are hernias in which organs prolapse (abnormally protrude) through the weakened tissues of the support structure. Common symptoms are a feeling of heaviness or pressure in the vaginal area, or a feeling that something is dropping out of the vagina. Symptoms tend to occur when the woman is upright and may be relieved when she is in the recumbent position. Dyspareunia is sometimes present. In mild cases, the woman may be asymptomatic. Some symptoms are specific to a certain type of prolapse. A cystocele may lead to urinary incontinence, whereas a rectocele may cause constipation.

Diagnosis of pelvic floor disorders is made during a pelvic examination. The practitioner asks the woman to cough or bear down during the examination. Then the exam is repeated with the woman in a standing position. Other tests may be done to test bladder or bowel functioning.

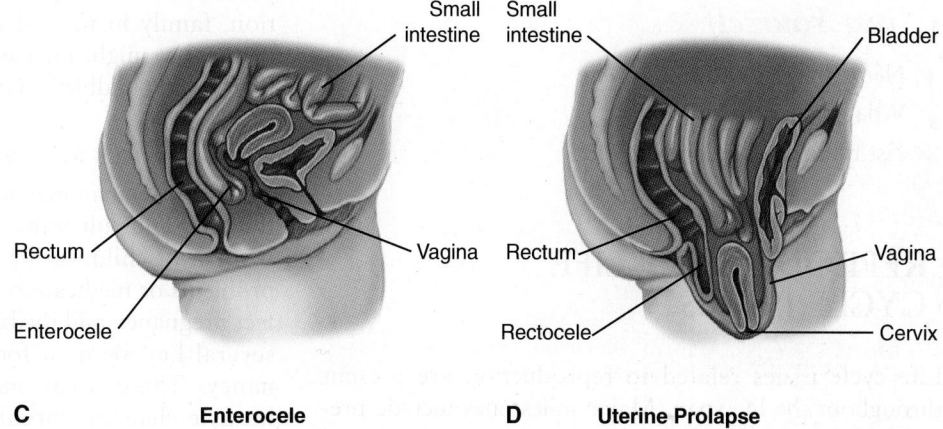

■ Figure 4-2 Types of pelvic support disorders. **(A)** Normal. **(B)** Rectocele and cystocele. **(C)** Enterocele. **(D)** Uterine prolapse.

Treatment

The type of pelvic floor dysfunction, the severity of the dysfunction, and symptoms the woman is experiencing dictate treatment options. For mild cases that are asymptomatic, no treatment may be necessary. If treatment is recommended, it is helpful to start with less invasive techniques and then progress to more invasive techniques, as needed.

Kegel exercises can strengthen pelvic floor muscles and improve tone. The woman can wear support garments that relieve some of the pressure. Another option is a pessary, which is a device that holds pelvic organs in place when inserted into the vagina. Pessaries are available in various shapes and sizes. The practitioner measures and fits the pessary to the woman, who must take it out periodically, clean it with soap and water, and then reinsert the device.

Surgical techniques are often necessary to treat pelvic support disorders. Hysterectomy is the classic treatment option for uterine prolapse. During a hysterectomy procedure, the surgeon can repair other pelvic support disorders. One new technique that avoids removal of the uterus is still under investigation. The surgeon uses a vaginal approach to create a mesh prosthesis that holds the pelvic organs in place (Nicita et al., 2005). For severe cases of prolapse in frail, older women who no longer engage in vaginal intercourse, vaginal closure is one surgical option (O'Dell & Jacelon, 2005).

Nursing Care

Teach the woman to do Kegel exercises regularly. The woman tightly squeezes the muscles used to stop the stream of urine. She then holds the squeeze tightly while she counts to 10. The woman repeats the exercise 10 to 20 times in a row several times per day. A woman can perform Kegel exercises discreetly wherever she happens to be. She can do the exercises while sitting, standing, or lying down.

Anything that increases intra-abdominal pressure can worsen the prolapse. Counsel the woman to lose weight, if needed. She should avoid lifting heavy objects, constipation, and chronic coughing. Smoking causes coughing, so advise her to quit smoking.

Teach the woman to recognize signs of urinary tract infection: pain or burning upon urination, urinary frequency and urgency, and cloudy urine. The woman with a cystocele is at higher risk for urinary tract infection. Other measures to prevent infection are to drink plenty of fluids, including fruit juices, to wipe from front to back after using the bathroom, and to get enough rest.

Age-Specific Considerations

Older women may not feel comfortable talking about subjects that involve private body parts, such as pelvic organ prolapse. They may avoid asking pertinent questions, or they may not report important symptoms. These women grew up in a culture that valued modesty, and it may be difficult for them to openly discuss these issues (Bates, 2006). Be patient and ask specific questions. Clarify any vague terminology the woman uses, such as "it."

Test Yourself

✔ Name five symptoms of PMS.
✔ What is endometriosis?
✔ List three ways to prevent PID.

REPRODUCTIVE LIFE CYCLE ISSUES

Life cycle issues related to reproduction are present throughout the life span. Major milestones include prenatal differentiation of reproductive organs, growth and development of reproductive organs during childhood, maturation of the reproductive system in adolescence, reproductive capability during early and middle adulthood, declining reproductive capability during middle adulthood, and the end of reproductive capability in late-middle to older adulthood. This section addresses issues directly related to reproductive functioning.

FAMILY PLANNING

Family planning consists of two complementary components: planning pregnancy and preventing pregnancy. Family planning gives the woman control over the number of children she wishes to have and allows her to determine when births will occur in relation to each other and in relation to her age and/or the age of the father. Women and couples can avoid unwanted pregnancies, bring about wanted births, and control the intervals between births. Family planning may be a component of the nurse's role for the nurse employed in a family planning clinic, physician or nurse—midwife practice, and in the acute care setting, such as in the postpartum or gynecology units.

Planning Pregnancy

For many women of childbearing age, a planned pregnancy occurs simply by discontinuing the use of contra-ception. However, pregnancy planning should include "pre-pregnancy" planning. The condition of the woman before pregnancy affects pregnancy outcome. Therefore, a healthy pregnancy begins well in advance of conception.

Good health and avoiding exposure to harmful substances are significant contributing factors for a successful pregnancy and a healthy baby. If the woman waits until she is pregnant to remedy factors that can put her or an unborn child at risk, it may be too late to prevent complications. Box 4-2 describes components of preconception care. Preconception care is especially important for the woman with a history of problems with a previous pregnancy, such as miscarriage or preterm labor or birth. In many cases, identification and treatment of causative factors can reduce the risk for problems in subsequent pregnancies. Preconception care is equally important for the woman with a chronic medical condition, family history of genetic disorders, or any other factor that might increase the risk associated with pregnancy and childbirth (Graham, 2006).

Areas of Focus for Pregnancy Planning

Because a woman may not realize she is pregnant during the early and vulnerable weeks of fetal development, any woman of childbearing age should be aware of health problems or medication regimens that may adversely affect pregnancy and the birth of a healthy baby. There are several key areas of focus while planning for a pregnancy. These areas include nutrition and exercise, lifestyle changes, chronic illness and genetic disorders, and medications.

Nutrition and Exercise

The woman should optimize her intake of folic acid several months before becoming pregnant. Folate occurs naturally in foods, such as dark green leafy vegetables and legumes. Ideally, daily dietary intake should supply a minimum of 400 mcg (Moos, 2006). If needed, the woman can take folic acid supplements to meet daily requirements.

Regular aerobic exercise conditions the heart, lungs, muscles, and other organs in preparation for the increased demands of pregnancy. Exercise can also be helpful in building up low-back and abdominal strength—two areas that can cause discomfort throughout pregnancy.

Lifestyle Changes

Smoking cessation is an important consideration when planning for pregnancy. Women who smoke are at higher risk for miscarriage, lower infant birth weight, sudden infant death syndrome, and infant respiratory illnesses (Edwards, 2006).

Alcohol intake can affect the developing child, especially in the earliest weeks of pregnancy. Fetal alcohol syndrome is a cause of serious and irreversible birth defects, particularly mental underdevelopment (Welch-Carre,

Box 4-2 ▌ WHAT IS PRECONCEPTION CARE?

Preconception care is not simply one pre-pregnancy visit to a physician. Preconception care involves almost every encounter with a woman of childbearing age. In the spring of 2006, a special advisory panel of the Centers for Disease Control & Prevention (CDC) met and made recommendations to improve the health of all women who might become pregnant. The following is a summary of the committee's recommendations.

- **Reproductive planning:** Everyone (men and women) should have a reproductive plan. This means that every person makes a conscious, informed choice about whether or not to have children, and the timing and spacing of pregnancy, if so desired.
- **Increasing patient awareness:** Health care providers should teach patients about the importance of preconception health.
- **Preventive health care:** Every encounter with a health care provider can be a preventive visit, if the provider (including nurses) considers the woman's future pregnancy before prescribing medications or giving health advice. For example, a postpartum nurse instructs a woman who does not have antibodies to rubella to talk to her physician about a rubella vaccine before becoming pregnant. Or a clinic nurse encourages a woman to decide if she wants children, and if so, when she wants to become pregnant.
- **Interventions for identified risks:** The woman with a chronic condition, such as asthma, epilepsy,

diabetes, or high blood pressure, should seek out preconception care well in advance of a planned pregnancy. She should be on a medication regime that balances the risks to an unborn child, and her chronic condition should be well under control before pregnancy occurs.
- **Interconception care:** The woman who has had a poor pregnancy outcome (e.g., preterm or stillborn infant) needs specialized care between pregnancies to help lower modifiable risk factors.
- **Pre-pregnancy checkup:** Every woman should get a health care checkup, well in advance of a planned pregnancy. The visit entails at a minimum determination of general health and immunization status.
- **Health coverage for low-income women:** Health coverage could be in the form of health insurance or other plans that encourage preconception wellness visits.
- **Public health programs:** These programs should incorporate preconception care.
- **Research:** The United States needs more research to determine the worth and cost effectiveness of preconception care.
- **Improvement monitoring:** If a program offers preconception care, someone should monitor pregnancy outcomes to evaluate improvement.

Adapted from Freda, M. C. (2006). Editorial: It's time for preconception health! *AWHONN Lifelines, 31*(6), 346.

2005). The level of alcohol intake that causes birth defects to occur is unknown, so women of childbearing age should abstain from alcohol before, as well as during, pregnancy.

Chronic Illness and Genetic Disorders

A woman with a chronic illness, such as diabetes, asthma, heart disease, or high blood pressure, is at higher risk for poor pregnancy outcome. Therefore, the woman with a chronic disorder will need to consult with her health care provider about possible risks related to medications or therapies (Edwards, 2006). Adjustment of medication regimens before pregnancy can decrease the risk to the woman and her fetus.

Some women need referral for genetic counseling for indications, such as the following (Kirkham, Harris, & Grzybowski, 2005):

- The woman or her partner has a genetic disorder.
- Either partner is a known carrier for a genetic condition.

- A previous child was born with a genetic syndrome or when there is a strong family history of a genetically transmitted disorder.

Medications

Many medications cross the placenta easily and can cause birth defects. Pre-pregnancy planning includes assessment of medications the woman is taking. This assessment allows for timely adjustments in dosage or alterations in choice of medication.

Nursing Care

Nurses, especially those working in settings such as clinics or doctors' offices or

Be very careful!
A woman should never stop taking her prescribed medications before discussing it with her primary care provider, even if she suspects she is pregnant. In some conditions, the risk to the baby or mother of an uncontrolled medical condition outweighs the risk of harm from medications.

in public health, play an important role in pregnancy planning and preconception care. A major nursing focus of preconception care is education and counseling, which you may offer through individual counseling or in traditional classroom settings. You also may be responsible for gathering the woman's and her partner's health histories, including current health status and lifestyle practices. Nursing interventions include anticipatory guidance or teaching, discussing issues such as lifestyle, risk behaviors, or risk factors and corrective or preventative measures. Encourage the woman who is trying to become pregnant to follow the recommendations in Family Teaching Tips: Pregnancy Planning.

Preventing Pregnancy

Part of planning pregnancy means that the individual must take steps to prevent pregnancy until desired. Serious negative health consequences may result from unplanned pregnancy. Up to one-half of unplanned pregnancies are terminated by induced abortion. Even so, approximately 50% of all pregnancies in the United States are unplanned (Shulman, 2006). Of those that are unplanned, more than half of the couples were using some form of contraception when conception occurred (Dirubbo, 2006).

Family Teaching Tips

PREGNANCY PLANNING

At least 3 months before attempting to conceive:
- Stop or considerably reduce smoking.
- Stop or considerably reduce alcohol consumption.
- Stop use of recreational drugs.
- Eat a healthy diet that is rich in protein, calcium, iron, and zinc.
- Avoid raw meats. Be sure to thoroughly wash your hands before and after handling raw meat.
- Take folic acid tablets (400 mcg/day) to supplement the folate in a diet that includes leafy green vegetables, beans, and whole-wheat breads. Vitamin B complex is also beneficial.
- Begin a regular exercise program that includes aerobic conditioning.
- Share with your primary care provider any family history of genetic disorders or history of recurrent pregnancy loss.
- Know your rubella and varicella (chickenpox) immunity status and get vaccinated several months in advance of conception, if susceptible to either disease.
- Avoid exposure to x-rays.
- Consult your primary care provider about existing medical conditions or medications.

When pregnancy happens despite contraceptive use, either the method is imperfect (method failure) or the individual does not use the method perfectly (user error). Effectiveness grading of contraceptive methods compares perfect use scores and typical use failure rates. Perfect use describes a contraceptive method used exactly as directed 100% of the time. Typical use accommodates humans' tendency to forget or make errors. Perfect use has a lower associated failure rate than typical use.

The woman who wishes to defer or avoid pregnancy has a wide variety of contraceptive options. An ideal method of contraception is one that is effective, easy to understand and use, and acceptable to both partners. There should be minimal side effects and low risk of long-term consequences. The best contraceptive does not directly interfere with lovemaking or sexual pleasure. It should be inexpensive and easy to maintain. Protection from STIs is an additional consideration. Reversible methods should allow the couple to conceive readily after discontinuing use of the method. Figure 4-3 compares major contraceptive methods.

Natural Methods

A natural contraceptive method refers to any method that does not use hormones, pharmaceutical compounds, or physical barriers that block sperm from entering the uterus. Natural methods of birth control include abstinence, coitus interruptus, and natural family planning or fertility awareness methods.

Abstinence

Abstinence, as related to birth control, means refraining from vaginal sexual intercourse. Abstinence can include other means of sexual stimulation, such as oral sex. Complete, or strict, abstinence refers to the avoidance of all sexual contact. Abstinence is a normal and acceptable alternative to sexual intercourse, especially for teens and singles in noncommittal relationships. The use of complete abstinence as a method of birth control has no cost, is readily available, and is the only 100% effective method for preventing pregnancy and STIs. A major drawback is that it can be difficult to maintain abstinence. A couple may make a rash decision during the heat of passion, which may leave the woman without a means of preventing pregnancy.

Coitus Interruptus

Coitus interruptus, also called withdrawal, requires the man to pull the penis out of the vagina before ejaculation to avoid depositing sperm in or near the vagina. However, the pre-ejaculate fluid may contain sperm, so pregnancy can occur. Effectiveness is dependent on the male partner's ability to withdraw his penis before ejaculation.

One advantage of coitus interruptus is that it provides some level of protection when no other method is available. However, the disadvantages are many. This is an unreliable method of birth control (the failure rate is

Your comparative guide to contraceptives

Between the polar opposites of contraception, abstinence (0 % failure rate) and doing nothing to prevent pregnancy (85 % failure rate), there are myriad choices. If sexually transmitted disease is a concern, only male and female condoms offer protection.

Method	Failure rate (pregnancies per 100 users per year)	Price	How it's used	How it works	Advantages	Disadvantages
Pill (estrogen & progestin)	<1 if used perfectly; 8 in typical use.	$20–$50 per 28-day cycle	Daily pill for 3 weeks, then an inactive pill for 1 week, producing withdrawal bleeding.	Prevents ovulation and thickens cervical mucus to prevent sperm from passing. *	Long-term use reduces lifetime risk of ovarian and endometrial cancers. Typically eases menstrual symptoms such as cramps.	Can cause nausea, breast tenderness, spotting, moodiness, and headaches. Estrogen raises blood-clot risk slightly for healthy users, and significantly for smokers or those with high blood pressure.
Three-month pill (Seasonale)	<1 if used perfectly. Method is too new for typical use statistics.	$115 for 3 months	Daily pill for 12 weeks, then inactive pill for 1 week, producing withdrawal bleeding.	Same as pill.	Same as for pill. Suppresses periods for 3 months at a time.	Side effects same as for pill. Irregular bleeding can occur during the first cycles.
Patch (Ortho Evra)	<1 if used perfectly. Method is too new for typical use statistics.	$40 per 28-day cycle	Patch put on buttocks, abdomen, upper torso, or arm weekly for 3 weeks, then left off for 1 week, producing withdrawal bleeding.	Same as pill, except that hormones do not pass through digestive system.	Same as for pill. No need to take a daily pill.	Side effects same as for pill. Can detach from or irritate skin. Less effective in women weighing more than 200 lb.
Ring (NuvaRing)	<1 if used perfectly. Method is too new for typical use statistics.	$38 per 28-day cycle	Hormone-impregnated polymer ring worn in vagina for 3 weeks, then removed for 1 week, producing withdrawal bleeding.	Same as pill, except that hormones do not pass through digestive system.	Same as for pill. No need to take a daily pill. Can remove for up to 3 hours without compromising effectiveness.	Side effects same as for pill. May cause vaginal irritation or discharge. If dislodged or removed for more than 3 hours, must use back-up contraception for 7 days.
Mini-pill (progestin only)	<1 if used perfectly; 8 in typical use.	$30–$50 per 28-day cycle	Daily pill for 3 weeks, then an inactive pill for 1 week, producing withdrawal bleeding.	Thickens cervical mucus to block sperm.	Can be used when health prevents use of pills with estrogen.	Possible irregular bleeding. May raise cholesterol levels. Must take pill at same time each day.
Injection (Depo-Provera)	<1 if used according to schedule; 3 in typical use.	$57 per injection plus cost of office visit	A progestin injection every 3 months, usually at the doctor's office.	Same as mini-pill.	Frequently suppresses periods completely.	Can cause weight gain. Should not be used for more than 2 years because of bone thinning risk. May take 1 year or more to regain fertility after stopping use.
Male condom	2 if used perfectly; 15 if used typically.	$0.25–$1 per use	Put over erect penis prior to or during foreplay.	Sheath prevents sperm from entering vagina and uterus.	Very effective in preventing sexually transmitted disease.	Interrupts foreplay. May interfere with sensation. May break or slip off during use.
Female condom	5 if used perfectly; 21 if used typically.	$3 per use	Insert into vagina prior to or during foreplay.	Sheath covers vagina and cervix, prevents sperm from entering uterus.	No hormonal side effects. Helps prevent sexually transmitted disease.	Interrupts sexual foreplay. Large and awkward to use.
Copper intrauterine device (ParaGard)	<1.	$250–$300 every 10 years plus cost of office visit	T-shaped copper device inserted into uterus at doctor's office. Can leave in place for up to 10 years.	Believed to inhibit passage of sperm and maturation of eggs.	Fertility returns soon after removal. No hormonal side effects.	Can occasionally fall out. May increase menstrual cramps and bleeding. Rarely, can perforate uterus.
Progestin intrauterine system (Mirena)	<1.	$300–$400 every 5 years plus cost of office visit	T-shaped plastic device, with progestin, inserted into uterus at doctor's office. Can leave in place for 5 years.	Same as mini pill.	Fertility returns soon after removal. May lessen menstrual cramps and bleedings, or stop periods.	Can occasionally fall out. Rarely, can perforate uterus. Irregular spotting for first 3–6 months.
Diaphragm	6 if used perfectly; 16 if used typically.	$30–$40, plus cost of fitting and spermicide	Rubber dome placed over cervix before intercourse and left in place for 6–24 hours. Used with spermicide.	Prevents sperm from passing from vagina into uterus.	Can be inserted prior to foreplay. No hormonal side effects. Does not interfere with normal menstrual cycle.	Must plan ahead for use. Must remember to have on hand if away from home.
Cervical cap	For women who have not delivered vaginally, 9 in perfect use, 16 in typical use. For others who have, 26 in perfect use and 32 in typical use.	$100–$200, plus cost of fitting and spermicide	Silicon or latex rigid covering placed over cervix before sex and left in place for 8–48 hours. Used with spermicide.	Prevents sperm from passing from vagina into uterus.	Can be inserted prior to foreplay. No hormonal side effects. Does not interfere with normal menstrual cycle.	Must plan ahead for use. Must remember to have on hand if away from home.
Surgical sterilization	<1.	$2,500–$4,000	Fallopian tubes cut, blocked, or tied off in laparoscopic surgery.	Prevents sperm from reaching eggs.	Does not affect hormones or menstrual cycle.	Irreversible. Inappropriate for women who may wish to have more children.
Transcervical sterilization (Essure)	<1.	$2,000–$3,000	Coils inserted into fallopian tubes using instrument passed through the cervix.	After 3 months, scar tissue forms that blocks tubes, preventing passage of eggs.	Does not affect hormones or menstrual cycle.	Irreversible. Inappropriate for women who may wish to have more children.
Spermicides	15 if used perfectly; 29 if used typically.	$1–$1.50 per use	Jelly, suppository, foam, or cream inserted into vagina no more than 1 hour before intercourse.	Chemicals block cervix and kill sperm.	Can buy without a prescription at drug stores and some supermarkets.	Can leak. High failure rate if not used carefully. Those with nonoxynol-9 may irritate penis or vagina and may raise risk of sexually transmitted disease.
Rhythm method	1–9 if used perfectly; 25 if used typically.	No cost	Abstention from intercourse during fertile days of the menstrual cycle.	Fertile period determined by examining menstrual cycle, cervical mucus, and/or resting body temperature.	Only acceptable method in some religions. No physical or hormonal side effects.	High failure rate if used incorrectly, or if woman has irregular cycle.
Vasectomy	<1.	$250–$1,000	Sperm tubes tied or sealed in outpatient surgery via incision in the scrotum.	Sperm blocked from mingling with ejaculate so cannot cause pregnancy.	Does not affect sexual performance. Does not require action by woman.	Irreversible. Not appropriate for men who may wish to father more children.

■ Figure 4-3 Comparative guide to contraceptives. © 2005 by Consumers Union of U.S., Inc. Yonkers, NY 10703-1057, a nonprofit organization. Reprinted with permission from the February 2005 issue of CONSUMER REPORTS® for educational purposes only. No commercial use or reproduction permitted. www.ConsumerReports.org.

approximately 19% with typical use), and it offers little, if any, protection from STIs (Samra & Wood, 2006). This method requires a great deal of self-control on the part of the male partner and is not effective if the man ejaculates prematurely.

Lactational Amenorrhea

Breast-feeding offers some level of contraceptive protection because elevated prolactin levels help suppress ovulation. The method works best during the first 6 months after childbirth. The woman must breast-feed frequently, every 2 to 3 hours without fail. Advantages of breast-feeding include promotion of weight loss, suppression of menses, and a more rapid return of the uterus to its pre-pregnant state. Disadvantages are that the woman will not know for sure when fertility returns, and frequent breast-feeding may be inconvenient. This method is not appropriate for the woman who is HIV positive (Samra & Wood, 2006).

Fertility Awareness Methods

Fertility awareness methods (FAM), also known as the rhythm method, refer to all methods that use the identification of fertile and infertile phases of a woman's menstrual cycle to plan or prevent pregnancy. Such methods involve observing and charting the signs and symptoms of the menstrual cycle (e.g., menstrual bleeding, cervical mucus changes, and variations in basal body temperature) using one or a combination of several methods to determine the woman's fertile period. The woman then uses abstinence or a barrier contraceptive method during days identified as fertile to reduce the risk of pregnancy. FAM is also effective to plan pregnancy.

FAM requires the cooperation of both partners. Many couples who prefer a natural, mutual method of preventing pregnancy find cooperation to be an empowering component of these methods, giving them control of their fertility and encouraging shared responsibility. Advantages of these methods are that they are inexpensive, do not require the use of artificial devices or drugs, and have no harmful side effects. Disadvantages include that the method requires discipline to use and can seem cumbersome for a woman or couple with a busy lifestyle. It also has a high failure rate during the first year with typical use (see Rhythm method in Fig. 4-3).

A foundational component for practicing FAM is knowledge about the menstrual cycle. Guidelines derive from the assumption that ovulation occurs exactly 14 days before the onset of the next menstrual cycle and that the fertile window extends 3 to 4 days before and after ovulation, or in other words, between days 10 and 17 of the menstrual cycle. Five methods used to anticipate the fertile window are:

1. Calendar method
2. Basal body temperature method
3. Cervical mucus method
4. Symptothermal method
5. Standard days method

In addition to these five methods, some couples use an ovulation predictor test to determine ovulation and thus the fertile period.

Calendar Method. With the calendar method, fertile days are determined by an accurate charting of the length of the menstrual cycle over a period of 6 months. The woman counts the number of days per cycle, beginning on the first day of menses. The beginning of the fertile period is determined by subtracting 18 days from the length of the shortest cycle. The end of the fertile days is determined by subtracting 11 days from the length of the longest cycle (Samra & Wood, 2006). Box 4-3 gives an example of how to calculate the fertile period using this method. To avoid pregnancy, the couple abstains from sexual intercourse or uses a barrier method during the identified fertile period.

The major drawbacks of this method are that the couple is using data about past cycles to predict what will happen in the future, and they are counting on the regularity of what can be an unpredictable event. In reality, the timing of the fertile period can be highly variable, even for women who think that they have regular cycles. The method is contraindicated for women who do not have regular cycles, such as women who are anovulatory (absence of ovulation), adolescents, women approaching menopause, and women who have recently given birth.

Basal Body Temperature Method. The basal body temperature (BBT) is the lowest normal temperature of a healthy person, taken immediately after waking and before getting out of bed. The BBT method relies on identifying the shift in body temperature that occurs normally around the time of ovulation.

Box 4-3 ▌ CALCULATION OF FERTILE WINDOW USING THE CALENDAR METHOD

A woman keeps track of the length of her menstrual cycles for at least 6 months. Then she calculates her fertile window by subtracting 18 days from her shortest cycle and 11 days from her longest cycle. For a woman whose shortest cycle is 24 days and longest cycle is 28 days, the calculation would be as follows:

Shortest cycle	Longest cycle
24	28
−18	−11
6	17

Therefore, the woman's fertile window would be days 6 to 17 of her menstrual cycle. She and her partner would then use abstinence or a barrier method to prevent pregnancy during the fertile window.

The BBT ranges from 36.2°C to 36.3°C during menses, and for about 5 to 7 days after. At about the time of ovulation, a slight drop in temperature may occur, followed by a slight rise (approximately 0.2°C–0.4°C) after ovulation, in response to increasing progesterone levels. This temperature elevation persists until 2 to 4 days before menstruation. The BBT then drops to the lower levels recorded during the previous cycle, unless pregnancy occurs.

To prevent conception, the couple avoids unprotected intercourse from the day the BBT drops through the fourth day of temperature elevation. The woman must chart the BBT daily on a graph for an entire month to accurately determine a pattern. Confounding factors such as fatigue, infection, anxiety, awakening late, getting fewer than 3 hours sleep, jet lag, alcohol consumption, and sleeping in a heated waterbed or using an electric heating blanket, may all cause temperature fluctuation, altering the expected pattern. Because so many factors can interfere, BBT alone is not a reliable method for predicting ovulation (Barron & Fehring, 2005). Using BBT along with the calendar or cervical mucus methods increases the effectiveness.

Cervical Mucus Method. The cervical mucus method requires recognition and interpretation of characteristic changes in the amount and consistency of cervical mucus through the menstrual cycle. Accurate assessment of cervical mucus requires that the mucus be free of contraceptive gel or foam, semen, blood, or abnormal vaginal discharge for at least one full cycle.

Before ovulation, cervical mucus is thick and does not stretch easily. This quality inhibits sperm from entering the cervix. Just before ovulation, changes occur that facilitate the viability and motility of sperm, allowing the sperm to survive in the female reproductive tract until ovulation. Cervical mucus becomes more abundant and thinner with an elastic quality. It feels somewhat slippery and stretches 5 cm or more between the thumb and forefinger, a quality referred to as **spinnbarkeit** (Fig. 4-4). These cervical mucus changes indicate the period of maximum fertility.

Observation begins on the last day of menses and repeats several times a day for several cycles. The woman obtains mucus samples at the vaginal introitus, so there is no need to attempt to reach into the vagina to the cervix. Confounding factors include the presence of sperm, contraceptive gels or foam, vaginal discharge, use of douches or vaginal deodorants, sexual arousal, and medications, such as antihistamines. Although self-evaluation of cervical mucus can help the woman to predict ovulation, this method is more effective when used in combination with the calendar and/or BBT methods. This method may be unacceptable for the woman who is uncomfortable touching her genitals.

Symptothermal Method. The symptothermal method is a combination of the calendar, BBT, and cervical

■ **Figure 4-4** Spinnbarkeit refers to the stretchable, distensible quality of cervical mucus around the time of ovulation. Some fertility awareness methods (FAM) rely on this quality to help determine when ovulation has occurred.

mucus methods, along with an awareness of other signs of fertility. The woman acquires fertility awareness as she begins to understand the secondary physiologic and psychological symptoms marking the phases of her cycle. These secondary symptoms include increased libido, mid-cycle spotting, mittelschmerz (unilateral lower abdominal pain in the ovary region associated with ovulation), pelvic fullness or tenderness, and vulvar fullness. The woman may palpate the cervix to assess for changes that normally occur with ovulation. The cervical os dilates slightly, the cervix softens and rises in the vagina, and cervical mucus becomes abundant with a slippery consistency. Calendar calculations and cervical mucus changes are useful to approximate the beginning of the fertile period. Changes in cervical mucus and BBT may predict the end of the fertile period. Some studies have demonstrated a lower failure rate when the woman uses multiple indicators to predict the fertile window.

Standard Days Method. Planned Parenthood (2005) discusses a new fertility awareness method, the Standard Days Method (SDM). This method does not require detailed record keeping or complicated ways to keep track of fertile days. Most women who practice SDM use a special ring of beads to track their cycles (Fig. 4-5). There are 32 beads, each representing a day in the menstrual cycle. The woman moves a rubber ring onto one bead each day. The red bead marks the first day of her period. Brown beads correspond to days when she is likely *not* to get pregnant. These are "safe" days in which to have sexual intercourse. White beads stand for days when she is likely to get pregnant. These are "unsafe" times to have unprotected vaginal intercourse.

For successful use of SDM, the woman must meet several criteria. She must have regular menstrual cycles. Her

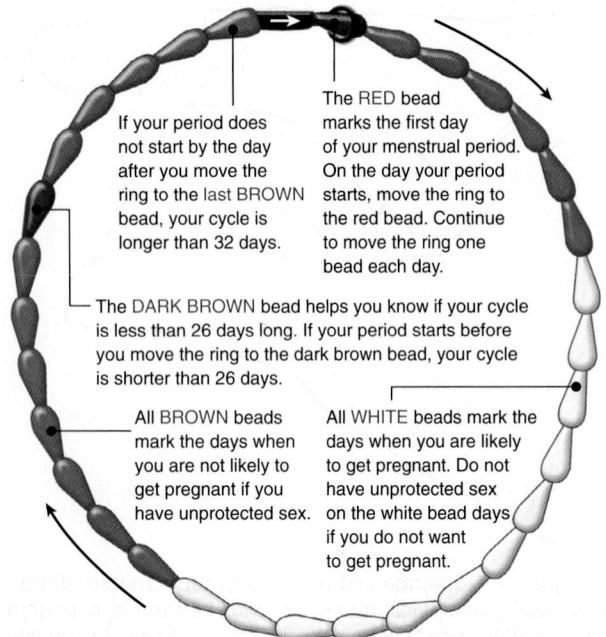

If your period does not start by the day after you move the ring to the last BROWN bead, your cycle is longer than 32 days.

The RED bead marks the first day of your menstrual period. On the day your period starts, move the ring to the red bead. Continue to move the ring one bead each day.

The DARK BROWN bead helps you know if your cycle is less than 26 days long. If your period starts before you move the ring to the dark brown bead, your cycle is shorter than 26 days.

All BROWN beads mark the days when you are not likely to get pregnant if you have unprotected sex.

All WHITE beads mark the days when you are likely to get pregnant. Do not have unprotected sex on the white bead days if you do not want to get pregnant.

■ Figure 4-5 CycleBeads help women use the Standard Days Method.

cycles must never be shorter than 26 days and never longer than 32 days. The beads help her determine if she meets the cycle length criteria. Of 100 women who use SDM perfectly for 1 year, five will become pregnant (Planned Parenthood, 2005).

Ovulation Predictor Test. The Ovulation Predictor Test is a handheld device that detects metabolites of LH and estrogen in the urine. LH levels surge during the 12 to 24 hours before ovulation, and the test detects the increase. The home kit supplies testing materials for testing the urine over several days during a cycle. An easily read color change indicates a positive reaction for LH. Currently in the United States, women use the device to determine ovulation to increase their chance of becoming pregnant. However, research is ongoing to determine the usefulness of the device as a contraceptive method.

Barrier Methods

Barrier methods of contraception provide a physical barrier, chemical barrier, or both to prevent sperm from entering the cervical os. Types of barrier methods of contraception include spermicidal gels or foams, condoms, diaphragms, and cervical caps. Spermicidal gels or foams used in conjunction with condoms, diaphragms, or cervical caps increase the effectiveness of barrier methods. Many barrier method contraceptives have the added benefit of providing at least some protection against STIs.

Spermicidal Agents

Vaginal spermicides provide a physical barrier that prevents sperm penetration and a chemical barrier that kills the sperm. The most commonly used chemical spermicide in the United States is nonoxynol-9 (N-9). Spermicides are available as aerosol foams, foaming tablets, suppositories, films, creams, and gels. Most of these products are designed to be inserted vaginally immediately before or within a few hours before engaging in vaginal sexual intercourse.

Advantages include that this method is readily available without a prescription. Because spermicides can be inserted several hours before vaginal sexual intercourse, the woman can use them discreetly. Some disadvantages are that effectiveness rates are highly variable (see Fig. 4-3) and current spermicides do not protect against (and may actually enhance) the transmission of STIs (Gupta, 2005). The effectiveness of spermicides greatly increases when combined with other physical barrier methods, such as the condom, diaphragm, or cervical cap.

Male Condom

The male condom is a thin, stretchable sheath that covers the erect penis during sexual intercourse. A condom functions as a contraceptive by collecting semen before, during, and after ejaculation to prevent sperm from entering the vagina and causing pregnancy. The majority of condoms are made of latex rubber, although a small percentage is composed of other substances, such as natural membrane or polyurethane. Additional features in condoms manufactured in the United States include different shapes, and the addition of lubricants and spermicides. One feature related to shape is the presence or absence of a sperm reservoir tip. Some condoms are contoured, rippled, or have a roughened surface to enhance vaginal stimulation. A thinner sheath increases heat transmission and penile sensitivity. Some condoms provide lubrication with a wet jelly or a dry powder, and some have spermicide added to the interior or exterior surface. Effectiveness is dependent upon correct and consistent application and usage (see Fig. 4-3). Family Teaching Tips: Safe Condom Use provides guidelines for use.

One significant advantage is the protection condoms afford against STIs. Individuals may use condoms as an additional protective measure against the transmission of HIV and other STIs, in conjunction with another method of contraception (such as oral contraceptives or barrier methods). Other advantages include low cost, easy availability (over-the-counter), and that application of condoms can be part of sexual play. Some men find condom use helpful in preventing premature ejaculation or maintaining an erection for a longer period.

There are also disadvantages. The condom can break, which decreases its effectiveness. Some couples find that condoms decrease sexual sensation. Some individuals perceive the use of condoms as inhibiting spontaneity, or the man may feel self-conscious. Another potential disadvantage is latex allergy; however, polyurethane condoms can be used instead.

Family Teaching Tips

SAFE CONDOM USE

PUTTING ON A CONDOM

Put the condom on as soon as the penis is erect and before any genital contact is made, following these steps:
- Retract the foreskin if not circumcised.
- Press out the tip of the condom to remove air bubbles and to leave a 1/2-inch space at the end (Fig. A).

- Holding the tip of the condom, carefully roll it down the shaft of the erect penis (Fig. B).
- Be certain that the condom covers the full length of the penis, with the rim of the condom at the base of the penis (Fig. C).

A   B   C

CONSIDERATIONS FOR USE

- Use a new condom each time.
- Heat can damage condoms. Store them in a cool, dry place out of direct sunlight.
- Handle condoms carefully to avoid damaging them with fingernails, teeth, or other sharp objects.
- Do not use a condom after its expiration date. Condoms in damaged packages or condoms that show obvious signs of deterioration (e.g., brittleness, stickiness, or discoloration) should not be used, regardless of the expiration date.
- The most effective type of condom for birth control is prelubricated latex with a tip or reservoir pretreated with nonoxynol-9 spermicide.
- If the condom is not pretreated, you may lubricate the inside by placing a few drops of water or water-based lubricant such as K-Y Jelly and a spermicidal jelly or foam containing nonoxynol-9 into the condom.

- Lubricate the outside of the condom as much as desired with a water-soluble lubricant.
- Do not use oil-based products such as mineral oil, massage oil, body lotions, cooking oil, shortening, or petroleum jelly for lubrication; they may weaken the latex.
- If the condom starts to slip during intercourse, hold it on. Do not let it slip off. Condoms come in sizes, so if there is a problem with slipping, look for a smaller size.
- After ejaculation, hold the rim of the condom at the base of the penis and withdraw before losing the erection.
- Remove the condom and tie a knot in the open end. Dispose of it so that no one can come in contact with semen.
- Immediately after intercourse, both partners should wash off any semen or vaginal secretions with soap and water.

Female Condom

The female condom, or vaginal sheath, is a thin tube made of polyurethane, with flexible rings at both ends (Fig. 4-6). The closed end is inserted into the vagina and anchored around the cervix. The open end covers the labia. Like the male condom, the female condom collects sperm before, during, and after ejaculation to protect against pregnancy and STIs. The woman can apply the condom before intercourse, a feature that may increase spontaneity. She can also add a spermicide, if not already present. The female condom comes in one size and, like the male condom, is available without a prescription.

A

Inner ring

Outer ring

B

A   Inserting the diaphragm

B   Positioning the diaphragm

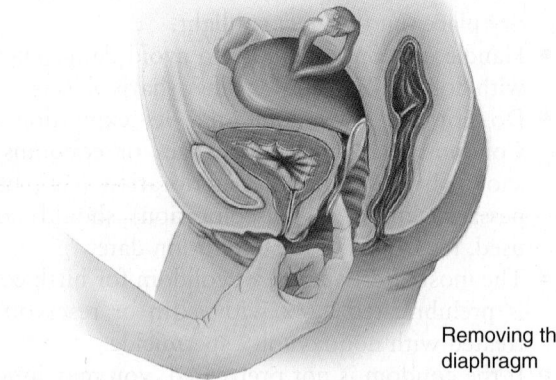

C   Removing the diaphragm

▮ Figure 4-6 **(A)** Female condom. **(B)** Insertion technique.

Advantages of the female condom are that it can be inserted before intercourse, an erection is not necessary to keep the condom in place, individuals who are allergic to latex can use it, and the external ring may supply clitoral stimulation. Reported disadvantages are that the condom may be difficult to apply, make noise, cause vaginal or penile irritation, or slip into the vagina during vigorous intercourse, a condition that decreases its effectiveness.

Diaphragm and Cervical Cap

The diaphragm is a shallow dome-shaped latex rubber device with a flexible, circular wire rim that fits over the cervix. The wire rim may be flat, coiled, arcing, or wide seal. A diaphragm works by mechanically blocking sperm from entering the cervix.

Diaphragms are available by prescription in a wide range of diameters. They require special fitting by a trained practitioner. The woman must apply spermicidal jelly or cream to the rim and center of the diaphragm before inserting and positioning the diaphragm over the

▮ Figure 4-7 Application of a diaphragm. **(A)** To insert, fold the diaphragm in half, separate the labia with one hand, then insert upwards and back into the vagina. **(B)** To position, make certain the diaphragm securely covers the cervix. **(C)** To remove, hook a finger over the top of the rim and bring the diaphragm down and out.

cervix (Fig. 4-7). A diaphragm may be inserted several hours before intercourse, and it must be left in place over the cervix for at least 6 hours afterward to allow the spermicide time to destroy the sperm. If the device is inserted and more than 6 hours passes before sexual intercourse, or if intercourse is repeated, the woman should leave the diaphragm in place and insert another application of spermicidal cream, jelly, or foam into the vagina. The woman should not leave a diaphragm in place for longer than 24 hours.

The cervical cap is much smaller than the diaphragm and is available in four sizes. Its rubber dome has a firm, pliable rim that fits snugly around the base of the cervix, close to the junction of the cervix and the vaginal fornices. The device should remain in place 6 to 8 hours after the last act of intercourse, but no longer than 48 hours. The seal of the cap provides a mechanical barrier. Spermicide applied in the center of the cap provides an additional chemical barrier.

Here's a teaching tip for diaphragm use. The woman must insert additional spermicidal jelly or cream into the vagina if she has intercourse again within 6 hours. With the cervical cap, using additional spermicide for repeated episodes of intercourse is optional.

The typical failure rates for both devices are similar for the woman who has never had a vaginal delivery. However, the failure rate of the cervical cap in the woman who has delivered children vaginally is quite high, even with perfect use (see Fig. 4-3). A practitioner must specifically fit the diaphragm or cervical cap to each woman. Both devices require refitting after pregnancy (whether it ends in miscarriage, abortion, or delivery), abdominal or pelvic surgery, and weight gain or loss of 10 lb or more. The woman must learn how to insert and remove the cap or diaphragm correctly and to verify proper placement. Before insertion, the woman should check either device for pinholes or weakened areas by holding it up to the light.

Typical advantages for the use of diaphragms and cervical caps are that both devices offer some protection against STIs and PID. Both may be inserted ahead of time and are not easily felt by either partner. Both methods are safe for use during breast-feeding and are immediately reversible.

Disadvantages unique to the diaphragm are that some sexual positions, penis sizes, and vigorous thrusting techniques can dislodge the device during intercourse, thus decreasing its effectiveness. Some women develop frequent bladder infections or cannot use the diaphragm because of poor vaginal tone. Disadvantages of both methods are that they can be difficult to insert, the woman must feel comfortable touching her genitals, and she must have the device on hand for all instances of vaginal intercourse. Also, there is a rare risk of TSS if the woman leaves either of these devices in for longer than recommended periods (Samra & Wood, 2006).

Hormonal Methods

Hormonal methods of contraception include oral contraceptives, implants, injections, vaginal ring, and transdermal patches. Depending on their hormonal composition, hormonal methods may prevent or suppress ovulation; thicken cervical mucus, making it resistant to sperm penetration; or create an inhospitable uterine environment, preventing implantation of any fertilized ovum, although this third mechanism of action occurs rarely.

Advantages of hormonal contraceptives are that they are highly effective in preventing pregnancy (see Fig. 4-3), when used consistently and correctly. Several hormonal methods provide noncontraceptive health benefits, such as menstrual cycle improvements, management of dysmenorrhea, and protection against certain cancers, ovarian cysts, ectopic pregnancy, PID, and acne (Rice & Thompson, 2006).

Although efficacious in preventing pregnancy, there are disadvantages to the use of hormonal methods of contraception. Many new users discontinue hormonal methods during the first year of use because of experienced or perceived side effects. In addition, hormonal contraceptives do not offer protection from STIs, including HIV, for either partner. Therefore, the couple must use condoms if they desire STI protection.

Combination Oral Contraceptives

Combination oral contraceptives (COCs), also known as "the pill," are the most commonly used reversible method of contraception (Alan Guttmacher Institute, 2006). COCs can be monophasic or phasic. Monophasic pills provide fixed doses of estrogen and progestin, whereas phasic pills (biphasic, triphasic, and multiphasic) are formulated to alter the amount of progestin, and in some cases, estrogen, within each cycle. Phasic preparations reduce the total dosage of hormones in a cycle, without sacrificing effectiveness. Typically, a pill is taken daily throughout the cycle (Fig. 4-8). The last 7 pills of the 28-pill pack are inert but help maintain the habit of taking the daily pill. Menstruation occurs during the time the woman takes the inert pills. Some practitioners prescribe longer regimens of COCs to suppress menstruation while also providing birth control. The woman must take the pill at the same time each day for it to be effective.

If taken daily as prescribed, COCs provide a high contraception effectiveness rate (see Fig. 4-3). In addition, COCs therapy offers many noncontraceptive benefits, in particular menstrual cycle improvements, including a decrease in menstrual blood loss, reduction in the occurrence of iron-deficiency anemia, regulation of irregular cycles, lessening of the symptoms of dysmenorrhea (painful menstrual periods), and lower incidence of premenstrual syndrome. COCs offer protection against endometrial adenocarcinoma and, perhaps, ovarian cancer. They are associated with a reduced incidence of benign breast disease, protection against the development of functional ovarian cysts and some types of pelvic inflammatory disease, and a decreased risk for ectopic pregnancy (Cunningham et al., 2005).

A

B

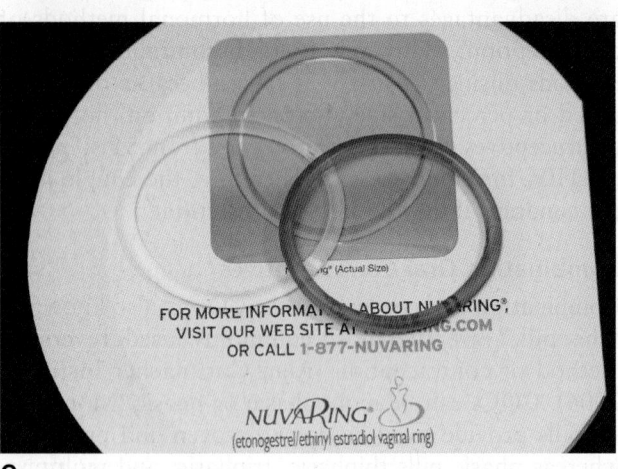

C

■ **Figure 4-8** Hormonal contraceptives. **(A)** Oral contraceptives. **(B)** Transdermal contraceptive patch. **(C)** Vaginal contraceptive ring.

Disadvantages of COCs include no protection from HIV and other STIs. In addition, the woman must remember to take the pill at the same time every day. A large percentage of women stop using COCs because of side effects. Common side effects include nausea, headache, breast tenderness, weight gain, break-through spotting or bleeding, and amenorrhea (Samra & Wood, 2006). These side effects usually decrease over time and are less common with lower-dose preparations. COCs may promote growth of breast cancer, although they probably do not cause breast cancer. Another disadvantage is the expense. COCs require a visit to the primary care provider or clinic and are available by prescription only.

Some women should not use COCs, or use them only with great caution. Box 4-4 outlines contraindications for their use. Instruct the woman to report any pre-existing health problems, any change in health that may affect her use of COCs, and the occurrence of any warning signs, including severe abdominal or chest pain, dyspnea, headache, weakness, numbness, blurred or double vision, speech disturbances, or severe leg pain and edema (Box 4-5).

Progestin-Only Pills

Progestin-only pills (POPs), also referred to as the "mini-pill," contain only one hormone: progestin. Its major

effect is to thicken the cervical mucus and make the endometrium inhospitable to implantation. POPs are slightly less effective than COCs in preventing ovulation.

Advantages include no estrogen side effects, so the woman is less likely to quit using the contraceptive. In addition, women for whom COCs are contraindicated

---

Box 4-4 ▪ CONTRAINDICATIONS FOR USING COMBINATION ORAL CONTRACEPTIVES (COCs)

Contraindications to the use of COCs include any of the following conditions or lifestyle patterns:

- Thromboembolic disorders
- History of heart disease or cerebral vascular accident
- Estrogen-dependent cancer or breast cancer
- Impaired liver function
- Undiagnosed vaginal bleeding
- A confirmed pregnancy or a strong suspicion of pregnancy
- A smoking pattern of more than 15 cigarettes per day in women older than 35 years

(e.g., those older than 35 years who also smoke and those who have a history of thrombophlebitis) may take POPs (Samra & Wood, 2006). There are no "hormone-free" days or inert pills to take, so the woman can maintain a daily routine of taking the same pill every day. The woman who is lactating can take POPs after the newborn is 6 weeks old. POPs decrease dysmenorrhea and the pain sometimes associated with ovulation.

Menstrual irregularities are one disadvantage of POPs, although periods are usually very short and scanty, which some women find desirable. The woman must take POPs every day at the same time of day without fail because their main action (thickening cervical mucus) lasts only 22 to 24 hours. As with COCs, POPs do not provide STI protection and require a primary care provider visit and a prescription.

Hormonal Injections

There are two types of hormonal injection therapies available: a progestin-only agent, depot medroxyprogesterone acetate (DMPA or Depo-Provera); and a combination estrogen/progestin product, medroxyprogesterone acetate with estradiol cypionate (MPA/E2C or Lunelle). Both products provide a level of contraceptive protection similar to that of COCs (see Fig. 4-3). As with other hormonal contraceptive methods, hormonal injections do not provide protection against STIs.

Depot Medroxyprogesterone Acetate: DMPA or Depo-Provera. Depo-Provera consists of a slow-release form of progestin that prevents ovulation. Intramuscular injections are administered four times a year (i.e., each injection provides 3 months of protection). The practitioner administers the first shot in the first 5 days of the menstrual period. After that, the woman must schedule appointments every 11 to 13 weeks for an injection. Currently a lower-dose subcu-

Take it easy!
When administering an injection of Depo-Provera, do not massage the site. This could hasten absorption of the hormone and cause a shorter period of effective contraception.

taneous form of Depo-Provera is available. This may give some women the ability to self-inject at home.

Advantages are that the woman does not have to remember to take a pill on a daily basis, and she does not have to use a product at the time of sexual intercourse. Depo-Provera provides the woman with a high level of privacy. No one has to know she is using this method of birth control, unless she chooses to share this information. Lactating mothers and women who cannot take estrogen products can use Depo-Provera (Planned Parenthood, 2005). Other advantages include decreased risk of endometrial cancer and improvement of premenstrual syndrome and the pain associated with endometriosis.

Disadvantages include prolonged amenorrhea. Many women stop menstruating after the third Depo-Provera injection. This effect is not harmful, and some women may even consider it an advantage. In addition to menstrual irregularities, the most common side effects are weight gain, headache, and nervousness. Sometimes depression and premenstrual symptoms worsen. Another potential disadvantage is the length of time it takes (an average of 10 months) before fertility returns after discontinuing the method. Some women have allergic reactions, although this is rare. Depo-Provera may lower the woman's estrogen levels, leading to loss of bone mineral density and increased risk of fractures. Some research has shown an increase in LDL ("bad") cholesterol and a decrease in HDL ("good") cholesterol levels. Contraindications for using Depo-Provera include pregnancy, history of breast cancer, stroke, or liver disease.

Combined Monthly Injection (Lunelle). Lunelle is a combination progestin/estrogen product given via monthly intramuscular injection. Lunelle works by preventing ovulation and by causing cervical mucus to thicken and the endometrial lining to thin. Advantages to Lunelle as compared with Depo-Provera are that a regular menstrual pattern continues, estrogen levels remain within normal limits, and fertility returns within 2 to 3 months after stopping the method. As with Depo-Provera, Lunelle provides privacy for the woman's contraceptive choice.

Disadvantages include repeated injections and returning for an office visit every month. Lunelle may cause breast tenderness and is not for use while breast-feeding. Some menstrual irregularities are normal at first but usually resolve after the first month or two of use. Weight gain has been reported but less than with Depo-Provera.

Hormonal Implants

The hormonal implant currently available in the United States is Implanon, a single etonogestrel (progestin-only) rod implant. The implant is a small, flexible, plastic rod about the size of a matchstick. The practitioner inserts the rod using local anesthesia just under the skin on the inside of the upper arm. Insertion takes approximately 1 minute. Removal requires a small incision and takes about 3 minutes. Implanon provides contraceptive protection for 3 years.

Implanon is an extremely effective method of birth control. Although no contraceptive method can claim to prevent pregnancy 100% of the time, in more than 10 different research studies to date there have been no pregnancies reported with this method (Samra & Wood, 2006). Advantages include there are no daily pills to remember and no interference with sexual activity to use the method. Fertility returns quickly (within a month) after the implant is removed (Szarewski & Hope, 2005). Implanon frequently improves symptoms of dysmenorrhea and appears to be safe for lactating women.

Disadvantages include weight gain, which is the most common reason women stop using this method of birth control. Irregular bleeding patterns, acne, breast pain, vaginitis, pharyngitis, and headaches are other side effects sometimes experienced with Implanon. The implant does not provide protection from STIs.

Transdermal Patch

The transdermal patch (Ortho Evra) supplies continuous levels of estrogen and progestin (see Fig. 4-8). It is available as a prescription. The woman places the patch on the lower abdomen, upper outer arm, buttock, or upper torso (excluding the breasts) on the first day of her menstrual period. She then applies a new patch every week for three weeks and then removes it for 1 week to allow menses to occur. The woman should apply each new patch on the same day of the week and should not wear more than one patch at a time.

Individuals who use the patch are more likely to be compliant with the method than with COCs or POPs because there is no daily requirement. It is a highly effective form of birth control (see Fig. 4-3). Disadvantages include decreased effectiveness in women who weigh more than 198 lb. The most common side effects include breast symptoms, application site reactions, and poor cycle control (Rice & Thompson, 2006).

Vaginal Ring

The vaginal ring contraceptive (NuvaRing) is a soft, flexible ring, approximately 2 inches in diameter that contains estrogen and progestin (see Fig. 4-8). The woman places the ring into the vagina once a month, during which time it releases low levels of hormones. Lower dosing is possible because it works in the vagina. After 21 days (3 weeks), the woman removes the ring to allow menstruation.

Advantages include low estrogen exposure with high effectiveness. There is a low incidence of hormone-related side effects such as headaches, nausea, and breast tenderness. It is easy to insert and generally discreet to use. Disadvantages include that a woman must feel comfortable touching her genitals, some women or their partners may be able to sense the ring during intercourse, the ring may slip out during intercourse, and the

Drug reservoir (progesterone)

Rate-controlling membrane

Monofilament thread (string)

■ Figure 4-9 An IUD in place in the uterus.

device may cause increased vaginal discharge (Samra & Wood, 2006).

Intrauterine Device

The intrauterine device (IUD) is a small T-shaped device that the practitioner inserts into the uterine cavity (Fig. 4-9). Currently, two types of IUDs are approved for use in the United States, each containing a chemically active substance (either copper or progestin). The copper-bearing device is effective for up to 10 years, and the progestin-releasing device for 5 years. As a safety measure, IUDs are radiopaque (can be seen on x-ray). Each month, the woman must check for presence of the string in the vagina to confirm continued placement of the device.

The copper-bearing IUD acts by damaging sperm in transit through the uterus. Few viable sperm are able to reach the ovum, thus preventing fertilization. The progestin-bearing device affects cervical mucus and endometrial development. The effect is local and typically causes no disruption of ovulation. The absence of estrogen makes the copper IUD a more appropriate contraceptive for women older than 35 years, heavy smokers, and for women with hypertension, vascular disease, or familial diabetes.

> **You can help dispel several myths!**
> The IUD does not work as a "mini-abortion" device. It does not increase the risk of ectopic pregnancy. There is no increased risk of infection or PID after the first 20 days following insertion.

The IUD offers continuous protection from unwanted pregnancy without the need to remember a daily pill or engage in other manipulations between coital acts. Placement of the IUD can occur at any time during the menstrual cycle after obtaining a negative pregnancy test. It is effective for use immediately after childbirth or after an abortion. When the woman wants to become pregnant, the practitioner removes the device and fertility returns. The progestin-bearing device offers the added benefits of decreasing dysmenorrhea and is useful for decreasing bleeding in women with menorrhagia (abnormally long or heavy menstrual periods). Both devices provide reduction in risk of endometrial cancer (Darney & Arias, 2006).

Side effects include cramping and bleeding upon insertion of the device. Common reasons for removal of the copper device include dysmenorrhea and increased menstrual flow. Headache, breast tenderness, and acne are common side effects of the progestin-releasing device. Risks include uterine perforation and accidental devise expulsion. The IUD offers no protection against STIs. Complications that may transpire should pregnancy occur include infection, spontaneous abortion, ectopic pregnancy, or preterm birth (Darney & Arias, 2006). Box 4-6 outlines signs of complications with IUD use.

Sterilization

Sterilization is a permanent method of birth control obtained via a surgical procedure. Although in some instances reversal may be accomplished, the procedure to do so is expensive and often not successful. Therefore, those who choose surgical sterilization procedures should consider them permanent.

Female Sterilization

Female sterilization, by tubal ligation or tubal occlusion, involves blocking or ligating (tying) the fallopian tubes. The procedure may be done immediately after giving birth (within 24–48 hours), at the time of an abortion, or during any phase of the menstrual cycle. It can be done using electrocautery or by application of bands or clips via a laparoscopic or mini-laparotomy technique. In 2002, the Food and Drug Administration (FDA) approved injection of an occlusive material into the tubes using a transcervical approach (nonsurgical sterilization, Essure).

During a mini-laparotomy, the surgeon makes a small vertical incision in the abdominal wall near the umbilicus. The surgeon brings each tube through the incision and cauterizes the tube, which destroys the tissue. An alternative is to ligate and then cut each tube. Regional or general anesthesia is required. Oral analgesics are usually sufficient to relieve postoperative discomfort. Although female sterilization is a minor surgical procedure, the postoperative recovery period is about 1 to 2 days. The woman should report bleeding or signs of infection.

Nonsurgical sterilization (Essure Permanent Birth Control System) is accomplished by using hysteroscopy to guide a tiny metallic implant through the vagina, uterus, and into each fallopian tube. Flexible coils hold the implant in place, and mesh material embedded in the coils of the device causes irritation in the tubes, which respond by causing scar tissue to grow and eventually completely occlude the tubes (Cunningham et al., 2005). Alternative methods of birth control are required for 3 months after the procedure to allow time for scar tissue to form and the method to be completely effective at preventing pregnancy.

Advantages of the Essure system include a less invasive procedure than a surgical approach, avoidance of general anesthesia, and the convenience of the physician's office or clinic. The most common side effects are cramping, nausea, and vomiting. Serious, but infrequently occurring, side effects include expulsion of the implant and uterine perforation.

Male Sterilization

Male sterilization, or vasectomy, can be performed using local anesthesia in an outpatient setting. The procedure takes about 20 minutes to perform. The surgeon makes a small incision on each side of the scrotum over the spermatic cord. The next step is ligation and cutting of each vas deferens. The surgeon may cauterize the cut ends of the vas deferens and then bury them in the scrotal fascia to reduce the chance of spontaneous reanastomosis. Closure of the skin incisions, often with a single suture, completes the procedure, and a dressing is applied.

The man should expect some pain, bruising, and swelling after the surgery. Rest, the application of an ice pack, scrotal support, and a mild oral analgesic are effective comfort measures. The surgeon usually recommends moderate inactivity for 1 to 2 days because of scrotal tenderness. Removal of the skin sutures occurs about 4 to 7 days after surgery. The man should report any signs of bleeding or infection.

The man may resume sexual intercourse as desired; however, with vasectomy, sterilization is not immediate because sperm remain in the system distal to the ligation. It takes approximately 1 month to completely purge sperm from the man's system. Therefore, it is necessary for the couple to use another method of birth control until a negative sperm count verifies sterility (Cunningham et al., 2005). Vasectomy has no effect on the man's ability to achieve or maintain erection or on the volume of ejaculate. In addition, there is no interference with the production of testosterone, so secondary sexual characteristics are not affected.

Emergency Contraception

Emergency contraception refers to methods used to prevent pregnancy after unprotected intercourse. The first use of emergency contraception was to protect rape victims from pregnancy. More recent uses include if a condom breaks or unplanned unprotected sexual intercourse occurs. Emergency contraception should not be the only method a sexually active individual uses to prevent pregnancy. It is much more effective to use a consistent form of birth control. It is also important to recognize that emergency contraception is not an "abortion pill." Emergency contraception works to prevent pregnancy from occurring.

An oral contraceptive or mifepristone (RU-486) prescribed as a "morning-after pill" reduces the risk of pregnancy in the event of unprotected intercourse. The woman takes the first dose within the first 72 hours after intercourse, followed by a second dose 12 hours after the first.

The practitioner can insert the copper IUD as long as 7 days after unprotected intercourse. One advantage of this method is that it is very effective at preventing pregnancy and it provides long-term protection (Darney & Arias, 2006). A woman who has an active STI or who is at high risk for STIs should not use this form of emergency contraception.

Nursing Process for Assisting the Couple to Choose a Contraceptive Method

Providing care related to contraception is a collaborative process, involving a variety of health care personnel. The nurse often works with a physician, certified nurse–midwife, nurse practitioner, family planning counselor, and social worker. Roles for each team member may vary across settings and may overlap within a specific setting. You may be involved in history taking, teaching, and counseling, as well as assisting during physical assessment. Communication among team members and clear protocols for physical assessment, counseling, and teaching are essential to provide quality care. The quality of all family planning care is dependent on the ability of health care team members to work together as professional colleagues.

Steps toward developing excellence in practice include clarifying your own feelings about family planning, maintaining a current knowledge base through independent study and continuing education activities, awareness of current standards of practice, evaluating current societal norms, and striving to avoid allowing personal prejudices to influence nursing care. Application of the nursing process provides a framework for working with women and their partners desiring a method of contraception.

Assessment

Assessment is an essential initial step for identifying the needs and desires of the woman and her partner, regarding contraception. Conduct the assessment in an unhurried and accepting atmosphere with adequate privacy to make the woman and her partner feel comfortable. It is important to treat the couple with respect, accepting their feelings and beliefs, even when these feelings and beliefs differ from your personal perspective. The assessment includes gathering physiologic, psychoemotional, sociocultural, and cognitive data related to the issue of preventing pregnancy.

The physician or nurse practitioner takes the patient's medical, reproductive, and contraceptive history. Examples of contraception-related questions include:

- What types of contraception were used in the past?
- What problems occurred?
- What did the couple like or dislike about the method?
- What were factors contributing to discontinuing use of the previous method?

The physician or nurse practitioner also performs a physical examination, which includes a general medical examination, a complete gynecologic examination, and routine diagnostic laboratory testing. This information assists in identifying any contraindications to a specific birth control method.

The nurse or family planning counselor often performs the psychoemotional, sociocultural, and cognitive assessments. Psychoemotional data should include information about the couple's feelings regarding their sexuality, family planning in general, and specific methods of contraception. To develop a long-range plan of care, it is important to discuss the couple's goals for their family, regarding the number of children they want and the preferred spacing of those children. Are both partners equally motivated? Studies have indicated that the woman's perception of her partner's support is a major predictor of her use or nonuse of any particular method. Other important issues helpful in identifying the optimal contraceptive method include the woman's self-image, level of comfort with her body, and willingness to touch her genitals.

Sociocultural issues such as family background, religious beliefs, or cultural taboos may influence the couple's compliance with a particular method for contraception. It is important to identify myths or sexual practices related to culture. Social data to identify include information about the nature of the woman's sexual activity, such as the number of partners and her desire for partner involvement in birth control. Assess the relationship between the woman and her partner(s) and the level/quality of communication they share because this influences the choice and subsequent use of contraception. Financial issues may also have an influence on the choice of contraceptive method.

Cognitive issues to assess include the couple's level of understanding about the reproductive cycle and their knowledge of varied types of birth control available. Many couples have a knowledge base regarding contraception gleaned from other sources, such as popular magazines, television, or the Internet. It is common for the lay media to disseminate new information before professional journals publish it. Identifying the couple's educational needs can be done as part of an interview or by using assessment questionnaires. Such assessment tools will help to quickly evaluate the couple's knowledge about birth control methods and identify educational needs, as well as personal preferences.

Selected Nursing Diagnoses

- Deficient Knowledge, lack of information related to reproductive cycle and birth control methods
- Decisional Conflict related to
  - contraceptive alternatives
  - unwillingness of sexual partner to agree on birth control method
  - possibility of contraceptive method side effects
- Ineffective Sexuality Patterns related to interference with normal sexuality patterns or discomfort caused by the contraceptive method

Outcome Identification and Planning

Appropriate goals may include that the woman and her partner will express adequate knowledge of the reproductive cycle and contraceptive methods; that they will choose a method of contraception suitable to their needs and lifestyle; and that the woman and her partner will express satisfaction with their pattern of sexual expression. Plan other goals and interventions according to the individual needs of the woman and her partner.

Implementation

Assessment data, goals, and plan of care dictate nursing interventions. The physician or nurse practitioner performs physical interventions, such as the fitting of diaphragms or cervical caps, or insertion of an IUD. Nursing interventions are concerned primarily with psychoemotional, sociocultural, or cognitive needs of the woman and her partner.

Providing Teaching

Present teaching in an unbiased manner, dispelling myths and misinformation, and providing needed information. Group teaching sessions or individual discussions are effective methods, depending on the needs and preferences of the couple. For example, if a couple has already decided on a specific method of contraception, a group session discussing all available methods may not be appropriate. In any case, it is imperative to provide complete and accurate information, regardless of the teaching format. Any discussion of contraceptive methods should include the following information:

- A description of the method, including an example or illustration
- The mode of action, showing how the method acts to prevent pregnancy
- The effectiveness or failure rate of the method and causes for method failure
- Requirements for use, such as how to obtain the method, implementation, and necessary compliance

- Possible effects on lovemaking, such as when the method should be implemented in relation to coitus, and possible effects on coitus
- Medical and emotional advantages and disadvantages
- Risks, contraindications, side effects, drug interactions, warning signs, and any factors related to safe use
- Effectiveness of the method to protect against STIs and HIV
- Costs of the method, both initially and for the long term
- Reversibility of the method, including how to discontinue the method and the length of time until the return of fertility

Addressing Emotional or Sociocultural Needs

Discussion of emotional or sociocultural needs should take place in private, individualized teaching sessions. This allows the couple to freely express feelings, opinions, and concerns, and ask questions about intimate, personal aspects of their lives. It is appropriate to explore religious, cultural, social, and financial concerns. This knowledge enables you to assess the couple's understanding and acceptance of the chosen method. Try to establish a trusting relationship with the couple, provide a warm and accepting atmosphere, and remain sensitive to their needs and concerns.

Assisting with Follow-Up

After the woman and her partner have chosen a method, follow-up is important to determine satisfaction with the method and ability to use the method correctly. Often a follow-up telephone call is appropriate. Ask the woman how things are going using the chosen method. Inquire regarding adverse effects or any problems she is having that might cause her to quit using the method. Each office visit is another opportunity to explore with the woman regarding how she is doing and her satisfaction level. Periodically ask the woman to explain the steps of the chosen method and correct any misperceptions.

Evaluation: Goals and Expected Outcomes

Goal: The woman and her partner will express adequate knowledge of the reproductive cycle and contraceptive methods.
Expected Outcomes: The woman and her partner

- describe the physical signs indicating fertile and infertile periods of the woman's menstrual cycle.
- verbalize understanding about contraceptive methods.

Goal: The woman and her partner will choose a method of contraception suitable to their needs and lifestyle.
Expected Outcomes: The woman and her partner

- discuss attitudes and feelings about contraception in general and about specific birth control methods.
- ask questions and express concerns related to using different birth control methods.

Goal: The woman and her partner will express satisfaction with their pattern of sexual expression using the chosen birth control method.

Expected Outcomes: The woman and her partner

- voice satisfaction with the chosen method.
- encounter no adverse reactions or complications related to the chosen birth control method.
- demonstrate successful use of the selected birth control method through prevention of unplanned pregnancy.

Test Yourself

✔ Name the two complementary components to family planning.

✔ List one advantage and one disadvantage to the use of coitus interruptus as a birth control method.

✔ List one fertility awareness method and one barrier method of birth control.

INDUCED ABORTION

An **induced abortion** is the purposeful interruption of pregnancy before 20 weeks' gestation. A **therapeutic abortion** is pregnancy termination performed for reasons related to maternal or fetal health or disease. The term **elective abortion** refers to an abortion performed at the woman's request that does not involve preservation of health. Most women who have elective abortions are Caucasian, younger than 24 years of age, and unmarried (Trupin, 2006). Approximately one half of women who have abortions report using a contraceptive method that failed (Dirubbo, 2006).

The type of abortion procedure used depends on the gestational age of the fetus. Before 8 weeks from conception, a woman may opt for medical or surgical procedures to terminate pregnancy (Table 4-1). Between the 8th and 12th week, surgeons elect to use dilatation and curettage. The procedure used for abortions after 12 weeks is dilatation and evacuation. After 20 weeks' gestation, there are many medical and surgical options available including methods used to induce labor (Trupin, 2006).

Table 4-1 ■ **SELECTED INDUCED ABORTION TECHNIQUES**

Method	Procedure	Special Considerations
Surgical Techniques		
Menstrual aspiration	Aspiration of the endometrial cavity with a flexible cannula and syringe	• Possible complications include implanted zygote missed (pregnancy continues), unrecognized ectopic pregnancy, and uterine perforation (rare). • Primary procedure used in United States.
Dilatation and curettage (D&C)	1. Dilation of the cervix with a blunt instrument or laminaria. 2. A sharp instrument, called a curette, scrapes the endometrium and removes uterine contents. 3. Suction to aspirate uterine contents, as needed.	• Possible complications include uterine perforation, cervical laceration, hemorrhage, incomplete removal of products of conception, and infection.
Dilatation and evacuation (D&E)	Procedure is similar to D&C; however, D&E requires wider dilation of the cervix to facilitate removal.	• Complications are the same as for D&C.
Medical Techniques		
Mifepristone (RU 486)	One oral dose given alone or in conjunction with prostaglandins. May require a repeat cycle of treatment.	• Used for very early terminations (under 8 weeks). • Common side effects are nausea, vomiting, and gastrointestinal cramping. • Complications include hemorrhage secondary to incomplete expulsion of pregnancy or rupture of an unrecognized tubal pregnancy.
Prostaglandins	Several routes of administration including oral, vaginal, intramuscular, or injection into the amniotic sac.	• Frequently used to induce second-trimester abortions. • Side effects include fever, vomiting, diarrhea, and uterine hyperstimulation.
Intra-amniotic hyperosmotic fluid infusion	Hyperosmotic saline or urea solutions injected into the amniotic sac.	• Used infrequently to induce second-trimester abortions. • High incidence of adverse side effects and complications, including death.

Nursing care roles and responsibilities vary, depending upon the setting, method of termination used, and the patient's needs. In some settings, the nurse and physician may be the only health care providers involved. In others, care providers may include social workers or counselors. In either situation, the nurse's role is central to achieving optimal patient care outcomes. It is important to examine your personal beliefs and values related to abortion before assuming responsibility for the care of women choosing to have an abortion. You must be able to provide compassionate and nonjudgmental care.

Document the amount and character of bleeding after the abortion procedure. Save anything that appears to be tissue or clots. A pad count with an estimation of pad saturation provides a more accurate record of blood loss. Assess the woman's vital signs frequently, as for other postoperative care, observe for signs and symptoms of hypovolemic shock. The practitioner usually orders hematocrit testing before discharge. The woman who is Rh negative needs a dose of Rh immune globulin.

Postabortion teaching should include information about signs and symptoms of possible complications, including elevated temperature, continued/excessive vaginal bleeding, malodorous vaginal discharge, and abdominal pain. The woman should report adverse effects immediately. Advise the woman to delay sexual intercourse for 1 to 2 weeks. Contraception counseling and instructions about follow-up care and appointments are important.

INFERTILITY

Infertility is the inability to conceive after a year or more of regular and unprotected intercourse, or the inability to carry a pregnancy to term. Infertility affects approximately 15% of couples in the United States, a rate that has remained stable for the past 50 years (Garcia & Nelson, 2006). There are two main types of infertility: primary and secondary. A couple who has never been able to conceive has primary infertility; whereas, a couple who has been able to conceive in the past but is currently unable to do so has secondary infertility.

For the majority of couples who engage in frequent, unprotected intercourse, the chance for conception is about 60% at 6 months, 90% at 12 months, and 95% at 24 months. Because the frequency of intercourse affects the chances of conception, if a couple has intercourse only one time per week for 6 months, there is only a 15% chance of pregnancy. If the couple increases intercourse frequency to four times a week around the time of ovulation, the chance of conception increases to 83%. Research has shown that the optimal timing of sexual intercourse for conception to occur is every 48 hours at midcycle. Counseling about the timing and frequency of intercourse and the expected time of ovulation often can resolve problems of infertility.

Causes of Infertility

For conception to occur, many factors have to work together perfectly. Viable sperm must enter the female reproductive tract. The passageway through the woman's cervix, uterus, and fallopian tubes has to be clear for sperm to negotiate the journey toward the egg. Ovulation has to occur. The egg must enter a fallopian tube. Fertilization of the egg must occur within 12 to 24 hours after ovulation, before it begins to disintegrate. After fertilization, the egg must travel down the fallopian tube to the uterus and implant. Any factor that prevents the sperm and egg from meeting or interferes with the fertilized egg traveling to and implanting in the uterine lining can result in infertility.

If a couple is having trouble conceiving, it is helpful for them to review their health histories to identify risk factors for infertility (Box 4-7). Female-specific risk factors include any condition or situation that interferes with ovulation, patency of the cervix or fallopian tubes, or ability of the fertilized ovum to implant in the uterine lining. Male-specific risk factors include anything that can cause decreased or abnormal sperm production or any factor that prevents sperm from being deposited in the female reproductive tract.

Initial Evaluation of Infertility

Frequently, the woman presents to her primary care provider with her concerns when she has been unable to conceive. The primary care provider or gynecologist

 A Personal Glimpse

My husband and I had been married 5 years when we decided to start a family. I tried to get pregnant for 8 months without success. My aunt advised me to get a physical examination. Reluctantly, I called to make an appointment. The physician couldn't see me for several months, so I booked the appointment with the women's health nurse practitioner. She performed a thorough physical exam. She told me that nothing appeared to be wrong with my reproductive tract. She said that many couples don't get pregnant right away. She instructed me that healthy living habits were good not only for a healthy heart, but also for a healthy reproductive tract. She advised me to start a regular program of exercise and to eat a well-balanced diet. She told me that stress can interfere with getting pregnant, and she referred me for yoga lessons after I indicated to her that I had always wanted to learn yoga. I followed her advice, and 6 months later I was pregnant.

Sylvia

Learning Opportunity: What advice can nurses give to couples who want to start a family? How does knowledge of the reproductive tract help nurses take care of women who want to get pregnant?

Box 4-7 ▪ **RISK FACTORS FOR INFERTILITY**

Risk Factors That Affect Both the Male and Female
Behavioral Factors
- Cigarette or marijuana smoking
- Alcohol use (even in moderation)
- Excessive exercise
- Being 10%–15% over or under ideal body weight
- Multiple sexual partners (increases risk for STIs)

Occupational and Environmental Factors
Exposure to
- High environmental temperatures
- Certain chemicals
- Radiation
- Heavy electromagnetic or microwave emissions

Emotional Factors
- High stress levels
- Depression

Female-Specific Risk Factors
Factors That May Interfere With Ovulation
- Advancing age*
- Chronic medical conditions and/or associated treatments; examples include
  - Diabetes mellitus
  - Thyroid dysfunction
  - Systemic lupus erythematosus (SLE)
  - Rheumatoid arthritis
  - Hypertension
  - Asthma
- Hormonal imbalance, signaled by any of the following
  - Menstrual irregularities
  - Menorrhagia (prolonged or excessive bleeding)
  - Hirsutism
  - Acne
- Ovarian cysts

Factors That May Interfere With Gamete Transport
- Surgical or invasive procedures involving the cervix or uterus, such as

- Cone biopsy
- Cryosurgery
- Dilatation and curettage
- Myomectomy
- In utero diethylstilbestrol (DES) exposure
- Any surgical procedure directly involving the fallopian tubes
- Any pelvic surgery
- Endometriosis
- Ectopic pregnancy
- History of STIs or pelvic inflammatory disease (PID)

Factors That May Interfere With Implantation
- More than one induced abortion
- Hormonal imbalance

Male-Specific Risk Factors
Factors That May Interfere With Sperm Viability
- Prescription medications for ulcers or psoriasis
- DES exposure in utero
- Exposure of the genitals to hot temperatures
  - Hot tubs
  - Steam rooms
  - Tight clothing
- Cryptorchidism
- Prostatitis
- Varicocele
- Genital tract infection
- Mumps after puberty

Factors That May Interfere With Sperm Deposition
- Erectile dysfunction
- Retrograde ejaculation
- History of hernia repair
- Hypospadias
- Vasectomy

---

*Female fertility declines with advancing age. A woman in her 30s is 30% less fertile than one in her 20s.

---

performs the initial evaluation. If complex problems exist, or the problem is not readily identifiable, the practitioner refers the woman and her partner to a reproductive endocrinologist for additional evaluation and treatment.

Because of the high incidence of multiple contributing factors, evaluation of infertility should include both partners, even when the problem seems to be "obvious." Evaluation begins with a thorough history and physical examination for both partners to identify evidence of conditions that may be affecting fertility. Important health history information includes:

- The woman's menstrual pattern
- Number of pregnancies with the current partner or any other partner, and the pregnancy outcomes
- Identification of any sexual dysfunction for both partners
- History of STIs or genital tract surgery or trauma for both partners
- Lifestyle issues, such as alcohol consumption, tobacco use, recreational drug use, occupation, and patterns of physical activity for both partners
- Chronic medical conditions and treatment for both partners

- The couple's pattern of intercourse as related to the woman's ovulatory cycle
- Length of time the couple has had unprotected intercourse
- Natural techniques or home tests the couple has already used

In addition to the above-mentioned health history, the practitioner will do a complete review of systems to help identify any endocrinologic or immunologic issues that might contribute to infertility. The practitioner then completes a thorough physical examination. A gynecologist may evaluate the female partner, whereas an urologist often performs the initial evaluation of the male partner.

The woman's physical examination includes a pelvic examination, Pap smear, cultures for gonorrhea and chlamydia, and a bimanual examination (see Chapter 6). A pelvic ultrasound is part of the initial examination. The male examination includes determining if any genital tract abnormalities are present. The practitioner discusses results of the initial evaluation with the couple, and explains plans for a more comprehensive evaluation, if needed.

Comprehensive Evaluation and Diagnostic Testing

Diagnostic testing for infertility usually begins with the simplest testing methods and moves toward the more complex and invasive methods. The timing of diagnostic testing is in relation to the woman's menstrual cycle. It may take up to two menstrual cycles to complete the testing (Garcia & Nelson, 2006).

Frequently, evaluation of male infertility factors takes place first because the testing is often simpler than that for female testing. The first diagnostic test is usually a semen analysis. For this procedure, the man must collect semen via masturbation or in a special condom during intercourse if masturbation is unacceptable to the couple. The man must abstain from sexual release for 3 to 5 days before the test to obtain optimal results. The man must deliver the entire ejaculate in a sterile container to the laboratory no later than 30 minutes after collection. The lab examines the sample for semen volume and quality, and for numbers, shape, motility, and viability of the sperm (Garcia & Nelson, 2006). Often adequate testing requires analysis of two to three samples, collected at least 2 to 3 days apart. If the semen analysis is normal, diagnostic testing then focuses on the female partner.

If the semen analysis results are abnormal, additional analysis 1 month later can rule out short-term causes or inadequate specimen collection. Additional tests of male fertility include endocrine hormonal analysis. Proper analysis includes examination of serum levels of four hormones—FSH, LH, testosterone, and prolactin. Transrectal (through the rectum) or scrotal ultrasonography can help identify structural abnormalities that could interfere with fertility. Sperm function tests can determine the ability of the sperm to penetrate and fertilize the egg. The practitioner may perform testicular biopsy to obtain testicular tissue for analysis. The results of this analysis can often pinpoint the cause of male infertility (Rubenstein & Brannigan, 2005).

Comprehensive fertility evaluation of the woman often begins with the least invasive techniques. The **post-coital test** evaluates the interaction of the man's sperm with the woman's cervical mucus. The timing of the test is critical for accurate results. The woman uses urine LH predictor kit to predict ovulation. When she determines that ovulation is near, the couple performs vaginal intercourse without lubricants. Several hours later, the practitioner collects a sample of cervical mucus and evaluates it for mucus characteristics, a sperm count, and evaluation of sperm motility. The clomiphene citrate challenge test detects decreased ovarian function, which has a poor prognosis for future pregnancy (Petrozza & Styer, 2006). Endocrine testing is useful. The practitioner orders serum hormone levels of estrogen, progesterone, thyroid-stimulating hormone, prolactin, and androgen to determine if endocrine abnormalities are present.

More invasive techniques include hysterosalpingogram, hysteroscopy, and laparoscopy. A hysterosalpingogram allows for identification of an obstruction anywhere along the tract. A hysteroscopy facilitates direct visualization of the endometrial cavity. This method can diagnose and treat some endometrial conditions. Laparoscopy is usually the last test performed because it involves surgical and anesthetic risk and cost. This procedure provides for direct visualization of the pelvic cavity, which frequently allows for accurate diagnosis of the cause of infertility (Garcia & Nelson, 2006).

Management of Infertility

The practitioner chooses appropriate therapy based on the underlying causes identified during diagnostic testing, duration of infertility, and the woman's age. As with testing, therapies begin with the simplest and least invasive and progress toward the more complex, as needed. Possible interventions include medication administration, surgical procedures, insemination techniques, advanced reproductive techniques, and other parenting/childbirth options.

Treatment of Cervical Factors

The easiest, most successful therapy for cervical abnormalities is intrauterine insemination. In this procedure, the physician inserts sperm directly into the uterus near the time of ovulation. Frequently, more than one insemination is required to ensure that insemination coincides with ovulation. Sperm can be from the woman's partner, homologous insemination, or from a donor, heterologous insemination. The woman assumes the dorsal lithotomy position, and the physician inserts a speculum into the vagina. After cleansing the cervix, the physician places the semen specimen in a 1-mL syringe attached to a thin, flexible catheter. The physician guides the catheter through the cervix until it reaches the upper uterus, taking care not to injure the endometrium or induce bleeding. The physician slowly injects the semen specimen into the uterus, and withdraws the catheter. The woman should remain supine for at least 10 minutes after the insemination.

Treatment of Endometrial and Tubal Factors

Most endometrial and tubal causes of infertility require various surgical techniques. Options include hysteroscopy, laparoscopy, or laparotomy, followed by a hysterosalpingogram to evaluate effectiveness of treatment. Discussion of treatment for endometriosis, a common cause of infertility, occurs earlier in this chapter.

Treatment of Ovarian Factors

Medications to stimulate ovulation, also known as fertility drugs, are the treatment of choice when lack of ovulation is the cause of infertility. All have side effects and potential complications, which can be severe. Multifetal pregnancy is common with these medications. Clomiphene citrate (Clomid, Serophene), human menopause gonadotropins (Pergonal, Humegon, Repronex), synthetic GnRH, and pure FSH are examples of fertility drugs used to treat ovarian dysfunction (Garcia & Nelson, 2006).

Treatment of Male Factors

If a varicocele is the cause of low sperm production, surgery is required. If the cause of a low sperm count is unknown and FSH, LH, and testosterone levels are normal, then the physician prescribes Clomid to increase sperm production. An alternate treatment is intrauterine insemination of the woman (Garcia & Nelson, 2006).

Assisted/Advanced Reproductive Therapies

The birth of Louise Brown in 1978 was the result of the first advanced reproductive therapy (ART) to be successful in humans, in vitro fertilization. Since that time, researchers have developed additional therapies, and indications for ART have expanded to include conditions that heretofore would have been impossible to treat.

The five leading ARTs are in vitro fertilization (IVF), gamete intrafallopian transfer (GIFT), zygote intrafallopian transfer (ZIFT), tubal embryo transfer (TET), and intracytoplasmic sperm injection (ICSI) (Petrozza & Styer, 2006). The nurse's role in this area is to provide the couple with balanced and accurate information regarding the risks and benefits of the technologies available to facilitate their decision-making process. Box 4-8 lists some ethical and legal questions associated with ARTs.

In Vitro Fertilization

IVF is a relatively common procedure used when the woman has absent or blocked fallopian tubes, when the man has a low sperm count, or when the etiology of infertility is unknown. IVF involves several steps. The procedure begins with administration of fertility drugs to the woman to stimulate ovulation. Then the physician harvests one or more ova (eggs) from the ovary, fertilizes

---

> **Box 4-8 ■ ETHICAL AND LEGAL ISSUES RELATED TO ADVANCED REPRODUCTIVE THERAPIES (ARTS)**
>
> Research in the area of ARTs has resulted in additional technologies that, while giving new hope to couples who once considered their infertility irreversible, are also creating ethical and legal dilemmas for all concerned. Common ethical and legal questions include:
> - Who should have the right to reproduce?
> - Should ARTs be limited to married couples?
> - Who owns the embryos produced?
> - Should embryos be frozen for later use?
> - Who are the parents?
> - Do the biologic donors or surrogates have custodial rights?
> - Should donors only be anonymous?
> - Should fetal reduction techniques be done when ARTs results in multifetal gestation?

the ova with sperm in the laboratory, and places the fertilized ova in a growth medium, where they develop for 48 to 72 hours. The physician then transfers the embryos to the uterus. Typically, the physician places two to four embryos in the woman's uterus.

Gamete Intrafallopian Transfer

In GIFT, the physician aspirates the harvested ova into a catheter containing prepared sperm. Then the physician transfers the gametes into the fallopian tube, where fertilization can take place. One prerequisite for the procedure is that the woman must have at least one patent fallopian tube.

Zygote Intrafallopian Transfer and Tubal Embryo Transfer

The ZIFT and TET procedures are a combination of IVF and GIFT. Fertilization of the ova occurs as in IVF; however, the physician returns the embryos to the fallopian tube versus the uterus. The difference between ZIFT and TET is the age of the fertilized egg at transfer.

Intracytoplasmic Sperm Injection

ICSI is the latest development to give hope to the male with very low sperm counts. Fertilization is possible with only one sperm. The man obtains the sperm specimen by masturbation, or the physician obtains the sperm by testicular biopsy or aspiration. The physician strokes the distal portion of the tail, which paralyzes the sperm. After the ovum is harvested, the sperm is placed into a microneedle (tail first), and then injected into the ovum. The physician then places the fertilized ovum into the woman's reproductive tract for implantation. An increased risk of congenital malformation and chromosomal abnormalities is associated with ICSI; however, some research studies do not demonstrate increased risk.

Surrogate Parenting

Surrogate parenting is a process by which a woman carries to term the infant of an infertile couple. A **gestational surrogate**, or surrogate mother, may donate only the use of her uterus, or she may also donate her ovum and agree to insemination with the male partner's sperm. Surrogate parenting has raised extensive legal and ethical issues that require counseling for both the infertile couple and the surrogate and possibly the surrogate mother's spouse and family.

Psychological Aspects of Infertility

Psychosocial consequences related to infertility include shock, guilt, isolation, depression, and stress. The partner who has the identified problem is at most risk for feelings of guilt. It is important to avoid using words that imply blame when discussing the problem of infertility.

A couple who is having difficulty conceiving may feel isolated and different from others who are able to conceive. They may separate themselves from others in an attempt to avoid emotional pain. Infertility will challenge the couple's self-image, self-worth, and sense of command over events in their life. They may experience a "roller coaster" of emotions, ranging from hope to despair with each ovulatory cycle.

Infertility places stress on the couple's relationship. One or both may develop poor self-esteem and feel unworthy or unlovable. A man may find it difficult to perform sexually or provide semen specimens on demand. Intimacy, love, and support, essential components of a couple's sexual relationship, may be lost because intercourse takes on a clinical and mechanical tone.

Failure to achieve pregnancy may lead the couple to consider adoption. Adoption is a viable option for parenting, but the couple must consider some realities about pursuing this route. Many couples have preferences regarding the health status, race, and possibly other characteristics they desire in an infant. A couple may need to reflect on their willingness to adopt an older child, a child of another race, or a child with special needs. How will they feel about having minimal information about the child's background? How would they feel about knowing the child's birth mother or father? The couple must consider these and other questions before deciding to adopt. Have information about adoption available and use positive language when discussing that option. Focus on sharing complete and balanced information and supporting the couples' feelings and decision.

Nursing Care

The major focus of nursing care related to infertility involves providing support for the couple as they undergo diagnosis and their chosen treatment option. Therapeutic communication skills are an essential component in nursing care. It is important to facilitate the couple's ability to communicate with each other and to encourage each partner to discuss his/her own feelings and be accepting of the other's. Reinforce the couple's coping strategies or assist them in exploring adaptive alternatives to poor coping, increasing their sense of control in this situation.

After the physician has told the couple about their diagnosis and potential treatment options, your major role as the nurse is to provide additional information, helping them to make an informed decision. Support the couple through the decision-making process and help them toward a resolution of infertility by either assisting with the grief process or through facilitating parenting. Providing emotional support is an essential component of care, especially when a treatment has been unsuccessful.

Test Yourself

✔ Define infertility.
✔ Which test of infertility is normally the first to be done?
✔ Describe two advanced reproductive technologies.

MENOPAUSE

Menopause, the cessation of menses, signals the end of the woman's reproductive capability. The climacteric, as defined in Chapter 3, refers to the gradual changes associated with declining ovarian function known as "the change of life." **Perimenopause** refers to the time before menopause when vasomotor symptoms (hot flashes, night sweats) and irregular menses begin. Menopause is a normal part of the life cycle and is not a disease, although associated symptoms may be distressing and require treatment.

> **Your perimenopausal patients will appreciate this tip!**
> Although fertility declines with age, pregnancy can still occur. The woman in perimenopause should continue to use a reliable form of birth control.

Menopause occurs when the ovaries no longer respond to stimulation from the pituitary. During the perimenopausal period, the woman begins to experience variable menstrual cycles and irregular bleeding (Curran & Bachman, 2006). Although these changes occur normally in response to hormonal changes, the woman should report all irregular bleeding to her primary care practitioner for evaluation.

Clinical Manifestations

The perimenopausal woman typically experiences a set of symptoms known as climacteric syndrome. These symptoms include hot flashes, insomnia, weight gain, bloating, emotional lability, irregular menses, and headache. Fluctuations in estrogen during perimenopause cause climacteric syndrome (Curran & Bachman, 2006).

A hot flash is a sudden feeling of warmth or intense heat sometimes accompanied by reddening of the skin on the upper body. The duration is anywhere from seconds to several minutes (Casper, 2006). The average length of symptoms in the perimenopausal woman is 2 years; however, some women experience hot flashes for 5 or more years. Although scientists do not completely understand the physiology, a hot flash corresponds to low estrogen levels and periodic surges of LH.

Physical changes associated with hormone depletion include changes to the reproductive organs. The vaginal mucosa thins and becomes pale and dry. Vaginal rugae disappear, and the vaginal walls become smooth. The uterus and ovaries decrease in size. Pelvic support muscles lose tone, and pelvic support disorders may become apparent. The skin loses its elasticity, and adipose tissue replaces dense breast tissue (Casper, 2006).

Decreased bone mineral density is one of the changes that can have life-threatening effects on the menopausal woman. The overall effect of decreased bone mineral density is loss of bone mass, with resulting reduction of bone strength and increased risk for fracture. This systemic condition is osteoporosis. It is important to know the risk factors for osteoporosis (Box 4-9) because this disease often has no symptoms until a serious bone fracture occurs.

Treatment

The gold standard for prevention and treatment of perimenopausal symptoms as a whole has historically been hormone replacement therapy (HRT). However, recent research is showing the HRT may not be the best option for many women. The Women's Health Initiative (WHI) study stopped early because of the adverse effects of HRT on women's health. HRT led to an increased risk for coronary heart disease, stroke, venous thromboembolism, and pulmonary embolism without a decrease in cardiovascular disease (one of the focuses of the study). Current recommendations for the use of HRT include control (not prevention) of perimenopausal symptoms. The practitioner should prescribe the lowest dose to control symptoms for the shortest time possible (AWHONN Lifelines, 2005). Benefits of HRT shown by the WHI study are a decreased risk for colorectal cancer and osteoporotic fractures.

Treatment for Hot Flashes and Sweats

Hot flashes and sweats are the most common reasons that the perimenopausal woman seeks medical treatment. To date, the most effective therapy for hot flashes continues to be HRT. Hormonal alternatives to HRT include progestins alone, which are beneficial in treating hot flashes. Nonhormonal options that show promise include the anticonvulsant gabapentin, and SSRI antidepressants, such as paroxetine (AWHONN Lifelines, 2005).

Treatment for Osteoporosis

HRT continues to be beneficial for reducing the risk of osteoporosis and fractures in the peri- and postmenopausal woman. However, other treatment options also lower the risk for fractures. These options include parathyroid hormone, raloxifene, calcitonin, and bisphosphonates. Calcium and vitamin D supplementation and regular weight-bearing exercise are preventive measures (Hobar, 2005).

Treatment for Vaginal Atrophy and Dryness

HRT continues to be an effective treatment, although the use of local applications of estrogen-containing vaginal creams, tablets, or suppositories brings relief of symptoms with minimal systemic absorption. If estrogen use is contraindicated, the woman may benefit from nonestrogenic vaginal lubricants.

Nursing Care

Nurses have a large role to play in health promotion for the perimenopausal and postmenopausal woman. It is important to develop rapport with the woman and to let her know that you are available to talk about her concerns. Reassure the woman of the normality of menopause.

Give the woman facts on HRT and other therapies. It may be helpful to give her a list of resources that she can read at home. It is important that the woman understand

---

Box 4-9 ▪ RISK FACTORS FOR OSTEOPOROSIS

- Female gender
- Caucasian or Asian ethnicity
- Slender build
- Advanced age
- Estrogen deficiency because of menopause (especially if early or surgically induced)
- Low bone mass density
- Family history of osteoporosis
- Personal history of fracture as an adult
- Smoking
- Excessive alcohol intake
- Low dietary intake of calcium
- Vitamin D deficiency
- Inactive lifestyle
- Use of glucocorticoids
- Use of anticonvulsants

the risks and benefits of any therapy so that she can make an informed decision.

Suggest lifestyle modifications to decrease the discomfort of hot flashes. These include dressing in lightweight clothing and dressing in layers. Regular exercise and setting the thermostat to a lower temperature may also be helpful. Suggest that she avoid spicy foods, caffeine, and alcohol.

Some common sense guidelines to prevent osteoporosis can be helpful as well. Encourage regular weight-bearing activity, such as walking and stair climbing, at least three to four times per week. The postmenopausal woman should continue to take calcium and vitamin D supplements. She should take her calcium supplements with orange juice (or another vitamin C source) and avoid caffeine, which tends to interfere with the absorption of calcium.

Safety instructions can help prevent fractures from falls inside the house. Encourage the postmenopausal woman to have her bed lowered, if possible; to eliminate throw rugs and clutter from the floors; and to use night-lights throughout the house. In the bathroom, it is helpful to install safety tread and safety rails. Suggest that she keep a cordless or mobile telephone close by to eliminate the temptation to run to answer the phone. All of her slippers and shoes should have tread and should provide traction and stability. To reduce falls outside the home, instruct the woman to take extra precautions after dark. Advise her to use railings whenever possible. She should clear walkways of debris and avoid walking on ice.

Review medications with the woman. She should understand how to take her medications and what side effects to report. She should also understand how often she should see her primary care practitioner and have required routine screening examinations, such as yearly mammograms and bone density measurements. Family Teaching Tips: Reducing the Discomfort of Menopause lists helpful tips to share with the woman and her family.

Family Teaching Tips

REDUCING THE DISCOMFORT OF MENOPAUSE

- Wear cotton clothes in layers.
- Avoid caffeine intake (e.g., colas, tea, coffee).
- Explore relaxation activities because stress exacerbates vasomotor symptoms.
- Discuss HRT with your caregiver.
- Consider nutritional supplements as recommended by your primary care practitioner to help reduce vasomotor symptoms.
- Use a water-soluble lubricant before intercourse.
- Nonprescription products, such as Replens and Lubrin, are effective for the relief of vaginal dryness.
- If using an estrogen vaginal cream, apply it at bedtime.
- Perform Kegel exercises to improve pelvic muscle tone.
- Drink at least 5 glasses of water per day. Do not count caffeine-containing drinks as part of this water intake.
- Urinate regularly; do not allow the bladder to become overdistended.
- Practice good hygiene, such as wiping from front to back, after toileting.

Test Yourself

✔ Define perimenopause.

✔ Name five symptoms that are part of the climacteric syndrome.

✔ Describe three things (nonpharmacologic) that you can teach the older woman to do to treat or prevent hot flashes.

Key Points

- ➤ Self-awareness of breast characteristics and yearly clinical breast examinations are appropriate for women of all ages. Women older than 40 years should have yearly mammograms as well.
- ➤ Sexually active women younger than 30 years should have annual Pap smears. The healthy woman older than 30 years should have Pap smears every 2 to 3 years.
- ➤ Dysmenorrhea is painful or difficult menses. Premenstrual syndrome (PMS) encompasses a constellation of symptoms that are cyclical in nature and progress with time.
- ➤ A classic symptom of endometriosis is cyclic pelvic pain that occurs in conjunction with menses. Therapy aims to suppress ovulation and induce an artificial menopause to curb growth of abnormal tissue and relieve symptoms. The nurse's role is to help the woman find pain relief and provide support.
- ➤ The major risk factor for development of pelvic inflammatory disease (PID) is untreated sexually transmitted infections (STIs). The woman and her partner should be treated with antibiotics.
- ➤ Weakening of the structures that support the pelvic organs causes pelvic support disorders.

➤ Major risk factors include pregnancy, vaginal delivery, and aging.

➤ Family planning involves the two components of planning pregnancy and preventing pregnancy. Family planning should include pre-pregnancy planning, which involves focusing on nutrition and exercise, lifestyle changes, counseling and treatment for chronic illness and genetic disorders, and evaluation of medications.

➤ Natural methods of contraception do not use hormones or other physical barriers to prevent conception. These methods include abstinence, coitus interruptus, and fertility awareness methods (FAM). Natural methods do not require the use of artificial devices or hormones but require a great deal of education and discipline to be effective.

➤ Barrier methods of contraception provide a physical or chemical barrier or both to prevent pregnancy. These include spermicides, male and female condoms, the diaphragm, and cervical cap. Many barrier methods have the advantage of decreasing the risk for STIs.

➤ Hormonal methods of contraception include combination oral contraceptives (COCs), progestin-only pills (POPs), hormonal injections, hormonal implants, transdermal patch, and vaginal ring. Hormonal contraceptives are highly effective but do not provide reliable protection against STIs.

➤ Intrauterine devices (IUDs) are small objects that provide long-term pregnancy protection. They must be inserted by a primary care provider and require removal every few years. They do not provide protection against STIs.

➤ Female and male sterilization techniques are highly effective, permanent methods of contraception.

➤ Emergency contraception refers to hormonal methods used to prevent pregnancy after unprotected intercourse.

➤ Infertility is the inability to conceive after a year of unprotected intercourse. Multiple factors contribute to infertility. Anything that interferes with the sperm and egg meeting or the fertilized egg from traveling to and implanting in the uterus can lead to infertility.

➤ Evaluation of infertility begins with the least invasive and complex and progresses to the more invasive and complex techniques. All infertility evaluations begin with a thorough history and physical examination of both partners. Usually the first test is a sperm analysis, and the second test is a postcoital examination.

➤ Treatment of infertility depends on the identified cause. Therapeutic insemination techniques, surgical techniques to correct structural problems, medication to stimulate ovulation, and advanced reproductive therapies (ART) may all be used in the treatment of infertility.

➤ A couple undergoing evaluation and treatment for infertility may feel guilt, shock, isolation, depression, and stress. It is very stressful on a relationship to perform sexually on demand, and intercourse often takes on a clinical and mechanical tone, rather than the desired traits of intimacy, love, and support.

➤ Menopause is a natural part of the life cycle. It is not a disease; however, the associated symptoms may need medication or other interventions.

➤ Hormone replacement therapy (HRT) used to be the gold standard of treatment for major menopausal-related symptoms; however, recent research has highlighted serious adverse effects that may be associated with HRT.

➤ Hot flashes, osteoporosis, and vaginal atrophy and dryness are the major symptoms for which women need and desire treatment and nursing care during menopause.

INTERNET RESOURCES

Endometriosis
www.aafp.org/afp/20060815/601ph.html (Patient teaching pamphlet)
www.endocenter.org
www.endometriosis.org

Family Planning
www.arhp.org/choosing
www.arhp.org/hormonalcontraception
www.plannedparenthood.org

Infertility
www.resolve.org

Osteoporosis
www.nof.org

Workbook

■ NCLEX-STYLE REVIEW QUESTIONS

1. An adolescent girl asks the nurse when she should have her first "Pap test." How should the nurse reply?

   a. "I don't know. Ask the doctor."
   b. "When you first start having sex."
   c. "As soon as possible and every year thereafter."
   d. "Three years after you first have sex, or age 21, whichever comes first."

2. A 35-year-old woman reports very heavy menstrual periods. How does the nurse chart this in the medical record?

   a. "Chief complaint: dysmenorrhea."
   b. "Complains of metrorrhagia."
   c. "Reports amenorrhea."
   d. "Reports menorrhagia."

3. A woman is having severe symptoms of PMS. She asks the nurse what she can do to obtain relief from these symptoms. What reply by the nurse is most likely to be helpful?

   a. "Antibiotics are necessary to treat the underlying infection."
   b. "Diuretics tend to be the most helpful medications for PMS treatment."
   c. "Don't worry. The medication the doctor has prescribed will take care of your symptoms."
   d. "In addition to taking medications, stress reduction and regular exercise are beneficial."

4. A woman with a pelvic support disorder reports all of the following. Which statement by the woman should alert the nurse to instruct the woman to come in immediately for examination by a physician?

   a. "My urine is cloudy."
   b. "I forgot to do my Kegel exercises today."
   c. "Every time I cough, a little bit of urine comes out."
   d. "I took my pessary out to wash it, and forgot to put it back in."

■ STUDY ACTIVITIES

1. Develop a 10-minute presentation on considerations a couple should make before deciding on a method of birth control.

2. Explain how natural family planning techniques can enhance the chance that a couple will get pregnant. Why do these methods work to both prevent and enhance pregnancy?

3. Using the table below, compare natural methods of contraception.

Methods	How It Works to Prevent Pregnancy	Special Nursing Considerations

■ CRITICAL THINKING: WHAT WOULD YOU DO?

Apply your knowledge of infertility and its treatments to the following situation.

1. Amanda Rodriguez is a 37-year-old woman who has never before been pregnant. She put off pregnancy to pursue her career as an attorney. Now she and her husband have been trying to conceive for 2 years without success. She has come to the clinic for initial evaluation.

   a. Explain to Amanda what she can expect from today's visit.
   b. The obstetrician asks you to assist her during the physical examination. What equipment and supplies will you gather?
   c. If Amanda is experiencing infertility, what type is it?
   d. Amanda confides in you that she thinks God is punishing her for waiting to start a family. She says that she should have tried to have children several years ago when all her friends were having babies. How would you reply to Amanda?

2. The physician tells Amanda that her husband will need to have a semen analysis and then a postcoital test will be done.

   a. Explain both of these procedures to Amanda.
   b. The semen analysis reveals a low sperm count. The physician recommends ICSI. Amanda asks how that procedure is done. How will you answer Amanda?

3. Apply your knowledge of menopause to the following situation: Cindy McFarland, a 52-year-old woman, comes to the clinic because she has been experiencing hot flashes. She tells you that the hot flashes are very intense and seem to last "forever." She says that her sweat drenches her clothes and she is embarrassed to go out in public.

   a. Explain the physiology of hot flashes to Cindy.
   b. What treatments will the physician likely recommend for Cindy?
   c. What other advice do you have for Cindy during this time of her life?

PREGNANCY

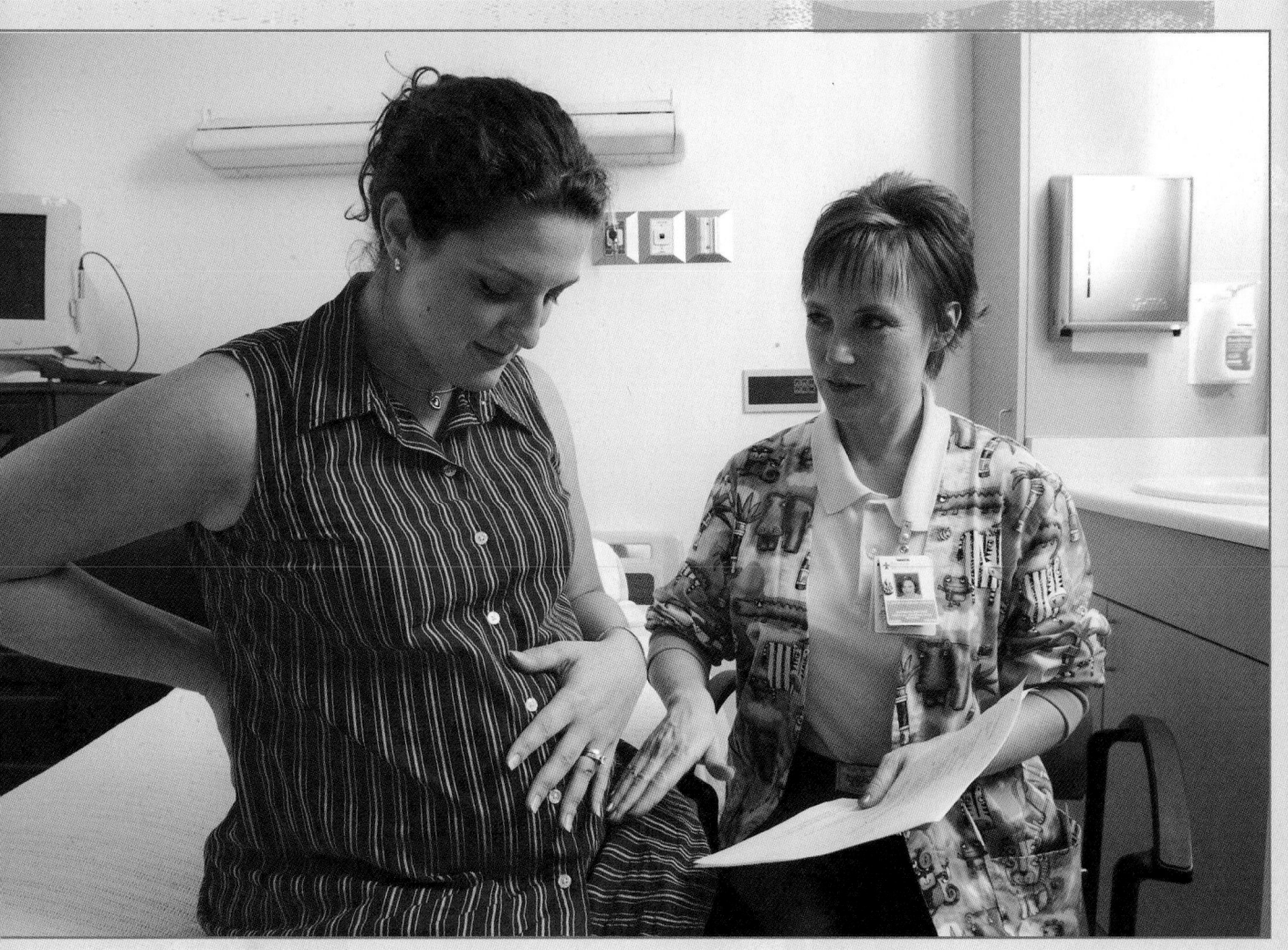

5 Fetal Development

KEY TERMS

amnion
amniotic fluid
blastocyst
chorion
chorionic villi
cleavage
decidua
dizygotic
ductus arteriosus
ductus venosus
ectopic pregnancy
embryo
fetus
foramen ovale
gametogenesis
monozygotic
morula
teratogen
Wharton's jelly
zygote

LEARNING OBJECTIVES

On completion of this chapter, you should be able to:

1. Explain mitosis and meiosis and differentiate between the two.
2. Describe the processes of spermatogenesis and oogenesis, and how they differ.
3. Explain how the sex of the conceptus is determined.
4. Describe the three developmental stages of pregnancy with regard to beginning and ending periods and major events occurring during each stage.
5. Describe the development of support structures during pregnancy.
6. Name four major functions of amniotic fluid.
7. Discuss three functions of the placenta.
8. List the steps in the process of the exchange of nutrients and wastes between the maternal and fetal bloodstreams.
9. Trace the path of fetal circulation, including the three fetal shunts.
10. Name three categories of teratogens and list examples of each kind.
11. Discuss the threat to pregnancy that occurs with ectopic pregnancy.
12. Differentiate between the types of multifetal pregnancies.

EVERY HUMAN being starts out as two separate germ cells, or gametes. The female gamete is the ovum, and the male gamete is the spermatozoon, or sperm for short. At conception, the gametes unite to form the cell that eventually becomes the developing fetus. Human development is an ongoing process that begins at fertilization and continues even after birth. Many factors affect development. Some of these factors can cause abnormalities and birth defects. Others are part of the normal process of human development, such as gender determination. This chapter discusses the major processes involved in human fertilization and development.

CELLULAR PROCESSES

It may seem contradictory to say that cellular division results in multiplication of cells, but that is exactly what happens in several stages of human conception and development. There are two major categories of cells and two major types of cellular division involved in the reproduction of human life.

Types of Cells

Cells are the building blocks of all organs. There are two major types of cells: Soma cells, which make up the organs and tissues of the human body, and gametes, also known as germ cells or sex cells. The gametes are found in the reproductive glands only.

The nucleus of each soma cell contains 46 chromosomes, arranged in 23 pairs. Each parent donates one chromosome of every pair. Each chromosome is composed of genes, which are segments of DNA that control hereditary traits. Twenty-two of the 23 pairs of chromosomes are autosomes; the remaining pair, the sex chromosomes, determines an individual's gender.

The ovum and the sperm are, respectively, the female and male gametes. Each gamete has 23 chromosomes, exactly half of the 46 required chromosomes needed for human development.

Cellular Division

There are two types of cellular division involved in the creation of human life: mitosis and meiosis (Fig. 5-1).

■ **Figure 5-1 (A)** Mitosis of the soma cell. **(B)** Gametogenesis. The various stages of spermatogenesis are indicated on the left; one spermatogonium gives rise to four spermatozoa. On the right, oogenesis is indicated; from each oogonium, one mature ovum and three abortive cells are produced. The chromosomes are reduced to one-half the number characteristic for the general body cells of the species. In humans, the number in the body cells is 46, and that in the mature spermatozoon and secondary oocyte is 23.

Mitosis

Mitosis is the process by which somatic (body) cells give birth to daughter cells. Each daughter cell contains the same number of chromosomes as the parent cell. The body grows and replaces somatic cells through the process of mitosis.

Meiosis

Meiosis is the process by which gametes undergo two sequential cellular divisions of the nucleus. This process reduces the number of chromosomes in the gametes by half. Remember, each gamete has only 23 chromosomes, which is half, also known as the haploid number, of the total number of chromosomes required for human cells. The female gamete, the ovum, undergoes meiosis in the ovaries just before ovulation. The male germ cell, the spermatozoon, divides in the seminiferous tubules of the testes.

The formation and development of gametes or germ cells by this process of meiosis is called **gametogenesis**. More specifically, the formation of the male gamete is called spermatogenesis, and the formation of the female gamete is called oogenesis.

Spermatogenesis

Spermatogenesis begins at puberty in the male. In the testes, primary spermatocytes, each containing 46 chromosomes, undergo the first meiotic division, which results in two secondary spermatocytes, each with 23 chromosomes. These spermatocytes then undergo a second meiotic division, resulting in a final number of four spermatids that contain the haploid number of chromosomes (23). The spermatids undergo a change in form to become mature spermatozoa but undergo no further meiotic divisions.

Oogenesis

Oogenesis begins in the ovaries before birth but is not fully complete until the childbearing years. At birth, the female ovaries contain primary oocytes, which have completed the prophase stage of the first meiotic division. The completion of the first meiotic division occurs before ovulation. The two cells that result from this division are not identical. They are the secondary oocyte and the first polar body. The secondary oocyte contains the haploid number of chromosomes. The first polar body soon disintegrates because it contains almost no

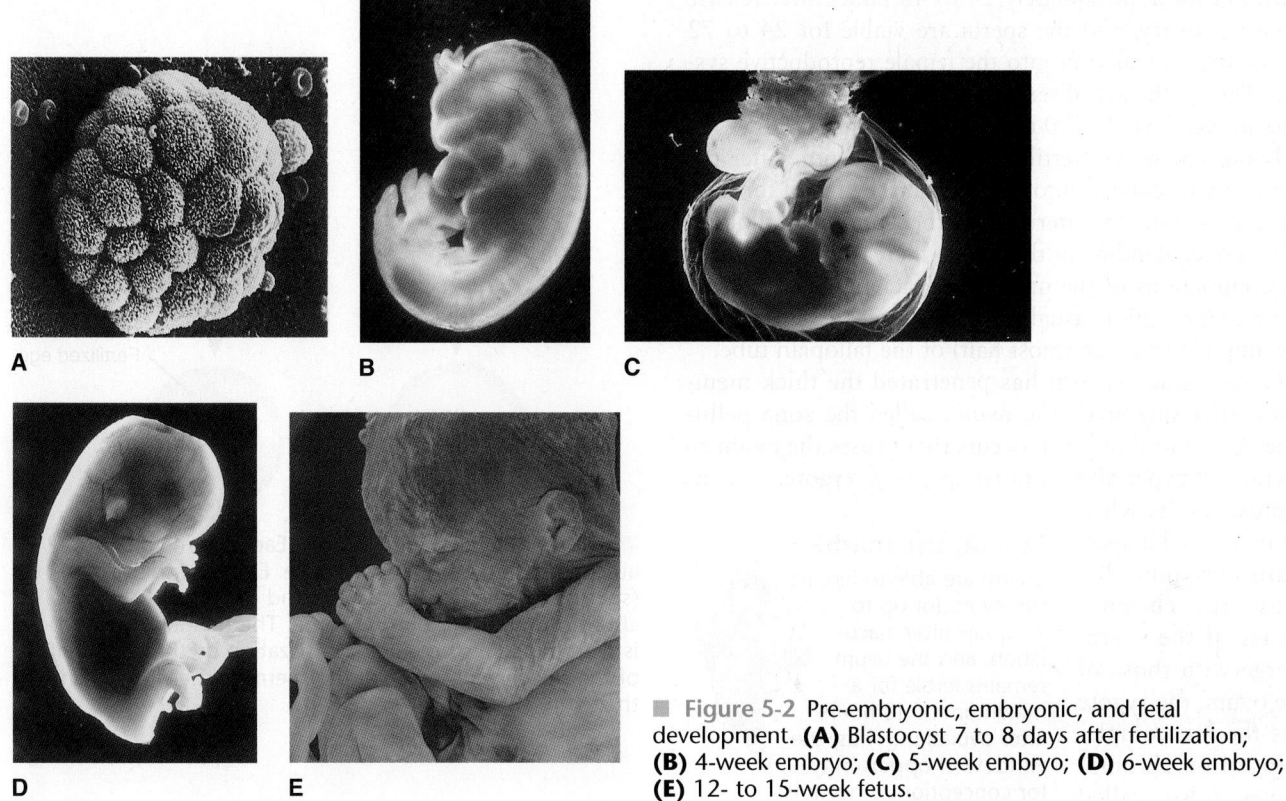

■ Figure 5-2 Pre-embryonic, embryonic, and fetal development. **(A)** Blastocyst 7 to 8 days after fertilization; **(B)** 4-week embryo; **(C)** 5-week embryo; **(D)** 6-week embryo; **(E)** 12- to 15-week fetus.

cytoplasm. The secondary oocyte begins its second meiotic division at ovulation, but does not complete the process unless a sperm fertilizes it.

STAGES OF FETAL DEVELOPMENT

The three stages of human development during pregnancy are

1. Pre-embryonic
2. Embryonic
3. Fetal

The pre-embryonic stage begins at fertilization and lasts through the end of the second week after fertilization. The embryonic stage begins approximately 2 weeks after fertilization and ends at the conclusion of the eighth week after fertilization. By the end of the embryonic stage, all of the organ systems have begun development and the conceptus is distinctly human in form. The fetal stage begins at 9 weeks after fertilization and ends at birth. However, birth is not the end of human development. Human development is an ongoing process of transformation that begins with fertilization and continues through the teenage years and beyond. Figure 5-2 illustrates pre-embryonic, embryonic, and fetal development.

In this chapter, fertilization age (number of weeks after fertilization) will be used rather than gestational age (number of weeks after the last menstrual period) when

discussing development during pregnancy. Table 5-1 compares postfertilization and gestational dates.

Pre-embryonic Stage

The pre-embryonic stage begins with fertilization and encompasses the first 2 weeks thereafter. Cellular division and implantation occur during this stage of development.

Fertilization

Fertilization, also called conception, occurs when the sperm penetrates the ovum. The ovum is receptive to fer-

Table 5-1 ■ COMPARISON OF GESTATIONAL AGE TO FERTILIZATION AGE

Stage of Development	Weeks After Fertilization	Gestational Age
Pre-embryonic	0–2 weeks	3–4 weeks' gestation
Embryonic	3–8 weeks	5–10 weeks' gestation
Fetal	9–38 weeks	11–40 weeks' gestation

tilization for approximately 24 to 48 hours after release from the ovary, and the sperm are viable for 24 to 72 hours after ejaculation into the female reproductive system. During the act of sexual intercourse, the man ejaculates approximately 300 to 600 million sperm. However, only one sperm will fertilize the mature ovum. After the sperm are ejaculated into the vagina, they travel through the cervix, into the uterus, and then into the fallopian tube. Prostaglandins in the semen increase smooth muscle contractions of the uterus that facilitate transport of sperm. Conception usually occurs when the ovum is in the ampulla (the outermost half) of the fallopian tube.

Once a single sperm has penetrated the thick membrane that surrounds the ovum, called the zona pellucida, a chemical reaction occurs that causes the ovum to become impenetrable to other sperm. A **zygote**, or conceptus, results when an ovum and a spermatozoon unite. Because the chromosomes of the sperm merge with those of the ovum, the zygote has the full complement of 46 chromosomes (also called the diploid number), arranged in 23 pairs.

> **You do the math!**
> Sperm are able to fertilize the ovum for up to 72 hours after ejaculation, and the ovum remains fertile for a maximum of 48 hours after ovulation. Thus, the window of opportunity for conception to occur is 5 to 3 days before until 2 days after ovulation.

Sex Determination

Sex determination occurs at the time of fertilization based on the inheritance of X or Y chromosomes. Because the spermatozoon can have either an X or a Y chromosome, the male gamete is responsible for fetal sex determination. The Y chromosome is smaller and contains mainly genes for maleness. The female ovum always contains an X chromosome, which carries several genes for other traits besides femaleness.

A female (XX) develops when the ovum (X) unites with a spermatozoon with an X chromosome. Conversely, fertilization with a spermatozoon that contains a Y chromosome will produce a male (XY) (Fig. 5-3). Research indicates that there is an approximately 50-50 chance of either occurrence.

> **This is worth noting!**
> Some couples mistakenly believe that they can influence sex determination by using certain sexual positions, ingesting particular foods before intercourse, or timing sex to occur at specific times during the menstrual cycle. These beliefs are often rooted in folklore and not based on scientific principles.

Cellular Reproduction

After fertilization, the zygote begins the process of mitotic division known as **cleavage**. As the cells divide, the

■ **Figure 5-3** Inheritance of sex. Each ovum contains 22 autosomes and an X chromosome. Each spermatozoon (sperm) contains 22 autosomes and either an X chromosome or a Y chromosome. The gender of the zygote is determined at the time of fertilization by the combination of the sex chromosomes of the sperm (either X or Y) and the ovum (X).

zygote transforms from one cell into two cells, and then each cell further divides to form four cells. Each of these cells in turn divides to form eight cells and so on. Each new cell contains the diploid number of chromosomes (46), beginning with the first mitotic division. While cleavage is occurring, the zygote is traveling through the fallopian tube toward the uterus.

At about 3 days after fertilization, the total cell count reaches 32. The solid cell cluster resembles a mulberry; hence, the name **morula** (Latin for mulberry). The morula continues its journey toward the uterine cavity while cleavage and transformation of the cells continue. By about 5 days after fertilization, the dividing cell mass develops a hollow, fluid-filled core and is now called a **blastocyst**. The blastocyst has an outer layer of cells called the trophoblast, a fluid-filled hollow core, and an inner cell mass. The trophoblast will go on to become the structures that nourish and protect the developing conceptus. By the end of the pre-embryonic period, the inner cell mass becomes the embryonic disk, which will eventually become the fetus.

Implantation

On about the sixth day after fertilization, the trophoblast develops fingerlike projections that help the blastocyst to burrow into the nutrient-rich endometrium. By the 10th day, the blastocyst has completely buried itself in the uterine lining. During the process of implantation, small cavities, called lacunae,

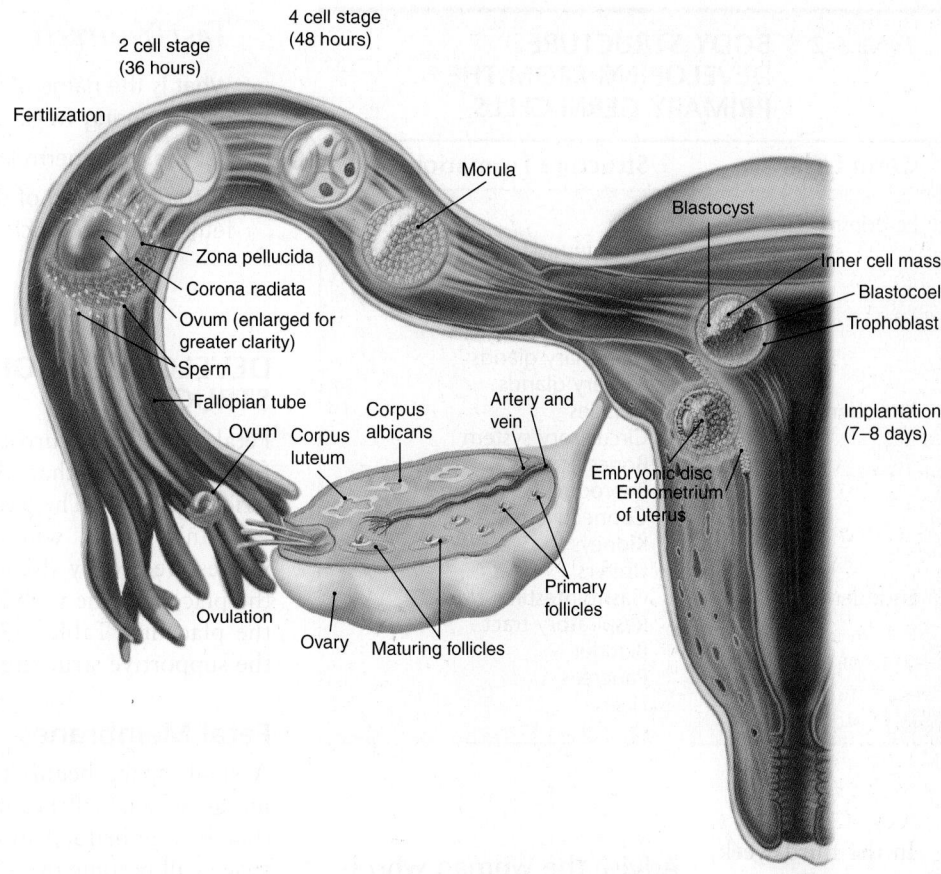

2 cell stage
(36 hours)

4 cell stage
(48 hours)

Fertilization

Morula

Blastocyst

Zona pellucida

Corona radiata

Ovum (enlarged for
greater clarity)

Sperm

Fallopian tube

Ovum

Corpus
luteum

Corpus
albicans

Artery and
vein

Inner cell mass

Blastocoel

Trophoblast

Implantation
(7–8 days)

Embryonic disc
Endometrium
of uterus

Primary
follicles

Ovulation

Ovary

Maturing follicles

■ **Figure 5-4** Fertilization and tubal transport of the zygote. From fertilization to implantation, the zygote travels through the fallopian tube, experiencing rapid mitotic division (cleavage). During the journey toward the uterus, the zygote evolves through several stages, including morula and blastocyst.

develop around the blastocyst. Maternal blood pools in the lacunae, which allows the exchange of nutrients from the woman for metabolic wastes from the blastocyst. The lacunae eventually become the intervillous spaces of the placenta. The tiny blastocyst begins to produce human chorionic gonadotropin (hCG), which signals the corpus luteum to continue producing progesterone to maintain the endometrial lining and the pregnancy.

At this point in the woman's menstrual cycle, the endometrium is ready to support the pregnancy. From this point through the end of pregnancy, the endometrium is called the **decidua**. The woman has not yet missed her menstrual period and is unaware of her pregnancy. Figure 5-4 illustrates the transport of the ovum from ovulation to fertilization and the transport of the zygote from fertilization to implantation.

Here is a teaching opportunity!

Some women have a small amount of bleeding during the time of implantation, which is known as implantation bleeding. This bleeding can be mistaken for a scanty menstrual period and can lead to miscalculation of fetal age.

Test Yourself

✔ Gametogenesis occurs by which type of cellular division: mitosis or meiosis?

✔ A male fetus carries which two sex chromosomes?

✔ What is the name of the single cell that results from fertilization?

Embryonic Stage

The embryonic stage lasts from the end of the second week after fertilization until the end of the eighth week. During this stage, the woman misses her first menstrual period, and the developing conceptus becomes the **embryo**. By the end of the embryonic stage, all of the organ systems and major structures are present, and the embryo is fully recognizable as human in form.

During the embryonic period, the cells of the embryo multiply, and tissues begin to assume specific functions, a process known as differentiation. It is through differentiation that tissues form rudimentary organs and organ systems.

Table 5-2 ■ BODY STRUCTURES DEVELOPING FROM THE PRIMARY GERM CELLS

Germ Layer	Structure Formation
Ectoderm	Skin
	Nervous system
	Nasal passages
	Crystalline lens of the eye
	Pharynx
	Mammary glands
	Salivary glands
Mesoderm	Muscles
	Circulatory system
	Bones
	Reproductive system
	Connective tissue
	Kidneys
	Ureters
Endoderm	Gastrointestinal tract
	Respiratory tract
	Bladder
	Pancreas
	Liver

In the third week, three germ layers develop in the embryo. These layers are the ectoderm, mesoderm, and endoderm. The germ layers will become the different organs and tissues of the developing embryo. The ectoderm, which is the outer layer of cells, develops to form skin, hair, nails, and the nervous system. The mesoderm is the middle layer, which will form the skeletal, muscular, and circulatory systems. Lastly, the endoderm, which is the inner layer, will form the glands, lungs, and urinary and digestive tracts (Table 5-2).

Advise the woman who is trying to become pregnant to be very careful!

Exposure to a teratogen (any substance or process that can lead to birth defects) during the embryonic stage produces the greatest damaging effects because cells are rapidly dividing and differentiating into specific body structures.

Fetal Stage

The fetal stage is from the beginning of the ninth week after fertilization and continues until birth. At this time, the developing human is called the **fetus**. During the fetal stage, there is additional growth and maturation of the organs and body systems. At the beginning of this stage, the fetus is about 50 mm long and weighs about 8 g. By the end of the fetal stage, the fetus will be about 36 cm long and weigh approximately 3,400 g. Box 5-1 summarizes and illustrates the highlights of growth during the embryonic and fetal stages.

Test Yourself

✔ What is the name of the stage of development that occurs during weeks 3 to 8?
✔ List the three germ layers in the embryo.
✔ At the beginning of the fetal stage, how long is the fetus and how much does it weigh?

DEVELOPMENT OF SUPPORTIVE STRUCTURES

Fetal membranes surround the fetus in a protective sac filled with fluid that allows for protection and unrestricted growth. The fetus receives its nutrition from the woman's blood, which also removes the metabolic wastes created by the fetus. This exchange happens at the placenta. The umbilical cord connects the fetus and the placenta. Table 5-3 summarizes characteristics of the supportive structures.

Fetal Membranes

A small space begins to form between the inner cell mass—which will become the embryo—and the tissue that has embedded into the endometrial lining. This space will become the amniotic cavity in which the fetus will grow. The amniotic cavity begins to develop around 9 days after conception. The **amnion** surrounds the amniotic cavity. The amnion is a thick fibrous lining, made

Table 5-3 ■ CHARACTERISTICS OF SUPPORTIVE STRUCTURES

Supportive Structure	Characteristics
Placenta	2–3 cm thick, thickness established by 20 weeks
	15–20 cm in diameter
	500–600 g in weight
	Made up of 15–20 lobes called cotyledons
Amniotic fluid	About 1 L at term
	Filtered and replaced every 3 hours
	Pale yellow to straw colored
Umbilical cord	50 cm long and 2 cm wide
	Blood flow through cord is about 400 mL/min
	Two arteries, which carry deoxygenated blood to placenta from fetus
	One vein, which carries oxygen and nourishment from placenta to fetus
	Formed from the amnion

Box 5-1 ▮ EMBRYONIC AND FETAL DEVELOPMENT

End of 4 Weeks

4 weeks

Chorionic villi form
The embryo is C-shaped
Length: 0.75–1 cm
Weight: 400 mg
Arms and legs are budlike structures.
Rudimentary eyes, ears, and nose are discernible.
Foundations for nervous system, genitourinary
  system, skin, bones, and lungs are formed.

End of 8 Weeks

8 weeks

Length: 2.5–3 cm (1 in)
Weight: 8 g
The head is disproportionately large as a result of
  brain development.
The heart, with a septum and valves, is beating
  rhythmically.
The fingers and toes are distinct and separated.
Sex differentiation begins.
Organogenesis is complete.

End of 12 Weeks

12 weeks

Length: 8 cm (3 in)
Weight: 25 g
Placenta is complete.
Divisions of the brain begin to develop.
The face is well formed.
The eyes are widely spaced and fused.
Heartbeat is audible by Doppler.
Kidney secretion has begun.
Spontaneous movements occur (may not yet be
  discernible by the woman).
Sex is discernible by outward appearance.

End of 16 Weeks

16 weeks

Second trimester

Length: 10–17 cm
Weight: 55–120 g
Lungs are fully shaped.
Fetus swallows amniotic fluid.
Skeletal structure is identifiable.
Downy lanugo hair present on body.
Liver and pancreas are functioning.
Sex can be determined by ultrasound.

End of 20 Weeks

20 weeks

Length: 25 cm
Weight: 220 g
Eyebrows and scalp hair are present.
Lanugo covers the entire body.
Vernix caseosa begins to form.
Heart sounds can be heard with a fetoscope.
Fetal movements are felt by the woman.

End of 24 Weeks

25 weeks

Length: 28–36 cm
Weight: 550 g
Eyelids are now open.

(*continues on page 106*)

Box 5-1 ▌ EMBRYONIC AND FETAL DEVELOPMENT *(continued)*

Pupils are capable of reacting to light.
Active production of lung surfactant begins.
Exhibits a startle reflex.
Skin is red and wrinkled, with little subcutaneous fat.
Vernix caseosa covers the skin.
May survive if born in a facility with a fully
  equipped neonatal intensive care unit (NICU).

End of 28 Weeks

29 weeks

Length: 35–38 cm
Weight: 1,200 g
Respiratory system is developed enough to provide
  gaseous exchange; however, the fetus needs care in
  a NICU in order to survive.
Adipose tissue begins to accumulate.
Male: The testes begin to descend into the scrotal sac.
Female: Clitoris is prominent and labia majora are
  small and do not cover the labia minora.

End of 32 Weeks

34 weeks

Length: 38–43 cm
Weight: 1,600 g

The lungs are not yet fully developed, but the fetus
  usually does well, if born at this time.
Active Moro reflex is present.
Steady weight gain occurs.
Male: Testes descend into the scrotum. The scrotal
  sac has few rugae.

End of 36 Weeks

37 weeks

Length: 42–48 cm
Weight: 1,800–2,700 g
Lanugo begins to thin.
Sole of the foot has few creases.
Birth position is usually assumed (vertex, head down).

End of 40 Weeks (Full Term)

Length: 48–52 cm
Weight: 3,000 g
Vernix caseosa is evident in body folds.
Lanugo remains on the shoulders and upper back
  only.
Creases cover at least two thirds of the surface of the
  sole of the foot.
Female: The labia majora are well developed.

Adapted from: Pillitteri, A. (2003). *Maternal and child health nursing: Care of the childbearing and childrearing family* (4th ed.). Philadelphia: Lippincott Williams & Wilkins; Mattson, S., & Smith, J. E. (Eds.). (2000). *Core curriculum for maternal–newborn nursing.* AWHONN publication (2nd ed.). Philadelphia: WB Saunders; Reeder, S. J., Martin, L. L., & Koniak-Griffin, D. (1996). *Maternity nursing: Family, newborn, and women's health care* (18th ed.). Philadelphia: Lippincott-Raven; The Visible Embryo website, http://www.visembryo.com.

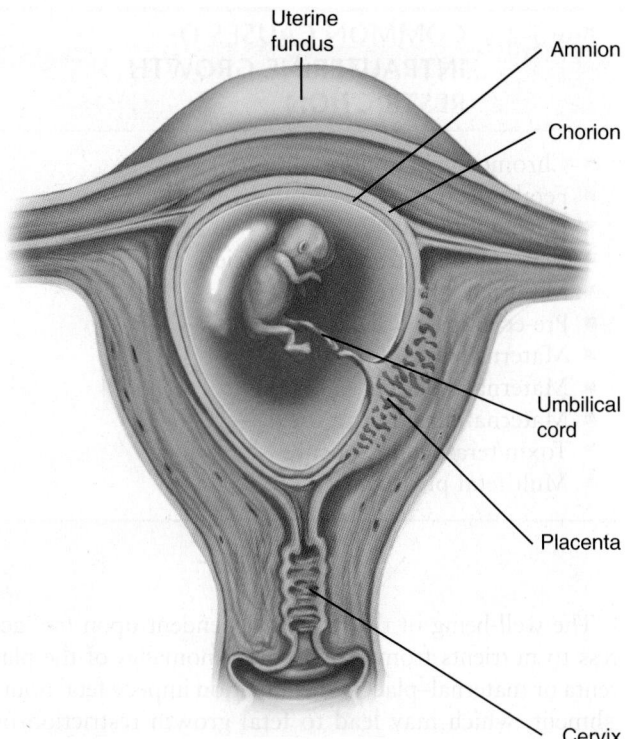

Uterine fundus

Amnion

Chorion

Umbilical cord

Placenta

Cervix

■ **Figure 5-5** The embryo is floating in amniotic fluid surrounded by the protective fetal membranes (amnion and chorion).

up of several layers, that helps to protect the fetus and forms the inner part of the sac in which the fetus grows. Amniotic fluid fills this sac. Lying against the amnion toward the exterior of the blastocyst is the **chorion**. The chorion is a second layer of thick fibrous tissue that surrounds the amnion. The amnion and chorion are not fused but lie in close contact with each other (Fig. 5-5). Together they make up the fetal membranes.

At the end of the second week after fertilization, **chorionic villi** begin to appear on the chorion. These are fingerlike projections that extend out from the chorion, giving it a rough appearance. Around 15 to 20 days after fertilization, cells in the chorionic villi form arterial-capillary-venous networks, which become fetal blood vessels. These capillaries pick up oxygen and nutrients from maternal blood that enters the intervillous spaces in exchange for waste products and carbon dioxide from the developing embryo.

Around the eighth week, some of the chorionic villi disintegrate, leaving a large area of the chorion that is smooth. The remaining chorionic villi increase in number and size and continue to branch out. The chorionic villi eventually become the fetal part of the placenta where the exchange of nutrients and wastes occurs.

Amniotic Fluid

A specialized fluid called **amniotic fluid** fills the amniotic cavity. Amniotic fluid serves four main functions for the fetus: physical protection, temperature regulation, provi-

sion of unrestricted movement, and symmetrical growth. Amniotic fluid also provides a medium for fetal evaluation because it collects substances from the fetal gastrointestinal, renal, and respiratory tracts. The fetal membranes produce amniotic fluid throughout pregnancy. It is produced from maternal blood, fetal urine, and secretions from the fetal respiratory tract. The fluid is composed mostly of water (98%–99%). Electrolytes, creatinine, urea, glucose, hormones, fetal cells, lanugo (fine downy hair), and vernix caseosa (a cheesy substance that protects fetal skin) make up the remaining 1% to 2% of the fluid.

Amniotic fluid acts as a cushion around the fetus. It protects the fetus from injury if the mother falls or if something hits her abdomen. It helps to maintain a constant temperature around the fetus because the fetus is not mature enough to regulate its own temperature. Amniotic fluid allows the fetus to move freely and aids in symmetrical growth. Lastly, it is a fluid source that the fetus drinks and then urinates. The fetal intestines absorb the swallowed amniotic fluid, and then the fetus urinates fluid back into the amniotic sac.

The fetus also takes in and releases amniotic fluid when it practices fetal breathing movements. During fetal exhalation, the lungs release surfactant into the amniotic fluid. The fetal lungs produce surfactant starting in the 28th week. Surfactant helps to decrease the surface tension in the alveoli. Sampling of the amniotic fluid can help to determine if the fetal lungs are mature enough for birth.

The fetus swallows its shed hair, epithelial cells, and sebaceous secretions. These substances form meconium as they gather in the fetal intestinal system. Meconium is the first bowel movement the infant has after birth. If an insult stresses the fetus during pregnancy or labor, the anal sphincter may relax and release meconium into the amniotic fluid. This action stains the fluid green. Meconium staining of the amniotic fluid has occurred if the amniotic fluid is green, instead of clear, at delivery. During the normal fetal process of swallowing and inhaling amniotic fluid in utero, the thick meconium particles can lodge in the fetal lungs. The newborn is then at risk for meconium aspiration pneumonia.

Did you know?

You can learn a lot from amniotic fluid! During pregnancy, a procedure called amniocentesis can obtain a sample of amniotic fluid. The practitioner can analyze the fluid to determine whether the fetal lungs are mature enough to support respiration outside of the womb. The fluid can also be used for genetic testing because the fluid contains fetal cells with fetal DNA.

Placenta

The placenta is the organ that sustains and nourishes the growing pregnancy. The placenta has three main functions: To provide for the transfer and exchange of substances, to act as a barrier to certain substances, and to function as an endocrine gland by producing hormones. The placenta begins to develop during the fifth week after fertilization at the site of implantation. Most of the placenta is of embryonic origin, but about 20% is maternal in origin.

Many lobes, or sections, called cotyledons compose the placenta. Each cotyledon consists of two or more main stem villi and their branches. A main stem villus consists of a branch of the umbilical vein and umbilical artery that branches out into the intervillous space. Maternal blood, from endometrial arteries, pools in the intervillous spaces.

The placenta is the exchange site for nutrients and wastes between the fetal and maternal circulatory systems. The maternal blood supply brings oxygen, water, electrolytes, vitamins, and glucose to the placenta. These nutrients enter the fetal circulation for use by the fetus. The fetal circulation brings carbon dioxide, carbon monoxide, urea, and uric acid to the placenta for removal by the maternal circulatory system. Simple or facilitated diffusion and active transport at the level of the chorionic villi move these substances across the placental membrane (Pridjian, 2005).

The fetus receives passive immunity from the mother by transfer of maternal antibodies. Maternal antibodies to diphtheria, smallpox, and measles travel across the placenta to the fetus. The fetus does not receive immunity to rubella, cytomegalovirus, varicella, or measles. If the woman encounters these pathogens during her pregnancy, fetal infection may ensue. Some diseases are teratogenic (able to cause birth defects).

The placenta acts as a barrier to some medications and hormones that are in the maternal blood supply. However, not all medications and substances are stopped by the placental barrier. Many of these substances cross over to the fetus.

Don't pass up this teaching opportunity!
The woman should consider that everything she takes in will pass to the fetus. Teach her to check with her primary care provider before taking any substance that is not specifically ordered for her. This warning extends to immunizations, as well.

The placenta also secretes hormones that help to sustain the pregnancy. These include progesterone, estrogen, human placental lactogen (hPL), and hCG. Progesterone is necessary to maintain the nutrient-rich endometrial lining (decidua). It also functions to keep the myometrium quiet, so that contractions do not occur prematurely, leading to loss of the pregnancy. Estrogen functions to provide a rich blood supply to the decidua and placenta. The main function of hCG is to sustain the corpus luteum at the beginning of the pregnancy. The main function of hPL is to regulate the glucose that is available for the fetus (Pridjian, 2005).

Box 5-2 ▌ COMMON CAUSES OF INTRAUTERINE GROWTH RESTRICTION

- Chromosomal abnormalities
- Fetal infection
- Placental infarcts
- Maternal nutritional deficiencies
- Maternal hypertension
- Pre-eclampsia
- Maternal renal disease
- Maternal smoking
- Maternal illegal drug use
- Toxin/teratogen exposure
- Multifetal pregnancy

The well-being of the fetus is dependent upon free access to nutrients from the mother. Anomalies of the placenta or maternal–placental circulation impede fetal nourishment, which may lead to fetal growth restriction or death. Intrauterine growth restriction (IUGR) indicates that fetal growth has slowed for some reason, resulting in a fetus that is smaller than expected for gestational age. IUGR can have many causes. Box 5-2 summarizes some of these common causes.

Maternal hypertension or infectious agents can cause areas of infarction and subsequent calcification in the placenta. These areas lead to a decreased surface area, which decreases the amount of nutrients that travel to the fetus at a given time. Vasoconstriction caused by hypertension, smoking, or illicit drug use also decreases the flow of blood to the fetus, which can lead to IUGR.

Umbilical Cord

The umbilical cord extends from the umbilicus of the fetus to the fetal surface of the placenta. In the cord are two arteries that bring deoxygenated blood from the fetus to the placenta and one vein that carries oxygenated and nourished blood from the placenta to the fetus. Connective tissue called Wharton's jelly surrounds these three vessels. **Wharton's jelly** is a clear gelatinous

Cultural Snapshot

Certain ethnic groups commonly produce offspring that are smaller than others are. The fetuses of these ethnic groups are not growth restricted (IUGR). It is important to take into account the ethnicity and stature of both the mother and the father when evaluating an infant for IUGR.

substance that gives support to the cord and helps prevent compression of the cord, which could impair blood flow to the fetus (Pridjian, 2005).

Test Yourself

✔ The fetal membranes are composed of what two main structures?

✔ Name two functions of amniotic fluid.

✔ List three hormones produced by the placenta.

FETAL AND PLACENTAL CIRCULATION
Fetal Circulation

Fetal circulation differs from the pattern of human circulation that is present after birth. While in utero, the fetus is dependent upon the maternal circulation for its oxygenation, and the fetus does not use its lungs to oxygenate blood. Because the level of oxygen that is in the fetus' bloodstream is lower than maternal levels, fetal circulation aids in streaming oxygenated blood from the placenta to the major organs, especially the brain, liver, and kidneys. Fetal circulation is possible because of three major shunts that are present in the fetus but that close shortly after birth. These shunts are the ductus venosus, foramen ovale, and the ductus arteriosus.

Fetal blood flows to the placenta via the umbilical arteries. Each umbilical artery serves one half of the placenta. The arteries branch off into main stem chorionic villi that then branch down toward the decidua basalis in the intervillous spaces. The exchange of oxygen and nutrients from the woman's bloodstream for waste products from the fetus occurs at this level.

Fetal blood returns to the fetus from the placenta via the umbilical vein. In the umbilical vein, the saturation of fetal blood with oxygen is about 80%. The umbilical vein enters the fetus at the site that will be the umbilicus after birth. Approximately half of the oxygenated blood circulates from the umbilical vein to the liver, and the other half of oxygen-rich blood shunts past the liver and flows directly into the inferior vena cava by way of the **ductus venosus**. The oxygenated blood in the inferior vena cava mixes with deoxygenated blood in the inferior vena cava that is returning to the heart from the lower limbs, abdomen, and pelvis, so that the oxygen saturation of the blood entering the right atrium is about 67%.

The majority of the blood in the right atrium flows into the left atrium via the **foramen ovale**. The foramen ovale is a hole that connects the right and left atria so the majority of oxygenated blood can quickly pass into the left side of the fetal heart and go to the brain and the rest of the fetal body. Blood entering the right atrium from the superior vena cava is mostly deoxygenated. In the right atrium, this blood mixes with some of the well-oxygenated blood from the inferior vena cava. This mixed blood then enters the right ventricle, which pumps it to the fetal lungs via the pulmonary trunk (Flanagan, Yeager, & Weindling, 2005).

In utero, the fetus does not oxygenate its own blood in the lungs; therefore, blood supplied to the fetal lungs is for nourishment of the tissues only. The fetal lungs are collapsed and filled with fluid, which leads to high resistance. Because of this resistance, only 5% to 10% of the blood in the pulmonary artery enters the fetal lungs. The remainder of blood coming from the right ventricle enters the **ductus arteriosus**. The ductus arteriosus is a fetal shunt that links the pulmonary artery with the aorta.

In the left atrium, the oxygenated blood mixes with some deoxygenated blood that is returning to the heart from the lungs. The blood then travels to the left ventricle, which pumps the blood to the aorta. The higher oxygenated blood from the ascending aorta flows to the heart, head, and upper limbs by way of the aortic arch branch. The lesser oxygenated blood from the pulmonary artery enters the aorta via the ductus arteriosus below the aortic arch branch.

Blood in the abdominal aorta divides so that half of the blood supply returns to the placenta for reoxygenation, while the other half goes to nourish the viscera and lower half of the body. The internal iliac arteries branch off to form the two umbilical arteries. The umbilical arteries then carry deoxygenated blood and waste products back to the placenta, which completes the fetal circulation circuit (Fig. 5-6).

At birth, fetal blood no longer flows to the placenta for oxygenation. Rapid physiologic changes occur to allow the newborn to oxygenate his own blood by his lungs. After birth, the ductus venosus, ductus arteriosus, and the umbilical vein and arteries constrict and eventually form ligaments, which remain present for the rest of the infant's life. It is possible for the ductus arteriosus to remain open, especially in premature infants or infants with hypoxia. When this shunt remains open, it is called patent ductus arteriosus; medications or surgery may be required to close the duct (Flanagan, Yeager, & Weindling, 2005). Refer to Chapter 13 for a detailed discussion of the circulatory changes that occur in the newborn.

Placental Circulation

The uterine arteries supply the uterus with maternal blood. The endometrial, or spiral, arteries then carry the blood to the intervillous spaces. In the intervillous spaces, maternal blood flows around the chorionic villi, where nutrients and oxygen from the maternal circulation are transferred by diffusion and active transport across a thin membrane into the fetal circulation. Likewise, fetal wastes diffuse into the maternal bloodstream. Blood leaves the intervillous spaces by the endometrial veins and returns to the maternal circulatory system (Pridjian, 2005).

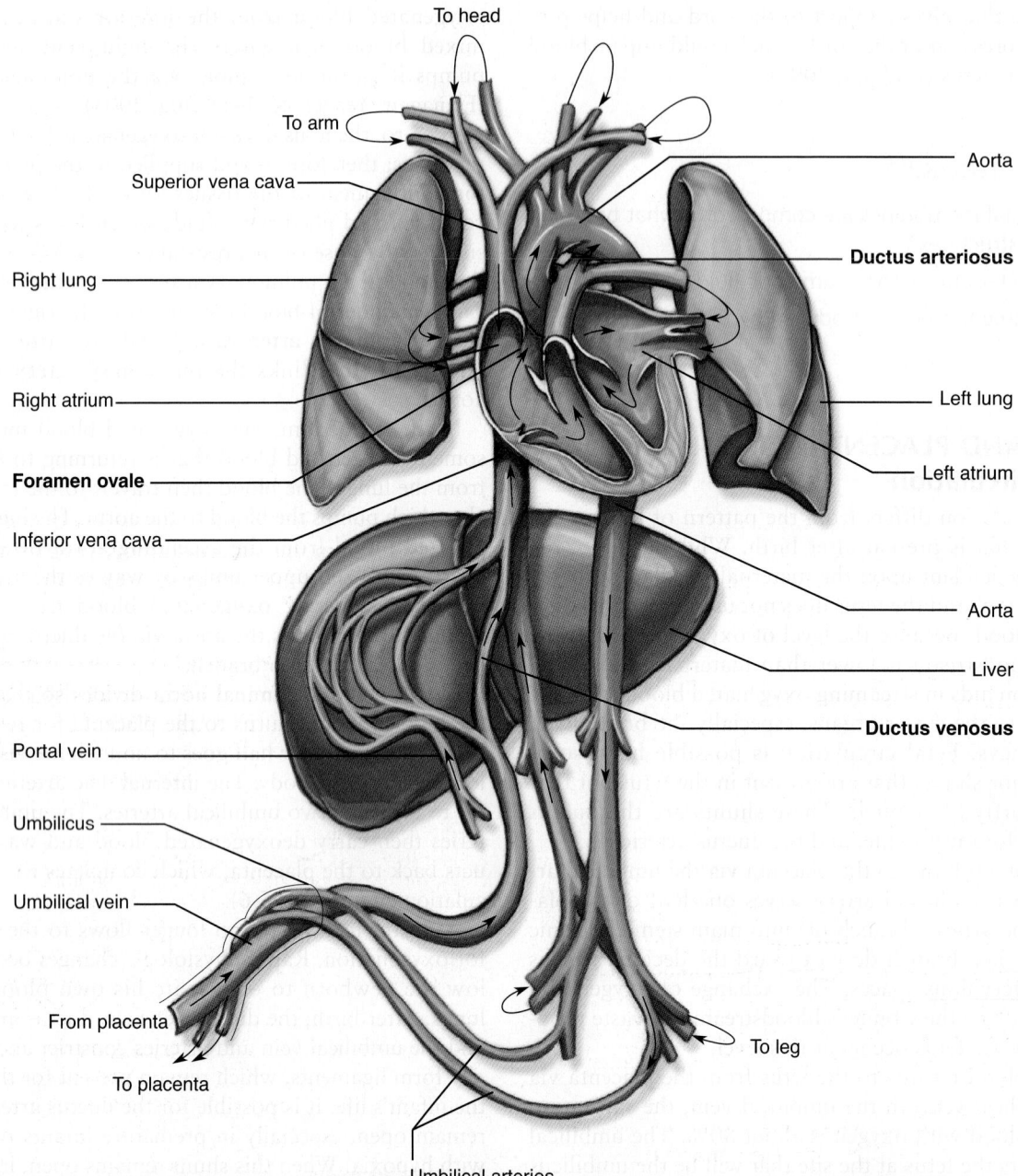

To head

To arm

Superior vena cava

Right lung

Right atrium

Foramen ovale

Inferior vena cava

Portal vein

Umbilicus

Umbilical vein

From placenta

To placenta

Umbilical arteries

Aorta

Ductus arteriosus

Left lung

Left atrium

Aorta

Liver

Ductus venosus

To leg

■ **Figure 5-6** Fetal circulation. Arrows indicate the path of blood. The umbilical vein carries oxygen-rich blood from the placenta to the liver and through the ductus venosus. From there it is carried to the inferior vena cava to the right atrium of the heart. Some of the blood is shunted through the foramen ovale to the left side of the heart where it is routed to the brain and upper extremities. The rest of the blood travels down to the right ventricle and through the pulmonary artery. A small portion of the blood travels to the nonfunctioning lungs, while the remaining blood is shunted through the ductus arteriosus into the aorta to supply the rest of the body.

SPECIAL CONSIDERATIONS OF FETAL DEVELOPMENT

Teratogens and the Fetus

As described earlier in this chapter, a **teratogen** is a substance that causes birth defects. The severity of the defect depends on when during development the conceptus is exposed to the teratogen (i.e., which body systems are developing at the time of exposure) and the particular teratogenic agent to which the fetus is exposed.

Effects of Teratogens on the Developing Fetus

During the pre-embryonic stage, exposure to a teratogen has an all-or-nothing effect. Either the exposure will cause death of the zygote, or there will be no effect because there is no connection between the maternal blood supply and the zygote.

Exposure to a teratogen during the embryonic stage produces the greatest damaging effects. It is during this time that development of the primary structure and function of organs and tissues occurs. Developing organs and body systems are highly susceptible to teratogens, and major abnormalities can result. Table 5-4 lists structures commonly affected by teratogen exposure during the embryonic period. Because the central nervous system (CNS) develops continuously throughout pregnancy, these structures are always vulnerable to teratogens.

Exposure to a teratogen during the fetal stage will have less of an effect on the fetus than exposure during the embryonic period. The effect of a teratogen during the fetal stage may cause physiologic defects and minor structural abnormalities. The CNS and brain continue to be susceptible to damage from teratogens during the fetal period.

Types of Teratogenic Agents

Teratogens usually fall into one of three categories: an ingested, infectious, or environmental substance. Table 5-5 summarizes some of the common teratogens and their effects.

Ingested Teratogens

Most substances ingested by the pregnant woman pass to the fetus from the maternal bloodstream through the placenta and then into the fetal circulation. Commonly

Table 5-4 ▌ STRUCTURES COMMONLY AFFECTED BY TERATOGENS DURING THE EMBRYONIC PERIOD

Week of Development (# of weeks after fertilization) in Which Exposure Occurs	Structures Commonly Affected
3	Heart and central nervous system (CNS)
4	Lip, heart, arm, leg, CNS
5	Heart, eye, arm, leg, CNS
6	CNS, heart, ear, teeth
7	CNS, ear, teeth, palate, heart
8	CNS, ear, palate, heart, external genitalia

Table 5-5 ▌ COMMON TERATOGENS AND ASSOCIATED EFFECTS

Teratogen	Possible Effect
Injested agents	
Dilantin	Cleft palate
Chemotherapy agents	Major congenital malformations, especially of the central nervous system
Tetracycline	Damage to developing dental and osseous tissue
Alcohol	Fetal alcohol syndrome with facial defects, low birth weight, affects brain
Infectious agents	
Varicella	Fetal varicella syndrome, which ranges in severity from generalized multiorgan damage to isolated defects, such as incomplete limb development or skin scarring
Rubella (German measles)	Cataracts, deafness, and cardiac malformations
CMV	Hearing loss, microcephaly
Environmental agents	
Mercury	Neurologic damage, blindness
Radiation	Congenital malformations, mental retardation (seen in large amounts of ionizing radiation)

ingested teratogens include prescription medications, illicit drugs, and alcohol. Some medications may be therapeutic for the mother but also have teratogenic properties. For example, phenytoin (Dilantin) is therapeutic for preventing seizures in the mother but can cause cleft palate and

Your sensitivity can make a big difference!

Guilt is a common feeling for the mother of an infant with a birth defect. Many defects happen before the woman knows she is pregnant. Avoid statements that imply blame. For example, don't say, "You shouldn't have been around x-rays while you were pregnant."

other abnormalities in the fetus. In such a circumstance, the practitioner weighs the risk to the mother against the risk to the developing fetus before prescribing a potential teratogen. Not all medications are teratogenic. Acetaminophen (Tylenol) is an example of a medication that, when taken as directed, is nonteratogenic. Some medications, such as heparin, are unable to cross the placental barrier and thus are safe to use during pregnancy.

In the 1950s, physicians prescribed thalidomide to pregnant women to help control morning sickness. Then physicians learned that thalidomide causes limb deformities in the developing fetus, and the drug was withdrawn from the market. The Food & Drug Administration recently approved thalidomide for the treatment of a complication of leprosy. Because physicians can now prescribe thalidomide, the March of Dimes strongly recommends warning women of childbearing age of the serious risk of birth defects (March of Dimes, undated).

One of the fetus' main body systems affected throughout the embryonic and fetal period is the brain and CNS. Alcohol and illicit drugs such as marijuana, cocaine, and heroin negatively affect the developing CNS. Infants exposed to these substances during pregnancy may be born with a physical dependence on the substance to which they were exposed. In addition, these substances can lead to decreased mental capacity and cause other defects and pregnancy complications. Therefore, ingestion of these substances is strongly discouraged during pregnancy.

Infectious Teratogens

If the pregnant woman develops an infection during her pregnancy, the infection can pass to the fetus and affect fetal development. Some common infections that have teratogenic effects include varicella, cytomegalovirus, and rubella.

Environmental Teratogens

Substances in the environment can have a teratogenic effect. Ionizing x-rays, radioactive substances, and certain chemicals can cause birth defects. The pregnant woman should take precautions to avoid these substances during her pregnancy. Avoiding unnecessary

A Personal Glimpse

The worrying began when I found out I was pregnant with my oldest child. We hadn't been officially trying to get pregnant, and so right away I started thinking about all the things I had ingested while already pregnant. I was a 3-cup-a-day coffee drinker; I had taken several doses of Tylenol for headaches; and I remembered celebrating my birthday with a few glasses of wine. To top it all off, I hadn't been taking prenatal vitamins. I started panicking about the harm I had caused my developing baby. I immediately stopped drinking caffeine completely (which gave me very bad headaches); swore off wine for the duration; avoided taking any kind of medication for pain; never missed a day taking prenatal vitamins; and avoided eating fish, hot dogs, and lunch meat (I had heard that these foods were bad to eat during pregnancy). I was also concerned about microwave rays (and stopped using the microwave completely); cats and cat litter; gardening; being around my friends' children (they might have some lurking virus); and mold in the house. I was starting to drive my husband and myself crazy.

At my first prenatal appointment, I talked with the staff at my primary care provider's office. They gave me a brochure that listed things to avoid completely during pregnancy; things to limit during pregnancy; and things that were OK during pregnancy. It also contained practical advice for maintaining a healthy home environment during pregnancy and child rearing. I remained careful during my pregnancy, but I learned to relax a bit more and just use common sense.

Allison

Learning Opportunity: How can the nurse help the woman of childbearing age be aware of possible teratogens without unduly scaring her? How should the nurse advise the woman who is very worried that she may have done something to harm her unborn child before she was aware of the pregnancy?

x-rays, or using a lead shield for unavoidable x-rays, and using gloves when handling chemicals are two ways the woman can help protect her developing fetus.

Ectopic Pregnancy

There are instances when the zygote implants in places other than the uterus. When the zygote implants outside the uterus, an **ectopic pregnancy** is the result. Of the implantations that occur outside of the uterine cavity, 95% occur in the fallopian tube. An ectopic pregnancy that occurs in a fallopian tube is a tubal pregnancy. Usually tubal pregnancies are caused by blockage or scarring of the fallopian tubes, from either infection or trauma, such as a tubal ligation reversal. Ectopic pregnancy occurs in 2% of all pregnancies (Sepilian & Wood, 2005).

As the embryo grows in the confined space of the fallopian tube, it causes the tube to dilate. The tube will

■ **Figure 5-7** Twin pregnancy. **(A)** Fraternal (dizygotic) twins with two placentas, two amnions, and two chorions (diamniotic dichorionic). **(B)** Identical (monozygotic) twins with one placenta, two amnions, and one chorion (diamniotic monochorionic).

eventually rupture if the condition remains undetected. If the tube ruptures, hemorrhage into the peritoneal cavity can lead to maternal death. Surgical removal of the affected tube and the products of conception is the most common treatment. Because there is no way to transplant the embryo into the uterine cavity and continue the pregnancy, tubal pregnancies always result in the death of the embryo (Sepilian & Wood, 2005). See Chapter 17 for a full discussion of ectopic pregnancy.

Multifetal Pregnancy

When a woman is carrying more than one fetus at the same time, it is called a multifetal pregnancy. Multifetal pregnancies can result in twins, triplets, or more. The overall prevalence of twin pregnancies in the United States is 12 per 1,000. Triplets naturally occur at a rate of 1 in 7,000 to 10,000 births. The overall rates of multifetal pregnancies have changed during the last few decades because of the increasing number of assisted reproductive procedures and the use of fertility medications (Zach & Pramanik, 2006).

Twins can be either identical or fraternal. Identical twins derive from one zygote (one egg and one sperm divide into two zygotes shortly after fertilization), so identical twins are **monozygotic** twins. They share the same genetic material and are always the same gender. Fraternal twins develop from separate egg and sperm fertilizations and are **dizygotic** twins. Fraternal twins may or may not be the same gender, and their genetic material is not identical. In pregnancies that have more than two fetuses, they may have all developed from a single fertilized egg, also referred to as monozygotic; or they may have developed from separate eggs; or they may be a combination of both types (Fig. 5-7).

Twins can be classified one of three ways—diamniotic-dichorionic, diamniotic-monochorionic, and monoamni-otic-monochorionic. Diamniotic-dichorionic twins each develop in their own amniotic sac. Their placentas do not share any vessels. Diamniotic-monochorionic twins each have their own amniotic sac but share a common chorionic sac. They each have a separate placenta, but the placentas share some vessels. These types of twins are at risk for developing a condition referred to as twin-to-twin transfusion syndrome. In this syndrome, one fetus gives the other fetus part of its blood volume but does not receive any in return. Lastly, twins can be monoamniotic-monochorionic. These types of twins have one amniotic cavity that they both share. The greatest risk to these twins is cord entanglement. They are also at risk for twin-to-twin transfusion syndrome (Zach & Pramanik, 2006), or to become conjoined (the popular term is "Siamese" twins).

Certain factors increase a woman's chance of becoming pregnant with dizygotic twins. She is more likely to have dizygotic twins if she is herself a twin or has twin siblings, if she recently stopped using oral contraceptives, if she is tall or has a large stature, or if she is of African American heritage. The use of fertility medications, such as clomiphene citrate (Clomid) or menotropins (Pergonal), increases a woman's chance of carrying a multifetal pregnancy. Multifetal pregnancies are at higher risk and require close monitoring (see Chapter 17).

Test Yourself

✔ Which organ system is susceptible throughout the pregnancy to teratogenic effects?

✔ Define ectopic pregnancy.

✔ Why are fraternal twins called dizygotic twins?

Key Points

- Mitosis is the process of cell division by which two daughter cells are produced that have the diploid number of chromosomes (46). Meiosis is a special type of cell division that results in the formation of cells with the haploid number of chromosomes (23).

- Spermatogenesis begins at puberty, whereas oogenesis starts during the fetal stage in the female infant and then stays in an arrested state until puberty. Spermatogenesis ends with four spermatids, each with 23 chromosomes. Oogenesis ends with one ovum containing 23 chromosomes.

- Sex determination occurs when the ovum and the sperm unite. The ovum always contributes an X chromosome, whereas the sperm contributes either an X or a Y chromosome. Two X chromosomes (XX) is female. An X and a Y chromosome (XY) is male.

- The pre-embryonic stage lasts from fertilization until the end of the second week after conception. During this time, the two sets of chromosomes combine, implantation occurs, and the beginning of maternal–fetal circulation occurs.

- The embryonic stage lasts from the end of the second week until the end of the eighth week. During this time, the organs and tissues begin to differentiate and assume specific functions. By the end of this stage, all organs are developed and the embryo is distinctly human in appearance.

- The fetal stage lasts from the end of the eighth week until birth. During this time, there is additional maturation and growth of already existing tissue.

- The close union of the amnion and chorion forms the fetal membranes. The amnion makes up the inner part of the membrane and is in contact with amniotic fluid and the fetus. The chorion is adjacent to (but not fused with) the amnion and has no contact with the fetus.

- Amniotic fluid serves as a cushion to protect the fetus from injury, a temperature control mechanism, and a medium that allows free movement and unrestricted growth.

- The placenta transfers nutrients, such as oxygen and glucose, to the fetus while removing waste products, such as carbon dioxide and urea. The placenta acts as a barrier to some harmful substances but does not prevent most substances from passing to the fetus. The placenta has an endocrine function in that it secretes hormones that help to sustain the pregnancy. These hormones include hCG, hPL, estrogen, and progesterone.

- Maternal blood rich in oxygen and nutrients reaches the placenta at the level of the intervillous spaces that are surrounded by the chorionic villi. The chorionic villi contain the fetal blood vessels. Exchange of nutrients for wastes occurs by simple diffusion or active transport across a thin membrane that separates the fetal and maternal bloodstreams.

- Fetal blood that contains newly oxygenated blood and nutrients leaves the placenta via the umbilical vein and enters the fetal inferior vena cava via the ductus venosus. From there it travels to the right atrium, where most of the blood crosses the foramen ovale into the left atrium. The blood then travels to the aortic arch to the brain and the upper body. Some of the blood enters the right ventricle and goes to the lungs to nourish the tissues. Most of the blood that leaves the right ventricle is shunted to the aorta via the ductus arteriosus. Deoxygenated fetal blood returns to the placenta via the two umbilical arteries.

- Teratogens are classified as ingested, infectious, or environmental. Ingested teratogens can be medications or illegal substances. Infectious teratogens include diseases such as cytomegalovirus, and rubella. Environmental teratogens include ionizing x-rays and chemicals.

- An ectopic pregnancy is one that develops outside of the uterus. Most ectopic pregnancies occur in a fallopian tube, which can rupture and lead to maternal hemorrhage and/or death. A tubal pregnancy always leads to death of the embryo, whether from tubal rupture or removal during surgery.

- Monozygotic twins are identical because they arise from one zygote and therefore share identical chromosomes. Dizygotic twins are fraternal because they arise from two separate zygotes and therefore do not share the same chromosomes.

INTERNET RESOURCES

Visible Embryo
www.visembryo.com

IUGR
http://familydoctor.org/313.xml

Teratogens
www.ibis-birthdefects.org/start/bd.htm
www.lpch.org/diseasehealthinfo/healthlibrary/genetics/terathub.html
www.modimes.org

Ectopic Pregnancy
www.aafp.org/afp/20000215/1080.html

Workbook

■ NCLEX-STYLE REVIEW QUESTIONS

1. During which time frame does the embryonic stage last?

   a. Ovulation to conception
   b. 1 to 14 days after conception
   c. 3 through 8 weeks after conception
   d. 9 through 38 weeks after conception

2. What is the main purpose of the chorionic villi?

   a. To adhere the blastocyst to the endometrial lining
   b. To form the tissues that will become the placenta
   c. To produce amniotic fluid
   d. To provide an exchange site for the exchange of nutrients and wastes

3. Which one of the following is a fetal shunt that aids in fetal circulation?

   a. Foramen primum
   b. Foramen ovale
   c. Ductus deferens
   d. Septum secundum

4. What is the classification of twins who share the same chromosomal material?

   a. Monozygotic
   b. Dizygotic
   c. Fraternal
   d. Trizygotic

5. A woman with epilepsy was on phenytoin (Dilantin) when she became pregnant. She is very worried that her baby will have a birth defect. Which reply by the nurse is most therapeutic?

   a. "All substances and medications increase the risk of birth defects when you are pregnant. It is very important for you to discontinue any medications or over-the-counter medications immediately. This is the best way you can protect your baby."
   b. "Please don't worry. Dilantin is a very safe medication and unlikely to cause a birth defect."
   c. "Yes, Dilantin increases the risk of certain defects in the fetus; however, overall the risk is low that your baby will be affected. Your doctor weighs the risk of untreated epilepsy on the fetus with the risk of the medication when making decisions about your treatment plan."

   d. "Yes, there is a very high risk that your fetus will have major birth defects. Your doctor will most likely switch you to a safer medication. Are you on any other medications?"

■ STUDY ACTIVITIES

1. Use the following table to compare major developmental milestones at each of the indicated gestational ages. Refer to this textbook and to the following Web site: www.visembryo.com

Gestational Age	Major Developmental Milestones
4 weeks	
8 weeks	
12 weeks	
16 weeks	
20 weeks	
28 weeks	
32 weeks	
36 weeks	

2. Talk to the following individuals in your community about teratogens. Have each person discuss several substances or processes that might be damaging to the fetus and how a pregnant woman can best protect her fetus from harm.

   a. Pharmacist
   b. Obstetrician
   c. Chemist
   d. Radiologist

3. Develop a teaching plan for a pregnant adolescent. Explain the processes of fertilization and development in language she will likely understand. Prepare the answers to three to four questions you anticipate she may ask you.

■ CRITICAL THINKING: WHAT WOULD YOU DO?

Apply your knowledge of fetal development to the following situation.

1. Rebecca, a 25-year-old woman, has just discovered she is pregnant for the first time. She missed her first menstrual period 4 weeks ago and came to the office for a pregnancy test, which was positive.

   a. Rebecca asks you what her baby looks like right now. What will you tell her?

   b. Rebecca is worried because she has taken Tylenol several times during the past week for tension headaches. How will you advise her?

2. Rebecca comes in for her 12-week checkup. She measures larger than expected for dates, so the physician orders a sonogram.

   a. Rebecca asks you to tell her what her baby looks like at this stage. How will you answer?

   b. The sonogram shows that Rebecca is carrying twins. She wants to know whether they are identical or fraternal. How will you answer her?

6 *Maternal Adaptation During Pregnancy*

KEY TERMS

ballottement
Braxton Hicks contractions
Chadwick's sign
chloasma
colostrum
couvade syndrome
cretinism
diastasis recti abdominis
glycosuria
Goodell's sign
Hegar's sign
linea nigra
lordosis
Montgomery's tubercles
pica
pyrosis
scurvy
striae
supine hypotensive syndrome

LEARNING OBJECTIVES

On completion of this chapter, you should be able to:

1. Differentiate between presumptive, probable, and positive signs of pregnancy.
2. Relate normal anatomy and physiology of the nonpregnant woman to that of the pregnant woman.
3. Explain expected changes in the major body systems during pregnancy.
4. Discuss maternal physiologic adaptation to pregnancy.
5. Discuss maternal psychological adaptation to pregnancy.
6. Describe changing nutritional requirements during pregnancy and outline components of a nutritious diet for a pregnant woman.

PREGNANCY IS a time of adaptation and change not only physically, but also psychologically as the woman and her partner prepare for parenthood. The body must adapt and accommodate the needs of the growing fetus. This chapter explores the signs of pregnancy, the physiologic and psychological changes associated with pregnancy, and the changing nutritional requirements of pregnancy.

SIGNS OF PREGNANCY

A woman wants confirmation of pregnancy whether she is trying to get pregnant or thinks she might be pregnant when she was not planning a pregnancy. The physician or certified nurse midwife uses a combination of signs to diagnose pregnancy (Box 6-1). These signs can be categorized as presumptive, probable, and positive. The presumptive, or subjective, signs are the symptoms the woman experiences and reports to the health care provider. Each of these signs, taken alone, can have causes other than pregnancy. The same is true for probable or objective signs. The only signs that are 100%

diagnostic of pregnancy are the positive signs, which are objective data noted by the examiner.

Presumptive (Possible) Signs

Presumptive signs of pregnancy are subjective data that the woman reports. The most common presumptive sign of pregnancy is a missed menstrual period, or amenorrhea. There are many causes of amenorrhea. Some women have irregular periods. Emotional distress can cause a woman to skip a menstrual period. Some disorders, such as anorexia nervosa, can lead to amenorrhea. Women who perform intense exercise, such as marathon running, may experience amenorrhea. Because so many factors, other than pregnancy, can cause a woman to miss a menstrual period, amenorrhea is classified as a presumptive or subjective sign of pregnancy.

Other presumptive signs include nausea; fatigue; swollen, tender breasts; and frequent urination. Nausea can be caused by emotional distress, a viral infection, gastritis, or a host of other problems. Anemia, lack of sleep, overexertion, or infection can lead to fatigue.

Box 6-1 ▮ SIGNS OF PREGNANCY

After each symptom, an alternative cause (if any) other than pregnancy is suggested. All symptoms and times can vary in occurrence between individuals.

Presumptive (Possible) Signs

- 3–4 weeks+: Early breast changes (e.g., prickling and tingling sensations). Could be caused by oral contraceptives.
- 4 weeks+: Amenorrhea (missed period). May be caused by hormonal imbalance, emotional stress, or illness.
- 4–14 weeks: Morning sickness. May be related to gastrointestinal disorders, pyrexial illness, and so on.
- 6–12 weeks: Bladder irritability. Can be associated with urinary tract infection or pelvic tumor.

Probable Signs

- 4–12 weeks: Presence of hCG in blood. May be caused by hydatidiform mole.
- 6–12 weeks: Presence of hCG in urine. Choriocarcinoma is a possible cause.
- 8 weeks+: Uterine growth. May be caused by tumors.
- 16 weeks: Braxton Hicks (painless contractions). May be caused by upset stomach.
- 16–28 weeks: Ballottement of fetus. May be elicited by a tumor.

Positive Signs

- 6 weeks+: Visualization of fetus by ultrasound.
- 20–24 weeks+: Fetal heart sounds by fetal stethoscope (fetoscope).
- 22 weeks+: Fetal movements palpable by a trained practitioner.
- Late pregnancy: Fetal movements visible.

Adapted from material by Ian Selth, BSc Midwife. Used with permission. Retrieved November 3, 2002, from http://www.midwifery.resources.btinternet.co.uk/midwifery.htm.

Breast tissue can become swollen and tender just before a woman starts her menstrual period in response to hormonal changes. Frequent urination can result from a urinary tract infection, nervousness, or from taking in substances such as caffeine and alcohol that either act as urinary irritants, or have diuretic properties.

Probable Signs

Probable signs of pregnancy are those detected by a trained examiner. These include objective data, such as **Chadwick's sign**, the bluish-purplish color of the cervix, vagina, and perineum. The examiner identifies **Hegar's sign**, softening of the uterine isthmus, and **Goodell's sign**, softening of the cervix, during the speculum and digital pelvic examinations. Other objective signs include a change in the shape of the uterus, an enlarging uterus, and Braxton Hicks contractions. **Ballottement** occurs when the examiner pushes up on the uterine wall during a pelvic examination, then feels the fetus bounce back against the examiner's fingers. The reason these signs are considered probable, rather than positive, is that pelvic tumors and some types of cancers can cause similar signs.

Another probable sign is the pregnancy test. Although pregnancy tests performed in a laboratory are highly reliable (from 97% to 99%), there is still the small possibility for error. Pregnancy tests measure the presence of human chorionic gonadotropin (hCG) in the urine or the blood. hCG levels can be elevated in conditions other than pregnancy, such as hydatidiform mole and choriocarcinoma.

Many women use home pregnancy tests to determine if they are pregnant. These home pregnancy tests are approximately 95% reliable when they are performed correctly and done at least 10 days after the last menstrual period. It is important for the woman to know that the home pregnancy test is more likely to be correct when it reveals a positive result than when a negative result is obtained. In other words, if the home pregnancy test is negative, she should still monitor for signs of pregnancy and repeat the test or schedule an appointment with her physician.

Several types of pregnancy tests can be done in the practitioner's office. The enzyme immunoassays utilizing monoclonal antibodies specific for hCG can be done in approximately 10 minutes and are reliable within 7 or 8 days after ovulation. Enzyme immunoassays can be done on urine or the woman's serum. If urine is used, it is best to have the first voided specimen of the morning because this urine is highly concentrated, making detection of hCG easier. Serum radioimmunoassay beta subunit (RIA-hCG-b) testing measures only the beta subunit of hCG. RIA testing is highly sensitive and can help diagnose pregnancy even earlier than the enzyme immunoassay method.

Positive Signs

Positive signs are diagnostic of pregnancy because no other condition can cause the sign. The positive sign that can be elicited earliest in the pregnancy is visualization of the gestational sac or fetus. With transvaginal ultrasound, the gestational sac can be seen as early as 10 days after implantation. The fetal outline and cardiac activity are visible by abdominal ultrasound at 7 to 8 weeks.

The fetal heartbeat, heard at 9 to 10 weeks with Doppler technology and by 18 to 20 weeks with a fetoscope, is a positive sign of pregnancy. Palpation of fetal movements by a trained examiner is a positive sign of pregnancy after the 20th week.

PHYSIOLOGIC ADAPTATION TO PREGNANCY

The woman's body must make tremendous changes to accommodate a pregnancy (Table 6-1). While she is pregnant, her body must maintain all her vital functions and those of the growing fetus. Some changes are structural and occur because of pressure exerted by the growing fetus and expanding uterus. Other changes are hormone related. The next section discusses the physiologic changes that occur during pregnancy by body system.

Reproductive Changes

Obviously, the reproductive system changes during pregnancy. Instead of shedding endometrial tissue every month,

---

Table 6-1 ▌ ANATOMY AND PHYSIOLOGY COMPARISON: NONPREGNANT TO PREGNANT WOMAN

System or Structure	Nonpregnant Characteristics	Pregnant Characteristics (At Term, Unless Otherwise Indicated)
Uterus	Weight: 70 g Uterine cavity capacity: 10 mL Structure: Almost solid Shape: Pear shaped Location: Pelvis Percentage of cardiac output supplying all abdominal organs combined: 24%	Weight: 1,100 g Uterine cavity capacity: 5 L average, but may expand to as much as 20 L Structure: Thin, muscular sac Shape: Globular Location: Fills the abdominal cavity Percentage of cardiac output supplying uterus/pelvic cavity alone: 20%
Breasts	Soft, nontender tissue Soft, nonprominent, relatively smooth areola	Tenderness in the first few weeks of pregnancy. Nodularity of breast tissue. Prominent areola with deepened pigmentation and prominent projections of Montgomery's tubercles.
Thyroid gland	Total gland volume: 12.1 mL	Total gland volume: 15.0 mL
Blood	Blood volume: 5 L Red blood cell volume: 2 L Plasma volume: 3 L Hemoglobin: 12–16 g/100 mL Hematocrit: 36%–46% White blood cell count: 4,500–11,000/mm^3	Blood volume increases by 40%–50% (could be as high as 7.5 L) Red blood cell volume increases by as much as 30% (2.6 L) Plasma volume increases by 50% (4.5 L) Hemoglobin: 11–12 g/100 mL Hematocrit: Decreases, particularly in the third trimester as plasma volume increases White blood cell (WBC) count: As great as 16,000 mm^3 (in labor the WBC count can reach as high as 25,000 mm^3)
Coagulation	Fibrinogen levels: 200–400 mg/dL Factors VII, VIII, and X: Normal	Fibrinogen levels: Values may be as high as 600 mg/dL Factors VII, VIII, and X: Increase by 20%–100% In general, pregnancy is considered to be a state of hypercoagulability.
Heart	Blood pressure in normal range: 90–140 mm Hg systolic and 60–90 mm Hg diastolic Heart rate 60–100 beats per minute Cardiac output: Approximately 5 L per minute	Blood pressure decreases slightly, particularly in the second trimester Heart rate increases by 10–15 beats per minute Cardiac output increases (as much as 40%–50%) beginning by the 5th week gestation
Respiratory	Respiratory rate: 16–20 breaths per minute Nasal mucosa thin and moist Tidal volume (the volume of air moved during normal inspiration and expiration): 500 mL Oxygen consumption normal for adult female PaCO$_2$: 35–45 mm Hg	Respiratory rate: Unchanged or increased by 2–3 breaths per minute Nasal mucosa edematous due to vasocongestion. Tidal volume: 700 mL Oxygen consumption increases by 14% Average PaCO$_2$: 32 mm Hg

Source: Cunningham, F. G., Leveno, K. J., Bloom, S. L., Hauth, J. C., Gilstrap, L. C. III, & Wenstrom, K. D. (2005). Maternal physiology. In *Williams obstetrics* (22nd ed., pp. 121–150). New York: McGraw-Hill Medical Publishing Division.

the uterus must maintain the decidua (the name for the endometrium during pregnancy). The myometrium (uterine muscle) must stay relatively relaxed. If it contracts too forcefully, the pregnancy will be lost. The uterus undergoes changes immediately after conception and continues to grow and change throughout the pregnancy. The cervix, vagina, perineum, and breasts also undergo changes.

Uterus

During the first weeks after conception, the uterine muscle cells begin to hypertrophy, causing the uterus to expand. It is thought that estrogen stimulates this muscle cell hypertrophy. At first, the uterine walls become thicker, but as the pregnancy progresses, the growing fetus and accessory structures begin to exert pressure so that the uterus enlarges and the uterine walls become thinner. By the end of the 12th week, the uterus expands upward into the abdominal cavity. At 16 weeks, the fundus can be palpated approximately halfway between the symphysis pubis and the umbilicus. At 20 weeks, the fundus reaches the level of the umbilicus. By the end of the pregnancy, the uterus occupies much of the abdominal cavity (Fig. 6-1).

Beginning in the first trimester, the uterus begins to contract sporadically. These contractions are usually painless and do not cause cervical changes. By the second trimester, these contractions are palpable. **Braxton Hicks contractions**, the painless, intermittent, "practice"

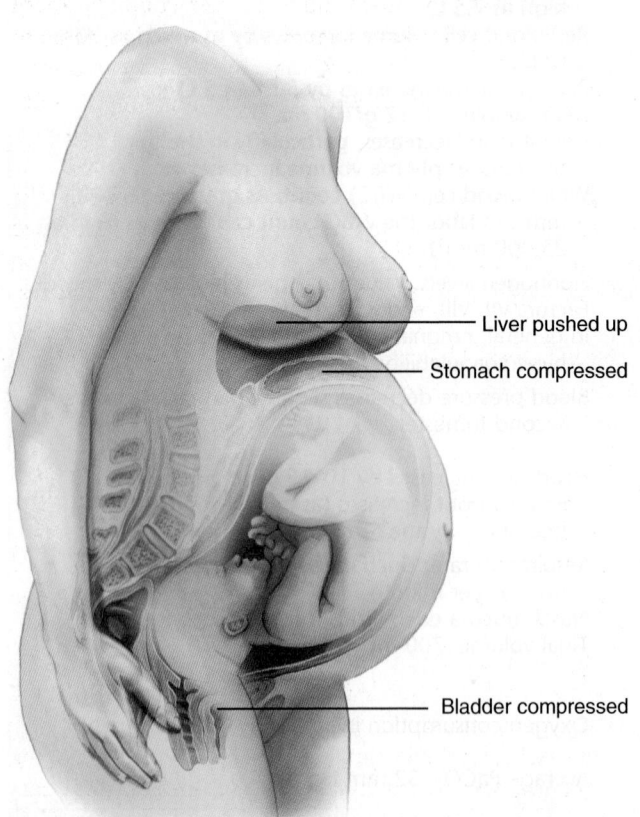

Liver pushed up

Stomach compressed

Bladder compressed

■ **Figure 6-1** The growing uterus in the abdomen.

contractions of pregnancy, are named after the physician who first wrote about them, Braxton Hicks. During the third trimester, as the pregnancy approaches term, Braxton Hicks contractions become more frequent and can sometimes cause discomfort. As the time for labor draws near, the contractions can become somewhat regular, causing the woman to think that she is in labor. This is the cause of so-called false labor.

Blood supply to the uterus increases dramatically throughout pregnancy. Under the influence of estrogen, new blood vessels grow in the placenta and uterine walls, and vasodilation occurs in maternal vessels to allow increased blood flow to the uterus and placenta. The diameter of the uterine artery increases during pregnancy. By 20 weeks, it doubles in diameter from the nonpregnant state.

Cervix and Ovaries

The cervix undergoes characteristic changes under the influence of estrogen and progesterone. Vascularity is increased, and glandular tissue multiplies during pregnancy. The vascular congestion and increase in glandular tissue is responsible for Goodell's, Hegar's, and Chadwick's signs. Shortly after conception, a thick mucous plug develops in the opening of the cervix, which helps to protect the uterine cavity from infection. The mucous plug is expelled shortly before, or at the beginning of labor. Small capillaries break when the plug is expelled, causing a bloody show.

Follicles in the ovaries do not mature during pregnancy, and ovulation stops. The corpus luteum continues to function and produces progesterone for approximately 6 to 7 weeks. If the corpus luteum stops functioning before that time, a spontaneous abortion (miscarriage) will occur. After 7 weeks, the placenta produces enough progesterone to maintain the pregnancy.

Vagina and Perineum

The vagina and perineum are affected by hormonal changes and increased blood supply to the area. The

You can help.
Encourage the woman who is less than 37 weeks' to report contractions that do not go away with rest, or are accompanied by cramping, pain, or low backache. These are signs of preterm labor.

This will reassure your patient.
Because the cervix increases in vascularity during pregnancy, a pelvic examination can rupture capillaries and cause spotting. After a pelvic exam, inform the woman that she can expect some spotting, particularly when she wipes after voiding.

vagina takes on a bluish-purplish hue, Chadwick's sign, because of vascular congestion. The vagina and cervix produce copious secretions because of the increased blood flow to the area.

Breasts

In the first few weeks of pregnancy, the breasts become tender and the woman may feel tingling sensations. As pregnancy progresses, the breasts increase in size under the influence of estrogen. Prolactin, an anterior pituitary hormone, stimulates glandular production, causing the breast tissue to feel nodular. The areolas darken. **Montgomery's tubercles**, sebaceous glands on the areolas, produce secretions that lubricate the nipple. Montgomery's tubercles become more prominent during pregnancy. Tiny veins become visible on the surface of the breasts. **Striae**, more commonly known as stretch marks, sometimes appear. Striae appear reddish at first, then gradually fade to a light silvery color after childbirth.

As the mammary glands develop, the breasts begin to produce and secrete **colostrum**, a thick, yellow fluid that precedes milk production. Colostrum is sometimes referred to as the "foremilk." During the first 3 days of breast-feeding, colostrum is the nourishment the baby receives. It is rich in antibodies and protein.

Endocrine Changes

The hormonal changes that occur in pregnancy are tremendous. Rising levels of certain pregnancy hormones cause changes in almost every body system. The placental hormones are discussed in Chapter 5. Changes in the endocrine system itself occur during pregnancy. The pituitary gland enlarges by 135%, compared with its nonpregnant size. In fact, pregnancy could not occur without the interaction of the pituitary hormones, follicle-stimulating hormone, and luteinizing hormone.

Prolactin levels increase progressively during pregnancy. Although this hormone is not necessary for the successful completion of pregnancy, it is crucial for the initiation of lactation (production of breast milk). Oxytocin, a posterior pituitary hormone, is responsible for the rhythmic uterine contractions of labor. Oxytocin stimulates the letdown reflex during breast-feeding and stimulates the uterus to continue contracting after delivery to control maternal bleeding.

Increased protein binding during pregnancy affects most endocrine glands. Hyperplasia of glandular tissue and increased vascularity cause the thyroid gland to increase in size. The need for insulin is increased. Some women have borderline pancreatic activity when they are not pregnant. During pregnancy, these women develop gestational diabetes because the borderline pancreas cannot handle the increased demands placed upon it.

Test Yourself

✔ List three positive signs of pregnancy.
✔ Describe three changes that occur in breast tissue during pregnancy.
✔ What is the purpose of the hormone prolactin?

Hematologic Changes

Blood volume increases by approximately 40% to 45% above pre-pregnancy levels by the end of the third trimester. Blood plasma and red blood cells (RBCs) both increase in volume, although plasma volumes increase at a higher percentage (50%) than do RBCs (30%). This physiologic hemodilution causes a slight decrease in hemoglobin and hematocrit levels. The average hemoglobin level at term is 12.5 g/dL. The hemoglobin level is considered normal until it falls below 11.0 g/dL. It is important to note that in the absence of sufficient iron, RBC volume increases by only 18%, rather than 30%.

Some blood clotting factors, such as fibrinogen and others, increase during pregnancy, making pregnancy a hypercoagulable state. However, clotting times and bleeding times remain within normal limits. The enlarging uterus inhibits blood return from the lower extremities, a situation that can cause venous stasis. A combination of venous stasis and hypercoagulability places the pregnant woman at risk for venous thrombosis (clot formation).

The increased blood volume and hypercoagulability of the blood serve protective functions during pregnancy. The expanded blood volume helps meet the needs of the enlarging uterus. It helps protect the woman and the fetus from harmful effects of decreased venous return when the woman is standing or lying supine, and enhances the exchange of nutrients and respiratory gases between the pregnant woman and fetus. The increased blood volume and hypercoagulable state serve to protect the woman from the blood loss that normally occurs during delivery.

Cardiovascular Changes

Pregnancy places tremendous demands upon the cardiovascular system. The heart has to handle the increased load of an expanded blood volume. It also must adjust to the demands of organ systems with increased workloads, such as the kidneys and uterus. In addition, the heart is physically pushed upward and to the left by the enlarging uterus, which may cause systolic murmurs.

Normally, the blood pressure decreases slightly during pregnancy, particularly in the second trimester. The heart rate rises by 10 to 15 beats per minute on average. Cardiac output increases, beginning in the early weeks of pregnancy and continuing throughout pregnancy.

A Supine position   **B** Side-lying position

■ **Figure 6-2** Supine hypotension can occur if a pregnant woman lies on her back. **(A)** The weight of the uterus compresses the vena cava, trapping blood in the lower extremities. **(B)** If a woman turns on her side, pressure is lifted off of the vena cava.

When the woman lies flat on her back in the latter half of pregnancy, the uterus and its contents compress the aorta and vena cava against the spine (Fig. 6-2). This compression decreases the amount of blood returned to the heart; therefore, the cardiac output and the blood pressure fall, leading to **supine hypotensive syndrome.** The woman may feel lightheaded and dizzy; her skin may exhibit pallor and clamminess. The cure (and prevention) is for the woman to rest on her side. The traditional position is left side-lying.

> **An ounce of prevention . . .**
> Advise the woman not to lie on her back in late pregnancy to prevent supine hypotension. If she wishes to lie on her back, instruct her to place a pillow under her right hip to enhance blood flow through the great vessels.

Respiratory Changes

The respiratory system must accommodate the changing needs and demands of pregnancy. Vasocongestion of the upper respiratory tract lining causes symptoms similar to that of the common cold. The nasal congestion and voice changes may persist throughout pregnancy. The nasal lining is more fragile, increasing the likelihood of nose-bleeds. It is thought that estrogen influences these characteristic changes.

As the uterus enlarges, it pushes up on the diaphragm. The body compensates for this crowding by increasing the anteroposterior and transverse diameters of the chest so that total lung capacity stays approximately the same as it was before pregnancy. Ligaments that loosen under the influence of hormones (probably progesterone) allow for the increased thoracic diameters.

The woman becomes more aware of the need to breathe and may feel short of breath even when she is not. In the third trimester, pressure exerted on the diaphragm from the expanding uterus can also cause the woman to feel dyspneic.

Musculoskeletal Changes

Lordosis, an increased curvature of the spine, becomes more pronounced in the later weeks of pregnancy (Fig. 6-3), as the expanding uterus alters the center of gravity. Lordosis helps counterbalance the effect of the protruding abdomen and keeps the center of balance over the lower extremities. The increased curvature can result in low backache. Hormonal influences on pelvic joints cause them to increase in mobility, which contributes to lower back discomfort and causes the characteristic waddling gait of pregnancy.

The enlarging uterus puts pressure on the broad and round ligaments that support it. Prolonged pressure can lead to round ligament pain. A woman who has been pregnant several times or a woman who is carrying twins is more likely to experience **diastasis recti abdominis,** separation of the rectus abdominis muscle that supports the abdomen.

> *Test Yourself*
> ✔ By what percentage does blood volume increase during pregnancy?
> ✔ By how much is cardiac output expected to increase?
> ✔ Define diastasis recti abdominis.

12 weeks   20 weeks   28 weeks   36 weeks   40 weeks

■ **Figure 6-3** Postural changes during pregnancy. Notice how the lumbar and thoracic curves become more pronounced as pregnancy progresses.

Gastrointestinal Changes

Nausea and vomiting are common in the first trimester under the influence of rising hCG levels. Occasionally a large increase in saliva production (ptyalism) occurs. The gums may become tender and bleed easily.

As the uterus expands upward into the abdominal cavity, the intestines are displaced to the sides and upward. The stomach is pushed upward and compressed (see Fig. 6-1). The lower esophageal sphincter relaxes under the influence of hormones. Pressures in the esophagus are lower than in the nonpregnant state, whereas pressures within the stomach increase. These changes lead to an increased incidence of **pyrosis**, heartburn caused by acid reflux through the relaxed lower esophageal sphincter.

Displacement of the intestines and possible slowed motility of the gastrointestinal tract under the influence of progesterone may lead to delayed gastric emptying and decreased peristalsis. As a result of these changes, the pregnant woman is predisposed to constipation. Constipation and elevated pressures in the veins below the uterus contribute to hemorrhoid development.

Progesterone interferes with normal gallbladder contraction, leading to stasis of bile. Cholestasis and increased cholesterol levels increase the risk of gallstone formation. Cholestasis can occur within the liver and lead to pruritus (itching).

Urinary Changes

Renal and ureteral dilation occur as a result of hormonal changes and mechanical pressure of the growing uterus on the ureters. The dilation causes an increase in kidney size, particularly on the right side. Peristalsis decreases in the urinary tract, leading to urinary stasis with a resultant increased risk for pyelonephritis.

The glomerular filtration rate rises by as much as 50% because of increased cardiac output and decreased renal vascular resistance. The rise in glomerular filtration rate occurs as early as the 10th week and is largely responsible for the increased urinary frequency noted in the first trimester. Urinary frequency is not a common complaint in the second trimester but occurs again in the third trimester because of the pressure of the expanding uterus on the bladder (see Fig. 6-1).

Glycosuria, glucose in the urine, may occur normally because the kidney tubules are not able to reabsorb as much glucose as they were before pregnancy. However, if the woman is spilling glucose in her urine, additional testing is warranted to rule out gestational diabetes. Protein is not normally found in the urine of a pregnant woman.

Integumentary Changes

Many skin changes in pregnancy result from hyperpigmentation. The so-called mask of pregnancy, **chloasma**, can appear as brown blotchy areas on the forehead,

■ **Figure 6-4** Linea nigra.

cheeks, and nose of the pregnant woman. This condition may be permanent, or it may regress between pregnancies. The skin in the middle of the abdomen may develop a darkened line called the **linea nigra** (Fig. 6-4). Striae (stretch marks) may appear on the abdomen in response to elevated glucocorticoid levels. As discussed in the section on breast tissue, the striae appear reddish and are more noticeable during pregnancy. After pregnancy, they tend to fade and become silvery-white in color.

Test Yourself

✔ List two reasons the pregnant woman is predisposed to pyrosis.

✔ Name two urinary changes normally experienced during pregnancy.

✔ List two conditions that result from hyperpigmentation during pregnancy.

PSYCHOLOGICAL ADAPTATION TO PREGNANCY

While adapting to rapid changes in physiology, the pregnant woman also must come to grips with her new role as parent. No matter how many children the woman has, each new pregnancy brings with it a role change. Adjusting to the role of parenting is a process that occurs throughout pregnancy and beyond.

Many factors influence how a woman adjusts to her role as parent. Societal expectations and cultural values may dictate the way a woman responds to pregnancy and the idea of parenthood. Family influences are usually very strong. The way the woman was raised and the values surrounding children and parenthood in her family of origin color the way a woman adapts to pregnancy. Her own personality and ability to adapt to change influences her response. Even her past experiences with pregnancy have an effect on the way she deals with the current pregnancy. For example, if she has a history of a stillbirth, she may not fully accept the pregnancy or begin to bond with the baby until he is born.

Social support is critical during pregnancy. If the woman is in a long-term relationship and feels supported, she will be much better prepared to handle the demands of pregnancy than if she feels alone and isolated without support. If the woman does not have a supportive partner, it is important for her to identify someone with whom she can share the experience of pregnancy. Often this will be a female friend, or perhaps the woman's own mother.

First-Trimester Task: Accept the Pregnancy

Pregnancy is a development stage, and as such, psychological tasks of pregnancy have been identified. The first task of pregnancy is to accept the pregnancy. This task is

A Personal Glimpse

When I first found out that I was pregnant, I started shaking. I couldn't believe that I was pregnant. My husband and I didn't plan for this to happen so soon. We had wanted to wait about 8 more months before beginning our family. We weren't ready; we had only been married 5 months. We still had some financial debt to pay off, and we had certain goals we wanted to meet.

We both wanted and loved children very much. In fact, we both wanted, and planned, to have three children. However, it was the timing that was wrong. I couldn't even tell my husband the news because he was away for several weeks. This added to my anxiety. Not only was I worried about my ability to be a mother, but I was worried that I may have eaten or been exposed to something harmful to my baby before knowing I was pregnant. I ended up confiding in my mother and best friends who truly helped me to calm down and get a grip.

I started to relax and accept the fact that, although my timing was off, this was pretty exciting. When I was finally able to tell my husband, he just beamed with joy. I knew in that moment that everything would be all right.

Sandra

Learning Opportunity: How would you advise this mother-to-be regarding her feelings when she found out that she was pregnant? How can the nurse help the woman and her family deal with the emotions that surround finding out about a pregnancy?

usually met during the first trimester, although some women have difficulty fully accepting the pregnancy until they can feel the baby move.

Initially the woman may be shocked that she is pregnant. Or she may be ecstatic or excited. There are a myriad of emotions that a woman may experience when she first hears the news that she is pregnant. Even if the pregnancy is desired intensely, a certain amount of ambivalence is a normal initial response to pregnancy. Ambivalence refers to the feelings of uncertainty most women must deal with in the early weeks of pregnancy. The woman may have tried to get pregnant for a while before conceiving, and now that the pregnancy has occurred, she may have second thoughts or doubts about her ability to be a good parent. Or the pregnancy may have been unplanned, so she must sort through her feelings about this unexpected demand that has been placed upon her. It may be helpful for her to hear that ambivalence is a healthy response because she may feel guilty about her uncertainty.

Acceptance can be healing.
Listen to your patient. If she wishes to talk, encourage her and use active listening skills. Tell her it is normal to experience a wide array of feelings during pregnancy.

As the woman experiences the early physiologic changes of pregnancy, she gradually comes to accept that she is pregnant. She is usually introverted and focused on herself during the first trimester. The nausea associated with early pregnancy may leave her feeling sick and irritable. She may be fatigued. Often, she is moody and sensitive.

It is important to be supportive of the woman's partner during this time. He (or she, if the woman is in a lesbian relationship) also must deal with feelings of ambivalence. In addition to accepting the pregnancy, the partner must learn to accept the pregnant woman as she changes with pregnancy. The mood swings, sensitivity, and irritability can make it difficult to cope. Jealousy of the unborn child can occur. It can be difficult to adjust to the introversion and self-focus of the woman. Often, the partner is relieved to learn that the changes his partner is going through are normal responses to pregnancy.

Second-Trimester Task: Accept the Baby

Generally, during the first trimester, the woman is focused on the pregnancy and on accepting this new reality as being part of her identity. Gradually, as the pregnancy progresses, she comes to have a sense of the child as his own separate entity. This acceptance may be enhanced when she first hears the fetal heart beat, when she feels the baby move inside her, or when she sees the fetal image during a sonogram.

As she comes to accept the uniqueness of her baby, she may begin to shop for baby clothes or prepare the nursery. When an ultrasound is done in the second trimester, it is generally possible to detect the sex of the child. The couple may name the baby once they know if it is a boy or a girl.

During the second trimester, the woman may become more extroverted. She often feels much better once the nausea and fatigue of the first trimester have passed. She starts to show so that the pregnancy becomes apparent to those around her, and she may have the glow of pregnancy. Frequently, the second trimester is a happy time. The woman may enjoy the extra attention and deference society gives to pregnant women.

It is important to remember that the partner is experiencing the pregnancy along with the woman. Some fathers actually experience some of the physical symptoms of pregnancy, such as nausea and vomiting, along with their partner. This phenomenon is called **couvade syndrome.** It may be easier for the man to accept his partner now that she is feeling better and is less introverted. In any event, it is important to encourage the couple to communicate their needs effectively to each other. Each needs the support of the other.

Third-Trimester Task: Prepare for Parenthood

Nesting instincts often begin in the third trimester. The couple may prepare the nursery and shop for baby furniture and clothes. A name may be chosen. The woman usually has a heightened interest in safe passage for herself and the baby during labor.

Toward the end of pregnancy, most women begin to feel tired of being pregnant. Many discomforts of pregnancy arise during the third trimester. It may be difficult to get comfortable at night, and so it may be hard to get a good night's sleep. Backache and round ligament pain may be bothersome. Urinary frequency often returns as the gravid uterus presses down against the bladder. Braxton Hicks contractions may become uncomfortable and more frequent. It is important to be supportive of the woman and listen to her concerns.

It is helpful for the couple to attend childbirth preparation classes, which are often offered in the third trimester. Not only does the couple learn techniques to help them prepare for labor, but they are also able to interact with other couples who are facing issues similar to their own. The social aspect of childbirth preparation can be a powerful source of support to the woman and her partner.

Be careful not to jump to conclusions!

Do not make the mistake of thinking that the woman has not yet accepted the baby if she does not name the baby during pregnancy. Some parents do not decide on a name until several days after the baby is born.

Test Yourself

✔ Describe two psychological characteristics normally associated with a woman in the first trimester of pregnancy.

✔ Which trimester of pregnancy is often the happiest for the woman?

✔ List two activities many women perform in the third trimester.

CHANGING NUTRITIONAL REQUIREMENTS OF PREGNANCY

Nutrition is an area that requires special attention during pregnancy, particularly during the second and third trimesters. The fetus needs nutrients and energy to build new tissue, and the woman needs nutrients to build her blood volume and maternal stores. There is an increased demand for energy and for almost every nutrient type. Most nutrient requirements can be met through careful attention to diet, although there are several nutrients that require supplementation during pregnancy. The U.S. Department of Agriculture and U.S. Department of Health and Human Services provide an interactive Web site, www.mypyramid.gov, where an individual can enter his or her personal information and receive an individualized nutrition plan based on MyPyramid. Figure 6-5 shows MyPyramid guidelines by trimester for the pregnant woman.

Energy Requirements and Weight Gain

Energy requirements increase during pregnancy because of fetal tissue development and increased maternal stores. During the first trimester, the recommended weight gain is 3 to 4 lb total. Subsequently, for the remainder of pregnancy the recommendation is roughly 1 lb/week, for a total weight gain of 25 to 35 lb for a woman who begins pregnancy with a normal body mass index (BMI).[1] Total weight gain recommendations vary depending upon the woman's prepregnancy BMI. A woman who is underweight when she enters pregnancy (low BMI) should gain 28 to 40 lb, whereas a woman who has a high BMI (overweight) is recommended to gain 15 to 25 lb during the pregnancy (March of Dimes, Undated).

Failure to gain enough weight, and in particular gaining less than 16 lb during pregnancy, has been associated with an increased risk of delivering a low-birth-weight baby (<2,500 g or 5.5 lb). Low birth weight has consistently been associated with poor neonatal outcomes. Conversely, a woman who gains too much weight is at

---

[1]BMI refers to body weight corrected for height of the person. Normal BMI is 18.5 to 24.9. An individual can calculate his or her BMI on-line at http://www.nhlbisupport.com/bmi/.

MyPyramid Plan for Moms

Food Group	1st Trimester	2nd and 3rd Trimesters	What counts as 1 cup or 1 oz?	Remember to...
	Eat this amount from each group daily.*			
Fruits	2 cups	2 cups	1 cup fruit or juice, ½ cup dried fruit	*Focus on fruits*—Eat a variety of fruit.
Vegetables	2½ cups	3 cups	1 cup raw or cooked vegetables or juice, 2 cups raw leafy vegetables	*Vary your veggies*—Eat more dark green and orange vegetables and cooked dry beans.
Grains	6 oz	8 oz	1 slice bread; ½ cup cooked pasta, rice, cereal; 1 oz ready-to-eat cereal	*Make half your grains whole*—Choose whole instead of refined grains.
Meat and Beans	5½ oz	6½ oz	1 ounce lean meat, poultry, fish; 1 egg; ¼ cup cooked dry beans; ½ oz nuts; 1 Tbsp peanut butter	*Go lean with protein*—Choose low-fat or lean meats and poultry.
Milk	3 cups	3 cups	1 cup milk, 8 oz yogurt, 1½ oz cheese, 2 oz processed cheese	*Get your calcium-rich foods*—Go low-fat or fat-free when you choose milk, yogurt, and cheese.

*These amounts are for an average pregnant woman. You may need more or less than the average. Check with your doctor to make sure you are gaining weight as you should.

■ Figure 6-5 MyPyramid adapted for pregnant women (From the U.S. Department of Agriculture and the U.S. Department of Health and Human Services).

increased risk for delivering a macrosomic (≥4,000 g or 8.5 lb) baby. High-birth-weight babies experience complications and poor outcomes more frequently than do babies with normal birth weights. A woman who gains too much weight also is at greater risk of requiring cesarean section (Gillen-Goldstein, Funai, & Roqué, 2007).

Many women assume falsely that eating for two requires a significantly increased caloric intake. In fact, the required caloric increase during the first trimester is negligible. During the second and third trimesters, approximately 300 kcal/day are required above the woman's prepregnancy needs. It is important that the diet supply enough calories to meet energy needs; otherwise, protein will be broken down to supply energy, rather than to build fetal and maternal tissue.

Protein Requirements

Protein needs are increased during pregnancy because of growth and repair of fetal tissue, placenta, uterus, breasts, and maternal blood volume. It is recommended that the pregnant woman obtain adequate protein from animal sources, including milk and milk products. Milk is an excellent source of protein and calcium for the pregnant and breast-feeding woman. As stated previously, it is important for the woman to have adequate caloric intake to preserve protein stores for tissue building and repair. When protein is used to supply energy, there is less available for fetal, placental, and maternal tissue growth needs.

During the average pregnancy, approximately 1,000 g of additional protein above the woman's basal needs are used. The fetus and placenta account for 500 g of added protein. The other 500 g is distributed among uterine muscle cells, mammary glandular tissue, and maternal blood in the form of hemoglobin and plasma proteins. The woman needs to take in 5 to 6 g of protein per day above her nonpregnant requirements in order to meet the additional demands (Gillen-Goldstein, Funai, & Roqué, 2007).

Mineral Requirements

The woman can obtain most minerals from a varied diet without supplementation, even during pregnancy. However, it is important for a pregnant woman to get sufficient amounts of minerals to prevent deficiencies in the growing fetus and maternal stores. Table 6-2 compares the Recommended Daily Dietary Allowances (RDA) of selected vitamins and minerals for nonpregnant, pregnant, and lactating women of childbearing age.

Iron

Iron is necessary for the formation of hemoglobin; therefore, it is essential to the oxygen-carrying capacity of the blood. If a woman's diet is iron deficient during pregnancy, her RBC volume will increase by only 18%; whereas, adequate supplementation of iron results in a 30% increase in RBC volume. This extra "cushion" of RBC volume increases the amount of oxygen available at the placenta for the fetus and helps protect the woman from the effects of blood loss after delivery.

Total iron requirements of pregnancy equal 1,000 mg. The fetus and placenta use 300 mg. Two hundred milligrams are lost through various routes of excretion, even when the woman is iron deficient. Five hundred milligrams are needed to supply the additional 450 mL of maternal RBCs. Almost all of these additional iron requirements are needed during the second half of pregnancy, so the need for iron increases dramatically after 20 weeks. If the woman is iron deficient, she will develop anemia. However, the fetus will get the iron needed to manufacture its RBCs. This is one instance in which nature robs from the woman to adequately supply the fetus.

It is almost impossible for the woman to receive an adequate amount of iron from diet alone. Therefore, it is recommended that the pregnant woman take iron supplementation. Sometimes the physician elects to omit the iron supplement during the first trimester because supplemental iron often intensifies the nausea and vomiting of early pregnancy. The dose varies depending on the individual needs of the woman. If she enters pregnancy with normal hemoglobin and hematocrit values, she will require lower doses of iron than if she is anemic when she becomes pregnant. A woman carrying twins or an obese woman will both require higher doses of supplemental iron.

Calcium

Calcium needs are not increased above pre-pregnancy levels (1,000 mg/day), mainly because pregnancy enhances calcium absorption. However, it is important for the pregnant woman to obtain sufficient amounts of calcium. Calcium is needed for a variety of bodily processes, including nerve cell transmission, muscle contraction, bone building, and blood clotting. Recent research has demonstrated that calcium supplementation during pregnancy can cut in half the risk of preeclampsia, a pregnancy-related condition that can lead to severe complications. Further studies are needed to determine the ideal dosage (Hofmeyr, Atallah, & Duley, 2007).

Calcium continuously moves between bone and blood because a precise amount is needed in the blood to maintain normal muscle contraction (including cardiac muscle contraction). Normally the movement of calcium in and out of bones is balanced—there is neither a net gain nor a net loss. However, if insufficient amounts are ingested, or if calcium is not absorbed from the gastrointestinal tract, the body will take calcium from the bones to maintain blood levels. This process will also occur to meet the calcium needs of the growing fetus.

Vitamin D is necessary for adequate absorption of calcium. The amount of vitamin D obtained from 10 to 20 minutes of exposure to sunlight per day is normally sufficient. If this source is not readily available, vitamin D is also present in fortified milk products.

Phosphorus

Phosphorus is readily available in a wide variety of foods. The pregnant woman normally has no trouble obtaining sufficient amounts of this nutrient. Intake of excessive amounts of phosphorus can inhibit calcium absorption. However, calcium metabolism requires a normal amount of phosphorus to build strong bones. The key to calcium and phosphorus consumption is to keep the two nutrients in balance.

Zinc

Zinc is needed during pregnancy to provide for fetal growth and during lactation for milk production. Because zinc is needed for nucleic acid synthesis and protein metabolism, adequate amounts are particularly important during early pregnancy when fetal body systems are developing. Milk production requires higher levels of zinc than the fetus demands during pregnancy; therefore, the RDA for zinc during lactation is higher than the RDA for pregnancy. Foods that contain zinc include meat, seafood, and to a lesser extent, whole grains.

Iodine

Iodine is needed for normal thyroid activity. Women with severe iodine deficiencies deliver infants with **cretinism,** a congenital condition marked by stunted growth and mental retardation. Recent studies have linked subclinical hypothyroidism with increased rates of mental retardation.

Table 6-2 ▌ COMPARISON OF RECOMMENDED DAILY DIETARY ALLOWANCES (RDA) FOR SELECTED VITAMINS AND MINERALS FOR NONPREGNANT, PREGNANT, AND LACTATING WOMEN AGES 19 TO 30 YEARS

Mineral/ Vitamin	Function	RDA for Nonpregnant Women	RDA for Pregnant Women	RDA for Lactating Women	Selected Food Sources
Calcium (mg/day)	Essential role in blood clotting, muscle contraction, nerve transmission, and bone and tooth formation.	1,000	1,000	1,000	Dairy products: milk, cheese, yogurt. Corn tortillas, calcium-set tofu, Chinese cabbage, kale, broccoli
Copper (mcg/day)	Component of enzymes in iron metabolism.	900	1,000	1,300	Organ meats, seafood, nuts, seeds, wheat bran cereals, whole grain products, cocoa products
Iodine (mcg/day)	Component of thyroid hormones and prevents goiter and cretinism.	150	220	290	Foods of marine origin, processed foods, iodized salt
Iron (mg/day)	Component of hemoglobin and numerous enzymes; prevents microcytic hypochromic anemia.	18	27	9	Fruits, vegetables and fortified bread and grain products, such as cereal (nonheme iron sources), meat and poultry (heme iron sources)
Vitamin A (mcg/day)	Required for normal vision, gene expression, reproduction, embryonic development and immune function	700	770	1,300	Liver, dairy products, fish (preformed Vitamin A sources); and carrots, sweet potatoes, mango, spinach, cantaloupe, kale, apricots (beta-carotene sources)
Vitamin B_1 (thiamin) (mg/day)	Coenzyme in the metabolism of carbohydrates and branched-chain amino acids	1.1	1.4	1.4	Enriched, fortified, or whole-brain products; bread and bread products, mixed foods whose main ingredient is grain, and ready-to-eat cereals
Vitamin B_2 (riboflavin) (mg/day)	Coenzyme in numerous redox reactions	1.1	1.4	1.6	Organ meats, milk, bread products, and fortified cereals
Vitamin B_3 (niacin) (mg/day)	Required for energy metabolism	14	18	17	Meat, fish, poultry, enriched and whole-grain breads and bread products, and fortified ready-to-eat cereals
Vitamin B_6 (pyridoxine) (mg/day)	Coenzyme in the metabolism of amino acids, glycogen, and sphingoid bases	1.3	1.9	2.0	Fortified cereals, organ meats, fortified soy-based meat substitutes
Vitamin B_9 (folacin, folate, folic acid) (mcg/day)	Coenzyme in the metabolism of nucleic and amino acids; prevents megaloblastic anemia; in pregnancy folate deficiency is linked to an increased risk for neural tube defects	400	600	500	Enriched cereal grains, dark leafy vegetables, enriched and whole-grain breads and bread products, fortified ready-to-eat cereals

(continued)

Table 6-2 ▌ COMPARISON OF RECOMMENDED DAILY DIETARY ALLOWANCES (RDA) FOR SELECTED VITAMINS AND MINERALS FOR NONPREGNANT, PREGNANT, AND LACTATING WOMEN AGES 19 TO 30 YEARS *(continued)*

Mineral/ Vitamin	Function	RDA for Nonpregnant Women	RDA for Pregnant Women	RDA for Lactating Women	Selected Food Sources
Vitamin B$_{12}$ (Cobalamine) (mcg/day)	Coenzyme in nucleic acid metabolism; prevents megaloblastic anemia	2.4	2.6	2.8	Fortified cereals, meat, fish, and poultry
Vitamin C (ascorbic acid) (mg/day)	Necessary for collagen synthesis and wound healing and as a protective antioxidant	75	85	120	Citrus fruits, tomatoes, tomato juice, potatoes, brussels sprouts, cauliflower, broccoli, strawberries, cabbage, and spinach
Vitamin D (calciferol) (mcg/day)	Maintain serum calcium and phosphorus concentrations	5	5	5	Fish liver oils, flesh of fatty fish, liver and fat from seals and polar bears, eggs from hens fed vitamin D fortified milk products, and fortified cereals
Zinc (mg/day)	Component of multiple enzymes and proteins; involved in the regulation of gene expression	8	11	12	Fortified cereals, red meats, certain seafood

Source for the RDAs: The National Academy of Sciences, (Eds.). (2004). Dietary reference intakes (DRIs): Recommended intakes for individuals, vitamins & elements. Retrieved October 13, 2007, from http://www.iom.edu/Object.File/Master/21/372/0.pdf

Most women in the United States get sufficient amounts of iodine, but during pregnancy, a woman loses larger amounts of iodine in the urine than when she is not pregnant. The current recommendation is for all pregnant women to use iodized salt versus routine supplementation (ICCIDD, 2007).

Vitamin Requirements

Vitamins are known catalysts for many chemical reactions in the body. A varied diet that includes adequate servings from each of the food groups on the MyPyramid food guidance system should supply sufficient amounts of most vitamins during pregnancy. A brief description of the function and selected food sources for each vitamin are highlighted.

Folic Acid (Vitamin B$_9$)

Folic acid is a B vitamin that can prevent up to 70% of birth defects of the central nervous system called neural tube defects. Because formation of the nervous system occurs during the first few weeks of pregnancy, before a woman knows she is pregnant, all women of childbearing age should take a daily 400-mcg supplement of folic

acid in addition to a nutritious diet. Recent studies suggest that intake of adequate folic acid can prevent other birth defects, such as cleft lip and palate and some heart defects (March of Dimes, 2006).

Vitamin A

Vitamin A is usually found in sufficient amounts in the diets of women who live in the United States. One concern is when a pregnant woman consumes too much vitamin A. In very large amounts (levels at or above 10,000 IU or 3,000 mcg) preformed vitamin A, found in meats (primarily liver) and some fortified foods, can cause birth defects. For this reason, pregnant women are encouraged to get the majority of their vitamin A intake from beta-carotene, a substance found in fruits and vegetables with yellow, orange, and red coloration, such as carrots and sweet potatoes. Beta-carotene is converted by the body to vitamin A and is much less toxic than preformed vitamin A. The key is balanced intake of this nutrient. Too much can be toxic to the fetus, but too little can stunt fetal growth and cause impaired dark adaptation and night blindness.

Vitamin C

Vitamin C is essential in the formation of collagen, a necessary ingredient to wound healing. **Scurvy**, a disease characterized by spongy gums, loosened teeth, and bleeding into the skin and mucous membranes, results from severe vitamin C deficiency. Less severe deficiencies lead to easy bruising. Vitamin C is necessary for normal fetal growth and bone formation. This vitamin also helps the body to absorb iron.

Fortunately, most women in the United States get adequate amounts of vitamin C in their diets. Vitamin C is found in most fresh fruits and vegetables. The best sources include citrus fruits, papaya, and strawberries. Broccoli and tomatoes are also good sources of vitamin C.

Vitamin B_6

Vitamin B_6, or pyridoxine, assists in the metabolism of the macronutrients (proteins, fats, and carbohydrates), helps convert amino acids to proteins, and forms new RBCs. This vitamin is necessary for the healthy development of the fetus' nervous system. Although increased amounts of the vitamin are needed during pregnancy, a varied diet should supply all that is needed.

Vitamin B_{12}

Vitamin B_{12}, or cobalamine, is needed to maintain healthy nerve cells and RBCs. It is also needed to form DNA. Vitamin B_{12} occurs naturally only in animal sources, such as fish, milk, dairy products, eggs, meat, and poultry. This vitamin can also be found in fortified breakfast cereals. Most Americans get sufficient amounts of vitamin B_{12} in their diet.

The two instances in which vitamin B_{12} deficiency generally occurs are when a person lacks intrinsic factor or she is a vegan (see discussion of vegetarianism that follows). Persons who lack intrinsic factor cannot absorb vitamin B_{12}. Without intramuscular injections of the vitamin, these individuals experience pernicious anemia.

Dietary Supplementation

Currently, the American Academy of Pediatrics and the American College of Obstetricians and Gynecologists do not recommend routine multivitamin supplementation during pregnancy. It is thought that a diet that includes a variety of food types is sufficient to meet the needs of the pregnant woman. There are several exceptions. The woman who has nutritional risk factors requires a daily prenatal multivitamin supplement. Nutritional risk factors include multiple gestation, substance abuse, vegetarianism, and problems with hemoglobin formation. Some health care providers still recommend a daily vitamin supplement for all pregnant women.

Iron supplementation is recommended for all pregnant women after 28 weeks' gestation. If the woman has low hemoglobin, is obese, or is carrying twins, higher doses of iron are needed. Folic acid supplementation is recommended during pregnancy to prevent neural tube defects.

There is some evidence that supplementation with antioxidants, such as vitamins C and E, may be helpful to reduce the risk for developing preeclampsia and having a low-birth-weight baby (Rumbold et al., 2005).

Dietary Restrictions During Pregnancy

There are several nutrition-related practices that the pregnant woman should avoid. It is not helpful for the pregnant woman to limit her intake to try to avoid weight gain. Often, this practice results in too few nutrients ingested to meet the increased demands of pregnancy. Consumption of unwashed fruits and vegetables, unpasteurized dairy products, raw eggs, or undercooked meats can be harmful to the growing fetus (Gillen-Goldstein, Funai, & Roqué, 2007).

Although seafood has many nutritional benefits, many types are contaminated with methylmercury, a metal that can irreversibly harm the developing fetal brain. Therefore, the Food and Drug Administration (FDA, 2005) gives specific recommendations regarding the type and amount of seafood a pregnant woman may consume. Family Teaching Tips: Food Safety During Pregnancy outlines the major points to cover (including the FDA recommendations regarding seafood consumption) when educating the pregnant woman about food safety.

Special Nutritional Considerations

Several situations require unique nutritional considerations. These include vegetarianism, lactose intolerance, and pica.

Vegetarianism

There are several different categories of vegetarians. The lacto-ovo-vegetarian does not eat any flesh meats, but does include milk, eggs, and dairy products in the diet. The vegan is a strict vegetarian who does not eat milk, eggs, or any dairy product. A fruitarian only consumes fruits and nuts.

A lacto-ovo-vegetarian can easily get all of the required nutrients for pregnancy by careful attention to a few basic principles. Protein has always been an area of concern for vegetarian diets. Fortunately, a lacto-ovo-vegetarian can get sufficient protein by drinking milk, eating eggs, cheese, yogurt, and other dairy products, and by combining foods. Although vegetables and grains do not contain all of the essential amino acids, when they are skillfully combined, all of the essential amino acids can be obtained. The general rule is to combine a grain and a legume. For instance, a corn tortilla (grain) eaten with pinto beans (legume) provides all of the essential amino acids and qualifies as a complete protein. Other combinations include lentils and whole grain rice, peanut butter on whole wheat bread, and whole grain cereal with milk.

A vegan will need to take extra care to get enough protein because she does not use milk or dairy products. Food combining, as discussed in the previous paragraph, is an important nutritional strategy for the vegan. It can also

Family Teaching Tips

FOOD SAFETY DURING PREGNANCY

FOOD PREPARATION GUIDELINES

Follow the FDA guidelines to clean, separate, cook, and chill food:

- Clean
  - Wash hands thoroughly with warm water and soap before and after handling food and after using the bathroom, changing diapers, or handling pets.
  - Wash cutting boards, dishes, utensils, and countertops with hot water and soap.
  - Rinse raw fruits and vegetables thoroughly under running water.
- Separate
  - Separate raw meat, poultry, and seafood from ready-to-eat foods.
  - If possible, use one cutting board for raw meat, poultry, and seafood and another one for fresh fruits and vegetables.
  - Place cooked food on a clean plate. If cooked food is placed on an unwashed plate that held raw meat, poultry, or seafood, bacteria from the raw food could contaminate the cooked food.
- Cook
  - Cook foods thoroughly. Use a food thermometer to check the temperature.
  - Keep foods out of the Danger Zone: The range of temperatures at which bacteria can grow, usually between 40°F and 140°F (4°C and 60°C).
  - 2-Hour Rule: Discard foods left out at room temperature for more than 2 hours.
- Chill
  - Place an appliance thermometer in the refrigerator, and check the temperature periodically. The refrigerator should register at or below 40°F (4°C) and the freezer at or below 0°F (−18°C).

- Refrigerate or freeze perishables (foods that can spoil or become contaminated by bacteria if left unrefrigerated).

LISTERIA PRECAUTIONS

Take precautions to avoid listeria, a harmful bacterium that can grow at refrigerated temperatures:
- Do not eat hot dogs and luncheon meats, *unless they are reheated until steaming hot.*
- Do not eat soft cheese, such as feta, Brie, Camembert, "blue-veined cheeses," "queso blanco," "queso fresco," and Panela, *unless it is labeled as made with pasteurized milk.* Check the label.
- Do not eat refrigerated pâtés or meat spreads.
- Do not eat refrigerated smoked seafood *unless it is in a cooked dish*, such as a casserole. (Refrigerated smoked seafood, such as salmon, trout, whitefish, cod, tuna, or mackerel, is most often labeled as "nova-style," "lox," "kippered," "smoked," or "jerky.")
- Do not drink raw (unpasteurized) milk or eat foods that contain unpasteurized milk.

SEAFOOD RECOMMENDATIONS

Follow the FDA recommendations about appropriate fish consumption to avoid mercury poisoning:
- Do not eat any shark, swordfish, king mackerel, or tilefish during pregnancy.
- Limit intake of other fish to no more than 12 oz (about 2–3 servings) per week.
- Limit consumption of fish caught in local waters to 6 oz (1 serving) per week.
- Do not eat more than one 6-oz can of white tuna or two 6-oz cans of light tuna.
- It is probably best to avoid tuna steaks because they often have high mercury levels. If you decide to eat tuna steak, do not eat more than 6 oz per week.

help to suggest adding fortified soy milk and rice milk to the diet. Larger amounts of nuts and seeds can help offset the protein requirements. Vitamin B$_{12}$ must be supplemented for the pregnant vegan.

A fruitarian will need intensive support from her health care provider and a dietitian to meet the nutritional requirements of a healthy pregnancy. Multivitamin supplementation is necessary in this situation.

Iron and zinc requirements are also of concern for the vegetarian. Nonmeat sources of iron are generally not absorbed as efficiently as meat sources. Therefore,

the iron requirement for the vegetarian is higher. The same is true for zinc absorption and requirements.

Lactose Intolerance

Individuals with lactose intolerance lack the enzyme lactase

Don't get confused!

A vegan can take oral forms of vitamin B$_{12}$. Only the woman who lacks intrinsic factor needs vitamin B$_{12}$ injections. Without intrinsic factor, the woman cannot absorb vitamin B$_{12}$ through the gastrointestinal system; therefore, she needs intramuscular injections.

that is necessary to break down and digest milk and milk products. Symptoms of lactase deficiency include abdominal distention, flatulence, nausea, vomiting, diarrhea, and cramps after consuming milk. Lactose intolerance occurs more frequently in individuals of African, Hispanic, Native American, Ashkenazic Jewish, and Asian descent.

Calcium deficiency is a major concern for the pregnant woman who is lactose intolerant. There are several ways to address this concern. Some lactose intolerant individuals are able to tolerate cooked forms of milk, such as pudding or custard. Cultured or fermented dairy products, such as buttermilk, yogurt, and some cheeses may also be tolerated. A chewable lactase tablet may be taken with milk. Lactase-treated milk is available in most supermarkets and may be helpful. Other options are to drink calcium-enriched orange juice or soy milk or to take a calcium supplement. If the woman is infrequently exposed to sunlight, she will need a vitamin D supplement (Marchiano & Ural, 2005).

Pica

Pica is the persistent ingestion of nonfood substances such as clay, laundry starch, freezer frost, or dirt. It results from a craving for these substances that some women develop during pregnancy. These cravings disappear when the woman is no longer pregnant. Pica is associated with iron-deficiency anemia, but it is unknown whether iron-deficiency is the cause or the result. Some women find that the cravings cease when they begin taking iron supplements (Mills, 2007). If

Cultural Snapshot

The practice of pica is rooted in more than 200 cultures worldwide (Mills, 2007). It is important to approach the woman who reveals pica behavior in a culturally sensitive manner. It would be inappropriate to abruptly tell her to stop the practice without first assessing for cultural implications.

you suspect or discover that a pregnant woman is practicing pica, tell the registered nurse or the practitioner immediately. Special counseling is indicated in this situation.

Test Yourself

✔ List the recommended weight gain (in pounds) for the woman with a normal body mass index.

✔ What are two reasons it is important for the pregnant woman to get adequate amounts of protein?

✔ State the recommendations of the American Academy of Pediatrics regarding multivitamin supplementation during pregnancy.

Key Points

➤ Presumptive signs of pregnancy, such as nausea and vomiting, can have causes other than pregnancy. Probable signs of pregnancy are objective signs the examiner detects that point to pregnancy; however, they are not 100% indicative of pregnancy. Pregnancy tests and changes in the reproductive organs, such as Chadwick's and Hegar's signs, are probable signs of pregnancy.

➤ A positive sign of pregnancy is diagnostic because no other condition can cause the sign. Positive signs include visualization of the gestational sac or fetus with ultrasound, hearing the fetal heart beat with Doppler or fetoscope, and palpation of fetal movements by a trained examiner.

➤ Changes in maternal anatomy and physiology during pregnancy include the change of the uterus from a solid, pear-shaped, pelvic organ to a thin, globular shaped, muscular sac that fills the abdomi-

nal cavity. The thyroid gland increases in volume. Blood volume increases by 40% to 50%. Coagulation factors increase. Cardiac output increases by as much as 50%.

➤ The woman's reproductive system undergoes significant changes during pregnancy. The uterus enlarges and the endometrial lining (decidua) is maintained. Blood supply to the uterus increases significantly. Increased vascularity to the reproductive tract is responsible for Goodell's, Hegar's, and Chadwick's signs.

➤ Endocrine system changes include enlargement of the pituitary gland, an increase in prolactin levels, and an increased need for insulin.

➤ Hematologic changes enhance the exchange of nutrients and gases between the woman and the fetus and protect the woman against blood loss during childbirth but predispose the woman to venous thrombosis.

➤ The heart must adapt to the increased demands of the greatly expanded blood volume. The woman should lie on her side and not lie on her back for prolonged periods late in pregnancy to avoid supine hypotensive syndrome, which taxes the cardiovascular system and decreases blood flow to the placenta.

➤ Respiratory system changes lead to nasal stuffiness and shortness of breath.

➤ Increasing lordosis, increased curvature of the spine, shifts the center of gravity and leads to a waddling gait in the last half of pregnancy.

➤ Gastrointestinal changes include nausea and vomiting in early pregnancy, pyrosis (heartburn) in mid and late pregnancy, constipation, and hemorrhoid formation.

➤ Changes in the urinary tract lead to an increased risk for pyelonephritis during pregnancy. Urinary frequency is common in the first trimester because of an increased glomerular filtration rate and again in the third trimester because of pressure of the gravid uterus on the bladder.

➤ Increased pigmentation, such as that seen in chloasma and the linea nigra, along with striae, are common integumentary changes.

➤ Psychological tasks of pregnancy include accepting the pregnancy (first trimester), accepting the baby (second trimester), and preparing for parenthood (third trimester). Ambivalence is a normal feeling when pregnancy is first diagnosed. Couvade syndrome occurs when the father experiences some of the physical discomforts of pregnancy along with his partner.

➤ Nutritional requirements change during pregnancy. The woman needs nutrients to build extra blood volume and tissue, and the fetus needs nutrients to grow. Energy requirements are increased. A woman who enters pregnancy at normal weight should gain 25 to 35 lb during pregnancy. A woman who is underweight should gain more, whereas a woman who is overweight should gain less. In no instance is it recommended for a woman to gain less than 15 lb during pregnancy.

➤ Protein requirements increase during pregnancy. Most vitamins and minerals can be obtained without supplementation if the diet is adequate.

➤ After the first trimester, it is generally recommended for a woman to take an iron supplement because it is difficult to get adequate amounts of this mineral from diet alone. Although calcium needs do not increase, it is important for the pregnant woman to get sufficient amounts of this mineral.

➤ Folic acid supplementation is recommended to help prevent neural tube defects. Vitamin A can be toxic in large amounts. It is best to use beta-carotene (plant) sources to meet vitamin A needs during pregnancy.

➤ Vitamin C deficiency can lead to scurvy (severe), easy bruising, and possibly gestational hypertension.

➤ The woman who lacks intrinsic factor must take intramuscular injections of vitamin B_{12}, and the vegan must supplement this vitamin orally.

➤ Routine multivitamin supplementation is not currently recommended; however, the woman with nutritional risk factors should take prenatal vitamins. Iron and folic acid supplementation is generally recommended for all pregnant women.

➤ Vegetarians can receive an adequate diet with close attention to combining foods. The lacto-ovo-vegetarian can use milk and dairy products to obtain sufficient protein. The vegan can carefully combine foods (legumes and grains) to supply all of the essential amino acids and should take vitamin B_{12} supplements. The fruitarian needs to be followed closely by a dietitian and must take multivitamin supplements.

➤ When individuals lack the enzyme lactase, they are lactose intolerant. To get sufficient dairy products, these individuals can try taking lactase when they consume dairy products, or sometimes they can tolerate cooked forms of milk.

➤ Pica is ingestion of nonfood substances. It can lead to iron-deficiency anemia and other nutritional deficiencies and requires follow-up.

INTERNET RESOURCES

Pregnancy Signs
www.thebabycorner.com/pregnancy/signs.html
www.fda.gov/cdrh/oivd/homeuse-pregnancy.html

Nutrition During Pregnancy
www.4woman.gov/pregnancy/pregnancy/eat.cfm
www.vrg.org/nutrition/pregnancy.htm

Workbook

▪ NCLEX-STYLE REVIEW QUESTIONS

1. Amanda is 2 weeks late for her menstrual period. She has been feeling tired and has had bouts of nausea in the evenings. What is the classification of the pregnancy symptoms Amanda is experiencing?

   a. Positive
   b. Presumptive
   c. Probable
   d. No classification

2. Amanda makes an appointment with an obstetrician. During the exam, the obstetrician notes that the uterine isthmus is soft. What is the name of this sign, and how is it classified?

   a. Chadwick's sign; presumptive
   b. Goodell's sign; presumptive
   c. Goodell's sign; probable
   d. Hegar's sign; probable

3. Amanda is now 16 weeks pregnant. If the pregnancy is progressing as expected, where would the practitioner find the uterine fundus?

   a. Just above the pubic bone.
   b. Halfway between the pubic bone and the umbilicus.
   c. At the umbilicus.
   d. The uterine fundus would not be palpable at 16 weeks.

4. You are teaching Amanda about a proper diet during pregnancy. If Amanda understands your instructions, how will she reply when you ask her approximately how many calories per day does she need over her normal pre-pregnant needs?

   a. "About 300."
   b. "Approximately 500."
   c. "I need to double my calories because I'm eating for two."
   d. "I should not increase my calories while I'm pregnant."

▪ STUDY ACTIVITIES

1. Devise a 3-day meal plan for a vegan who is pregnant. How will you meet her needs for protein, iron, calcium, and vitamin B_{12}?

2. Perform an Internet search using the key terms "pica" and "pregnancy." Share your findings with your clinical group.

3. Develop a teaching plan on the importance of folic acid for a group of women who wish to become pregnant. Be sure to address why women of childbearing age should get enough of this nutrient, how much is required, and examples of food sources.

▪ CRITICAL THINKING: WHAT WOULD YOU DO?

Apply your knowledge of maternal physiologic and psychological adaptation to pregnancy to the following situation.

1. Carla is 20 weeks pregnant. You are assisting the midwife during this prenatal visit.

   a. Where do you expect to find Carla's uterine fundus?

   b. You attempt to listen to the fetal heartbeat with a Doppler. Do you expect to be able to hear the heartbeat?

   c. Carla reports that she is excited about the pregnancy and that she and her husband have been shopping for the nursery. What do you chart regarding Carla's psychological adaptation? Is she showing evidence that she is completing the appropriate task for the trimester?

2. Carla is in the office for her 32-week checkup. She has gained a total of 20 lb so far during her pregnancy. When you enter the room to check her vital signs, you notice that she is lying on her back and she looks pale. Her blood pressure is 70/40 mm Hg.

   a. What is the likely cause of Carla's symptoms?
   b. What action do you take first, and why?
   c. How should you advise Carla regarding her weight gain?

3. Monica has just found out that she is pregnant. She is a vegan.

   a. How would you advise Monica to get enough protein in her diet?

   b. Monica complains that the iron pills her doctor prescribed are causing constipation. She asks you why she needs to take iron. How do you reply?

   c. Monica loves carrot juice, but she has heard that too much vitamin A could be unhealthy for the baby. How would you advise her?

7 Prenatal Care

KEY TERMS

amniocentesis
biophysical profile
chorionic villus sampling
cordocentesis
doula
estimated date of confinement
estimated date of delivery
gravida
microcephaly
multigravida
Nagele's rule
nulligravida
parity
percutaneous umbilical blood sampling
sonogram
teratogens

LEARNING OBJECTIVES

On completion of this chapter, you should be able to:

1. Explain the goals of early prenatal care.
2. Explain to a pregnant woman what to expect during the first prenatal visit.
3. List components of the history taken at the first prenatal visit.
4. Describe physical examination performed at the first prenatal visit.
5. List the laboratory tests completed during the first prenatal visit.
6. Describe methods for estimating the due date, and use Nagele's rule to calculate the due date.
7. Recognize factors that put the pregnancy at risk.
8. Describe components of subsequent prenatal visits.
9. For each fetal assessment test, outline the nursing care and implications.
10. Identify common nursing diagnoses for a pregnant woman.
11. Choose appropriate nursing interventions for the pregnant woman, including interventions to relieve anxiety, relieve common discomforts of pregnancy, teach self-care, maintain safety for the woman and fetus, and prepare the woman for labor, birth, and parenthood.
12. Evaluate the effectiveness of nursing care given during pregnancy.

EARLY PRENATAL care is crucial to the health of the woman and her unborn baby. In fact, the best strategy is for the woman to seek care before she conceives. A recent study found that birth outcomes for women who receive no prenatal care are two to four times worse than outcomes for the general population (Taylor, Alexander, & Hepworth, 2005). According to the National Center for Health Statistics (2007), 84% of mothers received prenatal care in the first trimester in 2004. Although this statistic falls short of the *Healthy People 2010* goal that 90% of pregnant women will begin care in the first trimester, it does show a significant increase compared with 1990, when only 75.8% of women received early prenatal care (Women's Health USA, 2005).

The goal of early prenatal care is to optimize the health of the woman and the fetus and to increase the odds that the fetus will be born healthy to a healthy mother. Early prenatal care allows for the initiation of strategies to promote good health and for early intervention in the event a complication develops. As a nurse and trusted health care provider, you play a large role in teaching women about the importance of early and continued prenatal care.

Assessment of maternal and fetal well-being is the focus of prenatal care. Nursing responsibilities include a heavy emphasis on teaching throughout the pregnancy. At each prenatal visit, it is the role of the nurse to screen the woman, monitor vital signs, perform other assessments as delegated by the primary care provider (PCP), answer questions, and provide appropriate teaching.

ASSESSMENT OF MATERNAL WELL-BEING DURING PREGNANCY
First Prenatal Visit

Ideally, the first prenatal visit occurs as soon as the woman thinks she might be pregnant. Often, the event that signals the woman to seek care is a missed or late menstrual period. She also may be experiencing some of the signs associated with pregnancy, such as nausea, fatigue, frequent urination, or tingling and fullness of the breasts. The utmost question on the woman's mind, regardless of whether the pregnancy was planned or not, is "Am I pregnant?" If the woman obtained a positive pregnancy test at home, she will want to confirm the results. If she did not, then she may feel anxious, nervous, excited, or any number of emotions until the practitioner confirms the diagnosis of pregnancy.

The first prenatal visit is usually the longest because the baseline data to which all subsequent assessments are compared are obtained at this visit. The woman may not be mentally prepared for all the questions and tests that must be done, particularly because her main goal at the first visit is to determine whether she is, in fact, pregnant. The major objectives of this visit are to confirm or rule out a diagnosis of pregnancy, ascertain risk factors, determine the due date, and provide education on maintaining a healthy pregnancy. These objectives are met through history taking, a physical examination, laboratory work, and teaching. Refer to The Nursing Process for Prenatal Care at the end of the chapter for discussion of teaching topics.

History

The history is one of the most important elements of the first prenatal visit. The woman may fill out a written questionnaire, and the nurse or physician will then confirm the answers. Some practitioners prefer to obtain the history exclusively by face-to-face interview. Whatever method is chosen, review the history thoroughly and report any abnormal or unusual details. There are several parts to the history, including chief complaint, reproductive history, medical–surgical history, family history, and social history.

Chief Complaint

The chief complaint is usually a missed menstrual period. Ask the woman about presumptive and probable signs of pregnancy.

Reproductive History

Note the time of menarche, as well as a summary of the characteristics of the woman's normal menstrual cycles. Common questions include, "Are your periods regular?" "How frequently do your periods occur?" Note the first day of the last menstrual period (LMP) if the woman knows this information.

The obstetric history is a part of the reproductive history. Review details of each pregnancy, including history of miscarriages or abortions and the outcome of each pregnancy (i.e., how many weeks the pregnancy lasted and whether or not the pregnancy ended with a living child).

Here's a tip

If another person accompanies the woman, find a tactful way to separate them for at least part of the history collection. There may be details in the woman's reproductive history that she won't be willing to reveal in the presence of others, such as history of abortion. Ensuring privacy will increase the accuracy of the history.

The obstetric history is recorded in a specific format that is a type of medical shorthand. The word "gravid" means pregnant. **Gravida** refers to the number of pregnancies the woman has had (regardless of the outcome). For example, a woman who has had one pregnancy is a gravida 1, whereas a woman who has had five pregnancies is a gravida 5. A woman who has never been pregnant is a **nulligravida**, whereas a woman who has had more than one pregnancy is a **multigravida**.

Once the total number of pregnancies has been determined and recorded, the next part of the obstetric history is parity. **Parity**, or para, communicates the outcome of previous pregnancies. If a gravida 1 delivers a live-born infant, or an infant who is past the age of viability (>20 weeks), her obstetric status is gravida 1, para 1. Nonviable fetuses that deliver before the end of 20 weeks' gestation are abortions (either spontaneous or induced) and do not count in the parity. For example, if a woman had a pregnancy that ended at 17 weeks, another at 26 weeks, and another at 40 weeks, and she is currently pregnant, her obstetric status is gravida 4 para 2 abortus 1. Parity refers to the outcome of the pregnancy and is counted as 1, even if the woman delivers twins or triplets.

One of the most common methods of recording the obstetric history is to use the acronym GTPAL. "G" stands for gravida, the total number of pregnancies. "T" stands for term, the number of pregnancies that ended at term (at or beyond 38 weeks' gestation); "P" is for preterm, the number of pregnancies that ended after 20 weeks and before the end of 37 weeks' gestation. "A" represents abortions, the number of pregnancies that ended before 20 weeks' gestation. "L" is for living, the number of children delivered who are alive at the time of history collection. Some PCPs further divide abortions into induced and spontaneous and note multiple births and ectopic pregnancies. Box 7-1 defines terms associated with the obstetric history.

It is important to obtain information regarding complications that may have occurred with other pregnancies. A problem the woman had in a previous pregnancy may manifest itself again in the current pregnancy or

---

Box 7-1 ∥ OBSTETRIC HISTORY TERMS

- *Gravida*: Total number of pregnancies a woman has had, including the present pregnancy.
- *Para*: The number of fetuses delivered after the point of viability (20 weeks' gestation), whether or not they are born alive.
- *Nulli* (null or none), *primi* (first or one), and *multi* (many): Prefixes used in front of the terms "gravida" and "para" to indicate whether or not the woman has had previous pregnancies and deliveries.
- GTPAL: Acronym that represents the obstetric history.
  Gravida
  Term deliveries
  Preterm deliveries
  Abortions
  Living children

increase the chance that she will develop another type of complication. For example, if a woman hemorrhaged after a previous delivery, she has a higher risk of hemorrhaging after subsequent deliveries. If she develops gestational diabetes with a pregnancy, she will likely develop the condition again with subsequent pregnancies. If she has a history of preterm delivery, she is at increased risk to deliver another baby prematurely. Any abnormality that presented itself in a previous pregnancy is an important part of the history.

Medical–Surgical History

After eliciting a thorough reproductive history, the practitioner must obtain a detailed medical–surgical history. If the woman has any major medical problems, such as heart disease or diabetes, she will require closer surveillance throughout the pregnancy. The prenatal record should list all medications the woman is taking, including over-the-counter medications and herbal remedies.

Part of the medical history involves determining if there are risk factors for infectious diseases. If the woman has been exposed to anyone with tuberculosis, she needs additional screening to rule out the disease. Determine the woman's immunization status. The woman who is nonimmune for a particular infection is at risk to contract that infection. Although most immunizations are contraindicated during pregnancy, the woman who is nonimmune can take precautions to decrease the chance she will contract infection during pregnancy. Determine risk factors for human immunodeficiency virus/acquired immunodeficiency syndrome (HIV/AIDS) and other sexually transmitted infections (Box 7-2).

Family History

A family history is important because it may highlight the need for genetic testing or counseling. Verify the health status of the father of the baby and any close relatives of the woman and her partner. If there is a family history for cystic fibrosis or hearing loss, the practitioner may recommend genetic screening. The ethnic background of the woman and relatives of the unborn child are important factors to consider. For instance, many people of African American descent are carriers for sickle cell anemia; people of Mediterranean descent are

---

Table 7-1 ▮ GENETIC DISORDER SCREENING CRITERIA BY ETHNICITY

Ethnicity	Genetic Disorders for Which Screening May Be Recommended
African American, Indian, Middle Eastern	Sickle cell anemia; thalassemia
European Jewish, French Canadian	Tay-Sachs disease
Mediterranean, Southeast Asian	Thalassemia
Caucasian	Cystic fibrosis

---

at increased risk for thalassemia. See Table 7-1 for examples of ethnic-related genetic diseases.

Social History

The social history focuses on environmental factors that may influence the pregnancy. A woman who has strong social support, adequate housing and nutrition, and greater than a high school education is less likely to develop complications of pregnancy than is a woman who lives with inadequate resources. The type of employment may influence the health of the pregnancy. A job that requires exposure to harmful chemicals is less safe for the woman and fetus than is a job that does not involve this type of exposure. Intimate partner violence can threaten the pregnancy; therefore, it is prudent to screen every woman for intimate partner violence.

Smoking, alcohol, and illicit and over-the-counter drug use can all potentially harm a growing fetus, so it is important to determine the woman's consumption patterns, particularly since conception. If the woman owns a cat or likes to garden, she is at increased risk for contracting toxoplasmosis, an infection that can cause the woman to lose the pregnancy or can result in severe abnormalities in the fetus.

Physical Examination

The practitioner performs a complete physical examination that covers all body systems. As the nurse, you may provide assistance as needed. The head-to-toe physical is done first. The examiner looks for signs of disease that may need treatment and for any evidence of previously undetected maternal disease or other signs of ill health. A breast examination is part of the physical. Although it is rare, breast cancer in a young pregnant woman is a possibility.

A vaginal speculum examination and a bimanual examination of the uterus follow the head-to-toe physical. During the speculum examination, the practitioner obtains a Papanicolaou test, or Pap smear (see Nursing Procedure 4-1 in Chapter 4), and notes signs of pregnancy, such as Chadwick's sign. The bimanual examination

---

Box 7-2 ▮ RISK FACTORS FOR SEXUALLY TRANSMITTED INFECTIONS

- Sex with multiple partners
- Sex with a partner who has risk factors
- Intravenous drug use (needle sharing)
- Anal intercourse
- Vaginal intercourse with a partner who also engages in anal intercourse
- Unprotected (no condom) intercourse

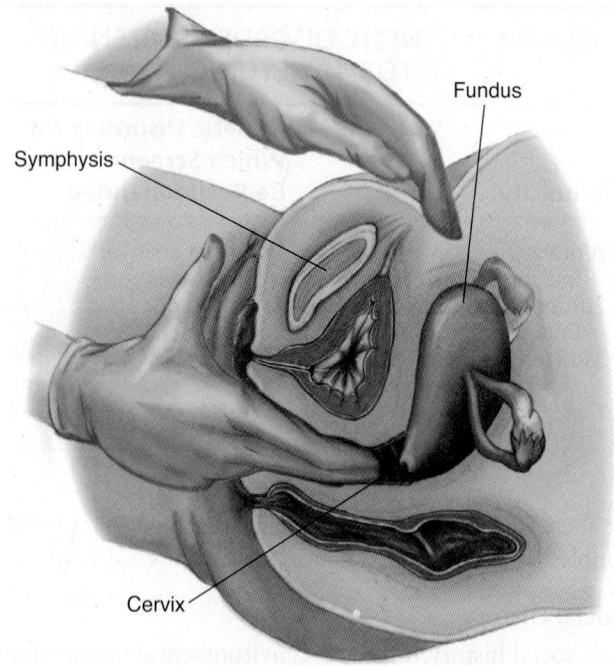

■ **Figure 7-1** Bimanual examination. The examiner palpates the fundus (top portion) of the uterus through the abdominal wall while the hand in the vagina holds the cervix in place. This examination can determine the size of the uterus, which helps date the pregnancy.

(Fig. 7-1) allows the practitioner to feel the size of the uterus and to elicit Hegar's sign.

Laboratory Assessment

Many laboratory tests are done during the course of the pregnancy. A complete blood count indicates the overall health status of the woman. Anemia manifests as a low blood count and low hemoglobin and hematocrit. Anemia is one indication of suboptimal nutritional status and is associated with poor pregnancy outcomes, unless caught and treated early. A woman who is at risk for sickle cell anemia or thalassemia is given a hemoglobin electrophoresis test.

Other laboratory tests routinely ordered include a blood type and antibody screen. This test helps identify women who are at risk of developing antigen incompatibility with fetal blood cells. A, B, and O incompatibilities can develop, as well as $Rh_o(D)$ incompatibilities. If an antigen incompatibility develops, the fetus may suffer from hemolytic anemia, as the mother's antibodies cross the placenta and attack his red blood cells (see Chapter 20 for further discussion of antigen incompatibilities).

Other tests screen for the presence of infection. The woman will undergo tests for hepatitis B, HIV, syphilis, gonorrhea, and Chlamydia. Each of these infections can cause serious fetal problems unless they are treated. A rubella titer determines if the woman is immune to rubella. If she is not, she will need a rubella immunization immediately after delivery because the rubella vaccine

cannot be given safely during pregnancy. A urine culture screens for bacteria in the urine, a situation that can lead to urinary tract infection and premature labor if it is not treated. The Pap smear screens for cervical cancer.

Traditionally, screening for hypothyroidism is done only when the woman has risk factors or symptoms. However, current research indicates that up to one third of the cases of hypothyroidism go undetected using this approach. Hypothyroidism can have devastating effects on the fetus' developing nervous system. Therefore, some experts now recommend that every pregnant woman receive thyroid function screening as part of routine prenatal care (Lockwood, 2007).

Due Date Estimation

One important aspect of the first visit is to calculate the due date, or the **estimated date of delivery** (EDD). An older term that is sometimes used is **estimated date of confinement** (EDC). Both terms refer to the estimated date that the baby will be born. This is critical information for the practitioner because he or she will manage problems that may arise during the pregnancy differently, depending on the gestational age of the fetus. Therefore, it is essential to have an accurate due date.

There are several ways to date a pregnancy. The most common way to calculate the EDD is to use **Nagele's rule**. To determine the due date using Nagele's rule, add 7 days to the date of the first day of the LMP, then subtract 3 months. This is a simple way to estimate the due date, but it is dependent upon the woman knowing when the first day of the LMP was. Sometimes this date is impossible to determine, particularly if the woman experiences irregular menstrual cycles, or if she cannot remember the date.

During the pelvic examination, the practitioner feels the size of the uterus to get an idea of how far along the pregnancy is. For instance, a uterus that is the size of a small pear is approximately 7 weeks. If the uterus feels to be the size of an orange, the pregnancy is approximately 10 weeks along, and at 12 weeks the uterus is the size of a grapefruit (MacKenzie, Stephenson, & Funai, 2006).

Other ways to validate the gestational age are to note landmarks during the pregnancy. Initial detection of the fetal heartbeat by Doppler ultrasound takes place between 10 and 12 weeks. Quickening typically occurs around 16 weeks for multigravidas and 20 weeks for primigravidas.

One of the most common and reliable ways to date the pregnancy is through an obstetric **sonogram**, a picture obtained with ultrasound (MacKenzie, Stephenson, & Funai, 2006). High-frequency sound waves reflect off fetal and maternal pelvic structures, allowing the sonographer to visualize the structures in real time. The sonographer measures fetal structures, such as the head and the femur. These measurements allow the practitioner to estimate the gestational age of the fetus, and thereby determine a due date. A sonogram obtained early in the pregnancy yields the most accurate due date. If there is a discrepancy between the EDD calculated using Nagele's rule and the EDD determined by sonogram, the results of the sonogram (if it is done in the first half of the pregnancy) are used to base treatment decisions.

Risk Assessment

The risk assessment takes into account all of the information gathered from the history, physical examination, and laboratory tests. Many factors put a pregnancy at risk. These factors include a negative attitude of the woman toward the pregnancy (e.g., an unwanted pregnancy), seeking prenatal care late in the pregnancy, and maternal substance abuse (alcohol, tobacco, or illicit drugs). A history of complications with previous pregnancies or poor outcomes, and the presence of maternal disease also put the current pregnancy at risk. Social factors that increase the risk of poor outcomes include inadequate living conditions and domestic violence or physical abuse. If the woman is unaware of the adverse effects of tobacco and alcohol, the benefits of folic acid, or the risk of HIV, the pregnancy is at increased risk for complications and poor outcomes. Age also plays a factor. Young teens and women older than 35 years of age are at higher risk for a complicated pregnancy. An unplanned pregnancy or a pregnancy when the woman is unsure of her LMP date may also be at risk.

Test Yourself

✔ Which obstetric term indicates the number of pregnancies a woman has had?

✔ List four laboratory tests that are routinely ordered during the first prenatal visit.

✔ Explain how to calculate the due date using Nagele's rule.

Subsequent Prenatal Visits

Traditionally, the practitioner sees the woman once monthly from weeks 1 through 32. Between weeks 32 and 36, prenatal visits are biweekly. From week 36 until delivery, the woman is seen weekly. Current research shows that fewer visits for low-risk pregnancies and more visits for at-risk pregnancies may be more beneficial overall than a rigid adherence to the traditional schedule of visits (Lockwood, 2007). In any event, encourage the woman to keep her appointments and maintain regular prenatal care throughout the pregnancy.

Most subsequent visits include specific assessments. Weight, blood pressure (Fig. 7-2), urine protein and glucose, and fetal heart rate (FHR) are all data that you may collect. At every visit, inquire regarding the danger signals of pregnancy (discussed in the Nursing Process for Prenatal Care). Ask the woman about fetal movement, contractions, bleeding, and membrane rupture. Normally the practitioner does not repeat the pelvic examination until late in the pregnancy, close to the expected time of delivery.

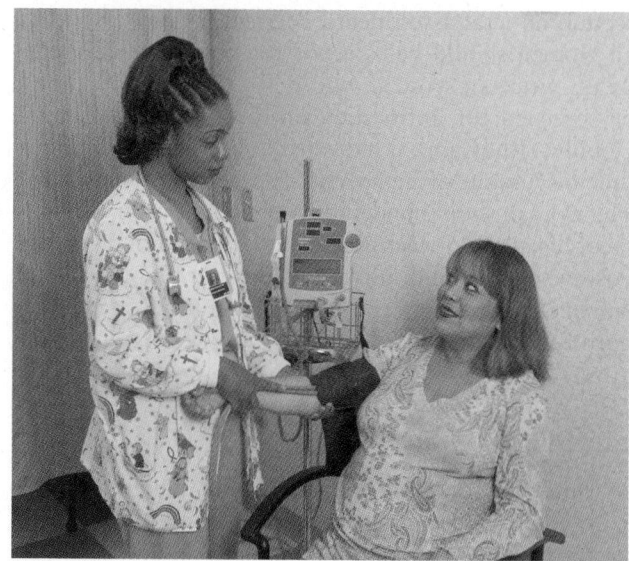

■ **Figure 7-2** The licensed practical/vocational nurse measures the blood pressure at a prenatal visit.

At each office visit, the practitioner measures the fundal height in centimeters (Fig. 7-3). This measurement provides a confirmation of gestational age between weeks 18 and 32. In other words, between weeks 18 and 32, the fundal height in centimeters should match the number of weeks the pregnancy has progressed. For example, if the woman is 18 weeks pregnant, the fundal height should measure 18 cm. If there is a discrepancy between the size and dates, the practitioner usually orders a sonogram to determine the cause of the discrepancy. A fundal height that is larger than expected could mean, among other things, that the original dates were miscalculated, that the woman is carrying twins, or that there is a molar pregnancy (see Chapter 17).

The woman undergoes screening at particular times during the pregnancy. Sometime between 15 and 20 weeks' gestation, a maternal serum alpha-fetoprotein (MSAFP) should be drawn (see the discussion in the

■ **Figure 7-3** The certified nurse midwife measures the fundal height.

section on fetal assessment). Between 24 and 28 weeks, all women should be screened for gestational diabetes. At 28 weeks, a woman who is $Rh_o(D)$-negative should be screened for antibodies and given anti-D immune globulin (RhoGam), if indicated (see Chapter 20 for further discussion of hemolytic disease of the newborn). The woman should undergo screening for group B streptococcus after 35 weeks and before the end of 37 weeks. Positive cultures indicate the need for antibiotics for the woman during labor and close observation of the newborn for 48 hours after birth.

Test Yourself

✔ How often does the woman with an uncomplicated pregnancy have prenatal office visits from weeks 1 through 32?

✔ What purpose does measuring the fundal height serve during prenatal visits?

✔ List the time during pregnancy when screening for gestational diabetes normally occurs.

ASSESSMENT OF FETAL WELL-BEING DURING PREGNANCY

Throughout the pregnancy, the PCP may order tests to assess the well-being of the fetus. Some are screening tests, which means they are not diagnostic. If an abnormal result occurs with a screening test, the practitioner orders additional diagnostic testing. The discussion that follows describes some of the most common tests and procedures. Not every woman will receive every test, although some screening tests are recommended for all pregnant women, at certain points during the pregnancy.

Fetal Kick Counts

A healthy fetus moves and kicks regularly, although the pregnant woman usually cannot perceive the movements until approximately gestational week 16 to 20. The practitioner or the nurse instructs the woman to monitor her baby's movements on a daily basis. Instruct the woman to choose a time each day in which she can relax and count the baby's movements. Each kick or position change counts as one movement. Using a special form or a blank sheet of paper, instruct the woman to note the time she starts counting fetal kicks and then keep counting until she counts 10 movements. A healthy fetus will move at

Don't forget.

"Routine" for you as a nurse is not at all routine for the woman. She will need careful explanation of all prenatal tests. This includes routine testing that occurs as part of prenatal care and tests performed for other reasons.

■ **Figure 7-4** Ultrasound is used to identify fetal and placental structures during pregnancy.

least 10 times in 2 hours (Wyatt & Rhoads, 2006). If it takes longer than 2 hours for the fetus to move 10 times, or if the woman cannot get her baby to move at all, she should immediately call her health care provider. The practitioner will order tests to determine the well-being of the fetus.

Ultrasonography

Ultrasound is the gold standard in the United States to determine gestational age, observe the fetus, and diagnose complications of pregnancy (Fig. 7-4). Because it appears to be a safe and effective way to monitor fetal well-being, the procedure is performed frequently. One result of monitoring virtually every pregnancy with ultrasound is that most parents know the gender of the child before he or she is born. Many sonographers take a still picture of the fetus and provide this to the parents, if desired.

As stated earlier in the chapter, ultrasound uses high-frequency sound waves to visualize fetal and maternal structures (Fig. 7-5). The developing embryo can first be

■ **Figure 7-5** Fetus viewed via ultrasound. The outline of the fetal head and trunk can be clearly seen in the transverse position.

Box 7-3 USES FOR ULTRASOUND TECHNOLOGY DURING PREGNANCY

- Diagnose pregnancy: intrauterine and ectopic (outside the uterine cavity).
- Diagnose multifetal pregnancies (twins, triplets).
- Monitor fetal heartbeat and breathing movements. The fetus makes "practice" breathing movements in utero as early as 11 weeks' gestation.
- Take measurements of the fetal head, femur, and other structures to determine gestational age or diagnose fetal growth restriction.
- Detect fetal anomalies.
- Estimate the amount of amniotic fluid that is present. Either too much (hydramnios) or too little (oligohydramnios) can indicate problems with the pregnancy.
- Identify fetal and placental structures during amniocentesis or umbilical cord sampling.
- Detect placental problems, such as abnormal placement of the placenta in placenta previa or grade the placenta (determine the age and functioning).
- Diagnose fetal demise (death). Absence of cardiac activity is used to diagnose fetal death.
- Verify fetal presentation and position.
- Estimate the birth weight, particularly if the fetus is thought to be abnormally large (macrosomic).

visualized at about 6 weeks' gestation. An ultrasound performed at this stage positively diagnoses the pregnancy. Ultrasound captures the fetus' cardiac activity and body movements in real time. Box 7-3 lists ways practitioners use ultrasound technology to monitor the pregnancy and fetal well-being.

Ultrasound can best detect most abnormalities of the fetus, placenta, and surrounding structures between 16 and 20 weeks' gestation. Detailed sonograms can diagnose severe congenital heart, spine, brain, and kidney defects. However, ultrasound cannot pick up all abnormalities. Some anomalies, such as Down's syndrome, have subtle characteristics that ultrasound often cannot pick up until late in the pregnancy. However, a skilled practitioner can detect 70% to 80% of Down's syndrome cases when observing for nuchal translucency (fetal neck thickness) on ultrasound between weeks 10 and 14 (Zindler, 2005). There are two main ways to perform an ultrasound—the transabdominal approach and the endovaginal approach.

Transabdominal Ultrasound

For the transabdominal method, the sonographer places a transducer on the abdomen to visualize the pregnancy.

In the past, it was recommended that the woman have a full bladder for transabdominal ultrasound. Current recommendations are that the woman does not need to have a full bladder (Shipp, 2006). In fact, a full bladder may actually distort anatomy. If the sonographer cannot see sufficient detail with the transabdominal approach, he or she will likely switch to the endovaginal technique.

If you are assisting during the procedure, place a small wedge (pillow or sandbag) under one hip to prevent supine hypotension. Explain to the woman that the sonographer will place a special gel on her abdomen and that it probably will be cold. She should not feel any discomfort during the procedure. A darkened room optimizes visualization of fetal structures during the procedure. Although the technician performing the sonogram can see fetal structures and obvious defects during the sonogram, it will take several hours to get the official results because the radiologist must review the films and dictate the diagnosis. After the procedure, clean the excess gel off the woman's abdomen and assist her to the bathroom.

Endovaginal Ultrasound

For the endovaginal method, the sonographer uses a specialized probe in the vagina. There are several advantages to this method. The endovaginal approach allows for a clearer image because the probe is very close to fetal and uterine structures. This method allows for earlier confirmation of the pregnancy than does the transabdominal method. The endovaginal method is superior for predicting or diagnosing preterm labor because the sonographer can measure and analyze the cervix for changes.

Assist the woman into lithotomy position (as for a pelvic examination) and drape her for privacy. A female attendant must be present in the room at all times during the procedure if the sonographer is male. The examiner covers the probe (which is smaller than a speculum) with a specialized sheath, a condom, or the finger of a glove; applies ultrasonic transducer gel to the covered probe; and inserts the probe into the vagina. Explain to the woman that she will feel the probe moving about in different directions during the test. The probe may cause mild discomfort, but it is generally not painful.

Doppler Flow Studies

Another test that uses ultrasound technology is a Doppler flow study, or Doppler velocimetry. A specialized ultrasound machine measures the flow of blood through fetal vessels. The ultrasound transducer on the woman's abdomen allows the sonographer to assess blood flow through the umbilical vessels and in the fetal aorta, brain, and heart. If the test shows that blood flow through fetal vessels is less than normal, the fetus may not be receiving enough oxygen and nutrients from the placenta, and the practitioner will order additional studies and interventions. Preparation and nursing care for a Doppler flow study are the same as for ultrasonography.

Maternal Serum Alpha-fetoprotein Screening

Alpha-fetoprotein is a protein manufactured by the fetus. The woman's blood contains small amounts of this protein during pregnancy. Many physicians recommend measuring MSAFP between 16 and 20 weeks' gestation because abnormal levels may indicate a problem and the need for additional testing (Natarajan & Klein, 2006).

MSAFP levels are elevated in several conditions. Higher-than-expected levels of MSAFP may indicate that the pregnancy is farther along than was predicted initially. When the woman is carrying multiple fetuses, such as twins or triplets, or when the fetus has died, MSAFP levels will be elevated. The main reason physicians screen MSAFP is to check for neural tube defects, such as anencephaly (failure of the brain to develop normally) or spina bifida (failure of the spine to close completely during development). MSAFP levels are usually elevated if the fetus has either of these anomalies. Omphalocele and gastroschisis (failure of the abdominal wall to close) are two other conditions that cause elevated MSAFP levels. Low MSAFP levels may also indicate a problem, in particular Down's syndrome.

It is important for the parents-to-be to understand the reasons for and implications of MSAFP testing. Even when the levels are abnormal, approximately 90% of the time the woman will deliver a healthy baby. However, abnormal results increase the likelihood that the fetus has an abnormality, and the practitioner will usually order additional diagnostic testing with ultrasound and/or amniocentesis. Even when the follow-up ultrasound is normal, there is no guarantee that the fetus will be healthy. An elevated MSAFP in the presence of a normal ultrasound increases the risk that the woman will develop a complication of pregnancy, such as preeclampsia or intrauterine growth restriction.

Some women want to have the test done so that they can decide whether to end the pregnancy before the age of viability. Other women feel strongly that abortion is not an option, but they may want to know if an anomaly is present so that they can deliver in a hospital with high-level care and have specialists immediately available to resuscitate and care for the baby. Other women may decide against testing because a false-positive test might be needlessly worrisome and lead to more invasive, riskier tests, such as amniocentesis, even though the baby might be healthy. Each woman must consider these issues in consult with her partner and practitioner. No matter what decision the woman makes regarding testing, it is critical to support her decision.

A little sensitivity goes a long way!

If a screening test result is "suspicious," or the practitioner orders further testing, the woman will need emotional support. It is scary not knowing what to expect while waiting for test results. Accept and let her talk through her feelings.

Triple-Marker (or Multiple-Marker) Screening

Measuring levels of two other hormones in conjunction with MSAFP increases the sensitivity of the test. When MSAFP, human chorionic gonadotropin (hCG), and unconjugated estriol levels are measured from the same maternal blood sample, the test is called a triple-marker screen. A low MSAFP, low estriol, and elevated hCG suggests that the baby has Down's syndrome, whereas low levels of all three hormones increases the risk the fetus has trisomy 18, a more severe and less common chromosomal defect. A fourth biochemical marker in maternal serum, inhibin A, has been found to increase the ability of blood tests to predict chromosomal abnormalities of the fetus, so some practitioners add this fourth screen. This test is a multiple-marker screen.

Sometimes the practitioner orders serial estriol levels in the third trimester to monitor the well-being of the fetus. Falling estriol levels in the third trimester may indicate that the fetus is in jeopardy, in which case an emergency cesarean delivery may save the fetus' life. Nursing care for MSAFP or triple marker screening is the same as that for any venous blood sampling of the woman.

Amniocentesis

An **amniocentesis** is a diagnostic procedure whereby a needle inserted into the amniotic sac obtains a small amount of fluid (Fig. 7-6). A variety of biochemical, chromosomal, and genetic studies are possible using the amniotic fluid sample.

The procedure is usually performed between 15 and 20 weeks' gestation, although early amniocentesis (at 12–14 weeks' gestation) may be preferable in some

■ **Figure 7-6** Amniocentesis. A pocket of amniotic fluid is located by sonogram. A small amount of fluid is removed by aspiration.

Box 7-4 ▌ **SELECTED INDICATIONS FOR CHROMOSOMAL STUDIES BY AMNIOCENTESIS OR CHORIONIC VILLUS SAMPLING**

- Advanced maternal age (generally accepted as older than 35)
- Previous offspring with chromosomal anomalies
- History of recurrent pregnancy loss
- Ultrasound diagnosis of fetal anomalies
- Abnormal MSAFP, triple-marker screen, or multiple-marker screen
- Previous offspring with a neural tube defect
- Both parents known carriers of a recessive genetic trait (such as cystic fibrosis, sickle cell anemia, or Tay-Sachs disease)

cases. Most practitioners will not perform amniocentesis before 12 weeks because of the increased risk for fetal foot deformities and pregnancy loss (Natarajan & Klein, 2006). Early and second-trimester procedures can determine the genetic makeup of the fetus because amniotic fluid contains fetal cells. Box 7-4 lists indications for first- and second-trimester amniocentesis. Third-trimester amniocentesis is usually done to determine fetal lung maturity, which allows for the earliest possible delivery in certain at-risk pregnancies.

Because amniocentesis is an invasive procedure that carries a small risk of spontaneous abortion, injury to the fetus, and chorioamnionitis (infection of the fetal membranes), the woman must give informed consent. The physician explains the procedure and risks and answers her questions. If you witness the consent, be certain that the woman has had all her questions answered before she signs. Explain the procedure to her so that she knows what to expect. Many women are worried that the procedure will be painful. Although pain is a subjective feeling that varies between individuals, most women find that the procedure is much less painful than they anticipated. Usually women report feeling a slight pinching sensation or vague cramping.

Just before the procedure, the practitioner uses ultrasound to locate a pocket of amniotic fluid. Without ultrasound to guide the needle, there is a high risk that the needle could puncture the placenta or the fetus. After locating the pocket of fluid (usually on the upper portion of the uterus), the practitioner prepares the site with povidone-iodine or alcohol, and places sterile drapes on the abdomen around the site. The sterile drapes also cover the ultrasound transducer. Next, the practitioner inserts a 20- to 22-gauge spinal needle into the chosen site. The practitioner watches the ultrasound picture and guides the needle along the chosen path into the pocket of fluid. The first 0.5 mL of fluid is discarded to avoid

contamination of the specimen with maternal cells. Then, 20 mL (less for early amniocentesis) of fluid is withdrawn, and the needle removed. The practitioner then monitors the FHR by ultrasound to ensure fetal well-being. The fluid sample, which is normally straw colored, is placed into sterile tubes, labeled, and sent to the laboratory for analysis. Results are usually available within 2 to 3 weeks and are highly accurate (approximately 99%).

The woman should remain on bed rest the day of the procedure. Attach continuous electronic fetal monitoring (EFM) to observe the FHR and contractions, if they should occur. Women who are Rh₀(D)-negative should receive RhoGam after the procedure. Observe the insertion site for leakage of amniotic fluid (a rare complication). Monitor the woman's temperature. Immediately report any temperature elevation, leaking of fluid from the site or from the vagina, vaginal bleeding, cramps, or contractions to the RN or the attending practitioner. After several hours of monitoring, the woman may go home. Instruct her to remain on bed rest for the rest of the day. The following day she may do light housework chores, and the third day she may resume regular activities. Warning signs she should immediately report to the attending practitioner include fever, amniotic fluid leakage, vaginal bleeding, and/or cramping.

As with any medical procedure that carries risk, amniocentesis has advantages and disadvantages that each woman and her partner must consider carefully. The most common reason for undergoing amniocentesis is to determine if there is a fetal abnormality so that the pregnancy might be ended (elective abortion) before the age of viability. Many women will not consider an abortion under any circumstances. In these cases, there are still benefits to amniocentesis. If the fetus does have a chromosomal abnormality, knowing in advance allows for the medical team and the parents to prepare for the birth. It also allows the physician to make better decisions about managing the pregnancy. Every woman who is contemplating amniocentesis should have genetic counseling. Then, no matter what decision the woman makes, it is critical that the health care team support her decision.

Chorionic Villus Sampling

Chorionic villus sampling (CVS) is a newer procedure that can provide chromosomal studies of fetal cells, similar to amniocentesis. Indications for CVS are the same as for amniocentesis (see Box 7-4). One advantage of CVS testing is that it is done earlier in the pregnancy than is amniocentesis, which allows decisions about elective abortion to be made sooner in the pregnancy. Elective abortions are safer for the woman the earlier they are performed. CVS is typically performed at 8 to 12 weeks' gestation (Natarajan & Klein, 2006). Because CVS is an invasive procedure, informed consent is required.

Just before the procedure, an ultrasound confirms fetal well-being, the location of the placenta, and gestational age. For the transcervical approach, assist the woman into lithotomy position in stirrups. The practitioner cleans her vagina and cervix with povidone-iodine or other antiseptic fluid. Using ultrasound guidance, the practitioner inserts a small catheter into the woman's vagina and through the cervix. Placental tissue is then extracted into a syringe to obtain fetal cells for chromosomal analysis. Sometimes the practitioner uses a transabdominal approach with a needle, similar to the procedure for amniocentesis. The woman usually experiences minimal discomfort and may resume normal activities after the test. RhoGam should be administered after the procedure to Rh$_o$(D)-negative women.

One advantage of CVS testing is that the results are available in 7 to 10 days, much faster than with amniocentesis. Another advantage is that testing can occur earlier in the pregnancy. However, there are disadvantages to this technique. First, some studies demonstrate a higher rate of pregnancy loss with transcervical CVS versus transabdominal CVS and second-trimester amniocentesis (Ghidini & McLaren, 2006). A second potential disadvantage is that there is no amniotic fluid in a CVS sample; therefore, the amniotic alpha-fetoprotein cannot be evaluated, as it can with amniocentesis. This means the woman would need to have MSAFP levels drawn at 16 to 18 weeks' gestation to test for neural tube defects. (A woman who has amniocentesis performed does not need the MSAFP test because amniocentesis results report the fetal alpha-fetoprotein level, which is a more accurate predictor of spinal defects than maternal serum levels.) The third disadvantage of CVS is that there is a small risk that the cells taken from the placenta will be different from fetal cells. If this happens, a situation called "placental mosaicism," the test results would be abnormal, even if the fetus were normal. Some authorities suggest that CVS performed before 9 weeks' gestation can cause fetal limb and digit deformations.

Percutaneous Umbilical Blood Sampling

Percutaneous umbilical blood sampling (PUBS), also known as cordocentesis, is a procedure similar to amniocentesis, except that fetal blood is withdrawn rather than amniotic fluid. The woman is prepared in the same manner as for amniocentesis and must give informed consent. Ultrasound locates the placenta and fetal structures and confirms gestational age and viability. The practitioner inserts a thin needle transabdominally under ultrasound guidance, and withdraws blood from the umbilical cord close to its insertion with the placenta. Alternatively, the practitioner can obtain blood from the fetal heart or from the umbilical vein within the liver, although these sites are not commonly chosen. The blood is then sent for testing.

Sometimes, PUBS is done specifically to diagnose and treat certain diseases of the blood, such as von Willebrand's disease, alloimmune thrombocytopenia, and hemolytic disease. It can also diagnose and treat cases of fetal infection such as toxoplasmosis, rubella, cytomegalovirus, varicella zoster, human parvovirus, and HIV. Through the technology of cordocentesis, the fetus with thrombocytopenia can receive weekly infusions of platelets until delivery. The fetus with hemolytic disease can receive exchange transfusions (part of the fetus' blood is withdrawn and the same amount replaced with healthy blood). The fetus with an infection can be treated with antibiotics or receive other therapies, depending upon the type of infection. The blood obtained from cordocentesis can also be sent for rapid chromosomal studies. Results are back within 48 to 72 hours. The risks associated with PUBS are approximately the same as those of amniocentesis.

Nonstress Test

The nonstress test (NST) is a noninvasive way to monitor fetal well-being. Usually around 28 weeks and onward, the fetal nervous system is developed enough so that the autonomic nervous system works to periodically accelerate the heart rate. Therefore, the practitioner can observe FHR accelerations using an EFM.

The woman requires no special preparation other than placement of EFM (see Chapter 10 for in-depth discussion of fetal monitoring). She may or may not have an event marker to hold.[2] If she uses one, she must push the button every time she feels the fetus move. The nurse or practitioner evaluates the fetal monitor tracing after 20 minutes. Generally, if there are at least two accelerations of the fetal heart in a 15 × 15 window (i.e., the fetal heart accelerates at least 15 beats above the baseline for at least 15 seconds), the NST is said to be "reactive," provided that the baseline and variability are normal and that there are no decelerations of the FHR. In the presence of a reactive NST, fetal well-being is assumed for at least the next week.

If, however, there are no accelerations or less than two occur within 20 minutes, the strip is said to be "nonreactive." In this case, the monitoring would continue for another 20 minutes in the hopes of obtaining a reactive NST. This is because fetal sleep cycles last for approximately 20 minutes. During fetal sleep, accelerations do not usually occur, so it is prudent to observe for an additional 20 minutes. Sometimes the practitioner attempts to stimulate the fetus. She may clap loudly close to the woman's abdomen or may manipulate the fetus through the abdomen with her hands, or she may give the woman something cold to drink. Any of these activities might stimulate a sleeping fetus to wake up, and result in a reactive tracing. If the tracing remains nonreactive or equivocal (results cannot be interpreted), additional testing is warranted. In these instances, the practitioner

---

[2]In the past, it was very important to monitor the FHR in conjunction with fetal movement. Now, it is generally felt that spontaneous accelerations with or without fetal movement are indicative of fetal well-being, so it is not necessary to have the woman track fetal movements, although some practitioners may prefer this.

frequently recommends vibroacoustic stimulation or a contraction stress test (CST).

Vibroacoustic Stimulation

For vibroacoustic stimulation, the practitioner places an artificial larynx a centimeter from or directly on the maternal abdomen. The sound stimulates the fetus to wake up, and a healthy fetus responds with a reactive NST. Some practitioners use vibroacoustic stimulation for all NSTs because it decreases the length of time needed to obtain a reactive tracing and decreases the number of false-nonreactive tracings. Other practitioners use vibroacoustic stimulation as the second step after obtaining a nonreactive NST.

Contraction Stress Test

Uterine contractions cause a momentary reduction of uteroplacental blood flow, which stresses the fetus. A CST monitors the fetus' response to contractions to determine his or her well-being. The woman is placed on EFM, as for the NST. There are three ways to obtain uterine contractions for a CST. The easiest way is if the woman is having spontaneous Braxton Hicks contractions because there is no need to induce contractions. Another way is to induce uterine contractions through nipple stimulation. Nipple stimulation causes release of oxytocin from the posterior pituitary gland. The oxytocin then stimulates the uterus to contract. The third way is to start an intravenous drip of Pitocin (synthetic oxytocin) to induce contractions.

The goal is to have three contractions of at least 40 seconds' duration within a 10-minute period. Then the practitioner reviews the fetal monitor strip to determine the reaction of the fetus to the stress of the contractions. If there are no late decelerations (decelerations that occur after the contractions; see Chapter 10) after any of the contractions, the CST is negative, which is a reassuring sign. A negative CST indicates that the fetus is not suffering from hypoxia and does not need immediate delivery. An equivocal CST occurs when there are late decelerations after some, but not all, of the uterine contractions. This result is suspicious of fetal hypoxia and may cause the physician to decide to perform a cesarean delivery of the fetus. A positive CST, late decelerations after every contraction, is indicative of fetal hypoxia and requires delivery of the fetus. An unsatisfactory CST occurs when there are insufficient contractions. The practitioner may repeat the test within 24 hours, or may order a biophysical profile.

Biophysical Profile

Biophysical profile uses a combination of factors to determine fetal well-being. Five fetal biophysical variables are measured. NST measures FHR acceleration. Then ultrasound measures breathing, body movements, tone, and amniotic fluid volume. Each variable receives a score of 0 (abnormal, absent, or insufficient) or 2 (normal or present) for a maximum score of 10. A score of 8 to 10 indicates fetal well-being. A score of 6 correlates with possible fetal asphyxia, whereas a score of 4 indicates probable fetal asphyxia. Scores of 0 to 2 are ominous and require immediate delivery of the fetus (Wyatt & Rhoads, 2006).

Test Yourself

✔ How many times should the fetus move in a 2-hour period of time?

✔ What three tests are included in the triple-marker screening test?

✔ What tissue is extracted for study when chorionic villus sampling is used?

THE NURSE'S ROLE IN PRENATAL CARE

Nurses are in a unique position to influence behaviors of the pregnant woman and to increase the chance she and her baby will stay healthy. Through consistent use of the nursing process, you can detect problems early in order to intervene, or assist the PCP to intervene, and support the woman through her pregnancy. Teaching remains the primary nursing intervention throughout pregnancy.

Nursing Process for Prenatal Care

Assessment

Ongoing assessment and data collection are essential components of prenatal visits. During the first prenatal visit, pay close attention to cues the woman may give regarding her feelings toward the pregnancy. Ambivalence is normal. The woman may express feelings of doubt about the pregnancy or her ability to be a good parent. These are normal reactions when a woman first finds out she is pregnant, and she needs reassurance that her responses are normal. Withdrawal or consistently negative remarks are warning signs. Report these observations to the registered nurse (RN) or PCP.

If you administer the initial questionnaire, show the woman all the pages and assist her to complete it, if necessary. Review the document carefully when she is done to ensure completeness. Look for answers that indicate the need for further assessment. Alert the RN or the PCP of possible risk factors identified in the history.

Assess for signs of nervousness and anxiety. The woman may express her nervousness by being restless or tense or by being quiet and withdrawn. Be attuned to signals she is giving regarding her comfort level. At every visit, inquire carefully regarding current medications, food supplements, and over-the-counter remedies she is using.

Note if the woman has been experiencing nausea and vomiting. Pay close attention to signs that might indicate poor nutritional status. Weight is an obvious clue. If the woman is overweight or underweight, she will need special assistance with nutritional concerns throughout the pregnancy. Other warning signs of poor nutritional status include dull, brittle hair; poor skin turgor; poor condition of skin and nails; obesity; emaciation; or a low hemoglobin level. Ask the woman to write down a typical day's food consumption pattern, and then compare her normal intake to MyPyramid to determine if her diet is adequate for her nutritional needs.

Determine her education level and knowledge of pregnancy and prenatal care. If she is highly knowledgeable, she may ask high-level questions that indicate an understanding of basic issues. Conversely, she may ask basic questions, or no questions at all, which could indicate a knowledge deficit.

During subsequent visits, you may assist with assessing for signs of fetal well-being. These assessments include obtaining fetal heart tones with an ultrasonic Doppler device (Fig. 7-7) beginning in week 10, and soliciting reports of active fetal movements after quickening. Pay close attention to vital signs, particularly the blood pressure. Monitor for danger signs of pregnancy (Box 7-5).

Don't make unfounded assumptions.

Don't assume that just because this is not the woman's first baby, or because she is educated, or even that she is a nurse, that she has the information she needs to maintain a healthy pregnancy. Assess her knowledge level by asking questions and entertaining her questions.

Selected Nursing Diagnoses

- Anxiety related to uncertainty regarding pregnancy diagnosis and not knowing what to expect during the office visit
- Health-seeking Behaviors related to maintaining a healthy pregnancy and concerns regarding the common discomforts of pregnancy

▮ **Figure 7-7** The nurse listens to fetal heart tones with a Doppler device.

> ### Box 7-5 ▮ DANGER SIGNS OF PREGNANCY
>
> Inquire regarding these warning signals at every visit. Instruct the woman to report any of these signs, if she should experience them, to her health care provider right away.
> - Fever or severe vomiting
> - Headache, unrelieved by Tylenol or other relief measures
> - Blurred vision or spots before the eyes
> - Pain in the epigastric region
> - Sudden weight gain or sudden onset of edema in the hands and face
> - Vaginal bleeding
> - Painful urination
> - Sudden gush or constant, uncontrollable leaking of fluid from the vagina
> - Decreased fetal movement
> - Signs of preterm labor
>   Uterine contractions (four or more per hour)
>   Lower, dull backache
>   Pelvic pressure
>   Menstrual-like cramps
>   Increase in vaginal discharge
>   A feeling that something is not right

- Deficient Knowledge of self-care during pregnancy
- Risk for Injury related to complications of pregnancy
- Fear related to the unknown of childbirth, concerns regarding safe passage of self and infant through the delivery experience, and concerns related to assuming the parenting role

Outcome Identification and Planning

Maintaining the health of mother and fetus is the primary goal of nursing care during the prenatal period. Specific goals are that the woman's anxiety will be reduced, she will manage the symptoms and discomforts associated with pregnancy; that she will feel confident in her ability to care for herself throughout the pregnancy; that she nor the fetus will experience injury from complications of pregnancy; that she will have sufficient knowledge to adequately meet her needs and those of the growing fetus throughout the pregnancy; and that she will express confidence in her ability to go through the labor and birth experience and assume the parenting role.

Implementation

Relieving Anxiety

Escort the woman to the examination room. Explain normal procedure and describe what she can expect during the visit. When the woman knows what to expect, she will be much less anxious. Maintain a calm, confident demeanor while giving care. Protect the woman's privacy during invasive examinations.

Try to understand the woman's perspective. Note if her anxiety level increases. Anticipate concern when fetal testing is required. Solicit questions and correct misconceptions the woman may have. Provide information concerning the treatment plan. Use active listening and encourage positive coping behaviors.

Relieving the Common Discomforts of Pregnancy

Pregnant women tend to experience similar discomforts because of the significant bodily changes they undergo. Some discomforts tend to occur in early pregnancy, some toward the end, and others continue throughout. Table 7-2 lists selected discomforts along with hints for helping the woman cope.

Nasal Stuffiness and Epistaxis. A pregnant woman is prone to nasal stuffiness and epistaxis (nosebleeds). Estrogen is the hormone most likely culpable for this discomfort because it contributes to vasocongestion and increases the fragility of the nasal mucosa. Sometimes the woman may have symptoms of the common cold that persist throughout pregnancy. Menthol applied just below the nostrils before bedtime might help relieve some discomfort from congestion. The woman should generally not use nasal decongestants, other than normal saline nasal sprays, and should consult her PCP before taking any medications, including over-the-counter remedies.

Avoiding vigorous nose blowing may prevent nosebleeds. It is also helpful to keep the nasal passages moist. Using a humidifier in the house and staying well hydrated can accomplish this. If a nosebleed occurs despite precautions, instruct the woman to pinch the nostrils and hold pressure for at least 4 minutes until the bleeding stops. Ice may help stop the bleeding. If the bleeding is heavy or does not stop with pressure, instruct the woman to consult her PCP.

Nausea. Morning sickness, or nausea, is a common complaint of early pregnancy, occurring in approximately 75% to 80% of pregnancies (Badell, Ramin, & Smith, 2006). Rising levels of hCG are thought to be part of the cause, although it is likely many factors that contribute. Although "morning sickness" is the lay term for the nausea of pregnancy, many women experience nausea at other times during the day, or even throughout the day. Fortunately, nausea generally subsides by the end of the first trimester.

Caloric intake during the first trimester is not as crucial as it is in the second and third trimesters, so nausea is usually not harmful to the pregnancy. However, severe nausea and vomiting can lead to nutritional deficiencies, dehydration, and electrolyte deficiencies, so preventive measures are important (Hunter & Young, 2007). Some helpful suggestions include advising the woman to place a high-carbohydrate, low-fat snack, such as Melba toast or saltine crackers, at the bedside before retiring. In the morning before getting out of bed, she should eat the snack. This can help prevent early morning nausea.

Other helpful hints are to encourage the woman to eat small amounts frequently throughout the day, instead of consuming three heavy meals hours apart, and never to let the stomach become completely empty. It also helps to avoid strong odors and spicy and fatty foods. Sometimes it is easier for the woman to eat when someone else prepares the meal. Brushing the teeth causes salivation, which can intensify nausea. In addition, the smell of the toothpaste may cause nausea, so the woman should wait for 1 hour after eating before brushing her teeth.

When the nonpharmacologic interventions described above do not sufficiently treat the nausea, there are several options. Two alternative therapies that have shown benefit are the herbal supplement ginger, at a dose of 250 mg by mouth 4 times per day or acupressure treatments. Sometimes taking a multivitamin supplement helps. Some studies have shown therapeutic benefit of taking 25 mg of pyridoxine (vitamin B_6) every 8 hours (Badell, Ramin, & Smith, 2006).

Persistent vomiting may be a sign of hyperemesis gravidarum, a complication of pregnancy that can lead to dehydration and electrolyte imbalances. If the vomiting is severe or prolonged, advise the woman to consult her PCP. She should call the practitioner if she is unable to retain any food or fluids for 24 hours (Hunter & Young, 2007).

Feeling Faint. Sometimes women feel faint during the first few weeks of pregnancy. Postural hypotension could be the cause. Low blood sugar levels aggravate the situation. Advise the woman to change positions slowly and to avoid abrupt position changes. Eating frequent high-carbohydrate meals helps to keep blood sugar levels up. If she feels faint, a walk outside might help. Alternatively, she might need to lie down with her feet elevated or sit with her head lower than her knees, until the feeling passes.

Frequent Urination. Frequent urination can be bothersome and interfere with sleep. One cause of frequent urination in the first trimester is the increasing blood volume and increased glomerular-filtration rate. Frequency usually diminishes during the second trimester, only to reappear in the third trimester because of pressure of the enlarging uterus on the bladder.

Increased Vaginal Discharge. Leukorrhea, or increased vaginal discharge, is common during pregnancy. Increased production of cervical glands and vasocongestion of the pelvic area contribute to the discharge. If the discharge causes itching or irritation, or if there is a foul smell noted, the woman should contact her PCP because these are signs of infection. She should avoid douching because douching can upset the normal balance of vaginal flora, increasing the risk of contracting an infection (Cottrell, 2006). Sanitary pads may help to absorb the discharge.

Shortness of Breath. Shortness of breath may occur during the first trimester because of the effects of progesterone. During the latter half of pregnancy, this symptom results from the pressure of the uterus pushing upward

Table 7-2 ▌ COMMON DISCOMFORTS OF PREGNANCY

Discomfort	Contributing Factor or Cause	Hints for Relieving the Discomfort
Bleeding gums	Stimulating effects of estrogen on the gums	• Visit the dentist • Use rinses and gargles to freshen the oral cavity • Use a soft-bristled toothbrush
Nasal stuffiness	Effects of estrogen on the nasal mucosa cause vasocongestion and stuffiness.	• Use a cool-air vaporizer • Try normal saline nasal sprays • Try to avoid commercial medicated nasal sprays because initial relief may be followed by rebound stuffiness
Nosebleeds	The tiny veins of the nasal lining are prone to breaking and causing nosebleeds. Dry nasal passages increase the risk.	• Avoid vigorous nose blowing • Use a humidifier • Drink plenty of fluids
Breast tenderness	Progesterone and estrogen are thought to contribute to the tingling or heavy sensations in the breasts that come and go throughout pregnancy.	• Wear a well-fitted support bra • Wearing a bra at night might be helpful if breast discomfort is interfering with restful sleep.
Nausea and nausea with vomiting	Rising levels of hCG probably contribute to nausea along with other factors.	• Begin the day with a high-carbohydrate food, such as melba toast, saltines, or other crackers. • Change positions slowly, especially when getting up in the morning. • Eat small high-protein meals frequently throughout the day. • If protein is not well tolerated, try high-carbohydrate, low-fat snacks to avoid hypoglycemia. • Wait at least 1 hour after eating to brush the teeth. • Drink small amounts frequently. Include electrolyte-replenishing liquids, such as Gatorade and AllSport. • Avoid noxious odors. • Take a walk outside in the fresh air. • Delay iron supplementation until the second trimester.
Feeling faint	Postural hypotension can easily develop with the hemodynamic changes that occur in a normal pregnancy as the blood vessels in the periphery relax and dilate.	• Change positions slowly. • Avoid abrupt position changes. • Eat small, frequent, high-carbohydrate meals.
Fatigue	Cause is unknown. Progesterone may contribute.	• Plan for daily naps. • Take frequent rest breaks throughout the day. • Go to bed early.
Shortness of breath	In early pregnancy, the effects of progesterone can create a sense of shortness of breath. In later pregnancy, the uterus pushes on the diaphragm.	• Sit up straight to increase diameter of the chest. • If shortness of breath is interfering with sleep, prop up with pillows.
Heartburn	Relaxation of the LES under the influence of progesterone and increased intra-abdominal pressure due to the growing uterus cause acid reflux into the lower esophagus.	• Eat small, frequent meals • Avoid substances that increase acid production, in particular cigarette smoking. • Avoid substances that cause relaxation of the LES, such as coffee, chocolate, alcohol, and heavy spices. • Avoid lying down after a meal. • Avoid lying flat.
Low back pain	Changes in the center of gravity and loosened ligaments	• Avoid gaining too much weight. • Avoid high-heeled shoes. • Always bend at the knees, not the waist. • Avoid standing for too long at one time. • Keep one foot on a stool when standing. Frequently change the foot that is resting on the stool.

(continued)

Table 7-2 ▌ COMMON DISCOMFORTS OF PREGNANCY *(continued)*

Discomfort	Contributing Factor or Cause	Hints for Relieving the Discomfort
Round ligament pain	Sharp, severe pain, usually on the right side brought on by stretching of the round ligaments that support the uterus.	• Avoid sudden changes in positions or sudden movements. • Apply heat. • Lie on the side opposite the pain.
Leg cramps	Not known.	• Avoid plantar flexion. • Rest frequently with the feet elevated. • When cramps occur, extend the affected leg and dorsiflex the foot. • Take magnesium lactate or citrate 5 mmol in the morning and 10 mmol at night.
Varicose veins	Increased pelvic pressure, vasodilation in the lower extremities and vagina, along with pooling of blood in the lower extremities can contribute to varicosities of the legs and vagina.	• Exercise daily. • Rest with the legs elevated several times daily. • Wear compression stockings. Put them on before getting out of bed in the morning. • Avoid prolonged periods of standing or sitting. Move around frequently. Stretch and take small walks. • When you must stand for a long time, frequently exercise the leg muscles and change positions frequently. • Keep within the recommended weight range during pregnancy.
Ankle edema	Progesterone effects, increased pressure in the lower extremities, increased capillary permeability	• Avoid prolonged periods of standing. • Rest frequently with the feet elevated. • Soak in a warm pool or bath. • Avoid constrictive garments on the lower extremities.
Flatulence	Relaxation of the gastrointestinal tract under the influence of progesterone, pressure of the uterus on the intestines, air swallowing	• Avoid gas-producing foods. • Chew foods thoroughly. • Get plenty of exercise. • Maintain regular bowel habits.
Constipation and hemorrhoids	Slowing of the gastrointestinal tract under the influence of progesterone and increased blood flow and pressure in the pelvic area	• Drink at least 8 glasses of noncaffeinated beverages per day. • Eat plenty of fiber. • Get adequate exercise. • Use a stool softener, if prescribed by the primary care provider. • Use topical anesthetic agents to treat the pain of hemorrhoids.
Trouble sleeping	Many discomforts of pregnancy, as well as the increase in size of the abdomen, can all contribute to sleepless nights in the third trimester.	• Get adequate exercise. • Try different positions and use pillows to support and wedge. • Try sleeping in a sitting position. • Drink a glass of warm milk before bed. • Have a late-night, high-carbohydrate snack. • Try progressive muscle relaxation or guided imagery.

on the diaphragm. Advise the woman to take her time and rest frequently. If shortness of breath occurs during exercise, she may need to decrease the level of intensity. During late pregnancy, shortness of breath may interfere with sleep. Propping up with pillows can help expand the chest and decrease the sensation of being unable to catch her breath. Shortness of breath accompanied by chest pain, coughing up blood, or a smothering sensa-

tion with fever is a danger sign that indicates the need for medical intervention.

Heartburn. Heartburn, or pyrosis, is a common complaint occurring in 30% to 50% of pregnancies (Richter, 2005). Several factors contribute to this discomfort. Progesterone causes a generalized slowing of the gastrointestinal tract and can cause relaxation of the lower esophageal sphincter (LES). When the LES is relaxed, acid content from the stomach can back up into the lower part of the esophagus and cause a burning sensation, known as heartburn. The increased pressure in the abdomen from the enlarging uterus contributes to the problem.

Prevention is generally the best way to treat heartburn. Several factors aggravate the condition. Smoking increases the acid content of the stomach. Certain foods and beverages, such as coffee, chocolate, peppermint, fatty or fried foods, alcohol, and heavy spices, can contribute to LES relaxation and exacerbate heartburn. Explain that the woman should avoid the particular substances that cause her discomfort. The pregnant woman should not smoke or drink alcohol because of the harmful effects on the fetus.

Advise the woman regarding interventions to help prevent heartburn or lessen its severity. The woman should eat smaller meals more frequently and avoid drinking fluids with meals. Filling the stomach with a heavy meal or with food and fluid increases the pressure and contributes to gastric reflux. It is best if the woman avoids lying down after meals. If she must lie down, suggest that she lie on her left side with her head higher than her abdomen. Placing 6-in blocks under the head of the bed or propping pillows at night to keep the chest higher than the abdomen may help. Chewing gum can help neutralize acid (Richter, 2005).

If nonpharmacologic interventions are not successful to prevent heartburn, medication may help. However, the woman should not take any over-the-counter medications or remedies without first consulting her PCP because several commonly used heartburn remedies, such as sodium bicarbonate, are not for use in pregnancy. The primary care provider may prescribe an antacid. If so, the woman should not take her vitamins within 1 hour of taking antacids.

Backaches. More than two thirds of all pregnant women experience low back pain at some point during pregnancy (Pennick & Young, 2007). Obesity and previous history of back pain are risk factors. Softening and loosening of the ligaments supporting the joints of the spine and pelvis can contribute to low back pain, as can the increasing lordosis of pregnancy and the changing center of gravity.

Teach the woman to prevent low back pain by using good posture, proper-body mechanics, such as bending the knees to reach something on the floor, rather than stooping over from the waist. She should also avoid high-heeled shoes. Good pelvic support with a girdle might be helpful for some women. Strengthening and conditioning exercises may be beneficial.

Treatment of mild backache includes heat, ice, acetaminophen, and massage. If the woman must stand for prolonged periods, she can put one foot on a stool. She should periodically switch the foot that is on the stool (Trupin, 2006). Severe back pain is usually associated with some type of pathology. The woman should consult her PCP for severe pain.

Round Ligament Pain. The round ligaments support the uterus in the abdomen. As the uterus expands during pregnancy, it applies pressure to the round ligaments, which respond by stretching and thinning. Because ligaments are pain sensitive structures, some women experience round ligament pain. The pain most frequently occurs on the right side and can be severe. The pain can occur at night and awaken the woman from sleep, or exercise can bring it on.

Helpful hints to treat round ligament pain include the application of heat. A heating pad or warm bath might be soothing. Sometimes lying on the opposite side can relieve some of the pressure on the ligament and reduce the pain. Avoiding sudden movements may help prevent round ligament pain. If fever, chills, painful urination, or vaginal bleeding accompanies the pain, the woman should seek emergency care because the pain is likely the result of a medical condition.

Leg Cramps. Leg cramps are a common occurrence during pregnancy, but researchers do not know the cause. Preventive measures include getting enough rest, resting several times per day with the feet elevated, walking, wearing low-heeled shoes, and avoiding constrictive clothing. Another preventive measure is for the woman to avoid plantar flexion (pointing the toes forward). A recent Cochrane Database meta-analysis found that there is little evidence to support supplementation with calcium, sodium, or multivitamins to prevent leg cramps. The supplement that helps most is magnesium lactate or citrate. The woman should take 5 mmol in the morning and 10 mmol at night (Young & Jewell, 2007). When cramps occur, the woman's partner can help by assisting her to extend her leg, then dorsiflex the foot so that the toes point toward the woman's head. If she is alone, she can extend her leg and dorsiflex the foot until the cramp resolves.

Constipation and Hemorrhoids. The natural slowing of the gastrointestinal tract under the influence of hormones can lead to constipation during pregnancy, and constipation can lead to hemorrhoids. The best way to treat constipation is to prevent it. The same common sense approaches to preventing constipation that are advisable under normal situations are also helpful during pregnancy. These include drinking at least eight glasses of noncaffeinated beverages each day. Advise the woman to get adequate exercise. Adding fiber to the diet or a bulk-forming supplement such as Metamucil to the daily routine are also helpful hints.

Hemorrhoids can become a problem during pregnancy because of the increased blood flow in the rectal veins and pressure of the uterus that prevents good venous return. Elevating the legs and hips intermittently throughout the day can help counteract this problem. Hemorrhoids can cause pain, itching, burning sensation, and occasionally bleeding. Applying topical anesthetics such as Preparation H or Anusol cream and compresses, such as witch hazel pads, can relieve the pain and swelling.

Trouble Sleeping. Many of the discomforts discussed previously, such as heartburn and shortness of breath, can contribute to restlessness at night and trouble sleeping. As the pregnancy progresses, it becomes increasingly difficult to find a position of comfort in bed. Suggest that the woman try lying on her side with plenty of pillows to support her back and legs. If that position does not help, she may find it easier to sleep in the sitting position in an armchair.

Urinary frequency returns during the third trimester and can contribute to sleeplessness because of frequent trips to the restroom. Drinking the majority of fluids early in the day and limiting fluids in the evening hours can reduce this problem. Heartburn can contribute to reduction in sleep, as can the movements of an active fetus. Some degree of sleeplessness and restlessness at night is an expected occurrence in the third trimester.

Teaching Self-Care During Pregnancy

The woman is usually too distracted during the first visit to absorb and retain much information. Keep teaching sessions brief and give her printed materials to read at home. The PCP should have a handout with a list of resources, such as books and Web sites to give to the woman. Tailor teaching topics to the individual needs of the woman during subsequent visits. Important self-care topics are discussed below. Family Teaching Tips: Major Components of Prenatal Self-Care highlights key topics to discuss with the pregnant woman during the course of prenatal care.

Maintaining a Balanced Nutritional Intake. During the first trimester, the fetus' demands on maternal stores are less than at other times during the pregnancy. This is helpful because sometimes it is difficult for the woman to eat a well-balanced diet when she is coping with nausea. Focus on assessing the adequacy of her diet and answering her questions during the first visit. Emphasize the importance of taking the prenatal vitamins the PCP ordered for her. On subsequent visits, assist the woman to assess her own diet for adequacy by using the MyPyramid Web site at http://mypyramid.gov/. This interactive Web site developed by the U.S. Department of Agriculture and U.S. Department of Health and Human Services allows the woman to enter personalized information and receive a nutrition plan tailor-made for her. Instruct her to go to the Web site and choose "For Pregnancy and Breastfeeding" on the left side menu.

The key to healthy nutrition during pregnancy is quality and variety. Detailed nutritional guidelines may overwhelm some women. In general, it is safe to counsel the pregnant woman about the following strategies. Make certain there is enough food to eat and then advise the woman to eat the amount and type of food that she wants, salting it to taste. MyPyramid can assist the pregnant woman achieve a balanced diet. Monitor weight gain throughout pregnancy. There should be a steady increase in weight throughout pregnancy, for a total increase of 25 to 35 lb. Sudden weight gain often is asso-

Family Teaching Tips

MAJOR COMPONENTS OF PRENATAL SELF-CARE

- Avoid alcohol. Alcohol harms the fetus; no amount of alcohol is safe during pregnancy.
- Avoid smoking. Smoking harms the fetus. It can lead to lower birth weight and increase the incidence of preterm labor.
- Eat a healthy, well-balanced diet. If you consume a variety of nutritious foods daily, you will likely get the nutrients you need.
- Consume approximately 300 calories more per day than before pregnancy.
- Take an extra 400 mcg of folic acid per day. If the doctor ordered prenatal vitamins, the recommended dose will be met.
- Avoid dieting during pregnancy. Every pregnant woman with a normal body mass index should gain 25 to 30 lb during the pregnancy.
- Continue to exercise during pregnancy. However, do not exercise to the point of exhaustion or start a grueling new workout that you were not doing before pregnancy.
- Avoid handling raw meat and cat litter. Wear gloves when gardening to prevent contracting toxoplasmosis from animal droppings, an infection that is very harmful to the baby.
- Handle cold cuts carefully. Heat thin slices of meat in the microwave until steaming hot. Wash hands with hot soapy water after handling deli meats to avoid listeriosis, a bacterial infection that is harmful to the baby.
- Avoid douching. Douching during pregnancy increases the risk for bacterial infection.
- Avoid taking any medication (other than acetaminophen) or over-the-counter herbal remedy unless your primary care provider has approved it.

ciated with fluid retention and may be a sign of developing preeclampsia. Periodically assess the diet by asking the woman to do a 1- to 3-day food recall. Encourage the woman to take her iron and folic acid supplement. Monitor the hemoglobin and hematocrit at the 28-week check-up for any decreases. (See Chapter 6 for more detail on prenatal nutrition.)

Dental Hygiene. A pregnant woman needs to continue regular dental checkups and practice excellent dental hygiene. This includes at least twice-daily brushing, once-daily flossing, and a nutritious diet. If pregnancy gingivitis is a problem, then regular dental checkups are necessary. Untreated gingivitis can damage the gums and result in bone and tooth loss.

Vomiting in association with morning sickness can be hard on teeth. Stomach acids in the vomitus can make the teeth more susceptible to injury from the toothbrush. To reduce the impact of this problem, instruct the woman to rinse with water after vomiting, followed by a fluoride rinse or sugarless chewing gum to help neutralize the stomach acid. She should avoid brushing her teeth for at least 1 hour after vomiting to decrease the risk of enamel loss.

Exercise. Exercise is healthy during pregnancy. A woman may generally maintain her normal exercise routine during pregnancy, as long as she does not become overheated or excessively fatigued. Conditioned women have safely run marathons during pregnancy. Some research indicates that women who exercise during pregnancy experience shorter labors, have fewer cesarean deliveries, and have fetuses that experience fewer episodes of fetal distress. Women who exercise often report having better self-esteem and fewer depressive symptoms than do their nonexercising counterparts. These women return to their prepregnancy weight faster than sedentary women (Kelly, 2005). Box 7-6 outlines the March of Dimes (2007) precautions to increase the safety of exercise for the pregnant woman.

The American College of Obstetricians and Gynecologists (2005) recommends that a well-conditioned woman continue her pattern of aerobic exercise during pregnancy. If the woman is sedentary before pregnancy, she should not start a vigorous aerobic routine. In this situation, walking is the preferred exercise after getting approval from her PCP. There are some high-risk conditions, such as premature rupture of membranes, preeclampsia, vaginal bleeding, or incompetent cervix, in which exercise is contraindicated.

General common sense guidelines include advising the woman to listen to her body. The woman can use the "talk test" to gauge exertion level; that is, she should not be too short of breath to carry on a conversation while exercising (Kelly, 2005). If she is feeling fatigued, she should slow down or stop. She should not allow her heart rate to exceed 140 beats per minute. In the last trimester as the center of gravity changes, she should take extra care to avoid injury during exercise.

Hygiene. Perspiration and vaginal discharge increase during pregnancy, making personal hygiene a concern for some pregnant women. In general, tub baths or showers can continue throughout pregnancy with an eye toward safety. Some general personal hygiene considerations for pregnancy follow.

■ Bathe in warm, not hot, water. Extreme temperature elevations associated with hot showers, baths, saunas, hot tubs, and fever are dangerous to the developing fetus.
■ Take care, particularly in the third trimester, when getting in and out of the tub or shower. Fainting can

---

Box 7-6 ■ PRECAUTIONS TO ENSURE A SAFE EXERCISE PROGRAM FOR THE PREGNANT WOMAN

The pregnant woman should avoid the following activities:

■ Contact sports and any activities that can cause even mild trauma to the abdomen, such as ice hockey, kickboxing, soccer, and basketball.
■ Activities with a high risk for falling, such as gymnastics, horseback riding, downhill skiing, and vigorous racquet sports.
■ Scuba diving, which puts the baby at increased risk for decompression sickness and may contribute to miscarriage, birth defects, poor fetal growth, and preterm labor.
■ Exercising on the back after the first trimester. Also, avoid prolonged periods of motionless standing. Both can reduce blood flow to the uterus.
■ Jerky, bouncing, or high-impact movements that may strain joints and cause injuries.
■ Exercising at high altitudes (more than 6,000 ft) because it can lead to reduced amounts of oxygen reaching the baby.
■ Overheating, especially in the first trimester. Drink plenty of fluids before, during, and after exercise. Wear layers of "breathable" clothing and do not exercise on hot, humid days.
■ Bathing in hot tubs, saunas, and Jacuzzis.

Source: March of Dimes, (Eds.). (2007, March). Fitness for two. *Professionals & Researchers Quick Reference and Fact Sheets.* Retrieved October 13, 2007, from http://www.marchofdimes.com/printableArticles/14332_1150.asp

---

occur, particularly if the water is too hot. Balancing can become problematic because the center of gravity changes. Handrails in the shower or tub are ideal. Rubber bath mats are also helpful.
■ Avoid douching during pregnancy. This practice increases the risk for bacterial infection. Gentle cleansing of the genital area with warm water and soap are sufficient to control discomfort from increased vaginal secretions.

Breast Care. A pregnant woman should wear a bra that fits well and supports the breasts. She should use only clean water to wash the nipples. Soap dries the nipples and can lead to cracking.

Some women wish to condition their nipples for breast-feeding. Exposing the nipples to air and sunlight for a portion of each day is helpful. Manually stimulating the nipples by rolling them between the fingers or oral stimulation of the nipple by the partner, as a part of sexual expression, are additional ways to toughen the nipples. These practices are acceptable as long as there is no history of preterm labor because nipple stimulation can stimulate labor.

Clothing. Clothing should be loose and comfortable. The woman should not wear garments that constrict the waist or legs. If finances are tight, the woman might try borrowing clothes from a friend or relative, rather than investing in expensive maternity clothes. She might also buy used maternity clothes. High heels exacerbate backache and can be a safety hazard for the pregnant woman who has problems with balance. Shoes should fit comfortably.

Sexual Activity. Many couples are fearful that sexual activity during pregnancy might hurt the fetus. Unless there is a history of preterm labor, vaginal bleeding, ruptured membranes, or other medical contraindication, the woman and her partner can safely continue intercourse and other sexual activities throughout pregnancy. Many factors influence the woman's desire for sexual activity. During the first trimester, she may feel nauseous and tired, so her interest in sex might be low. During the second trimester, she often feels better and may have a heightened interest in sex. The increased blood flow to the pelvic area can intensify the sexual experience for the pregnant woman. Some women experience orgasm for the first time during pregnancy. During the third trimester, fatigue may reduce her desire or she might fear hurting the fetus.

The partner's sexual desire is also dependent on several interrelated factors. Some men find the pregnant body sexually appealing and desirable. Others may have trouble adjusting to their partner's changing body shape. Some men are afraid of hurting their partner or the unborn child during intercourse. It may be helpful to have a tactful discussion regarding sexual concerns with the woman and the partner. During the third trimester, the male superior position may become difficult to accomplish. A side-lying or woman superior position might be easier. Vaginal penetration is less deep with the male facing the woman's back. This position might be more comfortable for the woman (Trupin, 2006).

Sometimes the woman might be content with kissing, cuddling, and caressing as forms of sexual expression. If her partner needs more release, the woman might stimulate him to ejaculation, or he may prefer to masturbate. The essential ingredient is ongoing respectful communication between the partners regarding their sexual needs and desires.

A word of caution: If the couple practices anal intercourse, they should not proceed to vaginal intercourse after engaging in anal intercourse. Doing so could introduce the bacterium *Escherichia coli* into the vagina that could cause an ascending infection.

Employment. How long a woman can remain safely employed during pregnancy depends on several factors. In general, a woman with a low-risk pregnancy can continue working until she goes into labor, unless there are specific hazards associated with her job. Research demonstrates that women in physically demanding jobs, such as working in the fields (day laborers), experience a higher incidence of low-birth-weight infants, preterm delivery, and hypertension during pregnancy. A woman who is required to stand for long periods as part of her job also is at increased risk for preterm delivery.

When a woman chooses to work during pregnancy, it is most helpful if she can take frequent rest periods. If she must stand for prolonged periods, suggest that she shift her weight back and forth, and that she take frequent breaks to walk around and to sit with her feet elevated. She should avoid excessive fatigue.

Exposure to **teratogens**, substances capable of causing birth defects, is always a concern when a woman works during pregnancy. Environmental hazards that might put the pregnant woman at risk in the work place include exposure to chemicals, metals, solvents, pharmaceutical agents, radiation, extreme heat, second-hand smoke, and infection (Fowler & Culpepper, 2007). The woman should investigate the type of chemicals or other substances to which she is exposed during the course of her work and then work with her employer to limit exposure to harmful substances.

Travel. Travel is generally not limited during the first trimester. The woman can travel safely in the second and third trimesters with careful planning. One concern when traveling long distances is the chance that labor will occur while the woman is away from her PCP. It is advisable for the woman to carry copies of her prenatal records with her when she travels. This practice will increase the odds that she will receive appropriate care if she must seek health care away from home.

When traveling by car, encourage the woman to make frequent stops (at least every 2 hours) so that she can empty her bladder and walk about. Sitting for prolonged periods in one position can predispose the woman to clot formation. She should not decrease fluid intake to avoid having to stop to void. Insufficient fluids can lead to dehydration and increase the risk for clot formation, constipation, and hemorrhoids. There is no increased risk with air travel, other than the risk of developing complications in an area remote from the help needed.

The greatest risk to the fetus during an automobile crash is death of the mother. Therefore, all pregnant women should use three-point seat belt restraints when traveling in the car (Fig. 7-8). Teach the woman to apply the lap belt snugly and comfortably. When driving, she should move the seat as far back as possible from the steering wheel. The airbag should be engaged with the steering wheel tilted so that the airbag releases toward the breastbone versus the abdomen or the head (Cesario, 2007).

■ **Figure 7-8** Proper application of a seat belt during pregnancy.

Test Yourself

✔ List three suggestions for reducing nausea in early pregnancy.

✔ Name three actions the pregnant woman can take to reduce heartburn.

✔ Why should the pregnant woman avoid hot showers or baths?

Medications and Herbal Remedies. The general principle regarding medication use during pregnancy is that almost all medications cross the placenta and can potentially affect the fetus. The woman should not take any medication, including over-the-counter medications and herbal remedies, during pregnancy without the express approval of the PCP. Before she takes any medication, the practitioner should make a careful appraisal of risk versus benefit. Treatment, including medications, for certain diseases and conditions must continue during pregnancy. Examples include epilepsy, asthma, diabetes, and depression (see Chapter 16).

The problem with most medications is that they cross the placenta, but their effect on the fetus or pregnancy is not always known. Because of ethical concerns, controlled trials of medication use during human pregnancy are usually not possible. The little that is known about medication effects during pregnancy comes from animal trials and from experience over the years in treating chronic maternal conditions. The problem with animal

---

Box 7-7 ▌ FDA PREGNANCY CATEGORIES OF MEDICATIONS

The Food and Drug Administration (FDA) has delineated five categories for medication use during pregnancy. Each category details the overall threat, if any, the drug in that category might pose to the fetus or pregnancy. The categories are differentiated according to the type and reliability of documentation available and the risk-versus-benefit ratio. The categories are as follows:

Category A: Adequate studies in pregnant women have not demonstrated a risk to the fetus in the first trimester of pregnancy, and there is no evidence of risk in later trimesters.

Category B: Animal studies have not demonstrated a risk to the fetus, but there are no adequate studies in pregnant women. Or animal studies have shown an adverse effect, but adequate studies in pregnant women have not demonstrated a risk to the fetus during the first trimester of pregnancy, and there is no evidence of risk in later trimesters.

Category C: Animal studies have shown an adverse effect on the fetus, but there are no adequate studies in humans; the benefits from the use of the drug in pregnant women may be acceptable, despite its potential risks. Or there are no animal reproduction studies and no adequate studies in humans.

Category D: There is evidence of human fetal risk, but the potential benefits from the use of the drug in pregnant women may be acceptable despite its potential risk.

Category X: Studies in animals or humans demonstrate fetal abnormalities or adverse reaction; reports indicate evidence of fetal risk. The risk of use in a pregnant woman clearly outweighs any possible benefit.

In any case, the woman should not take any medication during pregnancy unless there is a clear benefit for its use.

---

studies is that there is no guarantee that human pregnancies or fetuses will respond in the same way as the animal that is being studied responds. Box 7-7 describes the Food and Drug Administration's five pregnancy categories for medications.

Many women use herbal remedies. Some remedies are culturally determined, passed from mother to daughter from generation to generation. Some women believe that herbs and alternative therapies are safer than medications. Some studies are verifying the health benefits of certain herbs. However, certain herbs are contraindicated in pregnancy, so it is important for the pregnant woman to report all herbal and over-the-counter remedies to the PCP. Enhance communication by asking about herbal use in a nonthreatening way (Born & Barron, 2005).

Teaching About Substance Use and Abuse

Substance use is a term that simply refers to use of a substance, whereas the term *substance abuse* specifically indicates that a person has a problem with the use of the substance. Although many substances have the potential for abuse, this section covers caffeine, tobacco, alcohol, and recreational drug use. Chapter 20 provides more in depth coverage of the fetal/neonatal effects of alcohol and recreational drug use during pregnancy.

Caffeine. There is controversy and uncertainty regarding the role of caffeine use during pregnancy. Current recommendations are that the pregnant woman may safely consume coffee and caffeine in moderation. The March of Dimes (2005) defines moderate as one to two 8-oz cups of coffee per day. Although there is no definitive proof that caffeine in larger doses causes problems in pregnancy, there is some evidence that the woman who drinks three or more cups of coffee per day may be at increased risk for spontaneous abortion or delivering a low-birth-weight baby.

Tobacco. Smoking is contraindicated during pregnancy. Smoking increases the risk for low birth weight; preterm delivery; abortions; stillbirths; sudden infant death syndrome; birth defects, such as cleft lip and palate; and neonatal respiratory disorders, including asthma. Smoking poisons the fetus with carbon monoxide and nicotine, leading to fetal hypoxia. It also affects the placenta, causing it to age sooner than normal, a condition that reduces blood flow to the fetus, contributing to hypoxia and stunted growth. Despite these health hazards, approximately half a million women in the United States continue to smoke during pregnancy (Chen et al., 2006), and these figures may actually be much higher due to underreporting (Okah, et al., 2005). Although aids to stop smoking, such as nicotine gum and the new drug varenicline (Chantix), are pregnancy Category C drugs and the transdermal patch is in pregnancy Category D (see Box 7-7), the risk of injury caused by smoking may outweigh the risk of harm from these drugs.

Alcohol. There is no safe amount of alcohol consumption during pregnancy, but one in eight pregnant women consume alcohol (Krulewitch, 2005). A woman should not drink any alcoholic beverages during pregnancy because alcohol is a potent teratogen. Even one drink can cause an unborn baby long-term harm (Constantinou, 2005). For years, the risk of fetal alcohol syndrome has been linked to the use of large amounts of alcohol during pregnancy. Characteristics of fetal alcohol syndrome include **microcephaly** (a very small cranium), facial deformities, growth restriction, and mental retardation. Although smaller amounts of alcohol may not lead to a full-blown case of fetal alcohol syndrome, subtle features of the syndrome might present to include milder forms of mental retardation and learning disabilities.

Marijuana. There is conflicting data about the effects of marijuana on pregnancy. Some studies suggest that marijuana use in pregnancy may slow fetal growth and possibly increase the risk for premature delivery. Infants born to women who smoke marijuana during pregnancy show evidence of stressed nervous systems (March of Dimes, 2006). These infants tend to have high-pitched cries, tremulousness, and reduced response to visual stimuli. Researchers continue to study the long-term effects of marijuana use in pregnancy on the child.

Cocaine. Cocaine has many negative effects on pregnancy. Pregnancy increases the cardiovascular dysfunction associated with cocaine use. This puts the pregnant woman who uses cocaine at high risk for cardiac dysrhythmias and myocardial ischemia and infarction (Kuczkowski, 2005). Cocaine use is associated with a higher rate of spontaneous abortion and premature labor. Infants born to women who use cocaine during pregnancy tend to be small and have a higher incidence of low birth weight. Cocaine use during pregnancy can cause the placenta to pull away from the uterine wall prematurely (placental abruption), leading to fetal and maternal hemorrhage. These infants exhibit withdrawal behaviors after birth and must receive special treatment for the withdrawal (see Chapter 20).

Maintaining Safety of the Woman and Fetus

Monitor the pregnant woman at every visit for warning signs (see Box 7-5). If she reports experiencing any of the warning signs, notify the RN or PCP immediately. If at any time during the pregnancy an elevated blood pressure is noted, report this finding immediately to the RN or PCP, particularly if it is accompanied by a headache, epigastric pain, or blurred vision.

Preparing the Woman for Labor, Birth, and Parenthood

Being prepared for labor, birth, and parenting boosts the woman's confidence and increases her use of positive coping measures. Many women search the Internet and read books that address the birth and parenting experience. The PCP should also provide lists of resources available in the local community. Available resources may include classes on a variety of topics offered by private practice or not-for-profit educational organizations or by hospitals.

Packing for the Hospital or Birthing Center. As the woman prepares for the birth of her baby, she may begin to gather items she will need at the hospital or birthing center. She should pack one bag of articles she will need for labor and another bag of things for her postpartum stay and the trip home from the hospital (Box 7-8).

Communicating Expectations About Labor and Birth. It is important for the woman to feel comfortable

---

Box 7-8 ▮ WHAT TO PACK FOR THE HOSPITAL OR BIRTHING CENTER

Labor Items
- Lotion for massage or effleurage
- Sour lollipops (counteracts nausea, moistens mouth, gives energy)
- Mouth spray or toothbrush and toothpaste
- Chapstick or lip balm
- Socks
- Tennis ball, ice pack, back massager
- Picture or object for focal point
- Camera with good batteries and plenty of film (check with hospital regarding policies on cameras during delivery)
- CD player and CDs for relaxation music
- Contact lens case and solutions
- Hair brush and hair ribbon or band to get hair off neck
- Hand fan
- Favorite pillows

Postpartum Items
- Nursing gowns
- Robe and slippers
- Nursing bras
- Toilet articles (toothpaste and toothbrush, deodorant, tissues)
- Cosmetics
- Pen and paper
- Baby book
- Personal address book with telephone numbers
- Loose-fitting clothes for the trip home
- Socks for baby
- Clothes for baby to wear home
- Baby blankets appropriate for weather

---

communicating her desires regarding labor and birth. Some women feel very strongly about having natural childbirth or breastfeeding. Others want an epidural as soon as possible after they go into labor. These are only three examples of expectations a woman may have. Encourage the woman to write down her questions and expectations and to communicate these to her PCP. Some women develop written birth plans (Box 7-9) to communicate their desires. These can be helpful to the woman and the PCP.

Be careful.

It isn't helpful to make promises that you can't keep. If a woman or her partner discloses unrealistic expectations about the birth process, be honest and tell her it is unlikely her expectations will be met. This gives her the opportunity to decide if her plan is negotiable or if she needs to go elsewhere to get her needs met.

If the woman communicates her expectations early in the pregnancy, there is time for her to find another provider if her current provider cannot or will not meet her expectations.

Choosing the Support Person. The expectant mother may have choices involving her labor support team if she delivers in the hospital or birthing center. Some hospitals limit her to one or two persons for labor support. Other women may have the option of having more support persons for labor. The woman may choose the father of the baby as her main support person. In other situations, the primary support person might be her mother, sister, other family member, or friend.

The woman may choose to have a **doula** with her as a support person. The word *doula* is Greek for servant. Doulas of North America (DONA), founded in 1992, is an international association of doulas who are trained "to provide the highest quality emotional, physical and educational support to women and their families during childbirth and postpartum" (The DONA International Advantage, undated). The woman may contract with a doula to provide support for labor and birth and help with establishing breastfeeding. A doula can also provide support for the postpartum period. The doula's role may include assisting the woman and her partner in preparing for and carrying out their plans for the birth; providing emotional support, physical comfort measures, and an objective viewpoint; as well as helping the woman get the information she needs to make good decisions. A woman may choose to hire a doula because she wants to decrease the likelihood of needing pharmacologic pain management, oxytocin (Pitocin), forceps, vacuum extraction, or cesarean birth, and because she wants an advocate at a time when she may feel unable to vocalize her needs adequately.

Childbirth Education Classes. Since the 1970s, many parents have begun to prepare for labor and childbirth by attending classes. Today, childbirth educators offer classes in private practice, not-for-profit organizations, and hospitals. Some classes adhere to the philosophy of one method of unmedicated childbirth (Box 7-10). Others combine philosophies of two or more methods of childbirth. Still, others tend to teach the woman little about birthing a baby without medical pain management and focus on the medical procedures and routines that she can expect upon admission to the hospital. Some programs combine information about birth, baby care, and breastfeeding in one series of classes. Others offer separate classes for which the woman and her partner can register. Box 7-11 lists common topics included in childbirth education classes.

Pregnancy and Postpartum Exercise Classes. The purpose of these classes is to enhance endurance as well as to strengthen the arms, legs, pelvic floor, back, and abdomen. A certified childbirth educator or a nurse usually offers these classes. Some fitness centers also offer pre- and postnatal exercise classes. Basic pregnancy exercises,

Box 7-9 ▮ SAMPLE BIRTH PLAN

Birth plan for Rachel Thompson
Due date: March 23, 2010
Patient of Dr. Maria Martinez
Scheduled to deliver at Metropolitan Medical Center

January 10, 2010

Dear Dr. Martinez and Staff at Metropolitan Medical Center, ,

I have chosen you because of your reputations for working with parents who feel strongly about wanting as natural a birth as possible. I understand that sometimes birth becomes a medical situation. The following is what I would prefer as long as medical interventions are not indicated. I would appreciate you working with me to have our baby in the way described in our birth plan, if possible.

Sincerely,

Rachel Thompson

Laboring

I would prefer to avoid an enema and/or shaving of pubic hair.
I would like to be free to walk around during labor.
I prefer to be able to move around and change position at will throughout labor.
I would like to be able to have fluids by mouth throughout the first stage of labor.
I will be bringing my own music to play during labor.
I do not want an IV unless I become dehydrated.
I need to wear contact lenses or glasses at all times when conscious.

Fetal Monitors

I do not want to have continuous fetal monitoring unless it is required by the condition of my baby.

Stimulation of Labor

If labor is not progressing, I would like to have the bag of water ruptured before other methods are used to augment labor.
I would prefer to be allowed to try changing position and other natural methods before oxytocin is administered.

Medication/Anesthesia

I do not want to use drugs if possible. Please do not offer them. I will ask if I want some.

C-section

If a cesarean delivery is indicated, I would like to be fully informed and to participate in the decision-making process.
I would like my husband present at all times if my baby requires a cesarean delivery.
I wish to have regional anesthesia unless the baby must be delivered immediately.

Episiotomy

I am hoping to protect my perineum. I am practicing ahead of time by squatting, doing Kegel exercises, and perineal massage.
If possible, I would like to use perineal massage to help avoid the need for an episiotomy.

Pushing

I would like to be allowed to choose the position in which I give birth, including squatting.
Even if I am fully dilated, and assuming my baby is not in distress, I would like to try to wait until I feel the urge to push before beginning the pushing phase.

Immediately After Delivery

I would like to have my baby placed on my chest.
I would like to have my husband cut the cord.
I would like to hold my baby while I deliver the placenta and any tissue repairs are made.
I plan to keep my baby with me following birth and would appreciate if the evaluation of my baby can be done with my baby on my abdomen unless there is an unusual situation.
I would prefer to hold my baby skin to skin to keep her warm.
I want to delay the eye medication for my baby until a couple hours after birth.
I have made arrangements to donate the umbilical cord blood if possible.

Postpartum

I would like a private room so my husband can stay with me.
Unless required for health reasons, I do not wish to be separated from my baby.

Nursing My Baby

I plan to nurse my baby very shortly after birth if baby and I are OK.
Unless medically necessary, I do not wish to have any formula given to my baby (including glucose water or plain water). If my baby needs to be supplemented, I prefer an alternative method to using a bottle.
I do not want my baby to be given a pacifier.
I would like to meet with a lactation consultant.

Photo/Video

I would like to make a video recording of labor and/or the birth and want pictures of the doctor and the baby.

Labor Support

My support people are my husband, Owen, and friends Judy and Margaret, and I would like them to be present during labor and/or delivery.
I would like my other children (ages 4 years and 6 years) to be present at the birth. My physician has approved this. Judy and Margaret will take care of the other children during the birth.

Box 7-10 ■ METHODS OF PREPARED CHILDBIRTH

Dick-Read Method

The work of Dr. Grantly Dick-Read is fundamental to most methods of prepared childbirth. Dr. Dick-Read was a British obstetrician who practiced from 1919 to 1940. Dr. Dick-Read regarded fear as the basis of pain in childbirth and believed that civilization had culturally conditioned women to expect childbirth to be painful. He described a fear–tension–pain cycle. When labor began, the laboring woman tensed in fear at the beginning of each contraction. This tension resulted in the increase of pain; the pain reinforced the belief that labor was painful; and thus the cycle continued. He believed that pregnant women could interrupt this fear–tension–pain cycle with prenatal education and knowledge to reduce fear of the birth process and conscious relaxation during labor.

Lamaze Method

Dr. Fernand Lamaze built on Dick-Read's ideas and combined them with Pavlov's theory of conditioned response. The Lamaze instructor teaches the pregnant woman to rehearse conditioned positive responses (i.e., relaxation, breathing, and attention focusing) to a stimulus (i.e., beginning of a contraction). Then, when she is in labor, the goal is for her to respond with the helpful conditioned responses, instead of natural responses (e.g., panic, breath holding, and increased tension) that can slow the progress of labor and increase the woman's pain level. Her partner is trained to respond by supporting the laboring woman with encouragement and praise; providing focus and offering physical comfort measures, such as position changes, controlling the environment, massage, talking her through the contractions, enhancing her relaxation, and instilling confidence (Bing, 1994).

Bradley Method

Dr. Robert Bradley also based his obstetric practice on the work of Dick-Read. Dr. Bradley became convinced that the way to make childbirth an enjoyable experience was to copy what animals do naturally. He empowered the woman's partner to take an active role in the labor and birth process. The principles of the Bradley method include the need for:
- *Darkness and solitude.* Animals usually choose to birth babies in dark secluded places; therefore, labor and birth should occur in a darkened room.
- *Quiet.* Loud or unexpected noises are disturbing.
- *Physical comfort.* Comfort measures, such as controlling the room temperature, pillows for support, positioning, nonconstricting clothing, and familiar objects, contribute to the laboring woman's needs.

- *Physical relaxation.* Conscious relaxation on the part of the laboring woman increases her comfort and allows her uterus to work more effectively and quickly. Tensing up during contractions produces increased pain.
- *Controlled breathing.* Slow, deep, sleeplike breathing by mouth is encouraged throughout labor.
- *Closed eyes and the appearance of sleep.* Shutting the eyes enhances concentration on deep breathing by shutting out visual stimuli.

LeBoyer Method

Dr. Frederick LeBoyer's method recommends decreased stimulation for the newborn during the birthing process and immediately thereafter. He stressed turning down the lights, limiting noise and loud talking, warmth, and gentleness. One long-lasting effect of Dr. LeBoyer's methods is his emphasis on not separating the woman and her newborn.

Underwater Birth Method

During the 1980s, the concept of giving birth in water gained popularity. Those who encourage water births cite that humans begin life surrounded by liquid in the womb. Moreover, soaking in a warm bath enhances relaxation. Free from gravity's pull on the body, and with reduced sensory stimulation, the laboring woman's body is less likely to secrete stress-related hormones, thus allowing production of endorphins. Supporters of underwater birth believe that this release of endorphins has an analgesic effect on the laboring woman. Two benefits of birthing in water cited by proponents include a decrease in maternal blood pressure within 10 to 15 minutes of entering the water and increased elasticity of the perineum, which reduces the frequency of and severity in tearing of the perineum.

In 1989, Barbara Harper, RN, founded Waterbirth International/GMCHA (Global Maternal Child Health Association). This organization provides information and facilitates networking among those who are interested in learning more about birthing in water (http://www.waterbirth.org/).

Hypnobirthing

Hypnobirthing incorporates an eclectic approach to labor and birth. The fundamental belief is that the woman who is prepared physically, mentally, and spiritually can experience the joy of birth. Forms of hypnosis and deep relaxation are integral parts of the method. Some women use traditional hypnosis with posthypnotic suggestions during labor and delivery. Others use forms of self-hypnosis, incorporating the basics of Drs. Dick-Read and Lamaze, such as deep relaxation and breathing for each phase of labor.

Box 7-11 ▐ COMMON TOPICS INCLUDED IN CHILDBIRTH EDUCATION CLASSES

- Psychological and emotional aspects of pregnancy
- Anatomic and physiologic changes involved in pregnancy and childbirth
- Fetal development
- Communication with obstetrician/pediatrician: verbal and written birth plans
- Choosing a pediatrician
- The normal, natural process of labor and birth
- Stages/phases of labor: physical and emotional changes of each
- Partner's role in providing support for each stage/phase of labor
- Comfort measures for labor: relaxation, movement, breathing, focus, massage, pressure, encouragement, and support
- Medication and anesthesia options for labor and birth
- Back labor: causes, physical signs, and comfort measures
- Induction of labor: indications for induction and what to expect
- Possible complications of labor: prevention and management
- What to pack for the hospital
- Hospital admission routine
- Medical procedures and interventions, such as vaginal examinations, routine laboratory work, fetal monitoring, artificial rupture of membranes (AROM), IVs, vacuum extraction, and forceps
- Cesarean birth
- Breastfeeding
- Physical and emotional aspects of the postpartum period

Box 7-12 ▐ SUGGESTED ITEMS FOR THE LAYETTE

Clothes
- 4–6 "onesies"
- Gowns
- Sleepers
- 2–3 blanket sleepers
- 4–6 undershirts
- 4–6 pairs of socks
- 4–6 receiving blankets
- 3–4 hooded towels
- 4–6 washcloths
- 4–6 bibs
- 4–6 burp cloths
- Several packages of newborn size diapers and wipes or washcloths

Baby Supplies
- Baby lotion
- Baby shampoo
- Zinc oxide ointment
- Cotton swabs
- Rubbing alcohol
- Cradle or bassinet
- Crib
- Changing pad or table
- Sling
- Swing
- Stroller
- Baby bathtub

---

such as the pelvic tilt, Kegel, tailor sit and tailor stretch, and stretches as comfort measures to combat some of the discomforts of pregnancy, are included, as well as exercises that allow the woman to be able to utilize beneficial labor positions comfortably. Postnatal exercise classes strengthen muscles affected by the pregnancy. Sometimes, they incorporate the baby as part of the exercise.

Baby Care Classes. These classes are usually offered to the pregnant woman and her partner. Basics such as infant bathing, diapering, and feeding are featured. Parents-to-be receive information on newborn sleeping and waking patterns and infant comforting and rousing techniques. Safety information such as handling of the baby, car seat safety, and safety proofing the home is included. Signs of illness and guidelines for when to call the pediatrician are an important part of this class. Discussion

usually includes items needed for the nursery or the instructor provides a list in handouts (Box 7-12).

Breast-feeding Classes. An international board certified lactation consultant often teaches breast-feeding classes; however, certified breast-feeding educators or specially trained nurses may also conduct these classes. Usually offered in the last trimester of pregnancy, this class educates the woman and her partner on the benefits of breast-feeding, signs of good latch and position, and establishing a good milk supply. Selection of and using a breast pump and milk storage are topics of interest in this class, as many women plan to return to work and continue to nurse their infants. Attendance of this class by the woman's partner increases his support and ability to provide assistance, thus contributing to the success of breast-feeding. The instructor usually provides contact information for lactation support resources in the community.

Siblings Classes. Many hospitals provide siblings classes for children who are soon to be big brothers and big sisters. Siblings' class goals include preparing children for the time of separation from mother while she is in the hospital and helping the children accept the changes resulting from the arrival of the new baby in the family. The instructor demonstrates basic infant care, with emphasis on how the child can be included or help with the tasks related to baby care. The class usually includes tours of the maternal–child areas of the hospital. The instructor shares suggestions with parents on ways to help the older siblings accept changes in the household after the baby arrives.

In hospitals that allow siblings to attend births, siblings' classes may include information on how to help prepare the older child for being present at delivery. Most hospitals require an adult to be responsible for children at birth, in addition to the partner who is caring for the laboring woman.

Evaluation: Goals and Expected Outcomes

Goal: The woman's anxiety is reduced.
Expected Outcomes: The woman

- verbalizes a reduction in anxiety
- names at least two outlets for dealing with her anxiety

Goal: The woman's symptoms and discomforts of pregnancy are manageable.
Expected Outcomes: The woman

- voices feeling relaxed and confident in her ability to deal with the common discomforts of pregnancy
- demonstrates the use of effective strategies for coping with the discomforts of pregnancy

Goal: The woman will feel confident in her ability to care for herself throughout pregnancy.

Expected Outcomes: The woman

- verbalizes understanding of how to modify lifestyle to accommodate the changing needs of pregnancy
- answers questions regarding self-care appropriately
- asks informed questions

Goal: The woman and fetus remain free from preventable injury throughout the pregnancy.
Expected Outcomes: The woman

- schedules and attends prenatal visits
- describes warning signs to report
- calls with questions and concerns
- calls if warning signs are experienced

Goal: The woman will express confidence in her ability to go through the labor and birth experience and assume the parenting role.
Expected Outcomes: The woman

- expresses realistic expectations regarding plans for labor and birth
- schedules and attends childbirth education and/or parenting classes
- prepares the home for arrival of the baby

Test Yourself

- ✔ Identify at least five ways smoking increases pregnancy risk.
- ✔ How much alcohol is it OK for a pregnant woman to drink?
- ✔ What is a doula?

KEY POINTS

➤ The goal of early prenatal care is to increase the chances that the fetus and the mother will remain healthy throughout pregnancy and delivery.

➤ The main goals of the first prenatal visit are to confirm a diagnosis of pregnancy, identify risk factors, determine the due date, and provide education regarding self-care and danger signs of pregnancy.

➤ The history at the first prenatal visit includes chief complaint, reproductive history, medical–surgical history, family history, and social history. The reproductive history includes the obstetric history, which looks at previous pregnancies and their outcomes. Determining the gravida and parity of the woman is an important part of the obstetric history. The parity is usually further subdivided into the number of term deliveries, preterm deliveries, abortions (spontaneous or induced), and living children.

➤ A complete physical examination will be done during the first visit to include a breast exam, a speculum examination with a Pap test, and a bimanual examination of the uterus.

➤ The most common laboratory assessments (in addition to the Pap test) done on the first prenatal visit include a complete blood count, blood type and screen, hepatitis B, HIV, syphilis, gonorrhea, Chlamydia, rubella titer, and a urine culture.

➤ To calculate the estimated due date by Nagele's rule, add 7 days from the first day of the last menstrual period, then subtract 3 months to obtain the due date. Other methods for estimating the due date use uterus size, landmarks in the pregnancy, and ultrasonographic measurement of fetal structures.

➤ Any abnormal part of the history, physical examination, or lab work can put the pregnancy at risk. A history of difficult pregnancy or pregnancy complications puts subsequent pregnancies at risk.

➤ Subsequent prenatal visits are shorter and focus on the weight, blood pressure, urine protein and glucose measurements, fetal heart rate, and fundal height. Inquiry is made regarding the danger signals of pregnancy at each prenatal visit.

➤ Fetal kick counts are done by the woman at the same time each day. It should not take longer than 2 hours to get to 10 counts. If it does, the woman should call her primary care provider.

➤ Ultrasonography uses high-frequency sound waves to visualize fetal and maternal structures. Ultrasound is done to determine or confirm gestational age, observe the fetus, and diagnose fetal and placental abnormalities.

➤ Maternal serum alpha-fetoprotein testing is recommended for every pregnant woman between 16 and 18 weeks. Elevated levels are associated with various defects, in particular fetal spinal defects.

➤ Triple-marker screening involves a blood test to determine levels of three hormones, maternal serum alpha-fetoprotein, hCG, and unconjugated estriol. This test screens for chromosomal abnormalities, but an abnormal result does not mean that something is definitely wrong with the fetus. Further tests are needed.

➤ Amniocentesis involves aspiration of amniotic fluid through the abdominal wall to obtain fetal cells for chromosomal analysis. Amniocentesis is usually done between 15 and 20 weeks' gestation.

➤ Chorionic villus sampling is similar to amniocentesis, but it can be performed earlier, usually at 10 to 12 weeks. Placental tissue is aspirated through a catheter that is introduced into the cervix.

➤ Percutaneous umbilical blood sampling (PUBS) is similar to an amniocentesis; however, fetal blood is withdrawn from the umbilical cord for testing, rather than amniotic fluid.

➤ The nonstress test measures fetal heart rate acceleration patterns. A reactive NST is reassuring. The CST exposes the fetus to the stress of uterine contractions. A negative CST is reassuring. A positive CST indicates probable hypoxia or fetal asphyxia.

➤ Vibroacoustic stimulation is a method by which an artificial larynx is activated over the pregnant abdomen to stimulate the fetus to move. This is done in conjunction with an equivocal nonstress test.

➤ CST is a test done to determine how well the fetus can handle the stress of contractions. Three contractions are needed within a 20-minute period. These can occur spontaneously or they may be induced by nipple stimulation or oxytocin infusion. A "negative" (desired) result occurs when there are no decelerations during the test. If decelerations occur with one half or more of the contractions, this is a "positive" (undesirable) result.

➤ The biophysical profile combines the NST and several ultrasound measures, breathing, movements, tone, and amniotic fluid volume to predict fetal well-being.

➤ Common nursing diagnoses during the pregnancy are anxiety, health-seeking behaviors, risk for injury, and deficient knowledge.

➤ Nursing interventions are tailored to the needs of the individual woman and are focused on relieving anxiety and the common discomforts of pregnancy. Interventions include assisting the woman to maintain a balanced nutritional intake, monitoring the blood pressure and weight and inquiring regarding the danger signals at each visit, teaching throughout the pregnancy, and helping the woman prepare for labor, birth, and parenting. Refer the woman to community resources, such as childbirth education or sibling classes.

➤ Nursing care has been successful if the woman is less anxious, reports that pregnancy discomforts are tolerable, consumes a balanced diet, and verbalizes an understanding of self-care.

INTERNET RESOURCES

Pregnancy
www.marchofdimes.com

Prenatal Care
www.nlm.nih.gov/medlineplus/prenatalcare.html

Childbirth Education
www.icea.org

Nutrition
www.mypyramid.gov

Childbirth
www.childbirth.org
www.lamaze.org

Doulas
http://dona.org
www.doula.com
http://doulanetwork.com

Complementary and Alternative Medicine
http://nccam.nih.gov/news/newsletter
www.botanicalmedicine.org
www.herbalgram.org

Medications
www.cc.nih.gov/phar/updates

Workbook

■ NCLEX-STYLE REVIEW QUESTIONS

1. A woman reports that her LMP occurred on January 10, 2010. Using Nagele's rule, what is her due date?

    a. October 17, 2010
    b. October 17, 2011
    c. September 7, 2010
    d. September 7, 2011

2. A woman presents to the clinic in the first trimester of pregnancy. She has three children living at home. One of them was born prematurely at 34 weeks. The other two were full term at birth. She has a history of one miscarriage. How do you record her obstetric history on the chart using GTPAL format?

    a. G3 T2 P1 A1 L3
    b. G4 T3 P0 A1 L3
    c. G4 T2 P1 A1 L3
    d. G5 T2 P1 A1 L3

3. A woman who is 28 weeks' pregnant presents to the clinic for her scheduled prenatal visit. The nurse midwife measures her fundal height at 32 cm. What action does the nurse expect the midwife to take regarding this finding?

    a. The midwife will order a multiple-marker screening test.
    b. The midwife will order a sonogram to confirm dates.
    c. The midwife will schedule more frequent prenatal visits to monitor the pregnancy closely.
    d. The midwife will take no action. This is a normal finding for a pregnancy at 28 weeks' gestation.

4. A G1 at 20 weeks' gestation is at the clinic for a prenatal visit. She tells the nurse that she has been reading about "group B strep disease" on the Internet. She asks when she can expect to be checked for the bacteria. How does the nurse best reply?

    a. "I'm glad that you asked. You will be getting the culture done today."
    b. "The obstetrician normally cultures for group B strep after 35 weeks and before delivery."
    c. "You are only checked for group B strep if you have risk factors for the infection."
    d. "You were checked during your first prenatal visit. Let me get those results for you."

5. Results of an early CVS test show that a woman's baby has severe chromosomal abnormalities. When the obstetrician explains the findings to her, she becomes tearful. She shares with the nurse that it is against her religious beliefs to have an abortion. How would the nurse best respond to her?

    a. "Abortion is really the best thing for the baby. He has no chance of a normal life."
    b. "I agree with you. It is against my religious beliefs, too."
    c. "It is dangerous to carry a fetus with chromosomal abnormalities to term. You really should consider an abortion to protect your health."
    d. "You don't have to decide what to do today. Take some time to talk this over with your family. I will support you whatever decision you make."

■ STUDY ACTIVITIES

1. Do an Internet search on "genetic counseling." Make a list of at least three genetic counselors in your area to which a pregnant woman could be referred.

2. Using the following table, fill in key points for each topic regarding self-care during pregnancy. Note any special precautions for that topic that would be important to emphasize to the pregnant woman.

Topic	Key Points	Special Precautions
Nutrition		
Dental hygiene		
Exercise		
Hygiene		
Breast care		
Clothing		
Sexual activity		
Employment		
Travel		
Medication use		

3. Develop a teaching plan for pregnant women who are 20 weeks and greater. Address common discomforts of pregnancy that the women are likely to encounter during the last half of pregnancy.

■ CRITICAL THINKING: WHAT WOULD YOU DO?

Apply your knowledge of the nurse's role during pregnancy to the following situations.

1. Theresa Martinez presents to the clinic because she thinks she might be pregnant.

   a. What nursing assessments should be completed?
   b. During the history, Theresa reports that there is a history of type 2 diabetes in her family, and that her mother delivered large babies (10 and 11 lb). What should you do with this information?

2. Amanda Jones calls the clinic. She is a G2 P1 at 28 weeks' gestation. She is worried because she thinks the baby is moving less than usual.

   a. What should you tell Amanda to do first?
   b. Amanda comes to the office to be checked because she is still worried about the baby. What is the priority nursing assessment that should be completed at this time? Why?

   c. Because Amanda has decreased fetal movement, the physician orders a biophysical profile. How would you explain this test to Amanda? Which part of this test would you normally expect to be a nursing function?

3. Rebecca Richards is pregnant for the first time. She is 40 years of age. The obstetrician has suggested chromosomal studies.

   a. Explain the advantages and disadvantages of CVS versus amniocentesis.
   b. Rebecca tells you that she is opposed to abortion for any reason. She asks why she should go through CVS because she will not accept an abortion. How would you respond to Rebecca?
   c. Halfway through the pregnancy, Rebecca's fetus is diagnosed with thrombocytopenia. What therapy will likely be ordered for the fetus? Explain this therapy to Rebecca.

LABOR AND BIRTH

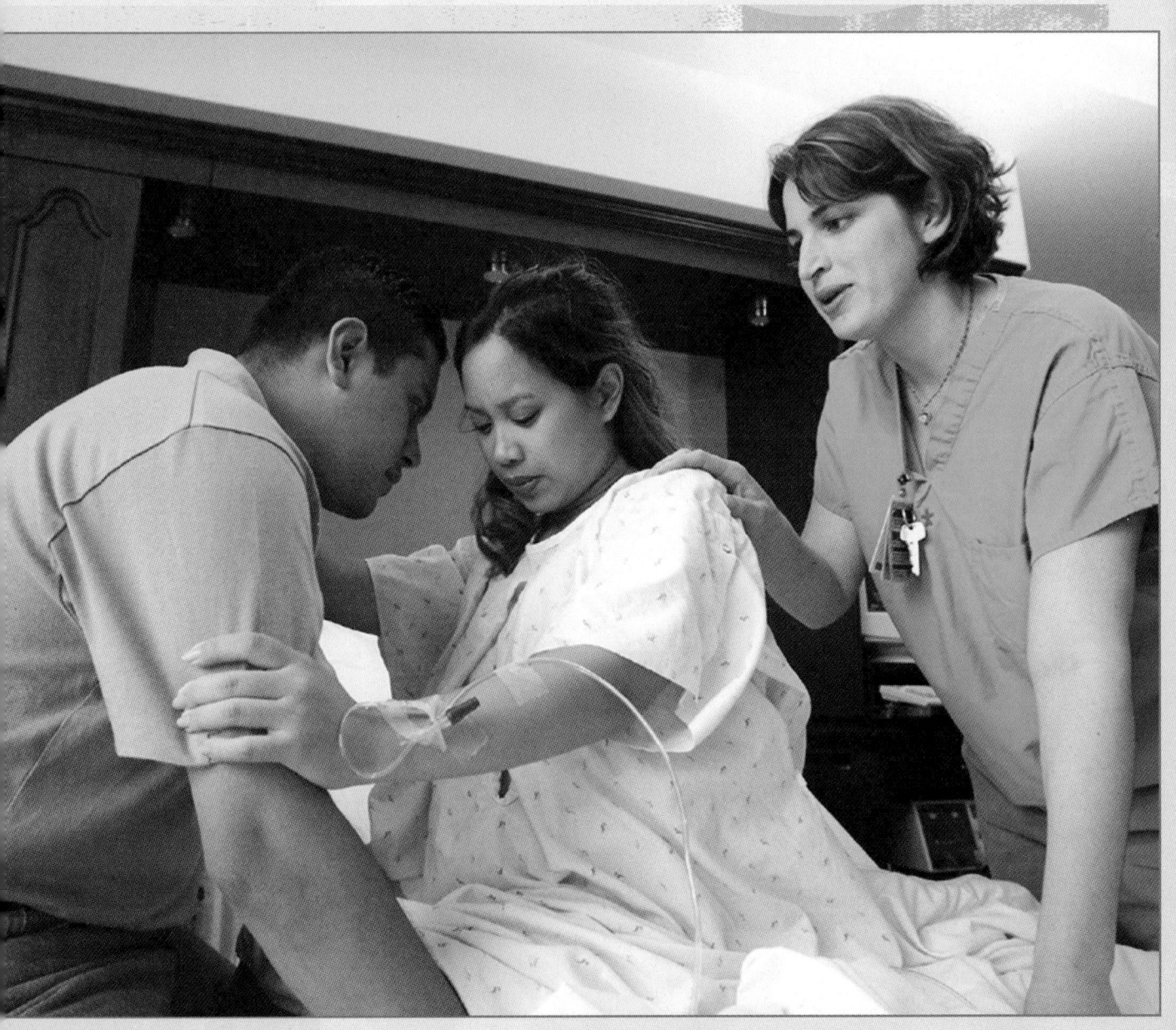

8 The Labor Process

KEY TERMS

android pelvis
anthropoid pelvis
caput succedaneum
cardinal movements
diagonal conjugate
effacement
engagement
false pelvis
fetal attitude
fetal lie
fetal presentation
gynecoid pelvis
molding
obstetric conjugate
platypelloid pelvis
station
true pelvis

LEARNING OBJECTIVES

On completion of this chapter, you should be able to:

1. Explain the four essential components of the labor process and how they work together to accomplish birth.
2. Discuss current theories regarding causes of labor onset.
3. List anticipatory signs of labor.
4. Differentiate between prodromal labor and true labor.
5. Outline the seven mechanisms or cardinal movements of a spontaneous vaginal delivery.
6. Classify the stages and phases of labor.
7. Discuss ways the woman physiologically and psychologically adapts to labor.
8. Describe fetal physiologic responses to labor.

AS A NURSE, it is essential for you to understand the components of labor, how these components work together in the process of labor, and how the woman and fetus adapt to labor (in normal situations). This knowledge allows you to support the laboring woman appropriately and assist her through a safe labor and delivery. This chapter explores each component of labor and birth separately and then discusses the combined components during the process of labor. Normal maternal and fetal adaptations to labor are examined.

FOUR ESSENTIAL COMPONENTS OF LABOR

There are four essential components of labor. These are known as the "four Ps" of labor: passageway, passenger, powers, and psyche. A problem in any of these four areas will negatively influence the labor process.

Passageway

The passageway consists of the woman's bony pelvis and soft tissues of the cervix and vagina.

Bony Pelvis

The bony pelvis forms the rigid passageway through which the fetus must navigate to deliver vaginally. The flared upper portion of the bony pelvis is the **false pelvis**.

The false pelvis is not part of the bony passageway. The portion of the pelvis below the linea terminalis is the **true pelvis**. The true pelvis is the bony passageway through which the fetus must pass during delivery. Important landmarks of the true pelvis include the inlet (entrance to the true pelvis), midpelvis, and outlet (exit point). Figure 8-1 illustrates important landmarks of the pelvis.

The basic shape and dimensions of the pelvis may favor a vaginal birth or may interfere with the ability of the fetus to descend.

Pelvic Shape

The shape of the inlet determines the pelvic type. There are four basic pelvic shapes: gynecoid, anthropoid, android, and platypelloid (Fig. 8-2). Most women have pelvises that are various combinations of the four types.

The **gynecoid pelvis** is most favorable for a vaginal birth. The rounded shape of the gynecoid inlet allows the fetus room to negotiate the dimensions of the bony passageway. The gynecoid pelvis is considered the typical female pelvis, although only about half of all women have a gynecoid pelvis (Cunningham et al., 2005a).

The **anthropoid pelvis** is elongated in its dimensions and is sometimes referred to as apelike. The anterior–posterior diameter is roomy, but the transverse diameter is narrow compared with that of the gynecoid

False pelvis

Ischial spines

Pelvic outlet

True pelvis

Linea terminalis

Pelvic inlet

Anterior view

Superior view

Inferior view

■ Figure 8-1 Important landmarks of the pelvis.

pelvis. However, a vaginal birth often can be accomplished in the approximately one third of women who have variations of an anthropoid pelvis (Cunningham et al., 2005a).

The **android pelvis** is the typical male pelvis. Approximately one third of white women and 16% of nonwhite women have an android pelvis (Varney, Kriebs, & Gegor, 2004). The heart shape of the android pelvis is not favorable to a vaginal delivery. Large babies often become stuck in the birth canal and must be delivered by

cesarean, whereas, a smaller baby may be able to navigate the narrow diameters.

The least common type is the **platypelloid pelvis**, occurring in less than 3% of women (Cunningham et al., 2005a). This pelvis is flat in its dimensions with a very narrow anterior–posterior diameter and a wide transverse diameter. This shape makes it extremely difficult for the fetus to pass through the bony pelvis. Therefore, women with a platypelloid pelvis usually must deliver the fetus by cesarean section.

A Gynecoid

B Anthropoid

C Android

D Platypelloid

■ Figure 8-2 Pelvic shapes.
(A) Gynecoid, **(B)** Anthropoid, **(C)** Android, and **(D)** Platypelloid.

Pelvic Dimensions

Early in the pregnancy, particularly if a woman has never delivered a baby vaginally, the practitioner may take pelvic measurements to estimate the size of the true pelvis. This helps to determine if the size is adequate for vaginal delivery. However, these measurements do not consistently predict which women will have difficulty delivering vaginally, so most practitioners allow the woman to labor and attempt a vaginal birth (Funai & Norwitz, 2006).

The most important measurement of the inlet is the **obstetric conjugate** because this is the smallest diameter of the inlet through which the fetus must pass. However, the obstetric conjugate cannot be measured directly; therefore, the practitioner must estimate the size. To obtain this estimate, the practitioner measures the **diagonal conjugate**, which extends from the symphysis pubis to the sacral promontory. The practitioner then subtracts 1.5 to 2.0 cm from the measurement of the diagonal conjugate to approximate the dimensions of the obstetric conjugate. An obstetric conjugate that measures 11 cm is considered adequate to accommodate a vaginal delivery.

The practitioner takes measurements of the midpelvis at the level of the ischial spines. If the ischial spines are prominent and extend into the midpelvis, they can reduce the diameter of the midpelvis and might interfere with the journey of the fetus through the passageway during labor. One important measurement of the outlet is the angle of the pubic arch. This angle should be at least 90 degrees.

Take note of this detail.
You cannot determine the shape and dimensions of the pelvic inlet by the size of the woman. A woman might be small in stature but have a roomy gynecoid pelvis. A larger woman may have a small, contracted platypelloid or android pelvis.

Here's an interesting fact.
A woman's pelvis might be roomy enough for a vaginal delivery in one portion but too small in another portion. Just because the inlet and the outlet are adequate for delivery does not mean that the midpelvis is adequate.

Soft Tissues

The cervix and vagina are soft tissues that form the part of the passageway known as the birth canal. In early pregnancy, the cervix is firm, long, and closed. As the time for delivery approaches, the cervix usually begins to soften. Then, when labor begins, uterine contractions affect the cervix in two ways. First, the cervix begins to get shorter and thinner, a process called **effacement**. Cervical effacement is recorded as a percentage. The cervical canal measures approximately 2 cm before effacement. At a length of 1 cm, the cervix is 50% effaced. When the cervix is paper thin, it is 100% effaced.

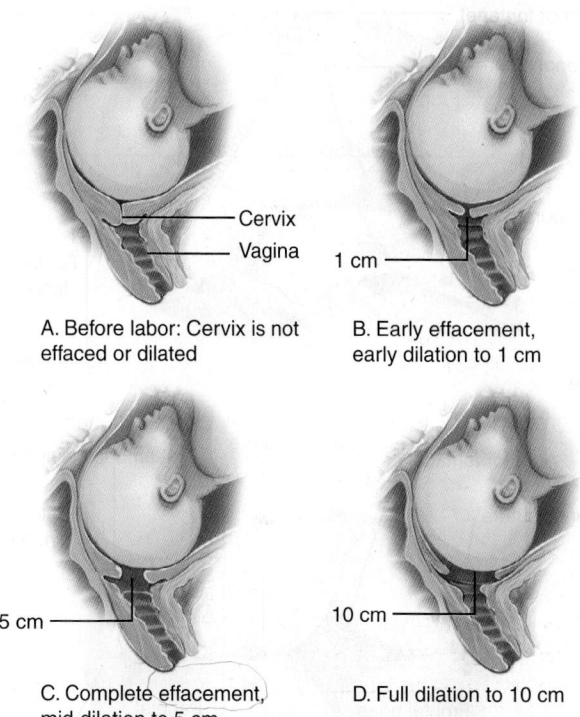

A. Before labor: Cervix is not effaced or dilated — Cervix, Vagina

B. Early effacement, early dilation to 1 cm — 1 cm

C. Complete effacement, mid-dilation to 5 cm — 5 cm

D. Full dilation to 10 cm — 10 cm

■ Figure 8-3 Cervical effacement and dilation.

The second cervical change that occurs during normal labor is dilation. The cervix must open to allow the fetus to be born. Dilation is measured in centimeters. When the cervix is dilated completely, it measures 10 cm. Normally, a primiparous woman experiences effacement before dilation. For a multiparous woman, both processes usually occur at the same time. Often, the multipara's cervix dilates 1 to 2 cm several weeks before labor begins. Figure 8-3 illustrates the processes of cervical effacement and dilation as they normally occur for the primipara.

The vaginal canal participates in childbirth via passive distention. During birth, the rugae of the vaginal walls stretch and smooth out, allowing for considerable expansion. The muscles and soft tissues of the primipara provide greater resistance to stretching and distending than do those of the multipara. This is one reason the first baby often takes longer to be born than do subsequent babies.

Test Yourself

✔ Which type of pelvis provides the most room to allow the fetus to be born vaginally?

✔ Which two pelvic types are least suited for a vaginal delivery?

✔ What structures other than the pelvis form the passageway?

A

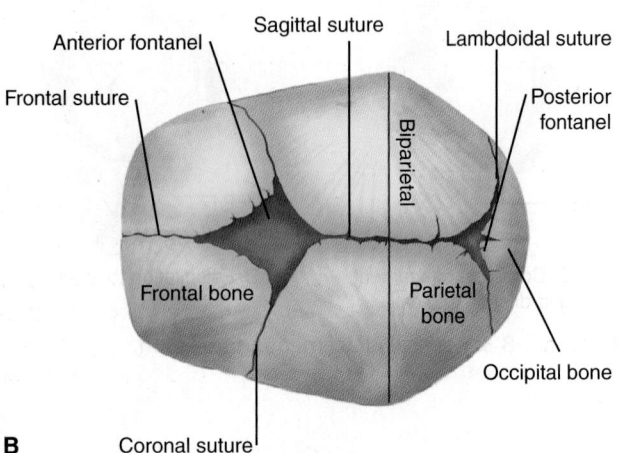

B

■ **Figure 8-4** Clinically important landmarks of the fetal skull. **(A)** Side view showing important diameters in a cephalic presentation. **(B)** Top view showing sutures and fontanels.

Passenger

The "passenger" refers to the fetus. The size of the fetal skull and fetal accommodation to the passageway (i.e., fetal lie, presentation, attitude, position, and station) can significantly affect labor progress. The next section defines and discusses each concept in relation to its influence on the progression of labor.

Fetal Skull

The skull is the most important fetal structure in relation to labor and birth because it is the largest and least compressible structure (Fig. 8-4). The diameters of the fetal skull must be small enough to allow the head to travel through the bony pelvis. Fortunately, the fetal skull is not entirely rigid. The cartilage between the bones allows the bones to overlap during labor, a process called **molding** that elongates the fetal skull, thereby reducing the diameter of the head. The newborn of a primipara often has significant molding.

Fetal Lie

Fetal lie describes the position of the long axis of the fetus in relation to the long axis of the pregnant woman. There are three basic ways that the fetus can lie in the

A Longitudinal lie

B Transverse lie

■ **Figure 8-5** Longitudinal versus transverse lie. **(A)** Longitudinal lie (the fetus lies parallel to the maternal spine). The fetus is in a breech presentation in a left sacrum posterior (LSP) position. **(B)** Transverse lie (the fetus lies crosswise to the maternal spine).

uterus: in a longitudinal, transverse, or oblique position (Fig. 8-5). A longitudinal lie, in which the long axis of the fetus is parallel to the long axis of the mother, is the most common. When the fetus is in a transverse lie, the long axis of the fetus is perpendicular to the long axis of the woman. An oblique lie is in between the two.

Fetal Presentation

Fetal presentation refers to the foremost part of the fetus that enters the pelvic inlet. There are three main ways that the fetus can present to the pelvis: head (cephalic presentation), feet or buttocks (breech presentation), or shoulder (shoulder presentation). Approximately 97% of fetuses are in a cephalic presentation at the end of pregnancy (Cunningham et al., 2005b).

Breech presentations occur in approximately 3% of term pregnancies (Cunningham et al., 2005b). Figure 8-6 illustrates different types of breech presentations. Shoulder presentations are the least common, occurring in less than 0.3% of all term pregnancies (Cunningham et al., 2005b). Shoulder presentation is associated with a transverse lie.

Fetal Attitude

Fetal attitude refers to the relationship of the fetal parts to one another. In a cephalic presentation, there are several different ways the head can present to the maternal pelvis, depending on fetal attitude. The most common attitude, and the one that is most favorable for a vaginal

■ **Figure 8-6** Breech presentations. **(A)** Frank breech. **(B)** Complete breech. **(C)** Single footling breech. **(D)** Double footling breech.

birth, is an attitude of flexion, also called a vertex presentation. When the fetus curls up into an ovoid shape, he or she presents the smallest diameters of her skull to the bony pelvis. When the fetus is neither flexed nor hyperextended, she is in a military presentation and a larger head diameter presents. If the fetus demonstrates an attitude of partial extension, the brow (or frontum) becomes the presenting part. In an attitude of full extension, the face presents. Figure 8-7 shows variations of cephalic presentation in association with fetal attitude.

Fetal Position

The fetal position is determined by comparing the relationship of an arbitrarily determined reference point on the presenting part of the fetus to the quadrants of the maternal pelvis (Table 8-1). To determine position, first establish the presenting part and locate the appropriate reference point. Then determine towards which pelvic quadrant the reference point is facing.

Document fetal position in the clinical record using abbreviations (Box 8-1). The first letter describes the side of the maternal pelvis toward which the presenting part is facing ("R" for right and "L" for left). The second letter or abbreviation indicates the reference point ("O" for occiput, "Fr" for frontum, etc.). The last part of the designation specifies whether the presenting part is facing the anterior (A) or the posterior (P) portion of the pelvis, or whether it is in a transverse (T) position. For instance, the occipital bone, or occiput, is the reference point in a vertex presentation. If the occiput is facing the right anterior quadrant of the pelvis, the position is recorded as right occiput anterior (ROA). Figure 8-8 illustrates examples of different positions in a vertex

Be careful!

A transverse position is not the same as a transverse lie. The lie refers to the general way the fetus' body is aligned in the uterus: longitudinal, oblique, or transverse, whereas position refers to the way the landmark on the presenting part presents to a specific quadrant of the pelvis (right/left, anterior/posterior/transverse, etc.).

■ **Figure 8-7** Fetal attitude affects the type of presentation in cephalic (head-first) presentations. The degree of fetal flexion affects whether the presentation is classified as **(A)** vertex, **(B)** military, **(C)** brow, or **(D)** face.

Table 8-1 ■ REFERENCE POINTS FOR DETERMINING POSITION	
Presenting Part	**Reference Point**
Vertex	Occiput
Brow	Frontum (brow)
Face	Mentum (chin)
Breech	Sacrum
Shoulder	Scapula (acromial process)

presentation and how the positions would be documented. The most favorable positions for vaginal birth are occiput anterior, ROA, and LOA.

Fetal Station

Station refers to the relationship of the presenting part of the fetus to the ischial spines of the pelvis (Fig. 8-9). When the widest diameter of the presenting part is at the level of the ischial spines, the station is zero (0). If the presenting part is above the level of the ischial spines, the station is recorded as a negative number and is read "minus." If the presenting part is below the level of the ischial spines, the station is recorded as a positive

Box 8-1 ■ RECORDING FETAL POSITION

For each presentation there are eight possible positions. Record the notation as an abbreviation using the following criteria:

First Designation
Refers to the side of the maternal pelvis in which the presenting part is found*
   Right (R)
   Left (L)

Second (Middle) Designation
Reference point on the presenting part
   ■ Occiput (O)—vertex and military presentations
   ■ Frontum or brow (Fr)—brow presentation
   ■ Mentum or chin (M)—face presentation
   ■ Sacrum (S)—breech presentation
   ■ Scapula (Sc)—shoulder presentation

Third (Last) Designation
Refers to the front, back, or side of the maternal pelvis in which the reference point is found
   ■ Anterior (A)—front of the pelvis
   ■ Posterior (P)—back of the pelvis
   ■ Transverse (T)—side of the pelvis

*This designation is not included in the notation if the reference point is exactly in the middle and is turned neither to the left nor to the right.

number and is read "plus." For example, in a cephalic presentation, if the vertex is 1 cm above the level of the ischial spines, the station is reported as a minus one and recorded as −1. If, on the other hand, the presenting part is 1 cm below the level of the ischial spines, the station is reported as a plus one and recorded as +1.

When the station is a minus four (−4) or higher, the fetus is said to be floating and unengaged. When the fetus is floating, the presenting part has not yet entered the true pelvis. When the presenting part has settled into the true pelvis at the level of the ischial spines, the fetus is at a station of zero (0) and engaged.

Think about this.

When the fetus is floating, he or she is high in the pelvis. A high station is recorded as a negative (minus) number. On the other hand, if the fetus has moved deep into the pelvis, his station is low and is recorded as a positive (plus) number. As the fetus is being born, his station is a plus four (+4).

Test Yourself

✔ What term is used to describe the fetal part that enters the birth canal first?
✔ When describing the relationship of fetal parts to one another, what term is used?
✔ How is fetal lie described if the fetus is lying perpendicular to the maternal spine?

Powers

The primary force of labor comes from involuntary muscular contractions of the uterus. These labor contractions cause effacement and dilation of the cervix during the first stage of labor. Secondary powers are voluntary muscle contractions of the maternal abdomen during the second stage of labor that help expel the fetus.

Each involuntary uterine contraction is composed of three phases—increment, acme, and decrement—followed by a relaxation period (Fig. 8-10). The increment, or building up of the contraction, is the longest phase. During the increment, the contraction gains strength until it reaches the acme, or peak, of the contraction. The decrement is the letting-up phase, as the contraction relaxes gradually to baseline.

Document the rhythmic, intermittent nature of contractions using three descriptors: frequency, duration, and intensity (see Fig. 8-10). Frequency refers to how often the contractions are occurring. Measure frequency by counting the time interval from the beginning of one contraction to the beginning of the following contraction. Duration is the interval from the beginning of a contraction to its end. Intensity refers to the strength of the contraction. Estimate intensity by palpating the fundus

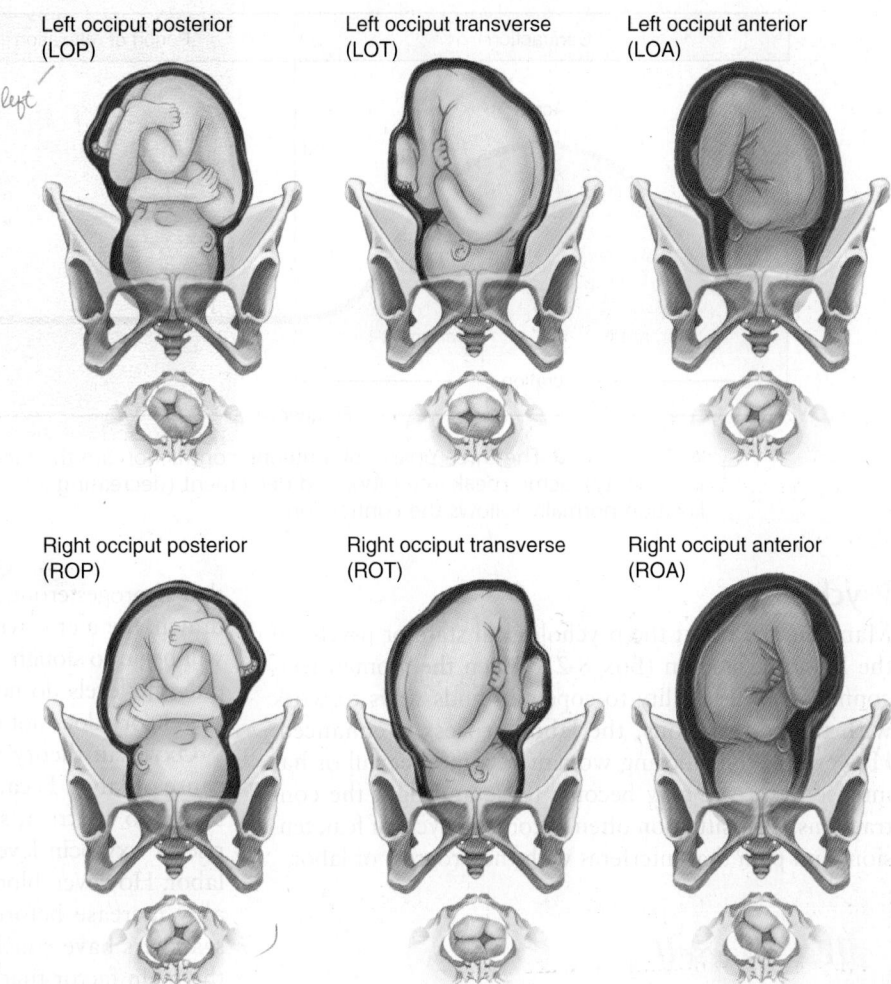

Left occiput posterior (LOP)

Left occiput transverse (LOT)

Left occiput anterior (LOA)

Right occiput posterior (ROP)

Right occiput transverse (ROT)

Right occiput anterior (ROA)

■ Figure 8-8 Examples of fetal position in a vertex presentation. In each illustration, the lie is longitudinal, and the attitude is one of flexion. Notice that the inset illustrations show the view that is seen with the woman in a dorsal recumbent position.

-4
-3
-2
-1
0
+1
+2
+3
+4

■ Figure 8-9 Fetal station.

at the peak of the contraction and record it as mild, moderate, or strong. Intensity can be measured directly with an intrauterine pressure transducer, although this technique is not used routinely.

It is extremely important to the well-being of the mother and the fetus that there is a period of relaxation between contractions (see Fig. 8-10). Each contraction squeezes the blood vessels that supply the placenta, thereby decreasing the amount of oxygen that flows to the fetus. The relaxation period allows the vessels to fill with oxygen-rich blood to supply the uterus and placenta. Relaxation is also necessary so that maternal muscles do not become overly fatigued and to allow the laboring woman momentary relief from the pain of labor.

This is an important point.

Because each contraction interrupts blood flow to the placenta temporarily, there is decreased oxygen available to the fetus. It is as if the fetus must hold his breath during each contraction. Obviously, the fetus cannot tolerate contractions that last too long, that are too strong, or that have no rest period between them for prolonged periods.

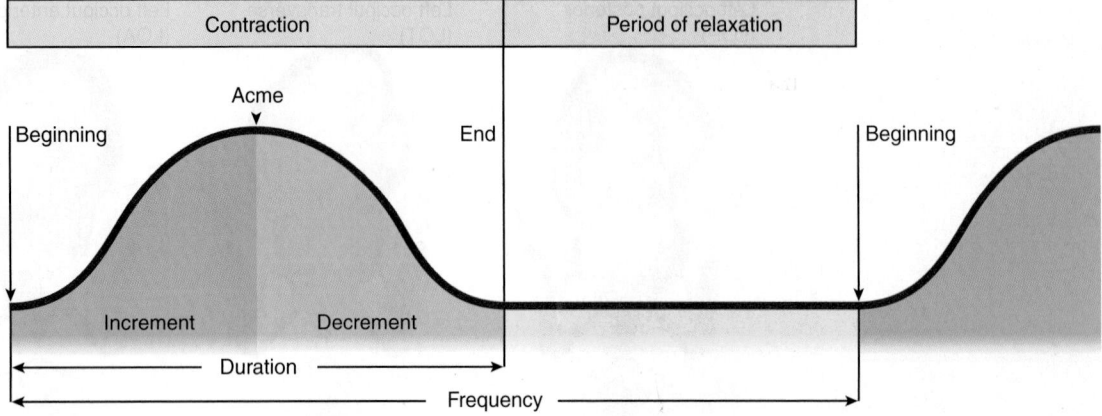

■ **Figure 8-10** The three phases of a uterine contraction are the increment (building up in intensity), acme (peak intensity), and decrement (decreasing intensity). A period of relaxation normally follows the contraction.

Psyche

Many factors affect the psychological state or psyche of the laboring woman (Box 8-2). When the woman feels confident in her ability to cope and finds ways to work with the contractions, the labor process is enhanced. However, if the laboring woman becomes fearful or has intense pain, she may become tense and fight the contractions. This situation often becomes a cycle of fear, tension, and pain that interferes with the progress of labor.

Test Yourself

✔ From where does the primary force of labor come?

✔ How is the frequency of uterine contractions measured?

✔ What is the purpose of the relaxation period between uterine contractions?

THE PROCESS OF LABOR

The discussion thus far has centered on the individual components of the labor process. However, it is the interplay between the components that causes labor to progress. The following section illustrates how the labor process works to accomplish birth.

Onset of Labor

Scientists often search for reasons why things work as they do. One question that intrigues scientists is, "What is the trigger that causes labor to begin?" As pregnancy nears term, the pregnant woman is more concerned with when labor will begin than with what causes labor to begin. She often asks the physician, "When will I go into labor?" This section explores both questions.

Theories Regarding Causes of Labor Onset

There are several hypotheses regarding what triggers labor to begin. The progesterone-withdrawal theory suggests that if progesterone (the hormone of pregnancy) is withdrawn, the uterus will begin to contract, the uterine lining will begin to slough, and labor will result. However, progesterone levels do not fall before labor (Smith, 2007), so this theory does not explain what causes labor to begin.

Oxytocin theory is another hypothesis regarding the cause of labor. Because the hormone oxytocin causes the uterus to contract, some scientists have proposed that a rise in oxytocin levels may be responsible for initiating labor. However, blood levels of oxytocin do not measurably increase before labor begins; therefore, some researchers have concluded that oxytocin is probably not the main factor that stimulates labor to begin.

The prostaglandin theory is another theory of labor initiation. Prostaglandins influence labor in several ways, which include softening the cervix and stimulating the uterus to contract. However, evidence supporting the theory that prostaglandins are the agents that trigger labor to begin is inconclusive.

Because a single causative factor of labor initiation has not yet been determined, the most likely answer seems to be that labor results from a combination of maternal and fetal factors working together in a cascade effect. During the cascade, factors that inhibit contractions, such as progesterone, are suppressed, and factors that promote contractions, such as prostaglandins, are engaged (Norwitz, 2006).

Anticipatory Signs of Labor

Nature usually provides clues as to the nearness of labor. Approximately 2 weeks before labor, the presenting part may settle into the pelvic cavity, causing the pregnant woman to sense that the baby has "dropped." This subjective feeling is called "lightening." The woman is able to breathe more easily, and she may need to urinate more frequently because of the pressure of the fetus on the urinary bladder. Not all women experience lightening before the onset of labor. Multiparous women often do not experience lightening until labor begins.

Box 8-2 ▌ FACTORS THAT MAY AFFECT THE MATERNAL PSYCHE

Factors that may affect the woman's psyche during labor include the woman's:

- Current pregnancy experience
  - Unplanned versus planned pregnancy
  - Amount of difficulty conceiving
  - Presence of risk factors
  - Complications of pregnancy
- Previous birth experiences
  - Complications of delivery
  - Mode of delivery (cesarean versus vaginal)
  - Birth outcomes (e.g., fetal demise, birth defects)
- Expectations for current birth experience
  - View of labor as a meaningful or a stressful event
  - Realistic and attainable goals versus idealistic views that conflict with reality (a situation that can lead to disappointment)
- Preparation for birth
  - Type of childbirth preparation
  - Familiarity with institution and its policies and procedures
  - Type of relaxation techniques learned and practiced
- Support system
  - Presence and support of a birth companion
    - Husband
    - Mother

- Lesbian partner
- Friend
- Doula
- Culture
  - A woman's culture influences and defines
  - The childbirth experience
    Shameful versus joyful
    Superstitions and beliefs about pregnancy and birth
    Prescribed behaviors and taboos during the intrapartum period
  - Relationships
    Interpersonal interactions
    Parent-infant interactions
    Role expectations of family members
    Support person involvement
  - Pain
    Meaning and context of pain
    Acceptable responses to pain
  - The significance of touch
    Soothing versus intruding
    May be a symbol of intimacy

Adapted from Mattson, S., & Smith, J. E. (Eds.). (2000). *Core curriculum for maternal–newborn nursing* (2nd ed., pp. 227–229). AWHONN publication. Philadelphia: WB Saunders.

Braxton Hicks contractions occur more frequently and are more noticeable as pregnancy approaches term. These irregular, practice contractions usually decrease in intensity with walking and position changes. The woman may experience gastrointestinal disturbances, such as diarrhea, heartburn, or nausea and vomiting, as labor approaches. Sometimes the mucous plug is expelled a week or two before labor begins. When the mucous plug passes, the woman will notice a one-time clear or pink-tinged discharge that is the consistency of jelly.

Frequently, the woman experiences a burst of energy 24 to 48 hours before the onset of labor. She may have the energy and desire to do heavy cleaning or some other big project in anticipation of the baby's arrival, a phenomenon known as the nesting urge. Caution the woman regarding the nesting urge, and advise her to conserve her energy for the work of labor.

Clinical signs that labor is approaching include ripening or softening and effacement (thinning) of the cervix. Dilation of the cervix may accompany softening and effacement, particularly in multiparous women. The practitioner informs the woman of these changes when a pelvic examination is done during a scheduled office visit.

Differences Between Prodromal and True Labor

Prodromal labor refers to the increase in Braxton Hicks contractions that occur toward the end of pregnancy. These practice contractions can be quite uncomfortable, making it difficult to distinguish true labor from "false" (prodromal) labor (Table 8-2). Sometimes the woman presents to the labor suite because she thinks she is in labor. After the initial assessment, instruct the woman to walk for an hour or two. Then, a vaginal examination is performed to determine any cervical changes. If there are changes, the practitioner diagnoses true labor and admits the laboring woman to the hospital. If there are no changes, the woman may go home with instructions to return if the contractions become stronger, more regular, or if other signs

Here's a helpful hint.

By definition, true labor results in progressive dilation and effacement of the cervix. If the woman is having contractions but the cervix is not getting thinner (effacing) or opening (dilating), she is not in true labor.

Table 8-2 ■ CHARACTERISTICS OF FALSE (PRODROMAL) VERSUS TRUE LABOR

	True Labor	False (Prodromal) Labor
Cervical changes	Progressive dilation and effacement	No change
Membranes	May bulge or rupture spontaneously	Remain intact
Bloody show	Present	Absent; may have pinkish mucous or may expel mucus plug
Contraction pattern	Regular (may be irregular at first) pattern develops in which contractions become increasingly intense and more frequent	Pattern tends to be irregular, although the contractions may seem to have a regular pattern for a time
Pain characteristics	Often starts in the small of the back and radiates to the lower abdomen; may begin with a cramping sensation	May be described as a tightening sensation; usually the discomfort is confined to the abdomen
Effects of walking	Contractions continue and become stronger	May decrease the frequency or eliminate the contractions altogether

of true labor occur, such as increased bloody show or rupture of the membranes.

Mechanisms of a Spontaneous Vaginal Delivery

For a vaginal birth to occur, the passenger must pass through the passageway. The turns and movements made during the journey are referred to as the mechanisms of delivery or the **cardinal movements.** These include engagement, descent, flexion, internal rotation, extension, external rotation, and expulsion (Fig. 8-11). Although the movements are discussed separately, it is important to understand that these mechanisms may overlap or occur simultaneously:

- *Engagement.* Initial descent of the fetal head may result in **engagement,** when the presenting part descends to the level of the ischial spines. Engagement may occur as early as 2 weeks before labor or not until after the onset of labor. Engagement is more likely to occur earlier in the primigravida and later in the multigravida.
- *Descent.* Descent may begin before labor when the fetus "drops." Descent is measured by station, relationship of the fetal presenting part to the maternal ischial spines. Descent continues throughout labor to varying degrees.
- *Flexion.* As the head descends during labor, the fetus encounters resistance from the soft tissues and muscles of the pelvic floor. This resistance normally coaxes the fetus to assume an attitude of flexion. Flexion is the attitude that presents the smallest diameters of the fetal head to the dimensions of the pelvis.
- *Internal rotation.* Frequently, in early labor, the fetal head presents to the pelvis in a transverse position because the inlet of the pelvis is widest from side to side. During active labor, the fetal head typically rotates 45 degrees from a transverse position to an

anterior position so that the head can accommodate the pelvic outlet, which is wider from front to back. This movement is called internal rotation. If the fetus does not rotate, the widest diameters of the fetal head present to the outlet of the pelvis, resulting in a less than optimal fit between the head and the bony passageway. This can prolong labor.

- *Extension.* Typically, the fetal head is well flexed with the chin on the chest as the fetus travels through the birth canal. When the fetus reaches the pubic arch, it must extend under the symphysis pubis.
- *External rotation.* As the head is born, external rotation (restitution) lines the head up with the shoulders.
- *Expulsion.* Expulsion (birth) occurs after delivery of the anterior and posterior shoulders.

Think this through.

If the fetus is in an occiput posterior position, the fetal head must rotate 90 degrees versus 45 degrees. The typical result is a prolonged and painful "back" labor.

Test Yourself

✓ List three anticipatory signs of labor.

✓ What is the main difference between true and false labor?

✓ List the cardinal movements of labor.

Stages and Duration of Labor

Labor is categorized into four stages, and the first stage is divided further into three phases. Each stage and phase of labor has unique characteristics that help the nurse and physician or midwife determine if labor is

1. Engagement, decent, flexion

2. Internal rotation

5. External rotation (restitution)

3. Extension beginning (rotation complete)

6. Delivery of anterior shoulder

4. Extension complete

7. Delivery of posterior shoulder, followed by expulsion of newborn

▮ **Figure 8-11** The cardinal movements (or mechanisms) of delivery.

progressing as expected. It is important to note that individual labors vary greatly with regard to length. Many factors affect the progress of labor, such as use of agents to soften the cervix, labor induction techniques, and type of anesthesia (if any) used. These factors are discussed in other chapters.

This can be confusing. Although technically a woman who has never delivered a viable child is a nullipara, when she goes into labor, she is usually referred to as a primipara.

The following discussion focuses on the physical characteristics of each stage of labor and approximate times of each stage. Because parity influences labor progress, typical differences between the primiparous woman and the

multiparous woman are noted. Table 8-3 summarizes the stages of labor.

First Stage: Dilation

The first stage of labor begins with the onset of true labor and ends with full dilation of the cervix at 10 cm. This stage is subdivided into three phases: latent, active, and transition.

Early Labor (Latent Phase)

Early labor begins when the contractions of true labor start and ends when the cervix is dilated 4 cm. Contractions during this phase are of mild intensity and typically occur at a frequency of 5 to 10 minutes (although they may occur as infrequently as every 30 minutes), with duration of 30 to 45 seconds. In a normal labor, the

Table 8-3 ▌ STAGES OF LABOR

	Definition	Contractions	Characteristics
First Stage: Dilation	Onset of true labor through full dilation of cervix at 10 cm		
Latent Phase	Contractions of true labor through dilation of cervix to 4 cm	*Frequency:* every 5–10 minutes *Duration:* 30–45 seconds *Intensity:* mild	Contractions may be irregular at first followed by increasing regularity. Cervical effacement (thinning) generally occurs before dilation for the primipara.
Active Phase	Cervical dilation of 4 cm to cervical dilation of 8 cm	*Frequency:* every 3–5 minutes *Duration:* 40–60 seconds *Intensity:* moderate to strong	Contractions are regular and progressively increase in frequency, duration, and intensity. Progressive cervical dilation. Fetal descent.
Transition Phase	Cervical dilation of 8 cm to cervical dilation of 10 cm (complete dilation)	*Frequency:* every 2–3 minutes *Duration:* 60–90 seconds *Intensity:* strong	Most difficult phase. Woman must resist if she has a strong urge to push.
Second Stage: Birth	Complete cervical dilation (10 cm) through birth	*Frequency:* every 2–5 minutes *Duration:* 60–90 seconds *Intensity:* strong	Fetal descent is most pronounced during second stage. Woman should push when she feels the urge.
Third Stage: Delivery of Placenta	From birth through delivery of the placenta	Variable	Signs of placental separation: gush of blood, lengthening of umbilical cord, fundus becomes globular.
Fourth Stage: Recovery	From delivery of the placenta through 2 to 4 hours postdelivery	Afterpains: variable	In general, afterpains are more noticeable for the multipara and for the breastfeeding woman.

pattern of contractions during the latent phase becomes increasingly regular with shorter intervals between contractions.

The latent phase lasts on average approximately 8 to 9 hours for a primiparous woman but generally does not exceed 20 hours in length. Multiparous women usually experience shorter labors (an average length of approximately 5 hours, with an upper limit of 14 hours).

Here's a tip for encouraging the woman.

The nulliparous woman may become discouraged during the early phase of labor if many hours have passed and the cervix is still dilated less than 3 cm. Explain to the woman that her cervix is making progress because it is effacing. Reassure her that the cervix will begin to dilate more rapidly with the contractions of active labor.

Active Labor (Active Phase)

The active phase begins at 4-cm cervical dilation and ends when the cervix is dilated 8 cm. Contractions typically occur every 2 to 5 minutes, last 45 to 60 seconds, and are of moderate to strong intensity. Progressive cervical dilation and fetal descent normally occur in this phase.

For primiparas, dilation should occur at approximately 1.2 cm/hour. Multiparas progress at a slightly faster pace of 1.5 cm/hour. These designations are only approximations and may vary a great deal if the woman receives medication, anesthesia, or other medical intervention during labor. Fetal descent is often slow in the first stage of labor, regardless of parity. Occasionally, the fetus does not descend during active labor.

Transition (Transition Phase)

Transition is the most difficult part of labor. This phase of the first stage of labor starts when the cervix is dilated 8 cm and ends with full cervical dilation. The contractions are of strong intensity, occur every 2 to 3 minutes, and are of 60 to 90 seconds in duration.

Frequently, the woman experiences a strong urge to push as the fetus descends. It is important for the woman to resist the urge to push until the cervix is dilated completely. Pushing against a partially dilated cervix can cause swelling, which slows labor, or the cervix can develop lacerations, leading to hemorrhage.

Second Stage: Birth

The second stage begins when the cervix is dilated fully and ends with the birth of the infant. Contractions usually continue at a frequency of every 2 to 3 minutes, last 60 to 90 seconds, and are of strong intensity. The average length of the second stage is 1 hour for primiparas and 20 minutes for multiparas, although it is normal for a primipara to be in this stage for 2 hours or longer.

During the second stage, the woman is encouraged to use her abdominal muscles to bear down during contractions while the fetus continues to descend and rotate to the anterior position. Fetal descent is usually slow but steady for the primipara, from the active phase of the first stage through the second stage. Frequently, the fetus of a multipara may not descend significantly during active labor but may rapidly descend during the second stage. In this scenario, the baby may be born with one or two pushes. When the fetus is at a station of +4, he or she proceeds to move through the cardinal movements of extension and external rotation, followed by delivery of the shoulders and expulsion of the rest of the body.

Third Stage: Delivery of Placenta

Stage 3 begins with the birth of the baby and ends with delivery of the placenta. This stage normally lasts from 5 to 20 minutes for both primiparas and multiparas. Signs that indicate the placenta is separating from the uterine wall include a gush of blood, lengthening of the umbilical cord, and a globular shape to the fundus.

The placenta usually delivers spontaneously by one of two mechanisms. Expulsion by Schultze's mechanism means that the fetal or shiny side of the placenta delivers first. Delivery by Duncan's mechanism specifies that the maternal or rough side of the placenta presents first.

Fourth Stage: Recovery

Because of the tremendous changes that the new mother's body goes through during the process of labor and delivery, the period of recovery after delivery of the placenta is considered to be a fourth stage of labor. This recovery stage may

This advice may be helpful on a test!

It is easy to confuse phases of the first stage of labor with stages of labor. Be sure you are able to clearly define each stage and phase so that you do not confuse phases with stages during an examination.

last from 1 to 4 hours. During this fourth stage, observe the woman frequently for signs of hemorrhage or other complications.

MATERNAL AND FETAL ADAPTATION TO LABOR
Maternal Physiologic Adaptation

Labor has an effect on the woman as if she were engaged in moderate to vigorous aerobic exercise. There is an increased demand for oxygen during the first stage of labor, attributable in part to the energy used for uterine contractions. To meet the demand, there is a moderate increase in cardiac output throughout the first stage of labor. During pushing (second stage), cardiac output may be increased as much as 40% to 50% above the prelabor level. Immediately after birth, it may peak at 80% above the prelabor level.

The pulse is often at the high end of normal during active labor. Dehydration and/or maternal exhaustion accentuate these normal increases in the heart rate. Blood pressure, however, does not change appreciably during normal labor, although the stress of contractions may cause a 15-mm Hg increase in the systolic pressure. The increased demand for oxygen and the pain of uterine contractions cause the respiratory rate to increase, which puts the laboring woman at risk for hyperventilation. Mouth breathing and dehydration contribute to dry lips and mouth.

Labor prolongs the normal gastric-emptying time. This change often leads to nausea and vomiting during active labor and increases the woman's risk for aspiration, particularly if general anesthesia is required. Traditionally, the laboring woman receives intravenous fluids while solid food and fluids are withheld. However, research shows that the risk for aspiration remains high, even if the woman maintains a nothing by mouth status because gastric secretions become more acidic during periods of fasting. Women tend to desire fluids and food during early labor, but the desire declines as labor progresses (Tranmer et al., 2005). Current recommendations are to allow the laboring woman to have clear liquids, unless there is a high likelihood that she will deliver by cesarean.

Pressure on the urethra from the presenting part may cause overfilling of the bladder, a decreased sensation to void, and edema. A full bladder is uncomfortable and slows the progress of labor. As the bladder fills, it rises upward in the pelvic cavity, which puts pressure on the lower uterine segment and prevents the head from descending. Sometimes the use of an in-and-out (straight) urinary catheter becomes necessary to empty the bladder.

Labor affects some laboratory values. The stress of vigorous labor may cause an increase in the white blood cell count to as high as 30,000 cells/microliter (mcL). This increase is the body's normal response to inflammation, pain, and stress. Frequently the urine specific gravity is high, indicating concentrated urine, and there may be a trace amount of urinary protein because of increased metabolic activity. Gross proteinuria is never normal during labor and is a sign of a developing complication.

Maternal Psychological Adaptation

Labor is hard work that puts a demand on the woman's coping resources. The woman's response changes as labor progresses. During early labor, the woman is often excited and talkative, although anxiety and apprehension are common responses. As labor becomes active, the woman becomes more introverted and focuses her energies on coping with the stress of contractions. Women who are unprepared psychologically for labor lose control easily during the active phase and may resort to crying, screaming, or thrashing about during contractions. This response may impede the labor process by causing muscular tension. Tense muscles work against cervical dilation and fetal descent.

Transition is the most intense phase of the first stage of labor, and many women, even ones who have had natural childbirth classes, have a difficult time maintaining positive coping strategies during this phase of labor. Many women describe feeling out of control during this phase of labor. A woman in transition needs support, encouragement, and positive reinforcement. Once pushing efforts begin, the woman usually feels more in control and is better able to cope.

Maternal responses to the actual birth vary widely. Many mothers are excited and eager to see and hold the baby. Others are exhausted and may doze intermittently. Most new mothers are anxious about the baby's health. When the woman holds the baby for the first time, it is normal for her to use fingertip touching and for her to explore the infant and count his fingers and toes.

Fetal Adaptation to Labor

Normal labor stresses the fetus in several ways. Intracranial pressure increases as the fetal head meets resistance from the birth canal. Sometimes this increased pressure results in a slowing of the fetal heart rate at the

---

> **Box 8-3 ▮ EVALUATING FETAL SCALP pH**
>
> Fetal pH
> - >7.25
>   - Reassuring
>   - Associated with normal acid-base balance
> - Between 7.20 and 7.25
>   - Worrisome
>   - May be associated with metabolic acidosis
> - <7.20
>   - Critical
>   - Represents metabolic acidosis
> - <7.0
>   - Damaging
>   - Frequently associated with fetal neurologic damage

---

peak of a contraction—a normal phenomenon described in Chapter 10. Placental blood flow, the source of oxygen for the fetus, is temporarily interrupted at the peak of each contraction. Pushing efforts interrupt placental blood flow for even longer periods. Because of these changes, even the healthy fetus experiences a slowly decreasing pH throughout labor. Box 8-3 describes normal and abnormal changes in fetal pH. Although labor stresses the fetal cardiovascular system, a healthy fetus is able to compensate and maintain the heart rate within normal limits (see Chapter 10). This ability to compensate demonstrates the presence of a well-oxygenated fetus with a healthy neurologic system.

The act of passing through the birth canal is beneficial to the fetus in two ways. The process of labor stimulates surfactant production to promote respiratory adaptation at birth, and as the fetus descends, maternal tissues compress the body, a process that helps clear the respiratory passageways of mucus. Infants who are born by cesarean section usually require more frequent suctioning because they have not had the benefit of this "vaginal squeeze."

Pressure on the fetus caused by progress through the birth canal may result in areas of ecchymosis or edema, particularly on the presenting part. Pressure on the vertex may cause formation of a **caput succedaneum**, swelling of the soft tissue of the head, or development of a cephalohematoma, collection of blood under the scalp.

Cultural Snapshot

The laboring woman's culture influences her response to pain. In some cultures, the woman is expected to accept pain stoically. In other cultures, loud expressions of pain are accepted. It is important to perform a careful assessment of a woman's discomfort and to determine measures the laboring woman thinks would be helpful to relieve the pain. Just because the woman is quiet during labor does not mean that she is not experiencing pain. (Refer to Chapter 9 for an in-depth discussion of pain management during labor.)

Test Yourself

✔ How many centimeters must the cervix dilate before a woman is in active labor?

✔ Which stage of labor requires the woman to help by pushing?

✔ In which stage of labor does birth occur?

Key Points

- Four essential components of the labor process are the passageway (maternal pelvis and soft tissues), passenger (fetus), powers (involuntary and voluntary muscle contractions), and psyche (psychological state of the woman).
- The bony pelvis is the rigid passageway through which the fetus must pass. There are four basic pelvic shapes: gynecoid, anthropoid, android, and platypelloid. The gynecoid type is the most favorable for vaginal birth. The diameters of the inlet, midpelvis, and outlet are important in determining the adequacy of the pelvis for vaginal delivery.
- The cervix, part of the soft tissue of the passageway, must completely efface (thin) and dilate (open) for the fetus to be born. Full dilation is equal to 10 cm.
- The fetal skull is the most important fetal structure because it is the largest and least compressible. A comparison of the diameters of the true pelvis to the diameters of the fetal skull is important when the physician is attempting to determine if a vaginal delivery is possible.
- Fetal lie refers to the relationship of the long axis of the fetus to the long axis of the mother. A longitudinal lie is the most favorable to a vaginal birth.
- The large majority of fetuses enter the pelvis head first, a condition referred to as a cephalic presentation. When the feet or buttocks present first, the fetus is in a breech presentation. Shoulder presentation is uncommon.
- A flexed fetal attitude presents the smallest diameters of the fetal head to the pelvis.
- The part of the fetus that is closest to the cervix is the presenting part. Presentation and attitude together determine the presenting part.
- To determine fetal position, first verify the presenting part and locate the reference point (occiput, frontum, mentum, sacrum, etc.). Then determine the relationship of the reference point to maternal pelvic quadrants to confirm fetal position.
- Station is a determination of the relationship of the presenting part to the ischial spines. Zero station occurs when the presenting part is at the level of the ischial spines. When the fetus is high in the pelvis (above the ischial spines), the station is recorded as a negative number. A low station (below the ischial spines) is recorded as a positive number.
- The primary power of labor comes from involuntary uterine contractions, which serve to efface and dilate the cervix. Maternal pushing efforts supply secondary powers during the second stage of labor.
- The contraction pattern (frequency, duration, and intensity) and the resting interval are important to assess because the fetus can become hypoxic if contractions are too close together, too strong, or do not have a rest period.
- Maternal psyche is an important influence on the labor process. Nursing interventions can help break the cycle of fear, tension, and pain that can interfere with labor.
- Theories of what causes labor to begin include progesterone withdrawal theory and the oxytocin and prostaglandin theories. Current research indicates that maternal and fetal factors work together in a cascade effect to initiate labor.
- Anticipatory signs of labor include gastrointestinal disturbances, expelling the mucous plug, lightening, Braxton Hicks contractions, a burst of energy, and cervical ripening and dilation.
- True labor results in progressive effacement and dilation. Contractions become progressively stronger and occur more frequently. Walking does not cause true labor contractions to stop.
- Engagement, descent, flexion, internal rotation, extension, external rotation, and expulsion are the mechanisms of delivery or cardinal movements by which the fetus is born.
- Labor occurs in four stages: first stage, dilation; second stage, birth; third stage, expulsion of placenta; and fourth stage, recovery. The first stage is composed of three phases: latent, active, and transition. Each phase and stage has unique characteristics that differentiate it from other phases and stages.
- Labor affects the mother in much the same way as vigorous exercise does. The heart rate, cardiac output, and respiratory rate increase to meet the body's increased oxygen need. Other systems, notably the gastrointestinal and urinary, are also affected.
- The healthy fetus is able to withstand the stress that labor places on the cardiovascular system. A vaginal birth helps mature the respiratory system and clears mucus from the respiratory tract.

INTERNET RESOURCES

www.emedicinehealth.com/labor_signs/article_em.htm
www.methodisthealth.com/pregnancy/labor.htm

www.childbirth.org/articles/labor/laborbasics.html
http://americanpregnancy.org/labornbirth/index.htm

Workbook

■ NCLEX-STYLE REVIEW QUESTIONS

1. A 32-year-old woman is dilated 4 cm. The physician states that she has a roomy pelvis and the baby is in a right occiput anterior (ROA) position at a +1 station. Her contractions are occurring every 10 minutes, lasting 30 to 40 seconds, and palpate mild in intensity. She is calm and relaxed. Given these data, the nurse knows which essential component of labor is unexpected and likely to slow the progress of labor at this time?

   a. Passageway
   b. Passenger
   c. Powers
   d. Psyche

2. A woman near the end of pregnancy comments to the nurse, "I'm curious. What causes labor to begin?" Which reply by the nurse is best?

   a. "It is a mystery. No one knows."
   b. "It is believed that several factors work together to stimulate labor to begin."
   c. "The pituitary gland in the brain releases a special hormone that signals labor to begin."
   d. "You don't need to worry about that. The baby will come when he is ready."

3. The fetus is in a cephalic presentation. His occiput is facing toward the front and slightly to the right of the mother's pelvis, and he is exhibiting a flexed attitude. How does the nurse document the position of the fetus?

   a. LOA
   b. LOP
   c. ROA
   d. ROP

4. A woman has just delivered a healthy baby girl, but the placenta has not yet delivered. What stage of labor does this scenario represent?

   a. First
   b. Second
   c. Third
   d. Fourth

■ STUDY ACTIVITIES

1. Using the table below, write a brief definition or explanation of each of the "four Ps" of labor. List critical nursing observations/assessments for each area and briefly describe what should be documented.

Four Ps of Labor	Definition or Explanation	Observations (What to Look for)	Documentation
Passageway			
Passenger			
Powers			
Psyche			

2. Develop a teaching aid or poster explaining the stages of labor to a first-time pregnant woman.

3. Have a discussion with your clinical group about the way culture affects behaviors and choices regarding labor and birth. Compare different rituals and taboos of which your classmates are aware that relate to labor and birth.

■ CRITICAL THINKING: WHAT WOULD YOU DO?

Apply your knowledge of the components of labor to the following situation.

1. Anna, a 25-year-old gravida 2, has been in labor for several hours, but her cervix is not dilating. The physician says that Anna's pelvis is roomy and adequate for a vaginal delivery.

   a. In what way do you anticipate the journey of the fetus through the passageway will be affected because Anna's cervix is not dilating?
   b. Discuss two possible causes of the failure of Anna's cervix to dilate.

2. Anna's midwife performs a vaginal examination and states the fetus is "occiput posterior."

   a. Anna asks you, "What does it mean that the baby is occiput posterior?" How would you explain this position to Anna?
   b. What will you tell Anna's partner regarding the probable progress of labor because the fetus is in a posterior position?

3. Anna has been in active labor for 7 hours. She has been quietly coping with contractions with the help of her partner. Now she begins to cry, "I can't stand it anymore!" She screams at her partner, "This is all your fault. You're not helping me at all!"

   a. The nurse performs a pelvic examination. How far do you expect Anna to be dilated? What stage and phase of labor is most likely represented in this scenario?
   b. How will you advise Anna's partner? How can he continue to be helpful and understanding during this difficult part of labor?

4. Anna progresses to the second stage of labor. The fetus has not rotated to an anterior position, so the baby is delivered face up.

   a. What does the physician document in the delivery note regarding the position of the baby at birth?
   b. How would you expect the baby's head to look after his long journey through the birth canal?
   c. How do you expect Anna will react to the birth of her baby?

9 *Pain Management During Labor and Birth*

LEARNING OBJECTIVES

On completion of this chapter, you should be able to:

1. Explain how the pain of labor and birth differs from other types of pain.
2. Describe sources of labor pain.
3. List factors influencing the woman's experience of labor pain.
4. Discuss principles of labor pain management.
5. Compare nonpharmacologic interventions to manage labor pain.
6. Explain various relaxation techniques that help a woman cope with labor.
7. Differentiate analgesia from anesthesia.
8. Describe advantages and disadvantages of opioid administration.
9. Compare methods of regional anesthesia.
10. Explain major complications associated with epidural and spinal anesthesia.
11. Discuss reasons general anesthesia is risky for a pregnant woman and her fetus.

PAIN IS AN individual, subjective, sensory experience. A complex interplay of physiologic, psychological, emotional, environmental, and sociocultural factors influences the way a person perceives and responds to pain. A woman's response to labor pain is influenced by all of these factors, including her expectations about labor and her confidence in her ability to cope with labor. As a licensed practical/vocational nurse (LPN/LVN), you assist the registered nurse (RN) to manage the pain associated with labor and birth.

THE PAIN OF LABOR AND CHILDBIRTH

Uniqueness of Labor and Birth Pain

The pain of labor and birth is different from other types of pain in several ways. In most instances, pain is a warning sign of injury, but labor pain is associated with a normal physiologic process. In other types of pain, greater intensity is often associated with greater injury. During labor, intensity increases as the woman approaches birth, which is the desirable and positive outcome. Although the pain of labor begins without warning, once labor is established it occurs in a predictable pattern with respite from pain between contractions. This characteristic is different from most other types of

pain. Because it is predictable, the woman can prepare for and better cope with the pain.

Physiology and Characteristics of Labor Pain

Pain sensations associated with labor originate from different places, depending on the stage of labor. During the first stage of labor, the stretching required to efface and dilate the cervix stimulates pain receptors in the cervix and lower uterine segment. During the second stage of labor, the main source of pain is from pressure on the perineum and birth canal as the fetus descends.

Labor pain in the first stage of labor has characteristics similar to other types of abdominal pain. It is often diffuse in nature, occurs in the lower abdomen, and may be referred to the lower back, buttocks, and thighs. Women often describe contractions as wavelike, with some "waves" more powerful than others. The contraction begins as a sensation of cramping in the lower abdomen or lower back and gradually increases in strength to the peak of the contraction, and then it slowly subsides.

Women sometimes describe the pain of birth as the most extreme sensation of pain. Most women experience an intense sensation of burning in the perineum as the tissues stretch in response to the fetus pressing against them during descent. Often the sensation is so powerful that the physician can perform an episiotomy (cut into the perineum) without anesthesia, and the woman does not feel it.

Factors Influencing Labor Pain

Many factors influence the pain of labor and birth, making it a multidimensional experience. Examples of psychosocial influences include the level of the woman's fear and anxiety, her culture, and the circumstances surrounding the birth experience, such as whether or not the pregnancy is planned or unplanned, the child is wanted or unwanted, the birth is preterm or term, and the fetus is living or dead.

There are two general concepts related to pain that are helpful to understand: threshold and tolerance. The pain threshold is the level of pain necessary for an individual to perceive pain. Pain tolerance refers to the ability of an individual to withstand pain once it is recognized. Each woman has her own pain threshold and tolerance of pain. Each woman responds to labor in a unique way, and women report the experience of labor differently. In addition, a woman experiences each labor uniquely with each subsequent birth.

Many variables affect the woman's perception of labor pain. The younger the woman, the more likely she is to report severe pain. Women bearing children for the first time also report more intense levels of pain. High levels of anxiety and fear correlate with high levels of perceived pain. A woman who is physically conditioned usually reports lower levels of pain during labor and birth.

Caution!

Don't assume that the woman who reports severe pain has low pain tolerance. Always do a thorough assessment because pain that is not controlled with normal interventions may be a signal that the woman is experiencing a complication of labor or a medical emergency.

Physiologic factors directly related to the birthing process also affect the perception of pain. In general, the longer the labor, the more likely the woman is to report extreme pain. In obstructed or dysfunctional labor, the woman usually reports more pain. Obstructed labor can result from fetopelvic disproportion and abnormal fetal positions. When labor contractions are induced with oxytocin, women report them as extremely strong. Women may describe induced contractions as intense and lacking the gradual ebb and flow of naturally occurring contractions. Back labor usually is perceived as being intensely painful, even excruciating. Some women report that back labor feels as if the back is literally breaking in two. In addition, when a woman experiences back labor, her pain may not completely resolve between contractions.

PAIN MANAGEMENT PRINCIPLES AND TECHNIQUES

There is no one "perfect way" to control labor pain. Each woman responds to the experience uniquely. Pain management during labor should be planned and implemented, keeping several principles in mind. The specific techniques used to manage pain can be divided into two major categories: nonpharmacologic interventions and pharmacologic interventions. Safety considerations for the woman and her fetus are an important part of the nursing care plan for both categories.

Principles of Pain Relief During Labor

Research has shown that women report higher levels of satisfaction with their labor experience when they feel a high degree of control over the experience of pain (Stuebe & Barbieri, 2005). Inform the woman of pain management options, and be supportive of the choices that she makes. Remember that the woman has the right to change her mind about the acceptability of any particular pain management technique at any time before or during labor.

Rarely is there a completely pain-free labor. Even when a woman plans for an epidural, she frequently reports severe pain before the epidural is administered. Caregivers commonly underrate the severity of pain when compared with the woman's ratings (Prkachin, Solomon, & Ross, 2007). It is important to accept the woman's description of the severity of the pain, even when she may not appear to be in pain.

Sensitivity and understanding go a long way!

It is important to be non-judgmental when assisting a woman to cope with pain. Some nurses feel strongly that a woman should have a "natural" childbirth without medication. Other nurses don't understand why any woman would want to "suffer" through labor without an epidural. In both situations, the nurse is in danger of not providing the support that the laboring woman needs and deserves.

Cultural Snapshot

A woman's cultural values influence the way that she responds to pain. Some women are very vocal. They may cry or moan with pain. Some women display a stoic response to pain. They may be very quiet or appear to be resting. Caregivers frequently underestimate the pain of both types of women. The woman who is vocal may be labeled a "difficult" patient who does not handle pain well. The stoic woman may be labeled a "good" patient. However, neither of them is likely to get the pain control that they need, unless the nurse does a careful pain assessment.

Ideally, the woman discusses labor pain management with her primary care provider during the pregnancy and attends prenatal classes. The woman who enters labor with realistic expectations usually copes well and reports a more satisfying labor experience than does a woman who is not as well prepared. However, if the woman is not prepared, teach the woman what to expect and assist her to cope when she presents in labor.

Nonpharmacologic Interventions

Almost every woman uses some type of nonpharmacologic pain intervention during labor, even when pharmacologic methods are used. Most commonly, a woman uses a combination of techniques to cope with labor. She may need assistance coping before medication is used or in conjunction with medication.

There are numerous methods of nonpharmacologic pain relief. Some interventions are evidence based. Other interventions need more research to demonstrate efficacy. In general, the intervention that works for the woman is frequently the best one to use. Typically, a woman needs a variety of interventions throughout labor. As labor becomes more intense, the woman may need to switch to a different method of coping. For example, effleurage and distraction are often helpful in early labor, but not as effective in active labor and transition. Table 9-1 compares selected nonpharmacologic interventions.

Continuous Labor Support

Continuous labor support with a trained nurse or doula (trained layperson, who supports and coaches a woman during labor) has been shown to be effective to increase the coping ability of the laboring woman. Additional benefits include fewer requests for pain medication, fewer obstetric interventions, and a lower rate of cesarean delivery. Women do not experience the same benefit when nurses provide intermittent labor support, as is typical for busy labor and delivery settings. You may encourage the woman to hire a doula, particularly if the woman desires childbirth with minimal medical intervention.

Comfort Measures

The need for comfort measures during labor should not be underestimated. Lip balm can help keep the lips hydrated during labor. Ice chips, lollipops, and clear liquids (if allowed) can be helpful to moisten the mouth. Mouth breathing during labor can lead to dry mouth.

Change linens soiled with perspiration or body fluids. Most facilities have pads to place under the buttocks to catch bloody show and amniotic fluid during labor. Explain to the woman that it will be impossible to keep her completely dry, but reassure her that you will change the pads frequently. Give perineal care with warm water after she uses the restroom and before changing the linens.

Relaxation Techniques

Relaxation is the objective of almost every nonpharmacologic intervention. When the woman becomes anxious or apprehensive, she tenses her muscles. This action can slow the labor process and decrease the amount of oxygen reaching the uterus and the fetus. When the woman maintains a state of relaxation during and between contractions, she is actually working with her body to facilitate the labor process. The following discussion highlights several techniques that may help the woman to relax during labor. Some of these methods require training and practice before labor to be most effective, although you can teach the woman and her partner some of the basic techniques when she presents to the delivery suite.

Patterned Breathing

In times past, childbirth educators encouraged the use of very structured breathing techniques for labor. Now the trend is to teach basic principles of patterned breathing without emphasizing strict patterns. Frequently, the woman begins with a slow-paced breathing pattern. She maintains the slow-paced pattern until it is no longer working to enhance relaxation, and then she switches to a higher level. Table 9-2 describes the basic breathing patterns often taught in childbirth preparation classes.

All breathing patterns should begin and end with the woman taking a cleansing breath. A cleansing breath is a deep, relaxed breath that signals the woman to relax and provides deep ventilation. Encourage the woman to breathe through the nose or through the mouth, whichever is most comfortable and natural for her. If she uses mouth breathing, pay particular attention to measures to keep the mouth moist.

Breathing should be comfortable and should not cause the woman to hyperventilate. If she feels short of breath, she may need to take deeper breaths. If she begins to tingle in her hands and around her mouth, she is probably hyperventilating. She should slow her breathing and breathe into her cupped hands or a paper bag until the tingling stops.

Attention Focusing

Many childbirth classes teach methods of attention focusing, or concentration. Women attending Lamaze-oriented classes are encouraged to focus internally or externally, whichever is more effective. Bradley classes advocate an internal focus because Dr. Bradley, the method's founder, believed that external focus distracts the woman from the job of "listening to her body" while laboring. Attention focusing, or concentration, helps the woman to work with her body, instead of panicking.

Another name for internal focus is imagery. Imagery is a technique used to help the woman associate positive thoughts with the birth process. The method engages the senses and promotes relaxation. The woman is encouraged to visualize a positive, healing situation during

Table 9-1 ▮ COMPARISON OF SELECTED NONPHARMACOLOGIC INTERVENTIONS FOR RELIEF OF LABOR PAIN

Intervention	Effectiveness to Relieve Labor Pain	Advantages	Disadvantages
Continuous labor support	Highly effective throughout labor. May increase the woman's perception of personal control, a factor that correlates with higher satisfaction with the labor experience.	• Low-technological/high-touch intervention • Addresses the emotional and spiritual aspects of labor and birth.	Most busy labor and delivery hospital settings cannot provide this level of support for the laboring woman, so the woman and her partner must usually hire a doula if they desire this level of support.
Patterned breathing	Can be very effective when the woman has practiced before labor and has an attentive labor coach.	• Does not require any special tools. • Promotes relaxation. • Basic patterns can be taught by the nurse when the couple presents in labor.	Requires training and practice before labor to be most effective.
Effleurage	Can be helpful during early labor to decrease the sensation of pain.	• Is easy to learn and simple to perform. • Does not require any special tools.	Is less effective during active labor as the contractions become more intense. Fetal monitor straps on the abdomen may interfere with the woman's ability to use this technique.
Water therapy	Highly effective to promote relaxation and decrease the sensation of pain, especially during the first hour or two of use.	• Many women find water very comforting during labor. • Promotes relaxation.	• Requires availability of a tub—equipment that is not always available in the hospital setting. • May slow labor if used too early. • The woman may notice decreased effectiveness over time.
Imagery	Can be very effective for some women.	• Is noninvasive. • Requires no special tools. • Incorporates spirituality with the birthing process.	• Requires discipline and practice to achieve maximum benefit. • May not be appropriate for individuals with mental illness or history of emotional trauma.
Hypnosis	Carefully selected women can benefit from hypnosis during labor.	• Requires no special tools. • Promotes the woman's sense of control over her pain. • Involves a holistic approach to labor.	• Special training by a therapist is required. • Can be expensive and may not be covered by insurance. • Does not work for all women. • History of psychosis is a contraindication.
Intradermal water injections	Very effective to relieve back pain during labor.	• Can be administered by the nurse.	• Invasive (requires an injection). • Not effective for abdominal discomfort associated with contractions.
Acupressure and acupuncture	Anecdotal reports suggest that these therapies may be helpful to reduce the pain of labor.	• Addresses the holistic nature of labor and incorporates spiritual and emotional aspects. • Acupressure is noninvasive.	• Requires a trained practitioner to perform. • Acupuncture is invasive and requires special needles.

Table 9-2 ▮ PATTERNED BREATHING TECHNIQUES FOR LABOR*

Breathing Pattern	Description
Slow-paced breathing	The woman takes slow, deliberate breaths while she focuses on maintaining a relaxed stance. She may use effleurage, music, or any technique that encourages relaxation while using slow-paced breathing. The rate is approximately 6 to 10 breaths per minute.
Modified-paced breathing	The woman begins taking slow, deep breaths at the beginning of the contraction. She then increases the rate while decreasing the depth of respirations as she reaches the contraction peak, after which she slows the rate and increases the depth.
Patterned-paced breathing or the "pant-blow" technique	This technique is similar to modified-paced breathing with the addition of a rhythmic pattern. There are several rhythms that can be taught; however, the 4-to-1 rhythm is a popular one. The woman takes 4 light breaths and then blows out through her lips, as if she is blowing out a candle. Different rhythms can be used, such as 4-to-1, followed by 6-to-1 and repeating through the peak of the contraction.

*Note that each pattern begins and ends with a cleansing breath.

contractions. For example, some childbirth educators encourage the woman to visualize each contraction as a wave. As the contraction strengthens, the tide rises. As the contraction fades away, the tide ebbs. Or, the woman may visualize her body opening and allowing the fetus to pass through. Sometimes, the woman visualizes herself at a favorite relaxing place, such as the beach or in a comfortable chair at a vacation cabin. Music used in association with imagery sometimes helps the woman focus and relax.

The woman who focuses externally opens her eyes and focuses on a picture, person, or object that is helpful to her. For example, one woman used a picture of her grandmother as her focus. As she looked into her grandmother's face during her contractions, she drew strength remembering that her grandmother had birthed 11 babies, all at home without medications. Another woman used a picture of a mountain she and her husband had climbed as her focus. As she labored, she remembered her feelings as she overcame the challenges of the ascent of the mountain and likened it to the challenge of her labor. Remembering the feeling of accomplishment when she reached the peak of the mountain, she felt strengthened knowing she would have a strong sense of achievement when she felt her baby slide from her body and held him in her arms. Focusing on sounds, music, voices, relaxation, and breathing may also benefit the laboring woman.

Movement and Positioning

Changing positions frequently can be helpful during labor. Current research suggests that ambulation and standing interspersed with other positions helps make early labor more tolerable (Simkin & Klein, 2007). Any position of comfort is acceptable, as long as the fetal heart rate stays within the normal range. If the woman wants to be on her back, be certain to place a pillow or a wedge under one hip to prevent supine hypotension. The woman may find a birthing ball to be

helpful. The ball allows her to rock and move to a position of comfort. Women who ambulate and reposition themselves, as needed, during labor tend to report higher satisfaction levels with the birthing process. Figure 9-1 illustrates several positions the woman can try during labor.

Touch and Massage

Effleurage, a form of touch that involves light circular fingertip movements on the abdomen, is a technique the woman can use in early labor (Fig. 9-2). The theory is that light touch stimulates the nerve pathways to the brain and keeps them busy, thereby blocking the pain sensation. As contractions become stronger during active labor, effleurage becomes less effective. At that point, the woman can use deeper pressure. Pressure is applied with the hands directly over the area of greatest pain intensity, often above the pubic bone or on the upper thighs. Either the woman or her partner/coach may apply deep pressure.

Massage can be used throughout labor as a way to provide support and comfort and promote relaxation (Zwelling, Johnson, & Allen, 2006). If the woman is experiencing intense back labor, it is often helpful for you or the partner to give the woman a massage over the lower back or to use the fists or palms of the hands to apply counter-pressure (Fig. 9-3). Alternately, a tennis ball can be used to massage the lower back.

Water Therapy

Exposure to warm water either by showering or bathing in a tub or whirlpool can significantly increase the ability of the laboring woman to cope with uterine contractions. In fact, some women use water not only to provide labor pain relief, but they also deliver in water.

Suggestions for using water safely during labor differ slightly between authors. Simkin & Klein (2007) recommend that the water temperature remain at or slightly

■ Figure 9-1 Various positions for use during labor: **(A)** ambulation, **(B)** leaning forward, **(C)** sitting in a chair, and **(D)** using a birthing ball.

above body temperature, and that the woman's temperature should be monitored. There are no restrictions mentioned regarding dilation, labor status, or duration in the water. Waterbirth International (undated) recommends using a water temperature of 95°F to 100°F (not to exceed 101°F). This organization also suggests that the woman get in the water whenever she chooses to do so, with the caveat that entering water before 5 cm of cervical dilation may cause labor to progress more slowly. There is no time limit given for bathing, although the organization does suggest that the first hour in the water is usually the most relaxing and helpful for the laboring woman.

There are differing opinions in the medical establishment regarding the safety and advisability of using water during labor and birth. In particular, the American Academy of Pediatrics Committee on Fetus and Newborn (2005) advises that waterbirth should only be accomplished under strict research conditions until its safety for the newborn can be validated. Current research is confirming the safety and efficacy of this intervention during labor even with ruptured membranes (Simkin & Klein, 2007). However, more research is needed to establish guidelines for practice, to determine the safety of waterbirth for the newborn, and to encourage more hospital settings to provide water therapy during labor.

■ **Figure 9-2** Effleurage. The woman uses her fingertips to lightly touch her abdomen using circular strokes. This form of light touch often decreases the sensation of pain in early labor.

Hypnosis

Hypnosis helps some women to relax and decrease the pain of labor. The woman attends several sessions with a trained therapist during pregnancy. At each session, she learns how to induce a trancelike state that she can

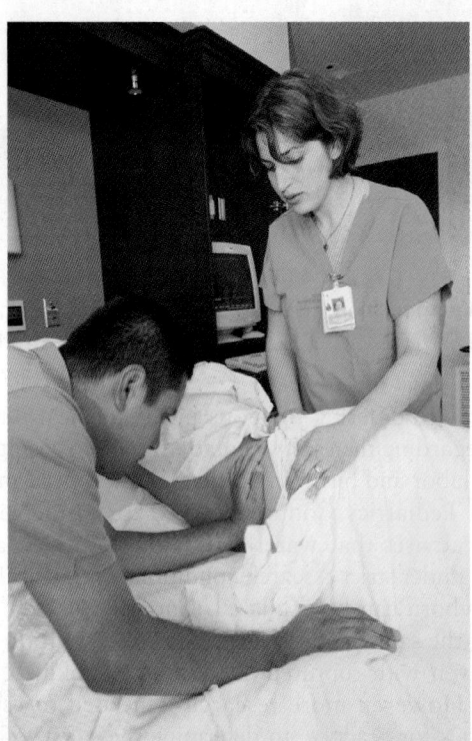

■ **Figure 9-3** The woman's partner uses the palm of his hand to apply counter-pressure to the woman's lower back.

■ **Figure 9-4** Location of intradermal water injections. The nurse administers four sterile water injections to relieve the pain of back labor.

use during labor. Currently, the limited research available on hypnosis and labor shows promising results (Smith et al., 2006). Hypnosis is contraindicated for women with a history of psychosis (Simkin & Klein, 2007).

Intradermal Water Injections

Intradermal injections of sterile water can effectively relieve the pain of back labor. Draw up four injections of 0.05 to 0.1 mL sterile water using a 1-mL syringe with a 25-gauge needle. Then inject the sterile water into the intradermal space in the lower back (Fig. 9-4). Explain before the procedure that the injections sting significantly for up to 1 minute, but they effectively reduce back pain for 45 to 120 minutes after they are given (Simkin & Klein, 2007). Injections may be repeated as needed.

Acupressure and Acupuncture

Acupressure and acupuncture are two similar techniques used in traditional Chinese medicine. The goal is to restore balance by promoting the flow of energy, which decreases muscle tension, promotes relaxation, and decreases the sensation of pain. Acupuncture involves the use of needles, whereas acupressure is a noninvasive form of massage. Both methods involve stimulating energy points. Current research shows promising results for the use of acupuncture to control labor pain (Smith et al., 2006).

> *Test Yourself*
>
> ✔ Name two general principles of pain relief during labor.
> ✔ List three nonpharmacologic methods of labor pain management.
> ✔ Describe three relaxation techniques that help increase the woman's ability to cope with labor pain.

Pharmacologic Interventions

There is currently no perfect method to relieve the pain of labor. The ideal pharmacologic method would provide excellent pain relief and still allow the woman to freely change positions and ambulate. The ideal method would not cross the placenta and would not have potentially severe side effects.

One reason women began to choose the hospital as a place to deliver babies was for the pharmacologic pain relief methods that were available. The pendulum has swung back and forth regarding the favor in which pharmacologic methods are viewed. In the 1950s, women were given strong medications that caused them to forget the pain of labor. Beginning in the 1960s and 1970s, women demanded to have more control and more say over the birth process, and natural childbirth came into favor as the "best" way to experience labor and birth. Currently, many women choose to deliver in hospitals so that they can get pain relief from epidural analgesia or anesthesia.

It is important to understand the difference between analgesia and anesthesia, although the terms are sometimes used interchangeably. **Analgesia** is the use of medication to reduce the sensation of pain. **Anesthesia** is the use of medication to partially or totally block all sensation to an area of the body. Anesthesia may or may not involve loss of consciousness. Table 9-3 compares pharmacologic medications used to relieve labor pain.

Analgesia and Sedation

Sedatives promote sedation and relaxation; however, they do not provide direct pain relief (analgesia). Barbiturates, such as secobarbital (Seconal) and pentobarbital (Nembutal), may be given in early labor to promote sleep. These medications can cause respiratory and central nervous system depression in the newborn if given within 12 to 24 hours of birth.

Opioids, medications with opiumlike properties (also known as narcotic analgesics), are the most frequently administered medications to provide analgesia during labor. Opioids, such as meperidine (Demerol) and fentanyl (Sublimaze), frequently assist the woman to better tolerate labor contractions by causing relaxation and sleep between contractions (Grant, 2006b). Opioids are most frequently given by the intravenous (IV) route because this route provides fast onset and more consistent drug levels than do the subcutaneous or intramuscular routes.

Be very careful!
Always warn the woman and her support person to call you before she tries to get up after receiving IV sedation. Women have fallen when attempting to ambulate after IV sedation, and have even delivered their babies unattended in the bathroom because they mistake the urge to push for the need to have a bowel movement.

Opioids given during labor are not without risk. These medications cross the placenta and cause changes in the fetal heart pattern. They stay within the fetal circulatory system and can cause respiratory depression in the newborn. In rare instances, opioids have led to maternal deaths by aspiration, inadequate ventilation, and overdosage (Cunningham et al., 2005).

Test Yourself

✔ What is the difference between analgesia and anesthesia?

✔ What is another name for opioids?

✔ Name two effects opioids have on the fetus and newborn.

Anesthesia

There are three basic types of anesthesia: local, regional, and general. Local anesthesia is used to numb the perineum just before birth to allow for episiotomy and repair. Regional anesthesia can provide excellent pain relief during labor and birth and is the preferred type of anesthesia for nonemergent cesarean births. General anesthesia is reserved for emergencies in which the baby must be delivered immediately to save the life of the baby or the mother, or both.

Regional Anesthesia

Regional anesthesia involves blocking a group of sensory nerves that supply a particular organ or area of the body. Local anesthetics and opioids are given to induce regional anesthesia/analgesia. The types of regional anesthetics that may be used during labor are pudendal block, paracervical block, epidural anesthesia, combined epidural/spinal anesthesia, and spinal block.

Anytime an anesthetic is administered using any of the techniques described, there is a chance that the local anesthetic agent will inadvertently enter the bloodstream and cause a toxic reaction in the woman. Fortunately, this situation rarely occurs; however, be prepared to assist with a full resuscitation, if one is needed. Every facility in which regional anesthetics are administered must have emergency equipment available, including oxygen, oral airway, equipment for emergency intubation and cardiac monitoring, and emergency medications.

It is the nurse's role to assist the anesthesia provider and to monitor the woman and her fetus during and after administration of anesthesia. Most of these techniques require IV access. Monitor vital signs frequently during the procedure and while the woman is under the effects of anesthesia.

Pudendal Block. A pudendal block is given just before the baby is born to provide pain relief for the birth.

Table 9-3 ▌ COMPARISON OF SELECTED PHARMACOLOGIC INTERVENTIONS FOR RELIEF OF LABOR PAIN

Medication Class	Advantages	Disadvantages	Associated Side Effects
Sedatives	• Promote sleep in the early stage of labor. • Decrease anxiety. • Promethazine (Phenergan) and hydroxyzine (Vistaril) may be administered with an opioid to decrease nausea and vomiting. • May increase effectiveness of uterine contractions.	• Do not provide pain relief. • Can produce neonatal respiratory depression if given within 12–24 hours of birth.	• Excessive sedation and/or central nervous system depression • Decreased FHR variability
Opioids (narcotic analgesics)	• Increase the woman's ability to cope with uterine contractions. • May be nurse administered.	• Reduce but do not eliminate pain sensations. • Associated with neonatal central nervous system and respiratory depression. • Inhibit neonatal sucking and delay effective feeding. • May decrease neonatal alertness.	• Nausea and vomiting • Pruritus • Delayed gastric emptying • Dysphoria • Drowsiness • Hypoventilation • Decreased FHR variability • Neonatal depression
Paracervical block	• Provides excellent pain relief for the first stage of labor. • Does not interfere with maternal mobility. • Is an alternative when epidural block is contraindicated.	• Requires multiple injections because the duration of pain relief is short. • Cannot be used for pain relief in the second stage of labor. • Rapidly crosses the placenta, which can lead to fetal central nervous system depression. • Can cause constriction of the uterine artery, with resultant decrease in blood flow to the placenta. • Is not used frequently because of the association with fetal bradycardia.	• Fetal bradycardia (occurs in approximately 15% of paracervical blocks [Cunningham et al., 2005])
Epidural analgesia/ anesthesia	• Provides more effective pain relief than opioid analgesia. • Often completely eliminates pain sensation. • Anesthesia can be continued indefinitely. • If the woman needs a cesarean section, the epidural can be used to provide anesthesia, which saves time in an emergency situation. • Serious side effects are rare.	• Often impairs motor function, which decreases the ability to walk during labor. • Women frequently require urinary catheterization. • Increases the need for labor augmentation with oxytocin, particularly when administered before 5 cm of dilation. • Increases the duration of the second stage of labor (Anim-Somuah, Smyth, & Howell, 2005). • Vacuum assistance and forceps are more frequently required (Anim-Somuah, Smyth, & Howell, 2005). • Increases the likelihood of maternal fever, which increases neonatal sepsis evaluation and antibiotic treatment (Courtney, 2007). • Must be administered by an anesthetist or anesthesiologist. • Requires complex nursing care.	• Hypotension, which often requires administration of medication to raise the blood pressure • Maternal fever • Shivering • Itching (if opioids are used) • Inadvertent injection of anesthetic into the bloodstream • Accidental intrathecal puncture ("wet tap") with possible spinal headache • Inadequate pain relief or failed block • Fetal distress

Table 9-3 ∎ COMPARISON OF SELECTED PHARMACOLOGIC INTERVENTIONS FOR RELIEF OF LABOR PAIN *(continued)*

Medication Class	Advantages	Disadvantages	Associated Side Effects
Intrathecal anesthesia (spinal block)	• Rapid onset of analgesia. • Provides excellent pain relief. • It is the anesthetic method of choice for planned cesarean birth.	• A complete block results in the woman's lower extremities being temporarily paralyzed. • Used alone for labor, the dose might wear off before labor is completed. • Must be administered by an anesthetist or anesthesiologist. • Requires complex nursing care.	• Hypotension • Shivering • Spinal headache
General anesthesia	• Especially useful in emergency situations because total anesthesia can be accomplished rapidly. • Provides total pain relief.	• Requires intubation, which is more challenging during pregnancy. • All agents used to induce and maintain general anesthesia cross the placenta and can cause severe neonatal depression.	• Hypertension during intubation • Hypotension during maintenance • Difficult or failed intubation • Aspiration of stomach acid/contents • Malignant hypothermia • Uterine atony

The physician injects a local anesthetic bilaterally into the vaginal wall to block pain sensations to the pudendal nerve. A pudendal block can be helpful for instrument-assisted deliveries and for repair of an episiotomy or perineal tear. This method is most effective when administered by an experienced practitioner. If an incomplete block occurs, the practitioner may have to inject additional local anesthesia for episiotomy repair. This method is not effective to relieve the pain of labor.

Paracervical Block. A paracervical block involves the injection of a local anesthetic in the area close to the cervix. This method provides significant pain relief during the first stage of labor but cannot be used once the cervix is completely dilated. One advantage of the technique is that it does not block sensation and movement in the lower extremities, as does epidural anesthesia. However, the procedure must be repeated frequently due to the short duration of action. Many practitioners do not perform paracervical blocks because of the risk of fetal bradycardia.

Test Yourself

✔ List three types of regional anesthesia.

✔ Why is it critical for all facilities in which regional anesthesia is provided to have emergency equipment available?

✔ Describe a pudendal block.

Epidural Anesthesia. Epidural anesthesia for the management of labor pain has become increasingly popular in the United States. This method usually provides excellent pain relief, often completely blocking pain sensation. The anesthesiologist or nurse anesthetist places a small catheter into the epidural space and then injects the catheter with local anesthetics or opioids to provide pain relief. Sometimes a one-time dose of medication is placed into the spinal fluid (in the subarachnoid space), which is called an **intrathecal** injection, in conjunction with epidural anesthesia. The advantage of the combined epidural/intrathecal technique is that the intrathecal dose is effective almost immediately. It provides pain relief until the epidural begins to work.

Although its use is popular, epidural anesthesia is not without risk. There is significant risk of maternal hypotension that often requires treatment with vasopressors (medication to raise the blood pressure). Before a woman receives epidural anesthesia, an IV line must be in place. A 500- to 2,000-mL IV fluid bolus is required before epidural medications are administered to reduce the risk of hypotension. Because it is an invasive procedure, informed consent is required.

The anesthetist must evaluate the woman before placing an epidural. The anesthetist reviews the medical history and laboratory results and interviews the woman. He or she explains the procedure, answers the woman's questions, and obtains informed consent. Assist the RN, as directed, with giving the IV fluid bolus and positioning the woman for epidural placement. The woman can be sitting up on the edge of the bed with her feet dangling, or she may be side lying. In either case, it is important for her to arch her spine because this position opens up the spaces between the vertebrae and allows for easier insertion of the catheter. The nurse holds the woman in position or assists the support person to do so (Fig. 9-5). The RN monitors the pulse and oxygen saturation continuously during

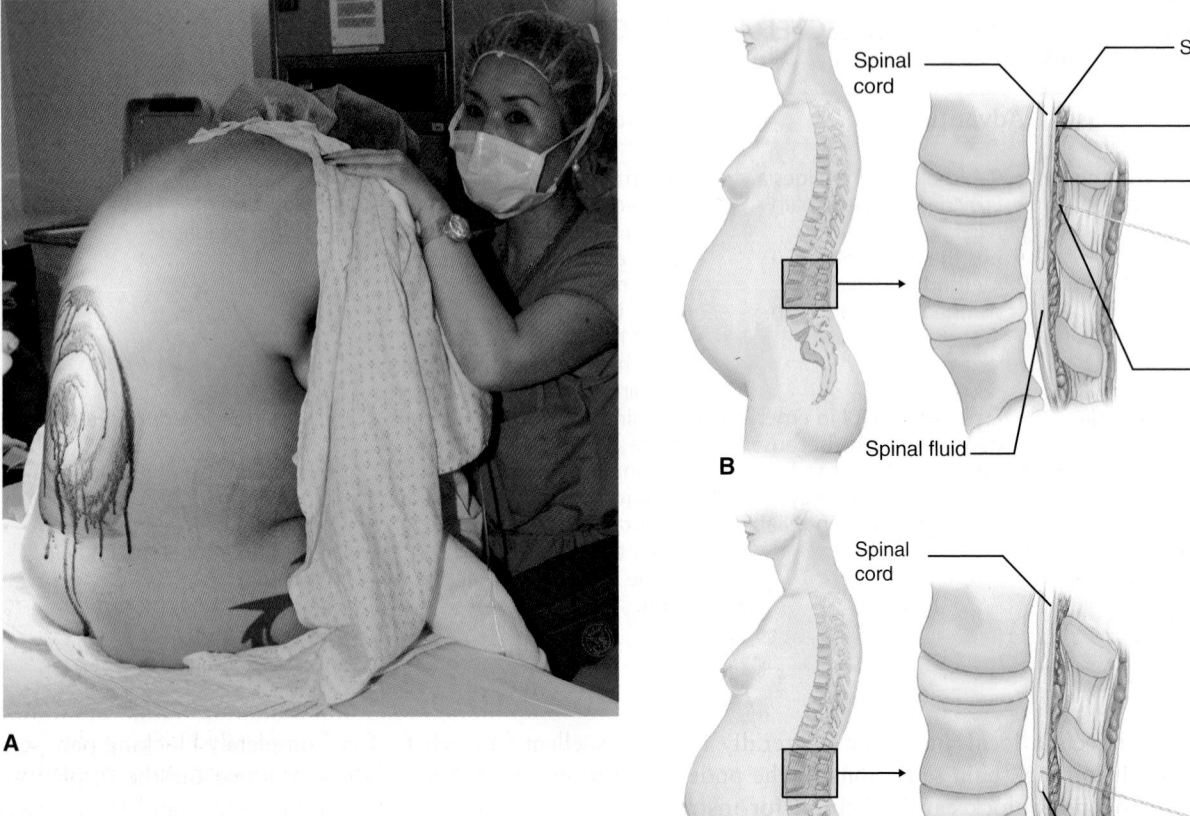

■ **Figure 9-5** Epidural or intrathecal anesthesia. **(A)** The woman is correctly positioned for epidural anesthesia. **(B)** Location of epidural catheter. Note that the epidural space is located just outside the dura mater. No spinal fluid is present in the epidural space. The epidural catheter is left in place to allow for intermittent or continuous infusion of medications to relieve the pain of labor and birth. **(C)** Location of intrathecal injection. Notice that the needle has a drop of spinal fluid at the hub to indicate the subarachnoid space has been entered. The local anesthetic or narcotic is then injected into this space.

the procedure using pulse oximetry. He or she also monitors the blood pressure frequently (sometimes every 3 to 5 minutes) during the procedure.

When the woman is in the proper position, the anesthetist prepares a sterile field with the supplies and medications that will be needed. The woman's back is prepared with alcohol and povidone-iodine. A local anesthetic is injected to numb the planned insertion area. The anesthetist inserts a special needle into the epidural space (just outside the dura mater) and administers a test dose (see Fig. 9-5). The anesthetist questions the woman regarding how she feels and what she is experiencing to detect any adverse reaction. If there is none, the anesthetist proceeds to place the epidural catheter, remove the needle, and tape the catheter securely to the woman's back. At this point, assist the woman to a position of

comfort. If the woman desires to be on her back, place a wedge under the right hip.

Once the epidural catheter is in place, the anesthetist may intermittently bolus the catheter when the woman begins to feel pain, or a continuous infusion can be set up and connected to the catheter. In either case, it is critical that the epidural catheter be clearly marked so that epidural medications are not administered inadvertently into the IV and vice versa. Management of the epidural is the role of the anesthetist. Monitor for and report any untoward effects.

After delivery, the RN stops the continuous infusion, removes the epidural catheter, and applies a sterile pressure dressing to the site. Nursing care during recovery from epidural anesthesia includes assessment of return of sensory and motor function to the lower extremities, and monitoring for urinary retention. Instruct the woman not to ambulate without assistance. Allow the woman to dangle her legs for a while, before she attempts to ambulate. Be available to provide immediate assistance, if needed, during initial ambulation attempts.

Intrathecal Anesthesia. Intrathecal anesthesia, also known as a spinal block, is similar to epidural anesthesia. The main difference is the location of the anesthetic. Instead of injecting local anesthesia and/or opioids into the epidural space, these medications are placed in the subarachnoid space into the spinal fluid (see Fig. 9-5). This type of anesthesia is used most frequently for planned cesarean deliveries. The disadvantage to using a spinal block during labor is that the anesthetic might wear off while the woman is still in labor. Nursing care is similar to that provided for epidural anesthesia.

Complications Associated With Epidural and Intrathecal Anesthesia. Hypotension is the most frequent side effect associated with epidural or intrathecal anesthesia. Low blood pressure occurs in approximately one third of women who receive epidural or spinal anesthesia (Cunningham et al., 2005). As noted, prehydration with IV fluids helps to prevent or decrease the severity of this side effect. If the blood pressure falls dramatically,

ephedrine may be given intravenously to raise the blood pressure.

Total spinal blockade is a rare, but potentially fatal complication that can occur with epidural or intrathecal anesthesia. The condition results from inadvertent injection of a local anesthetic into the intrathecal space instead of the epidural space or from the anesthetic traveling too high up the woman's body, causing paralysis of the woman's respiratory muscles. Without immediate supportive care, respiratory and cardiac arrest will occur. Another potentially fatal complication is accidental injection of a local anesthetic into a blood vessel. Seizures as well as respiratory and cardiac arrest can result.

Maternal fever is a side effect of epidural anesthesia. An elevated temperature during labor can lead the practitioner to suspect infection and order expensive tests and/or potentially unnecessary treatment.

Spinal headaches occur rarely because of advanced techniques and smaller needle sizes than those used in the past. A spinal headache is suspected when the woman has an intense headache in the upright position that is relieved when she lies still. IV caffeine can give temporary relief. An epidural blood patch provides lasting relief for severe spinal headache. In a procedure

A Personal Glimpse

I was 37 weeks' pregnant with my first baby. I started to have some contractions while I was at work. Nothing big; I wasn't even sure they were contractions because they didn't hurt, but I was able to time them at 10 to 15 minutes apart. I went home at lunchtime and called my husband to tell him that I thought I was in labor. He hurried home to be with me. I stayed home the rest of the day and did some light housework. Around 6 p.m., the contractions started to get more intense. I ran some warm water and soaked in the tub. It made me feel better for a while. My husband kept timing the contractions until they were 5 minutes apart. Then I called the hospital, and the nurse told me to come on in. We arrived at the hospital at about 8 p.m. The nurse checked me and said I was at 4 cm and 95% effaced. The nurse suggested that we walk the hallways to speed things along. Sure enough, 45 minutes later, I was a good 5 cm. She asked me if I wanted anything for the pain, and I said no. I was hanging in there just fine. The pain wasn't as bad as I thought it would be. After approximately 45 minutes, the contractions became more intense, and I begged my husband to call the nurse. The nurse checked me and I was 7 cm. By now, I was begging for an epidural. The anesthesiologist came in and asked me some questions and told me about some risks. I didn't care. I just wanted the epidural. I had to sit very still through several contractions while the doctor put in the epidural, but it was worth it because the pain went away right away. An hour after the epidural was inserted, I was dilated to 8 cm. I was very excited,

but then I got stuck at 8 cm for several hours. The doctor thought that the epidural must have slowed down my labor. They were having a hard time monitoring my baby with the external device, so they had to insert an internal monitor. Then the nurse started me on Pitocin to help me progress. Sure enough, after an hour of Pitocin, I was completely dilated and ready to push. For me, pushing was the hardest part. I still felt no pain because of my epidural, so the nurse had to tell me when I was having a contraction so that I could start pushing. I threw up several times from pushing so hard. However, the baby just didn't come down. After 2 hours, I was totally exhausted. The nurse asked if I wanted her to call the doctor and have her come and use the vacuum to help get the baby out. I was just so tired that I said yes. Elizabeth Michelle was born after just two pushes with the vacuum. She didn't cry at first, so the nurse rushed her to the warming table and gave her some oxygen. Then I heard the most beautiful sound in the world, a cry. My husband and I were thrilled. After the nurse dried the baby, I got to hold her for a while before they took her to the nursery. The baby weighed 7 lb even, and was 19½ inches long. She was worth everything I went through to have her.

Laura

Learning Opportunity: What questions should the nurse ask the woman about pain relief during labor? What should the nurse tell the woman about pain management options when she presents to the birthing facility in labor?

similar to that used to provide epidural anesthesia, the anesthesia provider injects 10 to 20 mL of the woman's blood into the epidural space. The headache usually resolves immediately (Cunningham et al., 2005).

When narcotics are used in addition to anesthetics, pruritus is a common side effect. Most women tolerate the itching, particularly because the pain relief is generally excellent for the first 24 hours after surgery. Nalbuphine (Nubain), an opioid agonist-antagonist; naloxone (Narcan), an opioid antagonist; and diphenhydramine (Benadryl), an antihistamine, are medications that may be ordered to treat severe pruritus.

Respiratory depression is another possible side effect when narcotics are used for spinal and/or epidural anesthesia. For this reason, IV naloxone (Narcan) should be readily available if respiratory depression occurs. Sometimes the anesthesiologist may order continuous pulse oximetry for the first 24 hours. In all cases, it is prudent to take vital signs at least every 2 hours and to check on the woman frequently during the first 24 hours after spinal or epidural narcotics have been administered. Nursing Care Plan 9-1: The Woman With Labor Pain describes pain management for a woman in labor.

General Anesthesia

General anesthesia is not used frequently in obstetrics because of the risks involved. The pregnant woman is at higher risk for aspiration. It requires more skill to intubate a pregnant woman because of physiologic changes in the trachea and thorax. In addition, general anesthetic agents cross the placenta and can result in the birth of a severely depressed neonate who requires full resuscitation.

When general anesthesia is to be used, the anesthetist usually orders preoperative medications to reduce the risk of harm should aspiration occur. Sodium citrate (Bicitra) 30 mL may be given orally. IV antacids often are given before surgery.

The anesthetist may use an inhalation agent, an IV agent, or more commonly both to induce anesthesia. The woman is preoxygenated with 100% oxygen and then rapidly put to sleep. The RN gives cricoid pressure (pressure with the thumb and forefinger over the cricoid cartilage in the trachea), which closes off the esophagus and decreases the risk of aspiration. Cricoid pressure is maintained until the woman is intubated and the cuff inflated (Grant, 2006a). The anesthetist then manages the airway and continues to administer anesthetic agents and muscle relaxants as needed throughout surgery. Every attempt is made to deliver the baby as quickly as possible after the woman is anesthetized to avoid neonatal de-

pression. Be prepared to assist in resuscitating the newborn, if necessary.

When the surgery is completed, the anesthetist removes the endotracheal tube when the woman is awake and has regained her protective reflexes (swallowing and gagging). The woman is transported to the postanesthesia care unit (PACU). The RN completes a full assessment; administers oxygen; and monitors oxygen saturation, vital signs, and the continuous electrocardiogram. The RN must be especially vigilant to monitor for hypoventilation after general anesthesia.

Malignant hyperthermia is a rare, but potentially life-threatening, complication of general anesthesia. It is an inherited condition that causes sustained muscle contractions in the presence of certain anesthetic agents. For this reason, a thorough history is important before general anesthesia is given. Ideally, a pregnant woman with a family history of malignant hyperthermia is identified in the prenatal period so the health care team can be prepared to care for the woman if general anesthesia becomes necessary. In these cases, it is best for the woman to receive epidural anesthesia during labor. This practice allows for safe anesthesia if a cesarean delivery is required. For planned cesarean delivery, the woman usually receives spinal anesthesia.

Be alert to the development of signs and symptoms of malignant hyperthermia. Early signs include severe muscle rigidity, tachycardia, irregular heart rhythm, decreased oxygen saturation, and cyanosis. Body temperature can rapidly increase to lethal levels; however, this may be a late sign. Dantrolene sodium given intravenously is the drug of choice to treat malignant hyperthermia. This medication must be readily available in any area in which general anesthesia is administered.

Postoperative nursing care of the woman who receives general anesthesia is similar to that of the woman who receives regional anesthesia. However, careful assessment for hypoventilation and uterine atony are indicated.

Test Yourself

✔ Describe the procedure for epidural placement.
✔ List four complications associated with epidural or spinal anesthesia.
✔ Name two ways to reduce the threat of maternal aspiration when general anesthesia is used.

THE WOMAN WITH LABOR PAIN

CASE SCENARIO
Patricia (Pattie) Smith is a 29-year-old gravida 1, para 0 at term. She attended childbirth preparation classes with her husband, Ed. Pattie says that she wants to try natural childbirth, but that she might change her mind and request an epidural if the pain becomes unbearable. She is admitted to the hospital in active labor at 4 centimeters dilation. Admitting vital signs are BP 120/76 mm Hg, T 98.7°F, P 70 bpm, R 20 per minute. She describes her pain as starting in the small of her back and then radiating to her lower abdomen with each contraction. She says that the intensity is strong, particularly at the peak of the contraction. Her contractions are occurring every 5 minutes, last 50 to 60 seconds, and palpate moderate intensity. The fetal heart rate is in the 140s to 150s and is reactive.

NURSING DIAGNOSIS
Acute Pain related to uterine contractions.

GOAL: Reports ability to tolerate the pain of labor.

EXPECTED OUTCOMES
- Uses nonpharmacologic interventions.
- Uses pharmacologic interventions, if desired.
- Expresses satisfaction with pain control.

Nursing Interventions	*Rationale*
Perform a pain assessment at least every hour during labor to include pain description, location, duration, and intensity (measured by a pain scale).	A thorough pain assessment will reveal the need for more intensive interventions to control the pain of labor.
Note reports of continuous, severe pain. If this occurs, report it to the RN in charge immediately.	Severe, unrelenting pain may be associated with a complication of labor.
Assess general comfort at least every hour. Note the condition of the lips and offer lip balm PRN. Offer ice chips and lollipops to relieve complaints of dry mouth. Give perineal care as indicated, and change the under-buttock pad frequently. Change the linen when it becomes moist with perspiration or other body fluids.	Comfort measures increase the ability of the woman to cope with labor. It is more difficult to cope if the woman has dry, cracked lips, a dry mouth, moist linens, and is in need of perineal care.
Encourage the use of relaxation techniques that are helpful for Pattie.	The more relaxed the woman can remain during labor, the better she will be able to cope with the pain of labor.
Reinforce the use of patterned breathing. Encourage her to switch to a more complex pattern of breathing when simpler patterns are no longer helpful.	Patterned breathing techniques are learned during childbirth classes. Use of these techniques can facilitate relaxation and increase the woman's ability to cope.
Assist Pattie to change positions frequently.	Position changes can help the woman to cope. If she remains "frozen" in one position, she is more likely to become tense, which increases the perception of pain.
Encourage the use of effleurage, for as long as it is helpful. Encourage the use of pressure when effleurage is no longer helpful.	The use of touch, such as effleurage and pressure, can interrupt the sensation of pain.

Pattie progresses to 8 centimeters dilation. At this point, she is having difficulty maintaining control. She thrashes about at the peak of contractions and says that nothing is helping the pain. She begs for an epidural. The obstetrician agrees, and the anesthesiologist is called.

NURSING DIAGNOSIS
Acute Pain related to advanced progress of labor.

GOAL: Enhanced ability to cope with labor.

(continues on page 198)

THE WOMAN WITH LABOR PAIN

EXPECTED OUTCOMES
- Uses nonpharmacologic and pharmacologic interventions.
- Expresses satisfaction with pain control.

Nursing Interventions	*Rationale*
Remain supportive of Pattie's decision to use an epidural for pain relief.	The woman has the right to change her mind about pain relief interventions and to choose interventions that will best help her to cope.
Reassure Ed that this is a normal response to this phase of the labor process, and that Pattie's request does not represent a failure on his part as her coach.	There is a danger that the coach may feel that he has somehow "failed" when pharmacologic interventions are requested.
Continue to perform a pain assessment every 30 minutes after the epidural is placed.	Frequent assessment of pain will allow for rapid detection of the onset of pain.
Report new complaints of pain to the anesthesiologist.	New reports of pain may signal the need for a bolus of medication through the epidural catheter.

NURSING DIAGNOSIS
Risk for Injury related to hypotension associated with epidural anesthesia.

GOAL: Maintenance of adequate blood pressure to support perfusion to vital organs, including the placenta.

EXPECTED OUTCOMES
- Blood pressure will not drop below 90/60 mm Hg.
- Oxygen saturation will remain above 96%.
- Fetal monitor strip baseline will remain above 120 with reactive patterns noted.

Nursing Interventions	*Rationale*
Prehydrate Pattie with 1,000 cc of lactated Ringer's solution, as ordered.	Prehydration with IV fluid will decrease the risk of hypotension.
Monitor oxygen saturation with pulse oximetry.	A decrease in oxygen saturation can be quickly detected and treated, which will help prevent adverse fetal affects.
Monitor fetal heart tones and reactivity.	Monitoring is done to detect non-reassuring changes, which may indicate inadequate placental perfusion.
Assist Pattie to a sitting position with her feet dangling over the side of the bed. Demonstrate to Ed how to hold Pattie in the proper position for catheter insertion.	When the woman is in the proper position, the epidural is placed more easily.
Monitor the blood pressure, pulse, and oxygen saturation every 3 to 5 minutes during the procedure.	Frequent monitoring allows for early detection of changes that may indicate the development of a complication.
Once the epidural catheter is taped in place, assist Pattie to a side-lying position.	The side-lying position enhances blood pressure and placental perfusion.
Monitor for signs of urinary retention and insert a Foley catheter, as ordered, if needed.	Epidural anesthesia frequently causes urinary retention, which may interfere with the progress of labor.
Check for progress of labor shortly after the epidural takes effect.	Rapid progress of labor sometimes occurs because the woman relaxes after the pain is relieved.
Monitor for ability to push effectively in the second stage of labor. Report this finding to the anesthesiologist.	Sometimes, epidural anesthesia can interfere with the ability to push effectively. The anesthesiologist may decrease the amount of medication given to allow for partial return of sensation with an increased ability to push.

EVALUATION:
Pattie pushes well and delivers a healthy baby boy 3 hours after she receives her epidural. Her blood pressure remains above 90/60 mm Hg. She reports that she is very satisfied with her labor experience and does not regret getting the epidural.

KEY POINTS

➤ Labor pain differs from other types of pain because it is associated with a normal physiologic process, increases in intensity as the desired outcome (birth) approaches, and is predictable.

➤ Sources of pain during the first stage of labor are the thinning and stretching of the cervix in response to uterine contractions. Sources of pain during the second stage of labor are the stretching of tissues in the perineum as the fetus descends.

➤ Factors that influence the woman's experience of labor pain include her threshold and tolerance to pain, age, parity, anxiety level, physical conditioning, length of labor, size and position of the fetus, induced versus natural labor, and whether or not the labor is dysfunctional.

➤ Major principles of labor pain management include that women are more satisfied when they have control over the pain experience; caregivers commonly underrate the severity of pain; and women who are prepared for labor usually report a more satisfying experience than do women who are not prepared.

➤ Nonpharmacologic interventions to relieve labor pain include continuous labor support, comfort measures, various relaxation techniques, intradermal water injections, and acupressure and acupuncture.

➤ Relaxation techniques that help a woman cope with labor include patterned breathing, attention focusing, movement and positioning, touch and massage, water therapy, and hypnosis.

➤ Most nonpharmacologic interventions are noninvasive, address emotional and spiritual aspects of birth, and promote the woman's sense of control over her pain. Disadvantages include that many of the interventions require special training and/or practice before birth, and these methods are not effective for every woman.

➤ Analgesia reduces the sensation of pain. Anesthesia partially or totally blocks all sensation to an area of the body.

➤ Advantages of opioid administration during labor include an increased ability for the woman to cope with labor, and the medications may be nurse administered. Disadvantages include frequent occurrence of uncomfortable side effects, such as nausea and vomiting, pruritus, drowsiness, and neonatal depression; and pain is not eliminated completely.

➤ Types of regional anesthesia include pudendal block, paracervical block, epidural anesthesia, combined epidural/spinal anesthesia, and spinal block. A pudendal block provides pain relief for the birth. Paracervical blocks and epidurals provide pain relief during labor.

➤ Complications associated with epidural and spinal anesthesia include hypotension, maternal fever, pruritus, high spinal block, inadvertent injection into the bloodstream, and spinal headache.

➤ General anesthesia is risky for the pregnant woman because of the increased risk for aspiration. It is risky for the fetus because the medications cross the placenta and may result in severe neonatal depression that requires intensive resuscitation.

➤ Malignant hyperthermia is a rare, life-threatening complication of general anesthesia. Dantrolene sodium is the treatment of choice for malignant hyperthermia.

INTERNET RESOURCES

www.childbirth.org/articles/labor/painrelief.html
www.americanpregnancy.org/labornbirth/epidural.html

Workbook

■ NCLEX-STYLE REVIEW QUESTIONS

1. A 22-year-old gravida 2, para 0 is in the doctor's office for a checkup at 36 weeks' gestation. Which comment by the woman indicates that she needs additional information about pain relief during labor?
   a. "I have discussed pain relief options with the doctor and my childbirth educator."
   b. "I'm so glad that I won't have any pain because I'm going to have an epidural."
   c. "I've been practicing the relaxation exercises I learned in my childbirth class."
   d. "I want to have medications through the IV if the pain gets so bad that I can't handle it."

2. The labor nurse reports to the nurse on the on-coming shift, "The woman in labor room 2 is handling her pain very well. She smiles whenever I go in to talk to her, and she doesn't complain at all!" What assessments by the on-coming labor nurse would best reveal if the off-going labor nurse's observations were correct?
   a. Asking the woman to describe her pain and rate it on a scale of 0 to 10.
   b. Observing for grimacing, moaning, and other nonverbal indicators of pain.
   c. Taking the woman's vital signs and observing her interactions with visitors.
   d. No additional assessments are indicated until the woman begins to report pain.

3. A woman asks the nurse during a prenatal office visit, "What pain relief method is best during labor?" What answer by the nurse best answers the question?
   a. "Epidurals are best because they provide complete pain relief."
   b. "Most women need IV pain medications at some point during labor."
   c. "It is best to learn and use several methods of pain relief to find the one that works best for you."
   d. "There is no one best way. However, natural childbirth is best for the baby."

4. A 34-year-old gravida 3, para 2 is experiencing severe back pain with each contraction. She is extremely un-comfortable and upset because she never had this type of pain with her other labors. What interventions are most likely to help in this situation?
   a. Comfort measures, intermittent labor support by the nurse, and reassurance that the pain is temporary
   b. Counter-pressure with a fist or tennis ball to the lower back and intradermal water injections
   c. Effleurage, ambulation, and frequent position changes
   d. Hypnosis, imagery, and slow chest breathing

5. The nurse is preparing a woman for epidural anesthesia. The woman asks, "Why is my IV running so fast? It feels cold!" What reply by the nurse is best?
   a. "Don't worry. This is a routine procedure in preparation for an epidural."
   b. "I'll slow the IV down so you won't feel so cold."
   c. "IV fluids help prevent spinal headaches."
   d. "IV hydration helps prevent the blood pressure from dropping too low."

■ STUDY ACTIVITIES

1. Use the following table to compare advantages and disadvantages of pain relief methods for labor.

Method	Advantages	Disadvantages
Natural childbirth		
IV analgesia		
Epidural anesthesia		
General anesthesia		

2. Develop a teaching plan on the advantages and disadvantages of epidural anesthesia to present to a childbirth education class.

3. Interview the following caregivers in the community regarding their recommendations for pain relief during labor: a doula, a nurse midwife, a family practice physician, and an obstetrician. What similarities did you find in their answers? In what ways did they disagree? Which argument did you find most convincing? Share your findings with your clinical group.

■ CRITICAL THINKING: WHAT WOULD YOU DO?

Apply your knowledge of pain management during labor to the following situation.

1. Betty, a 30-year-old gravida 1, reports that she wants to try natural childbirth.

   a. What recommendations will you make to increase the chances that she will be able to experience natural childbirth?

   b. About what will you caution her, to decrease the likelihood that she will have unrealistic expectations about pain relief during labor?

2. Betty presents to the labor suite in labor. She is 3 cm dilated, 90% effaced, and at a –1 station. Her contractions are every 3 to 5 minutes apart and of moderate intensity.

   a. What nonpharmacologic pain interventions are most helpful at this point in Betty's labor?

   b. Several hours later, Betty is 5 cm dilated, 100% effaced, at a 0 station. She is requesting IV analgesia. How will you reply?

   c. When Betty reaches 8 cm, she is screaming at the peak of contractions. She says, "I can't stand the pain anymore. I want an epidural." How will you reply?

10 Nursing Care During Labor and Birth

KEY TERMS

acceleration
amnioinfusion
early deceleration
episodic changes
late deceleration
lochia
nadir
open-glottis pushing
periodic changes
ritual
urge-to-push method
uteroplacental insufficiency
variability
variable deceleration
vigorous pushing

LEARNING OBJECTIVES

On completion of this chapter, you should be able to:

1. Discuss assessments and procedures the nurse performs during the woman's admission to the hospital.

2. Describe external and internal methods for monitoring uterine contractions.

3. Compare and contrast advantages and disadvantages of intermittent auscultation of fetal heart rate with that of continuous electronic fetal monitoring.

4. Compare and contrast advantages and disadvantages of external fetal monitoring with that of internal fetal monitoring.

5. Explain how to apply the external fetal monitor.

6. Identify the role of the practical (vocational) nurse in the interpretation of fetal heart rate patterns.

7. Define three major deviations from the normal fetal heart rate baseline.

8. Differentiate between early, variable, and late decelerations with regard to appearance, occurrence in relation to uterine contractions, causes, and whether or not the pattern is reassuring or nonreassuring.

9. Outline appropriate nursing interventions for each major periodic change: early, variable, and late deceleration patterns.

10. Discuss advantages and disadvantages of fetal stimulation, fetal scalp sampling, and fetal pulse oximetry for monitoring fetal status.

11. Determine data to collect when assessing a laboring woman for progress of labor and birth throughout each stage and phase of labor.

12. Identify common nursing diagnoses associated with each stage of labor and birth.

13. Choose appropriate nursing interventions for each stage of labor and birth to facilitate safe passage of the mother and fetus.

14. Evaluate the effectiveness of care given during each stage of labor and birth.

THE ONSET OF labor heralds the transition from pregnancy to motherhood, and the transformation of the fetus to a newborn. The woman experiences the process in many dimensions, including physiologic, psychological, social, and spiritual. When the powers, passageway, passenger, and psyche work together harmoniously, the miracle of birth progresses in an orderly and predictable sequence.

The licensed practical/vocational nurse's role in labor and delivery is to provide care to the laboring woman under the supervision of a registered nurse (RN). You must have a basic understanding of the processes of labor and birth to provide care to the woman and her family. It is important for you to be able to recognize deviations from the "normal" or expected sequence of labor and birth and to report deviations immediately. Your understanding will also help you answer the woman's and her support person's questions regarding labor and birth. Although you may not independently perform many of the procedures and assessments described in this chapter, a basic understanding of these procedures and assessments is necessary to effectively assist the RN or physician.

Your role as the obstetric nurse is central to the care of the laboring woman and her family. You facilitate the labor process and ensure safe passage of the laboring woman and fetus through this critical life event. To be an effective obstetric nurse you must maintain an attitude of acceptance of the mother's preferences during labor and birth, utilize supportive actions, and develop keen assessment skills to detect subtle changes in maternal or fetal status.

Although labor and birth are normal physiologic events, you must be prepared to recognize and manage complications that may arise during the process. It also is critical to be prepared to give intensive support to the laboring woman and her partner or coach. Assisting the family during the miracle of labor and birth is a challenging but ultimately satisfying and rewarding experience.

Every woman's labor is unique, and if a woman bears more than one child, she experiences each birth differently. This chapter focuses on the nursing care of a first-time mother undergoing normal progression of labor and birth who does not experience complications. Common deviations associated with the nursing care of the multiparous woman are noted. For purposes of this chapter, it is assumed that the delivery environment is a labor, delivery, and recovery room (LDR) in a hospital setting. Similar nursing interventions apply to other settings, and the labor process is the same regardless of the environment in which birth occurs.

THE NURSE'S ROLE DURING ADMISSION

The woman may present to the birthing suite at any phase of the first stage of labor. Therefore, it is important to assess birth imminence, fetal status, risk factors, and maternal status immediately. If birth is not imminent and the fetal and maternal conditions are stable, perform additional admission assessments, including the full admission health history, a complete maternal physical assessment, the status of labor, and labor and birth preferences.

Immediate Assessments
Birth Imminence

Nursing assessment for signs that birth is imminent begins from the moment the woman arrives in the labor and delivery unit. If the woman is introverted and stops to breathe or pant with each contraction, you can infer that she is in an advanced stage of labor. In addition, if the woman makes statements such as, "I feel a lot of pressure," or "The baby is coming," or "I want to have a bowel movement," it is likely the woman is in the second stage of labor, and the baby will be born soon. Other signs that birth is imminent include sitting on one buttock (if the woman presents to the unit in a wheelchair) and bearing down or grunting with contractions. When any of these signs is present, it is prudent to quickly move the woman to a labor bed, perform a vaginal examination if the presenting part is not yet visible, and be prepared to assist with the birth.

Occasionally, you may be the only person available to assist delivery of the baby. Figure 10-1 illustrates the steps to follow for an emergency birth. There may not be time to perform all the steps listed. Do the best you can with the time and equipment available. Instruct the woman to remain calm and reassure her that you know what to do to assist with the delivery. Instruct her to blow out through her lips in little puffs (as if she were blowing out candles) so that she will not forcefully expel the baby in an uncontrolled manner. Then follow the steps in Figure 10-1 to assist with the birth.

Once the baby delivers, it is not necessary to cut the cord immediately. However, in most facilities, the protocol is to double clamp the cord and cut between the clamps. Dry the infant thoroughly to prevent heat loss and place him under a radiant warmer for resuscitation, or place the newborn in skin-to-skin contact with his mother and cover them both with a blanket.

The birth attendant usually arrives before delivery of the placenta. However, if signs of placental separation occur (a gush of blood, lengthening of the cord at the introitus), allow the placenta to deliver, and then massage the uterus to help it contract. Another way to prevent excessive blood loss immediately after delivery of the placenta is to place the infant to the woman's breast. The suckling action of the newborn will stimulate the woman's body to release oxytocin, which helps her uterus to contract and control bleeding.

Fetal Status

When the woman arrives at the hospital, perform an immediate assessment of fetal status. In most delivery suites, the woman is placed on the fetal monitor for continuous monitoring, but it is within accepted standards of care to check the fetal heart rate (FHR) by fetoscope or by Doppler ultrasonography for the low-risk woman. The FHR should be strong and regular, with a baseline between 110 and 160 beats per minute[1] with no late decelerations and should remain so throughout all phases

Nursing judgment is in order.

If the woman presents to the hospital in an advanced stage of labor and it appears that delivery is imminent, the admission history and physical is abbreviated to focus on current status. The history can be completed later, even after delivery, if necessary.

---

[1]In the past, the baseline FHR was expected to be between 120 and 160 beats per minute. Newer standards list 110 as the lower acceptable limit of normal.

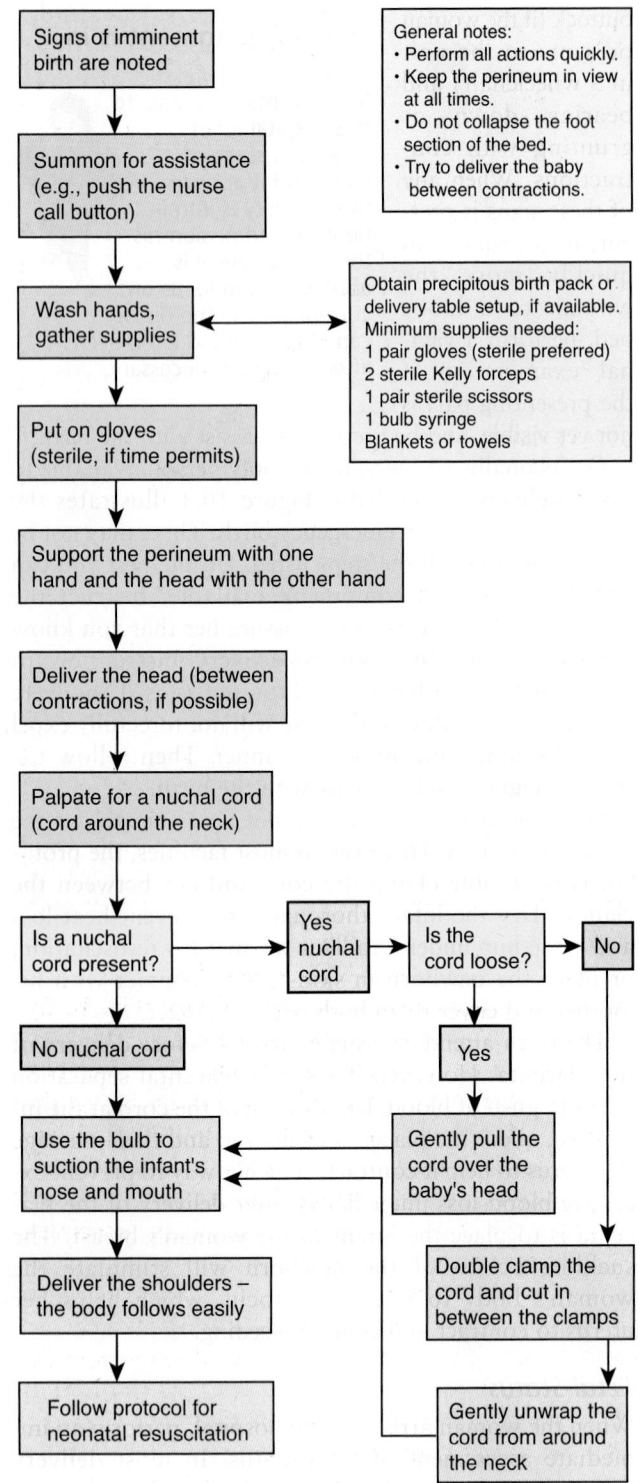

Figure 10-1 Emergency delivery by the nurse.

General notes:
- Perform all actions quickly.
- Keep the perineum in view at all times.
- Do not collapse the foot section of the bed.
- Try to deliver the baby between contractions.

Obtain precipitous birth pack or delivery table setup, if available. Minimum supplies needed:
1 pair gloves (sterile preferred)
2 sterile Kelly forceps
1 pair sterile scissors
1 bulb syringe
Blankets or towels

membranes have ruptured include reports by the woman of a gush or continual leaking of warm fluid from the vagina. Sometimes the woman will report intermittent leaking of fluid, and it may be unclear if the membranes have ruptured. In this instance, it is important to look for objective signs of rupture. The RN may use a speculum to check for pooling of fluid in the vagina. Alternatively, the RN may place nitrazine paper in the fluid to determine the pH. If the membranes have ruptured, the nitrazine paper will turn dark blue, indicating that the fluid is alkaline; this is a positive nitrazine test. If the status of the membranes is still in doubt, a fern test may be performed. The RN collects a fluid sample and smears it on a slide, which is then examined under a microscope. If a ferning pattern is present, the fern test is positive, and membrane rupture is diagnosed.

Other important factors to assess include the color, odor, and amount of fluid and the time of rupture. The fluid should be clear with specks of vernix caseosa and no foul odor. If several hours have passed since the membranes ruptured, assess the woman for signs of infection, such as elevated maternal temperature, cloudy or foul-smelling fluid, and fetal tachycardia. Green fluid signals the presence of meconium in the amniotic sac and may indicate that the fetus is distressed.

Assess for vaginal bleeding. The presence of bloody show is an expected finding, but heavy bleeding (heavier than a normal menstrual period) is not normal. Immediately report heavy bleeding to the charge nurse. In addition to the amount of bleeding, note other important characteristics, such as color (dark or bright red), amount and type of associated pain, and time that the bleeding began.

When delivery is imminent, it is important to ask the woman if she experienced any problems with this pregnancy, such as bleeding, high blood pressure, or diabetes. Determine if any prenatal fetal assessment tests were done and if any complications were diagnosed. Verify the expected due date. Ask if there were any complications in previous pregnancies. Establish the approximate number of times the woman saw the health care provider for prenatal care and during what month of pregnancy prenatal care began. Each of these assessments is important to determine if risk factors are present that might require a specialist to be present at the delivery.

Some nurses find this approach helpful.

If the woman presents to the labor unit complaining of "bleeding," ask her how many times she has changed sanitary napkins. Her answer will help you determine the approximate amount of bleeding.

and stages of labor. See the section "The Nurse's Role: Ongoing Assessment of Uterine Contractions and FHR" for in-depth information on assessment of FHR.

Risk Assessment

The status of the membranes is one of the initial risk assessments performed. Symptoms indicating that the

Maternal Status

A quick physical assessment of the woman's status upon admission to the hospital is crucial. Assess the woman's

---

Box 10-1 ▌ COMPONENTS OF THE ADMISSION HEALTH HISTORY

Obstetric History
- Number and outcomes of previous pregnancies in GTPAL (gravida, term, preterm, abortions, living) format (see Chapter 7 for a detailed explanation of these terms)
- Estimated delivery date
- History of prenatal care for current pregnancy
- Complications during pregnancy
- Dates and results of fetal surveillance studies, such as ultrasound or nonstress test
- Childbirth preparation classes
- Previous labor and birth experiences

Current Labor Status
- Time of contraction onset
- Contraction pattern
- Status of membranes
- Description of bloody show or bleeding
- Fetal movements during the past 24 hours

Medical–Surgical History
- Chronic illnesses
- Current medications
  - Prescribed
  - Over-the-counter
  - Herbal remedies

Social History
- Drug and alcohol use during pregnancy
- Amount of smoking during pregnancy
- Marital status
- Support system
- Domestic violence screen
- Cultural/religious considerations that affect care

Desires/Plans for Labor and Birth
- Presence of a partner, coach, and/or doula (see Chapter 7 for discussion of doulas)
- Pain management preferences
- Other personal preferences affecting intrapartum nursing care

Desires/Plans for Newborn
- Plans for feeding—breast or formula
- Choice of pediatrician
- Circumcision preference, if the infant is male
- Rooming-in preference

---

vital signs, including temperature, pulse, respiration, and blood pressure, for signs of infection, hypertension, or shock. If there is not enough time before delivery to do a full assessment of vital signs, the blood pressure is the most critical immediate measurement.

Additional Assessments

Maternal Health History and Physical Assessment

The admission health history is part of the initial assessment and includes an obstetric history, determination of status, a medical–surgical history, social history, desired plans for labor and birth, and desires/plans for the newborn. Box 10-1 lists examples of data that are obtained routinely for each category in the admission health history. Review the prenatal record to obtain baseline vital signs and weight and to identify other pertinent information.

This is critical to remember.
Always perform a quick assessment to determine if the woman has signs of preeclampsia, a serious complication of pregnancy. Report immediately blood pressure greater than 140/90 mm Hg, brisk reflexes or presence of clonus, protein in the urine, edema of the hands or face, sudden weight gain, and reports of headache or blurred vision.

Obtain the woman's current weight and compare it with her weight at her most recent prenatal visit (Fig. 10-2). Sudden weight gain indicates fluid retention and may signal the onset of preeclampsia (see Chapter 17). Measure vital signs, which should be similar to the woman's baseline. It is normal for the pulse to increase slightly during labor, but the blood pressure, measured during the relaxation phase of a contraction, should not be elevated. Collect a urine specimen to screen for the presence of protein, ketones, glucose, blood cells, or bacteria.

Assist the RN to perform a head-to-toe physical assessment. Critical measurements include lung sounds, the presence or absence of right upper quadrant (RUQ) pain or tenderness, deep tendon reflexes (DTRs), clonus, and amount and location of any edema.

Labor Status

Assess the woman's contraction pattern to include frequency, duration, and intensity (see the section "The Nurse's Role: Ongoing Assessment of Uterine Contractions and FHR" for in-depth information on monitoring uterine activity).

It also is important to determine fetal lie, presentation, attitude, position, and station when the laboring woman first presents to a birthing facility. This process begins with Leopold's maneuvers (Nursing Procedure 10-1). Fetal

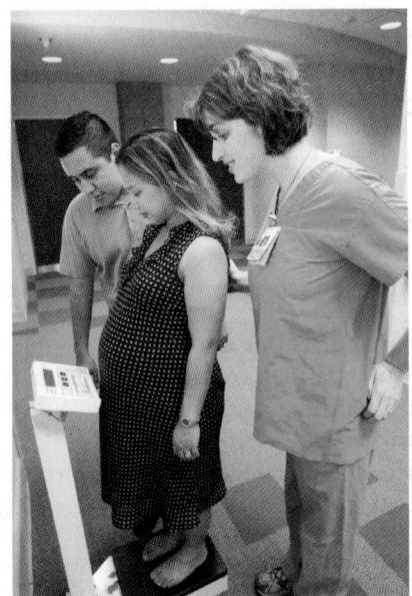

■ **Figure 10-2** The nurse measures the woman's weight during the admission process to labor and delivery. (Photo by Joe Mitchell.)

presentation, position, and attitude often can be determined using this technique.

The initial vaginal examination is done to assess dilation and effacement of the cervix and to determine specific information regarding the passenger's progress through the birth canal. The examiner can confirm presentation, position, attitude, and fetal station.

The LPN assists with vaginal examinations. There is no firm rule that establishes how frequently vaginal examinations should be performed during labor. The RN observes for cues that labor is advancing, so that vaginal examinations are done only as frequently as is necessary to evaluate labor progress. Because vaginal examinations are invasive, performing them too frequently increases the risk for infection. The RN performs a vaginal examination when other labor assessments indicate labor is advancing, before administering pain medications, when the water bag breaks, or for the sudden onset of deep variable decelerations. Vaginal examinations should never be done if the woman presents with bright red painless bleeding until placenta previa (see Chapter 17) is ruled out.

Balance is the order of the day.

Vaginal examinations should be done frequently enough to adequately assess labor progress but not so frequently as to increase the risk for infection.

Record the results of the initial vaginal examination in the woman's clinical record. Compare these results with the results of subsequent examinations to demonstrate progress of labor or to diagnose arrest of dilation or descent. One example of a form used to graph results of cervical examinations is the partograph (Fig. 10-3). This graph gives a visual representation of the progress of labor and allows for documentation of parameters indicating maternal and fetal status. Each time a vaginal examination is done, the examiner plots the cervical

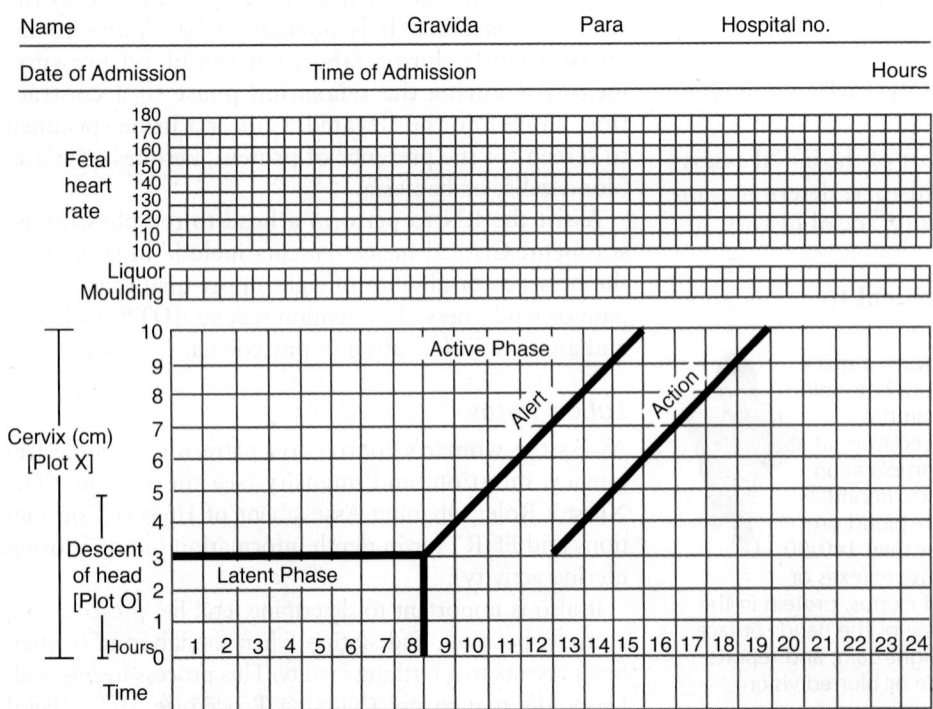

■ **Figure 10-3** Partograph for recording labor progress.

Nursing Procedure 10-1
LEOPOLD'S MANEUVERS

Leopold's maneuvers are a noninvasive method of assessing fetal presentation, position, and attitude. This technique can also be used to locate the fetal back before applying the fetal monitor.

EQUIPMENT

Warm, clean hands

PROCEDURE

1. Determine presentation.
   Stand beside the woman, facing her. Place both hands on the uterine fundus and palpate the contents of the fundus. If the buttocks are in the fundus (indicating a vertex presentation), you will feel a soft, irregular object that does not move easily. However, if the head is in the fundus indicating a breech presentation, you will palpate a smooth, hard, round, mobile object.

2. Determine position.
   Place both hands on the maternal abdomen, one on each side. Use one hand to support the abdomen while you palpate the opposite side with the other hand. Repeat the procedure so that you palpate both sides of the abdomen. Try to determine the location of the fetal back and extremities in relationship to the maternal pelvis. The back will feel hard and smooth and the extremities will be irregular and knobby.

3. Confirm presentation.
   Place one hand over the symphysis pubis and attempt to grasp the part that is presenting to the pelvis between your thumb and fingers of one hand. In the vast majority of cases, you will feel a hard, round fetal head. If the part moves easily, it is unengaged. If the part is not movable, engagement probably has occurred. If the breech is presenting, you will feel a soft, irregular object just above the symphysis.

4. Determine attitude.
   Begin the last step by turning to face the woman's feet. Using the finger pads of the first three fingers of each hand, palpate in a downward motion in the direction of the symphysis pubis. If you feel a hard bony prominence on the side opposite the fetal back, you have located the fetal brow, and the fetus is in an attitude of flexion. If the bony prominence is found on the same side as the fetal back, you are palpating the occiput, and the fetus is in an attitude of extension.

dilation and location of the fetal head on the graph. The "alert" line on the graph allows for the nurse or physician to determine if labor is not progressing as expected. No cervical change in 2 hours when the woman is in active labor is "arrest of dilation." Failure of the fetus to descend (the station does not change) in a primigravida is a sign that labor is not progressing as expected, even if cervical dilation is occurring. The fetus of a multigravida may not descend until full dilation has occurred and then may move down the birth canal rapidly. Notify the physician or nurse midwife when labor does not progress as expected.

Labor and Birth Preferences

One very important part of the assessment is to determine if the woman and her partner have special requests for labor and birth. Some women go to great lengths to plan the birth. Ask if the woman has a written birth plan. Ideally, she has reviewed the plan with her birth attendant well ahead of time and the birth attendant has approved the document. Read the plan and notify the RN of the contents. Birth plans often contain preferences regarding such things as mobility during labor, intravenous (IV) fluids during labor, episiotomy, presence of friends and family at the birth, fetal monitoring, pain management, and food and fluids during labor.

Many women do not have birth plans. However, it is very important to ask the woman specific questions regarding her preferences and needs. What expectations does she have about the labor process? How does she expect her pain will be managed? Did she attend childbirth class? Does she want to try natural childbirth? What individuals, if any, does she want in the delivery room with her? It is important to reassure her that she can change her mind at any time during labor. If some of her requests are outside the normal protocols and procedures used at the facility, inform the RN or the birth attendant.

Cultural Snapshot

A woman's culture has a tremendous impact on the type and quantity of support she needs and on her methods of coping with the stress of labor. Some cultures frown on the presence of men during the labor and birth process. In these cases, it would be counterproductive for the nurse to pressure the man to be the support person.

Ask the woman to identify who should provide support. Inquire regarding the relationship of the support person to the woman. Ask the woman to identify any special methods that might help her cope with labor. This information will help you to individualize care while taking into account the woman's culture.

Performing Routine Admission Orders

After the admission history and assessment is completed, a full report is given to the attending physician or nurse midwife. Sometimes additional observation is ordered to determine if the woman is in true labor, or if she should be sent home to wait until active labor ensues. If the woman is to be admitted, admission orders may include a perineal shave preparation or clip or Fleet enema if the membranes are intact. However, these procedures are no longer a routine part of labor care. In most facilities, some type of IV access is started. Usually, a liter of the ordered IV solution is hung and titrated to the specified rate. Alternatively, a saline lock may be inserted to allow for IV access if needed for medication administration or fluid bolus. Some practitioners and facilities do not routinely insert an IV as part of the admission procedure.

A little sensitivity is in order.
If the woman is not in true labor and is discharged home, she may feel embarrassed. Reassure her that it is normal for a woman to present several times to the hospital before she goes into true labor. Instruct the woman when to return to the hospital, and encourage her to call with concerns or questions.

Laboratory studies are part of the routine admission orders. Compare the results with the prenatal record to determine if changes have occurred during pregnancy. For example, a VDRL or RPR serology test is drawn to determine if the woman has developed a syphilis infection during pregnancy so that mother and baby can be treated, if necessary. Box 10-2 lists routine laboratory work for a woman admitted to the delivery suite.

Box 10-2 ▮ ADMISSION LABORATORY STUDIES

- Complete blood count (CBC)
  - Monitor hemoglobin and hematocrit for signs of iron-deficiency anemia (hemoglobin levels below 11 g/dL).
  - White blood cell count (WBC) may increase to 20,000/mm^3 with the stress of labor. Levels above 20,000/mm3 may indicate infection.
- Blood type and Rh factor
- Serologic studies, such as VDRL or RPR, to test for syphilis
- Rubella titer (not done if prenatal record indicates the woman is immune)
- ELISA to detect HIV antibodies
- Vaginal or cervical cultures
  - Gonorrhea
  - Chlamydia
  - Group B streptococcus
- Urinalysis (clean-catch specimen)

THE NURSE'S ROLE: ONGOING ASSESSMENT OF UTERINE CONTRACTIONS AND FHR

It is important to assess uterine activity and FHR frequently during labor. These assessments are necessary to determine adequacy of the labor pattern and to detect signs of fetal well-being or distress. Table 10-1 compares the advantages and disadvantages of each of the methods discussed in the text for monitoring uterine and fetal status during labor.

Monitoring Uterine Contractions

Evaluate the uterine contraction pattern every time you assess the FHR (see Box 10-5 for frequency of assessment). The contraction pattern can be evaluated using external or internal methods.

External Methods

If intermittent assessment techniques are used, use palpation to evaluate the contraction pattern. When using continuous electronic fetal monitoring (EFM), a tocodynamometer (toco) measures contraction frequency and duration. The toco is a transducer with a sensor that works like a moveable button. Place the toco on the fundus with the sensor facing down and then strap it securely to the abdomen with a belt (see Nursing Procedure 10-3). As the uterus contracts, the sensor is displaced; an action that sends a signal to the microprocessor. The microprocessor converts the signal into a graphic representation of the uterine contraction on the video display and printout along with the FHR pattern tracing. In this way, the health care provider can monitor the FHR pattern in conjunction with the uterine contraction pattern.

Contraction frequency and duration are determined by evaluating the EFM tracing. However, unless the woman has an internal uterine pressure catheter, you must palpate the contractions to evaluate intensity. As you will recall from Chapter 8, the height of the contraction is an estimate of its intensity. However, many factors affect the height of the contraction on an external tracing. For example, a small woman with minimal adipose tissue may be having mild contractions, but on the monitor strip, the contractions appear tall and pronounced. On the other hand, an obese woman may be having strong contractions that barely register on the tracing. For these reasons, palpation is the most accurate way to estimate intensity when using external monitoring. Nursing Procedure 10-2 describes how to palpate uterine contractions.

> **Here's a helpful hint.**
> It is difficult for inexperienced nurses to determine the intensity of uterine contractions by palpation. If the fundus feels like the tip of your nose at the peak of a contraction, the contraction is mild. If the fundus feels firmer, as when you touch your chin, the contraction is of moderate intensity. A fundus that cannot be indented, one that feels like you are pushing on your forehead, is indicative of a strong contraction.

Nursing Procedure 10-2

PALPATION OF UTERINE CONTRACTIONS

EQUIPMENT

Warm, clean hands

PROCEDURE

1. Explain procedure to the woman and her partner.
2. Wash hands thoroughly.
3. Locate and place one hand on the uterine fundus.
4. Use the tips of your fingers to feel changes in the uterus as it contracts.
5. At the beginning of the contraction, you will feel the muscle begin to tighten.
6. Note the time the contraction begins.
7. Use your fingertips to evaluate how strong the contraction gets before the muscle begins to relax. Intensity is measured at the strongest point (the acme) of the contraction.
8. Note the time the contraction ends to determine duration.
9. Continue with your hand on the fundus through the next three contractions. Note if the uterus completely relaxes by becoming soft between contractions.
10. Note the time from the beginning of one contraction to the beginning of the following contraction, to determine frequency. Frequency is documented as a range when appropriate (e.g., every 3–5 minutes, or every 2–3 minutes), unless they are occurring regularly (e.g., every 2 minutes, every 5 minutes).
11. Wash hands.
12. Chart the contraction pattern (frequency, duration, and intensity) in the labor record. Document whether or not the uterus is fully relaxing between contractions.

Note: It is best to time several contractions consecutively before charting frequency because it is rare for contractions to be exactly "x" minutes apart. It is more common that the contraction pattern occurs every "x" to "y" minutes apart (e.g., every 3–5 minutes). Palpation is a method that takes practice. It is best to learn to palpate contractions in conjunction with the use of EFM. In this way, you can see the contraction begin and concentrate on perceiving the tightening of the uterus with your fingertips. You can also see the acme, which lets you know when to evaluate intensity.

Table 10-1 ▌ COMPARISON OF MONITORING TECHNIQUES DURING LABOR

Technique	Description	Advantages	Disadvantages
Intermittent fetal heart rate (FHR) auscultation	Fetoscope, Doppler, or fetal monitor used to periodically check FHR	• Noninvasive • Increases maternal comfort and mobility • Focus of health care provider is the laboring woman, rather than technology	• Requires one-to-one nurse-to-patient staffing ratios • Subtle signs of distress may be overlooked
Continuous external electronic fetal monitoring (EFM)	External transducer placed on maternal abdomen with straps to detect the FHR via ultrasound technology	• Noninvasive • Provides a continuous tracing of FHR • Allows for detection of signs of fetal compromise	• An active fetus or maternal movement can interfere with the continuity of the tracing • Generally confines the laboring woman to bed, unless telemetry unit is used
Continuous external monitoring of uterine contractions	External toco placed on maternal abdomen with straps to detect uterine contraction	• Noninvasive • Shows the frequency and duration of uterine contractions • Allows for comparison of FHR pattern with uterine contraction pattern	• Does not accurately depict the intensity of uterine contractions • Tends to be confining and limits maternal movement
Continuous internal EFM	Electrode is placed on the fetal scalp and connected to a reference electrode on the maternal thigh to record electrical activity of the fetal heart	• Allows for continuous monitoring of active fetus • Allows for continuous monitoring even if laboring woman is restless and changes positions frequently	• Invasive; requires that the membranes be ruptured and the cervix be at least partially dilated • Requires a specially trained practitioner for insertion • Increased risk for complications, such as chorioamnionitis, fetal scalp cellulitis, or osteomyelitis (rare)
Continuous internal monitoring of uterine contractions	Intrauterine pressure catheter inserted into a pocket of amniotic fluid to detect pressure changes within the uterus and record the contraction pattern	• Allows for more accurate determination of contraction intensity than external techniques • Useful for labors in which there is a risk for uterine rupture (e.g., previous uterine incision or induction with oxytocics)	• Invasive; requires that the membranes be ruptured and the cervix be at least partially dilated • Requires a specially trained practitioner for insertion • Increased risk for complications, such as chorioamnionitis
Fetal scalp sampling	Small sample of fetal scalp blood is taken during a special vaginal examination and tested for pH level	• Gives direct evidence of fetal status • Allows for better practitioner decisions regarding continuation of labor	• Invasive; requires that the membranes be ruptured and the cervix be at least partially dilated • Requires a specially trained examiner to collect the specimen • Increased risk for infection, blood incompatibilities, and fetal anemia
Fetal scalp pulse oximetry	Sensor placed on the fetus' cheek or brow to detect oxygen saturation	• Does not require a blood sample to be taken • Allows for continuous reading of fetal oxygenation status	• Invasive; requires that the membranes be ruptured and the cervix be at least partially dilated • Requires a specially trained practitioner for insertion • Has fallen out of favor. The newest research indicates fetal pulse oximetry is not beneficial.

Internal Method

Infrequently, an intrauterine pressure catheter is used. The trained examiner places the catheter tip above the presenting part in a pocket of amniotic fluid and then connects the catheter to the fetal monitor. In addition to recording the frequency and duration of contractions, the internal catheter accurately measures the intensity of uterine activity. This information is particularly useful when the woman is undergoing labor after a previous cesarean delivery or when she is receiving an oxytocic to induce labor.

Test Yourself

✔ Name three signs that indicate that birth is imminent.
✔ List the four parameters that must be charted regarding ruptured membranes.
✔ How do you evaluate the uterine contraction pattern when external EFM is used?

Monitoring FHR

Labor is stressful not only for the woman but also for the fetus. If there is decreased blood flow to the placenta, or if the fetus is subjected to chronic hypoxia, the fetus may not be able to withstand the stress of labor. General characteristics of the FHR and changes that occur with uterine contractions give clues as to fetal status. For these reasons, the fetal heart rate is monitored in relation to the contraction pattern.

Intermittent Auscultation of FHR

An acceptable method for monitoring FHR in a low-risk pregnancy is to use intermittent auscultation (IA). The most common practice is to place the woman on an external fetal monitor for 20 minutes to get a baseline evaluation of the FHR. If the pattern is reassuring, then a fetoscope, hand-held Doppler device, or the external fetal monitor is used to monitor the FHR at intermittent intervals. Auscultation of the FHR occurs with the same frequency as is recommended for continuous monitoring methods (see Box 10-5). The FHR is monitored for at least one full minute and is auscultated throughout at least one uterine contraction. If any abnormalities are noted, or if there is slowing of the FHR with or after contractions, apply the fetal monitor for continuous monitoring.

There are several advantages to the use of IA. The woman has more freedom to move about than when she is strapped continuously to a fetal monitoring device, and nurses are encouraged to focus on the laboring woman and her support person, rather than on the technology (Tillett, 2007). In addition, the use of IA is associated with fewer medical interventions and fewer surgical deliveries than occur with continuous monitoring (Alfirevic, Devane, & Gyte, 2007).

There are also disadvantages to the use of IA. This approach takes more time than does continuous EFM, a situation that requires higher nurse staffing levels. Therefore, IA may not be practical in a busy labor and delivery unit. Many practitioners unaccustomed to using IA fear the potential of missing an ominous FHR pattern. However, research to date demonstrates similar neonatal outcomes for IA and continuous EFM (Young, 2007).

Continuous EFM

As with monitoring uterine contractions, there are two ways to monitor the FHR using a continuous fetal monitoring device. Continuous EFM can be accomplished using external (indirect) methods or by using internal (direct) monitoring techniques.

External EFM

The most common way to assess fetal status during labor is with the use of an external fetal monitor. Although fetal monitors are manufactured by several companies and vary in shape and size, the basic components are the same and include a microprocessor, transducer, tocodynamometer (toco), audio capability, and graphic printout. The external monitor works on the principle of ultrasound. The transducer releases ultrasonic waves that are intercepted by the movement of fetal heart valves as the heart beats. The microprocessor interprets the signal and sends the results to the recording units. Characteristics of the fetal heart rate pattern can then be monitored continuously via a video display and/or a continuous printout. As stated, the toco monitors the contraction pattern, which allows for monitoring of the FHR pattern in conjunction with the uterine contraction pattern. See Nursing Procedure 10-3: Application of External Fetal Monitors.

External EFM helps screen for signs of fetal compromise. It is noninvasive and used widely. However, it is sometimes difficult to get a consistent tracing if the fetus is small or extremely active or if the woman is obese. Maternal positioning can adversely affect the quality of the tracing, and many women find external monitoring uncomfortable and confining.

Some manufacturers of fetal monitors have developed telemetry units, which provide wireless transmission of FHR patterns and uterine activity to the monitoring device so that the woman is not attached by cables to the fetal monitor. These units allow for continuous EFM while the woman ambulates, alternates her position, or uses a birthing ball. There are telemetry units that even allow the woman to submerse her body in water to soothe the discomfort of labor.

Internal EFM

Internal EFM is an invasive procedure in which a spiral electrode is attached to the presenting part just under the skin (Fig. 10-4). A wire that extends from the spiral electrode is connected to a reference electrode that is placed on the laboring woman's inner thigh. The microprocessor

Nursing Procedure 10-3

APPLICATION OF EXTERNAL FETAL MONITORS

EQUIPMENT

Electronic fetal monitor
Tocodynamometer (toco)
Transducer
Two belts
Ultrasonic gel
Monitor paper

PROCEDURE

1. Thoroughly wash your hands.
2. Locate the fetal back through the use of Leopold's maneuvers (see Nursing Procedure 10-1).
3. Assist the woman to a position of comfort. If she wishes to be on her back, a wedge should be placed under one hip to tilt the uterus off of the great vessels.
4. Place ultrasonic gel on the transducer and turn on the power to the fetal monitor.
5. Place the transducer on the woman's abdomen over the fetal back.
6. Turn up the volume, and move the transducer over the abdominal wall until the heartbeat is clearly heard.
7. When the monitor is consistently recording the FHR, secure the transducer in place with a belt.

8. Next locate the hardest part of the uterine fundus.
9. Place the toco over the fundus and secure it to the maternal abdomen with a belt (see figure).
10. Check to make sure the paper is recording the FHR and uterine contraction pattern.

11. Label the EFM strip with the laboring woman's identification data, the date and time the EFM was applied, and maternal vital signs and position.
12. Be sure the call light is within reach before you leave the room.
13. Thoroughly wash your hands.

Note: It is important to position the woman comfortably before attempting to locate the fetal heart. If you wait until after you locate the FHR to reposition, you may lose the FHR and need to relocate the transducer.

---

interprets the signal and records a graphic representation of the electrical activity of the fetal heart. It is easier than with external monitoring to obtain a consistent tracing regardless of fetal activity, and maternal position changes usually do not cause interference. When internal techniques are used, the most common combination is that of internal fetal scalp electrode with an external toco to record the contraction pattern. Less frequently, an intrauterine pressure catheter is used to evaluate uterine contractions (refer to the previous discussion).

The fetal membranes must be ruptured and the cervix must be adequately dilated to use internal monitoring. Accordingly, these procedures increase the risk of maternal and fetal infection and injury.

This is important!

Because internal monitoring techniques are invasive, both the woman and the fetus can become ill with infection. Internal methods should be used only when the benefit clearly outweighs the risk.

Figure 10-4 Continuous internal EFM. The internal fetal scalp electrode is placed on the fetal scalp and connected to the reference electrode on the maternal thigh and to the fetal monitor.

Evaluating FHR Patterns

Baseline FHR

The obstetric nurse is responsible for monitoring FHR patterns. The RN not only must assess and interpret the pattern accurately, but also must know how to intervene and when to notify the physician or certified nurse midwife (CNM). The LPN is not expected to make a final decision about an FHR pattern; that is the responsibility of the trained RN. However, you must be able to differentiate reassuring and nonreassuring signs in order to get help when indicated.

When interpreting a fetal monitor tracing, the first element to evaluate is the baseline FHR. The baseline rate is measured between uterine contractions during a 10-minute period. The normally accepted baseline rate is between 110 beats per minute (bpm) and 160 bpm (Alfirevic, Devane, & Gyte, 2007).

Another element to evaluate is the baseline **variability**, fluctuations of the FHR from the baseline rate. In the re-

---

Box 10-3 ▮ FETAL HEART RATE (FHR) VARIABILITY DEFINITIONS

- Absent: No fluctuations of FHR
- Minimal: ≤5 bpm
- Moderate: 6–25 bpm (normal)
- Marked: >25 bpm

---

cent past, the definition of variability included two types: short-term and long-term. The Association of Women's Health, Obstetric, and Neonatal Nurses (AWHONN, 2006) no longer makes this distinction. Variability is evaluated visually as a unit. Baseline variability is normal if the fluctuations are greater than 6 bpm and less than 25 bpm (Fig. 10-5). Box 10-3 gives definitions of variability.

FHR variability results from the interplay between the sympathetic and parasympathetic branches of the fetal autonomic nervous system. The sympathetic division nudges the FHR higher, whereas the parasympathetic division tugs the FHR downward. Therefore, variability in the tracing is a reassuring sign that the fetal nervous system is intact. The presence of moderate variability reassures the practitioner that the fetus is well oxygenated (Acker, 2007).

There are three major deviations from a normal FHR baseline: tachycardia, bradycardia, and absent or minimal variability. By definition, fetal tachycardia is a baseline rate greater than 160 bpm. A baseline FHR below 110 bpm is fetal bradycardia. The abnormal rate must continue for at least 2 minutes for identification of tachycardia or bradycardia. The absence of variability also is a nonreassuring sign. Table 10-2 lists examples of conditions

A word of caution is in order.

Make certain that a nonreassuring pattern is not attributable to medical intervention. For example, fetal bradycardia may result from maternal hypotension secondary to epidural anesthesia, and some medications cause decreased variability. Often, correcting the maternal condition remedies the nonreassuring pattern.

Fetal heart rate (bmp)

Uterine activity (mm Hg)

Figure 10-5 The EFM tracing shows moderate (normal) variability.

Table 10-2 ▮ CONDITIONS THAT CAN INFLUENCE THE FHR BASELINE

Baseline FHR Deviation	Possible Causes
Tachycardia (>160 bpm) Mild 161–180 bpm Severe >180 bpm	• Maternal or fetal infection • Dehydration • Fever • Hyperthyroidism • Fetal hypoxemia (acute or chronic) or anemia • Premature fetus • Fetus with congenital anomalies • Certain medications given to the woman in labor, particularly tocolytics (medications used to stop preterm labor), and any drug that causes maternal tachycardia (e.g., caffeine, epinephrine, or theophylline) • Street drugs
Bradycardia (<110 bpm) Moderate 80–100 bpm Severe <80 bpm	• Maternal hypotension • Supine hypotensive syndrome • Vagal stimulation • Fetal decompensation

Decreased or absent variability	• Medications
	  • Narcotics
	  • Magnesium sulfate (to treat preterm labor or preeclampsia)
	  • Tocolytics (medications to stop labor)
	• Fetal sleep (normal fetal sleep cycle is 20 minutes)
	• Prematurity
	• Fetal hypoxemia

that can cause fetal tachycardia, bradycardia, and absent variability.

Periodic Changes

The next step after evaluating the baseline is to check for **periodic changes**, variations in the FHR pattern that occur in conjunction with uterine contractions, and **episodic changes**, variations in the FHR pattern *not* associated with uterine contractions. Because the clinical implications are the same for periodic and episodic changes, the text will refer to these changes as periodic changes. Periodic changes can be reassuring, benign, or nonreassuring. Figure 10-6 illustrates the appearance and causes of certain periodic changes.

Reassuring Periodic Changes. Spontaneous elevations of the FHR, **accelerations**, above the baseline by at least 15 bpm for at least 15 seconds (15 × 15 window) are considered to be reassuring. In fact, as stated in Chapter 7, accelerations are the basis for the nonstress test (NST).

Benign Periodic Changes. Sometimes, instead of accelerations, there is a slowing of the FHR. If the dip in the FHR tracing occurs in conjunction with and mirrors a uterine contraction, it is an **early deceleration**. This type of deceleration looks like a U on the fetal monitor tracing, like that of an upside down contraction. Three criteria classify the deceleration as early: (1) the FHR begins to slow as the contraction starts; (2) the lowest point of the deceleration, the **nadir**, coincides with the acme (highest point) of the contraction; and (3) the deceleration ends by the end of the contraction.

Current scientific evidence indicates that early decelerations are caused by pressure on the fetal head as it meets resistance from the structures of the birth canal. The contraction pushes the fetal head downward, causing pressure, which in turn leads to a slowing of the FHR. As long as the baseline remains within normal limits and the variability is good, early decelerations are benign. Therefore, no specific nursing intervention is indicated other than to continue to monitor the tracing and observe closely for the development of nonreassuring patterns.

Nonreassuring Periodic Changes. A **variable deceleration** may occur at any point during a contraction, and it has a jagged, erratic shape on the fetal monitor tracing. The FHR suddenly drops from the baseline and then recovers. A variable deceleration is variable in timing and in shape. It may resemble a U, V, or W.

The presence of variable decelerations, or *variables*, as labor and delivery personnel commonly call them, indicates some type of acute umbilical cord compression. When repetitive variables occur on the strip, the cause often becomes apparent at delivery when the umbilical cord is wrapped around a body part, such as the neck (nuchal cord) or foot. At other times, the cause of compression is oligohydramnios (decreased amount of amniotic fluid), or it results from an occult (hidden) cord prolapse (see Chapter 18). It is important to note that the cord compression is not continuous when variable decelerations are occurring. The compression occurs when the uterus contracts and squeezes the cord against the fetus. It is relieved when the uterus relaxes

| Onset | Recovery | Variable onset | | Onset | Recovery |

normal HR

Nadir

A. Early   B. Variable   C. Late

■ **Figure 10-6** Appearance and causes of periodic changes. **(A)** Early decelerations mirror uterine contractions and are caused by head compression. **(B)** Variable decelerations are variable in onset and shape; they are caused by cord compression. **(C)** Late decelerations are offset from uterine contractions and are caused by uteroplacental insufficiency.

between contractions. When compression is continuous, prolonged decelerations or bradycardia occur.

Variable decelerations require careful observation. If the baseline is within normal limits, variability is present, and the variables recover quickly (within the space of a normal contraction), there is no immediate cause for alarm. However, you should be aware that the cord compression stresses the fetus because the umbilical cord is his lifeline to oxygen. It is as if he is holding his breath while the cord is compressed during the contraction. Therefore, nursing interventions are aimed at relieving the compression.

First, assist the woman to change positions. Try to find a position that is comfortable for the woman that relieves the compression. If the variables stop after the position change, you will know that the compression has been relieved. However, if the variables continue, try a variety of position changes, including the knee-chest position.

Pay attention to the details!

Here's how to tell if variable decelerations indicate distress. Repetitive variable decelerations with loss of variability or that last longer than 1 minute or dip deeper than 60 bpm below the baseline are nonreassuring.

Other interventions for persistent or prolonged variables include stopping any oxytocic infusion, increasing the rate of IV fluids (if they are infusing), starting oxygen via face mask at 10 to 12 L/min, and notifying the charge nurse and physician. The charge nurse may perform a vaginal examination to rule out a prolapsed cord. Sometimes the physician will order an **amnioinfusion,** infusion of normal saline into the uterus, to cushion the umbilical cord and relieve compression.

Another type of nonreassuring periodic change is a pattern of **late decelerations;** these are the most ominous type of periodic change. Like early decelerations, these decelerations appear smooth and U shaped on the EFM tracing, but unlike early decelerations, they are offset from the contraction. Late decelerations begin late in the contraction and recover

Don't forget the importance of your observation skills.

It is easy to be so concerned about the fetal monitor tracing that you overlook or downplay the skills of inspection and palpation. Always begin your assessment by performing a quick visual inspection of the woman and her environment. If there are no immediate problems, then you may turn your focus to reading the EFM strip.

■ **Figure 10-7** An early deceleration mirrors the contraction, is caused by head compression, and is benign, requiring no intervention. A late deceleration is offset from the contraction and is caused by uteroplacental insufficiency; interventions are aimed at improving blood flow to the placenta.

after the contraction has ended. The slope and size of the deceleration mirrors the contraction. Figure 10-7 compares early and late decelerations on a fetal monitor tracing.

Late decelerations are associated with **uteroplacental insufficiency**, diminished or deficient blood flow to the uterus and placenta. This pattern occurs from chronic interruption of the blood supply to the placenta. This is a grave situation because the placenta is the fetus' sole source of oxygen. Interventions are aimed at improving blood flow to the placenta.

The following interventions are indicated for a pattern of late decelerations. Position the woman on her right or left side[2] to relieve compression on the maternal great vessels. Discontinue the infusion of oxytocics (if present). Apply oxygen via a face mask at 10 to 12 L/min. Immediately notify the charge nurse and physician. Sometimes the physician will order tocolytics (medications to relax the uterus) in an attempt to improve blood flow to the placenta. Box 10-4 lists signs of an increasingly distressed fetus.

Measures Used to Clarify Nonreassuring FHR Patterns

Because a nonreassuring FHR pattern may not truly reflect a compromised fetus, researchers continue to search for methods that can more accurately determine true fetal hypoxia and acidosis. Many of the techniques developed to date are not widely used. Some techniques practitioners may use include fetal stimulation, fetal scalp sampling, and fetal scalp pulse oximetry.

Fetal Stimulation

To see if the fetus is responsive, the practitioner or RN may elect to try fetal stimulation. For this procedure, the fetus is stimulated indirectly with an acoustic vibrator through the abdominal wall or is stimulated directly on the scalp by the gloved fingers of the examiner's hand during a vaginal examination. If the fetus responds by accelerating the heart rate, fetal acidosis is not present. If FHR accelerations do not occur after stimulation, fetal acidosis is a strong possibility (Young, 2007).

Test Yourself

✔ What are the components of the electronic fetal monitor?

✔ What is the baseline fetal heart rate?

✔ How does a late deceleration appear on the fetal monitor tracing?

✔ What interventions should be made when a pattern of late decelerations is detected?

---

[2]Research shows that positioning the woman on either side relieves pressure on the abdominal aorta and inferior vena cava and improves blood flow to the placenta. Previously, it was thought that positioning on the left side afforded the best blood flow. Some health care providers may still prefer to use the left side for a pattern of late decelerations.

Box 10-4 ■ SIGNS OF AN INCREASINGLY DISTRESSED FETUS

As the fetus becomes hypoxic, certain physiologic signs can be noted. These signs are listed in order of least distress to most distress. As you move down the list, the signs are indicative of ever-worsening hypoxia.

1. Absent accelerations
2. Gradual increase in FHR baseline
3. Loss of baseline variability
4. Late deceleration pattern develops
5. Decelerations gradually increase in length and take longer to recover to baseline
6. Persistent bradycardia
7. Death

Fetal Scalp Sampling

Fetal scalp sampling, a technique for checking fetal status, was developed in the late 1960s to verify fetal compromise in the presence of a nonreassuring FHR pattern. For this procedure, the practitioner places a lighted endoscope into the vagina through the dilated cervix and holds it on the fetal scalp. The practitioner then cleans the scalp with a special cotton swab, makes a tiny cut (like a finger stick to check for blood sugar), and collects a small amount of blood in a long, heparinized capillary tube. The blood sample is tested immediately to determine the pH (Cunningham et al., 2005a). A fetal pH within the normal range (≥7.25) is reassuring. If, however, the pH is abnormally low (≤7.15), the fetus almost certainly has acidosis[3] (Young, 2007). Fetal acidosis indicates that the fetus is truly in distress and needs to deliver quickly. Supplies and personnel are prepared in anticipation of resuscitation of the newborn, if needed.

Although the risk is low, complications can result from fetal scalp sampling. The fetus can get an infection from the cut on the scalp; fetal and maternal blood may intermingle, potentially leading to blood incompatibilities; and the fetus can experience anemia from blood loss. Many facilities have stopped using this technique due to the costs involved, the degree of technical skill required, maternal discomfort during the procedure, and equipment and laboratory needs (Young, 2007).

Fetal Scalp Pulse Oximetry

Because fetal scalp sampling has many drawbacks, a newer technique was developed to monitor fetal oxygenation: fetal scalp pulse oximetry. This technology uses the same principles of pulse oximetry as those used to measure oxygen saturation in adult patients. In this instance, the sensor is inserted into the uterus and placed next to the fetal cheek or temple. The sensor detects fetal oxygen saturation levels. A microprocessor interprets the signal, and sends the information to a monitor that gives a continuous readout. In this way, the physician or nurse midwife can make a better decision about fetal status than with EFM alone. Current research indicates that fetal pulse oximetry does not reduce the number of cesarean deliveries for nonreassuring fetal tracings, as was hoped. The current recommendation is that fetal pulse oximetry is not beneficial for use in labor (Bloom et al., 2006b).

Test Yourself

✔ Describe two techniques of fetal stimulation.

✔ What evidence does fetal scalp sampling reveal regarding fetal status?

✔ What is fetal scalp pulse oximetry?

---

[3]Interpretation and intervention for fetal scalp pH between 7.15 and 7.20 varies based on other fetal and labor assessments.

THE NURSE'S ROLE DURING EACH STAGE OF LABOR

Nursing Process During the First Stage of Labor: Dilation

The first stage of labor includes three phases: latent, active, and transition. The first stage begins with the onset of labor and ends when the cervix is 10 cm dilated and 100% effaced. The nurse's role during this stage of labor focuses on assessment, providing physical care to the mother and fetus, providing psychological care to the mother, and keeping the practitioner informed about labor progress (Box 10-5).

Latent Phase (Early Labor)
Assessment

During the latent phase of labor, assess fetal and labor status at least once every hour. Contractions during early labor are typically 5 to 10 minutes apart, last 30 to 45 seconds, and are of mild intensity. The cervix is dilated from 1 to 3 cm, and effacement has begun. Additional assessment parameters include maternal status and the status of the membranes.

It is also important to assess the woman's psychosocial state during the latent phase of labor. She may be talkative and express feelings of confidence and excitement. Conversely, she may be fearful, particularly if she feels unprepared for the event; or she may experience anticipatory anxiety.

Selected Nursing Diagnoses

■ Risk for Injury (fetal and maternal) related to possible complications of labor
■ Anxiety related to uncertainty of labor onset and insecurity regarding ability to cope
■ Acute Pain related to contractions
■ Deficient Knowledge of labor process related to inadequate preparation for delivery or unexpected circumstances of labor

Outcome Identification and Planning

Maintaining the safety of the laboring woman and her fetus throughout the latent phase of the first stage of labor are primary goals when planning care. Other goals and interventions are planned according to the individual needs of the laboring woman and her partner. Appropriate goals may include that no injury will occur to the fetus or mother, that the laboring woman's anxiety will be reduced and her pain will be manageable, and that the woman and her partner will have adequate knowledge of the labor process.

Implementation
Preventing Fetal and Maternal Injury

Monitor the woman's vital signs every hour. The temperature may be taken every 4 hours unless the water bag is ruptured, which requires hourly monitoring. Mild

Box 10-5 ▌ NURSING CARE FOR THE FIRST STAGE OF LABOR

Caring for the Woman

Assess the woman's vital signs.

- Temperature
  - If membranes are intact, monitor and record every 4 hours.
  - If membranes are ruptured, measure every 2 hours.
  - An elevated temperature may be associated with dehydration or infection.
- Blood pressure, pulse, and respirations
  - Measure every 60 minutes during the latent phase of labor.
  - Measure every 30 minutes during active labor and transition.
  - When certain procedures are done, such as induction of labor or placement of epidural anesthesia, take the vital signs more frequently.

Monitor hydration status.

- Maintain strict intake and output.
- Maintain and monitor IV fluids, if present.
- Offer ointment for dry lips.
- Provide frequent mouth care.
- Offer fluids and ice chips if allowed/desired.
- Encourage voiding every 2 hours.
- Check for the presence of glucose or protein in the urine.

Remain attuned to the maternal psyche.

- Provide ongoing assessment of maternal coping status.
- Assess effectiveness of partner, coach, or doula in supporting and comforting the woman.
- Promote positive coping.
  - Teach/reinforce patterned breathing techniques (Chapter 9).
  - Encourage frequent position changes.
  - Encourage rituals and creative approaches to dealing with contractions.
  - Administer analgesia appropriately, if desired by the woman.
  - Assist with the administration of anesthesia as ordered, if desired by the woman.
- Provide supportive care.
  - Provide privacy.
  - Provide a relaxing environment.
    - A fan may helpful if the woman is hot.
    - Soft lighting or darkening the room promotes relaxation.
  - Keep noise to a minimum.
    - Some women need absolute quiet during a contraction.
    - Some women find music to be soothing.
  - Provide for personal hygiene needs.
    - Absorbent pads placed under the hips and buttocks catch the continual drainage associated with labor.
    - Frequent perineal care and pad changes promote comfort.
    - Some women find a shower comforting.
  - Keep the woman and her partner or coach informed of labor progress and purpose of procedures.
- Be a role model for the support person.
  - Actively involve the partner or coach, if so desired by the laboring woman. Remember some cultures discourage participation by the father in the birthing process.
  - Encourage the support person to take breaks as needed.

Caring for the Fetus

Assess FHR* (*Note:* The frequency recommendations apply to both intermittent and continuous monitoring techniques):

- Evaluate the FHR of the low-risk laboring woman every
  - 1 hour during latent phase of the first stage of labor
  - 30 minutes during active phase of the first stage of labor
- Evaluate the FHR of the at-risk laboring woman every
  - 30 minutes during latent phase of the first stage of labor
  - 15 minutes during the active phase of the first stage of labor

Additional times for monitoring and documenting the FHR pattern:

- Immediately after artificial or spontaneous rupture of the membranes
- Before and after medication administration during labor and at time of peak medication action
- Before and after any invasive procedure (e.g., vaginal exam, enema expulsion, urinary catheterization, amnioinfusion)
- Before and after ambulation
- After any increase in frequency, duration, or intensity of uterine contractions

Management of the Labor Process

Observe for spontaneous rupture of the membranes, or assist when the birth attendant performs an artificial rupture of the membranes.

- Observe the color of the fluid (should be clear); report green or cloudy fluid.
- Record the time of rupture, the characteristics and amount of fluid, and an assessment of the FHR.

Monitor for signs of umbilical cord prolapse (see Chapter 18).

- Immediately after the membranes rupture, when the risk for prolapse is greatest, assess the FHR for 1 full minute.

Box 10-5 ▌ NURSING CARE FOR THE FIRST STAGE OF LABOR *(continued)*

- If fetal bradycardia is present, perform a vaginal examination to check for a prolapsed cord.
- Continue ongoing fetal assessments because prolapse can occur anytime after the membranes rupture.

Assess uterine contraction pattern each time the FHR is assessed.

- Pattern should generally correlate with the phase of labor.
- Uterus should relax completely between contractions.
- Report tetanic contractions (lasting longer than 90 seconds and of strong intensity) or failure of the uterus to relax.

Assess bloody show.

- An increase may be a sign of advancing labor.

- Heavy bleeding is a sign that a complication of labor is developing.

Assist the RN or childbirth attendant with vaginal examinations to determine progress of dilatation, effacement, and descent. To decrease the risk of infection:

- Sterile technique should be used.
- The number of examinations should be kept to a minimum.

Note maternal and fetal response to interventions.
Document all assessments and procedures.

---

*Recommendations of the American College of Obstetrics and Gynecology (ACOG) and Association of Women's Health, Obstetric, and Neonatal Nurses (AWHONN).

---

tachycardia may be associated with anxiety or the stress of labor contractions. Immediately report elevations in the blood pressure or temperature.

Check the fetal monitor tracing frequently. Record FHR and uterine contraction pattern at least hourly during the latent stage of labor. Report extended periods of reduced variability, FHR decelerations, or other signs of fetal compromise.

Relieving Anxiety

Anxiety causes the release of catecholamines (fight-or-flight hormones), which slow down the labor process (Hottenstein, 2005). Current research demonstrates that continuous labor support by a caring nurse or doula results in better birth outcomes (Campbell et al., 2006). As the LPN/LVN, you are in a wonderful position to provide supportive care during labor and influence birth outcomes in a positive way.

Encourage the woman to verbalize her fears and uncertainties. It may be helpful to ask what concerns her most about labor. Often, anxiety decreases when the woman verbalizes her fears. When the source of anxiety is determined, implement measures to decrease the anxiety based on the cause. For example, if the woman is unsure she will be able to withstand the pain of labor, a discussion of pain relief options may be helpful. If she does not know what to expect, she may benefit from a brief explanation of the normal process of labor.

The woman also may fear losing control. In this instance, it may be appropriate to involve the partner in developing a plan to assist her if she starts to lose control. Verbal cues and position changes may be part of the plan. Inquire regarding coping behaviors that have been helpful to her during other stressful situations. In this way, you can assist the couple to adapt previously successful coping strategies to assist coping efforts during labor.

Promoting Comfort

It is important to support the woman and her partner in their attempts to cope with the discomfort and stress of labor. If the membranes are intact, encourage the woman to ambulate. Even if the membranes are ruptured, she may ambulate with a support person or nurse, if the fetus is engaged and well applied to the cervix. Ambulation and upright positions are frequently helpful throughout the labor process. If the woman chooses not to ambulate, assist with comfort measures and position changes. However, do not allow the woman to remain flat on her back.

If the woman and her coach are well prepared for labor, they may decide to stay at home during the latent phase. This practice is permissible as long as the membranes are intact, and some nurses encourage it to allow the woman more control over the early labor process. Encourage distraction techniques. Engaging in conversation, watching television, and shopping are examples of diversionary activities that may be helpful during the latent phase of labor. Food and beverage intake during labor is a subject of debate (Box 10-6).

Providing Patient Teaching

The latent phase of labor is an excellent time to teach the woman and her partner or coach about the process of labor. Important teaching points include what the woman and her coach can expect to experience during each phase and stage of labor. Explain pain relief options and discuss appropriate timing of analgesia and anesthesia. Briefly describe the frequency and purpose of nursing assessments and interventions common to each stage of labor.

It is important that the woman and her partner understand how to work with the labor process and how to avoid fighting against it. If the woman has not attended childbirth preparation classes, use this time to teach basic relaxation techniques. Otherwise, review and

Box 10-6 ▊ FOOD AND FLUID INTAKE DURING LABOR

For the past 50 decades in the United States, the normal practice has been to withhold food and fluids from the laboring woman. The rationale for this practice was to prevent the woman from aspirating in the event that anesthesia was needed for a cesarean delivery. Now there are a wide range of practices and opinions on the issue (Funai & Norwitz, 2006).

Nurse midwives who deliver patients at home or in birthing centers often allow food and fluid intake during the latent phase of labor and then restrict the woman to clear fluids during active labor. The woman needs fluids during labor to prevent dehydration. Because the woman who delivers at home rarely has an IV, she is usually encouraged to take fluids by mouth. Many midwives who deliver in birthing centers give IV fluids to the woman in active labor. In this instance, the woman is usually allowed clear liquids as a comfort measure.

Practices regarding food and drink during labor vary widely at hospitals across the country (Tranmer et al., 2005). Many physicians prefer to give IV fluids to every woman in active labor and allow only ice chips, while others allow clear liquids. Currently, more research is needed before updated recommendations can be made. The nurse is well advised to follow the practitioner's recommendations regarding food and fluid intake during labor.

The fetus maintains signs of well-being. The fetal heart tracing shows

- FHR within the expected range.
- reactivity (accelerations with good variability).
- no decelerations or other signs of distress.

Goal: The woman's anxiety is reduced.
Expected Outcomes: The woman

- verbalizes confidence in her ability to cope with labor.
- uses relaxation techniques effectively.

Goal: The woman's pain is manageable.
Expected Outcomes: The woman

- verbalizes satisfaction with pain management.
- expresses the ability to cope with her pain.
- demonstrates the use of effective strategies for coping with labor.

Goal: The woman and her partner have adequate knowledge of the labor process.
Expected Outcomes: The woman and her partner

- express realistic expectations regarding the duration, intensity, and process of labor.
- work with the labor process (versus fighting against it).

Test Yourself

✔ What assessment findings would lead to keeping the low-risk laboring woman on bed rest?

✔ Describe four important nursing interventions during the latent phase of labor.

reinforce breathing and relaxation techniques that the couple learned in class (see Chapter 9 for discussion of techniques).

The partner or coach needs encouragement regarding the importance of his or her role during labor. Give information regarding measures the woman may find comforting during each stage of labor, and encourage the partner to take breaks periodically to conserve energy for the duration of labor. Explain the importance of using the nurse as a resource and source of support for the partner and the woman throughout labor. When the woman knows what to expect and receives support during labor, she has less anxiety and fear, which enhances the labor process (Campbell et al., 2006; Hottenstein, 2005).

Evaluation: Goals and Expected Outcomes

Goal: The woman and fetus remain free from injury.
Expected Outcomes: The woman

- has stable vital signs.
- maintains blood pressure that is not elevated above baseline levels.
- remains afebrile.

ACTIVE PHASE (ACTIVE LABOR)

Assessment

Assess the woman's psychosocial state. Note if the woman is becoming more introverted, restless, or anxious; if she is feeling helpless or fears losing control; or if distraction techniques are failing to promote coping. These behaviors signal that the woman is moving into the active phase of labor.

Assessment of Labor Progress

During the active phase, evaluate the contraction pattern every 30 minutes. Typically, contractions occur every 2 to 5 minutes, last 45 to 60 seconds, and are of moderate to strong intensity. The cervix should dilate progressively from 4 to 8 cm. The fetus should descend steadily, although descent does not typically progress as rapidly as does cervical dilation. As the fetus descends below the level of the ischial spines, station is described in positive numbers. Plot cervical changes and fetal descent on a labor graph to evaluate labor progress. It is also critical to assess whether the uterus is relaxing completely between contractions. An adequate relaxation period allows for sufficient blood flow to the placenta and promotes oxygenation of the fetus.

Assessment of Fetal Status

Assess and document fetal status at least every 30 minutes. Record the baseline FHR every 30 minutes, and evaluate the fetal monitor tracing for nonreassuring patterns. Variability should be present, except for brief periods of fetal sleep or when the mother receives narcotics or other selected medications, and no late decelerations should be present. Accelerations of the FHR are reassuring.

Assessment of Maternal Status

Assess maternal status with the same frequency as fetal status. The woman becomes more introverted during active labor because the contractions are closer together, of a stronger intensity, and last longer than during early labor. Blood pressure may rise slightly but should be lower than 140/90 mm Hg. It is important to take the blood pressure between contractions because the stress of a uterine contraction can cause the blood pressure to rise briefly, resulting in an inaccurate measurement.

Pulse and respirations may also increase with the work of labor. Monitor for signs of tachycardia and hyperventilation. A falling blood pressure and a rising pulse could indicate the onset of shock; immediately report this finding. Several labor complications can cause shock, including hemorrhage or uterine rupture.

Assess the presence and character of pain at least hourly during active labor. Ask the woman to rate her pain on a standardized pain scale to make pain assessments measurable. Anxiety and tension often decrease the woman's ability to cope with contractions; therefore, it is important to document how the woman and her partner are coping and to determine if the coping strategies are helpful. For example, if the woman is using patterned breathing techniques to manage contractions, she may hyperventilate and need assistance to regain control of her breathing technique.

Evaluate breathing patterns frequently. Assess for signs of hyperventilation, which include tachypnea, feelings of lightheadedness or dizziness, complaints of tingling around the mouth or in the fingers, and carpopedal spasms (Fig. 10-8).

Check for dry cracked lips, thick saliva, and a coating on the tongue that may be caused by mouth breathing and lack of oral intake (if restricted). Measure the temperature every 4 hours if the water bag is intact and hourly after the membranes have rup-

Exercise caution!
When the membranes rupture, whether spontaneously or artificially, check the FHR for one full minute immediately afterward. If fetal bradycardia or deep variable decelerations occur, assist the woman to the knee-chest position and call the RN immediately to perform a vaginal examination to check for a prolapsed cord.

■ Figure 10-8 Carpopedal spasms.

tured. Monitor for signs of infection such as elevated temperature, fetal and maternal tachycardia, and cloudy, foul-smelling amniotic fluid. Box 10-7 lists danger signs to watch for during labor.

Selected Nursing Diagnoses

- Risk for Trauma to the woman or fetus related to intrapartum complications or a full bladder
- Acute Pain related to the process of labor
- Anxiety related to fear of losing control
- Ineffective Coping related to situational crisis of labor
- Ineffective Breathing Pattern: hyperventilation related to anxiety and/or inappropriate application of breathing techniques

---

Box 10-7 ▌ DANGER SIGNS DURING LABOR

If any of the following signs occur during labor, immediately notify the RN, physician, or nurse midwife.
- Elevated maternal blood pressure (BP) (≥140/90 mm Hg)
- Low or suddenly decreased maternal BP (≤90/50 mm Hg)
- Elevated maternal temperature (>100.4°F)
- Amniotic fluid that is green, cloudy, or foul smelling
- Nonreassuring FHR patterns
- Prolonged uterine contractions (>90 seconds duration)
- Failure of the uterus to relax between contractions
- Heavy or bright red bleeding
- Maternal reports of unrelenting pain, right upper quadrant pain, or visual changes

- Impaired Oral Mucous Membrane related to dehydration and/or mouth breathing
- Risk for Infection related to invasive procedures (e.g., vaginal examinations) and/or rupture of amniotic membranes

Outcome Identification and Planning

In addition to maintaining maternal and fetal safety during the active phase of the first stage of labor, appropriate goals may include that the laboring woman's pain will be manageable, she will exhibit lessened anxiety, demonstrate effective strategies for coping with labor, display effective breathing patterns, maintain an intact oral mucosa, and remain free of signs of infection.

Implementation

Preventing Trauma During Labor

It is important to continue to monitor closely the EFM tracing during active labor. Immediately report any signs of nonreassuring FHR patterns that do not respond to position changes and other accepted interventions. Report abnormal maternal vital signs, heavy bleeding, or failure of the uterus to relax well between contractions.

Another source of trauma that can interfere with the progress of labor is a full bladder. Every 2 hours, palpate the area just above the symphysis pubis, feeling for a rounded area of distention, which indicates the bladder is full. Failure of the fetus to descend is another sign that the bladder might be full. Offer the bedpan every 2 hours or assist the woman to the restroom, if allowed. If the woman is unable to void, perform a sterile in-and-out catheterization procedure.

Check out this tip.
A full bladder may interfere with fetal descent. Encourage the woman to void at least every 2 hours during labor.

Providing Pain Management

The active phase of labor is the time when most women need pain relief measures. Epidural anesthesia may be initiated, or narcotic analgesia may be administered (see Chapter 9); however, it is critical to respect the woman's preferences for pain control. If the woman desires a natural childbirth, she will need intensive support throughout the active phase of labor.

Implementing general comfort measures can help to manage the pain and discomfort of labor. Work closely with the coach to demonstrate distraction and relaxation techniques, such as effleurage, back rubs, or application of pressure to the lower back during contractions (see Chapter 9). A cool, damp washcloth to the forehead is often comforting.

Perspiration, amniotic fluid, and bloody show frequently soil linen and gowns during active labor. Place linen savers, such as chucks or other under-buttocks pads, under the hips and replace as needed. Provide frequent perineal care. At a minimum, perform perineal care after any invasive procedure involving the vagina and after elimination.

Reducing Anxiety

During active labor, assist the woman and her partner to implement the anxiety reduction plan agreed upon during early labor. Continue to encourage the woman to verbalize her concerns. If her chosen method of pain relief is not working, remind her that she can change her mind about pain relief options. You may need to repeat earlier instruction and reassure the couple that it does not represent a failure on the woman's part if she chooses an alternate method of pain management. If she starts to lose control, assist the labor coach to use verbal cues and position changes to help the laboring woman regain control.

Promoting Effective Coping Strategies

It is important to support the woman and her partner in their attempts to cope. Some women do not benefit from the use of patterned breathing techniques. Frequently, these women will develop personalized "rituals" to help them cope with contractions.

A **ritual** is a routine, a repeated series of actions that the woman uses as an individualized way of dealing with the discomfort of labor. For example, one woman might find it helpful to close her eyes and attempt to visualize a peaceful scene during contractions. Another woman might involve her partner by squeezing his hands throughout each contraction. Still, another woman might assume a particular position during contractions. As long as these creative approaches to coping are helpful, encourage and support their use. When the ritual is not working to promote adaptation, assist the woman in trying other approaches.

Promoting Effective Breathing Patterns

Frequently reinforce breathing techniques appropriate to the active phase of labor (see Chapter 9). Often, it helps to make eye contact and perform the breathing patterns with the woman during her contraction to help keep her focused (Fig. 10-9). Vigorous application of breathing techniques can lead to hyperventilation. If hyperventilation occurs, breathing into cupped hands or a paper bag usually relieves the problem.

Maintaining Integrity of the Oral Mucosa

Frequent mouth care stimulates saliva production, which helps

Do you know the why of it?
Hyperventilation can cause respiratory alkalosis. Breathing into a paper bag retains CO_2, reverses alkalosis, and relieves associated symptoms.

■ **Figure 10-9** The nurse instructs the labor coach to maintain eye contact and breathe with his partner during contractions to help keep her focused. (Photo by Joe Mitchell.)

to keep the oral mucosa moist. Suggest that the woman brush her teeth or gargle with normal saline when her mouth feels dry. Chewing gum also stimulates saliva production and leaves a pleasant taste in the mouth. Providing ice chips, sips of clear liquids, flavored ice, or hard candy (if allowed) can be soothing. Lip balm is comforting if the lips are dry or chapped. If the woman does not have lip balm, the water-soluble lubricant available in most labor rooms effectively moistens the lips.

Preventing Infection

Hand washing remains the number one way to prevent the spread of infection. Wash your hands thoroughly before and after providing care. Encourage the woman and her partner to wash their hands before and after any contact with the perineum and after using the restroom.

Frequent vaginal examinations are discouraged, particularly if the membranes are ruptured. Nursing judgment determines frequency. Usually, it is best not to examine the cervix unless there is a clear indication that labor is progressing. Assist the examiner to maintain sterile technique when it becomes necessary to perform a vaginal examination.

Perform invasive procedures, such as the application of an internal fetal monitor or insertion of a urinary catheter, only if there are clear indications for their use. Strict adherence to sterile technique when performing an invasive procedure is critical.

Evaluation: Goals and Expected Outcomes

Goal: The fetus and woman remain free of trauma.
Expected Outcomes: The woman's

- vital signs are stable.
    - blood pressure is not elevated above baseline levels.
    - temperature is not elevated.

- bladder is not distended.
- uterus is relaxing well between contractions.

The fetus maintains signs of well-being. The fetal heart tracing shows

- FHR within the expected range.
- reactivity (accelerations with good variability).
- no decelerations or other signs of distress.

Goal: The woman's pain is manageable.
Expected Outcomes: The woman

- states that the pain of labor is tolerable.
- verbalizes that pain-relief techniques are effective.

Goal: The woman's anxiety is reduced.
Expected Outcomes: The woman

- reports decreased anxiety.
- relaxes between uterine contractions.

Goal: The woman copes effectively.
Expected Outcomes: The woman

- works with the labor process (versus fighting it).
- uses social supports (partner, coach, relative, or doula) to help her cope.
- modifies individualized rituals as labor progresses.

Goal: The woman uses effective breathing techniques.
Expected Outcomes: The woman

- uses slow and accelerated breathing techniques during contractions, as appropriate.
- does not hyperventilate.

Goal: The woman's oral mucosa remains intact.
Expected Outcomes:

- The woman's lips and oral mucous membranes remain moist and intact.

Goal: The woman and fetus exhibit no signs of infection.
Expected Outcomes: The woman

- remains afebrile.
- maintains a white blood cell count within expected parameters.
- has clear and odorless amniotic fluid.
- has no foul-smelling drainage.

The fetus

- does not develop tachycardia.
- continues to have a reactive tracing.

Test Yourself

✔ Why is it important for the laboring woman to void frequently?
✔ What assessment findings are associated with the nursing diagnosis Ineffective Breathing Pattern: hyperventilation?
✔ List five nursing interventions appropriate for the active phase of labor.

TRANSITION PHASE

Assessment

Assess for signs that the woman has reached the transition phase of the first stage of labor. Look for an increase in bloody show and a strong urge to push if fetal station is low. Assess the woman's ability to cope. She will often express irritability, restlessness, and will feel out of control. She may tremble, vomit, or cry. It is important to assess for hyperventilation during this phase.

Do you know the why of it?

Nausea and vomiting are common occurrences during labor because of decreased gut peristalsis and delayed gastric-emptying time. If vomiting occurs, assist the woman to turn to her side to help prevent aspiration.

Check the contraction pattern at least once every 30 minutes; contractions should occur every 2 to 3 minutes, last 60 to 90 seconds, and be of strong intensity. The uterus should relax completely between uterine contractions. Cervical examination during transition reveals dilation between 8 and 10 cm.

It is essential to continue to evaluate fetal status at least every 30 minutes. The FHR baseline should remain between 110 and 160 bpm and should not significantly increase or decrease. It may be normal to see variable decelerations as the fetal head descends. Variability should be present. There should be no late decelerations or other signs of fetal compromise.

Selected Nursing Diagnoses

- Acute Pain related to frequent, intense uterine contractions and pressure of the descending fetal head
- Ineffective Breathing Pattern: hyperventilation related to intense uterine contraction pattern and loss of control of breathing techniques
- Powerlessness related to intensity of the labor process
- Fatigue related to energy expended coping with the intense labor

Outcome Identification and Planning

Major goals for the transition phase of the first stage of labor include that the woman's pain will be manageable, she will exhibit effective breathing patterns, she will maintain a sense of control, and she will rest between uterine contractions.

Implementation

Managing Pain

Reassure the woman that although this period of labor is the most intense, it is usually short. Continue to assist the coach to provide comfort and support during uterine contractions. Frequent position changes, breathing with the woman during contractions, and providing other comfort measures may help decrease the intensity of the pain stimulus.

Narcotics are not given at this advanced stage of labor to prevent delivery of a neonate who is too sleepy to take his or her first breath (Briggs & Wan, 2006). Some women request epidural anesthesia during transition. This request is usually granted, although sometimes by the time the anesthetist has prepared for the insertion, the woman has rapidly progressed and birth is imminent. The woman should know that an epidural given during transition might delay effective pushing in the second stage of labor.

Promoting Effective Breathing Patterns

If the woman is using patterned breathing techniques, encourage her to switch to a more advanced technique when the pattern she is using is no longer working. Assist the coach to breathe with her and to assess for signs of hyperventilation. She may feel the urge to push. Explain the importance of resisting the urge to push until full cervical dilation.

Promoting a Sense of Control

Accepting behavioral changes of the laboring woman is an important nursing intervention during this forceful period of labor. You will need to provide intensive psychological support. If the woman falls asleep between contractions, awaken her at the beginning of a contraction so that she can begin her coping strategy before the contraction reaches full intensity.

This advice could save the day.

If the woman is feeling a strong urge to push, assist her to blow at the peak of the contraction when the urge is most intense. Pushing efforts before the cervix is fully dilated can result in cervical lacerations or can cause edema of the cervix and slow dilation.

Supporting the Woman Through Fatigue

Relaxing with contractions may be almost impossible; assist the woman to achieve relaxation or even sleep between contractions. Help her to find a comfortable position. Support her position with pillows. Placing a cool cloth to her forehead or giving her a back rub may help her relax between contractions (Fig. 10-10). Some women find music to be soothing. When the woman is able to relax between contractions, she conserves energy that she will need during the next stage in order to push effectively. The partner/coach is often fatigued as well; encourage him or her to take breaks as necessary.

Preparing the Room for Delivery

Often, you will prepare the room for delivery during the transition phase (Fig. 10-11). Many delivery units have physician preference cards so you can prepare the equipment and supplies most often needed by the attending physician. Prepare the table maintaining surgical asepsis

▪ **Figure 10-10** The labor coach provides comfort measures, such as a cool washcloth to the face and forehead, to help the woman relax as much as possible during the transition phase of labor. (© B. Proud.)

so that a sterile field is available during delivery. It is important to ensure that supplies and medications needed for the birth are readily available. Check the infant resuscitation area and replace any missing supplies or malfunctioning equipment.

Evaluation: Goals and Expected Outcomes

Goal: The woman's pain is manageable.
Expected Outcomes: The woman

- verbalizes ability to tolerate the pain of contractions.
- cooperates with support person and nurse to find effective strategies to manage the pain.

Goal: The woman's breathing pattern is effective.
Expected Outcomes: The woman

- uses accelerated breathing techniques during contractions.
- does not hyperventilate.

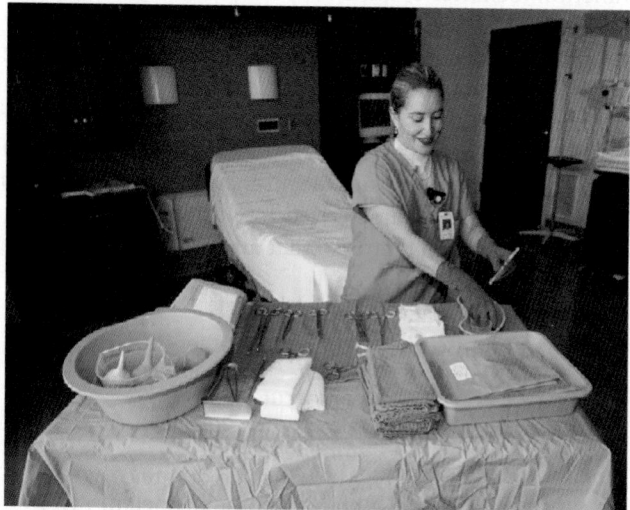

▪ **Figure 10-11** The nurse prepares the labor room for delivery. (Photo by Joe Mitchell.)

- uses pant-blow techniques to refrain from pushing despite pressure from the fetal head.

Goal: The woman maintains a sense of control.
Expected Outcomes: The woman

- expresses ability to deal with contractions.
- works with coach/support person to regain control if she loses control momentarily.

Goal: The woman rests between uterine contractions.
Expected Outcomes: The woman

- remains quiet and calm between uterine contractions.
- sleeps or rests with eyes closed between uterine contractions.

Test Yourself

✔ Discuss the five signs associated with the transition phase of labor.
✔ What responsibilities does the nurse have for supporting the partner or coach?
✔ Why is it important that the woman refrain from pushing until the cervix is completely dilated?

Nursing Process During the Second Stage of Labor: Expulsion of the Fetus

The second stage of labor begins when the cervix is 10 cm dilated and 100% effaced and ends with the birth of the newborn. Nursing care during this stage of labor focuses on providing physical and psychological support to the woman while she pushes the fetus through the birth canal. Assessment of maternal and fetal well-being during this stage is crucial.

Assessment

During the second stage of labor, close observation of the laboring woman and her fetus is indicated. Monitor the blood pressure, pulse, and respirations every 15 to 30 minutes. Cervical examination reveals that the cervix is fully dilated (10 cm) and completely effaced. The fetal station is usually 0 to +2.

Assess the contraction pattern every 15 minutes. The pattern will be similar to that found in the transition phase (i.e., contractions occur every 2 to 3 minutes, last 60 to 90 seconds, and are of strong intensity). Assess for the woman's report of an uncontrollable urge to push, which is caused by pressure from the descending fetal head.

Assessment of the fetus during the second stage is essential. As the fetus descends into the pelvis, the pressure on his head is very intense. There may also be pressure on the umbilical cord during contractions. Frequently, the fetal monitor strip reveals early or variable decelerations. Variables are usually not ominous at this stage as long as the FHR returns quickly to baseline as the contraction relaxes, the baseline remains between 110 and 160 bpm, and variability is present. Check the FHR every

15 minutes for the low-risk woman and every 5 minutes for the woman who is at risk for labor complications.

Evaluate the woman's psychosocial status; the laboring woman may find it less difficult to cope with the contractions now that she can push. Often, she is less irritable and more cooperative. Assess the woman's level of fatigue. If the second stage is prolonged, she may become extremely fatigued and experience difficulty finding the energy to push.

Selected Nursing Diagnoses

- Fatigue related to length of labor and pushing efforts
- Risk for Trauma related to pushing techniques and positioning for delivery

Outcome Identification and Planning

Appropriate goals for the second stage of labor include that the woman will push effectively despite fatigue and that she will give birth with minimal or no trauma to the fetus and herself.

Implementation

Promoting Effective Pushing Despite Fatigue

All of the comfort measures appropriate to active labor continue to apply during the second stage, particularly while the woman is pushing. Using comfort measures, such as applying a cool cloth to the forehead and offering ice chips and mouth care, can promote relaxation between contractions, which helps to conserve energy and prevent exhaustion.

Assist the woman to the chosen position for pushing and provide support throughout each pushing effort. For instance, if the woman is using the sitting position to push, you and the coach can assist her to the sitting position when the contraction starts and support her back while she pushes.

If the woman has experienced a prolonged labor and is having a difficult time pushing effectively, it may be appropriate to position her on her side for comfort and allow her to rest for 30 minutes to an hour in order to regain her strength. As long as the fetal monitor tracing remains reassuring, allowing for a break from pushing is acceptable. In fact, if the woman is able to push more effectively after the break, often the fetus will descend and birth will occur soon afterward.

Reducing the Risk for Trauma

Assist the RN to ensure the safety of mother and baby during the second stage by promoting effective pushing techniques and positions for pushing.

Effective Pushing Techniques. Once the cervix is fully dilated, the woman can begin pushing efforts. Traditionally, obstetric nurses have taught women to use vigorous pushing techniques. When **vigorous pushing** is used, the woman is told to take a deep breath, hold the breath, and push while counting to 10. She is encouraged to complete three "good" pushes in this manner with each

A Personal Glimpse

After 2 days of doctors trying to induce labor, I was about ready to request a cesarean section. Although I truly desired a vaginal birth, my husband and I were at our wits' end after having tried every measure available to start labor. During those frustrating days, the nurses I had were so supportive. They encouraged me to think positively and hold onto hope that I would eventually have a vaginal birth. When I was finally able to push, my labor and delivery nurse, Mary Ellen, was so supportive. Somehow, she convinced me that every push was the first one. With her gentle guidance, I believed I could get my baby out, even when it seemed it would never happen. I will never forget how helpful and tender she was. She told me time and again that I was "almost there" while my doctor shook his head in disagreement. Having spent more time with Mary Ellen than with the doctor who would eventually deliver my child, I believed her assessment far more than his! I don't think I even remember his name, but I will always remember Mary Ellen for her reassurance and gentle care.

Sara

Learning Opportunity: Describe three supportive nursing behaviors that can encourage a woman to not give up when labor seems overwhelming.

Why do you think the nurse's support is beneficial to prevent unnecessary cesarean deliveries?

---

contraction. However, recent research has revealed that vigorous pushing techniques that employ the Valsalva maneuver are associated with changes in the mother's heart rate and blood pressure, and fetal oxygenation may be adversely affected (Simpson, 2005; Simpson & James, 2005). Current research also suggests that vigorous pushing techniques result in more perineal lacerations and may contribute to long-term pelvic floor dysfunction (Schaffer et al., 2005; Simpson & James, 2005; Wenstrom, 2006). Even so, in the majority of delivery rooms, obstetric nurses continue to coach women to use vigorous pushing (Sampselle et al., 2005).

Researchers currently advocate two natural forms of pushing: open-glottis pushing and the urge-to-push method. You may instruct the woman to use **open-glottis pushing**, which is characterized by pushing with contractions using an open glottis so that air is released during the pushing effort. You also may encourage the woman to use the **urge-to-push method**, in which the woman bears down only when she feels the urge to do so using any technique that feels right for her. Contrary to conven-

> **Watch out!**
> When the mother is pushing effectively, delivery can occur rapidly. Monitor for signs of imminent delivery, which include grunting, bulging of the perineum, crowning of the fetal head, and exclamation that "the baby is coming!"

tional thinking, using the urge-to-push method does not appear to significantly lengthen the duration of the second stage of labor (Bloom et al., 2006a; Sampselle et al., 2005). No matter what pushing technique is used, never leave the woman alone during pushing efforts.

Positions for Pushing and Delivery. There are many different positions that are acceptable for pushing and for delivering the baby. However, in the United States, most women deliver in a modified dorsal recumbent position in which the woman's legs are on foot pedals and the head of the bed is elevated approximately 45 degrees. Occasionally, the practitioner will ask for the legs to be positioned in stirrups (lithotomy position). Dorsal recumbent and lithotomy positions allow for greater control by the attendant but may not be the most comfortable or effective positions for enhancing delivery.

One major disadvantage of the lithotomy position is that gravity does not assist the birth. Other positions use gravity to aid in the pushing process, which conserves energy during the second stage of labor. Some positions, such as hands and knees, encourage rotation of the fetus, which shortens the second stage of labor. The hands and knees position enhances blood flow to the placenta, resulting in fewer nonreassuring EFM tracings. Table 10-3 illustrates and compares positions used for pushing and delivery of the baby.

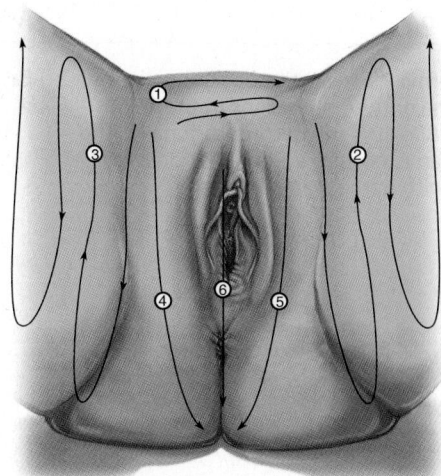

Don't forget!

Prevention of supine hypotension remains a priority during delivery. If a lithotomy position is used, place a wedge under the woman's hip to tilt the uterus away from the major vessels.

Preparing for Delivery of the Newborn

Nursing judgment is necessary to decide when to prepare the woman for delivery. You may observe bulging of the perineum (Fig. 10-12) or crowning of the fetal head, which indicate imminent delivery. Preparation of the primipara is typically done when the fetus is crowning, whereas preparation of the multipara may be done when the fetus reaches a +2 or +3 station. However, the RN may prepare sooner in both cases if the fetus is descending rapidly.

■ **Figure 10-12** Bulging of the perineum is an indicator of imminent delivery. (© B. Proud.)

■ **Figure 10-13** Perineal scrub in preparation for delivery. An antiseptic solution is used to clean the perineum just before delivery. The numbers represent the order in which each stroke is completed. The arrows represent the direction of the scrub. A new sponge is used for each stroke.

If the woman has been laboring in a birthing bed and she will deliver in the semisitting or lithotomy position, the bed is "broken"—the lower part of the bed is removed to allow room for the birth attendant to control the delivery. Often, you will place the woman's feet on foot pedals. If stirrups are used, take care to position the stirrups properly, then lift both legs together and place them in the stirrups. Clean the woman's perineum with an antiseptic solution (Fig. 10-13); a povidone-iodine scrub is often used. Position the instrument table close to the birthing bed and uncover it. If the urinary bladder is full, perform an in-and-out catheterization.

Prepare the equipment necessary to receive the baby in anticipation of the birth. This preparation involves turning on the radiant warmer and placing a warm blanket under the warmer. Be sure that the forms to begin the baby's chart are in the room, and check the resuscitation equipment once more before delivery.

The RN is responsible for overseeing events during the birth. Surgical terms describe the role of the RN; therefore, he or she is the circulator for the delivery. The RN should remain in the delivery room until after the infant is born, the placenta delivers, and mother and baby are stable. Box 10-8 lists the major responsibilities of the nurse in the delivery room, including immediate care of the newborn (see Chapter 13 and 14 for comprehensive coverage of newborn care). Figure 10-14 shows a delivery sequence from crowning through birth of the newborn.

This advice could be a lifesaver!

The risk for splashing of bodily fluids is high during a delivery. Eye shields, gowns, and gloves may be necessary for protection from contact with bodily fluids.

Table 10-3 ■ COMPARISON OF POSITIONS FOR PUSHING AND DELIVERY

Position	Advantages	Disadvantages
Lithotomy: This was the position used by the majority of physicians in the 1960s to 1980s. It is still used occasionally. The woman is positioned on a flat delivery bed with her legs in stirrups.	Easy access to the perineum and greater control of delivery by birth attendant	Greater risk of supine hypotensive syndrome and positioning injuries (e.g., clot formation from compression or muscle strain from improper placement in stirrups)
Modified dorsal recumbent or semisitting: This is a common pushing position. When it is time for delivery, the woman's feet are placed on foot pedals and the birthing bed is "broken" in preparation for delivery.	Easy access to the perineum and good control of delivery by birth attendant	May be uncomfortable for the woman. May not be the best position to facilitate expulsion of the baby.
Side-lying	May increase comfort of the woman.	Decreases access to the perineum by the birth attendant. Requires high degree of cooperation from the woman and possible assistance of the nurse or support person to hold the upper leg during delivery.
Squatting	Highly likely to increase the comfort of the woman. Uses gravity to facilitate expulsion of the baby.	Difficult access to the perineum. Requires a birth attendant who is flexible and willing to use this approach. The woman may lose her balance in this position. A pushing bar can help maintain balance, or a birthing stool may be used.

(continued)

Table 10-3 ▮ COMPARISON OF POSITIONS FOR PUSHING AND DELIVERY *(continued)*

Position	Advantages	Disadvantages
Hands and knees: The woman is assisted to her hands and knees on the birthing bed to push and deliver the baby.	Encourages rotation of the fetal head, which hastens delivery. Enhances placental blood flow, which decreases fetal stress. Allows for the perineum to stretch better than other positions so that an episiotomy is less often required. Allows for greater access to the perineum by the birth attendant than some of the other alternative positions.	May be more tiring for the woman. Does not allow for the use of instruments to assist delivery.

Box 10-8 ▮ RESPONSIBILITIES OF THE NURSE IN THE DELIVERY ROOM

Closely monitor the laboring woman.
- Record vital signs and status assessments per facility protocol.
- Assess for maternal response to anesthesia.

Closely monitor the fetus. Assess FHR
- Every 15 minutes for low-risk labors.
- Every 5 minutes for at-risk labors.

Maintain accurate delivery room records.
- Note and record the time of delivery.
- Record all nursing procedures performed and maternal/newborn response.

Provide immediate newborn care (refer to Chapters 13 and 14 for in-depth discussion of newborn adaptation and care).
- Maintain warmth.
  - Immediately dry the newborn on the woman's abdomen or under the radiant warmer.
  - Wrap the newborn snugly and place a cap on the head when not in skin-to-skin contact with the woman or when not under a warmer.
- Assess adaptation to extrauterine life.
  - Assess and record Apgar scores (see Chapter 14 for a discussion of Apgar scoring).
- Maintain a patent airway.
  - Position the newborn to facilitate drainage.
  - Suction secretions with a bulb suction device or with wall suction.

- Provide for safety and security. Before the newborn and the mother are separated after delivery
  - Obtain the newborn's footprints and mother's thumb or fingerprint (if part of the facility protocol).
  - Place identification bands with matching numbers on the infant and new mother. Two bands are placed on the infant and one on the new mother. In some facilities, a band is also placed on the new father or support person.

Promote parental-newborn bonding.
- Allow/encourage the woman and her partner to hold the newborn.
- Allow/encourage breast-feeding immediately after delivery.
- Encourage skin-to-skin contact with the newborn.
- Point out positive characteristics of the newborn.

Assist the birth attendant.
- Perform sponge and instrument counts.
- Ensure that supplies are available for episiotomy and repair, if needed.
- Obtain additional supplies as needed, such as forceps or vacuum extractor for difficult deliveries, or extra suturing material.

■ Figure 10-14 Delivery sequence from crowning through birth of the newborn. (A) Early crowning of the fetal head. Notice the bulging of the perineum. (B) Late crowning. Notice that the fetal head is appearing face down. This is the normal OA position. (C) As the head extends, you can see that the occiput is to the mother's right side—ROA position. (D) The cardinal movement of extension. (E) The shoulders are born. Notice how the head has turned to line up with the shoulders—the cardinal movement of external rotation. (F) The body easily follows the shoulders. (G) The newborn is held for the first time! (© B. Proud.)

A

B

▮ **Figure 10-15** A healthy placenta after delivery. **(A)** Notice the shiny surface of the fetal side. **(B)** The maternal side is rough and divided into segments (cotyledons). (Photos by Joe Mitchell.)

Evaluation: Goals and Expected Outcomes

Goal: The woman will push effectively despite fatigue.
Expected Outcomes: The woman

- pushes effectively with contractions and works with her partner or coach while pushing.
- rests between contractions.

Goal: The woman and fetus remain free from trauma.
Expected Outcomes: The woman

- uses open-glottis or natural-pushing techniques.
- maintains vital signs within expected ranges.

The fetus maintains signs of well-being. The fetal heart tracing shows

- FHR within the expected range.
- reactivity (accelerations with good variability).

Test Yourself

✔ What instructions should be given to the laboring woman regarding pushing?
✔ What are the major responsibilities of the nurse in the delivery room?

Nursing Process During the Third Stage of Labor: Delivery of Placenta

The third stage of labor begins with the birth of the newborn and ends with delivery of the placenta. During this stage of labor, nursing care focuses on monitoring for placental separation and providing physical and psychological care to the woman.

Assessment

Assess the woman's psychosocial state after she gives birth. Immediately after birth, the new mother often experiences a sense of relief that the birth has been accom-

plished and contractions have ceased. Monitor for signs of placental separation, which generally occur within 5 to 20 minutes of delivery. These signs begin with a uterine contraction, then the fundus rises in the abdomen, the uterus takes on a globular shape, blood begins to trickle steadily from the vagina, and the umbilical cord lengthens as the placenta separates from the uterine wall.

The placenta may deliver in one of two ways (Fig. 10-15). The most common way is for the smooth, shiny, fetal side to deliver first (Schultze's mechanism). Sometimes, the edge of the placenta appears at the introitus, revealing the rough maternal surface (Duncan's mechanism). The latter mechanism of delivery is more frequently associated with retained placental fragments. After the placenta delivers, the birth attendant inspects it for completeness. Palpate the fundus to make certain the uterus is firm and contracted. Monitor the perineum for excess bleeding.

Selected Nursing Diagnoses

- Risk for Deficient Fluid Volume related to blood loss in the intrapartum period
- Risk for Trauma: Hemorrhage, amniotic fluid embolism, retained placenta, or uterine inversion related to delivery of the placenta

Outcome Identification and Planning

The major goals during the third stage of labor are that the new mother will maintain adequate fluid volume and that she will remain free of trauma.

Implementation

Preventing Fluid Loss

Monitor the woman's vital signs at least every 15 minutes during the third stage of labor. Tachycardia and a falling blood pressure are signs of impending shock; immediately report these signs. Note how much time has passed since the birth of the newborn. The placenta normally separates within 20 minutes of delivery. If a longer period has passed, the woman may be experiencing retained placenta, which can lead to acute fluid loss from hemorrhage. Monitor intravenous fluids to ensure patency and prevent the development of dehydration.

Maintaining Safety and Preventing Trauma

Monitor the woman for any sudden change in status. Complaints of shortness of breath, chest pain, or tachypnea may indicate the development of an amniotic fluid embolism (see Chapter 18).

Oxytocin is given in the third stage of labor to prevent hemorrhage. Some practitioners prefer to give oxytocin before the placenta delivers to hasten its delivery, whereas others administer oxytocin as soon as the placenta delivers (Silverman, 2006). When the placenta separates from the uterine wall, it leaves an open wound that is subject to hemorrhage if the uterus does not contract effectively. When given after the placenta delivers, oxytocin causes the uterus to contract, which puts pressure on the open blood vessels at the former placenta site. The oxytocin is usually added to the IV fluids, but some physicians and midwives prefer intramuscular injection.

Try nature's way!
Encourage the mother to breastfeed immediately after delivery. Breastfeeding stimulates oxytocin release from the posterior pituitary, which helps control bleeding.

Evaluation: Goals and Expected Outcomes

Goal: The woman will maintain an adequate fluid volume.
Expected Outcomes: The woman

- maintains adequate vital signs: Her blood pressure does not fall; her pulse does not rise.
- does not experience excessive blood loss (no more than 500 mL).

Goal: The woman remains free of trauma.
Expected Outcomes: The woman

- delivers an intact placenta.
- does not lose more than 500 mL of blood.
- does not experience a life-threatening complication: respirations remain unlabored, lung sounds are clear, and fundus remains firmly contracted.

Nursing Process During the Fourth Stage of Labor: Recovery

The fourth stage of labor begins with delivery of the placenta and ends when the woman's physical condition has stabilized (usually within 2 hours). Nursing care during this stage focuses on continued assessment and care of the woman and promoting parental–newborn bonding.

Assessment

Continue to assess the woman for hemorrhage during the fourth stage of labor. The new mother is at highest risk for hemorrhage during the first 2 to 4 hours of the postpartum period. Monitor the woman's vital signs, and palpate the fundus for position and firmness. The fundus should be well contracted, at the midline, and approximately one fingerbreadth below the umbilicus immediately after delivery. Assess the **lochia** (vaginal discharge after birth) for color and quantity. The lochia should be dark red and of a small to moderate amount.

Monitor for signs of infection. The temperature may be elevated slightly, as high as 100.4°F, because of mild dehydration and the stress of delivery. Any elevation above that level may indicate infection and should be reported. The lochia should have a fleshy odor but should not be foul smelling.

The woman should void within 6 hours after delivery. Trauma from the birth may have caused edema in the perineal area or anesthesia may persist, leading to an inability to sense a full bladder. Both conditions can lead to urinary retention. Monitor for suprapubic distention and a high fundus displaced to the right. These signs indicate that the urinary bladder is full.

Assess the woman's comfort level. There are many sources of pain during the immediate postpartum period. Cramping from uterine contractions and perineal pain from edema or episiotomy repair are common sources of pain for the new mother. Ask the woman to describe the location of the pain and to rate it on a standardized pain scale.

Assess the mother's psychosocial state during the fourth stage. Typically, the mother is fatigued and ravenously hungry. It is normal for her to be self-absorbed and demonstrate dependent behaviors. She also has an intense need to talk about the labor and delivery experience.

Assess initial bonding behaviors of the new family. It is normal for parents to want to hold and touch the newborn as soon as it is born. You may notice that the parent begins initial inspection of the newborn with the fingertips; this is normal behavior and indicates positive beginning attachment.

Be careful not to be too hasty to diagnose inadequate bonding. Some mothers are so fatigued that they may not desire prolonged interaction with the newborn beyond the initial inspection. Behaviors that indicate a risk for inadequate attachment include turning away from the newborn or making disparaging comments about the newborn.

Selected Nursing Diagnoses

- Risk for Impaired Parent–Infant Attachment related to disappointment regarding the gender of the newborn or an unwanted pregnancy
- Risk for Deficient Fluid Volume related to possibility of hemorrhage from the former site of placenta attachment
- Risk for Infection related to invasive procedures and vaginal examinations during labor
- Impaired Urinary Elimination related to perineal trauma during delivery

- Acute Pain related to episiotomy, birth trauma, and/or afterpains
- Fatigue related to energy expended during labor

Outcome Identification and Planning

Appropriate goals for the new mother during the fourth stage of labor (recovery) are that the parents will begin a positive bonding process with their newborn and that the woman will maintain adequate fluid volume, remain without signs of infection, maintain adequate voiding patterns, not become extremely fatigued, and that her pain will be adequately managed.

Implementation

Providing Care Immediately After Delivery

After the birth attendant has completed his or her duties, inspect and cleanse the perineum. Remove the soiled drapes and linen, and place an absorbent pad under the buttocks with two sterile perineal pads against the perineum. Place a warm blanket (from a blanket warmer, if possible) over the new mother. Reassemble the birthing bed. If the woman is in stirrups, remove both legs from the stirrups at the same time.

Promoting Parent–Newborn Attachment

While the birth attendant is suturing any lacerations or episiotomy and making a final inspection of maternal tissues, it is important to promote parental bonding with the newborn. Hand the newborn to the woman as soon as it is determined that he does not need extraordinary resuscitation. If the father is present at the delivery, encourage him to hold and interact with the newborn (Fig. 10-16). This is a good time for the new mother to attempt breast-feeding for the first time. If the woman permits it, place the newborn skin-to-skin against her body and place several blankets over them. This technique (called kangaroo care) keeps the infant warm and promotes bonding.

■ **Figure 10-16** The father and mother bond with their newborn son soon after birth.

Maintaining Adequate Fluid Volume

Continue to monitor the woman for signs of fluid volume deficit or hemorrhage. Take vital signs every 15 minutes during the fourth stage of labor. Falling blood pressure and tachycardia may indicate fluid volume deficit or hemorrhage and should be reported. Massage the fundus every 15 minutes, and inspect the lochia for amount and color. The fundus should be firm or should quickly become firm when gently massaged. Continue to monitor IV fluids and offer food and fluids to the new mother.

Preventing Infection

Continue to use excellent hand-washing technique. Wash hands before and after care, between patients, and any time contact with bodily fluids occurs. It is critical to use standard precautions. Wear gloves at all times when you perform procedures anywhere near the perineum or dirty linens. Anything that comes in direct contact with the perineum should be sterile. Handle perineal pads from the ends, and do not touch the middle area that will be in contact with the perineum.

Promoting Urinary Elimination

If the woman has the urge to void, assist her to the bathroom unless she is still under the effects of anesthesia and does not have complete control of her legs. It is much easier for her to void sitting on a toilet than it is on a bedpan. Have her dangle her feet at the bedside for several minutes before assisting her to a standing position. Once she is safely in the bathroom, run water or let her soak her hands in warm water if she is having difficulty getting the stream of urine started. An in-and-out catheterization is usually not done unless there is significant suprapubic distention or discomfort from the full bladder or until 6 hours have passed without voiding.

Minimizing Pain

Nonsteroidal anti-inflammatory drugs (NSAIDs) and oral narcotic analgesics, such as codeine, often are prescribed for pain after delivery. The NSAIDs are quite effective at reducing painful uterine cramping. Many providers order large doses (600–800 mg) of ibuprofen to be given every 6 to 8 hours around the clock. This type of dosing is often more effective at keeping pain under control than is an "as needed" schedule in which the woman must ask for the medication before it is given.

Combination medications consisting of a mild analgesic, such as acetaminophen, with a narcotic, such as codeine, may be ordered on an as-needed basis for breakthrough pain. Sometimes, codeine is ordered for perineal pain, and NSAIDs are given to control cramping. Assess the woman's pain frequently and administer medications before the pain becomes intolerable.

Warmth to the abdomen may be helpful in reducing the discomfort of uterine cramping. Position changes may also be helpful. If the pain is from an episiotomy or edema of the perineum, it is helpful to apply ice packs. Most labor units have combination perineal pads/ice packs. These are convenient, but a clean glove filled with ice also works as an ice pack. If used, apply the glove between two perineal pads so that a nonsterile object does not come in direct contact with the perineum.

Watch out!

Extreme perineal pain may indicate the development of a perineal hematoma. Other signs of a hematoma include restlessness, inability to find a comfortable position, and tilting to one side when sitting.

Reducing Fatigue

After the initial bonding period, it may be helpful to discourage visitors and promote rest for the new mother. Her partner can stay with her to care for the newborn if the newborn is rooming-in or if the hospital provides couplet care. If the newborn is to be stabilized in a newborn nursery, this is a good time for both the new mother and her partner to get some much-needed rest and sleep, if possible.

Evaluation: Goals and Expected Outcomes

Goal: The parents begin a positive bonding process.
Expected Outcomes: The parents

- inspect the newborn immediately after birth.
- make positive comments about the newborn.

Goal: The woman maintains an adequate fluid volume.
Expected Outcomes: The woman's

- blood pressure and pulse remain within expected limits.
- fundus remains firm.
- vaginal bleeding remains small.

Goal: The woman remains free of signs of infection.
Expected Outcomes: The woman

- remains afebrile (temperature ≤100.4°F).
- has lochia with a normal fleshy odor that is not malodorous.

Goal: The woman will maintain adequate voiding patterns.
Expected Outcomes: The woman

- expresses the ability to void without difficulty.
- empties her bladder effectively.
- has no suprapubic distention.

Goal: The woman's pain will be adequately managed.
Expected Outcomes: The woman

- reports that interventions are effective at relieving pain.
- reports a tolerable pain level.

Goal: The woman does not become extremely fatigued.
Expected Outcomes: The woman

- reports the ability to rest and sleep in the immediate postpartum period.
- takes naps, as needed.
- reports feeling refreshed after sleeping.

Test Yourself

✓ Identify four signs of placental separation.
✓ How often are vital signs checked during the fourth stage of labor?
✓ Name three parameters that should be assessed with each vital sign check during the fourth stage of labor.

Key Points

➤ Continuous support of a skilled obstetric nurse facilitates the labor process and the woman's satisfaction with the birth experience.
➤ Throughout the labor process, monitor maternal and fetal status and labor progress. Frequent assessment of vital signs and FHR are critical nursing functions.
➤ When a woman arrives at the labor unit, immediate assessment involves observing for signs that birth is imminent, in which case admission procedures are abbreviated until after delivery, as well as assessing fetal status, risk factors, and maternal status.
➤ If the birth is not imminent, admission assessment includes a thorough obstetric, medical–surgical, and social history and a complete physical assessment. Also, assess labor status and the woman's labor and birth preferences.

➤ Evaluate the uterine contraction pattern using external or internal methods. External evaluation always involves palpation when using intermittent auscultation. Also, palpate to determine intensity when the external toco is used during continuous fetal monitoring. Internal evaluation requires the use of an internal pressure catheter. The internal pressure catheter measures intensity as well as frequency and duration.
➤ IA of FHR allows for freedom of maternal movement and focuses the nurse's attention on the woman, rather than the technology. Disadvantages are that IA requires higher staffing levels and some practitioners fear that subtle signs of fetal compromise may be missed. Continuous monitoring restricts maternal movement and tends to focus the nurse on the monitor versus the woman.

Advantages are that the nurse can take care of more patients and can detect immediately changes in fetal status.

➤ External fetal monitoring is noninvasive and allows for evaluation of FHR patterns. Internal fetal monitoring requires that the membranes be ruptured and the cervix be at least partially dilated.

➤ To apply the fetal monitor, first locate the fetal back, and then apply the transducer using ultrasonic jelly. Next, locate the fundus, and place the toco on the firmest part of the fundus. Both the toco and transducer are secured to the abdomen with straps.

➤ LPN/LVNs must be able to detect nonreassuring FHR patterns in order to notify the charge nurse and/or the practitioner, who then makes a final decision regarding care of the patient.

➤ Three major deviations from a normal FHR baseline are tachycardia (FHR >160 bpm), bradycardia (FHR <110 bpm), and absent or minimal variability (fluctuations ≤5 bpm).

➤ Early decelerations are gradual decreases in the FHR that mirror the contraction. Head compression is the cause, and the pattern is benign. Variable decelerations are abrupt decreases in the baseline that are variable in shape and timing (many are shaped like Vs or Ws) and are caused by cord compression. The pattern is nonreassuring when the decelerations are deep and repetitive and when other signs of fetal compromise are present (i.e., absent variability and changing baseline). Late decelerations are gradual decreases in the FHR that are offset from the uterine contraction (i.e., they are late in timing). Late decelerations indicate uteroplacental insufficiency and are nonreassuring.

➤ No intervention is required for early decelerations, other than continued monitoring. Nursing interventions for variable decelerations are aimed at relieving cord compression and include maternal position change or amnioinfusion. Late decelerations require aggressive management. The woman is positioned on either side, oxygen is started via face mask, and any oxytocin infusion is discontinued. Sometimes, tocolytics are prescribed to decrease the frequency and duration of uterine contractions, which improves blood flow to the placenta.

➤ Fetal stimulation is another way to measure how well the fetus is tolerating the stress of labor. It can be done noninvasively with an acoustic vibrator or invasively during a vaginal examination. An increase in the FHR with stimulation is reassuring.

➤ Fetal scalp sampling is an invasive procedure that provides direct evidence of fetal status via the pH. Disadvantages include that it requires that the membranes be ruptured and there is a small chance that fetal and maternal blood will intermingle and lead to incompatibilities.

➤ Fetal pulse oximetry gives direct evidence of fetal oxygenation without being directly invasive to the fetus; however, its use has fallen out of favor.

➤ The latent phase of the first stage of labor is marked by feelings of excitement as well as by anticipatory anxiety and fear. Teaching about the labor process can help reduce anxiety. Distraction techniques are helpful in facilitating coping.

➤ Contractions become more frequent and stronger during the active phase of labor. Distraction techniques typically do not help during active labor. Support of the woman and her partner include encouragement to continue behaviors that promote coping and assistance in finding alternative approaches when coping is ineffective. Reinforcing breathing techniques and rituals can be helpful.

➤ The transition phase is the most intense phase of labor. The woman becomes irritable and less cooperative. Assist the woman to rest between contractions and to avoid pushing efforts until the cervix is fully dilated.

➤ Full dilation of the cervix marks the beginning of the second stage of labor. Because the woman can now participate actively by pushing, she often feels re-energized to deal effectively with the labor. The open-glottis or natural method of pushing is recommended. Encouragement and reinforcement of pushing techniques are helpful nursing interventions.

➤ The placenta is delivered in the third stage of labor. Monitor for signs of placental separation and ensure that the fundus remains contracted after the placenta delivers. Risk for trauma from birth-related complications is an appropriate nursing diagnosis.

➤ During the fourth stage of labor, or the recovery period, the risk for hemorrhage is high. Close monitoring of the fundus, lochia, and vital signs is warranted. Risk for deficient fluid volume and risk for birth-related trauma are priority nursing diagnoses.

INTERNET RESOURCES

www.childbirth.org
www.childbirth.org/articles/labor.html
http://americanpregnancy.org/labornbirth/index.htm

www.thebabycorner.com (Click on the Pregnancy tab, then click on the Labor & Childbirth link.)
www.4woman.gov/pregnancy/childbirthandbeyond/laborandbirth.cfm

Workbook

■ NCLEX-STYLE REVIEW QUESTIONS

1. A woman presents to the labor suite and states, "I have water leaking down my legs." What assessment is most appropriate in this situation?

   a. Reflexes
   b. Fern test
   c. Blood pressure check
   d. Urine test for protein

2. A primipara is dilated 8 cm and is completely effaced at a +1 station. She tells the nurse, "I can't keep myself from pushing when I have a contraction." What intervention is most appropriate in this situation?

   a. Offer comfort measures.
   b. Reapply the fetal monitor.
   c. Assist the woman to blow at the peak of contractions.
   d. Tell the coach that it is not good for the baby if she pushes right now.

3. A G1 P0 is in the active phase of labor. She is a low-risk patient. You evaluate the fetal monitor strip at 10:00 a.m. Moderate variability is present. The FHR is in the 130s with occasional accelerations, no decelerations. At what time do you need to re-evaluate the FHR?

   a. 10:05 a.m.
   b. 10:15 a.m.
   c. 10:30 a.m.
   d. 11:00 a.m.

4. A G3 P2 with no apparent risk factors presents to the labor and delivery suite in early labor. She refuses the fetal monitor. She says that she delivered her second baby at home without a monitor and everything went well. How do you plan to handle this situation?

   a. Explain that she will need to be on the monitor for a few minutes to be certain this baby is doing well. After this initial assessment, the baby can then be monitored intermittently.
   b. Insist that the fetal monitor be used because there are not enough staff members to adequately monitor her using any other method.
   c. Request that the charge nurse reassign you to another patient because you do not want to be responsible if anything were to happen to her baby during labor.
   d. Tell her that it is her decision, but continuous EFM is the only recommended way to monitor how well her baby is doing during labor.

5. It is most likely that the physician would consider performing an amnioinfusion if the EFM tracing shows which of the following?

   a. Consistent early decelerations, variability present, and occasional accelerations.
   b. Flat line without variability and no decelerations.
   c. Occasional mild variable decelerations and moderate variability present.
   d. Deep variable decelerations with every contraction.

■ STUDY ACTIVITIES

1. Choose what you think are the three most important nursing assessments and interventions during labor. Using the table below, compare your top three picks for the laboring woman during the active phase, transition phase, and the second stage of labor. Include the frequency of the interventions. What similarities do you see? What differences are apparent?

Active Phase	Transition Phase	Second Stage
Major nursing assessments		
Major nursing interventions		

2. Run a search on the Internet using the key words "birth plans." How many sites returned? After exploring some of the sites, what are the main issues covered in a birth plan? Does a birth plan seem realistic to use if the woman intends to deliver in the hospital? Why or why not?

3. Interview a labor and delivery nurse. Ask her how her facility handles birth plans. Does she recall a time when parts of the birth plan could not be honored? How was the situation handled? What was the outcome?

■ CRITICAL THINKING: WHAT WOULD YOU DO?

Apply your knowledge of the labor process and the nurse's role during labor and birth to the following situation.

1. Priscilla, a 26-year-old G1 P0, presents to the birthing center because her "labor pains" have begun. She talks excitedly with her husband, who is to be her coach. She says that she is pleased that the happy day is finally here, but she is afraid that she will "lose it" when the contractions get stronger. She

and her husband have attended childbirth preparation classes.

a. What nursing assessments should be completed?
b. What phase/stage of labor do you suspect Priscilla is in?
c. What do you expect the vaginal examination will reveal?
d. What nursing interventions will you implement for Priscilla and her husband?
e. How would your care be different if the couple had not attended childbirth classes?

2. Several hours after admission to the birthing center, Priscilla is dilated 5 cm and the cervix is completely effaced. When a contraction begins, Priscilla kneels on the bed, rests her upper body against her husband, closes her eyes, and sways slowly while humming softly. At the end of the contraction, her husband gently places her on her side and she rests with her eyes closed until the next contraction begins.

a. What phase/stage of labor is Priscilla in?
b. What nursing assessments need to be completed at this time?
c. What is your assessment of Priscilla's coping technique?
d. What nursing actions are appropriate for Priscilla and her partner at this point in her labor?

3. Three hours later, Priscilla becomes agitated and snaps at her husband and the nurse. She exclaims, "I can't stand this anymore! I want to go *home*!"

a. What nursing assessments should be completed at this time? Why?

b. What nursing interventions are appropriate for Priscilla and her husband now?
c. How would you decide whether or not your interventions had been effective?

4. It is the beginning of your shift. The charge nurse gives you a report on Martha Brown, a 29-year-old G2 P1. The fetus is in a vertex presentation, and the water bag is intact. A vaginal examination was done 1 hour previously. At that time, her cervix was 4 cm dilated and 80% effaced. The station was +1, and the position was LOT. Continuous EFM is ordered, and IV fluids are infusing into her left arm.

a. What assessments do you make, in what order, when you enter Martha's room?
b. How do you evaluate the contraction pattern?

5. A few hours later, you go to check on Martha. You notice that she is much more restless than she has been. The fetal monitor tracing shows the FHR baseline in the 140s. Moderate variability is present. During each contraction, the FHR dips into the 120s. The dip is smooth with a gentle slope on both sides, like a contraction, only upside down. The FHR is back to 140 by the end of the contraction. You do perineal care because Martha has a lot of bloody show.

a. How do you interpret the FHR pattern? Is the pattern reassuring or nonreassuring? Defend your answer.
b. What should your next action be? Why?

11 Assisted Delivery and Cesarean Birth

KEY TERMS

amniotomy
Bishop score
cesarean birth
chorioamnionitis
elective induction
episiotomy
fetal fibronectin
forceps
laminaria
perioperative period
time out

LEARNING OBJECTIVES

On completion of this chapter, you should be able to:

1. Identify medical indications for induction of labor.
2. Explain methods practitioners use to determine labor readiness.
3. Contrast mechanical methods for hastening cervical readiness with pharmacologic methods.
4. Describe the procedure for artificial rupture of membranes.
5. Outline essential steps and possible complications associated with oxytocin induction.
6. Discuss important issues and considerations associated with episiotomy.
7. Compare mediolateral and midline episiotomies.
8. Describe indications, risks, and medical and nursing considerations for vacuum extraction and forceps-assisted delivery.
9. Name the most common and less common indications for cesarean birth.
10. Explain maternal and fetal complications of cesarean delivery.
11. Differentiate between vertical and transverse skin and uterine incisions.
12. List the responsibilities of each member of the surgical team throughout the perioperative period for a cesarean delivery.
13. Compare nursing interventions needed to prepare a family for a planned cesarean birth with those for a family who is to undergo emergency cesarean delivery.
14. Discuss the controversy surrounding vaginal birth after cesarean (VBAC).
15. Explain important medical and nursing considerations for a woman undergoing attempted VBAC.

THERE ARE many techniques and tools available to the birth attendant to decrease the risk of labor and/or birth to the woman and her fetus. Induction techniques are used to initiate labor, if delivery is indicated. Some tools allow the primary care provider to intervene during labor when conditions arise that threaten the safety of the woman or her fetus. The birth attendant also has tools to assist the delivery, if needed. Many of these options help avoid cesarean delivery, which subjects the woman and her fetus to all the hazards of major surgery.

Before the advent of surgical asepsis and antibiotics, if a laboring woman could not deliver a child vaginally, there were few options available to the physician or midwife. Sometimes, the woman died. Other times, extreme measures became necessary and the unborn child's life

was sacrificed to save the life of the mother. Today, cesarean birth is available if other options do not work or the risk of vaginal delivery outweighs the risk of surgical intervention.

All of the procedures discussed in this chapter carry risk. Many of these procedures are done to correct problems discussed in Chapter 18. Although many of these techniques are frequently used, they should never be considered routine.

INDUCTION OF LABOR

When a condition exists that could endanger the life of the woman or the fetus, the physician may elect to induce labor, rather than wait for nature to take its course. The rate of induced labors has risen dramatically over

Table 11-1 ▌ BISHOP SCORING SYSTEM

Score	Factor				
	Dilatation (cm)	Effacement (%)	Station*	Cervical Consistency	Cervical Position
0	Closed	0–30	−3	Firm	Posterior
1	1–2	40–50	−2	Medium	Midposition
2	3–4	60–70	−1.0	Soft	Anterior
3	≥5	≥80	+1, +2		

*Station reflects a −3 to +3 scale.
Adapted with permission from Bishop, E. H. (1964). Pelvic scoring for elective induction. *Obstet Gynecol,* (24), 266–268.

the past few years (Wing, 2007a). There are many reasons for this rise, although one contributing factor seems to be an increase in the number of elective inductions. An **elective induction** is one in which the physician and woman decide to induce labor in the absence of a medical reason to do so. Simpson and Thorman (2005) caution against elective induction unless the woman understands that elective inductions often result in more interventions, longer labors, higher costs, and possible cesarean birth.

Indications

Induction of labor is medically indicated when there is a condition that threatens the well-being of the woman or the fetus if the pregnancy were to continue. There are many such conditions. Postdate pregnancy, a pregnancy that persists beyond the expected due date, is probably the most common reason that labor is induced. Premature rupture of membranes, spontaneous rupture of membranes without the onset of spontaneous labor; **chorioamnionitis,** infection of the fetal membranes; gestational hypertension; and preeclampsia are obstetric complications that often require labor induction. Other examples include severe intrauterine fetal growth restriction or maternal medical conditions, such as diabetes mellitus or gestational diabetes. Sometimes, labor is induced in an attempt to avoid an unattended delivery. For example, a woman who has a history of rapid labors and who lives far away from the hospital or birthing center may have labor induced at or near term. In any case, the practitioner weighs the risks of allowing the pregnancy to continue against the risks of labor induction when trying to decide whether to induce labor.

Contraindications

Conditions in which spontaneous labor is contraindicated are also contraindications for the induction of labor. For example, complete placenta previa, history of a classical uterine incision, structural abnormalities of the pelvis, and invasive cervical cancer are maternal contraindications for both spontaneous and induced labor. Fetal contraindications include certain anomalies such as hydrocephalus, certain fetal malpresentations, and fetal compromise. Certain medical conditions that necessitate a cesarean delivery, such as active genital herpes, preclude labor induction (Briggs & Wan, 2006).

Labor Readiness

Cervical readiness is generally a prerequisite for successful labor induction. A cervix that is favorable for induction is called a "ripe" cervix. One commonly used scoring method to determine cervical readiness is the **Bishop score** (Table 11-1). Five factors are evaluated: cervical consistency, position, dilation, effacement, and fetal station. Each factor is given a score of 0 to 3: The higher the score, the greater the chance that induction will be successful. In general, a score of 8 or greater is associated with a favorable response to oxytocin-induced labor; that is the cervix is soft, in an anterior position, partially dilated and effaced, with an engaged fetus. A Bishop score of 5 or less indicates an unripe or unfavorable cervix, and labor induction is less likely to be successful (Briggs & Wan, 2006).

One relatively new method for predicting labor readiness is determination of cervical length by endovaginal ultrasound (see Chapter 7). A cervix that measures 27 mm in length (or less) is associated with a favorable induction rate, even in the presence of a low Bishop score (Daskalakis et al., 2006).

Another newer method for determining labor readiness is measurement of fetal fibronectin levels. **Fetal fibronectin** is a protein found in fetal membranes and amniotic fluid. Its presence in cervical secretions is associated with labor readiness. The test consists of swabbing the cervical area during a speculum examination to obtain a secretion sample. The sample is then sent to a laboratory to test for fetal fibronectin levels. However, this test is not done widely to determine labor readiness at term; it is more often used as a predictor of preterm labor risk.

In addition to cervical readiness, the fetus should be mature before labor induction, unless a condition exists in which the risks of continued pregnancy outweigh the risks of prematurity. Fetal maturity can be assessed in several ways. If the pregnancy has completed at least 38 weeks' gestation (as determined by reliable dating methods), the fetus is considered to be mature. The date that fetal heart tones were first audible and other pregnancy milestones can help validate fetal maturity. Fetal lung maturity is the major point of consideration. Measuring the lecithin/sphingomyelin (L/S) ratio via amniocentesis assesses lung maturity. An L/S ratio greater than 2.0 or a positive phosphatidyl glycerol test indicates fetal lung maturity.

Cervical Ripening

Frequently a medical reason exists for labor induction, but the cervix is not ready. In this situation, the practitioner may perform a procedure to ripen the cervix before induction with oxytocin. The following discussion explores mechanical and pharmacologic methods used to ripen a cervix in preparation for labor induction.

Mechanical Methods

One of the most common mechanical methods used to hasten cervical readiness is a procedure called "membrane stripping." The practitioner inserts a gloved finger through the internal cervical os and sweeps the finger 360 degrees to separate the membranes from the lower uterine segment. Plasma levels of prostaglandins (one substance associated with the onset of labor) are measurably higher after membrane stripping. Several research studies support the efficacy of membrane stripping at term to initiate spontaneous labor and decrease the use of oxytocin without increasing the risk of maternal infection or likelihood of cesarean birth (Wing, 2007a).

The practitioner may choose to dilate the cervix mechanically by inserting a catheter into the cervix and inflating the 30 to 80 mL balloon with normal saline. The practitioner pulls the catheter back until the balloon rests securely against the cervical os. Mechanical dilation can be accomplished with or without infusion of normal saline, a procedure known as extra-amnionic saline infusion, although the addition of saline does not increase the likelihood of success (Wing 2007c).

Laminaria, or cervical dilators, are sometimes used to soften and dilate the cervix. Laminaria are made from the root of seaweed. Synthetic products, a hygroscopic cervical dilator (Dilapan) and an osmotic cervical dilator (Lamicel), are also available. They work in much the same way as the seaweed laminaria. The practitioner places the cylindrical material in the cervix. The laminaria slowly expand as they absorb moisture, a process that dilates the cervix gradually. Synthetic dilators are removed in 6 to 8 hours, whereas laminaria stay in for 12 to 24 hours. The most common diagnoses for which laminaria are used are to induce abortion for therapeutic and elective reasons or to induce labor when the fetus has died in utero (Wing, 2007c). Few scientific studies have been done to evaluate the usefulness of laminaria for induction of labor at term, although some practitioners use them for this purpose.

Pharmacologic Methods

Locally applied prostaglandins are effective in preparing an unripe cervix for labor. There are two main preparations, although the only substance approved by the U.S. Food and Drug Administration (FDA) for this purpose is prostaglandin E_2 gel or vaginal inserts (dinoprostone). Prostaglandin E_1 (misoprostol) is used frequently for cervical ripening, although it is not approved for this use.

Prostaglandin E_2 (Dinoprostone)

There are two preparations of prostaglandin E_2 available for use: prostaglandin E_2 gel (Prepidil) and prostaglandin E_2 vaginal inserts (Cervidil). Prepidil comes in a 2.5-mL syringe that dispenses 0.5 mg of dinoprostone. The practitioner injects this preparation into the cervix. Cervidil is a time-release preparation available as a 10-mg vaginal insert that the practitioner places into the posterior fornix during a vaginal examination. The insert stays in place until spontaneous labor ensues, or for at least 12 hours. One advantage of Cervidil over Prepidil is that Cervidil can be removed by pulling on the string that is left in the vagina if uterine hyperstimulation occurs (Wing, 2007c).

The woman receiving dinoprostone should be in a facility that has continuous fetal monitoring capabilities. Assist the registered nurse (RN) to place the fetal monitor and run a tracing for at least 20 minutes to obtain a reactive nonstress test. When the practitioner is ready, bring the medication to the bedside and assist with a vaginal examination. Instruct the woman about the importance of lying in a recumbent position (do not forget to put a wedge under one hip) for at least 30 minutes. Continue the fetal monitor tracing, as ordered (usually for 30 minutes to 2 hours), and monitor for signs of uterine hyperstimulation or fetal distress.

Prostaglandin E_2 is usually administered in the evening. Sometimes the woman is allowed to go home and return when labor ensues. However, many practitioners prefer to keep the woman in the delivery suite overnight and begin oxytocin induction of labor in the morning (6–12 hours after dinoprostone is applied).

Prostaglandin E_1 (Misoprostol)

The synthetic prostaglandin E_1 analog misoprostol (Cytotec) is an antiulcer agent whose properties promote cervical ripening. It is available in a 100-mcg tablet that must be divided. The practitioner or a specially trained nurse places one quarter of the tablet (25 mcg) in the posterior vaginal fornix. The dose can be repeated every 3 to 6 hours. Sometimes a higher dosing protocol (1/2 tablet or 50 mcg) is used. However, the higher dose is associated with more cases of uterine hyperstimulation and fetal distress; therefore, many practitioners do not use it. The woman can also take misoprostol (Cytotec) orally. One 100-mcg tablet by mouth yields results similar to the 25-mcg vaginal dose. Research is ongoing into other routes of administration, such as buccal and sublingual (Wing, 2007c). Nursing care for the woman receiving misoprostol is similar to that described for dinoprostone.

Artificial Rupture of Membranes

Artificial rupture of membranes, also known as an **amniotomy,** can be done to induce labor or to augment labor that has already begun. The practitioner introduces a hard plastic instrument with a hook on the end, an Amnihook, into the vagina during a digital examination. The practitioner then guides the instrument through the cervix with two fingers and uses the hook to snag a hole in the membranes. At this point, amniotic fluid is usually expelled. This process causes the body to release prostaglandins, which enhances labor.

Oxytocin Induction

Intravenous oxytocin (Pitocin), a synthetic form of the posterior pituitary hormone that causes the uterus to contract, is the most common agent used for labor induction. The woman is admitted to a labor and delivery suite and the external fetal monitor is attached. After at least 20 minutes of fetal monitoring to obtain a baseline fetal heart assessment, a mainline intravenous (IV) line is started and oxytocin is connected as a secondary IV line. An infusion pump is required for oxytocin administration to ensure precise control of the dose. One common protocol is to place 10 U of oxytocin in 1,000 mL of IV fluid. Using this protocol, 6 mL/hr is equal to a dose of 1 mU/min. The practitioner usually orders upward titration of the dose by 1 to 2 mU every 15 to 20 minutes until an adequate contraction pattern develops.

Several potential complications are associated with the use of oxytocin for inducing labor. There is a higher risk that a cesarean birth will become necessary whenever labor is induced (Witter & Devoe, 2005). This is particularly true for primigravidas (Simpson & Thorman, 2005). There is also a risk that the uterus will be hyperstimulated. Hyperstimulation leads to contractions that occur one after the other without a sufficient rest period in between. This can lead to fetal distress and even uterine rupture. Another potential complication is water intoxication (Briggs & Wan, 2006). Because oxytocin is a posterior pituitary hormone, it is related chemically to antidiuretic hormone. Therefore, oxytocin can have an antidiuretic effect, causing the kidneys to retain water. Symptoms of water intoxication include hyponatremia, confusion, convulsions, or coma. Congestive heart failure and death also can occur.

Nursing Care

The licensed practical/vocational nurse's (LPN/LVN's) role during induction depends upon the procedure. The RN maintains responsibility for monitoring the woman and her fetus during pharmacologic cervical ripening procedures and oxytocin induction and augmentation. However, as the LPN/LVN, you may be asked to assist the birth attendant during a pelvic examination in which mechanical methods of cervical ripening are used (i.e., membrane stripping and laminaria insertion), or during amniotomy. When assisting with amniotomy, document the fetal heart rate before and after the procedure. Notify the RN or birth attendant if the rate drops precipitously. Sometimes, the birth attendant will ask for suprapubic or fundal pressure during the procedure. It is permissible to give this assistance, if you have been properly trained to do so.

Test Yourself

✔ Name two medical indications for the induction of labor.
✔ Which locally applied prostaglandin is approved by the FDA for cervical ripening?
✔ List two major complications associated with labor induction.

ASSISTED DELIVERY

Sometimes a problem develops in one of the essential components toward the end of labor. The fetus may descend to the pelvic floor without rotating to the anterior position, or the mother may become tired and stop pushing effectively. In cases such as these, the birth attendant may elect to use an operative technique or device to hasten the delivery. Types of assisted delivery include episiotomy, vacuum-assisted delivery, and forceps delivery. Another name for instrument-assisted vaginal delivery (vacuum and forceps) is operative vaginal birth. The surgeon may employ either instrument during cesarean birth as well, although the following discussion focuses on operative vaginal birth.

Episiotomy

An **episiotomy** is a surgical incision made into the perineum to enlarge the vaginal opening just before the baby is born. In the recent past, physicians performed episiotomies on virtually all primigravidas delivered in the United States. The American College of Obstetricians and Gynecologists (ACOG) discourages the routine use of this procedure. Even so, at least 25% of women who deliver in the United States have an episiotomy (ACOG, 2006b).

Previously, the pervasive medical opinion was that an episiotomy was less painful and healed faster than a jagged tear that might result without an episiotomy. However, research has not validated these assumptions (Viswanathan et al., 2005). In fact, research studies demonstrate that an episiotomy increases the risk that the perineum will tear into the anal sphincter, a condition

> ### Box 11-1 ▌ METHODS TO MINIMIZE THE NEED FOR EPISIOTOMY
>
> - Prenatal perineal massage
> - Using natural pushing techniques, particularly in the side-lying position
> - Patience with the delivery process
> - Warm compresses to the perineum during second stage of labor
> - Delivering the fetal head between contractions
> - Protection of the perineum immediately before birth (by the birth attendant) to avoid uncontrolled delivery of the fetal head

that increases maternal discomfort as well as the risk of infection and long-term consequences, such as anal incontinence. In addition, episiotomy increases the risk of blood loss immediately after delivery and contributes to painful sex in the months following delivery (Robinson, 2007). Box 11-1 lists several measures that can reduce the need for episiotomy.

However, episiotomy is appropriate in certain situations. These include:

- The baby's shoulders are stuck in the birth canal after the head is born (shoulder dystocia).
- The head will not rotate from an occiput-posterior position (persistent occiput-posterior).
- The fetus is in a breech presentation.
- Instruments (forceps or vacuum) are used to shorten the second stage of labor.

There are two basic types of episiotomies (Fig. 11-1). A median or midline episiotomy extends from the fourchette straight down into the true perineum. This type of episiotomy increases the risk for extension into the anal sphincter but is easier for the physician to repair than a mediolateral episiotomy, which angles to the right or left of the perineum.

The perineum requires repair after an episiotomy. If the woman had epidural anesthesia, she may not need additional anesthesia for repair. Frequently, the practitioner uses local anesthesia to numb the perineum for repair. Have suture readily available according to the physician or nurse midwife preference. Reassure the woman that the sutures are absorbable and do not need to be removed.

Vacuum-Assisted Delivery

A device sometimes used to hasten delivery is the vacuum extractor. In this procedure, the birth attendant places a suction cup (some are soft silicone cups and others are hard metal cups) on the fetal head and applies suction. The practitioner then uses the device to gently guide the delivery of the fetal head (Fig. 11-2). Nursing responsibilities include providing the necessary equipment, connecting and regulating the suction as instructed by the birth attendant, monitoring fetal status, and supporting the laboring woman during the procedure by keeping her informed of the procedure and progress.

Vacuum-assisted delivery is not without risk. Serious neonatal complications, such as scalp trauma, subgaleal and intracranial hemorrhage, and even death, can occur (Mahlmeister, 2005). The risk increases with the amount of pressure used and the number of times the suction cup suddenly loses suction, commonly called a "pop-off." One important nursing function is to keep the birth attendant apprised of the number of "pop-offs" and total length of time vacuum is in place. Pressures should not exceed 600 mm Hg, there should not be more than three to four pop-offs, and the vacuum should not be applied for longer than 20 to 30 minutes (Greenberg, 2006; Pope & O'Grady, 2006).

A

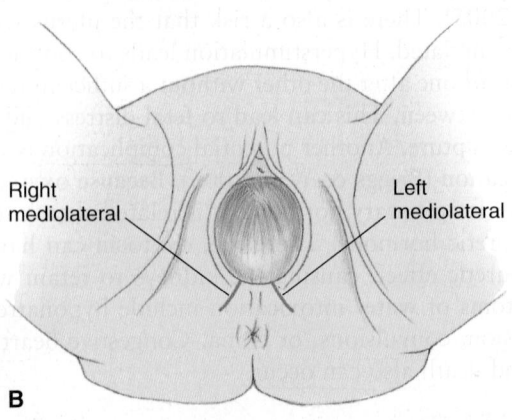

B

Right mediolateral

Left mediolateral

▌ **Figure 11-1** Two basic types of episiotomy. **(A)** Midline episiotomy extends straight down into the true perineum. **(B)** Mediolateral episiotomy angles to the right or the left of the perineum.

A   **B**

▮ **Figure 11-2** Delivery assisted by vacuum extraction. **(A)** The birth attendant has just placed the suction cup on the fetal head and is using the hand pump to increase the pressure. **(B)** Gentle traction is placed on the fetal head to assist it through the last maneuvers of delivery.

A Personal Glimpse

When I was pregnant with my second child, I re-read everything about the experience: the pregnancy, the delivery, the recovery, and nursing. Having had one healthy baby before this one, I felt like I was prepared for what was going to happen in the whole process of delivering a baby.

When my water broke at 4 a.m. on a Saturday, my husband and I rushed to the hospital. The vaginal delivery went well and quickly. However, after our little girl was born, I was told that I had been given an "episiotomy." Of course during the delivery, I was numb from the epidural, and I really had no idea what had gone on other than being told to push numerous times. The nurse left me some cotton pads and told me to keep myself clean until the stitches "melted."

The area of the episiotomy caused me a lot of pain. Every time I sat on the toilet to urinate, my vaginal area would hurt. I would avoid having bowel movements, as those were very painful as well. When I told the nurses about how much it hurt, they would tell me to clean myself better after urinating and got a doctor to prescribe me a stool softener to take home.

It wasn't until I was discharged and my mother was staying at home with me to help out that we figured out what the problem was. I asked my mother to look at my vaginal area, and she saw that one of the stitches had a knot that had irritated the skin around it and caused a sore.

It would have been better if one of the nurses had looked for me (with my giant belly after the delivery, I couldn't see a thing) and figured out what the problem was before I had left the hospital.

Shelly

Learning Opportunity: Discuss two actions the nurse could take to better prepare this new mother to understand how to take care of her episiotomy. What assessments do you think the nurse should make for a patient with an episiotomy?

Forceps-Assisted Delivery

Forceps are metal instruments with curved, blunted blades (somewhat like large hollowed-out spoons) that are placed around the head of the fetus by the birth attendant to facilitate delivery (Fig. 11-3). Low and outlet forceps are more common than are midforceps. Outlet forceps are applied when the fetal head can be seen at the introitus; low forceps are used when the station is equal to or greater than +2, but the head is not yet showing on the perineum; whereas, midforceps are used when the fetal head is well engaged but still relatively high in the pelvis (higher than +2). Midforceps are most often used to assist the fetus to rotate to an anterior position.

Prerequisites and indications for use of forceps and the vacuum extractor are similar. Prerequisites include complete cervical dilation, ruptured amniotic sac, engaged fetal head, satisfactory maternal anesthesia, and the

▮ **Figure 11-3** Forceps-assisted delivery.

woman consents to the procedure (Wegner & Bernstein, 2007). Any problem that causes the second stage of delivery to be prolonged or any situation of concern that is likely to be relieved by delivery of the infant may be an indication for assisted delivery. Maternal indications include fatigue (the woman may become exhausted while pushing); certain chronic conditions, such as heart or lung disease; and prolonged second stage of labor. If the fetal strip is nonreassuring and the woman is a candidate for forceps delivery, then the birth attendant may use forceps to deliver the infant rapidly.

Complications of Operative Vaginal Delivery

Because operative vaginal delivery is invasive, there are associated risks. Neonatal cephalhematoma, retinal, subdural, and subgaleal hemorrhage occur more frequently with vacuum extraction than with forceps. Facial bruising, facial nerve injury, skull fractures, and seizures are more common with forceps. The woman is at higher risk to have episiotomy and for extension of episiotomy into the anal sphincter with operative vaginal delivery. Other maternal complications include uterine rupture, perineal pain, lacerations, hematomas, urinary retention, anemia, and rehospitalization (Ross & Beall, 2007; Wegner & Bernstein, 2007).

Nursing Care

Nursing responsibilities during an assisted delivery include obtaining needed equipment and supplies; monitoring maternal and fetal status before, during, and after the procedure; assisting the birth attendant; providing support for the woman; and documenting the type of procedure, as well as maternal and fetal response. Be aware that use of a technique to assist vaginal delivery may not work and anticipate the possibility of cesarean delivery. Episiotomy care after delivery is discussed in Chapter 12.

For both vacuum-assisted and forceps-assisted deliveries (operative vaginal deliveries), inspect the infant carefully for signs of trauma. This could include cephalhematoma, retinal hemorrhage, bruising, edema, exaggerated caput (chignon), forceps mark, and transient facial paralysis. Reassure the parents that forceps marks and exaggerated caput (chignon) from vacuum-assisted deliveries will subside in a few days.

Maternal soft-tissue trauma may also result from an operative vaginal delivery. Inspect the perineum for bruising and edema. Monitor closely for excessive bleeding or development of a hematoma. (See Chapter 19 for

Tell the whole story!

It is critical to inform the postpartum and nursery nurses that the birth was instrument-assisted. Complications, although rare, may not appear until several hours after birth. Your report alerts caregivers to monitor for complications.

nursing care of the woman with postpartum hemorrhage.) Monitor for urinary retention.

Test Yourself

✔ Name two situations in which an episiotomy is helpful.

✔ List at least two fetal complications and one maternal complication of forceps or vacuum-assisted delivery.

CESAREAN BIRTH

A **cesarean birth** is the delivery of a fetus through abdominal and uterine incisions: laparotomy and hysterotomy, respectively. Cesarean comes from the Latin word "caedere," meaning, "to cut." Sometimes, the term "cesarean section" is used. This discussion uses the terms "cesarean birth" and "cesarean delivery" because the focus for the nurse and the woman is the birth experience.

Indications

There are many indications for cesarean birth. The majority (more than 80%) are done for the following four reasons (Capeless & Damron, 2007):

1. History of previous cesarean (or other uterine incision)
2. Labor dystocia (failure to progress in labor)
3. Nonreassuring fetal status
4. Fetal malpresentation

Other less common obstetric indications include placenta previa (placenta covers the cervix), abruptio placentae (placenta separates from the uterus before birth), cephalopelvic disproportion (fetal head cannot fit through the pelvis), active vaginal herpes lesions, prolapse of the umbilical cord, and ruptured uterus. Sometimes medical and obstetric conditions necessitate early delivery of the fetus and require cesarean delivery. Examples include maternal diabetes mellitus, preeclampsia, and erythroblastosis fetalis.

Incidence

Birth by cesarean was rare before the development of antibiotics and antiseptic surgical techniques because of high maternal mortality rates from infection. Currently, this method of delivery is highly accepted. The rate of cesarean deliveries quadrupled (from 4.5% to 22.8%) between 1965 and 1988 (Cunningham et al., 2005a). From 1988 to 1996, the rate fell, attributable in large part to a decrease in the rate of primary cesarean births and an increase in the number of vaginal births after cesarean (VBAC). From 1996 to the present, overall cesarean rates have been steadily rising. In 2006, 31.1% of births were by cesarean delivery, the highest rate ever reported in the United States (Hamilton, Martin, & Ventura, 2007). Box 11-2 lists some of the multiple contributing factors to this dramatic increase.

Box 11-2 ■ FACTORS CONTRIBUTING TO THE RISE IN CESAREAN DELIVERIES

- Change in perception of risk by physicians and patients
- Increase in the percentage of pregnant women who are carrying their first child
- Rise in the number of older pregnant women
- More labor inductions for nonmedical reasons
- Almost universal use of continuous electronic fetal monitoring, which carries with it high false-positive indications of fetal compromise (i.e., the tracing indicates compromise when none exists)
- Trend toward delivering breech presentation through the abdomen
- Return to the adage "once a cesarean, always a cesarean"
- Increasing concerns regarding malpractice litigation
- Increased prevalence of multiple gestations
- Increased prevalence of maternal obesity
- New phenomenon of cesarean by demand (women asking for planned cesarean without medical indications)

Risks

Cesarean birth is a major surgery and carries with it all the risks associated with surgery combined with the risks of birth itself. A woman who delivers by cesarean is up to three times more likely to die than is a woman who delivers vaginally (ACOG, 2006c), although death is a rare occurrence in obstetrics. Several recent studies have found that a low-risk woman who has a scheduled cesarean delivery is three times more likely to suffer severe morbidity (illness) and twice as likely to be rehospitalized within 30 days of discharge than a low-risk woman who plans to have a vaginal birth (Declercq et al., 2007; Liu et al., 2007). The normal physiologic changes of pregnancy amplify some surgical risk factors. For example, thrombophlebitis is a complication of both surgery and pregnancy, so the risk compounds with cesarean delivery. There are risks to the fetus as well. Inadvertent delivery of a premature fetus is one cesarean risk factor. In addition, a cesarean birth increases the incidence of neonatal respiratory distress. MacDorman et al. (2006) found that newborns delivered by cesarean were twice as likely to die as newborns delivered vaginally. For these reasons, ACOG (2006c) recommends that cesarean delivery be performed only when the risks of vaginal delivery clearly outweigh the risks of surgery.

Because of the higher morbidity and mortality rates associated with cesarean delivery versus vaginal delivery, it is a national goal to decrease the cesarean delivery rate. Much research has focused on determining safe vaginal delivery methods for a woman after a previous cesarean birth and on methods to treat labor dystocia.

Maternal Complications

Maternal complications that can occur during the operation include laceration of the uterine artery, bladder, ureter, or bowel; hemorrhage requiring blood transfusion; and hysterectomy. The most common postoperative complication associated with cesarean birth is infection (Liu et al., 2007). Two common infection sites are the uterus and the surgical wound, although sepsis, urinary tract infection, and other infections also can occur. Pneumonia, postpartum hemorrhage, thrombophlebitis, and other surgical-related complications can occur during the postoperative period.

Fetal Complications

The most common fetal complications are unintended delivery of an immature fetus because of miscalculation of dates and respiratory distress because of retained lung fluid. Because a fetus delivered by scheduled cesarean birth does not go through labor, he does not have the chance to get most of the amniotic fluid squeezed out of his lungs, as does a baby born vaginally. Therefore, respiratory distress happens more frequently in these newborns. In addition, general anesthesia given to the woman can depress the fetus' respiratory drive, making it difficult for the newborn to take his or her first breath. Less commonly, fetal injury can occur. For example, the scalpel cutting through the uterine wall can nick the baby. Usually, these wounds are superficial and require minimal intervention. The fetus can become wedged in the pelvis after a prolonged second stage with the woman pushing, which can make for a difficult extraction leading to bruising and possibly other injuries.

Incision Types

There are two major incisions made during cesarean birth: one through the abdominal wall and the other into the uterus.

Abdominal Incisions

Abdominal incisions can be vertical or low transverse (Fig. 11-4). Vertical abdominal incisions are located in the midline of the lower abdomen. A low transverse incision, *Pfannenstiel's* incision, is commonly known as a "bikini cut." Although a low transverse incision slightly increases the risk for bleeding, this is usually the preferred method for cosmetic reasons.

Uterine Incisions

Uterine incisions can also be vertical or low transverse (Fig. 11-5). There are two types of vertical uterine incisions: classical and low cervical. The classical incision (Fig. 11-5A) extends through the body of the uterus to the fundus. This incision is used only in severe

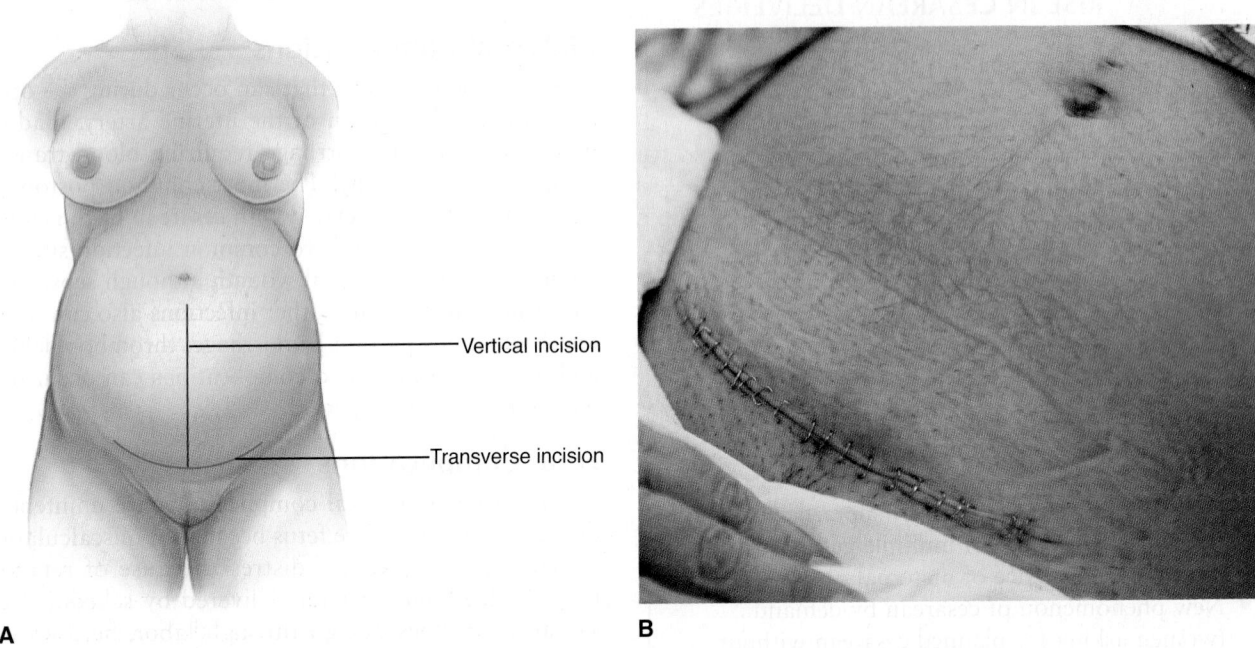

Vertical incision

Transverse incision

A

B

■ **Figure 11-4 (A)** Types of abdominal incisions used for cesarean delivery: vertical or low transverse. **(B)** Example of a low transverse abdominal incision.

emergencies, when it is critical to deliver the fetus immediately or when the fetus is unusually large. Bleeding during surgery is more likely with a classical uterine incision. It carries a higher risk for abdominal infection and the highest risk for uterine rupture in subsequent pregnancies. The low cervical vertical incision (Fig. 11-5B) is smaller and carries a lower risk for uterine rupture

than does the classical approach, but it is used infrequently because it is more complicated to perform, carries higher risk of maternal injury, and is associated with a higher risk of uterine rupture than is the low cervical transverse incision. It does have the advantage of allowing for extension of the incision into the body of the uterus, if the surgeon has difficulty extracting the fetus.

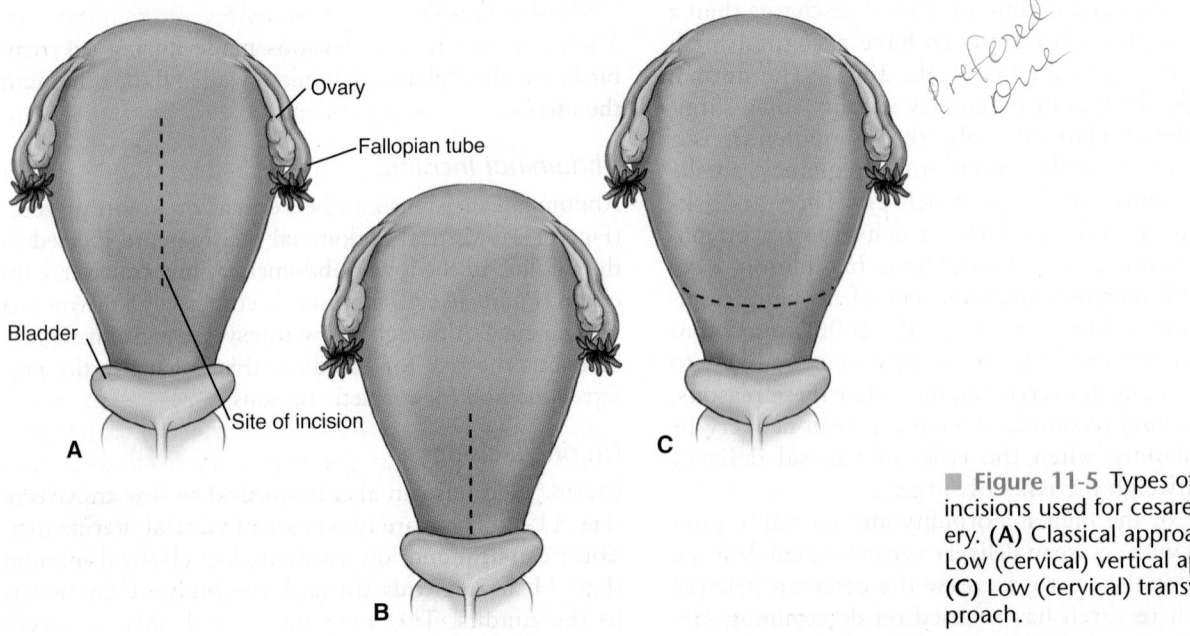

Ovary

Fallopian tube

Bladder

Site of incision

A

B

C

Preferred one

■ **Figure 11-5** Types of uterine incisions used for cesarean delivery. **(A)** Classical approach. **(B)** Low (cervical) vertical approach. **(C)** Low (cervical) transverse approach.

The low cervical transverse incision (Fig. 11-5C) is the preferred method. This incision is associated with the least risk of uterine rupture, is easier to repair, and is least likely to cause adhesions (Cunningham, 2005A).

Don't get confused.
The type of skin incision does not indicate the type of uterine incision. If the woman's obstetric history is unknown, the surgeon will ask to see the previous surgical record to determine the type of uterine incision.

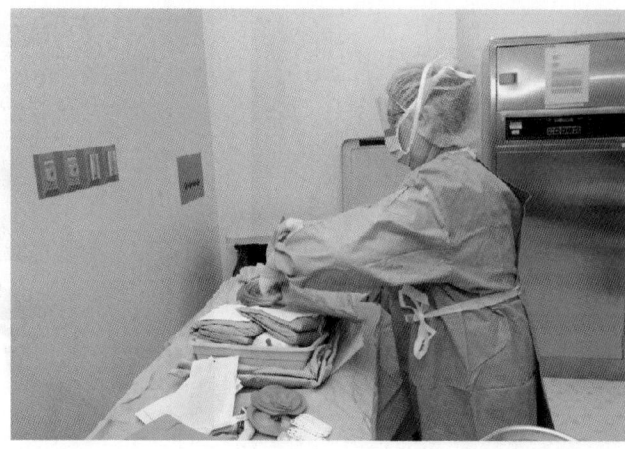

■ Figure 11-6 Cesarean birth: preoperative phase. The scrub nurse sets up the back table in preparation for cesarean delivery.

Test Yourself

✔ Cesarean delivery involves incisions into what two structures?
✔ Name three possible complications of cesarean birth.
✔ What is Pfannenstiel's incision?

Steps of a Cesarean Delivery

Because cesarean delivery involves major surgery, the period encompassing the procedure is the **perioperative period,** which has three phases: preoperative, intraoperative, and postoperative. Care of the woman during the preoperative and intraoperative phases requires a team approach, sometimes referred to as collaborative management. You may be involved in some of the preoperative care to prepare the woman for surgery. You may also be a part of the intraoperative care by functioning in the scrub nurse role. The RN usually carries out the immediate postoperative care in the postanesthesia care unit (PACU). You may assume care of the woman during the postoperative phase, after she has sufficiently recovered from anesthesia. The following sections describe and illustrate the major steps of a typical cesarean delivery. Some facilities and/or surgeons may perform the procedure slightly differently than the description that follows, but the basic principles remain the same.

Preoperative Phase

Preparing the woman for the cesarean birth is the focus of preoperative care. Nursing duties during the preoperative phase are discussed in the Nursing Care section. The anesthetist interviews the woman, explains the planned anesthesia to include risks, obtains verbal consent, reviews laboratory results, and orders preoperative medications, such as antacids and, less frequently, a sedative.

The scrub technician or nurse opens the sterile cesarean delivery pack and instruments, puts on a sterile gown and gloves, and proceeds to prepare the back table and mayo instrument stand (Fig. 11-6). The circulating RN fastens the back of the scrub nurse's gown, and together the circulating RN and scrub nurse perform an initial instrument, sponge, and sharp count. The initial and subsequent counts are extremely important to patient safety to help prevent foreign body retention (Simpson, 2007c). The scrub nurse holds accountability with the circulating RN for accuracy of counts during surgery.

The support person changes into attire (usually disposable scrub suit or a disposable gown that covers the clothes) appropriate for the operating room (OR). A surgical cap and mask complete the surgical apparel. The RN reviews the preoperative checklist and chart for completeness. A surgical cap is placed on the woman's head to cover her hair, and she is transported to the OR suite by wheelchair or stretcher, or she may ambulate to the OR.

Intraoperative Phase

The intraoperative phase begins once the woman enters the OR. The circulating nurse positions the woman on the operating table for regional anesthesia. The anesthetist may request the sitting position with the woman's legs dangling to one side, or the side-lying position. Support the woman so that her back remains in a C-shaped curve during placement of regional anesthesia by the anesthetist (Fig. 11-7A). (General anesthesia is uncommon; see Chapter 9 for nursing care for general anesthesia.)

The RN circulating nurse (circulator) and anesthetist assist the woman to the supine position on the OR table. At this point, the circulator places a wedge under one hip and inserts the Foley catheter, if one is not already in place. The circulator places a grounding pad on the woman's thigh, covers the woman's legs with a warm blanket, and secures a safety strap on the woman's legs. The circulator checks the fetal heart rate for at least 1 minute unless continuous fetal monitoring is in progress (Simpson, 2007a). The anesthetist places electrocardiogram leads, a blood pressure cuff, and pulse oximeter device and connects them to the monitoring equipment. The circulator and anesthetist position the woman's arms on arm boards and gently immobilize her wrists with soft restraints.

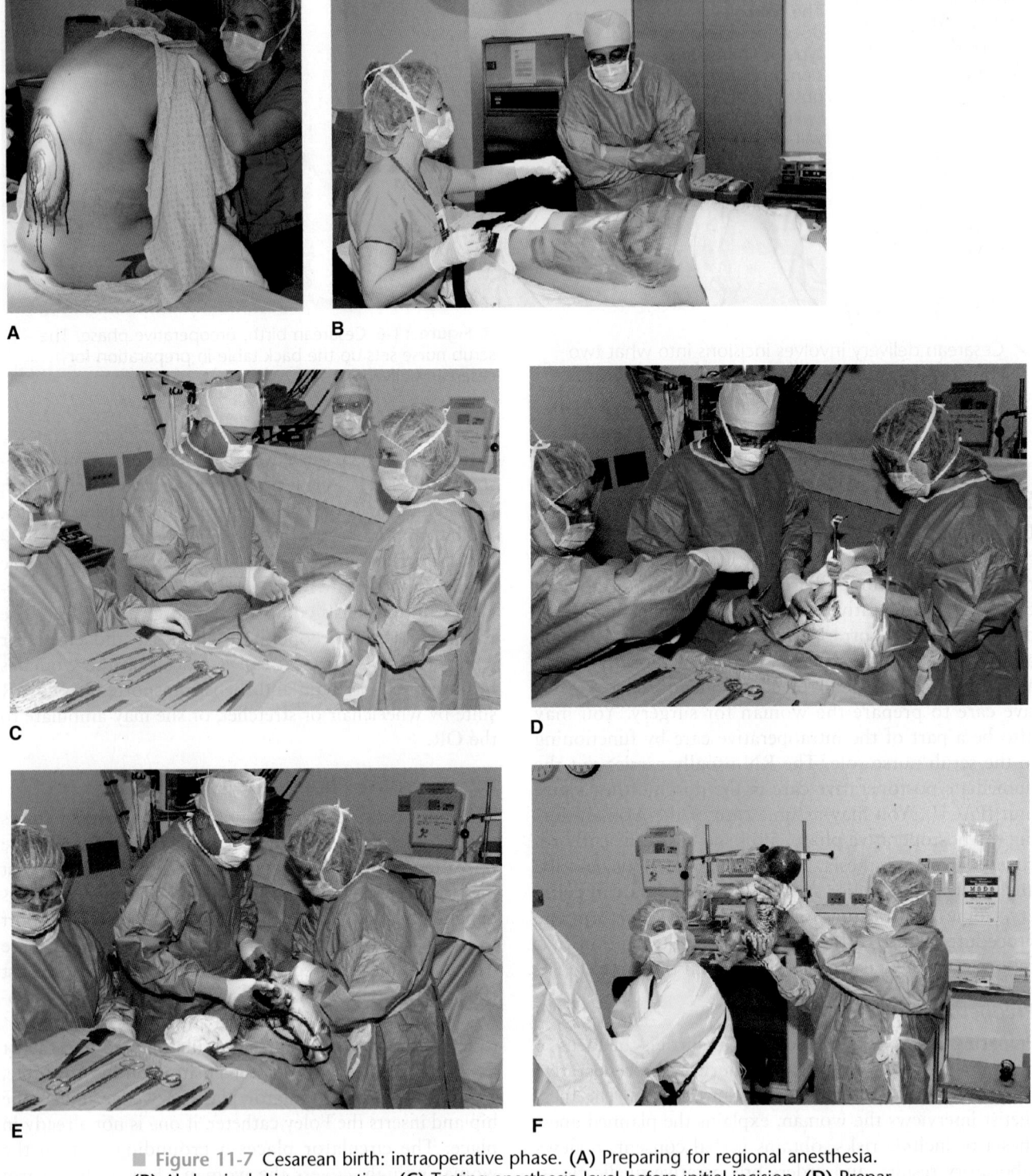

■ Figure 11-7 Cesarean birth: intraoperative phase. **(A)** Preparing for regional anesthesia. **(B)** Abdominal skin preparation. **(C)** Testing anesthesia level before initial incision. **(D)** Preparing for the uterine incision. **(E)** Delivery of fetal head. **(F)** Baby is quickly shown to the patient.

Meanwhile, the surgeon and the assistant complete a surgical scrub. The circulator performs a sterile abdominal preparation with alcohol, povidone-iodine, chlorhexidine, or other antiseptic, as per facility policy (Fig. 11-7B). The surgical team performs a **time out.** This procedure is part of the Universal Protocol developed to reduce the incidence of wrong site, wrong procedure, and wrong person surgery. The Universal Protocol emphasizes accurate patient and procedure identification and informed consent. During the time out, each member of the surgical team, which includes the patient, must agree and actively communicate his or her agreement that the right procedure is being performed on the right patient with documented informed consent before the procedure can begin.

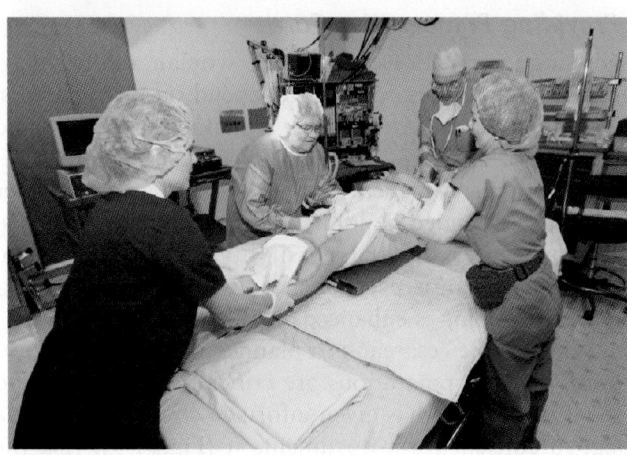

■ **Figure 11-7** *(Continued)* **(G)** The support person shows the mother her new baby. **(H)** The uterus is removed temporarily from abdominal cavity to make suturing easier. **(I)** A fallopian tube is ligated (the mother requested surgical sterilization). **(J)** Stapling the skin incision. **(K)** The surgical team moves the patient to a stretcher.

Then, the surgeon and assistant place sterile drapes on the woman. During the draping procedure, the circulator calls for the individuals who will be attending the newborn. The circulator also calls for the support person, who sits at the woman's head behind the surgical drapes.

The surgeon uses small pickup forceps to test the level of anesthesia before proceeding (Fig. 11-7C). Once the surgeon is satisfied that the anesthesia level is sufficient, the surgeon makes the initial cut and proceeds to cut

through the layers of skin, fascia, and muscle until the lower segment of the uterus is exposed (Fig. 11-7D). Then, the surgeon makes the incision into the uterus. The newborn's head is delivered (Fig. 11-7E), followed by the body. The surgeon double clamps and cuts the umbilical cord and then briefly shows the newborn to the mother and support person (Fig. 11-7F) before he or she is taken to the warmer for assessment and resuscitation, as needed. The surgeon delivers the placenta shortly after the baby is born.

When the newborn is breathing well and the skin color is pink, he is double wrapped in prewarmed blankets, a cap is placed on his head, and he is taken to the woman and support person for initial bonding (Fig. 11-7G).

The surgeon brings the fundus and body of the uterus through the incision (Fig. 11-7H) and cleans the inside thoroughly, then the uterine incision is sutured close. The circulating RN and scrub technician perform the second OR count. If the woman desires a tubal ligation, the surgeon performs the procedure at this time. The tubes are tied and ligated (Fig. 11-7I), and the specimens handed to the circulating RN, who labels them to be sent to the laboratory. The surgeon then replaces the uterus in the pelvic cavity.

Repair of muscle and fascia layers is done with absorbable suture while the third OR count is done. An x-ray should be done while the woman is still on the OR table if the counts were not done for any reason, or if there is a discrepancy between the initial and subsequent counts (Simpson, 2007c). The surgeon closes the skin with staples (Fig. 11-7J) or suture and applies a sterile dressing. Remove the drapes, massage the uterine fundus, and place a sterile perineal pad. The surgical team then moves the woman from the OR table to a stretcher (Fig. 11-7K) and transports her to the PACU for initial recovery from anesthesia.

Your voice is critical!

Never be afraid to speak up if the surgical counts are incorrect. Many patient injuries can be prevented by the scrub nurse voicing his or her concerns.

Postoperative Phase

The circulating RN gives report to the PACU RN (in labor and delivery units, the PACU RN and circulating RN may be the same individual). The RN places the woman on a cardiac monitor, an automatic blood pressure device, and a pulse oximeter (Fig. 11-8). The PACU RN performs a thorough assessment to include level of consciousness, cardiac and respiratory status, condition of the dressing,

■ Figure 11-8 Cesarean birth: postoperative phase.

fundal and lochia status, urinary output, condition and patency of IV site, pain status, and a full set of vital signs. The RN completes this assessment at least every 15 minutes for 1 hour or until the woman meets PACU discharge criteria, which varies by facility and anesthetist. The anesthetist writes orders for pain control in the PACU and usually for the first 24 hours after surgery.

Nursing Care
Providing Family Teaching for a Planned Cesarean Birth

The focus of nursing intervention for a planned cesarean is family education (see Family Teaching Tips: Preparing for a Planned Cesarean Birth). Each time you encounter the woman before surgery is an opportunity to explore with the woman and her partner what they know about cesarean delivery. Do they know the procedural steps to take, such as where to preregister, when and where to have laboratory work drawn, and when and where to present for surgery? Do they know what to expect during the surgical experience? Does the woman know how to help avoid complications in the postoperative period, such as the how and why of taking deep breaths and turning frequently while in bed, and why it is important to ambulate as soon as possible after surgery? Does she know the principles of postoperative pain control and the options that are available to her for pain relief? Teaching is more effective when it occurs over time, involves repetition of major concepts, and focuses on topics in which the family is interested.

Providing Preoperative Care

Nursing interventions to help the woman and her partner prepare for cesarean birth depend on many factors, including whether or not it is a planned procedure and whether or not the woman has experienced cesarean delivery in the past. Ideally, the woman and her partner will have attended childbirth classes. Part of class discussion centers on the possibility of cesarean birth. When a woman is psychologically prepared for the experience, coping is enhanced.

Whether the cesarean is a planned or emergent procedure, several preparations are critical. Always check to see if the woman has given informed consent and that a signed consent form documents it (Fig.11-9). Ask the woman when she last had anything to eat or drink. Follow facility and anesthetist orders regarding fasting times before surgery. Often, liquids are permissible closer to surgery time than are solids (Crenshaw & Winslow, 2006). Frequently, the anesthetist orders an antacid, such as Bicitra 30 mL, before surgery to reduce the risk of aspiration while the woman is under the effects of anesthesia. An IV must be in place with a large-bore (generally 18-gauge or lower) catheter. Lactated Ringer's is a commonly ordered IV fluid. Sometimes clippers are used to remove hair from the abdomen and perineal area. Clippers do not cause skin nicks like razors

■ **Figure 11-9** The nurse witnesses signing of the informed consent form.

can, so clippers are the preferred tool to use (Whitehouse & Sexton, 2007). A Foley catheter must be in place before the surgery begins to decrease the risk that the surgeon might inadvertently cut or puncture a full bladder during surgery. Sometimes the catheter is inserted in the preoperative area. Alternately, the circulating nurse may place it after anesthesia has been administered, which is more comfortable for the woman.

Ensure that required laboratory studies are completed. The routine complete blood count is important, as is the blood type and screen. When a type and screen is done, the laboratory holds at least 2 units of blood that matches the woman's blood type. In the event of an emergency, lab personnel complete the final steps of cross-matching so that the woman receives compatible blood if a transfusion becomes necessary. Most physicians also order other laboratory studies, such as electrolytes. When the woman is ready for surgery, assist the RN to transfer her to the operating suite and then to the operating table.

> **Remember**
> A patient can withdraw consent at any time. If she states she has changed her mind, she is not sure, or she needs more information, alert the charge nurse or physician immediately so that her concerns can be addressed.

Providing Support During an Unplanned or Emergency Cesarean Birth

When a cesarean birth becomes necessary because of an unplanned or emergency situation, move quickly to prepare the patient for surgery. The woman and her family are often anxious and worried about the baby. She may be fearful of the surgery or anesthesia, particularly if she has never had surgery before. There is usually not much time for education; therefore, support of the woman and her family becomes paramount (Nursing Care Plan 11-1).

Nursing Care Plan 11-1

THE WOMAN UNDERGOING AN UNPLANNED (EMERGENCY) CESAREAN DELIVERY*

CASE SCENARIO
Rene Truitt is a 28-year-old primigravida who went into spontaneous labor at 40 weeks' gestation. She received an epidural when her cervix progressed to 4 cm dilation and reported adequate pain relief. She progressed to full dilation and pushed for 2 hours, but the fetal head did not descend below 0 station. The fetal monitor tracing is now showing occasional late decelerations. The physician has ordered a primary cesarean delivery. Rene is voicing concern over the welfare of her baby and is crying softly. Her husband is attempting to comfort her.

NURSING DIAGNOSIS
Anxiety related to fetal status and unexpected surgical procedure.

GOAL: The woman will use positive coping strategies to decrease anxiety.

EXPECTED OUTCOMES: The woman
- Seeks information to reduce anxiety.
- Accepts her husband's offered support.
- Voices acceptance of the situation.

Nursing Interventions	*Rationale*
Remain with Rene while preparing her for surgery.	Presence of the nurse can be reassuring in a stressful situation.
Display a calm and confident manner.	Promotes trust.
Explain procedures as you perform them.	Understanding what is happening helps decrease anxiety.
Emphasize the qualifications of the surgical team (i.e., surgeon, circulating nurse, and anesthetist).	Promotes trust and confidence.
Briefly describe what Rene and her husband will experience throughout the procedure.	Understanding what to expect helps decrease anxiety.
Encourage Rene's husband to participate throughout (e.g., holding her hand, remaining with her whenever possible).	The presence of a support person can be comforting.

NURSING DIAGNOSIS
Risk for injury related to major surgical procedure.

GOAL: The woman will not experience preventable injury throughout the perioperative period.

EXPECTED OUTCOMES: The woman
- Gives informed consent for cesarean delivery.
- Maintains urinary output at 30 mL/hour or higher.
- Maintains clear yellow urine.
- Maintains adequate fluid volume.

Nursing Interventions	*Rationale*
Check the chart for signed informed consent for cesarean delivery. Obtain signed consent, if not already completed.	Although it is primarily the physician's responsibility to obtain informed consent, the signed form is evidence that the woman has consented.
Make certain that Rene and her husband have had any questions or concerns they have about the procedure addressed. If there are additional questions, notify the RN or physician immediately.	It is imperative that the woman understand the risks involved for cesarean delivery, as well as the risks involved for continuing to attempt vaginal birth.

(continued)

Nursing Care Plan 11-1 (continued)

THE WOMAN UNDERGOING AN UNPLANNED (EMERGENCY) CESAREAN DELIVERY*

Check the chart for laboratory results. If they are not on the chart, place them in the chart before surgery.	The surgical team will refer to lab results to help determine if extra safety precautions are needed.
Make certain that at least 2 units of packed red blood cells are on hold in the lab, as ordered. Alternatively, the blood should at least be typed and screened.	The woman is at increased risk for bleeding because she will be experiencing major surgery. It is imperative that blood be immediately available, in the event hemorrhage should occur.
Check the IV line for patency before surgery. Inform the RN immediately if the IV needs to be restarted.	A patent IV line with a large-bore needle must be in place before the woman can go to surgery.
Check to see if a Foley catheter is in place. If not, insert the catheter before transporting Rene to the OR suite.	A urinary catheter is necessary to keep the bladder drained. This will decrease the chance of bladder injury during surgery.

NURSING DIAGNOSIS
Risk for aspiration (maternal) related to gravid uterus pressing upward on the stomach and anesthesia for cesarean delivery.

GOAL: The woman will not experience respiratory compromise.

EXPECTED OUTCOMES: The woman
- Maintains a respiratory rate between 16 and 22 breaths/minute.
- Maintains a regular respiratory rhythm.
- Remains free from adventitious breath sounds.

Nursing Interventions	*Rationale*
Report to anesthetist the date and time of last oral intake (solid and liquid).	This information allows the anesthetist to plan how to best protect the airway during surgery.
Administer IV or PO antacids, as ordered before surgery.	Antacids decrease the acidity of stomach contents, which reduces the potential for injury from aspiration.
Assess respiratory status before and after surgery.	Preoperative assessment will determine baseline respiratory status. Postoperative assessment is done to detect changes that might be associated with aspiration.

*Note: This care plan addresses preoperative care of a woman who experiences an unplanned cesarean delivery. Postoperative nursing care is addressed in Chapter 12.

Support is shown in many ways. Explain procedures as you are doing them. If the RN or physician says the fetal monitor tracing is reassuring, reinforce this important fact to the woman and her partner. Explain what sensations she can expect to experience and what to expect next. Be empathic. Acknowledge her feelings and let her know that these feelings are normal considering the situation with which she must cope.

Providing Care in the Immediate Recovery Phase

Many factors influence nursing care in the postoperative period. Some of these factors are the type of anesthesia that was given, complications that occurred during surgery, the outcome and condition of the neonate, and stability of maternal condition.

Assist the RN to transfer the woman from the operative suite to the PACU. The RN will connect her to monitoring devices that will record the electrocardiogram, blood pressure, pulse, and oxygen saturation of the blood. The RN will also take vital sign and pulse oximetry readings every 5 minutes until the readings are stable, and then every 15 to 30 minutes until the patient has met predetermined criteria. The RN will monitor the patient's urinary output to make certain it is at least 30 mL/hr.

In addition to normal PACU activities, the RN must perform postpartum assessments. The RN evaluates the condition of the fundus and records his or her findings along with vital signs. The RN can use his or her hand or a pillow to support the incision while gently massaging the fundus to determine if it is firm. A firmly contracted uterus minimizes bleeding. In conjunction with the fundal check, the RN performs an assessment of the amount and type of lochia (discharge from the uterus after birth). The RN performs and records these assessments at the same time interval as the vital signs. (See Chapter 12 for a full discussion of postpartum assessment and nursing care.)

A word of caution is in order.
During cesarean birth, the surgeon thoroughly cleans inside the uterus. Therefore, there is less lochia flow than after a vaginal delivery. Check for postpartum hemorrhage if lochia flow is moderate or heavy.

The type of anesthesia, in large part, influences the timing and process of recovery. Chapter 9 discusses the different types of anesthesia, including recovery considerations.

VAGINAL BIRTH AFTER CESAREAN

In the past, the adage "once a cesarean, always a cesarean" guided the practice of obstetrics in the United States, and most women with a prior cesarean birth were scheduled for repeat cesareans. During the 1980s, efforts began to decrease the number of cesarean births in the United States by reducing the number of repeat cesarean births (Turner, Agnew, & Langan, 2006). Many obstetricians encouraged their patients to attempt a vaginal birth after one or more VBAC. Accordingly, the VBAC rate rose to a high of 28% in 1996. However, the rate has fallen since then to a new low of 10% in 2005 (Martin et al., 2007). Many obstetricians no longer offer this procedure for their patients due to safety and legal liability concerns. In addition, ACOG revised their VBAC position statement to more conservative wording, which likely contributed to the decline in VBACs (Welischar & Quirk, 2007). In any case, there is continued debate in the medical community regarding the safety and advisability of VBAC.

Prerequisites

ACOG recommendations regarding trial of labor for a woman who has previously delivered by cesarean include an adequate pelvis, no previous uterine ruptures, personnel and facilities available to perform an immediate cesarean delivery, and no more than one prior low transverse uterine scar (Cunningham et al., 2005b). Current ACOG guidelines stipulate that the woman must give informed consent after consultation with the practitioner regarding the benefits and risks of both trial of labor after cesarean and scheduled repeat cesarean delivery. The guidelines require the presence of a surgeon, anesthesia provider, and operating room personnel in the hospital throughout active labor. A practitioner (this is often the RN) should be at the bedside who can read and interpret electronic fetal monitor tracings and who can recognize the signs and symptoms of uterine rupture.

Contraindications

The risk for uterine rupture during VBAC is much higher when a woman has a classical uterine incision from a previous cesarean delivery; therefore, VBAC is contraindicated when this type of scar is present. Other contraindications include any complication that disqualifies the woman for a vaginal delivery such as placenta previa, history of previous uterine rupture, and lack of facilities or equipment to perform an immediate emergency cesarean (Welischar & Quirk, 2007).

Risks and Benefits

The greatest concern during trial of labor after cesarean is uterine rupture. Although the overall risk remains very low, a woman who has a uterine scar is more likely to suffer uterine rupture during labor, which can have catastrophic effects for the woman and her fetus. There are conflicting data concerning which mode of delivery is safer after one previous cesarean delivery (McDonagh, Osterweil, & Guise, 2005). In many studies, no uterine ruptures occurred in the women who opted for a scheduled repeat cesarean, whereas uterine ruptures did occur in the trial of labor groups. Most studies demonstrate that overall maternal morbidity is lower for women who experience successful VBAC than in women who have a scheduled repeat cesarean. However, when VBAC is unsuccessful and an emergency cesarean is performed, maternal and neonatal morbidity and mortality are much higher than for women who have a scheduled repeat cesarean (Kripke, 2007; Kwee et al., 2007; Macones et al., 2005; Richter, Bergmann, & Dudenhausen, 2007; Tan, Subramaniam, & Omar, 2007).

Several factors increase the likelihood of VBAC success. These include history of a prior vaginal delivery or successful VBAC and onset of spontaneous labor with a favorable cervix. Conversely, there are factors that decrease the likelihood of success. Maternal factors include obesity, short stature, and increased age. Fetal macrosomia and induction of labor are other variables that decrease the chance of vaginal delivery (AAFP, 2005; Caughey, 2006; Ebell, 2007).

Use of oxytocin and/or prostaglandins to induce or augment labor is another source of controversy. Many studies have shown that inducing labor with oxytocin increases the risk of uterine rupture (ACOG, 2006a; Ebell, 2007; Wing, 2007b), whereas other studies have not found this association (Locatelli et al., 2006). The risk of uterine rupture is amplified when prostaglandins are used to ripen the cervix before induction with oxytocin. On the other hand, it appears that augmenting a naturally occurring labor with oxytocin does not increase the risk of rupture (Crawford & Kaufmann, 2006; Macones et al., 2005). Most authorities recommend either prostaglandins or oxytocin, but not both, for labor induction in VBAC. Of course, the practitioner needs to counsel the woman regarding the increased risk with labor induction. Other risk factors for uterine rupture include history of more than one cesarean, short interval between pregnancies, and history of infection with the prior cesarean (Caughey, 2006).

Nursing Care

It is outside the scope of practice for the LPN/LVN to care for a laboring woman who has a history of a previous cesarean delivery. An experienced RN will manage the labor. Many facilities require written informed consent that outlines the risks and benefits of VBAC. You may help ensure that the woman truly understands the plan of care and may witness the woman's signature on the consent form. The woman may verbally withdraw her consent at any time during the course of labor. At the time she withdraws her consent, the trial of labor is discontinued, and the woman is prepared for a cesarean delivery.

During the labor, the RN continuously monitors the electronic fetal monitoring tracing. The RN immediately reports any nonreassuring patterns to the attending practitioner because a nonreassuring pattern is the most

---

Box 11-3 ▮ SIGNS OF UTERINE RUPTURE

- Dramatic onset of fetal bradycardia or deep variable decelerations
- Reports by the woman of a "popping" sensation in her abdomen
- Excessive maternal pain (can be referred pain, such as to the chest)
- Unrelenting uterine contraction followed by a disorganized uterine pattern
- Increased fetal station felt upon vaginal examination (e.g., station is now –3 when it has been –1)
- Vaginal bleeding or increased bloody show
- Easily palpable fetal parts through the abdominal wall
- Signs of maternal shock

---

significant sign of a ruptured uterus. Box 11-3 lists signs associated with uterine rupture. The specially trained LPN/LVN may function as the scrub nurse if a cesarean becomes necessary.

Test Yourself

✔ What is the primary focus of nursing intervention when a cesarean delivery is planned?

✔ What is the primary focus of nursing intervention when a cesarean birth is emergent?

✔ What is one contraindication for a trial of labor after previous cesarean delivery?

Key Points

➤ Medical indications for the induction of labor include postdate pregnancy, PROM, chorioamnionitis, gestational hypertension, intrauterine fetal growth restriction, or certain medical conditions, such as maternal diabetes.

➤ The Bishop score helps determine cervical readiness for labor. Five factors are evaluated: cervical consistency, position, dilatation, effacement, and fetal station. Newer methods to evaluate cervical readiness include measuring cervical length and fetal fibronectin.

➤ Mechanical methods to enhance ripening of the cervix include membrane stripping and mechanical dilation of the cervix with either a catheter or laminaria.

➤ Pharmacologic methods to ripen the cervix require closer monitoring of the woman and include local application of prostaglandin gel or vaginal inserts, or insertion of a prostaglandin tablet.

➤ Oxytocin induction requires continuous fetal monitoring, a mainline IV, and a secondary IV line that contains the oxytocin on an IV pump. Oxytocin is titrated up until an adequate contraction pattern develops.

➤ Complications associated with the use of oxytocin include higher risk for cesarean delivery, hyperstimulation of the uterus with possible fetal distress, and uterine rupture. Water intoxication is another potential complication.

➤ An episiotomy is a surgical incision made in the perineum to enlarge the vaginal opening just before delivery. A midline episiotomy extends straight downward into the true perineum. A mediolateral episiotomy angles to the right or the left of the perineum.

➤ Vacuum extraction involves a suction cup placed on the fetal head, which allows the physician to provide gentle traction to assist delivery.

➤ In a forceps-assisted delivery, hard metal tools shaped like large hollowed-out spoons are applied to the fetal head. Midforceps can help rotate the fetus to an anterior position. Low and outlet forceps can assist delivery when the fetus is at a low station and the woman is too fatigued to push effectively, pushing is contraindicated (e.g., maternal heart disease), the second stage of labor is prolonged, or the fetal monitor tracing is nonreassuring.

➤ The four most common indications for cesarean delivery are history of previous cesarean, labor dystocia, nonreassuring fetal status, and fetal malpresentation. Other, less common, indications include placenta previa, abruptio placentae, cephalopelvic disproportion, active vaginal herpes lesions, prolapse of the umbilical cord, ruptured uterus, and certain medical and obstetric conditions.

➤ Cesarean delivery is a major surgical procedure. It carries with it all the risks and complications associated with abdominal surgery, in addition to those associated with normal birth.

➤ Both skin and uterine incisions can be vertical or transverse. The uterine incision is the most important of the two. The classical uterine incision is associated with the highest risk for rupture in subsequent pregnancies. The low cervical transverse uterine incision is the preferred method.

➤ During the preoperative phase of a cesarean delivery, the LPN/LVN may assist the RN to prepare the patient for surgery. With special training, the LPN/LVN may perform in the role of surgical technician during the intraoperative phase. After the initial assessment by the RN, the LPN/LVN may provide postoperative care for the woman and the newborn after a cesarean delivery.

➤ Nursing interventions for a planned cesarean birth focus on education to prepare the family for the birth. Interventions for an emergency cesarean include mostly supportive behaviors, such as explaining procedures as they are done and providing appropriate reassurance.

➤ Much controversy surrounds the advisability of VBAC. The greatest concern is the higher risk for uterine rupture during labor. The woman most likely to have a successful VBAC has only had one previous cesarean, her age is less than 40, and she goes into labor naturally (does not require induction). History of a classical uterine incision or a previous uterine rupture is a contraindication for VBAC.

➤ The RN manages the care of the woman attempting VBAC. Interventions include ensuring that the woman has given informed consent, frequent monitoring of the woman and fetus for signs of uterine rupture during labor, and preparing the woman for immediate cesarean delivery if a complication occurs.

INTERNET RESOURCES

Labor Induction
www.acog.org (Enter the search phrase "labor induction," then click on the link to the patient education pamphlet "Labor Induction.")
http://familydoctor.org (Enter the search phrase "labor induction.")

Cesarean Birth
http://ican-online.net
www.emedicinehealth.com/cesarean_childbirth/article_em.htm
www.nlm.nih.gov/medlineplus (Enter the search term "cesarean.")
www.noah-health.org (Enter the search term "cesarean.")

VBAC
www.acog.org (Enter the search phrase "vaginal birth after cesarean," then click on the link to the patient education pamphlet "Vaginal Birth After Cesarean.")
www.vbac.com

Photos
http://pregnancy.about.com/library/blsection.htm

Workbook

▪ NCLEX-STYLE REVIEW QUESTIONS

1. Which of the following statements about episiotomies is true?

   a. An episiotomy is a routine procedure during a vaginal delivery.

   b. An episiotomy is always done to protect the woman's perineum from hard-to-repair tears.

   c. An episiotomy is an invasive procedure that has associated risks and benefits.

   d. An episiotomy is only indicated for certain extreme emergencies, such as shoulder dystocia.

2. A primigravida is tired of being pregnant. She asks the nurse, "Why can't my doctor just schedule a cesarean delivery? My friend had a cesarean and everything went very well." What is the best reply by the nurse?

   a. "A cesarean birth involves major surgery, which puts you and your baby at higher risk for complications. Your physician will discuss the options with you."

   b. "I will ask your doctor. Sometimes he will allow a first-time mother to have a cesarean birth if she wants to do so."

   c. "Oh no. This would not be good for the baby. Try not to think too much about it. It is always better to have a vaginal delivery."

   d. "It is always your choice to have a cesarean delivery if that is what you want to do. Would you like me to help you schedule a date for the surgery?"

3. A woman is dilated 9 cm and the fetus is in an anterior position at a +1 station. The bag of water is ruptured. She has been in labor for several hours and is exhausted, so she asks the nurse, "My friend was tired at the end of her labor, and the doctor used forceps to help deliver the baby. Could the doctor pull the baby out with forceps so I can get this over with?" What response by the nurse is best?

   a. "I don't know. Let me ask the doctor."

   b. "The cervix must be completely dilated before forceps can be applied safely."

   c. "No. Once the water bag ruptures, the doctor cannot apply forceps."

   d. "Forceps are too dangerous. I'll get a vacuum extractor ready for your delivery."

4. The LPN is the scrub nurse for a cesarean delivery. The surgeon asks for the scalpel to make the initial incision before a time out has been called.

What response by the scrub nurse is most appropriate?

   a. The nurse does not give the surgeon the scalpel and whispers to the circulating nurse to call the time out.

   b. The nurse hands the surgeon the scalpel and calls the time out.

   c. The nurse hands the surgeon the scalpel, but says not to start until the time out is done.

   d. The nurse states that he or she will hand the surgeon the scalpel as soon as the time out is completed.

5. A woman with history of previous cesarean is in labor. She has signed the consent form for a VBAC. She is dilated 7 cm and is making satisfactory progress in labor. She tells her nurse that she has changed her mind and she wants a cesarean. What response by the nurse is best?

   a. "Don't you want to do what's best for the baby? Your baby has a higher chance of having problems if you have a cesarean."

   b. "Ok. Since you no longer consent to a VBAC, I will let the physician know and we'll begin preparing you for a cesarean delivery."

   c. "There is no reason to do a cesarean right now. Let me ask your doctor for an epidural to help relieve your pain."

   d. "You certainly have the right to change your mind. Can you tell me more about your reasons for wanting a cesarean so that we can discuss this further with your physician?"

▪ STUDY ACTIVITIES

1. Develop a 15-minute presentation on cesarean delivery to give to a group of first-time mothers at a prenatal education class.

2. Discuss how care of the newborn during cesarean delivery is different from care of the newborn after vaginal delivery. What additional risk factors does the newborn delivered by cesarean have?

3. Using the table below, compare methods of cervical ripening.

Methods	How it Works to Ripen the Cervix	Special Nursing Considerations

■ CRITICAL THINKING: WHAT WOULD YOU DO?

Apply your knowledge of cesarean birth and assisted deliveries to the following situations.

1. Amy Jones is a 21-year-old gravida 1 who is attending a prenatal childbirth education class. She comments that she thinks she will not attend next week's class because cesarean delivery is going to be discussed, and she does not plan to have a cesarean. How would you reply to Amy's comment?

2. A woman who is close to term asks the nurse at a normal obstetric visit, "My doctor says I have a Bishop score of 4. What does that mean?"

a. How would you reply?

b. If the physician felt that the woman's labor needed to be induced, what recommendation would he or she likely make to the woman? Why?

3. You are going to assist the physician to perform a fetal fibronectin test. What equipment do you need?

4. Ellen Hess, a 30-year-old gravida 2, has chosen to attempt a VBAC. After 4 hours of labor, she reports to you severe pain and a "popping" sensation in her abdomen. What would you do?

POSTPARTUM AND NEWBORN

12 *The Postpartum Woman*

KEY TERMS

attachment
boggy uterus
bonding
breakthrough pain
colostrum
diastasis recti abdominis
dyspareunia
en face
grand multiparity
involution
lochia
postpartum blues
puerperium

LEARNING OBJECTIVES

On completion of this chapter, you should be able to:

1. Describe physiologic adaptation of the woman during the postpartum period.
2. Discuss major points related to psychological adaptation during the postpartum period.
3. Describe components of a postpartum assessment.
4. Discuss the responsibilities of the practical (vocational) nurse in caring for the woman in the early postpartum period.
5. Compare and contrast the postpartum nursing care of the woman who delivers vaginally with that of the one who delivers by cesarean.
6. Outline the nurse's role in preparing the postpartum woman for discharge.

THE PROCESSES of pregnancy and birth challenge the woman's psychological and physiologic coping mechanisms. During the postpartum period, sometimes referred to as the fourth trimester of pregnancy, the woman must adjust to the reality of her new role as mother while her body recovers from pregnancy and childbirth. The postpartum period, or **puerperium**, encompasses the 6 weeks after birth. For ease of discussion, the puerperium is subdivided into three categories: the immediate postpartum period, which covers the first 24 hours; the early postpartum period or first week; and late postpartum period, which refers to weeks 2 through 6. This chapter discusses the adaptations a low-risk woman makes during the puerperium and the nursing care that promotes healing and wellness.

MATERNAL ADAPTATION DURING THE POSTPARTUM PERIOD
Physiologic Adaptation

The woman's body undergoes tremendous changes to accommodate pregnancy. Every body system and organ is affected. During the weeks after pregnancy, the body recovers from the stress of pregnancy and returns to its normal pre-pregnancy state.

Reproductive System

The organs and hormones of the reproductive system must gradually return to their nonpregnant size and function. **Involution** is the process through which the uterus, cervix, and vagina shrink and/or return to the nonpregnant state.

Uterus

Uterine Contraction and Involution. Immediately after the placenta delivers, the uterus contracts inward, a process that seals off the open blood vessels at the former site of the placenta. If the uterus does not contract effectively, the woman will hemorrhage. The clotting cascade also is initiated, a process that causes clot formation to control bleeding. Large blood vessels at the former placental site degenerate and smaller ones form (Weydert & Benda, 2006). Gradually, the decidua sloughs off, new endometrial tissue forms, and the placental area heals without leaving fibrous scar tissue.

Uterine contraction also leads to uterine involution, which normally occurs at a predictable rate. Caregivers assess uterine involution by measuring fundal height. Immediately after delivery, the fundus is firm and located in the midline halfway between the umbilicus and symphysis pubis. One hour after delivery, the uterus should be contracted firmly, with the fundus midline at the level of the umbilicus. The day after delivery, the fundus is found 1 cm below the umbilicus. The normal process of involution thereafter is for the uterus to descend approximately 1 fingerbreadth (1 cm) per day until it has descended below the level of the pubic bone and can no longer be palpated. This occurs by the 10th postpartum day (Fig. 12-1).

Several factors promote uterine contraction and involution. Breast-feeding stimulates oxytocin release from the woman's posterior pituitary gland. Oxytocin stimulates the uterus to contract. Early ambulation and proper nourishment also foster normal involution.

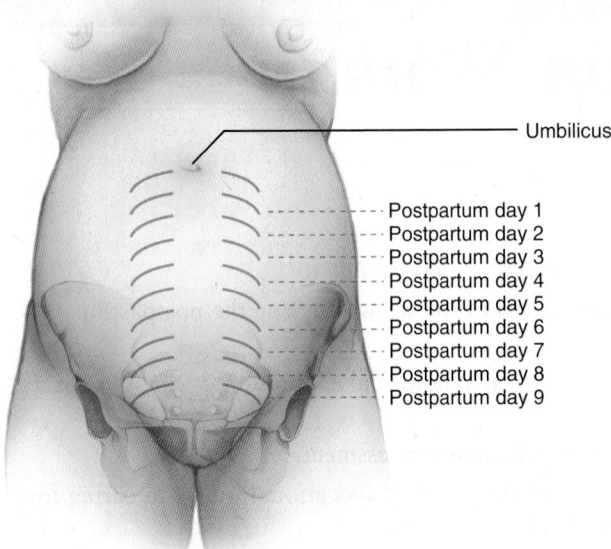

Umbilicus
Postpartum day 1
Postpartum day 2
Postpartum day 3
Postpartum day 4
Postpartum day 5
Postpartum day 6
Postpartum day 7
Postpartum day 8
Postpartum day 9

■ **Figure 12-1** Uterine involution.

In addition, there are factors that can inhibit or delay uterine involution. A full bladder impedes uterine contraction by pushing upward on the uterus and displacing it. Any condition that over distends the uterus during pregnancy can lead to ineffective uterine contraction after delivery. Examples include a multifetal pregnancy and hydramnios. Maternal exhaustion, excessive analgesia, and oxytocin use during labor and delivery also can hinder effective contraction of the uterus. Other factors include retained placental fragments, infection, and **grand multiparity**, five or more pregnancies. When the uterus does not contract effectively, blood and clots collect in the uterus, which makes it even more difficult for the uterus to contract. This leads to a **boggy uterus** and hemorrhage if the condition is not arrested. A boggy uterus feels soft and spongy, rather than firm and well contracted.

Afterpains. After a multipara delivers, the uterus contracts and relaxes at intervals. This leads to afterpains, which can be quite severe. For the primipara, the uterus normally remains contracted, and afterpains are less severe than that of the multipara. However, breast-feeding, because it causes the release of oxytocin, increases the duration and intensity of afterpains for both the primipara and multipara.

Lochia. The uterus must shed its lining that helped nourish the pregnancy. Blood, mucus, tissue, and white blood cells compose the uterine discharge, known as **lochia**, during the postpartum period. Lochia progresses through three stages:

- *Lochia rubra:* Occurs during the first 3 to 4 days; is of small to moderate amount; is composed mostly of blood; is dark red in color; and has a fleshy odor.

- *Lochia serosa*: Occurs during days 4 to 10; decreases to a small amount; and takes on a brownish or pinkish color.
- *Lochia alba*: Occurs after day 10; and becomes white or pale yellow because the bleeding has stopped and the discharge is now composed mostly of white blood cells.

Lochia may persist for the entire 6 weeks after delivery but often subsides by the end of the second or third week. Lochia should never contain large clots. Other abnormal findings include reversal of the pattern (e.g., the lochia has been serosa, then goes back to rubra), lochia that fails to decrease in amount or actually increases versus gradually decreasing, or a malodorous lochia.

> **Warning!**
> Normal lochia has a fleshy, but not offensive, odor. If the lochia is malodorous or smells rotten, suspect infection. Report this finding immediately to the RN or practitioner.

Ovaries

Ovulation can occur as soon as 3 weeks after delivery. Menstrual periods usually begin within 6 to 8 weeks for the woman who is not breast-feeding. However, the lactating woman may not resume menses for as long as 18 months after giving birth. Although lactation may suppress ovulation, it is not a dependable form of birth control. It is wise for the woman to use some type of birth control to prevent an unplanned pregnancy when she resumes sexual activity.

> **Did you know?**
> The return of ovulation and menstrual bleeding do not always occur together. Explain to the woman that she may be able to conceive even if the menses does not resume immediately.

Cervix

During labor, the cervix thins and dilates. This process does not occur without some trauma. Directly after delivery, the cervix is still partially open and contains soft, small tears. It may also appear bruised. The internal os closes after a few days. Gradually, the muscle cells regenerate and the cervix recovers by the end of the 6-week puerperium. The external os, however, remains slightly open and has a slitlike appearance, in comparison with the dimplelike appearance of the cervix of a nulliparous woman (Fig. 12-2).

Vagina and Perineum

The vagina may have small tears that will heal without intervention. Immediately after delivery, the walls of the vagina are smooth. Rugae begin to return to the vaginal walls after approximately 3 weeks. The diameter of the introitus gradually becomes smaller by contraction, but rarely returns to its pre-pregnant size (Berens, 2007).

■ Figure 12-2 Appearance of the cervical os. **(A)** Before the first pregnancy. **(B)** After pregnancy.

Muscle tone never fully returns to the pregravid state; however, Kegel exercises may help increase the tone and enhance sexual enjoyment. Because breast-feeding suppresses ovulation, estrogen levels remain lower in the lactating woman, which can lead to vaginal dryness and **dyspareunia**, painful intercourse.

The labia and perineum may be edematous after delivery and may appear bruised, particularly after a difficult delivery. If an episiotomy was done or perineal tears repaired, absorbable stitches will be in place. The edges of the episiotomy or repair should approximate. The episiotomy takes several weeks to heal fully. The labia tend to be flaccid after childbirth. Tone may improve over time but never completely returns to the pre-pregnant state.

Breasts

Colostrum, the antibody-rich breast secretion that is the precursor to breast milk, is normally excreted by the breasts in the last weeks of pregnancy and continues to be excreted in the first few postpartum days. Prolactin levels rise when estrogen and progesterone levels fall after delivery of the placenta. Suckling at the breast also causes prolactin levels to rise. Prolactin stimulates milk production by the breasts, and the milk normally comes in on the third day. See Chapter 15 for a detailed discussion of breast physiology, milk production, and breast-feeding.

Test Yourself

✔ Where is the fundus normally located on the day after delivery?

✔ Name three factors that can inhibit or delay uterine involution.

✔ Name the three stages, in order, through which lochia passes.

Cardiovascular System

In the early postpartum period, the woman eliminates the additional fluid volume that is present during the pregnancy via the skin, urinary tract, and through blood loss.

The woman who experiences a normal vaginal delivery loses approximately 300 to 500 mL of blood during delivery. If she has a cesarean delivery, normal blood loss is between 500 and 1,000 mL. As the blood volume returns to normal, some hemoconcentration occurs that causes an increase in the hematocrit.

> **You Do the Math**
> For every 250 mL of blood loss, the hemoglobin and hematocrit (H&H) fall by 1 and 2 points, respectively. So, if the woman's H&H were 12.0 and 34, then fall to 10.0 and 30, the approximate blood loss is 500 mL.

High plasma fibrinogen levels and other coagulation factors mark the postpartum period. This is protective against hemorrhage, but it also predisposes to the development of deep vein thrombosis (DVT), formation of blood clots in the deep veins of the legs. Dehydration, immobility, and trauma can add to the risk for DVT. (See Chapter 19 for discussion of DVT in the postpartum period.)

The white blood cell count is elevated to approximately 15,000 to 20,000/mL and may reach as high as 30,000/mL. Leukocytosis, high white blood cell count, helps protect the woman from infection, as there are multiple routes for infection to occur in the early postpartum period.

Immediately or very soon after delivery, the woman may experience a shaking postpartum chill. Hormonal and physiologic changes likely contribute to the cause. In any event, the chill is not harmful, unless accompanied by fever greater than 100.4°F or other signs of infection. The shivering normally resolves within minutes, especially if a prewarmed blanket is placed over the woman.

Vital Signs

The temperature may be elevated slightly during the first 24 hours because of the exertion and dehydration of labor. After the first 24 hours, a temperature of 100.4°F or greater is abnormal and may indicate infection.

The blood pressure should remain at the woman's baseline level. An elevated blood pressure could be a sign of developing preeclampsia (see Chapter 17) and should be promptly reported. A falling blood pressure, particularly in the presence of a rising pulse, is suggestive of hemorrhage. Assess the woman carefully for a source of blood loss if her blood pressure drops.

It is normal for the pulse to be slow in the first week after delivery. The heart rate may be as low

> **Here's a clinical tip.**
> For accurate blood pressure readings, have the woman sit on the edge of the bed for several minutes before measuring her blood pressure. If you take the blood pressure immediately after she sits up from a lying position, the reading may be falsely low due to orthostatic hypotension.

as 50 beats per minute. Occasionally the woman may experience tachycardia. This is more likely to occur after a difficult labor and delivery, or it may indicate excessive blood loss.

Musculoskeletal System

The most pronounced changes are evident in the abdominal muscles, although other muscles may be weak because of the exertion of labor. The abdomen is soft and sagging in the immediate postpartum period. Often the woman has to wear loose clothing for the first few weeks. The abdomen usually regains its tone with exercise. However, in some women, the abdomen remains slack. In this situation, if another pregnancy occurs, the abdomen will be pendulous and the woman will have more problems with backache. **Diastasis recti abdominis** is a condition in which the abdominal muscles separate during the pregnancy, leaving part of the abdominal wall without muscular support. Exercise can improve muscle tone when this condition occurs. A woman is predisposed to poor muscle tone and diastasis if she has weak muscles or is obese before the pregnancy, her abdomen is overdistended during the pregnancy, or she is a grand multipara.

Gastrointestinal System

Immediately after delivery, the postpartum woman is often very hungry. The energy expended during labor uses up glucose stores, and food has generally been restricted. Restriction of fluids and loss of fluids in labor, in the urine, and via diaphoresis often lead to increased thirst.

Constipation may be a problem. Intra-abdominal pressure decreases rapidly after childbirth, and peristalsis is diminished. These factors make it more difficult for feces to travel down the gastrointestinal tract. The woman may be afraid to defecate in the early postpartum period because of hemorrhoidal discomfort and perineal pain. Suppressing the urge to defecate complicates the problem of constipation and may actually cause increased pain when defecation finally occurs. Iron supplementation adds to the problem. However, by the end of the first postpartum week, bowel function has usually returned to normal.

Urinary System

The urinary system must handle an increased load in the early postpartum period as the body excretes excess plasma volume. Healthy kidneys are able to adjust to the increased demands. Urinary output exceeds intake. Transient glycosuria, proteinuria, and ketonuria are normal in the immediate postpartum period.

During the process of labor and delivery, trauma can occur to the lower urinary system. Pressure of the descending fetal head on the ureters, bladder, and urethra can lead to transient loss of bladder tone and urethral edema. Trauma, certain medications, and anesthesia given during labor can also lead to a temporary loss of bladder sensation. The result can be urinary retention. Sometimes, the woman voids small amounts but does not completely empty the bladder, or she may not be able to void at all. Voiding may be painful if the urethra was traumatized.

The urinary system is more susceptible to infection during the postpartum period. Hydronephrosis, dilation of the renal pelves and ureters, is a normal change that occurs during pregnancy because of hormonal influences. This condition persists for approximately 4 weeks after delivery. Hydronephrosis and urinary stasis predispose the woman to urinary tract infection.

Check this out!

If you palpate the fundus and find it above the umbilicus, deviated to the right side, and boggy, the most likely cause is a full bladder. Assist the woman to void, and then re-evaluate the fundus.

Integumentary System

Copious diaphoresis occurs in the first few days after childbirth as the body rids itself of excess water and waste via the skin. The woman notices the perspiration particularly at night. She may wake up and be drenched in sweat. This is a normal finding and is not a cause for concern.

The woman will likely have striae, stretch marks, on the abdomen and sometimes on the breasts. Immediately after birth, striae appear red or purplish. Over time, they fade to a light silvery color and remain faintly visible.

Weight Loss

Immediately after delivery, approximately 12 to 14 lb are lost with expulsion of the fetus, placenta, and amniotic fluid. The woman loses an additional 5 to 15 lb in the early postpartum period because of fluid loss from diaphoresis and urinary excretion (Berens, 2007). The average woman will have returned to her pre-pregnant weight 6 months after childbirth if she was within the recommended weight gain of 25 to 30 lb during pregnancy. Some women take longer to lose the additional pounds. In general, the breast-feeding woman tends to lose weight faster than the woman who does not breast-feed because of increased caloric demands.

Test Yourself

✔ A falling blood pressure and rising pulse in the early postpartum period is suggestive of _____.

✔ Name two factors that contribute to constipation in the postpartum period.

✔ How long does it take for the average woman to return to her pre-pregnant weight after delivery?

Psychological Adaptation

Role change is the most significant psychological adaptation the woman must make. This process occurs with each new addition to the family, but tends to be most pronounced for the first time mother. Each child is a unique being with his or her own temperament and needs who must be integrated into the existing family structure. Therefore, the whole family must adapt to the addition of a new member.

As the nurse, you can influence the development of positive family relationships in many ways. Careful assessment of maternal psychological adaptation and anticipatory guidance regarding postpartum blues and expected psychological adjustments can go a long way toward fostering positive transition for the woman and the new family.

Becoming a Mother

A woman begins the process of becoming a mother during pregnancy as she anticipates the birth of the baby. She fantasizes about and prepares for her newborn's arrival. After the birth, the woman must take on the role of mother to the baby. The two critical elements of becoming a mother are development of love and attachment to the child and engagement with the child. Engagement includes all the activities of care giving as the child grows and changes. This transition is a continuously evolving process throughout the woman's life (Fowles & Horowitz, 2006).

Although each woman takes on the mother role in her own way, influenced by her culture, upbringing, and role models, there are patterns of behavior that are similar for all women. The woman adapts to her new role as mother through a series of four developmental stages:

1. beginning attachment and preparation for the infant during pregnancy;
2. increasing attachment, learning to care for the infant, and physical restoration during the early postpartum period;
3. moving toward a new normal in the first 4 months; and
4. achieving a maternal identity around 4 months.

The stages overlap, and social and environmental variables influence their length (Mercer, 2006).

In the early puerperium, the new mother demonstrates dependent behaviors. She has difficulty making decisions and needs assistance with self-care. She tends to be inwardly focused and concerned about her own physical needs such as food, rest, and elimination. She relives the delivery experience and has a great need to talk about the details. This process is important for her to integrate the experience into her concept of self. She may remain in this dependent, reintegration phase for several hours or days. This is not an optimum time to teach detailed newborn care because the new mother is not readily receptive to instruction. Listen with an attitude of acceptance. No feeling the woman expresses is "wrong." Help her interpret the events of her birth experience.

Most women move quickly from the dependent stage to increasing independence in self- and newborn care. After she has rested and recovered somewhat from the stress of the delivery, the new mother has more energy to concentrate on her infant. At this point, she becomes receptive to infant care instruction. The first-time mother in particular needs reassurance that she is capable of providing care for her newborn. She may feel that the nursing staff is more adept than she is at meeting the newborn's needs. Therefore, it is important to encourage her to perform care for her newborn while providing gentle guidance and support. She responds well to praise for her early attempts at childcare during this phase. This phase lasts anywhere from 2 days to several weeks.

> **Be careful!**
>
> Assist the woman to take care of her newborn rather than do all the care yourself. The new mother needs guidance, practice, and praise to begin to feel confident in her new role.

Development of Positive Family Relationships

Attachment is the enduring emotional bond that develops between the parent and infant. However, this process does not happen automatically. Attachment occurs as parents interact with and respond to their infant. In the early postpartum period, the woman may have a wide range of emotions and responses to her newborn. Humans seem to respond to gains and losses in similar ways. Disbelief and shock are often the initial reactions. The mother may say repeatedly, "I can't believe I just had a baby." Ambivalence also is a normal response. The new parents may communicate uncertainty over their readiness to take on the parent role. Frequently, the new mother may experience negative feelings about the baby in the first few days after birth. However, she may not express these feelings because of the cultural expectation that "mothers always love their babies." If she does express negativity, such as, "I'm not sure that I like my baby," nurses or family members may reply in a way that denies or dismisses the emotion. "Oh, I'm sure you don't mean that," is one such dismissive response. It is important to remember that negative feelings are part of the process as mother and baby adjust to each other and become acquainted. Encourage the woman to express her feelings openly and then show acceptance and let her know that her feelings are normal (Hall & Wittkowski, 2006).

The initial component of healthy attachment is a process called **bonding**. This is the way the new mother and father become acquainted with their newborn (Fig. 12-3). The process begins with a predictable pattern of parental behavior. Initial inspection of the newborn begins with

A Personal Glimpse

I delivered my first child after 14 hours of intense labor. I went through my labor naturally without an epidural with the help of my doula. I pushed for 2 hours, so I was pretty exhausted after delivery. The midwife had to cut an episiotomy because she said it was a tight fit. My baby weighed 9 lb! The next day while the baby was in the room, I remember that everything felt so unreal. I kept telling myself that I should feel happy. But all I really wanted to do was to cry. The nurse came in and told me what a beautiful baby I had and asked me her name. I started to cry and said that I wasn't sure that I could be a good mother. I felt scared and confused and unready to take care of a baby. The nurse told me that the feelings I was having were very normal. She said that this was a huge change for me and that it takes time to get adjusted to the new mother role. She asked me if I had someone to help me at home. I told her that my sister was going to stay with me for several weeks. The nurse gave me a card with the phone number for the hospital. She wrote her name on it and told me that she would be happy to answer any questions I had after I went home. She said that I could talk to any of the nurses, if she wasn't on duty when I called. I felt relieved. The nurse then stayed with me a while and watched while I changed the baby's diaper. She told me that I was a quick learner and that I was very gentle with the baby. I felt so much better. I knew that it was going to be ok.

Holly

Learning Opportunity: Why do you think this new mother felt better after her interaction with the nurse? In what ways can you in your role as a nurse support the new mother when she expresses negative feelings about her baby or her abilities as a mother?

fingertip touching. The new mother explores her newborn's extremities, counting his fingers and toes. She then advances to using the palms of her hands to touch the newborn and begins to explore larger body areas. Eventually she enfolds the newborn with her hands and arms and holds her close. As bonding continues, she begins to spend more time holding the newborn in the **en face** position in which she interacts face to face with the newborn. She places the baby's face within her direct line of vision and makes full eye contact with the newborn. The new mother often talks to the baby using high-pitched tones. She smiles and laughs while she continues the en face posture. Box 12-1 lists the sequence of initial attachment.

You can do it!

If the new mother makes a negative comment, make your response accepting and supportive. You might reply, "It is natural to have feelings of uncertainty as you adjust to having a new baby." Be creative. I'm sure you can come up with some great supportive phrases.

One important component in the development of healthy attachment between the new parents and their baby is the amount and type of social support the new family has available to them. Access to supportive friends and relatives enhances attachment. When a new mother is isolated and without adequate social support, attachment is threatened. In this situation, it is important to assist the woman to find sources of support. Perhaps there is someone in her neighborhood or community who might be willing to provide support. Discuss the situation with the registered nurse (RN) in charge. A referral to social services may be in order.

▮ Figure 12-3 A mom and dad bond with their newborn immediately after birth.

Box 12-1 ▮ PROGRESSION OF INITIAL ATTACHMENT BEHAVIORS

The new mother and father both begin their interaction with the new baby in a fairly predictable sequence. Note that this process may take anywhere from hours to days.

1. Exploration begins with fingertip touching.
2. Next, the new parent explores the infant's extremities.
3. Fingertip touching gives way to touching with the palmar surface of the hands.
4. Then larger body surfaces are touched and caressed.
5. Soon the infant is enfolded with the hands and arms and cuddled closely to the parent.
6. Progressively more time is spent in the en face position talking to and smiling at the new baby.

Healthy bonding behaviors include naming the newborn and calling the newborn by name. Making eye contact and talking to the newborn are other indicators that healthy attachment is occurring. It is important to differentiate between a new parent who is nervous and anxious about her new role and one who is rejecting her parenting role. Warning signals of poor attachment include turning away from the newborn, refusing or neglecting to provide care, and disengagement from the newborn.

Traditional thinking assumed that the mother was the first and most important person to bond with the new baby. We now know that the baby can make many bonds. The father benefits from early contact with the newborn immediately after delivery. It is common for the father to describe strong emotions of pride, joy, and other positive emotions when he first holds his newborn. The father may be engrossed with the newborn. He progresses through a pattern of touching similar to that of the mother.

Siblings also bond with the new baby (Fig. 12-4). There are special considerations that the parents need to make for older siblings of a new baby. The birth of a new baby requires a role change for the sibling. Sometimes the new baby does not meet the sibling's expectations. For instance, the baby might be a boy, but the sibling wanted a sister. It is common for the sibling to regress for a few days after the birth.

Postpartum Blues

Approximately 40% to 80% of postpartum women experience the **postpartum blues**, sometimes called the "baby blues." The postpartum blues is a temporary condition that usually begins on the third day and lasts for 2 or 3 days. The woman experiences rapid mood swings, irritability, anxiety, and decreased concentration. She

■ **Figure 12-4** While the father bonds with his new son, big sister takes a first peak at her new baby brother.

may be tearful, have difficulty sleeping and eating, and feel generally let down (Lusskin & Misri, 2007). A combination of factors likely contributes to the baby blues. Psychological adjustment along with a physiologic decrease in estrogen and progesterone appear to be the greatest contributors. Additional contributing factors include too much activity, fatigue, disturbed sleep patterns, and discomfort. It is important for the woman and her family to know that this is a normal reaction; however, if the depression lasts for more than several days, or if the symptoms become severe, the woman should seek psychological evaluation. (See Chapter 19 for a discussion of postpartum depression.)

Test Yourself

✔ Name the four developmental stages through which a woman passes as she is becoming a mother.

✔ Define attachment.

✔ List the normal progression of interaction that occurs during the initial bonding experience between a new parent and the newborn.

THE NURSE'S ROLE IN POSTPARTUM CARE

Nursing Process for the Early Postpartum Period

Most women who deliver vaginally go home within 24 to 48 hours after delivery. Therefore, when caring for the woman in the early postpartum period, it is essential to do thorough assessments to detect any complications that might be developing, and to use every available opportunity to teach self- and newborn care.

Assessment

After the initial recovery period, the woman may be transferred to a postpartum room. If she delivered in a labor, delivery, recovery, and postpartum setting, she will stay in the room in which she delivered. Whatever the setting, it is important to do a thorough initial assessment if you are providing postpartum care.

Data Collection

Much of the data collection is done before the woman delivers and can be found on the initial admission assessment done in the labor and delivery unit. It is important to check the initial assessment and the prenatal record as part of the initial data collection. The labor and delivery nurse gives report to the postpartum nurse upon transfer. The report should include significant medical history, pregnancy history, labor and birth history, newborn data, and initial postpartum recovery data.

The medical and pregnancy histories are important because they alert the postpartum nurse to risk factors that might lead to postpartum hemorrhage or other complications and give clues as to bonding potential. The report includes the gravida and para, the estimated date of delivery, blood type and Rh, complications experienced during the pregnancy, group B streptococcus culture status, and any medical problems, including sexually transmitted infections.

The labor and birth history includes the length of labor, type and time of birth, type and timing of analgesia or anesthesia administered, type and timing of any intravenous (IV) medications given, and any complications experienced during labor. Important information regarding the newborn includes sex, Apgar scores, resuscitation efforts, congenital anomalies, current status, the mother's plans for feeding, and whether feeding was initiated in the delivery room. The labor and delivery nurse should report initial postpartum recovery data to include the following:

- Status of the fundus, lochia, and perineum
- Type of pain, if any, and success of analgesics and comfort measures to control the pain
- Whether or not the woman ambulated after delivery and how she tolerated it
- Type and amount of IV fluids infusing, if any
- Status of the bladder
- Response of the woman and her partner to the newborn

Initial Physical Assessment in the First Hour Following Delivery

If the woman is going to hemorrhage, she is most likely to do so within the first postpartum hour. For this reason, monitor her closely during this period. Measure her vital signs every 15 minutes during the first hour. With each vital sign check, determine the position and firmness of the uterine fundus, the amount and character of lochia, the status of the perineum, and monitor for signs of bladder distention. If the woman had a cesarean delivery, also check the incisional dressing for intactness and determine if there is any incisional bleeding. Measure the temperature and determine the status of the breasts once immediately after delivery and then again just before transfer to postpartum. Some institutions continue monitoring as above every 30 minutes for the second hour, then every 4 hours during the first 24 hours after delivery.

Complete Postpartum Physical Assessment

At least once per shift, perform a complete head-to-toe assessment. A quick visual survey and speaking to the woman reveals her level of consciousness and affect. Assist her to empty her bladder, if necessary, before beginning the full assessment. First, take the vital signs. Respirations should be even and unlabored. Be sure to rule out shortness of breath and chest pain. The heart rate should be regular without murmurs and may be as slow as 50 beats per minute. The lungs should be clear in all five lobes (Fig. 12-5). After the vital signs assessment,

■ Figure 12-5 The nurse auscultates the lungs as part of a complete postpartum assessment.

there are 11 main areas that must be assessed and monitored in the postpartum period:

- breasts
- uterus
- lochia
- bladder
- bowel
- perineum
- lower extremities
- pain
- laboratory studies
- maternal–newborn bonding
- maternal emotional status

Breasts. Inspect the breasts and nipples for signs of engorgement, redness, or cracks. Palpate the breasts gently to determine if they are soft, filling, or engorged with milk. Note if there are any painful areas. With a gloved hand, palpate the nipples to determine if they are erect or inverted. The breasts should be soft during the first postpartum day and begin filling on the second and third days. Engorgement may occur on the third day. There should be no reddened areas on the breasts, and the nipples should be intact without cracks or fissures.

Uterus. With the woman lying supine, palpate the fundus (Nursing Procedure 12-1). Note the position of the uterus and palpate the uterus to determine consistency, tone, position, and size. It should be firm, not boggy, located in the midline, and at the appropriate height in relation to the umbilicus, depending on what hour or day it is after delivery.

Lochia. Determine the amount and character of the lochia. Is it scant, small, moderate, or heavy? Is it rubra or serosa? Is there a foul smell? Be sure to check under her buttocks for pooling. Ask her how many times she has changed her sanitary napkins/pads since the previous assessment, and determine if she is saturating pads. The lochia should be rubra of small to moderate amount without large clots and no foul odor.

Nursing Procedure 12-1
FUNDAL PALPATION AND MASSAGE

EQUIPMENT

Warm, clean hands
Clean gloves

PROCEDURE

1. Explain procedure to the woman.
2. Instruct her to empty her bladder, if necessary.
3. Wash hands thoroughly.
4. Position her supine with the head of the bed flat.
5. Locate and place one hand on the uterine fundus. It should feel hard and rounded—something like a melon.
6. Place the other hand in a cupped position just above the symphysis pubis, as in the picture. Use this hand to gently support the uterus.
7. Gently massage the fundus, if it is soft or boggy.
8. Notice the location, height, and position of the uterus.
9. Wash hands.
10. Document the tone (soft, boggy, or firm) and the location of the fundus in finger breadths above or below or at the level of the umbilicus.

Note whether or not the fundus is midline or deviated to one side.

Note: Vigorous fundal massage or overstimulation can cause the uterus to become flaccid, rather than helping it to contract. Take measures to avoid overmassaging the fundus.

Bladder and Bowel. The woman should be voiding adequate amounts (more than 100 mL per each voiding) regularly. Voiding frequently in amounts smaller than 100 mL with associated suprapubic distention (a rounded area just above the symphysis pubis) is indicative of urinary retention. Next, visually inspect the abdomen and auscultate for bowel sounds. Bowel sounds should be present in all four quadrants. Ask the woman if she has had a bowel movement after delivery.

Perineum. Assist the woman to the Sims' position. Lift the top buttock, and with a good light source (such as a penlight or flashlight), inspect the perineum for redness, edema, and ecchymosis (Fig. 12-6). If the woman had an episiotomy or a tear, check the sutures and be certain the edges are well approximated. Determine if there is any drainage from the stitches. Palpate gently with a gloved hand to determine if there are any hematomas forming in the area. Note any hemorrhoids.

> **Notice this difference.**
>
> Expect less lochia after a cesarean delivery than after a vaginal delivery. This is because the surgeon wipes out the uterine cavity before suturing it closed, which removes much of the blood and debris. Report moderate amounts of lochia, as this may signal postpartum hemorrhage after a cesarean.

The perineum should be intact, with only minimal swelling and no hematomas.

Lower Extremities. Inspect the extremities for edema (Fig. 12-7A), equality of pulses, and capillary refill. Check for Homans' sign (Fig. 12-7B). Feel along the calf area for any warmth or redness. The calves should be of equal size and warmth bilaterally. There should be no reddened, painful areas, and there should be no pain in the calves when the feet are dorsiflexed (negative

■ **Figure 12-6** Postpartum perineal assessment. Notice that the woman is in the Sims' position. The nurse lifts the upper buttock and inspects the perineum.

A

B

■ Figure 12-7 Assessment of the lower extremities. **(A)** The nurse checks the right lower extremity for edema. **(B)** The nurse checks for Homans' sign. If the woman experiences pain in the calf of her leg when her foot is dorsiflexed, Homans' sign is positive, and the nurse should report this finding.

Homans' sign), or when the woman is walking. A positive Homans' sign and/or one calf with redness, warmth, and greater size than the other could indicate deep vein thrombosis (see Chapter 19) and should be reported.

Pain. Determine if the woman is experiencing any pain. If so, investigate the source (e.g., afterpains, episiotomy, painful urination, pain in the calves). Determine the characteristics, quality, timing, and relief after comfort measures.

Laboratory Studies. Monitor the hemoglobin and hematocrit (H&H). Note the H&H before delivery. Most practitioners order a postpartum H&H on the morning after delivery. If the values drop significantly, the woman may have experienced postpartum hemorrhage. Note the blood type and Rh. If the woman is Rh-negative, she will need a RhoGAM workup. Determine the woman's rubella status. If she is nonimmune, she will need a rubella immunization before she is discharged home.

Maternal–Newborn Bonding and Maternal Emotional Status. Anytime the newborn is in the room, note maternal–newborn interactions. Assess successfulness of breast-feeding attempts. Notice the quantity and quality of social support available to the woman. Monitor her mood and affect. Box 12-2 lists warning signs of poor attachment.

Test Yourself

✔ List five major components of the woman's history that are important to know when assuming care of the woman after delivery.

✔ Describe the appropriate way to perform an assessment of the episiotomy.

✔ Name three important laboratory studies to which you should pay attention after delivery.

Selected Nursing Diagnoses

■ Risk for Injury: Postpartum hemorrhage related to uterine atony, undetected lacerations, or hematoma formation
■ Acute Pain related to sore nipples, afterpains, or episiotomy discomfort
■ Risk for Infection related to multiple portals of entry for pathogens, including the former site of the placenta, episiotomy, bladder, and breasts
■ Risk for Injury: Falls related to postural hypotension and fainting
■ Urinary Retention related to periurethral edema, injury to the bladder during birth, or lingering effects of anesthesia
■ Risk for Constipation related to slowed peristalsis, inadequate fluid or fiber intake, and fear of pain during defecation
■ Risk for Injury: Thrombus formation related to increased coagulation factors and inadequate fluid intake

---

Box 12-2 ■ **WARNING SIGNS OF POOR ATTACHMENT**

■ Making negative statements about the baby
■ Turning away from the baby
■ Refusing to name the baby
■ Refusing to care for the baby
■ Withdrawing
■ Verbalizing disappointment with the sex of the baby
■ Failing to touch the baby
■ Limited handling of the baby

- Disturbed Sleep Pattern related to excess fatigue, overstimulation, or adjusting to newborn's frequent feeding needs
- Risk for Impaired Parent–Newborn Attachment

Outcome Identification and Planning

- Appropriate goals may include that the woman will not experience injury from postpartum hemorrhage, will express adequate pain control, will not exhibit signs and symptoms of infection, will not experience injury from falls, will have adequate urinary elimination without retention, will experience adequate bowel elimination, will not experience injury from DVT; will verbalize feeling rested after sleeping, and will exhibit behaviors that indicate the beginning of a healthy attachment with the newborn. Other goals and interventions are planned according to the individual needs of the woman and her partner.

Implementation

Promoting Hemostasis

As discussed earlier in the chapter, the postpartum woman is subject to hemorrhage from several sources. The cause of the most common type of postpartum hemorrhage is uterine atony. If the uterus feels boggy or soft to palpation, massage it until it firms up beneath your fingers. Monitor IV fluids and administer oxytocics, such as Pitocin, as ordered to prevent uterine atony. Teach the woman to perform periodic self-fundal massage.

The most likely cause of bright red bleeding that occurs in a steady stream in the presence of a firm fundus is a vaginal or cervical laceration that was not repaired. Report this finding to the RN or the primary care provider immediately. Report bleeding from or separation of the edges of the episiotomy. Monitor for and report any painful, soft, and possibly pulsing, masses palpable in the perineal area. These are signs of hematoma formation.

Be prepared.

When the woman gets up for the first time after delivery, it is normal for the lochia to seem heavy and to flow down her legs. Prepare her before she gets up that this is a normal occurrence caused by lochia pooling in the vagina while reclining and does not signify that she is hemorrhaging.

Providing Pain Management

There are several possible sources of pain during the postpartum period. To manage the pain adequately, you must first determine the source.

Breast Pain. Investigate breast pain to determine if it is unilateral and associated with increased warmth and redness. This could be a sign of mastitis, a postpartum complication discussed in Chapter 19. If the breasts are painful bilaterally because of engorgement, interventions will be chosen based on whether or not the woman is breast-feeding. If she is breast-feeding, warmth seems to help the most. Have her run warm water over her breasts in the shower, or place a warm washcloth as a compress on the breasts. If the engorgement is preventing the baby from latching on, assist the woman to express some milk before attempting to breast-feed.

If the breasts are engorged and the woman is bottle-feeding her newborn, instruct her to keep a support bra on 24 hours per day. Cool compresses or an ice pack wrapped in a towel will usually be soothing and help to suppress milk production.

If the nipples are painful during breast-feeding attempts, examine the nipples for cracks or fissures. Observe the woman when she puts her newborn to the breast and ensure that she is positioning the newborn properly to prevent sore, cracked nipples. Encourage the use of a lanolin-based cream to keep the nipples soft and promote healing. A mild analgesic may be helpful. (See Chapter 15 for additional breast-feeding interventions.)

Afterpains. If the source of pain is afterpains, ibuprofen or other nonsteroidal anti-inflammatory drugs are usually helpful. The primary care provider often will order 600 to 800 mg of ibuprofen every 6 to 8 hours as needed (PRN) for pain. For multiparas, it may be appropriate to schedule the medication around the clock, rather than waiting for the woman to ask for it. Timing administration of the drug so that the woman takes it 30 to 45 minutes before breast-feeding is also helpful because breast-feeding intensifies uterine cramping and associated afterpains. Nonpharmacologic methods that might be helpful include warm compresses to the abdomen, positioning for comfort, adequate rest and nutrition, and early ambulation.

Perineal Pain. If the pain is arising from the perineum, visually assess the perineum before taking measures to control the pain. Check that the episiotomy is well approximated and that there are no signs of a hematoma. Early interventions within the first 24 hours include ice packs to the perineum (Nursing Procedure 12-2). Ice helps reduce swelling and ease painful sensations. Most institutions use special perineal ice packs that incorporate the cold source into the perineal pad. The ice pack should be on for 20 minutes, then off for 10 to 20 minutes to be most effective.

After the first 24 hours, warm sitz baths can be especially comforting to a sore perineum (Nursing Procedure 12-3). Throughout the first few postpartum days,

Be careful.

When administering combination products for pain, be certain you know the dose of each product in the combination. Be particularly watchful that you do not exceed the maximum daily recommended dosage of acetaminophen when giving products that contain this medication.

Nursing Procedure 12-2
APPLICATION OF PERINEAL ICE PACKS

EQUIPMENT

A commercial ice pack or a clean glove and ice
Clean gloves

PROCEDURE

1. Explain procedure to the woman.
2. Wash hands thoroughly.
3. Position her in dorsal recumbent position.
4. Activate the commercial pack as instructed in the directions for use, or fill a clean glove with crushed ice and tie a knot at the opening at the top of the glove.

5. Cover the pack or the glove with a thin covering, such as a towel.
6. Place the pack on the perineum.
7. Assist her to a position of comfort.
8. Wash hands.
9. Leave in place for 20 minutes then remove for 10 minutes. Repeat as necessary for comfort during the first 24 hours postpartum.

Note: If the ice pack is allowed to stay next to the perineum continuously for prolonged periods, tissue damage could result.

---

mild analgesics combined with a narcotic are usually most helpful for perineal pain. Examples of combination products include acetaminophen with codeine (Tylenol No. 3) and hydrocodone with acetaminophen (Lortab, Vicodin). Local anesthetics, such as witch hazel pads or benzocaine sprays, may be helpful. Sitz baths, witch hazel pads, and/or

products that contain hydrocortisone can help reduce the pain associated with hemorrhoids.

Preventing Infection

There are multiple portals of entry for infection in the postpartum period. However, the number one way of

---

Nursing Procedure 12-3
ASSISTING THE POSTPARTUM WOMAN WITH A SITZ BATH

EQUIPMENT

New sitz bath in manufacturer's packaging with directions
Clean gloves

PROCEDURE

1. Explain procedure to the woman.
2. Instruct her to empty her bladder, if necessary.
3. Wash hands thoroughly.
4. Place the sitz bath in the toilet as per the manufacturer's instructions.
5. Place the tubing in the allotted slot and clamp the tubing.
6. Fill the bag with warm (102°F–105°F) water and hang it at a level of a few feet above the toilet.
7. Unclamp the tubing and allow the warm water to fill the basin.
8. Reclamp the tubing and refill the bag with warm water. Seal the bag with the locking mechanism provided.

9. Assist the woman to sit on the basin so that her perineum is submerged in the water.
10. Ensure that she can reach the emergency call bell.
11. Instruct her to unclamp the tubing periodically to allow water to run over the perineum and into the toilet.
12. Encourage the woman to stay on the sitz bath for at least 20 minutes.
13. Provide a clean towel with which to pat dry and clean sanitary napkins to apply when she is finished.
14. With clean-gloved hands, assist her to rinse out the basin, dry it, and store it for the next use.
15. Wash hands.

Note: Encourage the woman to use the sitz bath three times per day for at least 20 minutes per session, or as needed for comfort. Some women may prefer cooler water temperatures, which is an acceptable practice.

preventing infection continues to be hand washing. Wash your hands before and after caring for the patient, even if you will be wearing gloves. It is also important to teach the woman to wash her hands before touching her breasts or feeding the baby, before and after using the restroom or performing perineal care, and before eating. Early ambulation, adequate fluid intake, and good nutrition strengthen the immune system and help to prevent infection.

The best way to prevent mastitis (infection in the breast), in addition to frequent handwashing, is to avoid cracked nipples. Assist the woman to position the infant properly at the breast to prevent this complication. Other measures that help prevent cracked nipples are to rub the nipples with a few drops of expressed milk after breast-feeding and allow the nipples to air dry. Lanolin cream may also be a helpful measure. The woman should breast-feed at regular, frequent intervals. Milk stasis can lead to obstruction of a duct, which can lead to inflammation and then infection.

Endometritis, or infection of the uterine lining, is another type of infection that can occur in the postpartum period. Teach the woman that the best way to prevent this type of infection is to wash her hands before and after using the bathroom and/or performing perineal care. In addition, the woman should use a peribottle to perform perineal care and change her sanitary napkins/pads at least every 4 hours. Instruct her to fill the peribottle with warm water (she may add a gentle soap, if desired). After using the restroom, she should squeeze the bottle while aiming at the perineum so that the water flows from front to back. She can then use a washcloth or tissue to gently pat and dry the perineum from front to back. Instruct the woman to avoid touching the center part of the sanitary napkins/pads; she should handle the pads only by the ends. The part of the peripad that touches her perineum should be sterile. These measures can also help prevent infections of the episiotomy.

The postpartum woman is prone to bladder infections because of urethral trauma and perhaps from stasis related to incomplete bladder emptying. Urinary catheterization may be necessary to treat urinary retention; however, this invasive procedure increases the risk for urinary tract infection. Taking steps to avoid urinary catheterization, when possible, is helpful in decreasing the risk for urinary tract infection. Adequate fluid intake and measures to prevent retention are also helpful.

Preventing Injury From Falls

The first time the woman gets up, she is at risk for fainting and falling because of postural hypotension. When the woman is going to get out of bed for the first time after delivery, assist her to dangle her legs at the side of the bed for 5 minutes. If she is not feeling dizzy, assist her to the bathroom. Remain with her until she returns to bed. If she begins to feel dizzy at anytime, help her to sit down with her head forward for a few minutes. If she

begins to black out, gently support her to the floor until she comes to. Another time she is at increased risk for fainting is the first time she is in the shower. The warm water may cause peripheral dilation of blood vessels, which leads to hypotension and fainting. Stay in the woman's room while she is showering for the first time. Have a shower chair available for her to sit on if she begins to feel faint.

Promoting Urinary Elimination

The best way to assist the woman to empty her bladder is to help her up to the restroom to void. However, sometimes this is not possible because of incomplete recovery from regional anesthesia. In this instance, assist the woman to sit up on the bedpan, a position that may promote emptying of the bladder. Be certain that the woman has privacy. If she is having difficulty voiding, running water in the sink or using the peribottle to run warm water over the perineum may help. It also helps to give her plenty of time in which to void. If she feels rushed, this may contribute to urinary retention. If the woman cannot void on her first trip to the bathroom after delivery, it may be appropriate to allow her to wait for a while longer. If she is still unable to void and it has been longer than 6 hours, or there are signs of bladder distention, you may need to perform an in-and-out urinary catheterization to empty her bladder. Likewise, catheterization may be necessary if she is voiding small amounts (<100 mL) in frequent intervals.

Promoting Bowel Elimination

All of the normal measures that help prevent constipation are helpful in the postpartum period. Adequate fluid intake keeps the feces soft, facilitating passage. Early ambulation stimulates normal bowel peristalsis. Adding plenty of fruits, vegetables, and fiber to the diet also helps to prevent constipation. A bulk-forming agent, such as Metamucil, may also be helpful. Sometimes the primary care provider orders a stool softener for the first few days after birth. Encourage the woman not to suppress the urge to defecate.

Preventing Injury From Thrombus Formation

Assist the woman to ambulate as soon as possible after delivery. Early ambulation decreases the chance of thrombus formation by promoting venous return. Encourage liberal fluid intake. Dehydration contributes to the risk of thrombus formation.

Promoting Restful Sleep

Monitor the woman's sleep–wake cycle. Encourage her to continue presleep routines that she normally uses at home. Promote a relaxing, low-stress environment before sleep. Dim the lights and monitor noise and traffic near the woman's room during sleep time. Medicate for pain, if needed, at bedtime. Plan care activities so that she can sleep undisturbed for several hours at a time. For instance, if the postpartum recovery is going well and vital signs have been stable, consult with the RN about waiting until the 6 a.m. laboratory draw to obtain vital signs, rather than awaking the patient at 2 a.m. Or, instruct the woman to call you if she awakens in the night to use the restroom; you can perform the vital signs at this time.

Of course, it is challenging for a new mother to get enough sleep because newborns may awaken to feed every 2 to 3 hours. Encourage the woman to rest when the baby is sleeping. She may also wish to get in the habit of maintaining a quiet atmosphere and keeping the lights low when feeding the baby during the night. This practice helps to develop the baby's sleep–wake pattern so that it coincides with light and dark periods of the day. If the lights are on and the parents talk loudly and play with the baby in the middle of the night, he or she will think it is playtime and stay awake longer.

Promoting Parent–Newborn Attachment

It is important to allow as much parent–newborn contact as possible during the early postpartum period. Encourage the parents to cuddle the newborn closely. Encourage role model attachment behavior by talking to the newborn and calling the newborn by name. Point out positive features of the baby. Encourage the parents to participate in the care of the newborn. Provide privacy for the family to interact with the newborn. Assist the parents to learn the baby's cues that he or she is ready for interaction, that he or she is overstimulated, or that he or she is ready for sleep. Show the parents that a good time to interact with the newborn is during the alert state. Meet the woman's needs for pain relief, rest, and self-care so that she will have the energy to care for and interact with her newborn.

Evaluation: Goals and Expected Outcomes

Goal: The woman remains free from injury from postpartum hemorrhage.

Expected Outcomes:

- The fundus is firm and in the midline.
- The lochia flow is rubra (dark red in color) and small to moderate in amount.

Goal: The woman's pain is manageable.

Expected Outcomes: The woman

- reports pain before it becomes severe.
- verbalizes a tolerable pain level and a decrease in pain after interventions.

Goal: The woman remains free from the signs and symptoms of infection.

Expected Outcomes:

- The woman remains afebrile (temperature <100.4°F).
- There is no redness or heat in localized areas of the breast.
- Lochia has a normal fleshy scent without a foul odor.

- Episiotomy remains well approximated without purulent discharge.
- The woman does not report severe pain when voiding.

Goal: The woman does not experience injury due to fainting/falling.

Expected Outcomes: The woman

- does not fall during her postpartum stay.
- avoids head injury, bruises, or lacerations from fainting and falling unattended.

Goal: The woman does not experience urinary retention.

Expected Outcomes:

- The woman voids spontaneously within 6 hours of delivery.
- Urinary output is greater than 100 mL per episode, every 3 to 4 hours.

Goal: The woman has normal bowel elimination and avoids constipation.

Expected Outcome: The woman passes a soft, formed stool within the first 3 days after birth.

Goal: The woman does not develop DVT.

Expected Outcomes: The woman

- has a negative Homans' sign throughout her stay.
- has no unilateral swelling of the lower extremities.
- has no redness or heat in the calf area.

Goal: The woman experiences adequate amounts of restful sleep.

Expected Outcome: The woman verbalizes feeling rested with adequate energy to care for self and infant.

Goal: The woman and her partner demonstrate signs of healthy attachment to the newborn.

Expected Outcomes: The woman and her partner

- call the newborn by name.
- interact with the newborn in the en face position.
- talk to the newborn lovingly.
- make positive comments about the newborn.

Test Yourself

- ✔ Name two ways to promote hemostasis for the postpartum woman.
- ✔ List three nursing actions that can help a new mother avoid endometritis.
- ✔ What are three things you can do to help promote rest and sleep for a new mother?

Nursing Process for Postpartum Care After Cesarean Birth

The woman who has a cesarean birth faces the major postpartum challenges; however, she has also undergone major surgery. This section discusses how postpartum nursing care differs for the woman who has a cesarean birth. Remember that most of the nursing considerations discussed above for the postpartum woman also apply to the woman who delivers by cesarean section.

Assessment

The woman who has a cesarean has a significantly increased risk for death than does the woman who delivers vaginally. The top three causes of maternal mortality after cesarean are complications of anesthesia, postpartum infection, and thromboembolism (Deneux-Tharaux, Bouvier-Colle, & Breart, 2006). In addition to the normal postpartum assessment, the woman who has experienced a cesarean delivery requires close monitoring. Auscultate lung sounds at least every 4 hours in the first 24 hours and at least every 8 hours thereafter. The lungs should be clear without adventitious sounds and not diminished in any lobe.

Monitor the woman closely for signs of respiratory depression if a narcotic, such as Duramorph, was used in conjunction with the spinal or epidural anesthesia. Many anesthesiologists have preprinted orders that include how often the nurse should monitor respirations after this type of anesthesia. The orders may be to count the respiratory rate every 1 to 2 hours for the first 24 hours. Report respiratory rates of 12 per minute or less. Pulse oximetry, either continuous or intermittent, is often ordered. The oxygen saturation should remain above 95%.

Monitor the IV for rate of flow and correct solution. Check the IV site at least every 2 hours for redness, swelling, and pain. The IV usually remains in place for the first 24 hours after delivery. At that time, the practitioner usually gives an order to remove the device or to convert the IV to a saline lock.

The sources of pain and discomfort for the woman who delivers by cesarean are similar to those of a woman who has delivered vaginally. Usually, a woman who experiences cesarean birth does not have an episiotomy, although rarely this may be the case. However, she does have an abdominal incision that is an additional source of pain. The buildup of intestinal gas and referred shoulder pain are other sources of pain. Pruritus, (itching), is a common side effect of narcotic administration during regional anesthesia. This can be a source of discomfort for the woman who had a cesarean birth.

The abdominal incision is a site for possible hemorrhage and infection. Monitor for drainage on the dressing in the first 24 hours. Assess the incision at least once every 8 hours after removing the dressing. The incision should remain well approximated with sutures or staples. A small amount of redness is normal. An increase in the amount of redness, edema, or drainage from the site is an abnormal finding.

Monitor bowel sounds at least every 4 hours. Check closely for abdominal distention and pain associated with gas formation. It may be difficult for the woman to pass flatus after cesarean delivery because of decreased peristalsis. Ask the woman if she is passing gas. Instruct her to report bowel movements.

Observe the Foley catheter for urinary output. The catheter usually remains in place for the first 24 hours after cesarean birth. Output should be at least 30 mL/hr. The urine should be clear yellow or a light straw color. Cloudy urine is associated with infection. After removing the Foley catheter, observe the woman for the first few voids to make certain she is voiding adequately without retention.

Assess for signs of thrombus formation. The calves should be of equal size without redness, warmth, or pain. Remember, the woman who delivers by cesarean is at even higher risk for thrombus formation than is the woman who delivers vaginally.

Selected Nursing Diagnoses

- Ineffective Breathing Pattern related to respiratory depression from narcotics
- Risk for Injury: Hemorrhage from the normal postpartum routes and from the incision
- Risk for Infection related to postpartum status, stasis of secretions in the lungs, abdominal incision, and presence of the Foley catheter
- Acute Pain related to incision, discomfort from pruritus, or inability to pass flatus
- Risk for Injury: Thrombus formation related to postpartum status, bed rest, and lowered activity levels

Outcome Identification and Planning

Appropriate goals include that the woman will maintain an adequate respiratory rate, will not experience injury from hemorrhage, will remain free from signs of infection, will verbalize a tolerable pain level, and will remain free of injury from thrombus formation.

Implementation

Monitoring for an Adequate Respiratory Pattern

If the woman has had narcotics administered via the spinal or epidural routes, monitor her closely for respiratory depression. Monitor the respirations at least every 2 hours for the first 24 hours post–spinal narcotic administration. Have naloxone (Narcan) readily available. The anesthesiologist orders naloxone administration if the respiratory rate falls below 10 to 12 per minute. Monitor oxygen saturation, as ordered. Report continuous oxygen saturation levels below 95%.

Preventing Injury From Hemorrhage

Do not forget to check the fundus. It is not necessary to massage the fundus unless it is soft and the woman is bleeding vaginally. Any manipulation of the fundus increases pain. However, it is important to note fundal position, height, and tone.

Assess the dressing for drainage. Mark any areas of drainage so that you can tell if the area is increasing during subsequent assessments. If the dressing becomes saturated, reinforce it and apply pressure to the site. Notify the RN or primary care provider for further orders.

Preventing Infection

One major difference between care of the woman who has delivered vaginally and one who has had a cesarean is that of lung status. Assess the lungs of a woman who has experienced cesarean birth carefully at least every 4 hours during the first 24 hours. Also assist the woman to turn, cough, and deep breathe at least every 2 hours. It will not be easy for her to take deep breaths or to cough. Assist her to splint her incision with a pillow while she coughs. This stabilizes the area and reduces pain. The practitioner usually orders an incentive spirometer. Assist the woman to use it hourly for the first 24 hours when she is awake.

The incision is another possible site for infection. During the first 24 hours, the original dressing usually covers the incision. After the physician removes the dressing, assess the incision for increasing redness, edema, or drainage. Proper incision care includes washing the hands thoroughly before touching the incision for any reason. Instruct the woman to wash the incision with soap and water, and then pat it dry thoroughly. Nothing wet should remain against the incision.

The continuous Foley catheter that is in place during the first 24 hours is another potential source of infection. Provide frequent perineal and Foley care. Monitor IV fluids to ensure adequate infusion of fluids. As long as the woman remains well hydrated, her kidneys will produce enough urine to keep a steady flow. The flow helps to wash out bacteria. When you discontinue the catheter, assist the woman to void within 6 hours of removal.

Providing Pain Management

Pain management for the woman after cesarean birth is a challenge when providing postpartum care. During the first 24 hours, the anesthesiologist usually manages the pain. Generally, if the woman had a spinal narcotic administered, she will have orders for a PRN medication for **breakthrough pain**. Breakthrough pain occurs when the basal dose of analgesia does not control the pain adequately.

Another form of pain control that may be ordered is patient-controlled analgesia (PCA). This type of analgesia allows the woman to control how often she receives pain medication. The PCA pump delivers an opioid (usually morphine) into the IV line. The pump locks to prevent tampering. The physician orders describe how much narcotic the woman receives when she pushes the button. The orders include a lockout interval so that the woman cannot accidentally overdose herself. Many

A word of admonition!

Do not push the PCA button yourself, even if the woman does not push the button. Pushing the PCA button for the woman is called analgesia by proxy. This practice is dangerous because you or a family member could inadvertently cause respiratory arrest.

women require reassurance that they cannot self-administer too much medication when using PCA.

Infrequently, the anesthetist orders narcotics at PRN intervals after cesarean birth. In this instance, consult with the RN to administer the narcotic around the clock for the first 24 hours. Research has shown that it is easier to control pain before it becomes severe and that adequate pain control in the first 24 hours after surgery reduces the total amount of pain medication required. The woman who is breast-feeding may be reluctant to take pain medication. Inform her that adequate pain control is necessary so that she can ambulate well and for her to provide self- and newborn care (Karlstrom et al., 2007).

Pruritus is a common side effect of narcotics given by the spinal or epidural routes. This side effect can become quite uncomfortable and can lead to scratching and excoriation. Often the anesthetist prescribes an antipruritic, usually diphenhydramine (Benadryl), to help control this side effect. Current research demonstrates promising results with small doses of naloxone (Narcan) added to continuous epidural infusions of morphine to prevent pruritus (Jeon et al., 2005; Kim et al., 2007). If nothing is ordered, notify the anesthetist. Other comfort measures include applying lotion, administering a back rub, and using cool compresses or diversion to help control the itching.

Another common source of pain for the woman who delivers by cesarean is gas pain. The woman is at increased risk for gas formation after a cesarean because of decreased peristalsis, the lingering effects of anesthesia and analgesia, and manipulation of the intestines during surgery. If gas builds up and the woman cannot release it, she becomes bloated and can experience severe pain.

This pain is usually not relieved by analgesics. Many surgeons order simethicone (Mylicon) prophylactically. If this is the case, the surgeon orders simethicone around the clock. PRN is an alternate schedule. Frequent and early ambulation stimulates peristalsis and passing of flatus. Instruct the woman to avoid very hot or very cold beverages, carbonated beverages, and drinking through straws. All of these things can increase the formation and discomfort of gas. Other medical interventions may become necessary, such as rectal suppositories or enemas. Encourage the woman to lie on her left side. This position facilitates the release of gas.

Preventing Injury From Thrombus Formation

Many women come back from surgery with thromboembolic disease stockings (TEDS) already in place. If not, there will be an order to apply them. Pneumatic compression devices also may be ordered during the first 24 hours. These devices stimulate venous return to the heart, an action that helps prevent pooling and thrombus formation. Once the woman can get out of bed and ambulate, advise frequent ambulation. This is the best way to prevent a thrombus from forming. Another important nursing action is to ensure adequate fluid intake.

Evaluation: Goals and Expected Outcomes

Goal: The woman's respiratory pattern is not compromised.

Expected Outcomes:

- The woman maintains an adequate respiratory pattern (16 to 20 breaths per minute).
- Oxygen saturation remains above 95%.

Goal: The woman does not sustain injury from hemorrhage.

Expected Outcomes: The woman's

- fundus remains firm in the midline.
- lochia flow remains scant to small.
- incision remains free of drainage and bleeding.

Goal: The woman remains free from signs and symptoms of infection.

Expected Outcomes: The woman's

- temperature remains below 100.4°F.
- lungs remain clear to auscultation.
- incision is clean, dry, well approximated without redness or drainage.
- lochia does not have a foul odor.
- urine remains clear.

Goal: The woman's pain is manageable.

Expected Outcomes: The woman

- reports pain before it becomes severe.
- uses PCA, as ordered.
- voices adequate pain relief after interventions.
- states pruritus is at a tolerable level.

Goal: The woman remains free from thrombus formation.

Expected Outcomes: The woman maintains

- a negative Homans' sign.
- no unilateral swelling, redness, or warmth in the lower extremities.
- no shortness of breath or chest pain.

Nursing Process for Preparing the Postpartum Woman for Discharge

Discharge planning for the new mother begins upon admission and continues until she returns home. Most interventions related to discharge focus on teaching the woman to care for herself and the baby when she goes home. Observe how the woman and her partner are adapting to their new role as parents and support healthy adaptation behaviors.

Assessment

Bearing a child is a life-changing event. Observe how the parents interact with each other and with the baby. Watch for interactions between other members of the family, such as grandparents and siblings of the new baby. Determine what behaviors are helping the new family adjust, and note if any actions are getting in the way of positive adjustment.

Because teaching is the focus of most nursing interventions when planning for discharge, it is important to determine the woman's knowledge base. Do not assume that a woman knows how to take care of herself and the baby just because she may be educated, she is a nurse, or she has other children, and so on. The only way to know what a woman knows about self-care and baby care is to ask and to observe. This section focuses on maternal self-care at home. Newborn care is discussed in Chapter 14].

Selected Nursing Diagnoses

- Health-Seeking Behaviors
- Risk for Injury related to Rh negative blood type and/or non-immunity to rubella
- Deficient Knowledge of self-care

Outcome Identification and Planning

Appropriate goals include that the woman and her partner will demonstrate positive adjustment to the parental role; no injury will occur related to Rh status or rubella nonimmunity; and the woman will verbalize danger signs that should be reported immediately. Another goal is that the woman will demonstrate the ability to perform self-care to include breast care, fundal checks and massage, care of lochia and the perineum, pain management, and prevention of constipation and fatigue.

Implementation

Supporting Health-Seeking Behaviors

Reinforce positive family behaviors. Take particular care to praise the woman and her partner for positive parenting skills. When the parents require assistance as they learn new skills, provide positive verbal support. If the woman makes a mistake, it is not helpful to focus on the mistake in a negative way. For instance, it is not supportive to tell the mother, "No. That's not the way to do it. Do it like this." Instead, focus on the things she is doing well and use positive language to guide her when she is having difficulty with the task. Use words that convey acceptance, such as, "Some women find it helpful to do it this way." Or, "the baby might find this to be soothing."

Anticipatory guidance is helpful when siblings are involved. Explain to the parents that it is normal for the older sibling to regress in the first few days after the birth of the baby. Tell them it helps if they do not focus undue attention on regressive behaviors, such as a return to bedwetting, sucking the thumb, or clinging to a favorite toy or blanket. It is particularly important for the parents not to criticize or belittle the older child for regressive behaviors. Explain that the behavior is temporary and will pass as the child adjusts to his new role in the family. Suggest that the parents set aside time every day that is just "big brother or sister" time. The sibling will find it easier to adjust if he feels that his parents still care for and value him. Another helpful suggestion is to provide the older child with a doll and allow the child to take care of the doll, as the parent is caring for the baby.

This activity helps the older child to feel included and can help to develop nurturing skills.

Preventing Injury From Rh-Negative Blood Type or Nonimmunity to Rubella

Before the woman leaves the hospital, it is important to check to see if the woman who is Rh-negative is a candidate for $Rh_o(D)$ immune globulin (RhoGAM). If the woman is Rh-negative and the baby is Rh-positive, the woman will need an injection of RhoGAM to prevent the development of antibodies to Rh-positive blood. The woman must receive the RhoGAM within 72 hours of delivery to be most effective. If the baby is Rh negative, the woman does not need RhoGAM. Box 12-3 highlights nursing considerations for administering RhoGAM.

You must also determine the woman's rubella status. If she is nonimmune to rubella, the rubella titer is less than 1:8, she will need to receive the rubella vaccine before she is discharged. It is important for her to know that she should not get pregnant for at least 3 months after receiving the vaccine. Box 12-4 discusses nursing considerations for giving the rubella vaccine.

Providing Patient Teaching

Because the postpartum stay is very short, it is important to grab every available opportunity for teaching. On the day of discharge, give the woman written self-care instructions. It is best to ask her questions regarding how she plans to care for her breasts, perineum, pain, and so on; to determine how much information she has retained; and to reinforce areas she may not have absorbed. Instruct the woman that she needs to make an appointment with her primary care provider for a 6-week postpartum checkup. It is important for the woman to know danger signs that she should report to the primary care provider. Box 12-5 lists these danger signs.

Breast Care. Teach breast care as you are assisting the woman to breast-feed or when she takes a shower. Explain that plain water is sufficient to clean the nipples because soap is drying and can contribute to sore, cracked nipples. Encourage the use of lanolin cream on the nipples. After a feeding, teach the woman to express a drop of breast milk, rub it into each nipple, and allow the nipples to air dry. She should wear a good support bra at all times.

Fundal Massage. Teach self-fundal massage when you are assessing the fundus. Assist her to touch the top of the uterus and to massage it gently as she makes certain it stays firmly contracted. Explain to her that the uterus should no longer be palpable by the 10th day.

Perineum and Vaginal Care. Instruct the woman on proper perineal care the first time she gets up to use the bathroom. As described earlier, teach her how to clean the perineum using a peribottle and to handle sanitary napkins to avoid contaminating the center of the pad.

Box 12-3 ▌ PREVENTION OF ANTIBODY DEVELOPMENT

Medication: $Rh_o(D)$ immune globulin (RhoGAM)
Method of action: Prevents development of antibodies to $Rh_o(D)$-positive blood, if given to the $Rh_o(D)$- negative woman within 72 hours of abortion, invasive procedure such as amniocentesis, or delivery of an $Rh_o(D)$-positive infant.
Usual dosage and administration: One vial given via the intramuscular route
Antidote: None
Nursing interventions:

1. Ensure that the woman is a candidate for RhoGAM. She is a candidate if she meets all of the following criteria. She
   a. Is $Rh_o(D)$-negative
   b. Has never been sensitized to $Rh_o(D)$-positive blood
   c. Has had an abortion, ectopic pregnancy, or delivered an $Rh_o(D)$-positive infant within the past 72 hours
2. Explain that the woman is receiving RhoGAM to prevent her from becoming sensitized to $Rh_o(D)$-positive blood. This will prevent hemolytic disease of the newborn in subsequent pregnancies.
3. Inform the woman that RhoGAM is a blood product. Although RhoGAM is screened, tested, and treated to reduce the risk of disease transmission, there is still a slight possibility that she could get an infection from the product.
4. Explain that there may be soreness at the site.
5. Ask the woman which site she prefers for the intramuscular injection. The deltoid and gluteal muscles are both acceptable sites.
6. Instruct the woman to call her doctor immediately if she has fever, chills, shaking, back pain, a change in the color or amount of her urine, sudden weight gain, or swelling in her extremities. She should not take any vaccines for 3 months after treatment with RhoGAM because the medication can weaken the vaccine.
7. Give the woman a card indicating her Rh status and the date of RhoGAM administration. Instruct her to carry the card with her at all times.

Explain the importance of these instructions to help prevent bladder and episiotomy infections. Explain that she will need to continue to use sanitary napkins until the lochia stops. She should not use tampons because they contribute to uterine infection until the placental site has healed. Reinforce that she should continue perineal care after every voiding and defecation until the lochia stops.

Box 12-4 ▮ DEVELOPMENT OF IMMUNITY TO RUBELLA

Medication: Live rubella vaccine
Method of action: Causes the body to produce antibodies against the rubella virus, thereby stimulating the development of immunity to rubella.
Usual dosage and administration: One vial given subcutaneously in the upper, outer aspect of the arm.
Antidote: None
Nursing interventions:

1. Determine whether there are any contraindications for administering the vaccine. Contraindications include that the woman
   a. Is sensitive to neomycin
   b. Is immunosuppressed
   c. Has received a blood product (including RhoGam) within the past 3 months
2. Explain possible adverse reactions.
   a. Discomfort at the injection site.
   b. Development of rash, sore throat, headache, and general malaise within 2 to 4 weeks of the injection.
3. Obtain informed consent before administering the vaccine.
4. Instruct the woman on the importance of avoiding pregnancy for at least 3 months. Because the rubella vaccine is a live virus, it could be teratogenic to the fetus.
5. Inform the breast-feeding woman that the rubella vaccine crosses over into the breast milk. The newborn benefits from short-term immunity but may become flushed, fussy, or develop a slight rash. Suggest that the woman speak to the pediatrician if she has concerns.

Box 12-5 ▮ POSTPARTUM DANGER SIGNS

- Fever ≥100.4°F
- Shaking chills
- Localized reddened, painful area on one breast
- Frequency, urgency, and painful urination
- Sudden onset of shortness of breath and/or chest pain
- Severe unremitting abdominal or back pain that is unrelieved by normal pain measures
- Foul smelling lochia
- Increased or heavy lochia flow or passage of clots
- Return to lochia rubra after it has been serosa or alba
- Severe pain, redness, or swelling in the episiotomy or cesarean incision
- Swollen, reddened, painful area on the calf
- Prolonged or severe depression
- Thoughts of harming the baby or self (suicidal thoughts)

additional trauma and infection. Healing is indicated when the lochia flow stops and there is no discomfort when two fingers are placed inside the vaginal opening. Hormonal changes associated with breast-feeding sometimes contribute to vaginal dryness and associated dyspareunia. For this reason breast-feeding mothers may find it helpful to use a water-soluble jelly (e.g., KY jelly) for lubrication during sexual intercourse.

Pain Management. Teach the woman about pain management as you provide pain management for her. Explain that it is more effective to control pain before it becomes severe. Many women are afraid to take pain medication when they are breast-feeding. Reassure her that the analgesics the primary care provider has ordered will not harm her baby. Clarify that it is easier to breast-feed when the mother is comfortable and pain free. Tell her the name of the medication that you are giving her and briefly describe its benefit. For instance, when the woman complains of afterpains, administer the ordered ibuprofen, and explain that ibuprofen is usually very effective in controlling the pain of cramping. If she complains that her stitches hurt, administer the ordered analgesic-narcotic combination and make clear that this medication is most effective at controlling episiotomy or incisional pain. Tell her how frequently she can have each medication and why it is important not to take pain medication more frequently or at higher dosages than what is ordered.

Explain the benefits of using non-medicinal ways of easing pain, such as applying warmth to the abdomen to help soothe afterpains. When you assist her with the sitz bath, encourage her to continue using it at home until the episiotomy has healed. Some women worry that the

Encourage handwashing before and after performing perineal care.

Remind the woman that lochia flow should become progressively lighter. Lochia rubra generally lasts for approximately 2 to 3 days. This is followed by lochia serosa for the remainder of the first week after delivery. After the first week, the flow should be lochia alba. She should not saturate peripads, and there should not be any large clots.

Teach the woman to avoid sexual intercourse, tampons, or introduction of any substance into the vagina until the placental site and episiotomy or tear have healed to prevent

Here's a teaching tip.

If the woman engages in vigorous exercise during the postpartum period, the amount of lochia will temporarily increase. This is a normal finding.

stitches will have to be removed and anticipate that this will be painful. Reassure her that the body absorbs the stitches and they do not need to be removed.

Nutrition. Nutrition is an important aspect of self-care. Meal times are a good time to discuss nutrition with the woman. Determine what her normal pattern of intake is. Give her brochures that explain MyPyramid. Discuss with her how to use MyPyramid to plan meals. Instruct the woman who is not breast-feeding to decrease her caloric intake by approximately 300 kcal per day (i.e., she should reduce her intake to pre-pregnancy levels). The lactating woman will need to add an additional 200 kcal above the pregnancy requirement of 300 kcal per day, for a total of 500 kcal above pre-pregnancy requirements.

Constipation. As you are caring for the woman, explain how different activities contribute to or prevent constipation. Describe how activity helps the bowel to regain its tone, which helps prevent constipation. When you fill her water pitcher, explain that she needs to drink liberally of noncaffeinated fluids to help keep the stool soft. Explain that caffeine is a diuretic, so it is best to limit caffeinated fluids. Encourage her to drink fluids that she enjoys. If she does not like water, explore alternatives with her, such as noncaffeinated herbal tea, juice, and sugar-free gelatin. Explain to her the importance of heeding the urge to defecate. Ignoring the urge can contribute to constipation. Teach her about high fiber foods when you serve her a meal or bring her a snack. If the practitioner has prescribed a stool softener, tell her the name of the medication and its intended effect when you administer it. Offer her a large glass of water when she takes the stool softener and emphasize the importance of adequate hydration when taking a stool softener.

Proper Rest. It is important for the woman to know that it is easy to over do it in the first few days after having a baby. Explore the possibility of asking a friend or relative to help out for the first few days. Reassure her that her health and that of her baby are the most important concerns while she is recovering from childbirth. Give her hints such as, "When you are tired, rest. If you are exhausted, you will not have the energy to care for your baby." It might be helpful to suggest that she rest with her feet up when the baby is napping during the day. Reassure her that house-cleaning chores can wait if she is too tired to do them. The woman should not do heavy lifting. Teach the woman the good rule of thumb not to lift anything heavier than the baby for the first 6 weeks after delivery.

When the father is present, explain to him how much energy it takes for the body to repair itself after childbirth. If he was present at the birth, he probably readily understands this concept. If appropriate, encourage him to help with household chores and older sibling care while the woman recuperates.

Evaluation: Goals and Expected Outcomes

Goal: Both parents demonstrate positive adjustment to the parental role.

Expected Outcomes: The woman and her partner

- care for the newborn with confidence.
- demonstrate positive attachment behaviors with the newborn.

Goal: The woman will not experience injury from Rh incompatibilities or rubella nonimmunity.

Expected Outcomes: The woman

- receives RhoGAM within 72 hours after delivery, if eligible.
- receives rubella vaccine (or instructions as to where to obtain the vaccine) if nonimmune.

Goal: The woman demonstrates adequate self-care behaviors.

Expected Outcomes: The woman

- explains danger signals that need to be reported.
- demonstrates the ability to perform self-care to include breast care, fundal checks and massage, perineal care, pain management, constipation prevention, and avoidance of fatigue and sleep deprivation

Test Yourself

✔ Describe four major ways that assessment of the woman after cesarean delivery differs from that for a woman who delivers vaginally.

✔ Explain the proper way to perform perineal care.

✔ List four signs of infection that the new mother should report.

Key Points

- The reproductive system organs gradually return to the nonpregnant size and function in the process of involution.
- Fundal height decreases at a rate of 1 fingerbreadth (1 cm) per day until the uterus is no longer palpable on the 10th postpartum day.
- Multiparas more frequently experience afterpains than do primiparas.
- Lochia progresses from rubra to serosa to alba as the uterine lining and other cells are cast away from the uterus.
- Kegel exercises can help the postpartum woman regain tone in the perineal area, although the size and tone of the introitus never fully return to the prepregnant state.
- The extra fluid volume that builds up during pregnancy is eliminated in the early postpartum period, leading to high urinary output and diaphoresis.
- The woman's temperature may be slightly elevated during the first 24 hours after delivery because of dehydration and exhaustion. After the first 24 hours, temperature should be under 100.4°F. Blood pressure should remain at the level it was during labor. Mild bradycardia (50–60 bpm) in the early postpartum period is normal.
- The woman is often very hungry and thirsty after delivering a baby. Allow her to eat and drink unless medically contraindicated.
- Trauma to the lower urinary tract can lead to urinary retention in the postpartum period.
- The most significant psychological adaptation a woman must make is role change as she becomes a mother. She usually does this in four overlapping stages: beginning attachment and preparation for the baby; increasing attachment, learning to care for the baby, and physical restoration; moving toward a new normal; and achieving maternal identity.
- Bonding is the initial component of healthy attachment between a parent and the newborn. It generally occurs in a predictable sequence.
- Postpartum blues is a temporary mood disorder that manifests itself through tearfulness and other signs of mild depression.
- Postpartum assessment involves (1) data collection to include pregnancy history, medical history, and labor and birth history; and (2) a thorough head-to-toe physical assessment with focus on expected postpartum changes.
- Nursing interventions in the early postpartum period focus on preventing and detecting hemorrhage, treating pain, preventing infection, preventing falls, detecting and treating urinary retention, preventing constipation, preventing and detecting thrombus formation, promoting sleep, and promoting healthy parental–newborn attachment.
- The woman who has a cesarean birth requires additional nursing considerations because she has undergone surgery. Possible complications include respiratory compromise and pain, infection, and hemorrhage from abdominal incision.
- Helping the woman to turn, cough, and deep breath and encouraging early and frequent ambulation after cesarean delivery are necessary measures to help prevent respiratory compromise and thrombus formation.
- Prepare the woman for discharge by teaching her to perform self- and infant care. Self-care includes breast care, fundal massage, assessment of lochia, perineal care, pain management, prevention of constipation, and prevention of fatigue.

INTERNET RESOURCES

Postpartum Resources
www.childbirth.org/articles/postpartum.html

Helping Dads Support the New Mom
www.dona.org/PDF/DadsandPostpartumDoulas.pdf

Workbook

■ **NCLEX-STYLE REVIEW QUESTIONS**

1. An 18-year-old primipara is getting ready to go home. She had a third-degree episiotomy with repair. She confides in the nurse that she is afraid to go to her postpartum checkup because she is afraid to have the stitches removed. Which reply by the nurse is best?

   a. "It doesn't hurt when the midwife takes out the stitches. You will only feel a little tugging and pulling sensation."

   b. "It is very important for you to go to your checkup visit. Besides, the stitches do not have to be removed."

   c. "Many women have that fear after having an episiotomy. The stitches do not need to be removed because the suture will be gradually absorbed."

   d. "Oh, you mustn't miss your follow-up appointment. Don't worry. Your midwife will be very gentle."

2. A woman has just delivered her third baby. Everything has progressed normally up to this point. When the nurse tries to take the woman's blood pressure, she notices that the woman is shaking and that her teeth are chattering. Which action should the nurse take first?

   a. Finish taking the vital signs, and then decide what to do

   b. Notify the RN immediately

   c. Place two prewarmed blankets on the woman

   d. Put on the call bell to summon for help

3. The night shift LPN is checking on a woman who had a cesarean delivery with spinal Duramorph anesthesia several hours earlier. The nurse counts a respiratory rate of 8 in 1 minute. What should the nurse do first?

   a. Administer naloxone (Narcan), per the preprinted orders

   b. Awaken the woman and instruct her to breathe more rapidly

   c. Call the anesthesiologist from the room for orders

   d. Perform bag-to-mouth rescue breathing at a rate of 12 per minute

4. The nurse is performing the initial postpartum assessment for her shift on a woman who had a cesarean delivery the day before. The nurse notices that the woman is scratching her face and her arms. What action by the nurse is indicated?

   a. Administer naloxone (Narcan) immediately, per the preprinted orders

   b. Ask the woman if she wants something for the itching, and then call the anesthesiologist for orders

   c. Determine the severity of the itching and offer to give diphenhydramine (Benadryl), as ordered

   d. Observe and wait until the woman complains about the itching before treating it

5. A woman who has chosen to bottle-feed says that her breasts are painful and engorged. Which nursing intervention is appropriate?

   a. Assist the woman into the shower, and have her run warm water over her breasts

   b. Assist the woman to place ice packs on her breasts

   c. Encourage the woman to breast-feed because she is producing so much milk

   d. Provide a breast pump and assist the woman in emptying her breasts

■ **STUDY ACTIVITIES**

1. With your clinical group, develop a one-page postpartum instruction sheet to send home with the new mother that covers all of the essential information she needs for self-care at home.

2. Explain how nursing care of a woman after cesarean birth differs from that of a woman who delivers vaginally. What additional risk factors does the woman have after cesarean?

3. Using the table below, compare the different sources of postpartum pain.

Pain Source	Possible Causes	Nursing Care to Prevent and Treat
Breast		
Afterpains		
Perineal pain		
Gas pain and distention after cesarean		
Cesarean incision		

■ CRITICAL THINKING: WHAT WOULD YOU DO?

1. You enter the room of Heather, a 22-year-old primipara, and find her on the floor looking a little dazed. When you ask her what happened, she tells you that she remembers trying to get up to go the restroom and that she started feeling a bit dizzy and faint. The next thing she knew she was on the floor.

   a. What is the likely cause of Heather's fall? What nursing actions could have prevented this occurrence?

   b. Later that day, Heather reports that she feels like she just "dribbles" when she tries to urinate and she feels like she is bleeding too much. What assessments should you make first? What do you expect to find?

   c. What measures can the nurse take to help relieve Heather's urinary retention?

   d. On the third postpartum day, Heather says that she is experiencing chills and thinks she is coming down with a fever. In addition to taking the temperature, what other assessments should you make? Why?

2. Marla delivered her fifth child yesterday after a difficult labor that lasted almost 24 hours. The baby weighed 7 lb 6 oz, and she is breast-feeding.

   a. What factors put Marla at risk for postpartum hemorrhage?

   b. While you are checking Marla's lochia, you notice that her lochia has saturated through two sanitary napkins/pads since you last checked on her an hour ago. What do you think is causing the bleeding? What is your first action and why? What would you do next? Justify your answer.

3. Mindy had a cesarean delivery. This is her second postoperative day. She is in her bed when you come in to take vital signs. She looks miserable, and she says that she just cannot get comfortable.

   a. What assessments should you make first?

   b. You determine that Mindy is suffering from incisional pain and gas pain. What remedies should you offer for these two sources of pain?

   c. You perform a complete assessment and discover that Mindy has a positive Homans' sign. What action should you take?

13 Nursing Assessment of Newborn Transition

KEY TERMS

brown fat
caput succedaneum
cephalhematoma
cold stress
epispadias
Epstein's pearls
Harlequin sign
hyperbilirubinemia
hypospadias
jaundice
lanugo
meconium
molding
mottling
phimosis
physiologic jaundice
pseudomenstruation
simian crease
smegma
surfactant
thermoregulation
thrush
vernix caseosa

LEARNING OBJECTIVES

On completion of this chapter, you should be able to:

1. Identify respiratory adaptations the newborn makes as he or she transitions to life outside the womb.
2. Outline cardiovascular changes that occur immediately after birth.
3. Explain thermoregulatory capabilities of the newborn.
4. Discuss the role of the liver in the newborn's adaptation to extrauterine life.
5. Describe expected behavioral characteristics of the newborn.
6. Describe how an Apgar score is assigned.
7. Define newborn hypoglycemia.
8. Explain the major steps of the initial nursing assessment of the newborn.
9. Define expected weights and measures of the newborn.
10. Compare and contrast expected versus unexpected assessment parameters of the newborn.
11. Explain how to elicit each newborn reflex.

THE NEWBORN is a unique individual different than the fetus, older infant, child, and adult. The newborn's anatomy and physiology change immediately after birth and continue to change as he or she grows. As the nurse, it is essential for you to be aware of adjustments the newborn must make as he transitions to life outside the womb. It is important to know the characteristics of a normal newborn in order to make accurate assessments. This knowledge also enables you to answer appropriately parents' questions and concerns about their newborn. This chapter explores the immediate and ongoing adaptation of the normal newborn to life outside the womb and describes initial nursing assessments.

PHYSIOLOGIC ADAPTATION

The fetus is fully dependent upon the mother for all vital needs, such as oxygen, nutrition, and waste removal.

At birth, the body systems must immediately undergo tremendous changes so that the newborn can exist outside the womb. Table 13-1 compares the anatomy and physiology of the fetus and newborn.

Respiratory Adaptation

Fetal lungs are uninflated and full of amniotic fluid because they are not needed for oxygen exchange. Immediately after birth, the newborn's lungs must inflate, the remaining fluid must be absorbed, and oxygen exchange must begin.

One factor that helps the newborn clear fluid from the lungs and take his or her first breath begins during labor. The process of labor stimulates surfactant production, and much of the fetal lung fluid is squeezed out as the fetus moves down the birth canal. This so-called vaginal squeeze is an important way nature helps to clear the

Table 13-1 ▌ ANATOMIC AND PHYSIOLOGIC COMPARISON OF THE FETUS AND NEWBORN

Comparison	Fetus	Newborn
Respiratory system	Fluid-filled, high-pressure system causes blood to be shunted from the lungs through the ductus arteriosus to the rest of body	Air-filled, low-pressure system encourages blood flow through the lungs for gas exchange; increased oxygen content of blood in the lungs contributes to the closing of the ductus arteriosus (becomes a ligament)
Site of gas exchange	Placenta	Lungs
Circulation through the heart	Pressures in the right atrium greater than in the left; encourages blood flow through the foreman ovale	Pressures in the left atrium greater than in the right; causes the foreman ovale to close
Hepatic portal circulation	Ductus venosus bypasses; maternal liver performs filtering functions	Ductus venosus closes (becomes a ligament); hepatic portal circulation begins
Thermoregulation	Body temperature maintained by maternal body temperature and warmth of the intrauterine environment	Body temperature maintained through a flexed posture, muscle activity, and metabolism

airway in preparation for the first breath. The vaginal squeeze also plays a role in stimulating lung expansion. The pressure of the birth canal on the fetal chest releases immediately when the infant is born. The lowered pressure from chest expansion draws air into the lungs.

Chemical changes stimulate respiratory centers in the brain. The newborn's lifeline to oxygen is cut off when the umbilical cord is clamped. Oxygen levels fall and carbon dioxide levels rise causing the newborn's pH to fall. The resulting acidosis stimulates the respiratory centers of the brain to begin their lifelong function of regulating respiration.

It is critical for the newborn to make strong respiratory efforts during the first few moments of life. This effort is best demonstrated and stimulated by a vigorous cry because crying helps to open the small air sacs (alveoli) in the lungs. Immediate sensory and thermal changes stimulate the newborn to cry. Inside the uterus, it is warm and dark, sounds are muffled, and the fetus is cradled by the confines of the womb. The environment changes drastically at the moment of birth. The temperature is colder, it is brighter and louder, the security of the uterus is lost, and the newborn is touched directly for the first time.

Another important factor in the newborn's respiratory adaptation is surfactant. **Surfactant,** a substance found in the lungs of mature fetuses, keeps the alveoli from collapsing after they first expand. The work of breathing increases greatly when the lungs lack surfactant. The

Think about this.

A newborn delivered by cesarean does not always have the benefit of the vaginal squeeze. This newborn often has more fluid in his/her lungs, making respiratory adaptation more challenging. Closely monitor this newborn's respirations.

newborn without enough surfactant expends large amounts of energy to breathe and quickly becomes exhausted without medical intervention. By the end of 35 weeks' gestation, the fetus usually has enough surfactant to breathe without lung collapse. Maturity of the respiratory system can be determined prenatally by measuring the lecithin/sphingomyelin (L/S) ratio of amniotic fluid. Box 13-1 lists signs of respiratory distress in the newborn; report these signs promptly.

Cardiovascular Adaptation

The cardiovascular system also must make rapid adjustments immediately after birth. Fetal circulation differs from newborn circulation in several important ways. As you will recall from Chapter 5, only a small amount of blood flows to the fetal lungs. The rest flows away from the lungs through fetal shunts. Remember, the placenta oxygenates fetal blood, so only the blood needed to supply oxygen to the lung tissue goes to the lungs. Because the lungs are small and noncompliant in utero, they are resistant to blood flow and characterized

---

Box 13-1 ▌ SIGNS OF RESPIRATORY DISTRESS IN THE NEWBORN

- Tachypnea (sustained respiratory rate >60 breaths per minute)
- Nasal flaring
- Grunting (noted by stethoscope or audible to the ear)
- Intercostal or xiphoid retractions
- Unequal movements of the chest and abdomen during breathing efforts
- Central cyanosis

by high pressures. The high pressures in the lungs cause the pressures in the right atrium to be higher than are those in the left atrium. These pressure differences help route blood through the foramen ovale and ductus arteriosus, away from the nonfunctioning lungs, back into the general circulation. The ductus venosus shunts fetal blood away from the liver because the woman's liver performs most of the filtering and metabolic functions necessary for fetal life.

Newborn circulation is similar to adult circulation. After birth, deoxygenated blood that enters the heart must go to the lungs for gas exchange; therefore, the fetal shunts must close. Several factors contribute to their closing. The lungs fill with air, causing the pressure to drop in the chest as soon as the newborn takes his first breath. This change results in a reversal of pressures in the right and left atria, causing the foramen ovale to close, which redirects blood to the lungs. The first few breaths greatly increase the oxygen content of circulating blood. This chemical change (i.e., higher oxygen content of the blood) contributes to the closing of the ductus arteriosus, which eventually becomes a ligament. The ductus venosus also closes, allowing nutrient-rich blood from the gut to circulate through the newborn's liver.

Thermoregulatory Adaptation

Thermoregulation is the process by which the body balances heat production with heat loss to maintain adequate body temperature. The newborn has difficulty with thermoregulation because of two key factors. First, the newborn is prone to heat loss. The newborn's ratio of body mass to body surface area is much smaller than that of an adult. In other words, the amount of heat-producing tissue, such as muscle and adipose tissue, is small in relation to the amount of skin exposed to the environment. Second, the newborn is not readily able to produce heat by muscle movement and shivering. These factors make the newborn vulnerable to **cold stress,** exposure to temperatures cooler than normal body temperature so that the newborn must use energy to maintain heat.

There are four main ways that a newborn loses heat—conduction, convection, evaporation, and radiation (Fig. 13-1). Conductive heat loss occurs when the newborn's skin touches a cold surface, causing body heat to transfer to the colder object. Heat loss by convection happens when air currents blow over the newborn's body. Evaporative heat loss happens when the newborn's skin is wet. As the moisture evaporates from the body surface, the newborn loses body heat along with the moisture. Heat loss also occurs by radiation to a cold object

A. Conduction

B. Convection

C. Evaporation

D. Radiation

■ **Figure 13-1** Mechanisms of heat loss. **(A)** Conduction. **(B)** Convection. **(C)** Evaporation. **(D)** Radiation.

that is close to, but not touching, the newborn. An example of this type of heat loss is when the newborn is close to a cold windowpane, causing body heat to radiate toward the window and be lost.

A word of caution is in order.

It takes oxygen to produce heat. If the newborn becomes cold stressed, he or she will eventually develop respiratory distress. This is one important reason to protect the newborn from heat loss.

The normal newborn is not entirely without protection from heat loss. The newborn naturally assumes a flexed, fetal position that conserves body heat by reducing the amount of skin exposed to the surface and conserving core heat. The newborn can also produce heat by burning **brown fat,** a specialized form of heat-producing tissue found only in fetuses and newborns. Deposits of brown fat are located at the nape of the neck, in the armpits, between the shoulder blades, along the abdominal aorta, and around the kidneys and sternum. Unfortunately, brown fat is not renewable; once depleted, the newborn can no longer use this form of heat production.

Test Yourself

✔ Name two ways a vaginal birth assists the newborn's respiratory adaptation.

✔ What is the function of surfactant?

✔ Describe two factors that make it difficult for a newborn to maintain his body temperature.

Metabolic Adaptation

Throughout life, a steady supply of blood glucose is necessary to carry out metabolic processes and produce energy. Glucose is also an essential nutrient for brain tissue. *Neonatal hypoglycemia* occurs when blood glucose levels drop to 50 mg/dL or lower (Karlsen, 2006). It is important to be familiar with risk factors for hypoglycemia (Box 13-2). Any condition that adversely affects blood flow to the placenta during pregnancy puts the newborn at risk. If the mother's blood sugar was elevated during the latter part of the pregnancy, such as in maternal diabetes, or if she received medications that elevate her blood sugar, the newborn also is at risk for hypoglycemia. Any condition that puts physiologic stress on the fetus, such as prolonged labor or maternal infection, may deplete glycogen stores, putting the newborn at risk for low blood sugar. Respiratory distress and cold stress are also two stressors that often lead to neonatal hypoglycemia.

Early signs of hypoglycemia in the newborn include jitteriness, poor feeding, listlessness, irritability, low temperature, weak or high-pitched cry, and hypotonia. Respiratory distress, apnea, seizures, and coma are late signs.

Box 13-2 ▮ RISK FACTORS FOR HYPOGLYCEMIA

History of any of the following during the pregnancy increases the risk that the newborn will develop hypoglycemia.

- Gestational hypertension
- Maternal diabetes (pre-existing or gestational)
- Prolonged labor
- Fetal distress during labor
- Ritodrine or terbutaline administered to mother

Newborn characteristics that increase the risk for hypoglycemia. Note that many of these conditions result from an at-risk pregnancy.

- Intrauterine growth restriction
- Macrosomia (a very large baby)
- Large-for-gestational age
- Small-for-gestational age
- Prematurity
- Postmaturity
- Respiratory or cardiovascular depression requiring resuscitation

---

Hepatic Adaptation

Although immature, the newborn's liver must handle a heavy task. The fetus has a high percentage of circulating red blood cells to make use of all available oxygen in a low-oxygen environment. After birth, the newborn's lungs begin to function, and more oxygen is available immediately. Therefore, the "extra" red blood cells gradually die and circulate to the liver to be broken down.

Bilirubin (a yellow pigment) releases as the blood cells are broken down. Normally the liver conjugates bilirubin (i.e., makes it water soluble), and then bilirubin is excreted in the feces. However, the newborn's liver is immature and overwhelmed easily by the large volume of red blood cells. When this happens, the unconjugated bilirubin, which is fat soluble, builds up in the bloodstream, crosses into the cells, and stains them yellow. **Hyperbilirubinemia,** high levels of unconjugated bilirubin in the bloodstream (serum levels of 4–6 mg/dL and greater), can lead to **jaundice,** a yellow staining of the skin. Jaundice appears first on the head and face; then as bilirubin levels rise, jaundice progresses to the trunk and then to the extremities in a cephalocaudal manner.

In approximately one half of all term newborns, a condition known as **physiologic jaundice** occurs. Physiologic jaundice is characterized by jaundice that occurs after the first 24 hours of life (usually on day 2 or 3 after birth); bilirubin levels that peak between days 3 and 5; and bilirubin levels that do not rise rapidly (no greater than 5 mg/dL per day). Only jaundice that occurs within the first 24 hours is considered pathologic.

However, anytime jaundice is present, document and report it. See Chapter 20 for more in-depth discussion of jaundice and its treatment.

The liver manufactures clotting factors necessary for normal blood coagulation. Several of the factors require vitamin K in their production. Bacteria that produce vitamin K are normally present in the gastrointestinal tract. However, the newborn's gut is sterile because normal flora have not yet taken up residence. Therefore, the newborn cannot produce vitamin K, which in turn causes the liver to be unable to produce some clotting factors. This situation could lead to bleeding problems, so newborns receive vitamin K (AquaMEPHYTON) intramuscularly shortly after birth to prevent hemorrhage (see Chapter 14 for discussion of the vitamin K administration procedure).

Behavioral and Social Adaptation

Each newborn has a unique temperament and personality that becomes readily apparent. Some newborns are quiet, rarely cry, and are consoled easily. Other newborns are frequently fussy or fretful and are more difficult to console. There are as many variations and characteristics as there are newborns.

In 1973, Dr. T. Berry Brazelton developed the Neonatal Behavioral Assessment Scale based on research he had done on the newborn's personality, individuality, and ability to communicate. Dr. Brazelton's key assumptions include that the newborn is a social organism capable of communicating through behavior and controlling his or her responses to the environment (The Brazelton Institute, undated).

Dr. Brazelton identified six sleep and activity patterns that are characteristic of newborns. It is important to remember that individual infants display uniqueness in their sleep–wake cycles. Brazelton's states of reactivity are as follows (Adapted from Cheffer & Rannalli, 2004, p. 440):

1. *Deep sleep:* quiet, nonrestless sleep state; newborn is hard to awaken
2. *Light sleep:* eyes are closed, but more activity is noted; newborn moves actively and may show sucking behavior
3. *Drowsy:* eyes open and close and the eyelids look heavy; body activity is present with intermittent periods of fussiness
4. *Quiet alert:* quiet state with little body movement, but the newborn's eyes are open and he or she is attentive to people and things that are in close proximity; this is a good time for the parents to interact with their newborn
5. *Active alert:* eyes are open and active body movements are present; newborn responds to stimuli with activity
6. *Crying:* eyes may be tightly closed, thrashing movements are made in conjunction with active crying.

NURSING ASSESSMENT OF THE NORMAL NEWBORN
Initial Assessments at Birth

Immediate assessments of the newborn are concerned with the success of cardiopulmonary adaptation. A strong, healthy cry is usually the newborn's first response to external stimuli. A vigorous or lusty cry, heart rate greater than 100 beats per minute (bpm), and pink color are associated with effective cardiopulmonary adaptation. The registered nurse (RN) makes these assessments rapidly during the first seconds after birth.

A traditional immediate assessment of cardiopulmonary adaptation is the Apgar score. Dr. Virginia Apgar developed the Apgar score as a means of quickly assessing the success of the newborn's transition to extrauterine life. The score is not used to guide newborn resuscitation; however, it is useful to evaluate the effectiveness of resuscitation efforts and to help determine the intensity of care the newborn will require in the first few days of life.

Five parameters determine the total Apgar score: heart rate, respiratory effort, muscle tone, reflex irritability, and color. Each factor receives a score of 0 to 2 points, for a maximum total score of 10 (Table 13-2). The RN attending the birth assigns the Apgar score at 1 and 5 minutes after birth. If the newborn receives a score of less than 7 at 5 minutes, the RN continues to assign a score every 5 minutes until the score is 7 or above, the newborn is intubated, or until the newborn is transferred to the nursery.

Scores of 7 to 10 at 5 minutes are indicative of a healthy baby who is adapting well to the extrauterine environment. These newborns typically do well in the regular newborn nursery or rooming-in with their mothers. Scores between 4 and 6 at 5 minutes after birth indicate that the newborn is having some difficulty in adjusting to life outside the womb and needs close observation. These newborns usually go to a special nursery where they may receive oxygen and other special monitoring until their condition improves. Newborns who receive a score of 0 to 3 at 5 minutes are experiencing severe difficulty in making the transition to extrauterine life. These infants usually require observation and care in a neonatal intensive care unit.

Continuing Assessments Throughout Newborn Transition

During the transition period, continue to observe the newborn for signs of respiratory distress (see Box 13-1) or cardiovascular compromise. Observe for excess mucus, which could obstruct the airway. Measure the heart and

Table 13-2 ▌ APGAR SCORING

Apgar scoring is done at 1 and 5 minutes after birth. The newborn is considered to be "vigorous" if the initial scores are 7 and above. If the 5-minute score is <7, scoring is done every 5 minutes thereafter until the score reaches 7. The numbers in the left-hand column represent the number of points that are assigned to each parameter when the criteria in the corresponding column are met.

	Heart Rate	Respiratory Effort	Muscle Tone	Reflex Irritability	Color
2	Heart rate >100 beats per minutes (bpm)	Strong, vigorous cry	Maintains a position of flexion with brisk movements	Cries or sneezes when stimulated*	Body and extremities pink
1	Heart rate present, but <100 bpm	Weak cry, slow or difficult respirations	Minimal flexion of extremities	Grimaces when stimulated	Body pink, extremities blue (acrocyanosis)
0	No heart rate	No respiratory effort	Limp and flaccid	No response to stimulation	Body and extremities blue (cyanosis) or completely pale (pallor)

*Stimulation is provided by suctioning the infant or by gently flicking the sole of the foot.

respiratory rates at least every 30 minutes during the first 2 hours of transition.

Observe the newborn closely for cold stress. Use a thermal skin probe for continuous temperature assessment while the newborn is under the radiant warmer. Measure the axillary temperature at least every 30 minutes until the temperature stabilizes above 97.6°F (36.5°C).

Hypoglycemia is a potential problem that can, if prolonged, have devastating effects on the newborn. Therefore, it is critical for you to be able to recognize signs and symptoms of hypoglycemia in the newborn. These signs include:

- Jitteriness or tremors
- Exaggerated Moro reflex
- Irritability
- Lethargy
- Poor feeding
- Listlessness
- Apnea or respiratory distress
- High-pitched cry

The main sign of hypoglycemia is jitteriness, which the newborn often exhibits as an exaggerated Moro reflex. Conversely, the hypoglycemic newborn may have no symptoms. If hypoglycemia is prolonged without treatment, the newborn may have seizures or lapse into a coma. Permanent brain damage can result, leading to lifelong disability.

This is a critical point.
Never mistake jitteriness in the newborn for "shivering." If the newborn has shaky movements or startles easily, immediately check the blood sugar. Remember, newborns can develop hypoglycemia even when there are no recognizable risk factors for its development.

If a newborn is exhibiting signs of, or is at risk for (see Box 13-2), hypoglycemia, check the glucose level using a heel stick to obtain a blood sample for testing (see Chapter 14 for heel stick procedure). Blood levels between 50 and 60 mg/dL during the first 24 hours of life are considered normal. Levels less than 50 mg/dL are indicative of hypoglycemia in the newborn (Karlsen, 2006).

Initial Admitting Assessment

The RN completes the initial nursing assessment (sometimes called the admissions assessment) within the first 2 hours after birth. The RN, nurse practitioner, or pediatrician is responsible for the full assessment, but the licensed practical nurse may assist with portions of the examination. Therefore, you should be familiar with the procedure and expected findings.

Review of the woman's history is an important part of a complete newborn nursing assessment. The maternal family, medical–surgical, prenatal, and obstetric histories reveal clues to neonatal conditions.

The RN conducts the examination in a warm area that is free from drafts to protect the newborn from chilling. There should be plenty of light available to facilitate visual inspection. Indirect lighting works best. All equipment (neonatal stethoscope and ophthalmoscope) should be functioning properly and should be readily available to allow for economy of motion. An experienced practitioner can complete a thorough examination in a short time, which is ideal because newborns become easily fatigued when overstimulated by prolonged examination.

The general order of progression is from general observations to specific measurements. Least disturbing aspects of the examination, such as observation and auscultation, are completed before more intrusive techniques, such as deep palpation and examination of the hips. It is generally advisable to proceed using a head-to-toe approach. The overall physical appearance of the newborn is evaluated first, followed by measurement of vital signs, weight, and length. Then a thorough head-to-toe assessment follows, ending with assessment of neurologic reflexes and the gestational age assessment. The behavioral assessment is integrated throughout the examination as the practitioner notes how the newborn responds to sensory stimulation.

General Appearance, Body Proportions, and Posture

A healthy term newborn's appearance is symmetrical and well nourished without cyanosis. Typically, the newborn has a head that is large in proportion to the rest of his or her body. The newborn's neck is short, and the chin rests on the chest. The newborn maintains a flexed position with tightly clenched fists. The abdomen is protuberant (bulging or prominent) and the chest is rounded. Note the newborn's sloping shoulders and rounded hips. The newborn's body appears long with short extremities.

Vital Signs

Vital signs are important because they yield clues as to how well the newborn is adapting to life outside the uterus. The RN determines respiratory effort and character at the beginning of the examination while the newborn is quiet. Respirations are activity dependent. The respiratory rhythm is often irregular, a characteristic known as episodic breathing. Momentary cessation of breathing interspersed with rapid breathing movements is typical of an episodic breathing pattern. Extended periods of apnea are not normal. The abdomen and chest rise and fall together with breathing movements. The normal respiratory rate is 30 to 60 breaths per minute and should be counted for a full minute when the infant is quiet. The RN then auscultates the breath sounds.

The RN auscultates the heart rate apically for a full minute. The normal heart rate is the same for the newborn as it is for the fetus, ranging between 110 and 160 bpm, depending on activity level. When the newborn is sleeping, the heart tends to beat in the lower range of normal, and is not considered problematic as long as it stays above 100 bpm. The newborn's heart rate increases with activity and may increase to the 180s for short periods during vigorous activity and crying. The rhythm should be regular. Listen for any abnormal sounds or murmurs. Although most newborn murmurs are benign, always report a murmur to the primary care provider for further evaluation.

The axilla is the preferred site for newborn temperature measurement (Fig. 13-2). Normal temperature range is between 97.7°F (36.5°C) and 99.5°F (37.5°C). Blood pressures are not taken routinely. If they are measured, the cuff must be an appropriate size, and the pressure may be measured on an arm or leg. Table 13-3 outlines the expected vital signs of the term newborn.

■ Figure 13-2 Measuring the newborn's axillary temperature.

It's not so confusing!

To remember normal newborn heart rate and blood pressure values, think about this. A newborn starts with a low blood pressure (60/40 mm Hg) and a high pulse (120–160 bpm). By the time he or she grows up, the opposite is true: The blood pressure is high (120/80 mm Hg) and the pulse is low (60–80 bpm).

Table 13-3 ■ **EXPECTED VITAL SIGNS OF THE TERM NEWBORN**

Vital Sign	Expected Range	Characteristics
Heart rate	110–160 beats per minute (bpm); during sleep as low as 100 bpm and as high as 180 bpm when crying	Rhythm regular; murmurs may be normal, but all murmurs require medical evaluation
Respiratory rate	30–60 breaths per minute	Episodic breathing is normal; chest and abdomen should move synchronously
Axillary temerature	97.7°F–98.6°F (36.5°C–37°C)	Temperature stabilizes within 8–10 hours after delivery
Blood pressure	60–80/40–45 mm Hg	Not normally recorded for the normal newborn

Physical Measurements

Weight and length of a newborn are dependent on several factors, including ethnicity, gender, genetics, and maternal nutrition and smoking behaviors. The normal weight range for a full-term newborn is between 5 lb 8 oz and 8 lb 13 oz (2,500–4,000 g). The average length is 20 inches, with the range between 19 and 21 inches (48–53 cm). Length can be difficult to measure accurately because of the newborn's flexed posture and resistance to stretching. Nursing Procedure 13-1 lists the steps for obtaining the newborn's weight and length.

It is normal for the newborn to lose 5% to 10% of his birth weight in the first few days. For the average newborn, this physiologic weight loss amounts to a total loss of 6 to 10 oz, and the cause is a loss of excess fluid combined with a low fluid intake during the first few days of life. The newborn should regain the weight within 7 to 10 days, after which he or she begins to gain approximately 2 lb every month until 6 months of age.

Head and chest circumference are two additional important newborn measurements. Obtain the head circumference (Fig. 13-3A) by placing a paper tape measure around the widest circumference of the head (i.e., from the occipital prominence around to just above the eyebrows). To measure the chest circumference, place the infant on his or her back with the tape measure under the lower edge of the scapulae posteriorly and then bring the tape forward over the nipple line (Fig. 13-3B). The

---

Nursing Procedure 13-1
OBTAINING INITIAL WEIGHT AND MEASURING LENGTH

EQUIPMENT

Calibrated scale
Paper to place on the scale
Tape measure
Marker or pen
Clean gloves

PROCEDURE

Weighing the Newborn

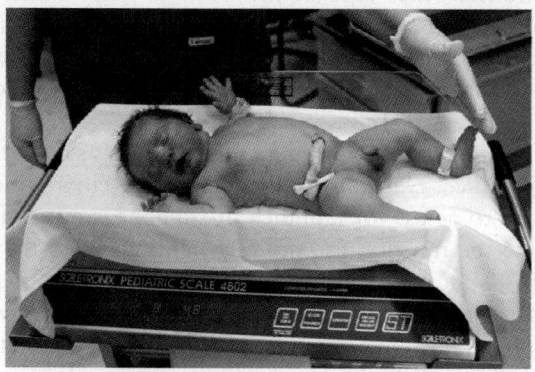

1. Thoroughly wash your hands.
2. Don a pair of clean gloves.
3. Place a paper or other designated covering on the scale to prevent direct contact of the newborn's skin with the scale.
4. Set the scale to zero.
5. Remove the newborn's clothes, including diapers and blankets, and place the newborn on the scale.
6. Hold one hand just above the newborn's body. Avoid actually touching the newborn.
7. Note the weight, in pounds and ounces and in grams.

Measuring the Newborn

8. Use the marker to place a mark on the paper at the top of the newborn's head.
9. Use one hand to firmly hold the newborn's heels together and straighten the legs.
10. Place a second mark on the paper at the newborn's heel.
11. Measure the area between the two marks with a tape measure. This is the newborn's length.
12. Remove your gloves and thoroughly wash your hands.
13. Record the newborn's weight and length in the designated area of the chart.
14. Be sure to report your findings to the mother, her partner, and other family members, as appropriate.

Note: Gloves are only necessary when handling the newborn before the first bath because of traces of blood, mucus, vernix, and other secretions on the body. Use universal precautions to protect yourself from blood-borne pathogens. To avoid inaccurate results, do not leave clothes, including diapers, on the newborn when he is weighed.

A

B

■ Figure 13-3 **(A)** Measuring the head circumference. **(B)** Measuring the chest circumference.

average head circumference is between 13 and 14 inches (33 and 35.5), approximately 1 to 2 inches larger than that of the chest.

Table 13-4 summarizes normal ranges for physical measurements of the term newborn.

Head-to-Toe Assessment

Skin, Hair, and Nails

The normal newborn's skin is supple with good turgor, reddish at birth (turning pink within a few hours), and flaky and dry. **Vernix caseosa** (or vernix), a white cheeselike substance that covers the body of the fetus during the second trimester, normally is found only in creases of the term newborn. Vernix protects fetal skin from the drying effects of amniotic fluid. **Lanugo** is fine downy hair that is present in abundance on the preterm infant but is found in thinning patches on the shoulders, arms, and back of the term newborn. The hair should be silky and soft. Fingernails are present and extend to the end of the fingertips or slightly beyond.

Common newborn skin manifestations are described in Box 13-3. Milia on the face are a frequent finding. These tiny white papules resemble pimples in appearance. Reassure parents that these are harmless and will subside spontaneously. Acrocyanosis, blue hands and feet with a pink trunk, results from poor peripheral circulation and is not a good indicator of oxygenation status. The mucous membranes should be pink, and there should be no central cyanosis. Birthmarks and skin tags may be present. These are not a cause for concern and can generally be removed easily if the parents desire. **Mottling** is a red and white lacy pattern sometimes seen on the skin of newborns who have fair complexions. It is variable in occurrence and length, lasting from several hours to several weeks. Mottling sometimes occurs with exposure to cool temperatures. **Harlequin sign,** also referred to as Harlequin coloring, is characterized by a clown suit–like appearance of the newborn. The newborn's skin is dark red on one side of the body while the other side of the body is pale. Dilation of blood vessels causes the dark red color, whereas constriction of blood vessels causes the pallor. This harmless condition occurs most frequently with vigorous crying.

It is important to evaluate the newborn's skin for signs of jaundice. Natural sunlight is the best environment in which to assess for jaundice. If sunlight is not available inside the nursery, use indirect lighting. Press the newborn's skin over the forehead or nose with your finger and note if the blanched area appears yellow. It is also helpful to evaluate the sclera of the eyes, particularly in dark-skinned newborns. A yellow tinge to the sclera indicates the presence of jaundice.

Table 13-4 ■ **AVERAGE PHYSICAL MEASUREMENT RANGES OF THE TERM NEWBORN**		
Measurement	**Average Range Metric System**	**Average Range U.S. Customary System**
Weight	2,500–4,000 g	5 lb 8 oz–8 lb 13 oz
Length (head-to-heel)	48–53 cm	19–21 in
Head circumference	33–35.5 cm	13–14 in
Chest circumference	30.5–33 cm	12–13 in

Box 13-3 ▌ COMMON SKIN MANIFESTATIONS OF THE NORMAL NEWBORN

Milia

Teaching tip: Small white spots on the newborn's face, nose, and chin that resemble pimples are an expected observation. Do not attempt to pick or squeeze them. They will subside spontaneously in a few days.

Erythema Toxicum or Newborn Rash

Teaching tip: This rash appears commonly on the chest, abdomen, back, and buttocks of the newborn. The rash is harmless and will disappear without treatment.

Mongolian Spot(s)

Teaching tip: These bluish black areas of discoloration appear commonly on the back, buttocks, or extremities of dark-skinned newborns. These spots should not be mistaken for bruises or mistreatment and gradually fade during the first year or two of life.

Telangiectatic Nevi or "Stork Bites"

Teaching tip: These pale pink or red marks sometimes occur on the nape of the neck, eyelids, or nose of fair-skinned newborns. Stork bites blanch when pressed and generally fade as the child grows.

Nevus Flammeus or Port-wine Stain

Teaching tip: This dark reddish purple birthmark most commonly appears on the face. A group of dilated blood vessels causes the mark. It does not blanch with pressure or fade with time. Cosmetics are available to help cover the stain if it is disfiguring. Physicians have had success fading port-wine stains with laser therapy.

Some skin characteristics are attributable to birth trauma or operative intervention. Bruising may occur over the presenting part or on the face if the labor or delivery was unusually short or prolonged. A chignon (knot or bump) may form on the newborn's head from vacuum extraction. A forceps mark on the face or cheek is common after a forceps-assisted delivery. Occasionally there will be a nick or cut on the infant born by cesarean, particularly if the surgery was done rapidly under emergency conditions.

Be careful!

Nursing assessment plays an important role in detecting early (i.e., pathologic) jaundice. If you notice jaundice, report it immediately. However, assessing for jaundice using the naked eye is not a reliable way to screen for hyperbilirubinemia. Most facilities use transcutaneous bilirubinometers or blood samples to screen for this purpose.

Test Yourself

✔ Name the major nursing actions to take while weighing and measuring a newborn.

✔ What is the significance of acrocyanosis?

✔ How would you explain the presence of milia to the parents?

Head and Face

The head may be misshapen because of **molding** or **caput succedaneum** (caput). Molding is an elongated head shape caused by overlapping of the cranial bones as the fetus moves through the birth canal (Fig. 13-4). Caput is swelling of the soft tissue of the scalp caused by pressure of the presenting part on a partially dilated cervix or trauma from a vacuum-assisted delivery. These conditions are often of concern to new parents. Reassure them

■ **Figure 13-4** Molding in the newborn's head.

that the molding and/or caput will decrease in a few days without treatment.

A **cephalhematoma** is swelling that occurs from bleeding under the periosteum of the skull, usually over one of the parietal bones. A cephalhematoma is caused by birth trauma, usually requires no treatment, and will spontaneously resolve. However, the practitioner should evaluate the newborn for signs of anemia (pallor) or shock from acute blood loss. It also is important to make certain the cephalhematoma does not cross over suture lines. If it does, it suggests a skull fracture. Sometimes it is difficult for the inexperienced practitioner to tell the difference between a cephalhematoma and caput. Figure 13-5 compares features of these conditions.

Sutures occur in the place where two cranial bones meet. The normal newborn's sutures are palpable with a small space between them. It may be difficult to palpate sutures in the first 24 hours if significant molding is present. However, it is important to determine that the sutures are present. Rarely sutures will fuse prematurely (craniostenosis). It is important to detect this condition

You may notice this relationship.

Molding and caput are more common or more pronounced in a first-born baby than in the newborn of a multipara. In addition, many newborns delivered by cesarean do not experience molding or caput unless the fetus is in the birth canal for a prolonged period of time before delivery.

A Personal Glimpse

The doctor was just about to use the vacuum extractor because I had been pushing for 3 hours. I gave one additional strong push and felt the absolute relief of my baby sliding out of my body. The doctor said, "It's a girl." My husband was crying, and I couldn't wait to see our little girl. I wanted to examine her, touch her, feel her, and look into her eyes. They laid our tiny baby girl on my chest, and the first thing I noticed was her very long, pointy head. "Oh, my poor little girl," I thought, "that looks so painful and awful." I had heard and read about molding but had no idea it would be so pronounced. I must have had a look of serious concern on my face because the nurse touched my arm and said, "Don't worry, her head will be back to a normal size and shape in just a day or two." The nurse then covered my sweet baby's pointy head with a soft pink cap, and my baby and I began to get to know each other.

Isabel

Learning Opportunity: How can nurses' knowledge of normal newborn assessment findings provide assurance to new parents?

Describe how a nurse's reaction to a common newborn finding could encourage or discourage parents.

❚ **Figure 13-5** Comparison of caput succedaneum and cephalhematoma. **(A)** Caput is a collection of serous fluid (edema) between the periosteum and the scalp caused by pressure of the fetal head against a partially dilated cervix. Caput often crosses suture lines. **(B)** Cephalhematoma is a collection of blood between the periosteum and the skull. It does not cross suture lines, unless there is a skull fracture, which is a rare occurrence.

because it will require surgery to allow the brain to grow.

Fontanels occur at the junction of cranial bones where two or more sutures meet. The anterior and posterior fontanels are palpable. The anterior fontanel is diamond shaped and larger than the posterior fontanel, which has a triangular shape. The posterior fontanel closes within the first 3 months of life, whereas the anterior fontanel does not close until 12 to 18 months of life. When the newborn is in a sitting position, the anterior fontanel should be flat, neither depressed nor bulging. It is normal to feel pulsations that correlate with the newborn's heart rate over the anterior fontanel. Bulging fontanels may indicate hydrocephalus or increased intracranial pressure, and sunken fontanels are a sign of severe dehydration.

Facial movements should be symmetrical. Facial paralysis can occur from a forceps delivery or from pressure on the facial nerve as the fetus travels down the birth canal. It is easiest to assess for facial paralysis when the newborn is crying. The affected side will not move, and the space between the eyelids will widen. Facial paralysis is usually temporary, but occasionally the deficit is permanent.

Eyes

The eye color of a newborn with light-skinned parents is usually blue-gray, whereas a darker skinned infant usually has a dark eye color. It is normal for the eyelids to be swollen from pressure during birth. A chemical conjunctivitis may develop after instillation of eye prophylaxis in the delivery room (see Chapter 14 for discussion of eye prophylaxis).

The sclera should be clear and white, not blue. The pupils should be equal and reactive to light. A red reflex should be present. The practitioner elicits the red reflex by shining an ophthalmoscope onto the retina of the eye. The normal response is a red reflection from the retina. Absence of the red reflex is associated with congenital

cataracts. Small subconjunctival hemorrhages may be present. These usually disappear within a week or two and are not harmful.

Eye movements are usually uncoordinated, and some strabismus (crossed eyes) is expected. A "doll's eye" reflex is normal for the first few days; that is, when the newborn's head is turned, the eyes travel to the opposite side. Persistence of this reflex after the second week requires evaluation.

The newborn is able to perceive light and can track objects held close to the face. He or she likes shapes and colors and shows a definite preference for the human face. Crying is usually tearless because the lacrimal apparatus is underdeveloped.

Nose

The newborn's nose is flat, and the bridge may appear to be absent. The nostrils should be bilaterally patent because the newborn is an obligate nose breather. The newborn clears obstructions from the nose by sneezing. There should be no nasal flaring, which is a sign of respiratory distress. The sense of smell is present, as evidenced by the newborn's turning toward milk and by turning away from or blinking in the presence of strong odors.

Give this a try.
To assess for bilateral nostril patency, use your finger to occlude one naris. The naris on the opposite side is patent if the newborn can breathe easily. Repeat the test on the other side.

Mouth

The mucous membranes should be moist and pink. Sucking calluses may appear on the central part of the lips shortly after birth. The uvula should be midline. Place a gloved finger in the newborn's mouth to evaluate the suck and gag reflexes and to check the palate for intactness.

The suck reflex should be strong, the gag reflex present, and both the hard and soft palates should be intact. Well-developed fat pads are present bilaterally on the cheeks.

Epstein's pearls are small white cysts found on the midline portion of the hard palate of some newborns. They feel hard to the touch and are harmless. Precocious teeth may be present on the lower

Don't forget!
A cleft palate can be present even in the absence of a cleft lip. Check the roof of the mouth carefully to be sure it is intact.

central portion of the gum. If the teeth are loose, removal is recommended to prevent the infant from aspirating them.

A fungal infection (caused by *Candida albicans*) in the oral cavity, called **thrush,** may be present. The newborn can contract the infection while passing through the birth canal. The fungus causes white patches that resemble milk curds on the oral mucosa, particularly the tongue. It is important not to remove the patches because doing so will cause bleeding in the underlying tissue. An oral solution of nystatin (Mycostatin, Nilstat) is the treatment of choice for thrush.

Ears

The pinna should be flexible with quick recoil, indicating the presence of cartilage. The top of the pinna should be even with, or above, an imaginary horizontal line drawn from the inner to the outer canthus of the eye and continuing past the ear (Fig. 13-6). Low-set ears are associated with congenital defects, including those that cause mental retardation and internal organ defects.

In recent years, most hospitals have developed newborn hearing screening programs in accordance with recommendations of the American Academy of Pediatrics (AAP) for universal screening. There are two main ways that a newborn's hearing can be tested satisfactorily using current technology: evoked otoacoustic emissions and auditory brain stem response. Both methodologies are noninvasive, take less than 5 minutes, and are easy to perform. Each method assesses hearing differently, and each has unique advantages and disadvantages. The important task for the nursery nurse is to make certain that each newborn receives the hearing screen before discharge.

Neck

The newborn's neck is short and thick. The head should move freely and have full range of motion. There should be no masses or webbing. Significant head lag is present when the newborn is pulled to a sitting position from a supine one (Fig. 13-7). Newborns can hold up their heads slightly when placed on their abdomens.

The clavicles should be intact. Occasionally, a clavicle fractures during a difficult delivery. Signs of a fractured clavicle include a lump along one clavicle accompanied

A

B

■ **Figure 13-6 (A)** In normal ear alignment, the top of the pinna should be even with, or above, an imaginary horizontal line drawn from the inner to the outer canthus of the eye and continuing past the ear. **(B)** Low-set ears may be seen in children with chromosomal abnormalities.

■ **Figure 13-7** The newborn exhibits significant head lag when pulled to a sitting position from lying on his back.

by crepitus (a grating sensation) at the site. An asymmetrical Moro reflex (discussed later in the chapter) is another indication.

Chest

The anteroposterior and lateral diameters of the chest are equal, making the chest appear barrel shaped. The xiphoid process is prominent. Chest movements should be equal bilaterally and synchronous with the abdomen.

Breast enlargement and breast engorgement is normal for both sexes. A thin milky secretion, sometimes called "witch's milk," may be secreted from the nipples. The breasts should not be squeezed in an attempt to express the liquid. Assess for supernumerary (accessory) nipples below and medial to the true nipples.

Abdomen

The newborn's abdomen is dome shaped and protuberant. Respirations are typically diaphragmatic, which make them appear abdominal in nature. Peristaltic waves should not be visible. Bowel sounds should be audible within 2 hours of birth. The abdomen should be soft to palpation without palpable masses. A normal umbilical cord is well formed and has three vessels. The base of the cord should be dry without redness or drainage, and the umbilical clamp should be fastened securely.

Genitourinary

The newborn should void within the first 24 hours of life. Vigorous newborns may urinate for the first time in the delivery room minutes after birth. The stream of a male newborn should be strong enough to cause a steady arch during voiding, and the female should be able to produce a steady stream. The kidneys are not able to concentrate urine well during the first few days, so the color is light, and there is no odor. It is normal to find a small amount of pink or light orange color in the diaper for the first few times the newborn voids. Excess uric acid in the urine causes this so-called "brick dust."

Both male and female genitalia may be swollen. **Smegma,** a cheesy white sebaceous gland secretion, is often found within the folds of the labia of the female and under the foreskin of the male. It is best to allow the secretion to gradually wear away because vigorous attempts at removal can irritate the tender mucosa. Immediately report the presence of ambiguous genitalia (i.e., it is difficult to tell if the newborn is male or female).

Female. The labia and clitoris may be edematous. In the term newborn, the labia majora cover the labia minora. A hymenal tag may be present. An imperforate hymen (a hymen that completely covers the vaginal opening) should be reported. A blood-tinged mucous discharge from the vagina, **pseudomenstruation,** results from the sudden withdrawal of maternal hormones. Reassure the parents that this condition is not cause for alarm.

Male. The urinary meatus should be positioned at the tip of the penis. If the opening is located abnormally on the dorsal (upper) surface of the glans penis, the condition is called **epispadias. Hypospadias** occurs when the opening to the urethra is on the ventral (under) surface of the glans. **Phimosis,** tightly adherent foreskin, is a normal condition in the term newborn. The tissue should not be forced over the glans penis. Monitor the urinary stream for adequacy. If phimosis interferes with urination, intervention will be needed. Spontaneous erections are a common finding.

The male scrotum is pendulous, edematous, and covered with rugae (deep creases). Dark-skinned newborns have deeply pigmented scrotum. Both testes should be descended. Using a thumb and forefinger, the RN gently palpates the scrotal sac while pressing down on the inguinal canal with the opposite hand. The procedure is repeated on the opposite side. *Cryptorchidism* results when the testes do not descend into the scrotal sac during fetal life. This condition requires medical evaluation. A hydrocele, fluid within the scrotal sac, may be present and should be noted.

Extremities

The term newborn maintains a posture of flexion. He has good muscle tone, and his extremities return quickly to an attitude of flexion after they are extended. The extremities are short in relation to the body and without deformities. Full range of motion is present in all joints, and movements are bilateral and equal.

The full complement of fingers and toes should be present without webbing between the digits and without extra digits. Syndactyly refers to fusion or webbing of the toes or fingers, while polydactyly is the medical term for extra digits. The palms of the hands should have creases. A single straight palmar crease, a **simian crease,** is an abnormal finding that is associated with Down's syndrome. Brachial pulses should be present and equal.

The legs are bowed and the feet flat due to fatty pads in the arch of each foot. Creases should cover at least two thirds of the bottom of the feet. The femoral pulses should be equal and strong bilaterally. A strong brachial pulse with a weak femoral pulse is abnormal and should be reported (Fig. 13-8).

You may be asked to assist the RN while he or she attempts

You can easily identify a hydrocele.

Take a penlight and hold it against the scrotal sac. If fluid is present (hydrocele), the light will transilluminate the scrotum. If there is no hydrocele, the light will not shine through solid structures.

Practice makes perfect.

Practice taking the femoral pulse on newborns that are resting quietly. Be patient and take your time. You will gain confidence as you are consistently able to find the pulse.

A   **B**

■ **Figure 13-8 (A)** Palpating the femoral pulse. **(B)** Palpating the brachial pulse.

to elicit Ortolani's maneuver and Barlow's sign (Nursing Procedure 13-2) to evaluate the hip for signs of dislocation or subluxation (partial dislocation). A positive sign is associated with subluxation. Other signs of a dislocated hip included uneven gluteal folds and one knee that is lower than the other when the newborn is supine with both knees flexed.

The feet may appear to turn inward because of the way the fetus was positioned in the womb or birth canal. If the feet are easily reducible, that is they can be easily moved to a normal position, the "deformity" is positional and will resolve spontaneously. If the feet do not move to a normal position, true clubfoot may be present. A specialist should evaluate this condition.

Back and Rectum

The newborn's spine is straight and flat. The lumbar and sacral curves do not appear until the infant begins to use his back to sit and stand upright. Feel along the length of the spine. There should be no masses, openings, dimples, or tufts of hair. Any of these findings may be associated with spina bifida (an opening in the spinal column).

The anus should be patent. **Meconium,** the first stool of the newborn, is a thick black tarry substance composed of dead cells, mucus, and bile that collects in the rectum of the fetus. Passage of meconium should occur within the first 24 to 48 hours and confirms the presence of a patent anus.

Test Yourself

✔ Name two differences between caput succedaneum and cephalhematoma.
✔ What is pseudomenstruation?
✔ Define subluxation of the hip.

Neurologic Assessment
General Appearance and Behavior

The first part of the neurologic examination involves quiet observation of the general appearance and behavior of the newborn. The newborn should maintain an attitude of flexion. Hypotonus (decreased tone) is an abnormal finding, as is hypertonus, distinct tremors, jitteriness, or seizure activity. Any of these states may be associated with neurologic dysfunction, hypoglycemia, hypocalcemia, or neonatal drug withdrawal. The cry should be vigorous and of medium pitch. A high-pitched, shrill cry is associated with neurologic dysfunction.

Reflexes

Normal newborn reflexes (Fig. 13-9) are assessed at the end of the examination. Although the list is not exhaustive, the reflexes discussed here are the most commonly assessed reflexes. In addition, the newborn should demonstrate the protective reflexes of sneezing, coughing, blinking, and withdrawing from painful stimuli.

Rooting, sucking, and swallowing reflexes are important to the newborn's nutritional intake. Gently stroking the newborn's cheek brings out the rooting reflex. The newborn demonstrates this reflex by turning toward the touch with an open mouth. Teach the new mother to use this reflex to help the newborn begin breast-feeding (see Chapter 15). Place a gloved finger in the newborn's mouth to test the sucking reflex. The suck should be strong. Swallowing is evaluated when the infant eats. Listen and watch for coordinated swallowing efforts.

Evaluate the palmar and plantar grasp reflexes by placing a finger in the palm or parallel to the toes. The digits will wrap around the finger and hold on. The grasp should be equal and strong bilaterally. Check the stepping reflex by supporting the newborn in a standing position on a hard surface. He or she will lift the legs up and down in a stepping motion. Babinski's sign is

Nursing Procedure 13-2
ORTOLANI'S MANEUVER AND BARLOW'S SIGN

EQUIPMENT

Warm, clean hands
Flat surface

PROCEDURE

1. Wash hands thoroughly.
2. Position the newborn flat on his back on a firm surface.
3. Position the knees together and flex the knees and hips 90 degrees.
4. Place your middle fingers over the greater trochanter of the femur and your thumbs on the inner aspect of the thigh.
5. Apply upward pressure and abduct the hips. A clicking or a clunking sound is a positive Ortolani's sign, which is associated with dislocation of the hip.

6. Next apply downward pressure and adduct the hips. Continue to maintain 90 degrees flexion. If you feel the head of the femur slip out of the acetabulum, the joint is unstable, and Barlow's sign is positive.

7. Position the newborn comfortably on the back or side.
8. Wash hands thoroughly.
9. Document your findings.

Note: In this instance, a positive Ortolani's or Barlow's sign is not wanted. It is not normal to hear clicking or clunking or to feel the femoral head slip out of the hip socket.

positive (normal) if the newborn's toes fan out and hyperextend and the foot dorsiflexes when a hard object (such as the blunt end of a writing pen) is traced from the heel along the lateral aspect of the foot up and across the ball of the foot. After the infant starts walking, this reflex should disappear and the toes should curl inward (negative Babinski), rather than fanning outward.

The Moro reflex is also known as the startle reflex. When the newborn is startled, he or she extends the arms and legs away from the body and to the side. Then the arms come back toward each other with the fingers spread in a "C" shape. The arms look as if the newborn is trying to embrace something. The Moro reflex should be symmetrical. This reflex disappears at approximately 6 months of age.

The tonic neck reflex is another total body reflex. With the newborn lying quietly on his or her back, turn the head to one side without moving the rest of the body. The newborn responds by extending the arm and leg on the side he or she is facing and flexing the opposite arm and leg. This position has been called the "fencer's position" because it looks as if the newborn is poised to begin fencing.

Behavioral Assessment

It is important to note how the parents react to the newborn's behavior states and how the parents talk about the newborn. Newborns who demonstrate self-quieting behaviors may be considered "good" babies. Parents usually respond positively to cuddly and sociable newborns. When a newborn resists cuddling or is difficult to console, the parents may feel rejected, and bonding can be adversely affected.

Teach the parents to watch the newborn for cues as to when he or she wants to interact. The quiet alert state is

■ Figure 13-9 Normal newborn reflexes. **(A)** Suck reflex. **(B)** Palmar grasp. **(C)** Stepping reflex. **(D)** Moro reflex. Notice the "C" shape of the arms. **(E)** Tonic neck reflex (fencer's position). Notice how the extremities on the side the newborn is facing are extended, whereas the opposite extremities are flexed.

a good time for focused interaction with the newborn. When the newborn is in the active alert stage, he or she likes to play. The drowsy state lets the parents know the newborn needs rest. Crying signals that the newborn has a need. Teach the parents to check for physical problems first such as a wet diaper, hunger, or need to burp. If the newborn is still crying, the parents can try soothing actions,

This is vital!
Teach the parents *never* to shake an infant. Shaking can cause permanent brain damage. If the parent is frustrated because a crying infant is inconsolable, encourage the parent to take a minute to stop and count to 10 or ask a friend for help.

such as walking, rocking, or riding in the car. Reassure the parents that, contrary to popular opinion, you cannot spoil a newborn by picking him up when he is crying. Holding reassures and comforts the newborn.

Gestational Age Assessment

The gestational age assessment is a critical evaluation. The RN is ultimately responsible for performing the gestational age assessment; however, as the licensed practical nurse, you should be familiar with the instruments used and be able to differentiate characteristics of the full-term newborn from those of the premature newborn. Chapter 20 details gestational age assessment and compares the preterm with the full-term newborn.

Key Points

➤ The newborn must adapt rapidly to life outside the womb. Respiratory adaptation occurs when the newborn fills his lungs with air, absorbs remaining fluid in the lungs, and begins oxygen exchange.

➤ All the fetal shunts (foramen ovale, ductus arteriosus, and ductus venosus) must close so that blood will travel to the lungs for gas exchange and to route blood through the liver.

➤ The newborn exhibits poor thermoregulation because he or she is prone to heat loss through the skin and because he or she cannot produce heat through muscle movement and shivering. Heat is lost through the processes of convection, conduction, evaporation, and radiation. The newborn conserves heat by maintaining a flexed position and produces heat by metabolizing brown fat.

➤ The newborn's immature liver may not be able to handle the heavy load from the breakdown of red blood cells, and physiologic jaundice appears. This condition is harmless if bilirubin levels do not rise dramatically and if jaundice is not present before the newborn is 24 hours old. Not all of the necessary blood coagulation factors are manufactured directly after birth, and the gut is sterile, so vitamin K is given intramuscularly to stimulate appropriate clotting.

➤ Each infant is unique, but all infants have similar sleep and activity patterns. These include deep sleep, light sleep, drowsiness, quiet alert state, active alert state, and crying.

➤ The RN performs immediate assessments in the delivery room, including assigning the Apgar score. The Apgar score is a way of determining how well the newborn is transitioning to life outside the womb. Five parameters (respiratory effort, heart rate, muscle tone, reflex irritability, and color) are used to assign a score at 1 and 5 minutes of life. A healthy, vigorous newborn has a 5-minute score of 7 or greater.

➤ Newborn hypoglycemia is a blood glucose level less than 50 mg/dL. Newborns can have no symptoms or may demonstrate multiple signs. The most common sign is shakiness or jitteriness.

➤ The nursing assessment is an important way to determine how well the newborn is adapting to life outside the womb. The least disturbing aspects of the examination are completed first. Respiratory rate and heart rate are taken early in the examination, while the newborn is quiet. Then examination proceeds in a head-to-toe manner, covering vital signs, physical measurements, and assessment of each body part.

➤ The expected weight range is 5 lb 8 oz to 8 lb 13 oz (2,500–4,000 g). Length is 19 to 21 inches (48–53 cm). Head circumference is 13 to 14 inches (33–33.5 cm) and chest circumference is 12 to 13 inches (30.5–33 cm).

➤ The skin should be supple with good turgor and have a pink color to it. Many variations are normally present on newborn skin.

➤ Head and face: Molding may be present. The newborn is an obligate nose breather. The hard and soft palates should be intact.

➤ Neck and chest: The neck is short and thick. Webbing should not be present. Periodic breathing episodes are normal.

➤ Abdomen: The abdomen is protuberant. The cord should be clamped and drying at the base with three vessels present.

➤ Genitourinary: The newborn should void within the first 24 hours. Genitalia of both sexes may be swollen.

➤ The back should be straight and free of hairy tufts, dimples, or tumors. The newborn should pass meconium, the first stool, within the first 24 hours.

➤ The main reflexes assessed to determine neurologic status are rooting, sucking, swallowing, grasping, Moro, Babinski's, and tonic neck or the fencer's position.

INTERNET RESOURCES

The American Academy of Pediatrics

www.aap.org

Workbook

■ NCLEX-STYLE REVIEW QUESTIONS

1. An infant is born by cesarean delivery. In what way is respiratory adaptation more difficult for this infant than the one who is born by vaginal delivery?

   a. More fluid is present in the lungs at birth.
   b. Surfactant is missing from the lungs.
   c. The respiratory centers in the brain are not stimulated.
   d. There is less sensory stimulation to breathe.

2. A new mother says, "I think something is wrong with my baby. She has a milky fluid leaking from her nipples!" What is the nurse's best response?

   a. "I don't know. Let me have the charge nurse check the baby."
   b. "It's nothing to worry about. That's a normal finding."
   c. "This is a normal occurrence. You may clean her with a damp washcloth, but be careful not to squeeze the nipples."
   d. "This means the baby was exposed to an infection during birth. I'll notify the doctor at once!"

3. Baby Boy Alvarez is 5 minutes old. The nurse performs a quick assessment and determines that the newborn has a heart rate of 110 bpm, a weak cry, and acrocyanosis. His extremities are held in partial flexion, and he grimaces when a catheter is placed in his nose. What Apgar score does the nurse record?

   a. 5–The newborn is having extreme difficulty transitioning.
   b. 5–The newborn is having moderate difficulty transitioning.
   c. 6–The newborn is having moderate difficulty transitioning.
   d. 6–The newborn is vigorous and transitioning with minimal effort.

4. The nurse is assessing a 1-day-old newborn and notices a small amount of white drainage and redness at the base of the umbilical cord. Which of the following is the best response by the nurse?

   a. Call the doctor immediately to ask for intravenous antibiotics.
   b. Carefully clean the area with a damp washcloth and cover it with an absorbent dressing.
   c. Notify the charge nurse because this finding represents a possible complication.
   d. Show the mother how to clean the area with soap and water.

5. A newborn's axillary temperature is 97.4°F. His T-shirt is damp with spit-up milk. His blanket is loosely applied, and several children are in the room running around his crib. The room is comfortably warm, and the bassinet is beside the mother's bed away from the window and doors. What are the most likely mechanisms of heat loss for this newborn?

   a. Conduction and evaporation
   b. Conduction and radiation
   c. Convection and radiation
   d. Convection and evaporation

■ STUDY ACTIVITIES

1. Do an Internet search using the key words "newborn crying." How many Internet sites returned? List three to four that would be good references for new parents. Compare your list to that of your clinical group.

2. Use the table below to describe important newborn assessments for each body system.

Body System	Critical Parameters to Assess	Expected Findings and Deviation From Normal
Respiratory		
Cardiovascular		
Gastrointestinal		
Metabolic		
Hepatic		
Skin		

3. Research resources in your community designed to help first-time parents in their new role. How many sources did you find? Were you surprised? Share your findings with your clinical group. Discuss ways the community might be more supportive of new parents.

■ CRITICAL THINKING: WHAT WOULD YOU DO?

Apply your knowledge of normal newborn adaptation to the following situation.

1. Mary, a 28-year-old woman, delivered her first baby several hours ago. She and the father of the baby had joyful interaction with the baby immediately after delivery. The newborn breast-fed well with assistance from the delivery room nurse. You are coming on duty for the evening shift and have just entered the room to assess the baby.

   a. You find the baby sleeping with only a diaper on in an open bassinet. The bassinet is located against the wall under a window. The baby's skin is mottled, and her extremities feel cool to the touch. What is your initial assessment of the situation? What actions should you take?

   b. What instructions should you give to the parents?

2. On day 3 of life, you notice that Mary's newborn's skin is a light yellow color.

   a. What is the likely cause of the yellow color?

   b. Mary asks you if the yellow color indicates illness. How do you reply?

3. Mary says she is frustrated. She has been trying to "play" with the baby, but he keeps looking away and yawning. She is worried that her baby does not "like" her.

   a. How should you reply to Mary?

   b. Mary expresses concern about a blue-black spot she found on the baby's back. She is worried that he received a bruise in the nursery. How do you explain this finding to Mary?

14 Nursing Care of the Normal Newborn

KEY TERMS

circumcision
kangaroo care
ophthalmia neonatorum
thermoneutral environment

LEARNING OBJECTIVES

On completion of this chapter, you should be able to:

1. Explain how to support immediate transition from fetal to extrauterine life.
2. Outline principles of thermoregulation for the newborn.
3. Discuss appropriate interventions for the newborn with hypoglycemia.
4. Describe immediate care of the newborn to include eye prophylaxis and administration of vitamin K.
5. Explain the nurse's role in protecting the infant from misidentification in the hospital.
6. Identify effective infection control procedures in the nursery.
7. Describe when and how the newborn receives his or her first bath.
8. Describe strategies hospitals can take to protect the newborn from abduction.
9. Name signs of pain in the newborn.
10. Compare the care of the uncircumcised newborn male with that of the circumcised newborn.
11. List immunizations and newborn screening tests that should be done before the newborn is discharged home.
12. Develop a teaching plan for the parents regarding normal newborn care.

AS YOU LEARNED in Chapter 13, the newborn must make rapid adjustments to adapt successfully to life outside of the womb. Your role is to support the newborn as he adapts to these changes, quickly recognize the development of complications, and report changes in condition to the RN to facilitate rapid intervention. Teaching the parents the skills needed to care for their newborn is another critical role you will play. This chapter discusses the basic nursing care required for newborns and their families.

NEWBORN STABILIZATION AND TRANSITION

The current standard of care for resuscitation of the newborn immediately after birth is outlined in the Neonatal Resuscitation Program (NRP) (American Academy of Pediatrics NRP Steering Committee, 2006).[1] The basic principles of newborn resuscitation are reviewed here. Refer to an NRP textbook for detailed guidelines on newborn resuscitation. The licensed practical nurse (LPN) normally is not responsible for a complete resuscitation; however, you must be able to initiate resuscitation and assist throughout the process.

Nursing Process in Immediate Stabilization and Transition of the Newborn

The first 6 to 12 hours after birth are a critical transition period for the newborn. The healthy newborn may stay with the mother immediately after delivery and be cared for by the same nurse who is overseeing the mother's recovery. In some facilities, the newborn is taken to a transition nursery after a short initial bonding period with his parents. In either case, when caring for the newborn during the transition period, you must be alert to early signs of distress and be ready to intervene quickly to prevent complications and poor outcomes.

---

[1]Developed and maintained by the American Heart Association (AHA) and the American Academy of Pediatrics (AAP).

Assessment

Immediate assessments of the newborn are concerned with the success of cardiopulmonary adaptation, as discussed in Chapter 13. The newborn requires close observation during the first 6 to 10 hours of life, the transition period. Measure the heart and respiratory rates at least every 30 minutes during the first 2 hours of transition. Monitor the axillary temperature every 30 minutes until it stabilizes in the expected range (between 97.7°F [36.5°C] and 99.5°F [37.5°C]). Be alert for signs of hypoglycemia.

A full physical assessment (see Chapter 13), including gestational age assessment (detailed in Chapter 20), is completed within the first few hours of life.

Selected Nursing Diagnoses

- Impaired spontaneous ventilation related to ineffective transition to newborn life
- Risk for injury: Hypoglycemia related to immature metabolism and/or presence of risk factors
- Ineffective thermoregulation related to immature heat-regulating mechanisms
- Risk for infection related to immature immune system, possible exposure to pathogens in the birth canal or in the nursery, and umbilical cord wound
- Risk for imbalanced fluid volume related to immature blood clotting mechanisms
- Risk for injury: Misidentification related to failure of delivery room personnel to adequately identify the newborn before separation from the parents

Outcome Identification and Planning

Maintaining the safety of the newborn during transition from intrauterine to extrauterine life is the primary goal of nursing care immediately after delivery and in the first 6 to 12 hours of life. Appropriate patient goals include that the newborn will experience adequate cardiovascular, respiratory, thermoregulatory, and metabolic transitions to extrauterine life. Additional goals are that he or she will remain free from signs and symptoms of infection, maintain hemostasis, and be adequately identified before separation from the parents.

Implementation

Supporting Cardiovascular and Respiratory Transition

Nursing interventions to support newborn vital functions begin before the birth occurs. If you will be assisting in the immediate care of the newborn, ensure that adequate supplies are present for a full resuscitation and that all equipment is functioning properly. Most delivery settings have a newborn resuscitation board or cabinet that contains needed supplies. Check that oxygen is readily available and that there is a functioning suction source. Ensure that a warmer is in the delivery area, and turn it on several minutes before the delivery is expected.

Observe the newborn carefully at birth. The delivery attendant will usually suction the mouth and nose with a bulb syringe and clamp and cut the umbilical cord. If the newborn cries vigorously, you may drape a blanket over the mother's abdomen and support the infant there when the birth attendant hands the newborn to you. Quickly palpate the base of the umbilical cord and count the pulse for 6 seconds. Multiply that number by 10 to calculate the heart rate. A pulse above 100 beats per minute and a vigorous cry are reassuring signs that indicate the newborn is making a successful transition.

If the newborn does not cry immediately, transport him to a preheated radiant warmer for prompt resuscitation. Dry him quickly to prevent heat loss from evaporation and to provide stimulation to encourage a first breath. If the newborn still does not make adequate breathing efforts, a bag and mask connected to 100% oxygen are used to provide respiratory support until spontaneous breathing occurs.

Most newborns do not require resuscitation, and the ones who do generally respond well to a short period of positive-pressure ventilation with a bag and mask. However, a very small number of infants also require chest compressions, intubation, and medications. Refer to the NRP for complete resuscitation guidelines.

Give constant attention to the airway. Newborns often have abundant secretions. The initial intervention is to position the newborn on the side or with the head in a slightly lower position than the body to help prevent aspiration of secretions. A bulb syringe is used to suction the mouth first and then the nose (Fig. 14-1). Keep the bulb syringe with the newborn, and teach the parents how and when to suction the baby. If copious secretions are present that do not resolve with a bulb syringe, a small suction catheter connected to a suction source may be used. Be careful not to apply suction for longer than 5 seconds at a time and to minimize suction pressures to avoid damaging the delicate respiratory structures.

> **Did you know?**
> It is important to suction the mouth of a newborn before the nose. If the nose is suctioned first, the newborn may gasp or cry and aspirate secretions in the mouth.

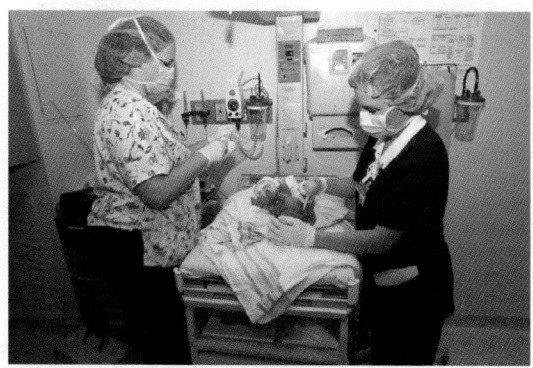

▌ **Figure 14-1** The nurse uses a bulb syringe to suction the mouth of the newborn before suctioning the nares.

Maintaining Thermoregulation

It is critical to protect the newborn from chilling. Cold stress increases the amount of oxygen and glucose needed by the newborn. He or she can quickly deplete glucose stores and develop hypoglycemia. The newborn can also develop respiratory distress and metabolic acidosis if exposed to prolonged chilling. If the newborn cries vigorously and has an adequate heart rate, he or she may stay with his mother. Quickly dry the newborn on the mother's abdomen, swaddle him snugly, and apply a cap to prevent heat loss. Another way to maintain the newborn's temperature and promote early bonding is to dry the newborn quickly, place a diaper or blanket over the genital area and a cap on the head, then place the newborn skin to skin with the mother or father and cover them both with blankets. This method of keeping the newborn warm is called **kangaroo care** (Fig. 14-2). Kangaroo care is an excellent way to meet the needs of the newborn and provide family-centered care.

It is important to support thermoregulation in the newborn, particularly in the first 24 hours of life. The environmental temperature necessary to maintain a **thermoneutral environment**, an environment in which heat is neither lost nor gained, is slightly higher for the newborn than that required for an older child or adult. Take care to prevent unnecessary heat loss in the nursery. For example, drafts of air can cause convective heat loss, and placing a newborn on a cold surface can lead to conductive heat loss (see Chapter 13 for discussion of these terms).

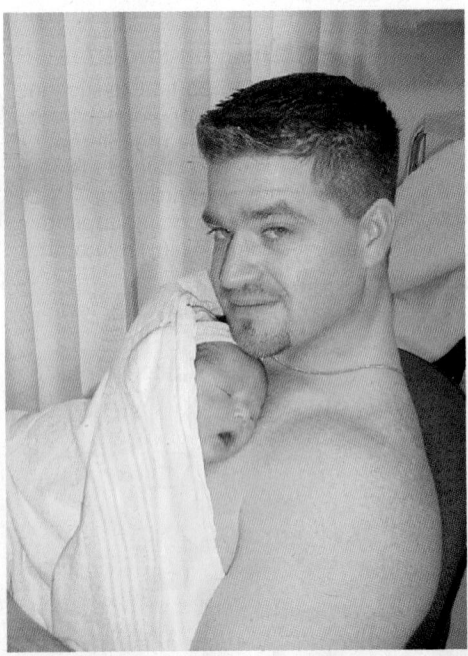

◼ Figure 14-2 A new father practices kangaroo care, keeping his newborn warm using skin-to-skin contact. Kangaroo care is also an excellent way for parents to bond with their newborn.

Conversely, do not allow the newborn to become overheated. Hyperthermia can be just as harmful as hypothermia. A skin temperature probe should be in place on the skin anytime the newborn is under the radiant warmer, and alarms should be set to signal if the skin temperature becomes too hot.

Preventing Injury from Hypoglycemia

The best way to prevent injury from hypoglycemia is to prevent the condition altogether. If the mother is breast-feeding, encourage early and frequent feedings. If she is experiencing difficulty, it may be necessary to have a lactation consultant assist the mother. See Chapter 15 for detailed information on breast-feeding and nutrition. If the newborn is to be bottle-fed, initiate early feedings.

When a newborn displays signs of hypoglycemia (see Chapter 13), perform a heel stick (Nursing Procedure 14-1) and use a bedside glucose analyzer to check the blood sugar level. If a heel stick specimen reveals a glucose level of less than 50 mg/dL, draw a venous blood sample and send it to the lab for confirmation because it is common for bedside glucose analyzers to under read glucose results. It is critical, however, that you immediately initiate treatment. Follow institutional policy for frequency of testing asymptomatic newborns at risk for hypoglycemia.

Most facilities have protocols to guide nursing care in the treatment of hypoglycemia. Many pediatricians have preprinted orders that can be initiated if the glucose level falls below a predetermined level (usually 40–50 mg/dL). In the past, glucose water was used to treat low blood glucose levels, but most authorities now recommend feeding breast milk or formula to the alert newborn. If the infant's symptoms are severe enough to interfere with regular feeding, intravenous dextrose solutions are administered (Karlsen, 2006).

Preventing Infection

Within the first hour after birth, an antibiotic ointment must be placed in the newborn's eyes (Fig. 14-3) to prevent **ophthalmia neonatorum**, a severe eye infection contracted in the birth canal of a woman with gonorrhea or chlamydia. There are three ophthalmic agents approved for eye prophylaxis: 1% silver nitrate, 0.5% erythromycin, and 1% tetracycline. Silver nitrate is used infrequently because it is irritating to the eyes. In some facilities, it is the practice to instill the eye drops in the delivery area immediately after birth, but it is recommended that the instillation be delayed up to 1 hour to allow the newborn and parents to bond while the infant is in a quiet alert state.

Another possible infection site is the umbilical cord stump. Practice careful handwashing, and use strict aseptic technique when caring for the cord. Often an antiseptic solution such as triple dye, bacitracin ointment,

Nursing Procedure 14-1
PERFORMING A HEEL STICK

EQUIPMENT

Alcohol wipe (or other antiseptic, per institution policy)
2 × 2 square gauze
Tape
Adhesive bandage
Lancet or other puncturing device
Device to read the glucose level and all supplies needed for its use
Clean gloves

PROCEDURE

1. Thoroughly wash your hands.
2. Don a pair of clean gloves.
3. Hold the foot so that it is well supported with your thumb or finger covering the flat surfaces of the foot to avoid puncturing this area and causing damage to nerves or blood vessels. The highlighted areas on the lateral aspects of the foot in the illustration are appropriate areas from which to perform a heel stick.

Lateral plantar artery
Lateral plantar nerve
Calcaneous
Safe areas for puncture
Medial plantar artery
Medial plantar nerve
Medial calcaneal nerve

4. Locate a fat pad on either side of the foot. Palpate the chosen site to ensure there is enough padding to avoid puncturing the bone, which could lead to infection.
5. Clean the site with alcohol (or other antiseptic, per institution policy) and allow to air dry.
6. Using the lancet, puncture the site to a depth of no greater than 2 mm. If using a commercial

puncturing device, follow the manufacturer's guidelines for use. Place the lancet in a sharps container.

7. Wipe away the first drop of blood. Do not squeeze the tissue close to the puncture site or the reading may not be accurate.
8. Collect the specimen from the second drop of blood. Follow the manufacturer's instructions regarding processing the specimen.

9. Make a pressure dressing from the gauze and tape it over the puncture site. An alternative is to hold pressure for a few moments and then apply an adhesive bandage when the bleeding stops.
10. Remove the gloves and thoroughly wash your hands.
11. Record the glucose level in the designated area of the chart.

Note: Current research does not support the use of warmth to prepare the heel (Folk, 2007).

■ **Figure 14-3** The nurse administers antibiotic ointment to the eyes of the newborn to prevent ophthalmia neonatorum.

or povidone-iodine is used initially to paint the cord to help prevent the development of infection.

Preventing Imbalanced Fluid Volume

One possible cause of hemorrhage and fluid volume loss is an immature clotting mechanism. Vitamin K is necessary in the formation of certain clotting factors. In the adult, normal flora manufacture vitamin K in the gut, but the gut of the newborn is sterile; symbiotic bacteria have not yet colonized it. Therefore, it is necessary to supply the newborn with vitamin K to prevent possible bleeding episodes. Within the first hour after birth, 0.5 to 1 mg of vitamin K (AquaMEPHYTON) is given intramuscularly (Nursing Procedure 14-2).

One potential source of hemorrhage is the clamped umbilical cord. An unusually large cord may have large amounts of Wharton's jelly, which may disintegrate faster

---

Nursing Procedure 14-2
ADMINISTERING AN INTRAMUSCULAR INJECTION TO THE NEWBORN

EQUIPMENT

Warm, clean hands
Clean (nonsterile) exam gloves
Syringe
0.5-inch 23- to 25-gauge safety needle
Alcohol pad
Flat surface

PROCEDURE

1. Wash hands thoroughly.
2. Check physician order for medication and dose.
3. Follow normal nursing procedure for drawing medications from a vial or ampule. Do not draw more than 0.5 mL for intramuscular (IM) injection to a newborn.
4. Identify the newborn by identity band. Place the newborn on a flat surface with good lighting.
5. Select an injection site on the vastus lateralis (anterior lateral aspect of the thigh) or rectus femoris (midanterior aspect of the thigh) muscle.
6. Apply clean gloves.
7. Clean the site with an alcohol pad. Use a circular motion from the center of the chosen site outward in ever-widening circles. Hold the alcohol pad between two of your fingers.
8. With your nondominant hand, hold the leg in place.

9. Using your dominant hand, insert the needle at a 90-degree angle with a quick darting motion.
10. Stabilize the needle with your nondominant hand and pull back gently on the plunger to aspirate for blood.
11. If no blood is noted, slowly inject the medication.

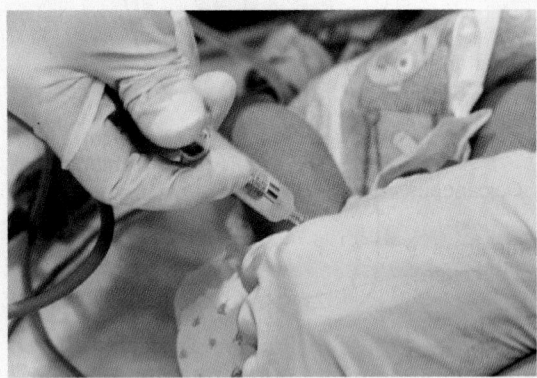

12. Use the alcohol pad to stabilize the skin as you withdraw the needle.
13. Discard the syringe and needle in a sharps container. Discard the gloves in a trash receptacle.
14. Wash hands thoroughly.
15. Document on the medication administration record.

Note: If blood is aspirated in step 10, withdraw the needle to avoid intravenous (IV) injection. Discard the syringe, needle, and medication in a sharps container. Go back to step 1 and begin again.

than the cord vessels and cause the clamp to become loose. This situation could lead to blood loss from the cord. Another cause could be an improperly applied or defective cord clamp. Inspect the umbilical cord for signs of bleeding.

Preventing Misidentification of a Newborn

Fortunately, it is a rare occurrence for newborns to be switched in the hospital and go home with the wrong parents, but it has happened. When the mistake is uncovered years later, the situation often results in heartache and heart-wrenching choices for all parties involved. Because of the serious consequences of mistaken identity, the delivery room nurse must take the utmost care to positively identify the newborn before he or she is separated from his parents.

Many facilities footprint the newborn and fingerprint the mother, but this practice is in decline because footprints are not often useful to identify infants. Most hospitals use some form of bracelet system. Three to four bracelets with identical numbers on the bands are prepared immediately after delivery and before the newborn is separated from his parents. Information included on the bands is the mother's name, hospital number, and physician, and the newborn's sex and date and time of birth. Two bands are placed on the newborn, one on the arm and one on the leg. A matching band is placed on the mother and another band may be placed on the father or other designated adult. Instruct the parents to always check the bands when the newborn is brought to them to ensure they are receiving their newborn.

Evaluation: Goals and Expected Outcomes

Goal: The newborn experiences adequate cardiovascular and respiratory transition.
Expected Outcomes: The newborn

- sustains a heart rate above 100 beats per minute.
- maintains a respiratory rate between 30 and 60 breaths per minute without signs of distress.
- retains a patent airway.

Goal: The newborn experiences thermoregulatory transition.
Expected Outcome:

- The newborn's body temperature stabilizes between 97.7°F (36.5°C) and 99.5°F (37.5°C).

Goal: The newborn experiences adequate metabolic transition.
Expected Outcome:

- The newborn's blood glucose level stays above 50 mg/dL.

Goal: The newborn remains free from the signs and symptoms of infection.
Expected Outcomes: The newborn remains free from

- purulent conjunctivitis.
- purulent drainage from the umbilical cord.

- other signs of sepsis, such as poor suck reflex and lethargy.

Goal: The newborn maintains adequate hemostasis.
Expected Outcomes:

- The newborn has no bleeding episodes.

Goal: The newborn is adequately identified before separation from the parents.
Expected Outcomes: The newborn

- possesses a permanent form of identification before he is separated from his parents.
- can be positively identified by his parents.

Test Yourself

✔ What is the normal temperature range for a newborn?
✔ Describe kangaroo care. List two purposes that it serves.
✔ What is the purpose of eye prophylaxis?

GENERAL NEWBORN CARE

Nursing care of the normal, stabilized newborn is directed toward controlling risk and early detection of developing complications.

Nursing Process in Providing Care to the Normal Newborn

Assessment

When caring for newborns, it is important to be familiar with signs that indicate the newborn needs special care. One common problem is the potential for aspiration from secretions and mucus that are present in the airways during the first few days of life. Monitor the newborn closely for excessive secretions. Gagging and frequent regurgitation are normal in the first few hours of birth. Signs of respiratory distress or central cyanosis should not be present.

Another potential problem is that of infection. Carefully monitor the newborn for signs of infection. An infected umbilical cord will show signs of redness and edema at the base and may have purulent discharge. Early signs of sepsis in the newborn include poor feeding, irritability, lethargy, apnea, and temperature instability. Late signs are an enlarged spleen and liver, jaundice, and petechiae.

Perform a thorough skin assessment. Turgor should be present, and the skin should be intact. Inspect the diaper area for signs of rash or breakdown. Assess for signs of jaundice. As you will recall from Chapter 13, jaundice that occurs within the first 24 hours of life is associated with abnormal lysis of red blood cells and is pathologic in nature.

Box 14-1 ■ PROFILE OF A TYPICAL INFANT ABDUCTOR

- Is usually female of "childbearing" age (12–50), and is often overweight.
- Usually is compulsive and frequently relies on manipulation, lying, and deception to gain access.
- Usually states she has lost a baby, or is incapable of having a child.
- Is often married or is cohabiting with a male companion.
- Usually, the companion has a desire to have a child, or the abductor has a desire to provide her companion with "his" child. Often, that is the motivation for the abduction.
- Frequently, the abductor lives in or is familiar with the community where the abduction takes place.
- Usually visits the nursery or maternity ward at more than one health care facility prior to the abduction, and asks detailed questions about procedures and the maternity floor layout.
- Frequently uses a fire exit stairwell for her escape, and may also try to abduct from the home setting.
- Although the abductor usually plans the abduction ahead of time, she does not necessarily target a specific infant and frequently seizes any opportunity present.
- Frequently impersonates a nurse or other allied health care personnel.
- Frequently becomes familiar with health care staff, staff work routines, and victim parents.
- Demonstrates a capability to provide "good" care to the baby once the abduction occurs.

Note: The typical abductor profile was developed from an analysis of 248 cases occurring between 1983 and 2007. Source: National Center for Missing & Exploited Children.

Between 1983 and 2006, 247 cases of infant abduction by a nonfamily member were reported in the United States (Burgess et al., 2008). Although infant abduction is a rare event, it has devastating effects on hospital personnel and family members of the victim. Studies of the problem have led to a "typical abductor" profile (Box 14-1). When taking care of newborns, be especially alert to any suspicious activity by visitors or persons unknown to you.

The newborn encounters numerous startling and noxious stimuli at birth. The womb is dark, confined, and warm. The abdominal and uterine walls muffle sounds. During labor and delivery, this situation is reversed. Suddenly the newborn meets a world that is bright, cold, and loud. The newborn's extremities flail out when he or she is startled with seemingly nothing to stop them. He does not know his boundaries. In addition, the newborn is exposed to invasive and sometimes painful procedures. These early experiences have the potential to cause the newborn to respond to the environment in a disorganized way.

Selected Nursing Diagnoses

- Ineffective airway clearance related to mucus and secretions
- Risk for infection related to cross-contamination of equipment, poor hand washing, poor hygienic practices, transmission from mother to baby
- Risk for impaired skin integrity
- Risk for injury: newborn abduction
- Risk for disorganized infant behavior related to pain, invasive procedures, or environmental overstimulation

Outcome Identification and Planning

Monitoring for and preventing complications is the aim of most newborn care interventions. After the newborn has had a successful transition, appropriate goals include that the newborn will maintain a clear airway, be free of infection; have clean intact skin, not be abducted from the hospital, and respond to the environment in an organized way. The goal of maintaining an adequate body temperature is addressed throughout the hospital stay. Interventions to meet that goal are interwoven throughout the following implementation section. The goal of maintaining adequate nutrition and hydration is covered in detail in Chapter 15.

Implementation

Keeping the Airway Clear

Keep the bulb syringe in the bassinet with the newborn at all times. Turn the newborn on the side and suction frequently as secretions and mucus accumulate. Teach both parents how to use the bulb syringe. Position the newborn on his or her back to sleep, as recommended by the American Academy of Pediatrics Task Force on Sudden Infant Death Syndrome (2005), to decrease the risk of sudden infant death syndrome (see Chapter 20).

Preventing Transmission of Infection

A newborn may contract infection from his mother, visitors, nursery personnel, or the environment. Infection can be particularly devastating for a newborn because the immune system is immature and the newborn has not yet developed effective defenses against invading pathogens. Therefore, it is essential to practice good infection control techniques when caring for newborns. Handwashing remains the mainstay of infection control, even in newborn nurseries. Many nurseries require a 3-minute surgical-type scrub at the beginning of the shift. Follow the protocol of the facility in which you are working. The hands should be washed thoroughly before and after caring for a newborn. In no instance should you care for a newborn and then proceed to handle or give care to another newborn without washing your hands in between. Many newborn nurseries have waterless hand sanitizer available. Hand sanitizer is acceptable to use between newborns when visible soiling of the hands has not occurred.

Other methods for reducing the transmission of infection include keeping all of the newborn's belongings together in the bassinet and not sharing items between newborns. This practice reduces the possibility of cross-contamination. Wipe reusable equipment, such as a stethoscope, with alcohol between uses. Rooming in also reduces the likelihood of cross-contamination.

It is necessary to use universal precautions for your protection. Do not handle a newborn without gloves until after the bath. After the bath, you may provide care for the newborn without gloves unless contact with bodily fluids is likely, such as during diaper changes and when drawing blood for testing.

Providing Skin Care

The first bath (Nursing Procedure 14-3) is delayed until the newborn's temperature is stable. Warm water is usually sufficient for bathing; however, a mild soap is permissible. The sponge bath is given under a radiant warmer to minimize heat loss. If a radiant warmer is not used, it is important to keep the infant wrapped and expose only the body part being washed.

Be careful
Do not use harsh soaps when bathing newborns because they can irritate the skin. Hexachlorophene in particular should not be used because it can be absorbed through the skin and cause central nervous system damage.

Nursing Procedure 14-3
GIVING THE FIRST BATH

EQUIPMENT

Clean exam gloves
Basin of warm water (98°F–100°F)
Mild soap and shampoo
Washcloth
Towel
Comb
Cap
Clean diaper
Shirt
Two receiving blankets

PROCEDURE

1. Assemble equipment.
2. Wash hands.
3. Use only clear water (no soap) on the eyes first (proceeding from inner canthus to outer canthus), then the rest of the face.
4. Hold the newborn with your nondominant arm using the football hold. Use the washcloth with the other hand to wipe off visible blood.
5. Lather the hair with shampoo and rinse thoroughly.

(continues on page 312)

Nursing Procedure 14-3
GIVING THE FIRST BATH *(continued)*

6. Comb through the hair to remove dried blood and to facilitate drying.
7. Place the infant back in the crib or under the radiant warmer (per the facility policy).
8. Bathe and rinse the neck and chest. Be sure to remove blood from the creases of the neck and armpits.

9. Proceed to the abdomen. Take care not to soak the cord in water (a wet cord increases the risk for infection).
10. Wash the extremities, then the back.

11. Next, bathe the genital region. For boys, do not force the foreskin over the glans. For girls, wash from front to back, avoiding contamination of the urethral and vaginal areas with bacteria from the rectum.
12. Last, bathe the anal region.
13. Apply a clean cap, t-shirt, and diaper.
14. Double wrap the newborn with two receiving blankets.
15. Rinse and dry the basin. Store unused soap and shampoo containers and comb in the basin in the storage area of the bassinet.
16. Place the towel and washcloth in the dirty linen hamper.
17. Remove gloves.
18. Wash hands.

Note: The room should be warm, approximately 75°F (24°C) to prevent chilling. In many facilities, the first bath is given under the radiant warmer. Bathing should proceed from the cleanest part of the body (face) and end with the dirtiest areas (diaper area). Each body area should be washed, rinsed, and then dried before proceeding to the next area to prevent heat loss from evaporation.

Be careful to wash off all traces of blood to minimize transmission of infection. Combing the hair helps to remove dried blood. Vernix serves as a lubricant and is protective against infections; therefore, it is best to gently massage the vernix into the skin and allow it to wear off naturally. However, in many facilities vernix is wiped away completely at the first bath to make the baby more presentable.

Encourage the parents to participate in the bath (Fig. 14-4). This is an excellent time to allow them to interact with their baby and help them gain confidence in parenting skills. When the bath is finished, check the axillary temperature. If it is within the expected range (see previous section), dress the newborn in a shirt, di-

aper, and cap. Swaddle the newborn in a blanket and place him in an open crib. If the temperature is below 97.5°F (36.4°C), return the newborn to the radiant warmer.

Use warm water to clean the perineal area and buttocks at diaper changes. Frequent diaper changes will help prevent diaper rash and skin breakdown. No special oils or ointments are necessary on clean, intact skin. Do not use talc powders because they can cause respiratory irritation when particles are inhaled. Fold the diaper down in the front so that the cord is open to air (Fig. 14-5). This action protects the cord area from irritation when the diaper is wet and promotes drying of the cord.

■ **Figure 14-4** The new father dries his newborn son after giving him his first bath.

Family Teaching Tips

KEEPING THE NEWBORN SAFE

- Never leave the newborn unattended.
- Do not remove the identification bands on the newborn until he or she is discharged from the hospital; alert the nurses if an identification band falls off or becomes illegible for any reason.
- Do not release the newborn to anyone who does not have a hospital photograph ID that matches the specific security color or code chosen by the facility to identify personnel authorized to transport and handle newborns.
- Know the nurses caring for you and your newborn.
- Question anyone who does not have the proper identification, or whose picture does not match the identification tag he or she is wearing, even if he or she is dressed in hospital attire.
- Alert the nurses immediately if you are suspicious of any person or activity.
- Know when the newborn will be taken for tests, what health care provider authorized the test, and how long the procedure is expected to last.

Providing Safety

Education and watchful vigilance are the keys to preventing infant abductions. Each facility that cares for newborns should have specific policies and procedures in place that address this problem. Review these policies and know the protocols for the facility in which you will be working.

Most nurseries and mother–baby units are in a part of the hospital that has some security features to discourage abductions. Most nurseries are locked from the outside, and a security code is necessary to gain entrance. Security cameras are usually placed strategically near entrances and exits. Some facilities use security bracelets

■ **Figure 14-5** The diaper is folded down so that it does not cover the drying umbilical cord.

that set off an alarm if someone attempts to remove it, or it may trip an alarm when a person exits the unit with a newborn. The matching identification bands for newborns and parents also are part of the security plan. In many facilities, identification photos are taken of each newborn. Cooperation of the parents is essential to the effectiveness of any security plan, especially because most infants who are abducted are taken from the mother's room. Family Teaching Tips: Keeping the Newborn Safe lists key points to discuss with parents regarding the safety and security of their newborn while in the hospital.

Enhancing Organized Infant Behavioral Responses

Newborns respond to the environment in more predictable and organized ways when caregivers anticipate their needs. The psychosocial task of infants is developing a sense of trust. Newborns begin to develop trust when the adults around them consistently meet their needs. Feeding the newborn, keeping him dry and comfortable, and holding him are actions that promote trust. Kangaroo care with either parent provides comfort and encourages attachment. Swaddling a newborn snugly is comforting and promotes sleep. Nonnutritive sucking on a gloved finger or pacifier can also be comforting.

Evaluation: Goals and Expected Outcomes

Goal: The newborn will maintain a patent airway.

Expected Outcomes: The newborn

- maintains a respiratory rate between 30 and 60 breaths per minute while at rest.
- has no signs of respiratory distress.

Goal: The newborn will maintain a normal body temperature.

Expected Outcomes:

- The newborn maintains axillary temperature above 97.5°F (36.4°C) and below 99.5°F (37.5°C)

Goal: The newborn remains free of the signs and symptoms of infection.

Expected Outcomes: The newborn maintains

- strong, coordinated suck and swallow reflexes[2].
- vigorous feeding behaviors.
- a drying umbilical cord without purulent drainage or foul odor.

Goal: The newborn maintains skin integrity.

Expected Outcomes:

- The newborn has clean, intact skin.

Goal: The newborn is not abducted from the hospital.

Expected Outcomes:

- The newborn remains safely in the company of family members and/or nursery personnel at all times.

Goal: The newborn responds to the environment in an organized way.

Expected Outcomes: The newborn

- begins to develop predictable sleep/wake patterns.
- interacts with caregivers with sustained alertness during interaction.

Test Yourself

- ✔ Name three characteristics of a "typical" infant abductor.
- ✔ List four things you can do as the nurse to decrease the spread of infection to newborns.
- ✔ Describe three steps parents can take to reduce the risk of infant abduction while in the hospital.

DISCHARGE PREPARATION

Risk management and promoting healthy adaptation to newborn life continue to guide nursing care when planning for discharge of a healthy newborn.

Nursing Process in Preparing the Newborn for Discharge

Assessment

Continue to assess respiratory, cardiovascular, thermoregulatory, nutritional, and hydration status. Monitor for signs of infection. Check vigilantly for developing jaundice.

Watch for signs of pain in the newborn, particularly if he or she is scheduled for a painful procedure. Until recently, little thought was given as to how newborns perceive pain and what, if any, long-term effects there might be if pain is prolonged or untreated. Many research studies now support the real physiologic pain responses experienced by the newborn. It appears that untreated pain in the newborn can lead to increased sensitivity to painful experiences later or result in more immediate consequences, such as illness during the neonatal period.

The newborn may experience pain and discomfort from any number of routine procedures carried out in a newborn nursery. Injections and heel sticks are two such sources of painful stimuli. One common procedure that causes pain is **circumcision**, surgical removal of the foreskin of the penis. Because the newborn cannot express pain verbally, other measures must be used to evaluate pain. Pain can be assessed in the newborn by paying attention to behavior, such as crying, sleeplessness, facial expression, and body movements. Changes in heart and respiratory rates, blood pressure, and oxygen saturation can also be used to determine physiologic responses to pain.

It also is important to assess the adaptation of the mother and father to the parenting role. Experienced parents may feel very comfortable in their role and carry out newborn care without difficulty. New parents may ask many questions, or may appear afraid to handle the newborn. Assess for signs of positive bonding with the newborn. Refer to Chapter 12 for an in-depth discussion of bonding.

Selected Nursing Diagnoses

- Pain related to painful procedures such as injections, heel sticks, and circumcision
- Risk for infection related to inadequate immunity in the neonatal period
- Risk for injury from undetected metabolic and hearing disorders
- Deficient knowledge (parental) related to normal newborn care

Outcome Identification and Planning

Prevention of, and relief from, pain are applicable goals throughout the newborn's stay in the hospital; however, these goals become particularly important when the newborn is scheduled for an invasive procedure, such as circumcision. Protection from infection and injury from preventable diseases by immunizing against and screening

---

[2]Poor feeding behaviors may be a sign of sepsis in the newborn.

for hepatitis B, phenylketonuria, and other metabolic disorders is a critical goal during this time. It also is important to evaluate parental knowledge and ability to care for the newborn throughout the hospital stay, but as the time draws near for discharge, this task becomes particularly important.

Implementation

Preventing and Treating Pain

It is the ethical responsibility of the nurse to prevent and treat pain. Enough research exists to document the adverse effects of unnecessary and untreated pain in the neonate. The best treatment is prevention. When possible, avoid situations that may be painful or distressing to the newborn. If there is a choice between an invasive versus noninvasive procedure, choose the noninvasive procedure whenever practical. Use common sense and make suggestions to the charge nurse or physician as appropriate. For instance, it may be less painful to insert an intravenous device than to give multiple intramuscular injections, or it might be more tolerable for the newborn to have laboratory specimens drawn by venipuncture than to undergo numerous heel sticks.

Provide for a quiet, soothing environment as often as possible. Simple comfort measures can be initiated that decrease the amount of pain perceived by the newborn. Swaddling and holding the infant securely are soothing measures. Nonnutritive sucking on a pacifier can be comforting. Placing sucrose on the pacifier, if allowed by hospital policy, adds the benefit of analgesia suitable for minor pain stimulus.

Assisting With Circumcision

There has been much debate concerning whether or not circumcision should be performed routinely. In the 1970s and 1980s, the American Academy of Pediatrics (AAP) held to a strict policy of strongly discouraging circumcisions based on the rationale that there were no valid medical indications for the procedure. Since that time, the AAP (2005) has softened its stance, currently stating, "Existing scientific evidence demonstrates potential medical benefits of newborn male circumcision; however, these data are not sufficient to recommend routine neonatal circumcision." The procedure is contraindicated in newborns who:

- Are still in the transition period
- Are preterm or sick
- Have a family history of bleeding disorder until the disorder is ruled out in the newborn
- Have received a diagnosis of a bleeding disorder
- Have a congenital genitourinary disorder, such as epispadias or hypospadias

The AAP advises that parents should be given enough information to make an informed choice and that pain relief measures should be provided if the procedure is done. Box 14-2 compares the advantages and disadvan-

Box 14-2 ▌ ADVANTAGES AND DISADVANTAGES OF MALE CIRCUMCISION

Advantages
- Lower rates of urinary tract infections. (Note that the overall rate of urinary tract infections in newborn male infants is very small.)
- Risk of penile cancer, a rare disease, is reduced if circumcision is performed in infancy.
- Significant reduction in sexually transmitted infections. (This is an important medical benefit of circumcision; however, practicing safe sexual behaviors remains the best way to prevent these infections.)
- Circumcision for the newborn has fewer complications than when the procedure is performed in adulthood, although medical necessity for adult circumcision is rare.
- Easier hygiene. (Good hygiene of the uncircumcised penis may be as protective as circumcision; however, most uncircumcised boys do not perform adequate hygiene under the foreskin.)

Disadvantages
- Neonates experience pain during circumcision.
- All anesthetic methods to block or reduce the pain of circumcision have side effects and possible complications.
- Circumcision can lead to the complications of hemorrhage and infection (infrequent occurrences, but potentially life threatening), and genital mutilation (extremely rare).

Note: The religious and cultural values of the parents may play a large role in the decision on whether or not to circumcise. These values must be respected.

tages of male circumcision. Whatever the parents decide, you must be supportive of their decision.

If the parents decide to have their male newborn circumcised, informed consent is necessary. It is the physician's responsibility to obtain informed consent, although you may be responsible for witnessing the parents' signatures to a written documentation of that consent. If the parents have unanswered questions, notify the physician before the procedure is done. Because of the overwhelming evidence regarding the adverse effects of pain on the newborn, many physicians recommend that language be put into the written consents informing the parents that anesthesia will not be used (if the physician does not use anesthesia) and listing the possible harmful effects of doing the procedure without anesthesia.

After the parents sign the written consent, prepare for the procedure by gathering all necessary supplies and equipment. Check the physician preference card to

A Personal Glimpse

The nurse walked into my room and found me crying and holding my newborn son. She asked me if I was in pain or if something was wrong with the baby. I said, "No." She asked if I needed to talk and I nodded my head. I blurted out, "I just don't know if I should circumcise my son or not. My husband thinks we should, but I don't want my baby to be in pain. I just don't know that it is a necessary procedure."

She sat down on the side of my bed and calmly explained that there was no right or wrong decision. She assured me that she and the other nurses and doctors would support us in any decision that we made for our son. Then she gave me several pamphlets to read explaining the pros and cons of circumcision, the pros and cons of choosing not to circumcise, and the latest recommendations from the American Academy of Pediatrics. I felt much better after our talk, and my husband and I were able to make an informed decision about whether or not our son would have this procedure.

Heather

Learning Opportunity: What things can the nurse tell parents about pain control for painful procedures? In what ways can the nurse act as an advocate for parents when they are trying to decide on whether or not to allow procedures on their newborn?

determine what procedure the physician uses and what special materials are required. Medical immobilization is usually provided with a padded circumcision board (Fig. 14-6). If the board is not padded, add blankets or other soft material to the board. Swaddle the infant's upper body during the circumcision.

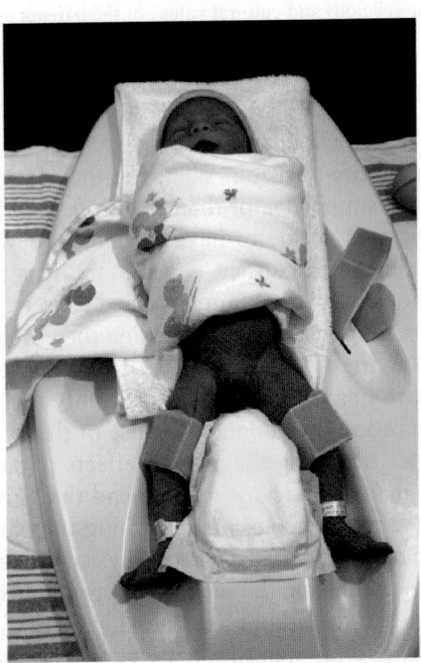

■ **Figure 14-6** Medical immobilization in preparation for circumcision.

Check the orders for preprocedure pain relief methods. Acetaminophen may be given within 1 hour before the procedure and then every 4 to 6 hours afterward during the first 24 hours per physician orders or facility protocol. If an anesthetic cream, such as EMLA, is to be used for the procedure, it must be applied approximately 1 hour before the procedure to adequately numb the area. The type of anesthesia that provides the best pain relief appears to be a dorsal penile nerve block. The physician performs the nerve block with buffered lidocaine at least 5 minutes before the circumcision to allow for complete anesthesia in the area. Other methods that can decrease the pain sensation include dimming the lights during circumcision, playing soft music or prerecorded intrauterine sounds for the newborn, and offering a sucrose-dipped pacifier to the infant before and throughout the procedure.

Immediately after the procedure, place a petrolatum gauze dressing, as ordered by the physician (Fig. 14-7). Then hold and comfort the newborn. If the parents are not readily available or cannot perform this action, you must step in to soothe the newborn. Position the newborn on the back or side to avoid excess pressure and pain on the circumcision site. Administer analgesics as ordered on a schedule for pain. Monitor the newborn for signs of unrelieved pain.

Assess the newborn every hour for the first 12 hours after circumcision for evidence of bleeding. If bleeding occurs, apply gentle pressure as needed. Carefully observe for return of voiding and observe the urine stream. Failure to void indicates a complication of circumcision. Report this situation to the charge nurse and physician. Refer to Family Teaching Tips: Uncircumcised and Circumcised Penis Care for important teaching points to discuss with parents after circumcision or, if circumcision is not done, how to care for the uncircumcised penis.

Preventing Infection Through Neonatal Immunization

Hepatitis B virus (HBV) vaccination is recommended by the Centers for Disease Control and Prevention for all

■ **Figure 14-7** A petrolatum gauze dressing applied after circumcision.

Family Teaching Tips

UNCIRCUMCISED AND CIRCUMCISED PENIS CARE

CARE FOR THE UNCIRCUMCISED NEWBORN

- Wash the penis with each diaper change.
- Avoid forcing the foreskin to retract because bleeding, infection, and scarring can result.
- Teach the child, when he is old enough, to wash under the foreskin daily by gently retracting the foreskin as far as it will go (without using forcible retraction).

CARE FOR THE CIRCUMCISED NEWBORN

- Inspect the circumcision site each time the diaper is changed. Call the doctor if more than a few drops of blood are present in the diaper.
- Wash the penis with warm water dribbled gently from a washcloth at each diaper change.
- Reapply petroleum jelly at each diaper change for the first 24–48 hours unless a Plastibell was used.
- Fasten the diaper loosely to prevent unnecessary friction and irritation.
- Remember that yellow crusting over the area indicates normal healing. The crust should not be removed.
- Hold and comfort your baby frequently while the site is healing. Nonnutritive sucking with a pacifier may be soothing.
- Call the physician if a Plastibell does not fall off within 5–8 days.
- Report the following warning signs after circumcision:
  - Bleeding spot larger than a quarter in the diaper.
  - No wet diapers within 6–8 hours after circumcision.
  - Fever, low-grade temperature, bad smell to the drainage, pus at the site.
  - Plastibell falls off before 5 days or is displaced.
  - Scarring after the area has healed.

newborns before they leave the hospital, regardless of the mother's hepatitis B surface antigen (HBsAg) status (all pregnant women who receive prenatal care are tested for HBsAg). The HBV vaccine requires parental consent. Be sure to obtain the parents' written consent before injecting the vaccine. Instruct the parents to follow up with the recommended vaccination schedule for all immunizations, starting at 2 months and continuing throughout infancy.

The HBV vaccination is especially important in newborns of mothers who are infected with hepatitis B or in whom infection is suspected. Many newborns who contract HBV from their mothers become chronic carriers of the disease. In some cases, the newborn develops an acute case of HBV and dies of the infection. In other cases, the newborn has no symptoms but has an increased risk for developing cirrhosis or hepatocellular carcinoma later in life. If the woman is HBsAg positive, bathe the newborn thoroughly after birth (to remove traces of blood and decrease the risk of transmission from the mother's blood on his skin when he receives his vaccination). In addition, the newborn is given the HBV vaccination and one dose of hepatitis B immunoglobulin within 12 hours of birth. This dosing schedule is 98% to 99% effective in preventing transmission of HBV from an infected mother to her newborn. If the mother's HBsAg status is unknown, the HBV vaccine is given, and the hepatitis B immunoglobulin dose can be postponed as long as 1 week while awaiting the mother's results.

Preventing Injury Through Neonatal Screening

It is crucial to screen newborns for several disorders that have the potential to cause lifelong disability if diagnosis and treatment are delayed (Box 14-3). The laws in most states require this initial screening, which is done within 72 hours of birth. The ideal time to collect the specimen is after the newborn is 36 hours old and 24 hours after he has his first protein feeding. Use a heel stick to draw blood from the newborn and collect a specimen on a special collection card. The card has five rings, and each ring must be filled with the newborn's blood (Fig. 14-8). The specimen is then labeled and sent to a special laboratory for testing. A second test is performed at 1 to 2 weeks of age. The mother must be instructed on where and when to take her newborn for the follow-up screening test.

A hearing screen is now encouraged for all newborns before they are discharged home. There are two tests that are used to screen a newborn's hearing: the Auditory Brainstem Response and Otoacoustic Emissions. Both

---

Box 14-3 ▌ NEWBORN SCREENING

Disorders for which newborn screening is commonly done:

- Phenylketonuria (PKU)
- Congenital hypothyroidism
- Galactosemia
- Maple syrup urine disease
- Homocystinuria
- Biotinidase
- Sickle cell disease
- Congenital adrenal hypoplasia
- Cystic fibrosis

Note: According to the National Newborn Screening and Genetics Resource Center, all 50 states mandate screening for PKU, congenital hypothyroidism, and galactosemia.

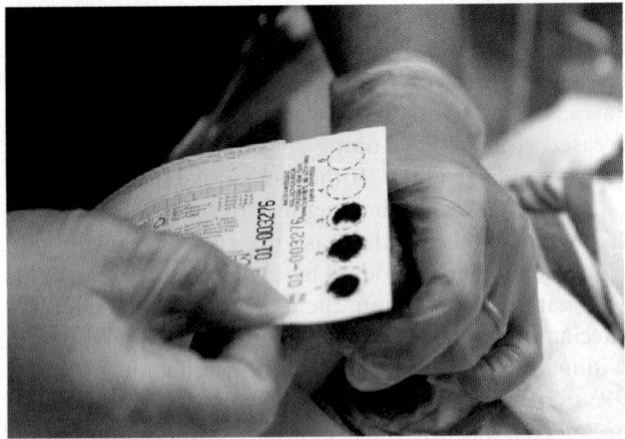

■ **Figure 14-8** The nurse collects a blood specimen on a special card to screen the newborn for treatable disorders that otherwise might cause mental retardation, disability, or even death.

tests use clicks or tones played into the newborn's ear. The Auditory Brainstem Response measures how the brain responds to sound through electrodes placed on the newborn's head. Otoacoustic Emissions measures sound waves produced in the inner ear. A probe is placed inside the newborn's ear canal, and the response or echo is measured. Both tests are effective screening devices. An abnormal screening result is followed-up with more extensive testing.

Because significant costs are involved for equipment and follow-up, it is mandated that insurance companies pay for this service. Early diagnosis and treatment results in better outcomes, including better chances for healthy attachment with parents, for newborns who have hearing disorders.

Supporting the Parent's Role through Discharge Teaching

Parent education is an essential part of normal newborn care. The parents need to know many things to meet the needs of their infant effectively. Because hospital stays are short, it is difficult to teach parents everything they need to know and to give them time to absorb the information and ask questions. At the very least, instructions should be written so that the parents can refer to them as needed. Family Teaching Tips: General Tips for Newborn Care at Home provides helpful information for new parents.

Some hospitals have newborn teaching videos that the parents can take home. Newborn care classes often are available that can be started before discharge and continued for several weeks or months afterward. Some hospitals have

Pay close attention.

If the parents are inexperienced, they need to feel confident in their ability to care for their child. Tactfully role model newborn care then let them develop their skills while you are available to assist. Sincerely compliment them when they do well.

home visitation programs in which a nurse or clinical nurse specialist follows up with the new family at home. All of these are ways to extend the teaching time and allow parents to absorb the material and formulate questions. Return demonstrations and home visits allow for direct observation of the parents' ability to care for their child. Several important topics that you will need to discuss with parents are covered in this section.

Handling the Newborn. New parents are often anxious about picking up their newborn for the first time. Assist them to slide one hand under the neck and shoulders and place the other hand under the buttocks or between the legs before gently lifting the newborn. Because newborns cannot support their head for the first few months, it is necessary for parents to provide this support when holding the baby.

Demonstrate different ways to hold the newborn (Fig. 14-9). The football hold is one position that allows the parent to support the head and body with one hand because the body is tucked under the arm. This leaves one hand free for other tasks. Instruct the parents to use the football hold judiciously while walking because the head is largely unprotected with this hold. Cradling the baby is familiar to most parents, as is the shoulder hold, which is sometimes comforting for a colicky baby. Newborns should always be placed on their backs to sleep to reduce the risk for sudden infant death syndrome.

Teach the parents to swaddle the newborn. Swaddling gives the newborn a sense of security and is comforting. Demonstrate and then let the parents give a return demonstration. Place the blanket in such a way that the newborn is positioned diagonally on the blanket. Fold down the top corner of the blanket under the infant's head. Pull the left corner around the front of the infant and tuck it under his arm. Pull up the bottom corner and tuck it in the front. Pull the right corner around the front of the infant and tuck it under the left arm (Fig. 14-10).

Hand washing before and after handling the baby is the best way parents can protect their newborn from infection. They should also encourage visitors to wash their hands before touching the baby. Anyone with obvious illness should not visit until he or she is well again.

Clearing the Airway. Teach the parents how to use the bulb syringe. Depress the bulb first and then place it in the newborn's mouth if excess secretions are noted. Suction the nose last. Clean the bulb with warm water and a mild soap. Sneezing is a normal response to particles in the air and is not indicative of a cold. Yellow or green nasal drainage are signs of illness that the parents should report to the physician. If the baby turns blue or stops breathing for longer than a few seconds, the parents should seek immediate emergency care (call 911).

Maintaining Adequate Temperature. Teach the parents to protect their newborn from drafts and to adequately dress the infant. However, sometimes the

Family Teaching Tips

GENERAL TIPS FOR NEWBORN CARE AT HOME

FEEDING

- Most newborns eat every 2–4 hours. Feeding patterns become fairly regular in approximately 2 weeks.
- Regurgitation ("spitting up") is expected. Vomiting should be reported to the pediatrician. Frequent vomiting can quickly lead to dehydration. Projectile vomiting may indicate an obstruction.

SLEEPING

- Newborns sleep approximately 16–20 hours per day.
- If you are caring for the newborn, it is a good idea to rest frequently throughout the day and sleep when the baby sleeps.
- For the first 3–4 months, it is difficult for infants to fall asleep by themselves. It is helpful to rock, walk, cuddle, or otherwise comfort the infant as he or she tries to fall asleep. After 4 months of age, you can help the baby learn to fall asleep at predictable times.
- There are wide variations of "normal" as to when babies sleep through the night. Some are able to do so by 6–7 weeks of age. Others may not until they are 3 or 4 months old.
- It does not help a baby sleep through the night to introduce solid foods too soon. A newborn's digestive system is immature and not ready to handle large protein molecules until approximately 4 months of age.

CRYING

- It is normal for a newborn to cry approximately 2 hours per day for the first 6–7 weeks of life.
- A "fussy period" during the day is to be expected.
- Crying is the way a baby communicates. First, check the baby for physical causes of discomfort, such as a wet or dirty diaper or hunger. Then, try all or some of the following suggestions to help quiet the baby:
  - Rock the baby.
  - Carry the baby and walk.
  - Take the baby for a stroll in the stroller.
  - Put the baby in a baby swing or a rocking cradle.
  - Gently pat or stroke the baby's back.
  - Swaddle the baby.
  - Take the baby for a ride in the car.
  - Turn on some white noise—washing machine, vacuum cleaner, air conditioner, radio not tuned to a station, etc.
- Never shake a baby for any reason. If you have tried everything and the baby continues to cry, put the baby down in a safe place and take a time-out. It won't hurt the baby to cry for a short time alone. Also, you could ask someone else to take over for awhile.

SENSORY INPUT

- Babies' brains need stimulation to develop. Use the five senses to communicate with the baby.
- Visual stimulation can be as simple as making faces with your baby during periods of alertness. Mobiles are another means of visual enrichment.
- Talking, singing, and reading give the baby auditory stimulation.
- Holding and cuddling the baby and letting him or her touch different textures and shapes develops the sense touch.
- Pay attention to your baby's cues. He or she will let you know when she has had enough stimulation and needs rest.

HEALTH MAINTENANCE

- Be sure to make an appointment with the pediatrician within the time frame given to you at discharge; usually at 2 weeks of age.
- Be sure to take the baby for follow-up screening and for immunizations at the appropriate times.
- Recognize signs of illness and follow up with the physician if these signs are present:
  - Fever
  - Vomiting
  - Unusually fussy
  - Diarrhea (frequent, watery stools)
  - Yellow or blue color to the skin
  - Breathing that appears stressed
  - Refuses to eat or has a poor suck
  - Appears listless

A

B

C

■ Figure 14-9 **(A)** The nurse teaches the new mother to support the newborn using the football hold. **(B)** The new father demonstrates the shoulder hold. **(C)** The grandfather is using the familiar cradle hold.

■ Figure 14-10 The nurse shows the new mother how to swaddle her newborn.

temptation is to overdress the newborn. The best advice is to instruct the parents to dress the newborn in the amount and quality of clothes that would keep the parents comfortable in the environment. Check the baby's temperature if he seems ill. Temperatures less than 97.7°F or greater than 100°F should be reported to the physician.

Monitoring Stool and Urine Patterns. It is normal for the newborn to have 6 to 10 wet diapers per day after the first day of life. Instruct the parents to report if the newborn does not void at all within a 12-hour period. Frequent, regular voiding indicates the newborn is getting enough milk.

Newborn stools initially are dark greenish black and tarry. The name for these stools is meconium. Transitional stools are lighter green or light green-yellow and are looser in character than is meconium. Most babies are having transitional stools by the time they are discharged home. In general, breast-fed babies have softer, less formed stools that have a sweetish odor to them. Bottle-fed babies tend to have more well-formed stools that are a little darker in color with a more unpleasant odor.

Signs of constipation are infrequent hard, dry stools. Babies normally turn red in the face and strain when passing stools. These signs do not indicate constipation. Diarrhea is defined as frequent stools with high water content. Because newborns dehydrate quickly, it is important for parents to notify the physician if the newborn has more than two episodes of diarrhea in one day.

Providing Skin Care. Teach new parents about normal, expected skin changes, such as Mongolian spots and newborn rash (see Chapter 13). Until the cord falls off (approximately 10–12 days after birth), the parents should give the baby sponge baths. Newborns need protection from chilling when they are bathed. It also is important for parents to monitor the water temperature to prevent scalding the newborn's tender skin. Daily tub baths are not necessary and may dry the skin. Some physicians want the parents to cleanse the cord site with alcohol several times daily.

Maintaining Safety. Newborns quickly learn to roll over and can move around on surfaces, even if unintentionally. For this reason, newborns and infants should never be left unattended on high surfaces, such as on dressing tables or beds. They also should not be left unattended around any amount of water to avoid the possibility of drowning. Plastic should not be used to cover infant mattresses or on any object to which the newborn has contact, to protect from suffocation. Pillows are not needed and may be dangerous for the young infant.

Parents need to be able to differentiate normal from abnormal newborn observations and behaviors. A yellow tint to the skin is indicative of jaundice and should be reported to the physician promptly. Untreated jaundice can lead to permanent brain damage. Listlessness and poor feeding behaviors are signs of illness that should be reported. Teach the parents normal behavior states of newborns, and help them learn to read the special cues their baby gives regarding when and how much interaction he can tolerate (see Chapter 13).

Proper use of car seats is a critical skill for new parents to learn. Car seats save lives, and infants should never be transported in a car without one. Most states have laws regarding their use, and parents must be familiar with these laws. Newborns are safest in rear-facing seats placed in the middle of the back seat of the car.

Parents should never place car seats in the front seat of cars equipped with air bags because death and injury have occurred when air bags deploy and infants are strapped into the front seat. If it is absolutely necessary to place the infant in a car seat in the front seat, there must be no air bag or the air bag must be professionally disabled. Parents should be thoroughly familiar with the operation of the car seat they choose.

Evaluation: Goals and Expected Outcomes

Goal: The newborn maintains an adequate level of comfort during the hospital stay.
Expected Outcomes: The newborn
- shows signs of contentment.
- is not overly fussy.
- does not show other signs of pain, particularly during and after painful procedures.

Goal: The newborn remains free from signs and symptoms of preventable diseases.
Expected Outcomes: The newborn
- is immunized against HBV.
- receives mandatory screening for metabolic and hearing disorders.

Goal: The parents will be able to care adequately for their newborn at home.
Expected Outcomes: The parents
- demonstrate the skills needed to care for their newborn.
- explain what follow-up is necessary and what to do if the screens are abnormal.
- describe when to take the newborn for repeat vaccinations for all childhood diseases.
- verbalize signs that should initiate a call to the physician.
- verbalize when follow-up is needed.
- verbalize how to find answers to questions that come up during the care of their newborn.

Test Yourself
- Name one advantage and one disadvantage of circumcision.
- What substance, in addition to the vaccination, is given to a newborn whose mother is positive for the HBsAg?
- List three ways parents can deal with newborn crying.

Key Points

- The delivery room should be prepared for resuscitation of the newborn before birth. Resuscitation supplies should be checked and the warmer turned on in anticipation of the birth. If resuscitation is needed, Neonatal Resuscitation Program guidelines should be followed.
- Steps should be taken to prevent the newborn from becoming overly cold or overly hot. A thermoneutral environment is ideal in which the temperature is maintained at a level so that heat is neither gained nor lost.
- Eye prophylaxis to prevent eye infection from gonorrhea and chlamydia should be instituted within the first hour after birth. Vitamin K is given intramuscularly to prevent bleeding problems.
- Identification bands are placed immediately in the delivery room before newborn and parents are separated. The identification bands are checked each time the baby is taken to or from his or her mother.
- Hypoglycemia is best prevented and treated with early and regular feedings. If the newborn cannot or will not eat, intravenous glucose may be necessary.
- Maintaining the newborn with his own crib and supplies, using excellent hand washing technique, and minimizing exposure to sick people are all measures nurses take to decrease the risk for cross contamination and infection in the newborn.
- Nurses must be vigilantly on guard for suspicious activity in and around a nursery. The risk for abduction is a real threat. Teach the parents to ask to see identification before releasing their newborn to anyone.
- Newborns show behavioral and physiologic responses, such as crying, grimacing (or making other faces), and increased heart and respiratory rates, to painful procedures.
- Circumcision remains a controversial procedure. The AAP strongly recommends the use of analgesia and anesthesia for the procedure. If the parents choose not to circumcise, they must be taught proper hygiene for the uncircumcised penis.
- All newborns should receive a HBV vaccination and screening for metabolic diseases, such as phenylketonuria and congenital hypothyroidism, that can lead to profound mental retardation and disability if left untreated.
- Parents need to learn how to hold and position their infant, how to clear the airway, maintain adequate body temperature, monitor stool and urine patterns, provide skin care, and maintain safety of their newborn.

INTERNET RESOURCES

Newborn Care
www.nlm.nih.gov/medlineplus/infantandnewborncare.html

Cord Care
www.nlm.nih.gov/medlineplus/ency/article/001926.htm

Vitamin K
http://newborns.stanford.edu/VitaminK.html

Preventing Newborn Abductions
www.cybertipline.com/missingkids/servlet/ServiceServlet?LanguageCountry=en_US&PageId=199

Workbook

■ NCLEX-STYLE REVIEW QUESTIONS

1. The delivery room nurse has just brought a 10-lb newborn to the nursery. The nurse monitoring the newborn during the transition period recognizes that which of the following assessment parameters will most likely inhibit this newborn's transition?

   a. Apgar score
   b. Blood sugar
   c. Heart rate
   d. Temperature

2. The newborn has just been delivered. He is placed in skin-to-skin contact with his mother. A blanket covers all of his body except his head. His hair is still wet with amniotic fluid, etc. What is the most likely type of heat loss this baby may experience?

   a. Conductive
   b. Convective
   c. Evaporative
   d. Radiating

3. A woman dressed in hospital scrub attire without a name badge presents to the nursery and says that Mrs. Smith is ready for her baby. She offers to take the baby back to Mrs. Smith. What response by the nurse is best in this situation?

   a. "I don't know you. Are you trying to take a baby?"
   b. "Leave immediately! I'm calling security."
   c. "May I see your identification, please?"
   d. "You must be Mrs. Smith's sister. She said her sister is a nurse."

4. A new mother is not sure if she wants her baby to be circumcised. Which response by the nurse is best?

   a. "Circumcision is best in order to protect the baby from diseases like cancer."
   b. "If you do not circumcise your baby, he will always have difficulty maintaining adequate hygiene."
   c. "It is best not to circumcise your baby because the procedure is very painful."
   d. "There are pros and cons to circumcision. Let me ask the pediatrician to come and talk to you about the procedure."

■ STUDY ACTIVITIES

1. Develop a poster that shows nurses ways to prevent transmitting infections in the nursery.

2. Develop a handout for nurses with helpful tips on preventing infant abductions. Use an Internet search to help find material for the handout.

3. Make a discharge teaching handout for parents of a newborn.

■ CRITICAL THINKING: WHAT WOULD YOU DO?

Apply your knowledge of the nurse's role in newborn care to the following situations.

1. A neighbor calls to tell you that his wife just delivered her newborn in the living room. The ambulance is on the way but is not yet there. You run to the house and find the baby loosely wrapped in a blanket. The neighbor says the baby was born approximately 2 minutes before you arrived.

   a. What actions do you take first and why?
   b. The newborn becomes jittery and irritable. What do you suspect may be the problem?
   c. What two interventions will need to be carried out as soon as the newborn and mother can be safely transported to a health care facility?

2. Mrs. Mathias just delivered a baby boy. He cries immediately and is pink. The newborn's cry sounds "wet" and "gurgly."

   a. What action should the nurse take first?
   b. If the respirations continue to sound wet, what step would the nurse take next?

3. Newborn Boy Hinojosa is crying and thrashing about after a circumcision.

   a. What is the likely cause of his crying?
   b. What should the nurse do in this situation?

4. A new mother calls the nursery from home. She and her newborn were discharged 2 days ago. She is worried about a small amount of yellow crust she notes at the circumcision site. She is also worried because the baby has been crying and fussy for the last hour.

   a. How would you advise the mother regarding the yellow crusting?
   b. What suggestions could you give her for the crying?

15 *Newborn Nutrition*

KEY TERMS

artificial nutrition
colostrum
engorgement
foremilk
hind milk
lactation
lactation consultant
mastitis

LEARNING OBJECTIVES

On completion of this chapter, you should be able to:

1. Describe factors that influence the woman's choice of feeding method.
2. Identify advantages of breast-feeding for both the woman and the newborn.
3. Discuss situations for which breast-feeding would not be recommended.
4. Discuss the physical and hormonal control of the breast during lactation.
5. Describe the role of the nurse when assisting a woman to breast-feed.
6. Outline appropriate teaching topics for the breast-feeding woman.
7. Outline appropriate nursing interventions for common problems the breast-feeding woman might encounter.
8. List signs that a newborn is not breast-feeding well.
9. Differentiate between breast milk and formula.
10. Name situations in which formula-feeding would be beneficial.
11. Compare the various types of formulas available to feed newborns and infants.
12. Outline appropriate teaching topics for the formula-feeding woman.
13. List several questions the nurse should ask the parents of a newborn who is not tolerating formula.

IN UTERO, the fetus obtains all of its nutrition in a passive manner. The nutrients cross from the maternal circulation, across the placenta, and enter the fetus' circulation. The nutrients then circulate to the tissues for use at the cellular level. At birth, the passive intake of nutrition ends, and the newborn must actively consume and digest food.

The newborn has unique nutritional needs. The healthy term newborn requires 80 to 100 mL/kg/day of water to maintain fluid balance and growth. He or she needs 100 to 115 kcal/kg/day to meet energy needs for growth and development (Gregory, 2005). Breast milk, or an iron-fortified infant formula, provides the newborn with all the calories and fluids necessary. In addition, breast milk and infant formulas are balanced to meet the carbohydrate, protein, and fat needs of the newborn. Table 15-1 summarizes some of the specific nutritional needs of the newborn.

SELECTION OF A FEEDING METHOD

There are two main types of nourishment suitable for the healthy term newborn: breast milk and commercially prepared formula. There are also two delivery methods: breast and bottle. The woman can choose to exclusively breast-feed; breast-feed and supplement with expressed breast milk in a bottle; breast-feed and supplement with formula; or she may choose to formula-feed exclusively.

Factors That Influence Choice of Method

Many factors influence the woman's decision about whether to breast-feed or bottle-feed. Some of these factors are culture, sociodemographic factors, prior experience with or exposure to breast-feeding, and intent or need to return to work or school.

Culture

A woman's culture often strongly influences newborn feeding choice. One culturally influenced issue is the acceptability of breast-feeding in public. Bottle-feeding rates are higher in women from cultures that frown upon breast-feeding in public or where there is a taboo against breast-feeding when men are present. The amount and quality of family and community support for breast-feeding is a strong culturally influenced predictor of the type of feeding the woman is more likely to choose.

The question is not only whether to breast-feed or bottle-feed. If breast-feeding is chosen, then culture

Table 15-1 ▌ DAILY NUTRITIONAL NEEDS OF THE NEWBORN

Nutrient	Amount Needed Daily
Protein	2.2 g/kg/day
Vitamin A	400 mcg/day
Vitamin C	40 mg/day
Vitamin D	5 mcg/day
Vitamin E	4 mg/day
Vitamin K	2 mcg/day
Calcium	210 mg/day

influences when the woman initiates breast-feeding (e.g., immediately versus after the "milk comes in"), how many times per day the woman breast-feeds, whether or not she supplements, and when to stop breast-feeding (i.e., wean the baby). In every culture, there are circumstances in which a woman cannot breast-feed or chooses not to breast-feed for many reasons.

In the United States, women receive mixed messages regarding infant feeding methods, with a general bias toward bottle-feeding. The media often send subtle messages, such as picturing babies bottle-feeding versus breast-feeding. Advertising by formula companies suggests that formula is of equal composition to breast milk. Health care professionals often contradict one another when giving advice to new mothers. Health care workers may promote breast-feeding verbally, but their actions may discourage breast-feeding initiation (e.g., separating the woman and baby immediately after birth, supplementing with formula in the nursery, etc.).

Breastfeeding rates vary by ethnicity. In the United States, the highest breast-feeding initiation rates (83.6%) are among women of Asian or Pacific Islander decent, whereas the lowest rates (58.7%) occur for non-Hispanic African American women. Hispanic or Latino women have higher initiation rates (80.6%) than do white women at 76.8% (CDC, 2008). Hispanic women are more likely to breast-feed if they are of Mexican descent and have not completely acculturated (Hernandez, 2006).

Sociodemographic Factors

Breast-feeding rates differ by age, amount of education, and socioeconomic status. Women older than 30 years of age have higher breast-feeding initiation rates than younger women do. Almost half of mothers younger than 20 years of age choose to bottle-feed their newborns. Higher levels of education correlate with higher breast-feeding initiation rates. Fewer women who live in poverty choose to breast-feed compared to women with higher income levels (CDC, 2008).

Past Experiences of the Woman and Her Support System

A woman's past experience with or exposure to breast-feeding greatly affects her decision whether to breast- or bottle-feed. The feeding experiences and attitudes of the individuals who compose the woman's support system strongly influence the woman's choice of feeding method. The woman's mother, her partner, and/or friends frequently have strong feelings about which method is best for the newborn. These attitudes may cause these individuals to put pressure on the new mother to choose a particular feeding method.

Intent to Return to Work or School

The need to return to work or school soon after the newborn's birth plays an important role in the woman's feeding choice. A woman who chooses to breast-feed in the hospital can continue to breast-feed and pump while at work or school, breast-feed when the infant is present and offer formula while she is away, or she can elect to stop breast-feeding. Some women prefer not to begin breast-feeding because of their work or school obligations and choose to feed formula from the newborn's birth.

Nursing Considerations

As the nurse, your role in assisting the new mother to choose a feeding method is to

1. provide education so that the woman can make an informed choice, and
2. support the woman to provide nutrition to her newborn according to the method that works for her.

Although it sounds simple, performing this role can be challenging. On one hand, providing a supportive environment is crucial to the success of the woman who chooses to breast-feed. However, the challenge is to provide this support without making the woman feel guilty if she chooses to bottle-feed her baby. Exclusive breast-feeding requires a huge commitment from the woman. Often, women without adequate support at home have difficulty maintaining the commitment.

Don't let the issue get lost in the emotion! The issue is nutrition for the baby. The mother's choice of method is not a reflection of her ability to be a good parent.

BREAST-FEEDING

Breast-feeding is the recommended method for feeding newborns because breast milk is superior nutritionally to commercial formulas. Many organizations, including the American Academy of Pediatrics; the World Health Organization; and the Association of Women's Health, Obstetric, and Neonatal Nurses; actively encourage breast-feeding. Each of these organizations has a policy statement that defines their position on breast-feeding and their recommendations for infant feeding.

The American Academy of Pediatrics recommends exclusive breast-feeding until 6 months of age and continuation of breast-feeding until at least 12 months of age. The American Academy of Pediatrics leaves it up to the woman to decide how long to continue breast-feeding after 12 months. One of the *Healthy People 2010* goals is to increase the proportion of women who breast-feed their babies; Box 15-1 lists the specific targets.

Advantages and Disadvantages of Breast-Feeding

Breast-feeding confers short- and long-term benefits on the woman, her newborn, and the society-at-large with very few (if any) disadvantages.

Advantages

Immediate advantages for the woman include more rapid uterine involution and less bleeding in the postpartum period. The woman's stress levels decrease during breast-feeding, and her immune function may actually be enhanced (Groer & Davis, 2006). One study found that both parents benefitted from more sleep when the woman breast-fed the infant at night versus supplementing with formula (Doan et al., 2007). The woman who breast-feeds loses weight faster, on average, than does the woman who formula-feeds.

Long-term advantages for the woman include decreased incidence of ovarian and premenopausal breast cancers. Breast-feeding may also have a protective effect against osteoporosis (Schanler, 2006). Other maternal benefits reported in the literature include decreased incidence of type 2 diabetes, rheumatoid arthritis, and heart attacks (Gribble, 2008).

The advantages of breast-feeding for the newborn are numerous. Breast milk contains substances that facilitate critical periods of growth and development, particularly of the brain, immune system, and gastrointestinal tract

(Wagner, 2006). Breast milk provides immunologic properties that help protect the newborn from infections and strengthen his or her immune system. Breast-fed infants tend to have lower incidences of otitis media, diarrhea, and lower respiratory tract infections. Breast-feeding also provides a possible protective effect against certain conditions or diseases such as sudden infant death syndrome, insulin dependent diabetes, and allergic diseases. There is a decreased risk for childhood obesity when the infant breast-feeds. One possible explanation is that breast-feeding allows the infant to self-regulate feeding based on his or her internal cues. Finally, there is a possible correlation between enhanced cognitive development and breast-feeding (Schanler, 2006).

There are also benefits for the family and society. Breast-feeding is economical. The breast-feeding woman does not need to purchase formula, bottles, or nipples. Breast milk is always available, needs no preparation or storage, and does not require cleanup of utensils or dishes after the feeding. When away from home, the woman does not need to carry extra equipment or supplies to feed her newborn. Breast-feeding reduces health care costs because breast-fed infants are healthier and are ill less frequently than formula-fed infants (Schanler, 2006). Breast-feeding could possibly decrease the risk for child abuse and neglect because it enhances maternal–newborn bonding.

Disadvantages

There are no physiological disadvantages to either the woman or the newborn during breast-feeding, although there may be perceived cultural barriers for some women. There are certain maternal conditions or situations in which breast-feeding is contraindicated. Examples of these conditions include:

■ Illegal drug use
■ Active untreated tuberculosis
■ Human immunodeficiency virus infection
■ Chemotherapy treatment
■ Herpetic lesions on the breast

In addition, certain newborn conditions are contraindications for breast-feeding. Galactosemia, an inborn error of metabolism, requires a specialty formula because the newborn lacks one of the necessary enzymes to breakdown the sugar in breast milk. With phenylketonuria, another inborn error of metabolism, the newborn requires a special diet that can include breast milk in limited amounts. Other medical conditions may necessitate that the newborn receive formula. In some situations, the woman may produce little to no breast milk. In this instance, a physician or specialist should complete a thorough assessment before advising the woman to supplement or switch over completely to formula.

There may be misperceptions or perceived barriers to breast-feeding. Some women feel that breast-feeding excludes others from caring for or feeding the newborn. Some fathers express an interest in wanting to feed the newborn and feel that breast-feeding might take away this opportunity. In this circumstance, you can suggest that for some feedings, the woman can pump her breast milk, and the father or other caregiver could then feed the newborn the breast milk with a bottle. This way the newborn still receives the superior nutrition of breast milk while allowing the father or other caregiver feeding time with the newborn. This also gives the woman a respite from feeding.

There are other perceived cultural or psychological barriers to breast-feeding. Some women feel that they will be unable to return to work or school if they breast-feed. Others feel that breast-feeding is too difficult or uncomfortable. The woman and/or partner may perceive that breast-feeding is sexual in nature, or that it detracts from the woman's sexuality. Some women feel restrained by breast-feeding in that it ties them to the baby, or they think it will make the baby "too clingy."

Test Yourself

✔ Name four factors that influence a woman's decision to breast-feed.

✔ List three advantages of breast-feeding for the woman and three advantages for the infant.

✔ What are the advantages to the community when a woman breast-feeds?

✔ Name two contraindications to breast-feeding.

Physiology of Breast-Feeding
Newborn Features That Facilitate Breast-Feeding

The newborn possesses several unique characteristics that make breast-feeding physiologically possible. Specifically, the newborn is born with a uniquely shaped nose and mouth, the rooting reflex, and the innate ability to suck. These characteristics disappear as the infant gets older.

Newborn Facial Anatomy

The newborn is designed uniquely for breast-feeding. The design of the nose, which looks flattened after birth, creates air pockets when up against the breast. This allows the newborn to eat without obscuring the nasal opening. Because newborns are nose breathers, they can breathe while their mouth is full. They do not have to release the breast to take a breath. The newborn's mouth is designed to compress the milk ducts located behind the nipple under the areola. The tongue, pharynx, and lower jaw are unique in shape when compared to those of the older child or adult. The newborn also has fat pads on each cheek that aid in the sucking process.

Rooting and Sucking Reflex

The newborn's reflexes also assist in breast-feeding. The newborn demonstrates the rooting reflex by turning his or her head towards the stimulation when the cheek is brushed lightly. Rooting is a feeding cue that lets the woman know her newborn is ready to nurse. When the newborn's lips are lightly touched, the newborn will respond by opening his or her mouth.

The sucking reflex occurs when the nipple is placed into the newborn's mouth and the newborn begins to suck. The term newborn has the ability to coordinate his or her sucking, swallowing, and breathing in a manner that facilitates nursing and prevents choking. The newborn sucks in a burst pattern; sucking several times and then pausing to rest. The length of the pause should be equal to the time the newborn sucks. The type of sucking also changes during the feeding. At the beginning of the feeding, the newborn nurses with rapid, short sucks. These sucks stimulate the breast to release the milk. When the milk is flowing freely, the newborn nurses with longer, slower sucks.

The Breast and Lactation

The female breast is a unique organ designed to provide the newborn with nourishment through **lactation**, the production and secretion of milk. The breast is very vascular, with a rich lymphatic and nervous supply. Each breast consists of 15 to 20 lobes containing the milk-producing alveoli. The alveoli are clustered together and empty into ducts. Smooth muscle cells surround the alveoli, which help to eject the milk into the ducts. The ducts lead to the nipple, where the milk is released. Figure 15-1 illustrates the anatomy of the female breast.

The breast makes milk in response to several different stimuli. These include the physical emptying of the breast, hormonal stimulation, and sensory stimulation.

Physical Control of Lactation

When the breast is emptied, either by the newborn sucking or by use of a breast pump, the breast responds by replenishing the milk supply. If the breast is emptied incompletely, it will not make as much milk the next time. This is why it is important for the newborn to nurse long enough and often enough to establish a good milk supply. If the woman is pumping, she should allow sufficient time for the pump to drain both breasts. She should not stop pumping until the flow of milk has stopped. If the newborn completely empties the breast and then nurses again shortly after the feeding, the breast is stimulated to increase milk production.

Hormonal Control of Lactation

The breast also is under hormonal control. When the newborn sucks on the breast, the woman's pituitary gland releases prolactin and oxytocin. Prolactin stimulates the alveoli to produce milk and then to release it. Oxytocin causes contractions of the muscle cells that

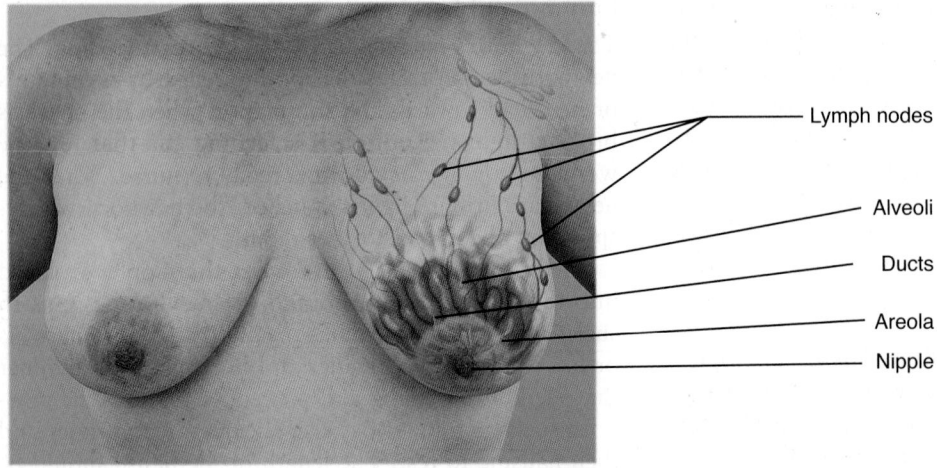

Lymph nodes

Alveoli

Ducts

Areola

Nipple

■ **Figure 15-1** Anatomy of the female breast.

surround the alveoli in the breast, which push milk downward toward the nipple (Fig. 15-2).

During the first few days, frequent nursing activates receptor sites in the breasts that respond to lactogen, which aid milk production. If the breast is not stimulated by the newborn's sucking or by a breast pump, the number of receptor sites is reduced. This change can reduce the quantity of the woman's milk supply. Encourage the woman to feed her newborn every 1.5 to 3 hours until her milk supply is established. If she is unable to nurse her newborn, she should pump at least every 3 hours around the clock.

Did you know?

The most common reason for insufficient milk supply is infrequent nursing. Help your patients avoid this common pitfall.

Sensory Stimulation

In addition to the physical emptying of the breast and hormones, the woman's body responds to sensory information from her newborn. As the woman holds her newborn and the newborn touches her breast or grasps her finger with his hand, the woman's skin is stimulated. As the woman looks at her baby, his or her feeding cues produce visual stimulation. When the baby cries or makes sucking noises, auditory stimulation occurs. Finally, the baby's scent stimulates the woman's sense of smell. The woman's brain processes all of these sensations and then sends messages to the breasts to produce the let-down reflex, which allows milk to flow to the newborn during breast-feeding.

Here's a quick tip.

Maternal alcohol consumption can inhibit the let-down reflex, so the breast-feeding woman should avoid drinking alcoholic beverages.

Composition of Breast Milk

Breast milk is a unique substance that commercial formulas have been unable to duplicate, especially with regard to the immunologic factors in breast milk. The woman's breast does not produce milk until approximately 3 to 5 days after birth. Until this time, the newborn receives a substance called **colostrum** during the nursing sessions. The breast begins to produce colostrum, a thick, yellowish gold substance, during the second trimester. Colostrum is higher in antibodies, lower in fat, and higher in protein content than is breast milk. There is between 2 and 20 mL of colostrum available for each feeding until the woman's milk comes in around the third day after birth.

Breast milk supplies 20 calories per ounce on average. There are two different compositions of breast milk: foremilk and hind milk. **Foremilk** is very watery and thin and may have a bluish tint. This is the first milk the baby

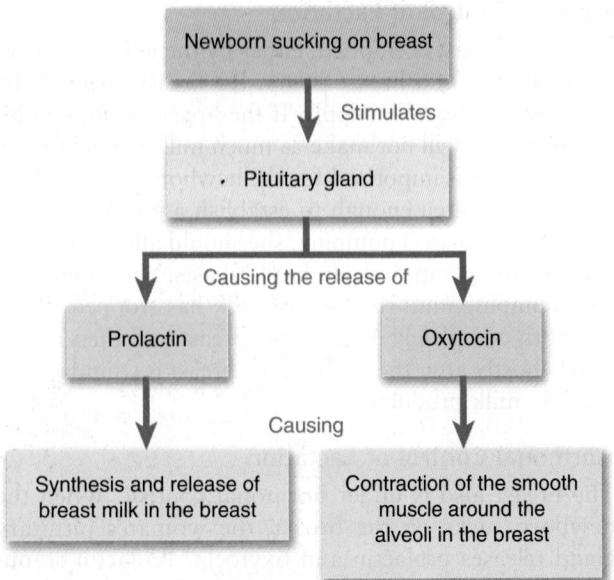

■ **Figure 15-2** Diagram of the hormonal effect on lactation.

receives during the nursing session. As the session progresses, the foremilk is replaced by hind milk. Hind milk is thicker and whiter. It contains a higher quantity of fat than foremilk and therefore has a higher caloric content. The **hind milk** satiates the infant between feedings. If the infant is thirsty and not very hungry, he or she will not nurse very long and will receive only the foremilk. The hungry infant nurses longer to get the hind milk.

It's OK to reassure the woman.
Until her milk comes in, the woman may feel that her newborn is not getting enough to eat. Assure the woman that her newborn is getting enough calories and that the frequent nursing will aid in establishing an ample milk supply.

Nutritional Needs of the Breast-Feeding Woman

The breast-feeding woman does not need to radically increase the amount of food she eats to produce milk for her infant. However, in order to meet the energy requirements of lactation, she does need to consume approximately 500 kcal/day above her pre-pregnant needs. The lactating woman needs plenty of fluids. If the woman does not consume enough fluids to satisfy her thirst or does not rest and eat a balanced diet, she may notice that she stops producing breast milk or that the quantity of her breast milk diminishes. A daily multivitamin will not make her breast milk more nutritious but will help ensure she obtains sufficient vitamins and minerals for her own body.

Nursing Care of the Breast-Feeding Woman

As the nurse, you have several roles when assisting a woman who is breast-feeding. These roles include assessing breast-feeding readiness, assisting with and assessing breast-feeding technique, assessing newborn fluid intake, and providing teaching about special breast-feeding topics.

Assessing Breast-Feeding Readiness

Certain situations or conditions require extra planning and nursing support. Assess the woman for flat or inverted nipples, history of breast surgery, attitudes toward breast-feeding, and quality of support for breast-feeding. A **lactation consultant** is a nurse or layperson who has received special training to assist and support

the breast-feeding woman. Be sure to ask one of these specialists to consult with the breast-feeding woman who has special needs or unusual difficulty nursing her baby.

Although she will need extra support in the beginning until she and the newborn become comfortable with nursing, the woman with flat or inverted nipples can still breast-feed. She may need to use a breast pump for a few minutes before nursing to help pull out and harden the nipples so the newborn can make a good latch. She may also need to use a nipple shield to assist the newborn in latching on.

The woman who has had breast augmentation or reduction surgery may still be able to breast-feed, depending on the type of surgery. She needs to be emotionally prepared for the possibility that she may not be able to exclusively breast-feed or that she may not be able to breast-feed at all (Chamblin, 2006). It is best to obtain a copy of the medical records of her surgery, if possible. This gives a starting point to evaluate her likelihood of being able to breast-feed. This woman will need the services of a lactation consultant.

Some women are opposed to or repulsed by the thought of the newborn sucking on the breast. The woman with this concern may choose to pump and feed her newborn expressed breast milk from a bottle once she understands the benefits of breast milk for herself and her newborn.

Assess the woman's support systems. If the woman has family members or friends who have breast-fed before or are supportive of her decision to breast-feed, the woman is more likely to continue to breast-feed. On the other hand, if the woman's support systems are opposed to breast-feeding, she may become discouraged and stop breast-feeding or not even begin to breast-feed because of the negative influences and comments.

Assisting with and Assessing Breast-Feeding Technique

While assisting the woman, provide support and encouragement because many breast-feeding women are unsure of their ability to breast-feed. If the newborn will not nurse after you have provided assistance, contact the registered nurse in charge and take steps to contact the hospital lactation consultant for additional help.

Beginning the Breast-Feeding Session

Ideally, the first breast-feeding should be in the delivery room within an hour after birth, unless the newborn's or woman's condition prevents this. Thereafter, the newborn should breast-feed on demand at least every 1.5 to 3 hours. If the newborn does

Be careful!
It is not helpful to give supplemental water or glucose solutions. Supplements give the newborn a feeling of fullness, so he or she will not nurse as frequently, which may in turn decrease the woman's milk supply.

A Personal Glimpse

Todd is my second baby. My husband and I hadn't been planning for another child when I found out that I was pregnant. The pregnancy was completely normal with a few more aches and pains than I remembered with my first child, Richard. Right after the delivery, I felt completely exhausted and ravenous. The nurse was insisting that I breast-feed and kept giving me a lot of information. I just couldn't deal with it. It seems like such a blur. I feel guilty that I didn't listen more. They whisked the baby away an hour after he was born. I was kind of relieved because I was so tired. But then when they brought him back to my room the nurse said, "They told me that you breast-fed in the delivery room. And since this is your second child, I'm sure you remember how to do it. He should feed for 5 to 10 minutes on each breast." I just looked at her. She handed me the baby and told me to call if I needed anything. Todd was fussy. I kept trying to get him to latch on but couldn't seem to figure out how to do it. I was sitting up in bed and having trouble getting comfortable. My stitches were hurting. But I didn't want to ask the nurse for help because I was afraid she would think I was dumb for not remembering how to get started with breast-feeding. The truth is I was very sick with my first child, so I only breast-fed for a couple of weeks, and it seemed so long ago. I finally gave up and called the nursery for a bottle. Todd immediately gulped down an ounce and a half. After that, he didn't seem interested in breast-feeding. Now that he is a year old, I sometimes wish I had tried a little harder to breast-feed. I feel that somehow I missed out on a very special experience.

Rowena

Learning Opportunity: What assumptions did the nurse make that discouraged the mother from asking for help? How could the nurse have approached this situation to give the new mother the help that she needed?

not wake up by 3 hours, the woman should wake the newborn and encourage him or her to feed.

Some women may become discouraged if their newborn is sleepy, will not latch immediately, or is crying vigorously and will not latch. Reassure the woman that the newborn will nurse. Take steps to rouse a sleepy newborn: change the diaper, gently rub the back or head, and wash the newborn's face with a wet washcloth. If the newborn is crying and not exhibiting signs of hunger, check for other causes of crying, such as a wet or dirty diaper or constricting clothing. Try to calm the newborn before attempting to put the newborn to the breast.

In the hospital when you bring the newborn to the woman for feedings, first check the newborn's and the woman's identification bands and make sure they match. After confirming identity, provide privacy by pulling a curtain around the bed or closing the door. Then, assist the woman into a comfortable position. The woman

Cultural Snapshot

Some cultures place a high importance on privacy and/or modesty. The breast-feeding woman may not want to expose herself completely to breast-feed, or she may not want to breast-feed in your presence, especially if you are a male.

should sit up in bed or in a chair or lie on her side in bed. Use pillows as needed to support the woman's back and arms. Make sure there is nothing constricting or obstructing the breast, such as a too-tight bra or a cumbersome hospital gown that is in the woman's line of sight or falling between her and the newborn.

Positioning the Newborn

There are three basic positions for a woman to hold her newborn while nursing. These are the cradle hold, football hold, and side-lying position (Fig. 15-3). Women who have breast-fed before may already know these three basic holds. However, a woman who does not have experience breast-feeding or who has just had surgery needs more help with positioning her baby correctly. Correct positioning and latching on of the newborn will help avoid nipple tissue trauma and sore nipples.

Cradle Hold. In the cradle hold, the newborn's abdomen is facing and touching the woman's abdomen. Make sure the newborn is not lying on his back and turning his head toward his shoulder to reach the breast. He or she should be on his side and "tummy-to-tummy" with the woman. Assist the woman to tuck the newborn's lower-arm between her arm and breast. In this position, the woman should use her free hand to support the breast that she is offering to the newborn (Fig. 15-3A).

Football Hold. For the football hold, the woman sits, and the newborn lies on a pillow beside her. The woman turns the newborn slightly on his side and supports his or her back with her arm. She supports the head with the palm of her hand. This is a good position for the woman who has undergone surgery or the woman with large breasts. It also facilitates an unobstructed view between the newborn and woman (Fig. 15-3B).

Side-Lying Position. For the side-lying position, both the woman and the newborn lie on their sides facing each other. A blanket roll behind the newborn's back provides support so he or she does not roll backward during the feeding. As with the cradle hold, the woman's and newborn's abdomens should be touching. The newborn should not be on his or her back with the head turned to the side during the nursing session (Fig. 15-3C). The side-lying position facilitates maternal rest and is good for a woman who has undergone surgery.

A

B

C

■ **Figure 15-3 (A)** The nurse is teaching the woman to use the cradle hold to breast-feed her newborn (photo © B. Proud). **(B)** The nurse is teaching the woman to use the football hold to breast-feed her newborn. **(C)** In the side-lying position, the woman can rest while feeding her newborn.

Latching On

After correctly positioning the newborn, the next step is latching onto the breast. The newborn's mouth needs to be wide open with the tongue down at the floor of the mouth, as during a yawn. When the newborn latches onto the breast, he or she must take the entire nipple and part of the areola into the mouth (Fig. 15-4). If only the nipple is in the mouth, the newborn will not compress

■ **Figure 15-4** Newborn with all of nipple and areola in mouth, correctly compressing milk ducts.

sufficiently the milk ducts in order to empty the breast. It will also cause the woman's nipple to become sore and/or cracked and bleeding.

Have the woman make a "C" shape with her free hand and grasp the breast with four fingers underneath and the thumb on top. Make sure that the woman's hand does not bump into the newborn's jaw or prevent the jaw from making a good latch. The woman may need to reposition her hand so that it is closer to the chest wall and farther from the newborn's jaw.

When the newborn is latched onto the breast, make sure the woman does not dimple the breast near the newborn's mouth and nose. Many women do this because they think they are providing breathing space for the newborn. However, this action can interfere with breast-feeding in several ways. It can cause the nipple to be pulled out of the mouth completely. It can cause the nipple to be pulled to the front of the mouth and lead to sore nipples. It can put pressure on the milk ducts, thereby reducing the flow of milk to the newborn, and preventing the breast from emptying completely.

Assessing the Breast-Feeding Session

Once the newborn is nursing, evaluate the effectiveness of the latch and sucking. A newborn that is correctly latched onto the breast will resist being pulled off of the breast. Audible swallowing and rhythmic jaw gliding are positive signs that the newborn is sucking effectively.

After the newborn has been nursing for a few minutes, many women report an increase in the flow of lochia or uterine cramping. This is a good indication that the newborn is nursing well because effective sucking causes the release of oxytocin from the posterior pituitary, which in turn causes uterine contractions. After her milk has come in, the woman may report leaking from the opposite breast or a let-down reflex. This is another good indication that the newborn is latched on and sucking well at the breast.

Ending the Breast-Feeding Session

The nursing session should last approximately 10 to 20 minutes per breast. When the newborn stops sucking vigorously (i.e., moves to nonnutritive sucking), the woman should remove him or her from the breast by placing her finger in the newborn's mouth between the gums and cheek to break the suction. She should then gently pull the newborn away from the breast. The woman should leave the flaps of her nursing bra open to allow her nipples to air dry.

After the feeding session, the woman may wish to burp her newborn. A breast-fed baby may not always burp after eating because he or she swallows less air at the breast than when drinking from a bottle. There are three ways for the woman to hold the newborn while burping: by placing him or her over her shoulder, sitting him or her upright, or lying the baby across her lap with the head elevated slightly above the level of the stomach.

> **This tip may help prevent sore nipples.**
>
> Tell the woman that it is important for her to break the suction before pulling the newborn from the breast. If she does not, tissue damage can occur, resulting in sore, cracked nipples.

Assessing Newborn Fluid Intake

There are several ways to assess the newborn's fluid intake. A small bit of milk left in the mouth after the feeding is a good indication the newborn is sucking well. The newborn should be satiated between feedings and after nursing appear to be drowsy or asleep. By the end of the third day of life, the newborn should have at least six wet diapers and about three bowel movements per day. Newborns that are breast-fed exclusively will have a yellow or mustard colored seedy type of bowel movement that is very loose and not formed. Explain to the woman that this is normal for the breast-fed newborn. Many breast-fed newborns will have a bowel movement during the nursing session.

Monitor the newborn's weight daily during the hospital stay. The breast-feeding newborn should lose no more than 10% of his birth weight and should return to birth weight by 7 to 14 days of age. Evaluate the newborn's weight and feeding status, and notify the registered nurse and the primary care provider if problems exist.

Teaching About Breast-Feeding Special Concerns

Nurses play a crucial role in teaching the breast-feeding woman. Items to be covered include tips on relieving common maternal breast-feeding problems; signs that the newborn is not feeding well; normal increases in the newborn's feeding schedule to accommodate for growth spurts; available resources for the breast-feeding woman; using supplements; breast-feeding amenorrhea; contraception while breast-feeding; and pumping and storing breast milk.

Relieving Common Maternal Breast-Feeding Problems

The breast-feeding woman needs information regarding problems she may encounter at home. Some of the most commonly reported problems include sore nipples, engorgement, a plugged milk duct, or mastitis.

Sore Nipples. Some nipple sensitivity is normal during the first few days of breast-feeding. It is normal for the nipples to feel sensitive during the first 30 seconds to 1 minute after the baby begins sucking (Hopkinson & Schanler, 2005). Incorrect latch is the most common cause of tissue trauma leading to sore nipples. If the woman reports sore nipples or cracked and bleeding nipples, observe how the newborn latches on. The newborn's mouth must open wide, and he or she must take all of the nipple and part of the areola into the mouth. Other reasons for sore nipples are that the newborn may be a vigorous breast-feeder or the woman may have sensitive or tender skin.

Some women find rubbing a few drops of expressed breast milk onto their nipples after the nursing session helpful. A purified lanolin ointment (Lansinoh) may help other women. Contact the lactation consultant if the woman continues to have sore nipples despite correct positioning and latch.

Engorgement. **Engorgement** refers to swelling in the breast that first occurs when the breast starts producing milk. The breasts may become hard and warm to the touch and can be quite painful. Frequent breast-feeding is the best way to prevent and treat engorgement, as long as the newborn is emptying the breast with each feeding. First, check to see that the newborn is able to obtain a good latch. A poor latch does not allow for complete emptying of the breast and can exacerbate engorgement. If the nipple is hard and this is interfering with a good latch, the woman may need to express a small amount of milk to soften the nipple before putting the newborn to the breast. Treatments to alleviate discomfort include cold packs to the breast and taking a mild analgesic such as ibuprofen (Motrin, Advil) or acetaminophen (Tylenol). It may help the woman to stand in a warm shower several times per day and let the water flow over her breasts. This may stimulate milk release and relieve some of the pressure. Reassure the woman that engorgement is temporary and will go away within a few days (Hopkinson & Schanler, 2005). Tell the woman not to empty her breasts by pumping between feedings, as this will increase her milk supply beyond the newborn's needs.

Plugged Milk Ducts. A plugged milk duct is a common problem. This happens when one of the milk ducts becomes obstructed, causing a backup of the milk. The woman usually notices a sore, reddened, hard lump in one area of her breast. Teach the woman to continue nursing. Sometimes it helps to position the infant with the chin close to the lump to facilitate drainage. She should avoid constricting clothing or bras, including underwire bras. Interventions to treat discomfort are the same as those to treat the discomfort of engorgement. If the site does not improve within a few days, she should contact her health care provider.

This is helpful advice.
Milk may leak from the breasts during engorgement. If the woman uses bra pads to help absorb the leaking milk, advise her to change the pads as they become damp to avoid maceration or possible infection of the nipple and/or areola.

Mastitis. Another common problem associated with breast-feeding is **mastitis**, an infection of the breast tissue. Women with mastitis usually describe having a rundown feeling or flulike symptoms and a low-grade fever. Tell the woman not to ignore these signs and symptoms but to report them immediately to her health care provider. Treatment consists of antibiotics, analgesics, bed rest, and fluids. The woman needs to know that she can continue to breast-feed during this time. Mastitis will not affect her milk quality, and the antibiotics prescribed usually do not affect the newborn or infant. If the health care provider prescribes medication that is contraindicated for breast-feeding and there is no alternative medication, the woman can pump and dump her breast milk and resume breast-feeding when the medication course is completed.

Signs the Newborn Is Not Feeding Well

The woman also needs to know how to evaluate how well her newborn is nursing and when to call for help. Dry mouth, not enough wet diapers per day, difficulty rousing the newborn for a feeding, not enough feedings per day, or difficulty with latching on or sucking are signs that the newborn is not receiving enough breast milk. Explain to the woman that if she notices any of these signs, she should immediately contact the newborn's

health care provider and a lactation consultant. Newborns can become dehydrated and suffer from a lack of nutrition very quickly and may need hospitalization.

Growth Spurts

Another important teaching topic for the breast-feeding woman is information on how the newborn increases the milk supply. Newborns have growth spurts in which they will nurse longer and more frequently for a few days and then space out their feedings after those few days. This causes the woman's breasts to increase their milk volume to match the growing newborn's needs. A woman who does not understand that the newborn increases the frequency and duration of feedings over a period of days to increase the milk supply may misinterpret the situation and think that she does not have enough milk to feed her newborn. This may cause the woman to stop breast-feeding unnecessarily.

Available Resources for the Breast-Feeding Woman

The breast-feeding woman needs to be aware of the many resources available to assist her and her newborn with breast-feeding. Lactation consultants, the La Leche League, and breast-feeding support groups in the community can give both practical and emotional support to the breast-feeding woman.

Lactation consultants work in the hospital, in the community, and sometimes in the primary care provider's office. In the hospital, lactation consultants can help the woman with positioning and getting the newborn latched on and sucking. After discharge, the hospital may provide follow-up visits or telephone calls to the woman to help ensure that the newborn is breast-feeding as expected. The newborn's pediatrician may have an agreement with a lactation consultant who can provide assistance to the breast-feeding woman.

The La Leche League is a national organization that provides support, education, and literature to the breast-feeding woman. The woman can find the League listed in the telephone book, or the hospital may provide the woman with the telephone number of the local chapter. In addition, the hospital may have a list of breast-feeding support groups the woman can join. These groups can provide both breast-feeding support and socialization.

Using Supplements

Many women have questions about supplements for their nursing newborn. The newborn who is breast-fed does not need supplemental bottles of water. Exclusive breast-feeding provides the newborn with all fluid needs. In the hospital, newborns are not started on any vitamin or iron supplements. The follow-up health care provider will instruct the woman on when and what types, if any, of supplements the newborn may need.

Table 15-2 ▌ CONTRACEPTIVE CHOICES FOR THE BREAST-FEEDING WOMAN			
Nonhormonal		**Hormonal**	
Permanent	Temporary	Nonestrogen	Estrogen
Tubal ligation Vasectomy	Abstinence Condom Diaphragm Spermicide	Mini-pill Depo-Provera	Birth control pill

The woman needs to know that her breast milk is nutritionally superior to any other newborn food and that she should not introduce any solids, including rice cereal, until the infant is at least 6 months of age. If there is a family history of allergies, solids should be delayed even longer.

Breast-Feeding Amenorrhea

A very important topic for the lactating woman is breast-feeding amenorrhea. The return of the woman's menstrual cycle occurs between 6 to 10 weeks after delivery. Approximately 75% of women do not ovulate during the first postpartum menstrual cycle. The woman who is breast-feeding exclusively (i.e., without providing any supplemental bottles or solids) may experience breast-feeding amenorrhea. Some women who exclusively breast-feed may not have a return of their menstrual cycle for several months. The woman needs to know that ovulation can happen in the absence of a menstrual period, and she can become pregnant. It is important for her to use contraception during this time.

Contraception While Breast-Feeding

The breast-feeding woman needs information about her choices in contraception. Contraception that contains hormones, especially estrogen, can lead to a decrease in the milk supply in the breast-feeding woman. The woman should be informed of this and make alternative contraceptive choices if breast-feeding is to continue. The first choice of contraception for the breast-feeding woman should be nonhormonal. If she chooses a hormonal type of contraception, a nonestrogen type, such as the mini-pill, is preferred over one that contains estrogen. Table 15-2 summarizes different contraceptive choices for the breast-feeding woman.

Pumping and Storing Breast Milk

Teach the woman to wash her hands before pumping her breasts and to use clean equipment. Before beginning pumping, it may be necessary for the woman to use techniques to aid the let-down reflex, which include bilateral breast massage and applying warm packs. The woman may also find that looking at a picture of her infant and mentally thinking about her infant's smell, texture, and sounds help induce a let-down reflex. At home, the woman may want to pump one breast while having the infant nurse on the opposite breast. The breast-feeding will stimulate the let-down reflex and allow her to collect more breast milk.

It is recommended the woman use a hospital-grade, dual electric breast pump, which pumps both breasts at the same time (Fig. 15-5). Pumping of both breasts at the same time increases the quantity of milk expressed at one sitting. The woman should be encouraged to pump until the flow of milk has stopped, usually about 15 to 20 minutes. When she is finished, she can refrigerate, freeze, or feed her infant the expressed breast milk immediately. She also needs to clean the equipment right after pumping. Tap water and a small amount of dish soap are usually sufficient to clean the equipment.

After pumping, she may want to rub a small amount of breast milk onto her nipples and allow them to air dry before covering them with a bra. If the woman experiences soreness with the breast pump, check to make sure she is using it properly and starting the pumping session at the lowest suction necessary.

Breast milk should be stored in hard plastic bottles or breast milk bags, not in glass containers or plastic bottle liners. The leukocytes in breast milk adhere to the glass,

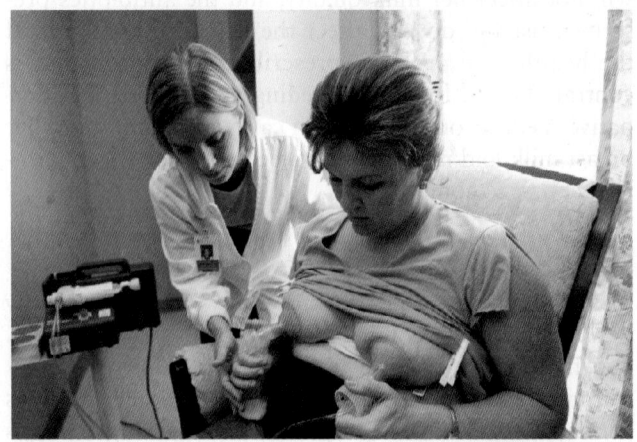

■ Figure 15-5 The nurse is assisting the woman to use a hospital pump to pump milk from both breasts at the same time.

Table 15-3 ▮ BREAST MILK STORAGE

Location of Storage	Duration of Storage
Room temperature (19°C–22°C)	Up to 10 hours
Refrigerator (0°C–4°C)	Up to 8 days
Freezer with door opening frequently	2 weeks
Separate freezer compartment with door opening frequently	4 months
Separate deep freeze	6 months
Thawed after being frozen	24 hours

and this decreases the bacteriostatic properties of the milk. The proper way to reheat breast milk is to place the bottle/bag into a pan of hot water. Heating in the microwave kills the antibodies in breast milk. In addition, milk reheated in the microwave may have hot spots that could burn the newborn's mouth and esophagus. Table 15-3 provides a timetable for breast milk storage.

Returning to Work

Just because the woman returns to work or school after giving birth does not mean that she must give up breast-feeding. The woman should breast-feed exclusively for at least 6 weeks before introducing the bottle. After 6 weeks if she has established a good milk supply and the newborn is nursing well, she should introduce one feeding per day of expressed breast milk. She should pump her breasts during this bottle-feeding so she will not reduce her milk supply.

Test Yourself

✔ In what three positions can a woman hold her newborn to breast-feed?

✔ How can you assess the effectiveness of the newborn's breast-feeding?

✔ What common problems might a breast-feeding woman encounter?

FORMULA-FEEDING

Artificial nutrition, that is infant formula or another type of animal milk, has been given to infants since ancient times. In the United States, commercially prepared infant formula has been available since the early 1900s. Today there are several brands available to women who choose not to breast-feed or who need a supplemental formula. There are also alternative formulas to meet specific infant needs.

Advantages and Disadvantages of Formula-Feeding

Infant formulas are helpful in certain circumstances. Many women choose to forgo breast-feeding and feed their infant only formula. No one should attempt to make the woman who chooses to do so to feel guilty regarding her decision. However, make sure that the woman has made an informed decision and has heard the advantages of breast-feeding before feeding her infant formula.

Advantages

There are specific circumstances in which formula-feeding is necessary. These include adoption or cases in which breast-feeding would be harmful to the infant, as discussed earlier in the chapter. In some cases, the woman may need to temporarily stop breast-feeding, such as for surgery or while taking a medication that can pass to the infant through the breast milk. Sometimes the woman's breast milk supply dries up sooner than expected or she does not produce enough milk to meet her infant's needs.

For many women, it is easier to quantify how much the infant has consumed with formula-feeding than with breast-feeding, which reduces their worries about the infant getting enough to eat. Some women feel it is easier to formula-feed than to breast-feed their infant. Formula-feeding also allows others to be involved in the infant's care by feeding the infant and preparing the formula and bottles for feeding.

Disadvantages

Formula-feeding has several disadvantages. It is inferior nutrition and has none of the immunologic properties provided by breast milk. Formula is harder for the newborn to digest than breast milk. There is a higher correlation between infants who are formula-fed and some illnesses, such as otitis media and allergies.

Infant formula is expensive. If the family is on a limited budget, formula-feeding creates additional financial needs. In addition to buying the formula, the family will need to purchase bottles, nipples, and the equipment needed to clean these items.

There are more steps involved in formula-feeding the newborn than in breast-feeding. With formula-feeding, the woman or caregiver must mix the right amount of powder or formula concentrate to water, store the mixed preparation, warm it when the newborn is ready to eat, and then wash all of the utensils afterward.

Make sure the woman is informed!

If the woman is on the Women, Infants, and Children's program, the woman will need to purchase 25% of the formula because the Women, Infants, and Children's program is only a supplemental program.

Formula is available for purchase in three forms: ready to feed, concentrate, and powder. Because of the differences in formulation, there can be errors with the proper dilution of the formula. Errors in preparation can lead to under- and overnutrition of the newborn. These errors can result in serious illness and even death.

Composition of Formula

There are three main types of formula: milk-based, soy-based, and hypoallergenic formulas. Most term newborn formulas are derived from cow's milk, and the main carbohydrate source is lactose or corn syrup solids. The protein used is a whey-casein blend to simulate that found in breast milk. The iron composition in infant formula is either high or low. Iron-fortified formulas contain 1.2 mg of iron per 100 mL. Iron-fortified, or high-iron formula, is the preferred formula to give to the healthy term newborn. Some women are reluctant to feed their newborn iron-fortified formula, thinking it will cause constipation. Studies have shown that there is no significant difference in constipation rates between infants fed iron-fortified and low-iron formulas.

Alternative formulas are available for newborns with special medical needs. Soy-based infant formulas are for newborns who are allergic to cow's milk or when there is a strong family history of cow's milk allergies. Hypoallergenic formulas are for newborns with allergy or malabsorption problems. The proteins are partially or completely broken down in these formulas. There are also a variety of formulas specially designed for specific medical conditions, including carbohydrate intolerance, impaired fat absorption, cystic fibrosis, congestive heart failure, and intestinal resection or short gut problems. The newborn should not receive these formulas unless specifically ordered by the primary care provider. Some pediatricians treat esophageal reflux with a formula thickened with some rice cereal or a specialized formula that already has rice cereal added to it.

There are many different compositions of formulas in the hospital. Formulas vary based on the needs of the newborn. Preterm formulas differ from term formulas in the amounts of vitamins and minerals and caloric and iron content. Preterm formulas have higher levels of sodium, potassium, calcium, and iron than do term infant formulas. Term formula, like breast milk, has 20 calories per ounce, whereas preterm formulas have 22 or 24 calories per ounce. See Table 15-4 for a comparison of different brands of formulas.

Nursing Care of the Formula-Feeding Woman

As the nurse, you have three major roles when assisting the bottle-feeding woman in the hospital. These are assisting with formula-feeding technique, assessing the

---

Table 15-4 ▌ COMPARISON OF COMMON FORMULAS

Category	Formulas (Manufacturer's Name)	Newborn Population/Medical Condition for Which Formula Designed
Milk-based formulas	Enfamil (Mead-Johnson), Good Start (Nestle), Similac (Ross)	For full-term healthy newborns
Soy-based formulas	Isomil (Ross), ProSobee (Mead Johnson), Soyalac (Loma Linda)	Milk protein allergy, lactose intolerance, lactase deficiency, or galactosemia
	Lactofree (Mead Johnson)	Lactose intolerance, lactase deficiency
Specific medical conditions	RCF (Ross Carbohydrate Free) (Ross)	Carbohydrate intolerance
	Portagen (Mead Johnson)	Impaired fat absorption, intestinal resection, lymphatic anomalies
	Nutramigen (Mead Johnson)	Protein sensitivity, galactosemia, malabsorption problems
	Pregestimil (Mead Johnson)	Malabsorption syndromes, cystic fibrosis, intestinal resection, short gut syndrome
	Alimentum (Ross)	Food protein sensitivity, cystic fibrosis
	Lonalac (Mead Johnson)	Congestive heart failure, reduced sodium intake
	Similac PM 60/40 (Ross)	Infants predisposed to hypocalcemia and infants with impaired renal, digestive, and cardiovascular functions
	Lofenalac (Mead Johnson), Phenyl-free (Mead Johnson), Phenex-1 (Ross), Phenex-2 (Ross), Pro-Phree (Ross)	Phenylketonuria
	Similac Special Care (Ross), Premature Enfamil (Mead Johnson), Neosure (Ross)	Premature infants

Note: This is not an exhaustive list of all of the types of formulas available or conditions for which formulas may be used.

formula-feeding woman and newborn, and teaching about special concerns of formula-feeding.

Assisting With Formula-Feeding Technique

In the hospital, standard infant formula comes ready to feed. This means that you do not need to mix or add any additives to the formula before feeding the newborn. The first step in feeding the formula-fed newborn is to check the primary care provider's order. Many primary care providers have a preference regarding which formula the woman should feed her newborn. Check the label on the formula bottle before taking it to the woman to feed her newborn. Make sure the brand, caloric content, and iron composition matches that of the primary care provider's order.

Compare the newborn's and woman's identification bands to ensure a match. Use pillows as needed to ensure the woman is in a comfortable position and can hold and see her newborn easily. Make sure the woman is in a comfortable position sitting upright. The formula-feeding woman should not feed her newborn in a lying down position. The newborn should be in a semireclined position in the woman's or other caregiver's arms. An angle of at least 45 degrees is preferred (Fig. 15-6).

Teach the woman to assess her newborn's hunger cues and her newborn's ability to suck, swallow, and breathe during the feeding. The woman should

> **This tip could save a life!**
> It is easier for the newborn to aspirate while sucking from a bottle. Instruct the woman to keep the light on in the room so that she can observe her newborn during the whole feeding.

also observe her newborn's color while eating. Instruct the woman on what to do if the newborn starts to choke during the feeding. Make sure the nasal aspirator and a burp cloth are within the woman's reach.

Gently shake the bottle of formula because some settling of contents may occur. Attach a sterile nipple and ring unit to the bottle. The woman should feed 1 to 2 oz per feeding in the immediate newborn period. She should burp her newborn after every 0.5 oz. As the newborn grows, she should advance the feeding amount slowly, no more than 0.5 to 1 oz per feeding. Instruct the woman regarding cues that the newborn is satiated and finished eating. If the newborn consumes too much formula at one time, emesis or diarrhea may result.

> **Teach the woman not to prop!**
> Propping the bottle increases the newborn's risk of aspiration and can lead to overfeeding and baby bottle syndrome. This practice also decreases opportunities for positive bonding with the baby.

You may assist the bottle-feeding woman by feeding the newborn if the woman is unable to (e.g., she is having surgery) or if she is sleeping and requests her newborn to be fed in the nursery during the night.

Assessing the Formula-Feeding Woman and Newborn

Assess the newborn's feeding ability, amount of formula consumed at each feeding, tolerance of the infant formula, and the woman's comfort level with formula-feeding. Also, assess the newborn's bowel movements. Explain to the woman that her newborn's stool should progress from meconium to transitional and then to a pasty yellow solid consistency (see Chapter 14).

Report signs of difficulty to the charge nurse immediately. These signs include that the newborn is not sucking well, has difficulty swallowing and breathing, or is not tolerating the formula. Emesis and diarrhea may indicate that the newborn is not tolerating the formula.

Teaching About Formula-Feeding Special Concerns

Teaching topics include how to prepare bottles of formula, adding supplements to the bottle, maternal breast care, and managing common problems in the formula-fed newborn.

Preparing Bottles of Formula

Teach the woman about the different forms of formula and how to mix each type. Powder formula is the least expensive and requires the addition of water. Concentrate also requires the addition of water but is more costly than the powder form. Ready-to-feed formula is the most expensive but does not require the addition of any water to the formula before feeding.

■ **Figure 15-6** A newborn receives a formula-feeding from her father. Notice the correct positioning.

Warn the woman that the newborn could be injured if formula is not mixed according to the package directions. Some women may be unable to afford formula and try to make the formula last longer by adding more water than the directions specify. This will cause malnutrition in the newborn. If too much powder is added to the water, the newborn will receive more calories per ounce. This can lead to an overweight infant or formula intolerance, with resulting diarrhea or emesis.

The woman will need to know what type of water to add to the powder or concentrate type of formula. This depends on what type of water she has available (e.g., city tap, well, or purified bottled water). She should mix only as much formula as the newborn needs in 24 hours. After mixing, the formula needs to be refrigerated. After 24 hours, she should discard unused formula.

Teach the woman how to warm cold formula. She should place the bottle containing the formula in a pan of hot water until the formula is warm, then she should shake the bottle before feeding the newborn. Warn the woman never to use the microwave to warm the formula because it can create hot spots that could burn the newborn. When the newborn has finished eating, teach the woman to discard any remaining formula. This is because as the newborn sucks, saliva mixes with the formula and remains in the bottle and then digestive enzymes in the saliva begin to break down the remaining formula. Teach the woman to wash the feeding utensils in hot soapy water or in the dishwasher after every feeding. Sterilizing the bottles and nipples is not necessary after each feeding.

Adding Supplements

The newborn's primary care provider will determine if and when the newborn needs any type of supplementation, such as multivitamins or fluoride. Teach the woman that the newborn does not need any other type of nutrition. Instruct her not to add anything to the formula. Some pediatricians tell parents to offer infant cereal mixed with formula, but not juice, around 4 to 6 months. The woman should not begin to feed solid foods until the infant's primary care provider has recommended it, usually around 6 to 8 months of age. Around 12 months of age, the infant's primary care provider will discuss weaning the infant from the formula.

Maternal Breast Care

Women who choose to formula-feed exclusively need to know how to care for their breasts in the immediate postpartum period. Explain to the woman that she will produce milk, even though she is not nursing, and that this is a normal physiologic process in response to giving birth. The woman will experience engorgement when her milk comes in. She should not express any milk because this will stimulate milk production. She should wear a tight bra; the constriction will help prevent leaking and aid in the drying up of the milk supply. In addition, a tight bra will help lessen discomfort from the full breasts. Some women benefit from having their breasts bound tightly with an elastic-type bandage. In the past, some primary care providers prescribed medications that would aid in the drying up of the woman's milk supply. However, it was determined that the benefit of their use did not outweigh the associated risks.

Common Problems in the Formula-Fed Newborn

The woman needs to monitor for problems in the formula-fed newborn. These include the newborn not wanting to eat, not tolerating the formula, and dental caries.

The woman who is formula-feeding is able to accurately determine how many ounces per feeding and per day the newborn is receiving. Table 15-5 lists the amount of formula and other foods the newborn and infant should be receiving at different ages. If the newborn or infant is not taking in enough formula for his age and weight, dehydration may result, and the infant may not gain sufficient weight to develop appropriately and be healthy. If a newborn or infant is refusing to eat, the woman should contact the pediatrician because there may be an underlying medical condition.

Some newborns take in the recommended amount of formula and then have large amounts of emesis after or during feedings. The woman should report this situation to the newborn's primary care provider because this is not an acceptable situation for growth and nutrition. This may be a symptom of overfeeding, gastroesophageal reflux, formula intolerance, or an underlying medical condition. Ask the woman the following questions: How much formula is the newborn taking per feeding and per day? When does emesis occur (during or after the feeding, with burps, or with repositioning)? How much emesis does the newborn have per episode? What is the consistency of the emesis? Which formula is the infant eating, and how is it prepared? What other foods are included in the infant's diet? The answers to these questions will assist the registered nurse and the primary care provider to determine the probable cause of the emesis.

Diarrhea also requires investigation. Again, ask specific questions: How much and what type of formula is the newborn eating, and how is it prepared? How many episodes of diarrhea has the newborn had in the past 24 hours? What is the consistency of the bowel movement, and is there blood present in the stool? It is important to assess the newborn's intake and output to check for

Contradict a wives' tale!

Some women add rice cereal to the formula because they have heard that doing so will make the newborn sleep longer. This should only be done if recommended by a primary care provider for a specific reason, such as reflux.

Table 15-5 ▮ AMOUNT OF FORMULA AND OTHER FOODS THE NEWBORN AND INFANT SHOULD RECEIVE

Age	Amount of Formula	Other Foods
Birth to 4 months	2–6 oz/feeding 20–24 oz/day	None
4–6 months	4–6 oz/feeding 24–32 oz/day	Infant cereal mixed with formula
6–8 months	6–8 oz/feeding 24–32 oz/day	Baby cereal, soft mashed fruits and vegetables, no more than 3–4 oz of fruit juice
8–10 months	7–8 oz/feeding 21–32 oz/day	Same as 6–8 months and begin to add pureed meats
10–12 months	16–32 oz/day	Same as 8–10 months but consistency may be firmer and portions may be slightly bigger

dehydration, and to perform a physical exam. Possible causes are overfeeding, illness, formula intolerance, or an underlying medical condition.

Inform the parents that newborns and infants can dehydrate much more quickly than adults can. For this reason, the parents must report quickly any cases of emesis or diarrhea.

Infants can develop dental caries from frequent sucking on a milk- or juice-filled bottle. This situation is known as "baby bottle syndrome" or "bottle-mouth caries." Often this happens when parents give the infant a bottle at bedtime and the infant sucks on the bottle throughout the night. The frequent exposure of the immature teeth to high levels of sugars found in the milk or juice leads to dental caries. The parents should not give the infant a bottle when he or she is in the crib. They also should not allow the toddler to carry a bottle around; this practice of continual drinking of formula increases the risk of damage to the infant's teeth and is associated with a higher incidence of aspiration and otitis media.

Test Yourself

✔ What different types of formula are available?

✔ Name two advantages of formula-feeding.

✔ What topics should you cover when teaching a woman to formula-feed?

Key Points

➤ The woman's decision to breast-feed is influenced by several factors including culture, age, education, past experience with breast-feeding, and the woman's intent to return to work or school.

➤ Maternal advantages of breast-feeding include more rapid uterine involution, less bleeding in the postpartum period, and less ovarian and premenopausal breast cancers. Newborn advantages to breast-feeding include a strengthened immune system, less risk of becoming overweight, and lower incidences of certain infections such as otitis media, diarrhea, and lower respiratory tract infections.

➤ Maternal contraindications to breast-feeding include a woman actively using illegal drugs, one who has untreated tuberculosis, one with human immunodeficiency virus, or a woman receiving chemotherapy medications. A newborn condition

that would exclude breast-feeding includes galactosemia.

➤ The breast is under both physical and chemical control to stimulate lactation. The hormones prolactin and oxytocin stimulate milk production and release from the breast. The newborn sucking on and emptying the breast also leads to milk production.

➤ Teach the breast-feeding woman about common problems, signs the newborn is not feeding well, growth spurts, available resources, supplements, contraception, and pumping and storing breast milk.

➤ When assisting a woman to breast-feed, provide for privacy, help the woman into a comfortable position, help the woman to hold her newborn correctly, and assess the newborn for correct latching on and positioning on the breast. Assess the woman's breasts and nipples, her comfort level with breast-feeding, her support systems, and the newborn's feeding ability.

➤ When caring for a woman with sore nipples, observe the latching on and the positioning of the newborn during nursing. A few drops of expressed breast milk or a purified lanolin treatment applied to the nipples after breast-feeding may help with soreness.

➤ When caring for a woman with engorgement, assess for a good latch and advise the woman to breast-feed frequently. Cold packs to the breast and taking a mild analgesic help alleviate discomfort. Letting warm water flow over her breasts several times per day may stimulate milk release and relieve some of the pressure.

➤ When caring for a woman with a plugged milk duct, advise the breast-feeding woman to apply warm packs to the site, take a warm shower, take acetaminophen (Tylenol), nurse in different positions, avoid constrictive clothing or bras, and massage the site.

➤ When caring for a woman with mastitis, advise the breast-feeding woman to contact her health care provider, take the antibiotics as prescribed, and continue to breast-feed even on the affected side. If breast-feeding is too uncomfortable on the affected side, she should pump the milk at each feeding so her milk supply does not diminish.

➤ Signs that a newborn is not breast-feeding well include dry mouth, fewer than expected wet or dirty diapers, difficulty rousing the newborn for feedings, and not enough feedings per day.

➤ Breast milk is superior to formula because it is easier to digest and has immunologic, bacteriocidal, and fungicidal properties that cannot be duplicated in artificial nutrition. Breast milk is economical and ready to feed and requires no special preparation or storage.

➤ There are many types of formulas available. The ingredients vary by protein source, caloric content, and mineral and electrolyte concentration. The primary care provider considers the newborn's gestational age and medical needs before recommending a specific formula.

➤ Formula-feeding is beneficial in cases in which the woman is unavailable to breast-feed, such as adoption, surgery, or if she is taking a medication that passes through the breast milk and would be harmful to the newborn. Formula-feeding also is beneficial when the newborn has certain medical conditions, such as galactosemia.

➤ Teach the formula-feeding woman how to feed her newborn and how much and when to increase feedings, how to prepare and store the formula and care for the equipment, how to care for her breasts after delivery, and when to notify the nurse or pediatrician.

➤ For the formula-fed newborn who is having emesis or diarrhea, ask: What type of formula is the newborn on and how is it prepared? How much is the newborn eating per session and per day? What does the emesis/bowel movement look like? What other foods is the newborn eating? How much emesis is there per episode? How many episodes has the newborn had in the last 24 hours?

INTERNET RESOURCES

Baby Friendly Hospital Initiative
http://babyfriendlyusa.org/eng/index.html

International Lactation Consultant Association
http://ilca.org/

La Leche League International
www.llli.org

Government Sources
www.cdc.gov/breastfeeding
www.4women.gov/breastfeeding

Promotion of Mothers Milk, Inc.
www.promom.org

Women, Infants, and Children
www.fns.usda.gov/wic

American Academy of Pediatrics
http://aappolicy.aappublications.org

National Guideline Clearinghouse
www.guideline.gov

World Health Organization
www.who.int/nutrition

Workbook

■ NCLEX-STYLE REVIEW QUESTIONS

1. A woman tells the nurse, "I don't need to use any contraception because I plan on breast-feeding exclusively." On which fact should the nurse base her response?

   a. Women who exclusively breast-feed do not ovulate.

   b. Ovulation can occur even in the absence of menstruation.

   c. The birth control pill is the best form of contraception for breast-feeding women.

   d. Breast-feeding women should not use contraception because it will decrease their milk supply.

2. During a prenatal visit an 18-year-old gravida 1, para 0 in her 36th week says to the nurse, "I don't know if I should breast-feed or not. Isn't formula just as good for the baby?" On what information should the nurse base her response?

   a. The benefits of breast-feeding are equal to those of formula-feeding.

   b. It is ultimately the woman's choice whether she wants to breast-feed or not.

   c. The immunologic properties in breast milk cannot be duplicated in formula.

   d. The economic status of the woman is an important breast-feeding consideration.

3. The nurse is assessing the breast-feeding woman during a feeding session. What assessment has priority during the feeding session?

   a. Assess the position, latching on, and sucking of the newborn.

   b. Assess the woman's visitors and their opinions regarding breast-feeding.

   c. Check the woman's perineal pad for increased lochia flow.

   d. Determine if the woman needs a visit from the lactation consultant.

■ STUDY ACTIVITIES

1. Use the following table to compare information contained in your nursing pharmacology reference with information the hospital lactation specialist has on medications and their use during breast-feeding. If the two references disagree, from where did the lactation specialist get her information? Which information do you think is more accurate? Why?

Medication	Pharmacology Reference	Lactation Specialist
Magnesium sulfate		
Phenobarbital		
Depo-Provera		
Vicodin		
Coumadin		

2. Call your local Women, Infants, and Children's clinic. Interview the nurse to determine what she does to encourage the woman to breast-feed the newborn.

3. Interview the lactation consultant at the local hospital. What foods does she tell the woman to avoid when she is breast-feeding, and why? How many calories should the woman consume? How much liquid should she drink? Share your findings with your clinical group.

■ CRITICAL THINKING: WHAT WOULD YOU DO?

Apply your knowledge of newborn nutrition to the following situations.

1. You are working in the prenatal clinic. Here is a list of several of the patients you encounter and the questions they ask you.

   a. Sally is a 20-year-old gravida 1, para 0. She tells you she is unsure about feeding her baby and asks you if she should breast-feed or bottle-feed. How would you respond?

   b. Betsy, a gravida 3, para 1, states she needs to return to work 6 weeks after the baby is born. "I don't know if it's even worth it to begin to breast-feed when I know I'll just have to stop in 6 weeks. It seems like a lot of work." How would you respond?

   c. Elizabeth is a 15-year-old gravida 1, para 0. She asks you, "I don't want to breast-feed, but I heard you still make milk after the baby is born. How do you stop it from happening?" How would you respond to Elizabeth's question?

2. You are working the mother–baby unit at the hospital. Here are some of your patients for the day and the questions they ask you.

   a. Susan is a 24-year-old gravida 3, para 1. She delivered 1 day ago and wants to breast-feed. When you examine her newborn, she tells you that she thinks she doesn't have enough milk to feed her baby and asks you to give her baby a bottle so he doesn't starve. How would you respond?

   b. It has been 3 days since Alicia's cesarean delivery, and she is formula-feeding her newborn a milk-based formula. She tells you her baby spits up with every feeding. What questions would you ask her and why?

   c. Lanya is a 30-year-old gravida 2, para 2 who had a postpartum tubal ligation earlier today. It is time to breast-feed her baby, but her abdomen is sore. How would you suggest Lanya feed her newborn and why?

   d. Tricia is a 28-year-old gravida 1, para 1 who is formula-feeding. She asks you how to mix formula and how she should care for the bottles and nipples. What information would you give her and why?

   e. Maria is a 24-year-old gravida 1, para 1. She has some questions for you about how long her breast milk is good for after she pumps it. How would you respond?

CHILDBEARING AT RISK

16 Pregnancy at Risk: Conditions That Complicate Pregnancy

KEY TERMS

dermatome
diabetogenic effect of pregnancy
gestational diabetes
hyperglycemia
hyperinsulinemia
hypoglycemia
macrosomia
polyhydramnios
pregestational diabetes
status asthmaticus
status epilepticus
TORCH

LEARNING OBJECTIVES

On completion of this chapter, you should be able to:

1. Compare and contrast the pathophysiology of the three major classifications of diabetes in the pregnant woman.
2. Explain treatment goals for the pregnant woman with diabetes.
3. Differentiate between the care of the pregnant woman with pregestational diabetes and one with gestational diabetes.
4. Describe typical nursing concerns for the pregnant woman with diabetes.
5. Explain the goals of treatment and nursing care for the pregnant woman with heart disease.
6. Differentiate between pregnancy concerns for the woman with iron-deficiency anemia and one with sickle cell anemia.
7. List treatment considerations for the pregnant woman with asthma.
8. Detail the risk to pregnancy from epilepsy and its treatment.
9. Describe the impact on pregnancy from the TORCH infections.
10. Differentiate between common sexually transmitted infections according to cause, treatment, and impact on pregnancy.
11. Outline treatment for the pregnant woman with human immunodeficiency virus/acquired immunodeficiency syndrome (HIV/AIDS).
12. Describe nursing considerations for the pregnant woman with a sexually transmitted infection.
13. Describe nursing concerns and treatment for the pregnant woman who is the victim of intimate partner violence.
14. Delineate special concerns associated with adolescent pregnancy.
15. Describe the impact of delayed childbearing on pregnancy.

IN THE VERY recent past, many women with chronic conditions were unable to successfully accomplish pregnancy and/or childbirth. Now that there are effective treatments available for many of these conditions, more women are entering pregnancy with chronic medical conditions. Consequently, the obstetric nurse must stay abreast of current research findings to intervene appropriately and to educate the woman carrying an at-risk pregnancy. As the licensed vocational/practical nurse, you will assist the registered nurse (RN) to provide care for the pregnant woman at risk.

Physicians need highly specialized knowledge to successfully manage the at-risk pregnancy. Maternal–fetal medicine is a branch of medical science that focuses on the perinatal period. Another name for a maternal–fetal medicine specialist is perinatologist. This physician specialist is an obstetrician who has received advanced training and specializes in the care of at-risk pregnancies. The maternal–fetal medicine specialist is competent in the diagnosis and treatment of the pregnant woman who presents with a pre-existing medical condition or who experiences a complication of pregnancy. The specialist sometimes provides consultations for the obstetrician who is managing the pregnancy. Alternatively, he or she may co-manage the woman's pregnancy with the obstetrician or be the primary care provider.

PREGNANCY COMPLICATED BY MEDICAL CONDITIONS

Chronic medical conditions and acute infections are risk factors for the pregnant woman. There are several ways in which pregnancy and medical conditions are interrelated. Pregnancy can affect the underlying medical disorder. The normal physiologic changes of pregnancy sometimes alleviate and at other times intensify the symptoms of illness. On the other hand, medical conditions can affect the progress and outcome of pregnancy. Frequently, chronic medical conditions of the woman adversely affect the fetus.

DIABETES MELLITUS

Diabetes mellitus (DM) is a chronic disease in which glucose metabolism is impaired by lack of insulin in the body or by ineffective insulin utilization. DM, particularly if it is poorly controlled, can adversely affect pregnancy outcomes. Conversely, pregnancy affects glucose metabolism, which makes the disease challenging to manage.

DM complicates approximately 3% to 10% of pregnancies (Moore & Warshak, 2005), and the rates are rising. The incidence of diabetes in pregnancy increased by 40% between 1990 and 2003 (Finegold, 2006). Factors contributing to the increase include sedentary lifestyles, dietary changes, immigration from high-risk populations, and the obesity epidemic in the United States (Moore & Warshak, 2005).

Specialists should be involved in the care of the pregnant woman with DM. Sometimes the obstetrician consults with an endocrinologist, who then manages the woman's DM throughout her pregnancy. At other times, the obstetrician consults with the perinatologist, or the perinatologist manages the woman with DM during her pregnancy. A team approach to the management of DM during pregnancy results in the best outcomes. At a minimum, the team should include the primary care physician, an RN, a certified diabetic educator, and a registered dietitian. Endocrinologists, social workers, and pastoral care may be team members.

Classification of Diabetes Mellitus

There are three overall categories of DM that occur during pregnancy: type 1, type 2, and gestational diabetes (GDM). Type 1 and type 2 DM are very different in nature. They both affect glucose metabolism, but type 1 is characterized by a lack of insulin in the body, whereas type 2 is most often associated with insulin resistance. A woman who enters pregnancy with either type 1 or type 2 DM has **pregestational diabetes.** Traditionally, type 1 DM has been associated with women of childbearing age. However, the incidence of type 2 DM in younger women is increasing (Homko & Reece, 2006). **Gestational diabetes** (GDM) is unique to pregnancy but in many respects mimics type 2 DM. The large majority (90%) of pregnant women with DM have GDM (Scollan-Koliopoulos, Guadagno, & Walker, 2006).

Pregestational Diabetes Mellitus

Historically, the woman with pregestational type 1 DM had a higher incidence of spontaneous abortions (miscarriages). If the woman was able to carry the pregnancy to term, the fetus was at high risk for congenital anomalies and/or stillbirth. Fortunately, outcomes have improved greatly with early monitoring and strict control of blood glucose levels. However, poorly controlled DM, particularly in the early weeks of pregnancy, is highly likely to lead to a less than optimal outcome for the fetus, such as a serious birth defect or stillbirth (Jovanovic & Nakai, 2006). Other pregnancy-related complications associated with pregestational DM include hypertensive disorders, **polyhydramnios** (excess levels of amniotic fluid), preterm delivery, and shoulder dystocia (Homko & Reece, 2006). The diabetic woman is more likely to experience a cesarean birth than a woman who does not have DM.

Some women who have had DM since childhood have damage to the blood vessels. Pregnancy has a tendency to speed up this damage (Hofmanova, 2006). For example, if a woman has diabetic retinopathy (damage to the retina that can cause blindness), her vision may deteriorate during pregnancy. Fortunately, by approximately 6 months after delivery, vision often returns to the pre-pregnant state, particularly for those with mild to moderate retinopathy (Jovanovic, 2007b). The most serious consequences of circulatory insufficiency occur in the kidneys, which can lead to renal damage and hypertension.

The placenta tends to be smaller, and maternal–fetal circulation is often decreased in longstanding DM, which may lead to chronic fetal hypoxemia and growth retardation, although, as with GDM (see discussion below), the fetus may be exceptionally large because of elevated maternal blood glucose levels (Moore & Warshak, 2006). Any type of DM increases the incidence of placental insufficiency, regardless of infant weight (Hall et al., 2006). (Refer to Chapter 20 for a more detailed description of the newborn of the woman with diabetes.)

Gestational Diabetes Mellitus

The woman who develops GDM is at increased risk for developing type 2 DM after pregnancy. In fact, more than half of these women will go on to develop type 2 DM within 20 years. It may be that the pancreas of the woman with GDM has sufficient resources to sustain normal blood sugars when she is not pregnant; however, the stress of pregnancy may be enough to bring on GDM. She then experiences sustained periods of high blood sugar, **hyperglycemia,** and elevated insulin levels, **hyperinsulinemia,** which puts her and the unborn child at risk.

As with type 2 DM, the underlying pathophysiology of GDM is insulin resistance, which is present even in normal pregnancy. During pregnancy, tissues become resistant to insulin to provide sufficient levels of glucose for the growing fetus. Although scientists do not know the exact cause of insulin resistance in pregnancy, they

Box 16-1 ▌ SELECTED RISK FACTORS FOR GESTATIONAL DIABETES MELLITUS (GDM)
▪ History of a large-for-gestational age infant ▪ History of GDM ▪ Previous unexplained fetal demise ▪ Advanced maternal age (>35 years) ▪ Family history of type 2 DM or GDM ▪ Obesity (>200 lb) ▪ Non-Caucasian ethnicity ▪ Fasting blood glucose >140 mg/dL ▪ Random blood glucose >200 mg/dL

Box 16-2 ▌ DIAGNOSTIC VALUES FOR THE ORAL GLUCOSE TOLERANCE TEST (OGTT)
Normal values are ▪ Fasting: <95 mg/dL ▪ 1 hour: <180 mg/dL ▪ 2 hours: <155 mg/dL ▪ 3 hours: <140 mg/dL GDM is diagnosed if two or more values meet or exceed the levels listed above.

think that the hormones estrogen, progesterone, and human placental lactogen are at least partially responsible. As these pregnancy hormones rise, insulin resistance increases (Petraglia & D'Antona, 2006). The result in a normal pregnancy is threefold (Endo et al., 2006):

1. Blood glucose levels are lower than normal (mild hypoglycemia) when fasting.
2. Blood glucose levels are higher than normal (mild hyperglycemia) after meals.
3. Insulin levels are increased (hyperinsulinemia) after meals.

Together these changes compose the **diabetogenic effect of pregnancy.** GDM develops when the woman cannot tolerate this normal pregnancy change. Box 16-1 lists selected risk factors for GDM.

The greatest risk for the fetus of the woman with GDM is excessive growth, resulting in **macrosomia** (birth weight >4,500 g [9.9 lb] or >90th percentile for gestational age) and birth trauma (shoulder dystocia). Insulin does not cross the placenta; however, blood sugar does. Large amounts of glucose cross the placenta when the woman's blood sugar levels are elevated. The fetus does not have insulin resistance, so his or her pancreas produces increased levels of insulin to handle the high sugar load. As with any disproportionate intake of sugar, the excess calories are stored in the fetus' body in the form of fat. The fetus is also at risk for delayed lung maturity and other complications seen in the newborn of the woman with DM (refer to Chapter 20). Research indicates that long-range complications for the infant include risk for obesity and type 2 DM (Ogata, 2005).

Most women who develop GDM do not experience symptoms, although they may notice increased thirst, urinary frequency, hunger, or fatigue. Therefore, screening for GDM is a standard of obstetric care. Most obstetricians screen for GDM at approximately 24 to 28 weeks of pregnancy, although physicians in states that have high rates (>5%) of insulin resistance may screen as early as 20 weeks. If the woman has a history of GDM, screening occurs at the first prenatal visit. The diagnosis

of GDM depends on the results of the oral glucose tolerance test, also known as the glucose challenge test. Box 16-2 outlines normal and diagnostic values of the oral glucose tolerance test.

Treatment

Pre-pregnancy Care

The woman who has pregestational DM should consult with her physician before she becomes pregnant. Persistent maternal hyperglycemia (elevated blood glucose levels) is harmful to the growing fetus, particularly during the first 8 weeks of pregnancy, when organogenesis is occurring. Therefore, it is important for the woman to attain a state of euglycemia (normal blood glucose levels) in the months before becoming pregnant (Jovanovic, 2007b). Several months before becoming pregnant, the woman with diabetes should start taking a daily multivitamin supplement that contains at least 1 mg of folic acid. Adequate folic acid intake is the best way to prevent neural tube defects, for which the woman's fetus is particularly susceptible (Moore & Warshak, 2006).

Monitoring Glycemic Control

It is important to track the pattern of glycemic control before pregnancy. Average blood sugar levels during the past 4 to 8 weeks are determined by measuring glycosylated hemoglobin (HbA_1C). This blood test determines the percentage of red blood cells (RBCs) that have glucose incorporated in the hemoglobin. Sustained periods of hyperglycemia result in higher HbA_1C levels. Because elevated glucose levels are the most damaging to the fetus during the first trimester, the goal is for the HbA_1C to be less than 6% for 2 to 3 months before the woman becomes pregnant (ACOG, 2005). At this level, the risk of congenital anomalies is equal to that of the general population (1%–2%). As a comparison, when the HbA_1C is greater than 8.5%, the risk of fetal deformity increases to 22.4% (Moore & Warshak, 2006). The physician monitors HbA_1C levels throughout the pregnancy.

During pregnancy, because of the increased challenge of managing blood sugar, the woman with DM must monitor her blood sugar many times during the day. Frequently

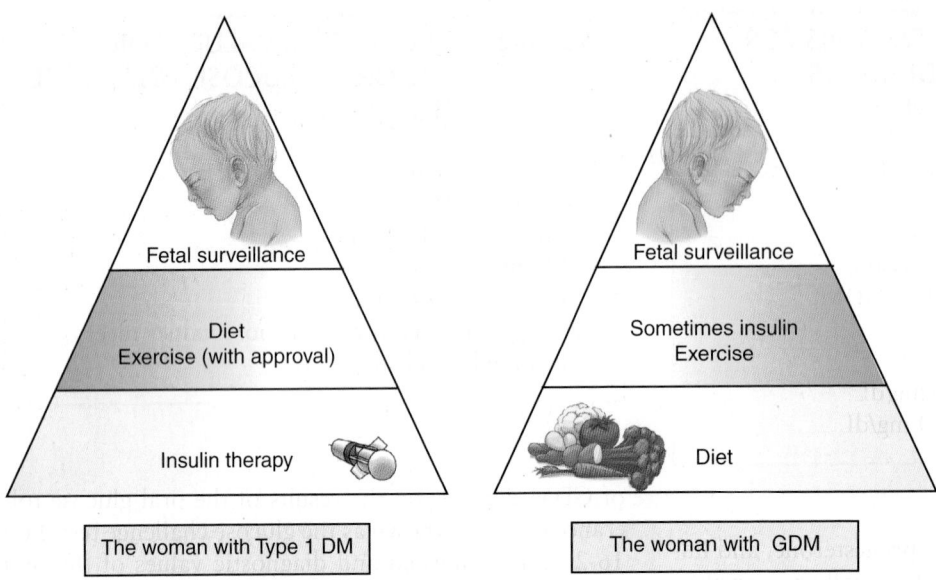

Fetal surveillance

Diet
Exercise (with approval)

Insulin therapy

The woman with Type 1 DM

Fetal surveillance

Sometimes insulin
Exercise

Diet

The woman with GDM

■ **Figure 16-1** Treatment overview for diabetes in pregnancy. For women with pregestational type 1 DM, the foundation of glycemic management is insulin therapy along with dietary management, exercise, and fetal surveillance. For the woman who develops gestational diabetes (GDM), dietary modification is generally the foundation of treatment. Some women with GDM require insulin therapy, and others do not. Exercise and fetal surveillance are also important facets of care.

she will need to check her glucose levels seven times per day: upon awakening, after breakfast, before and after lunch, before and after dinner, and before bedtime. The goal is to maintain fasting blood glucose levels of less than 95 mg/dL. Glucose levels should not exceed 120 mg/dL 2 hours after meals, and should average 100 mg/dL between meals (ACOG, 2005).

Maintaining Glycemic Control

The most important goal of treatment is for the woman to maintain tight glycemic (blood sugar) control before and throughout pregnancy. There are three main facets to glycemic control for the woman with pregestational DM: insulin, diet, and exercise (Fig. 16-1). Glycemic control for the woman with GDM focuses heavily on diet therapy and exercise; if these modalities fail to control the diabetes, the woman begins insulin therapy.

Insulin Therapy

Blood glucose levels vary with advancing gestation. In the first few months of pregnancy, the woman's insulin requirements fluctuate widely, and she is at risk for episodes of **hypoglycemia,** low blood glucose levels, particularly between meals. This phenomenon occurs because the rapidly growing embryo requires a constant supply of glucose, which may deplete maternal blood sugar levels. At the beginning of the second trimester, insulin requirements stabilize, and then begin to increase at approximately 24 weeks' gestation, continuing to increase until term (Cunningham et al., 2005). During labor, insulin needs are variable, and in the first 24 hours after delivery, insulin requirements fall dramatically. Because the pancreas of a woman with type 1 DM does not produce insulin, she must be on an insulin regimen. Orders may include two to three daily baseline doses of insulin to be self-administered subcutaneously. Often the

order calls for a combination of regular and intermediate and/or long-acting insulin (Jovanovic & Nakai, 2006).

The woman may use an insulin pump to administer insulin in low doses throughout the day. An insulin pump is a small device, approximately the size of a pager that the woman can wear with a belt or place in a pocket. A flexible tube placed in the subcutaneous tissue of the abdomen delivers the insulin (Fig. 16-2). The pump has several advantages. Its action mimics that of a healthy pancreas. The woman gets a continuous basal flow of insulin, which helps keep her blood sugar stable throughout

■ **Figure 16-2** Using an insulin pump during pregnancy is the best administration method to keep insulin levels constant.

the day. She can give herself an insulin bolus by pushing a button before eating or if her glucose level is elevated above a predetermined level. Some women find the pumps more comfortable and less intrusive than self-administering insulin several times per day.

Insulin therapy is recommended for women with GDM when, despite diet and exercise, fasting blood sugar levels cannot be maintained lower than 95 mg/dL or 2-hour postprandial (after meals) sugars below 120 mg/dL (Jovanovic, 2007d). When insulin becomes necessary, the woman may be hospitalized to titrate the dose and to provide education on self-administration.

Oral Hypoglycemic Agents

Historically, physicians told their patients not to take oral hypoglycemic agents during pregnancy due to the fear that these medications were teratogens. The use of oral hypoglycemic agents during pregnancy remains controversial. However, authorities are now cautiously recommending glyburide (Micronase) and metformin as possible insulin alternatives for the pregnant woman with diabetes. It does not appear that either of these agents crosses the placenta. The newest research indicates that the risk of fetal malformation from persistently elevated blood glucose levels is likely higher than the risk from oral hypoglycemic medications (Homko & Reece, 2006).

Diet Therapy

Another important part of diabetes management during pregnancy is diet therapy. In fact, the cornerstone of treatment for GDM is diet therapy, although insulin may be required, depending upon the severity of glucose intolerance. The goals of dietary intervention for any type of DM during pregnancy, in addition to supplying the nutritional needs of the woman and her fetus, are to maintain blood sugar levels in the normal range and to prevent ketoacidosis. Authorities recommend consultation with a registered dietitian, preferably one who is also a certified diabetic educator, because diet requirements are individualized.

The objective is to eat to avoid surges and dips in blood sugar. The recommended diet includes a total caloric intake of 30 to 35 kcal/kg of ideal body weight per day for the woman who enters pregnancy at a normal weight. Recommendations are for 40% to 50% of dietary intake to be composed of complex, high-fiber carbohydrates; 20% protein; and 30% to 40% fat (mostly unsaturated fat). Ideally, the woman spreads her food intake over the day by eating three regular meals interspersed with three snacks (ACOG, 2005).

Exercise

Exercise is another way to help control blood sugar for the woman with DM. However, the pregnant woman should always consult with her physician before exercising, particularly if her diabetes is poorly controlled or she has diabetes complications, such as vascular damage, hypertension, or renal insufficiency. It is ideal for the practitioner to give the woman an exercise prescription delineating the type, intensity, duration, frequency, and progression of difficulty over time (Artal, 2007).

Fetal Surveillance

Fetal surveillance is critical for the woman with DM. An initial sonogram during the first trimester determines gestational age and fetal viability. A more detailed, high-level sonogram follows at 18 to 20 weeks to look closely for structural defects in the fetus. The sonogram enables careful assessment of fetal anatomy for abnormalities, and measurement of amniotic fluid volume. Maternal serum alpha-fetoprotein levels measured at 16 to 20 weeks, screen for neural tube defects. If HbA$_1$C levels were elevated in early pregnancy, a fetal echocardiogram is recommended in the second trimester. Serial sonograms, done every 4 to 6 weeks in the third trimester (from approximately 26 weeks), measure fetal growth (Moore & Warshak, 2005).

Give your patient the "why" of it.

It is important to monitor fetal growth because macrosomia occurs more commonly in women with gestational DM. Conversely, for the woman with longstanding DM or vascular disease, the fetus may be growth restricted.

Third trimester fetal surveillance is vital to help detect signs of fetal stress that precede fetal death. The mother initiates daily fetal activity counts at 28 weeks' gestation. At 28 to 34 weeks' gestation, twice-weekly nonstress testing (NST) begins. Authorities generally recommend a weekly biophysical profile (BPP). The woman may need contraction stress tests (CSTs) if the NST is nonreactive or the BPP is nonreassuring (Moore & Warshak, 2005). (Refer to Chapter 7 to review prenatal fetal testing.)

Determining Timing of Delivery

Determining the optimum time and method of delivery is a consideration in the care of the pregnant woman with DM. The challenge for the obstetrician is to schedule the delivery to avoid fetal death, while giving the fetus time to mature fully. Elevated maternal glucose levels can delay fetal lung maturation, which predisposes the newborn to respiratory distress. Therefore, third trimester amniocentesis may be done to document fetal lung maturity (a lecithin-to-sphingomyelin ratio of at least 2:1). Many women with DM have labor induced at 39 weeks' gestation if the cervix is favorable and the fetal lungs are mature. If the pregnancy progresses for too long, there is an increased chance for delivery complications, such as shoulder dystocia and fetal demise (Moore & Warshak, 2005). Many physicians attempt to prevent shoulder dystocia by inducing labor in the woman as soon as amniocentesis verifies fetal lung maturity. Alternatively, the physician may elect to perform a cesarean delivery if he or she suspects macrosomia.

Nursing Process for the Pregnant Woman with DM

Assessment

Diagnosis of type 1 DM usually occurs during childhood or adolescence. Therefore, the woman may be accustomed to monitoring her blood glucose levels and self-administering insulin. However, she will likely need to increase the number of times she monitors daily. Have her do a return demonstration of self-glucose monitoring and recording of results. Be sure that she has a log and understands the importance of recording each blood sugar level.

Once GDM has been diagnosed, assess for understanding of therapeutic regimen management. Instruct the woman to bring her blood sugar log to every prenatal visit. Review the log with her and discuss blood sugar patterns noted. Assess her ability to self-manage her condition. Inquire regarding signs and symptoms of urinary tract infection (UTI) and/or candidiasis. In the third trimester, institute fetal surveillance as ordered by the physician.

During labor, frequent monitoring of blood glucose levels is required, sometimes as frequently as every hour. If the woman is unable to maintain normal glucose levels, an intravenous (IV) insulin drip may be initiated, with the insulin dose titrated to maintain glucose levels within a predetermined range. Chapter 20 covers care of the infant of the woman with diabetes.

Selected Nursing Diagnoses

- Ineffective Therapeutic Regimen Management
- Risk for Injury (maternal) related to unstable glucose levels: hypoglycemia or hyperglycemia and increased risk for obstetric complications
- Risk for Infection: Vaginal candidiasis and/or UTI related to elevated blood glucose levels
- Risk for Injury (fetal): Fetal demise or birth trauma related to unstable maternal blood sugars or fetal hyperinsulinemia
- Risk for Disproportionate Growth: Fetal macrosomia related to maternal hyperglycemia

Outcome Identification and Planning

Appropriate goals may include that the woman will manage the therapeutic regimen successfully; the woman will avoid injury from hypoglycemia, hyperglycemia, and obstetric complications; and the woman will remain free from infection. Fetal goals may include that the fetus will maintain health status, will be appropriate size for gestational age at birth, and will avoid birth trauma. Plan other goals and interventions according to the individualized needs of the woman throughout pregnancy, birth, and the postpartum period.

Implementation

Monitoring Management of Therapeutic Regimen

Information obtained regularly by self-monitoring or blood testing at home with a portable glucose monitor gives immediate feedback on effect of diet, activity, and medications on glucose levels. At every office visit, carefully review the woman's blood sugar log. If she is having difficulty maintaining her blood glucose levels within the expected parameters, explore with her possible reasons.

Dietary recall for the past 3 days may be helpful for identifying patterns of food intake that interfere with blood sugar control. Refer the woman for a consult with a registered dietitian if she is having difficulty following the prescribed dietary regimen. Review with the woman her exercise patterns to determine if improved blood sugar control might result from implementation of an exercise regimen.

Carefully explore the woman's compliance with insulin administration. If she is having difficulty controlling her blood glucose levels, ask her to do a return demonstration by having her check her blood sugar levels. If possible, request that she do a return demonstration of insulin preparation and/or administration. Assist her to correct her technique, if necessary.

The cause of frequent episodes of hypoglycemia may be too much insulin or too little food. Explore the woman's pattern of food intake in conjunction with insulin administration. Be certain she is eating three regular meals and three snacks daily. Food intake should follow insulin administration. A pattern of regular exercise may decrease insulin needs. Notify the physician of frequent episodes of hypoglycemia, particularly if the woman began a regular exercise program 3 to 4 weeks previously.

Preventing Maternal Injury

The woman with DM is at risk for unstable blood sugar levels and the associated risks. Take particular care to review the signs and symptoms of hypoglycemia (Box 16-3) with the woman and her family. Explain that it is important to pay attention to the warning signals because she is more prone to hypoglycemia during pregnancy.

Pay close attention!
Hypoglycemia can be deadly. The woman needs a ready source of glucose (e.g., a candy bar or glass of milk) close by. A family member must administer glucagon if the woman loses consciousness.

Although any woman with DM is at risk for developing diabetic ketoacidosis (DKA), the woman with type 1 DM during pregnancy is at highest risk. She should know the signs of hyperglycemia and avoid triggers for DKA (Box 16-4).

The woman with DM is at increased risk for pregnancy-related hypertension (see Chapter 17). In the third trimester, the physician will likely recommend weekly blood pressure and urinary protein measurements. At every office visit, carefully screen the woman for signs of the severe pregnancy complication, preeclampsia (see Chapter 17). Signs of preeclampsia include headache, visual disturbances, epigastric pain, generalized edema,

Box 16-3 ▌ SIGNS OF HYPOGLYCEMIA

It is particularly important for the pregnant woman and her family to be familiar with the signs and symptoms of hypoglycemia because she is more vulnerable to the condition during pregnancy. Sometimes it helps to remember that the symptoms of hypoglycemia mimic those of the fight-or-flight response. The woman may experience any of the following symptoms.

- Anxiety
- Shakiness
- Confusion
- Headache
- Tingling sensations around the mouth
- Hunger
- Sudden behavior change
- Pale skin
- Cold, clammy skin
- Increased pulse
- Seizure
- Unresponsiveness

urinary protein, and elevated blood pressure. Inform the woman to immediately call the physician if she should experience any of these symptoms.

Monitoring for and Preventing Infection

The woman with diabetes is at increased risk for UTI because of elevated blood sugar levels. Review with the

Box 16-4 ▌ DIABETIC KETOACIDOSIS (DKA) AND PREGNANCY

The onset of DKA is marked by the classic symptoms of hyperglycemia, which include

- Polydipsia (excessive thirst)
- Polyuria (increased frequency and amount of urine)
- Polyphagia (excessive hunger)

As DKA develops, the following symptoms appear

- Glucose >300 mg/dL
- Ketonuria
- Kussmaul respirations
- Acetone (like alcohol) breath
- Sleepiness
- Language slurring
- Decreased consciousness

Triggers for DKA include (but are not limited to) the following

- Too little insulin or too much food
- Infection
- Tocolytic therapy (to prevent preterm labor)
- Corticosteroid use
- Insulin pump failure

woman the signs of a UTI, which include increased frequency, voiding small amounts, burning with urination, and cloudy urine. Teach her to drink 8 to 10 glasses of noncaffeinated beverages every day to help prevent UTI and to wipe from front to back after using the restroom. Frequent hand washing (before and after meals and using the restroom) continues to be the best way to prevent infection. Remind the woman that if a UTI occurs, prompt treatment is essential because UTI can cause premature labor.

Candidiasis is another problem the woman with diabetes is more likely to develop. Signs of vaginal candidiasis include white, cheesy-type vaginal discharge, severe itching, and discomfort. The discharge does not have a foul odor but is highly irritating to tender vaginal tissue. Fluconazole (Diflucan) is an oral tablet sometimes prescribed for the woman with vaginal candidiasis. Normally, however, authorities do not recommend the use of fluconazole during pregnancy. Occasionally, the benefits of treatment with this medication outweigh the possible risks to the fetus. The physician will discuss these risks with the woman. Most frequently, the physician recommends treatment with over-the-counter vaginal creams and suppositories to control the symptoms of vaginal candidiasis during pregnancy. Verify that the woman understands treatment advice.

Monitoring Fetal Status

It is very important for the pregnant woman with DM to understand the risk of fetal demise, particularly if blood sugar levels are difficult to control and/or the woman requires insulin to manage her diabetes. The third trimester is generally the time of greatest danger. Institute fetal surveillance per the physician's orders. It is always appropriate to teach the woman to monitor fetal activity and kick counts, starting at approximately 26 to 28 weeks' gestation. Perform twice-weekly NSTs in the physician office, or as ordered. Give the fetal monitor tracing to the RN to assess and report results to the physician. If the NST is nonreactive, anticipate follow-up with a CST and/or a BPP.

Estimating Fetal Weight

The fetus of the woman with DM is at risk for disproportionate growth, resulting in fetal macrosomia. Assist the physician or RN to measure fundal height at each prenatal visit. Report findings that do not correlate with gestational age (refer to Chapter 7 to review fundal height assessment). Larger-than-expected size may be related to a large fetus or polyhydramnios.

Instruct the woman on the importance of serial sonograms to estimate the fetal weight. The macrosomic infant is much more likely to experience shoulder dystocia (difficulty delivering fetal shoulders after delivery of the head) during birth, leading to birth trauma.

Evaluation: Goals and Expected Outcomes

Goal: The woman will successfully manage the therapeutic regimen.

Expected Outcomes: The woman

■ monitors and records blood sugar levels as ordered.

■ adjusts her diet to recommendations by the physician and dietitian.

■ exercises at least three times per week using recommended exercises.

■ self-administers insulin, if ordered.

Goal: The woman will not suffer injury from hypoglycemia or hyperglycemia.

Expected Outcomes: The woman

■ recognizes and treats hypoglycemia promptly.

■ recognizes hyperglycemia and takes measures to prevent DKA.

Goal: The woman will remain free from infection.

Expected Outcomes: The woman

■ does not experience a UTI (or if she does, seeks prompt treatment).

■ seeks prompt treatment for vaginal candidiasis.

Goal: The fetus will maintain health status.

Expected Outcomes:

■ Fetal activity counts are within normal limits.

■ NST is reactive.

■ BPP score is greater than 7.

■ CST is negative.

Goal: The fetus will avoid birth trauma.

Expected Outcomes:

■ Fetal weight is appropriate for gestational age.

■ No birth injury results from shoulder dystocia.

Test Yourself

✔ What test is used to monitor long-term glucose control during pregnancy for the woman with diabetes?

✔ What term is used to describe the fetus whose weight exceeds 4,500 g?

✔ What are the three cornerstones of therapy for the pregnant woman with diabetes?

CARDIOVASCULAR DISEASE

Heart disease is the third leading cause of death in women of childbearing age and complicates approximately 1% of all pregnancies (Cunningham et al., 2005). In the past, most cases of heart disease during pregnancy resulted from rheumatic heart disease. Now, however, congenital heart disease is the underlying problem in at least 50% of pregnancies complicated by heart disease (Kilpatrick & Purden, 2007).

Significant cardiovascular changes occur in a normal pregnancy. Blood volume and cardiac output increase. Systemic vascular resistance drops. The normal healthy woman tolerates these cardiovascular changes with minor notice. However, for the woman with heart or vessel disease, the increased demands of pregnancy can lead to cardiac failure. Previously undiagnosed heart disease can be unmasked or cardiac symptoms can worsen in the woman with pre-existing disease. The periods of greatest risk for the pregnant woman with cardiac disease are at the end of the second trimester (when blood volume peaks), during labor, and in the early postpartum period secondary to fluid shifts (Perloff & Waksmonski, 2006a).

The New York Heart Association's classification system rates the severity of heart disease in the pregnant woman (Table 16-1). Generally, women with Class I or

Table 16-1 ▮ NYHA'S CLINICAL CLASSIFICATION OF HEART DISEASE

Class	Amount of Compromise	Symptoms	Physical Limitations	Pregnancy Prognosis
I	Uncompromised	Asymptomatic	None	Good
II	Slightly compromised	• Asymptomatic at rest • Symptomatic with normal physical exertion	Slight	Good
III	Markedly compromised	Symptoms occur with minimal activity	Marked	Moderate; may need hemodynamic monitoring and special anesthetic management during labor
IV	Severely compromised	Symptoms occur at rest	Unable to perform any physical activity without discomfort	Poor; will need hemodynamic monitoring and special anesthetic, management during labor

II heart disease have a good prognosis for pregnancy. However, women with Class III or IV are at much higher risk for poor pregnancy outcomes and require more extensive monitoring and treatment throughout the pregnancy. In addition, the risk of maternal and fetal complications increases if the woman has any of the following conditions: cyanosis, pulmonary hypertension, history of arrhythmia, or is currently taking anticoagulants (Perloff & Waksmonski, 2006a).

Clinical Manifestations and Diagnosis

Preconceptual counseling is imperative for the woman with cardiac disease. This allows for a complete history, physical, and workup to determine the risk to pregnancy and to initiate treatment to optimize pregnancy outcomes. The physician generally orders a 12-lead electrocardiogram, echocardiogram, and Doppler studies (Dobbenga-Rhodes & Prive, 2006). Measurement of maternal oxygen saturation levels gives one of the most important predictors of maternal and fetal outcomes. Resting oxygen saturation levels below 85% are particularly ominous (Perloff & Waksmonski, 2006a).

Signs and symptoms (Box 16-5) vary depending on the underlying cause of heart disease. Tachycardia that lasts for more than several minutes accompanied by dizziness or light-headedness suggests a tachyarrhythmia and requires further investigation. The woman with an existing stenotic valve tends to have an increase in symptoms during pregnancy, whereas the woman with incompetent valves tends to experience fewer symptoms during pregnancy. Pregnancy is particularly dangerous for the woman with severe (>80 mm Hg systolic) pulmonary hypertension.

The earliest warning sign of cardiac decompensation is persistent rales in the bases of the lungs. The woman will probably notice a nocturnal cough. A sudden decrease in the ability to perform normal duties, exertional dyspnea, and attacks of coughing with a smothering feeling are serious signs of heart failure. Upon physical examination, tachycardia, edema, and hemoptysis may be noted.

Treatment

A team approach to management of the pregnancy complicated by heart disease is ideal. The obstetrician, cardiologist, perinatologist, and other specialists often collaborate in the care of the pregnant woman with heart disease. Treatment varies depending on the etiology of the heart condition; however, there are general principles for management. These principles involve activity levels, stress management, diet, and medication. No matter what the underlying cause of the condition, the main goal is prevention, early detection, and early treatment of cardiac decompensation.

Activity Levels

Activity is allowed as tolerated. The woman is cautioned to rest frequently and not allow herself to become overly fatigued. Because pregnancy greatly increases the workload of the heart, complete bed rest is sometimes necessary, particularly for the woman who is severely compromised (see Table 16-1).

Stress Management

Any unusual stress that increases demands upon the cardiovascular system can precipitate heart failure. Examples include infection, anemia, underlying medical disorders, and excessive emotional or physical stress. The physician carefully screens for any condition that might precipitate the stress response. Authorities recommend pneumococcal and influenza vaccines because infection is particularly harmful for the pregnant woman with heart disease. Antibiotic prophylaxis to prevent endocarditis is necessary before some high-risk procedures (e.g., some dental work and other invasive procedures) for the woman with moderate to severe heart disease.

Diet and Medications

Diet is individualized. In some cases, sodium restriction is helpful. The woman usually can continue to take her cardiac medications during pregnancy, with the exception of warfarin (Coumadin), angiotensin-converting enzyme inhibitors, and angiotensin II receptor blockers. Warfarin crosses the placenta and increases the risk of congenital anomalies. An alternative is treatment with heparin. The large molecules of this anticoagulant do not cross the placental barrier. Angiotensin-converting enzyme inhibitors and angiotensin II receptor blockers can lead to intractable renal failure in the fetus and increase the risk of newborn mortality (DeCara, Jacobs, & Lang, 2006).

Box 16-5 ▌ SIGNS AND SYMPTOMS OF HEART DISEASE

The woman may complain of
- Dyspnea
- Orthopnea
- Nocturnal cough
- Dizziness
- Fainting
- Chest pain

Physical examination may reveal
- Cyanosis
- Clubbing of the fingers
- Neck vein distention
- Tachycardia
- Heart murmurs
- Edema

Management During Labor and the Postpartum Period

Labor requires special precautions for the woman with cardiac disease. During labor, cardiac output increases an additional 10% to 40% over pregnancy values, placing the woman with cardiac disease at risk for decompensation (Witcher & Harvery, 2006). Although no pregnant woman should be flat on her back during labor, it is particularly important for the woman with heart disease to avoid supine hypotensive syndrome. Supine hypotensive syndrome can lead to decreased placental perfusion with resultant fetal compromise. The condition can also increase maternal cardiac output and quickly lead to maternal compromise.

Don't do it!
Do not place the pregnant woman with heart disease flat on her back. Always use a pillow or wedge under one hip when she is semirecumbent.

The woman who is at risk for endocarditis needs antibiotic prophylaxis. The antibiotic therapy begins when labor begins. Administration continues through the first postpartum day (Perloff & Waksmonski, 2006a).

Vaginal birth is preferred, if possible. Benefits of vaginal versus cesarean birth include decreased oxygen demands, minimal blood loss, less chance of postoperative complications, such as infection and pulmonary dysfunction (Dobbenga-Rhodes & Prive, 2006). There are certain conditions, such as aneurysm or aortic dissection, in which cesarean delivery is preferable (Witcher & Harvey, 2006).

The stress and pain of labor greatly increases demand on the heart, making pain relief a crucial part of labor management for the woman with heart disease. Epidural analgesia is the pain relief option of choice during labor (Witcher & Harvey, 2006). During the second stage of labor, vigorous pushing using Valsalva maneuver can lead to cardiac decompensation; therefore, the fetus should descend without maternal pushing. The physician often assists the birth process with low forceps or vacuum extractor (Perloff & Waksmonski, 2006a). The woman remains at risk for heart failure in the postpartum period. Postpartum hemorrhage, anemia, infection, and thromboembolism are complications that greatly increase the risk of cardiac decompensation.

Nursing Care

Excellent nursing assessment and reporting of abnormal findings is critical for the pregnant woman with heart disease. Monitor for and report jugular distention, clubbing, and slow capillary refill time. If an irregular pulse is noted, compare it with the apical pulse.

The most important nursing action is to monitor for and teach the woman to recognize signs of cardiac decompensation. Listen to breath sounds at each office visit and during labor. Report rales in the bases of the lungs and complaints of nocturnal coughing. Elevated blood pressure and tachycardia are other warning signs that require immediate reporting. Increased respiration, shortness of breath, and productive coughing may indicate the development of pulmonary edema or pulmonary emboli, either of which is life threatening.

It is especially important for the pregnant woman with heart disease to protect herself from infection. Instruct her to avoid crowds and anyone with signs of respiratory infection, even the common cold. Explain that cigarette smoking increases the risk of contracting an upper respiratory infection. Advise her of the importance of frequent hand washing. Administer pneumococcal and influenza vaccines, as ordered. Remind the woman of the importance of reporting her heart condition to all health care providers, including the dentist.

Explain that the woman must take precautions to avoid clot formation. Encourage her to lie on her side when she is in bed or resting. If she must lie on her back, instruct her to put a wedge under one hip to avoid compromising the great vessels. She should minimize the amount of time she spends standing in one position or sitting with her knees flexed and legs dependent (Perloff & Waksmonski, 2006a).

Advise the woman to get adequate rest and to avoid strenuous physical activity. Discuss the importance of avoiding overheating. A cool, dry environment is therapeutic. It is also helpful to give the woman information about what to expect throughout the pregnancy and during labor. This intervention can relieve anxiety and decrease the risk for cardiac decompensation (Perloff & Waksmonski, 2006a).

Inquire regarding illicit drug use and cigarette smoking in a nonjudgmental way. Explain that many illicit drugs and cigarette smoking adversely affect the heart and increase the risk for decompensation. Make clear that intravenous (IV) drug use increases the risk for infective endocarditis, a potentially lethal complication.

Assist the woman with tests for fetal well-being. Explain that serial ultrasound measurements allow the physician to monitor growth of the fetus. Instruct the woman to do fetal kick counts in the second and third trimesters. She should immediately report decreased fetal movement. Assist with amniocentesis, as indicated. The physician may perform amniocentesis to determine fetal lung maturity in anticipation of early delivery if the woman's cardiac status begins to deteriorate in the third trimester.

Monitor the woman particularly closely during labor. Position her so that the gravid uterus does not compress the major blood vessels. Assess pain levels frequently. Administer IV analgesia as ordered. Assist with epidural anesthesia administration. Avoid rapid infusion of IV fluids. Maintain strict intake and output. Monitor vital signs as recommended for the at-risk pregnancy (see Chapter 10). Do not encourage active maternal pushing during the second stage of labor. Anticipate forceps or vacuum-assisted delivery. Continue to observe for signs of cardiac decompensation in the postpartum period. Immediately report fever, increased bleeding, and any signs of decompensation.

ANEMIA

Anemia is a condition in which the blood is deficient in RBCs, hemoglobin, or in total volume. Anemia is not itself a disease. Rather, it is a symptom of an underlying disorder. There are three main causes of anemia: blood loss, hemolysis (increased RBC destruction), and decreased production of RBCs. There are multiple etiologies associated with each category. Iron-deficiency anemia is the most common anemia experienced during pregnancy. Other anemias that could complicate pregnancy include megaloblastic anemia from folate deficiency, pernicious anemia from vitamin B_{12} deficiency, sickle cell anemia, and thalassemia. This section focuses on iron-deficiency and sickle cell anemia.

Iron-Deficiency Anemia

Reduced production of RBCs characterizes iron-deficiency anemia. This situation occurs because the body does not have enough iron to manufacture the hemoglobin molecule. The RBCs that are produced are smaller (microcytic) and are pale in color (hypochromic). Because the pregnant woman has increased iron requirements, she is particularly vulnerable to iron-deficiency anemia.

Clinical Manifestations and Diagnosis

Common signs and symptoms of iron-deficiency anemia in the pregnant woman are tachycardia, tachypnea, dyspnea, pale skin, low blood pressure, heart murmur, headache, fatigue, weakness, and dizziness. Pica (ingestion of nonfood substances, such as clay and laundry starch) and pagophagia (frequent chewing or sucking on ice) are both associated with severe iron-deficiency anemia. Hemoglobin levels less than 10 g/dL define anemia during pregnancy (Cunningham et al., 2005).

Treatment

Treatment for iron-deficiency anemia includes a diet rich in iron and folate in addition to iron and folate supplementation. Recent studies have shown that folate supplementation increases the effectiveness of iron therapy. If the woman refuses to take oral iron supplements, the physician orders iron injections (Cunningham et al., 2005). Rarely does the pregnant woman with anemia require a blood transfusion.

Sickle Cell Anemia

Sickle cell anemia is a hemolytic anemia that is caused by an abnormal hemoglobin molecule called hemoglobin S (Hgb S). Individuals who have sickle cell anemia inherit two copies of the genetic mutation for Hgb S, one from the father and one from the mother. Some people are carriers of the trait because they inherit only one copy of the mutation. Individuals who are carriers have sickle cell trait. In the United States, sickle cell anemia most commonly occurs in African American individuals. Every year, 1 in 625 African American newborns is born with sickle cell anemia, and approximately 1 in 12 African Americans has sickle cell trait (Curran & Poggi, 2007).

Sickle cell anemia is a chronic condition characterized by acute exacerbations of the disease called "crises." Stress typically triggers a crisis, in which the abnormal hemoglobin causes RBCs to "sickle" when oxygen is released from the hemoglobin. The abnormal cells are sticky and clump together in such a way that they cannot flow easily through the capillaries. If enough of the cells clump, the clumping blocks blood flow to the area, causing tissue ischemia and pain at the site of blockage. The reticuloendothelial system removes the damaged cells. Unfortunately, the bone marrow cannot produce enough RBCs to replace the damaged ones, so anemia results.

The pregnant woman with sickle cell anemia is at risk for decreased renal function, stroke, heart dysfunction, leg ulcers, and sepsis. Newborns of the woman with sickle cell anemia are more likely to be born prematurely or to be small for gestational age. Although outcomes have improved in recent years, the woman with sickle cell anemia and her fetus remain at risk for death (Curran & Poggi, 2007).

Clinical Manifestations and Diagnosis

The woman with sickle cell trait rarely experiences symptoms, and when she does, the symptoms are generally mild. The woman with sickle cell anemia, however, is at risk for a sickle cell crisis at any time during the pregnancy. In fact, pregnancy often increases the occurrence of sickle cell crises (Cunningham et al., 2005). Dehydration and infection are two examples of conditions that predispose the woman to a crisis. Depending upon which area of the body is affected, the woman may experience recurrent bouts of pain in the joints, bones, chest, and abdomen (Curran & Poggi, 2007). She also may experience nonspecific symptoms of anemia, such as fatigue, tachycardia, and dyspnea. Physical examination may reveal enlarged lymph nodes, enlarged spleen (splenomegaly), hematuria (bloody urine), or jaundice.

Treatment

Prevention of crises, if possible, is the focus of treatment for the pregnant woman with sickle cell anemia. Maintaining adequate hydration, avoiding infection, getting adequate rest, and eating a balanced diet are all common sense strategies that decrease the risk of a crisis. Hydroxyurea (Hydrea), a medication that decreases the frequency and severity of crises, is teratogenic in animals. For this reason, the physician carefully weighs the risk and benefits before ordering this medication (Cunningham et al., 2005).

The initial prenatal visit requires additional laboratory work for the woman with sickle cell anemia to include hemoglobin electrophoresis, serum iron, total iron binding capacity, ferritin levels, liver function tests, electrolyte analysis, kidney function tests, urinalysis, and urine culture. Hepatitis B vaccine may be administered if the woman does not have hepatitis B. Asymptomatic bacteriuria is treated with antibiotics to prevent a full-blown UTI.

The practitioner may instruct the woman to return for more frequent than normal prenatal visits. The recommended schedule for prenatal visits is every 2 weeks in the second trimester and every week throughout the second trimester. The practitioner orders ultrasound examinations to measure fetal growth and amniotic fluid at every visit in the latter part of pregnancy (Cunningham et al., 2005).

When the woman experiences a painful crisis, the physician orders a CBC, type and cross match, and sometimes arterial blood gas measurements. Infusion of IV fluids hydrates the patient and decreases blood viscosity. Narcotics are generally required to control the pain of an attack. If the fetus is viable, continuous fetal heart rate monitoring is necessary. The woman may require supplemental oxygen by face mask if her oxygen saturation is low. Antibiotics treat infection, if it is present. Occasionally the practitioner may order an exchange transfusion to reduce the amount of sickled RBCs in the circulation (Curran & Poggi, 2007). (For an exchange transfusion, a predetermined amount of blood is withdrawn from the patient [typically 500 mL], and 2 units of packed RBCs are transfused.)

Nursing Care

The woman with iron-deficiency anemia needs counseling regarding foods that are high in iron. These include animal protein, dried beans, fortified grains and cereals, dried fruits, and any food cooked in cast iron cookware. Instruct her that vitamin C enhances iron absorption. Therefore, she should try to eat foods high in vitamin C along with iron-rich foods. Drinking orange juice when she takes her iron supplement will increase absorption. Her diet should also contain adequate amounts of folate. Foods high in folic acid include fortified grains, dried beans, and leafy green vegetables.

At the initial visit, ask for a 1- to 3-day diet recall to help identify patterns of food intake for the pregnant woman with any type of anemia. She may be embarrassed to give an accurate recall. In these instances, it may be helpful for a family member to assist with the dietary recall. Request that the woman keep a food diary for the day or two before each visit. Draw blood as ordered to monitor hemoglobin and hematocrit.

Iron supplements predispose to constipation. The pregnant woman may be tempted to stop taking iron supplements because of constipation. Instruct her regarding the importance to her and her baby of continuing iron supplementation. All of the normal measures that help prevent constipation, such as maintaining adequate fluid intake, getting enough exercise, and establishing regular bowel habits are helpful for the pregnant woman taking iron supplements.

The woman with sickle cell anemia needs support and teaching throughout her pregnancy. Emphasize the importance of using common sense approaches to prevent crises. Instruct the woman to wash her hands frequently and to avoid highly crowded areas to decrease her risk of contracting an infection. Adequate fluid intake and rest are important for maintaining health in the pregnant woman with sickle cell anemia. Assist her to make and keep her prenatal appointments.

Test Yourself
✔ What is the earliest sign of cardiac decompensation?
✔ List the signs of supine hypotensive syndrome.
✔ Describe two conditions or situations that might trigger a crisis for the woman with sickle cell anemia.

ASTHMA

Asthma is a chronic, inflammatory disease of the airways characterized by acute exacerbations of reversible airway obstruction. Asthma complicates 3.7% to 8.4% of all pregnancies (Barclay & Vega, 2007). This condition, also known as reactive airway disease (RAD), can be a severe threat to the health of the woman and her fetus, especially if the disease is severe and/or uncontrolled. Pregnant women with poorly controlled asthma experience a higher incidence of preeclampsia-eclampsia, hemorrhage, premature labor, respiratory failure, and death. Fetal complications include intrauterine growth restriction (IUGR), fetal demise, and preterm birth (Curran, 2006). If the condition is well controlled throughout pregnancy, perinatal outcomes are similar to those of the general population.

Clinical Manifestations and Diagnosis

The course of the disease varies during pregnancy. Physical examination during remission may be completely normal. During an acute asthma episode, the respiratory rate increases and the woman feels short of breath and anxious. An expiratory wheeze is characteristic. Other auscultation findings may include diffuse rhonchi, bronchovesicular sounds, or bronchial sounds throughout the lung fields. Retractions of the respiratory muscles may be noted. Complaint of nocturnal awakening is a classic symptom. Other symptoms frequently include a cough and chest tightness. Pulsus paradoxus, a pulse that weakens during inspiration, is often noted.

Treatment

The goals of asthma management are prevention of acute episodes, control of symptoms, maintenance of normal pulmonary function, and avoidance of emergency department visits and hospitalizations. These goals are important for the pregnant woman because they serve to maximize the health of the woman and her fetus.

Here's an opportunity to correct a myth.
Explain to the woman with asthma that it is much safer for her baby if she takes her asthma medications. Poorly controlled asthma is not good for the pregnant woman or her baby.

The initial prenatal visit includes a thorough history of the course of the woman's asthma before pregnancy and in prior pregnancies, if applicable. The health care provider inquires as to the frequency of acute episodes, the severity of the disease, history of hospitalizations, and any known environmental stimuli that are asthma triggers for the woman. The practitioner elicits a careful medication history. Baseline spirometry measurement determines pulmonary function (Curran, 2006). The pregnant woman with asthma requires at least monthly prenatal visits (Schatz & Weinberger, 2007).

Maintenance care at home includes self-monitoring of lung function, proper control of the environment to reduce asthma triggers, and medication therapy. The woman monitors her lung function by measuring her peak expiratory flow rate (PEFR) or forced expiratory volume in 1 minute ($FEVR_1$) twice a day. Decreases in either value points to asthma exacerbation. In order to control asthma triggers, the woman must first identify her triggers and then take measures to reduce them. Inhaled medications, such as albuterol and corticosteroids are the frontline treatment agents. The practitioner reserves oral medications for severe cases (Curran, 2006).

Management of an Acute Exacerbation

Management of an acute attack often requires hospitalization for the pregnant woman. Treatment may take place on a 23-hour observation status, or her condition may necessitate a full admission. Spirometry and arterial blood gas measurement determine the severity of the attack (Curran, 2006).

Orders may include oxygen by nasal cannula to maintain the PO_2 above 70 mm Hg and the oxygen saturation greater than 95%. The woman receives IV fluids for hydration, which helps to loosen mucus in the airways (Schatz & Weinberger, 2007). Frequent metered dose inhaler (preferred method) or nebulizer treatments with a beta-agonist such as albuterol help to bring the attack under control. The woman may need inhaled anticholinergics, oral or IV corticosteroids, and/or IV magnesium sulfate, if she does not show significant improvement with the beta-agonist (Fanta, 2007).

The health care provider assesses fetal well being with continuous external fetal monitoring after 20 weeks' gestation. Other measures of fetal well-being, such as ultrasound or biophysical profile, may also be ordered.

Status asthmaticus, the most severe form of asthma, is a potentially fatal complication of an acute asthma attack. The pregnant woman in status asthmaticus receives aggressive treatment, with early intubation and mechanical ventilation in the intensive care setting (Cunningham et al., 2005).

Labor and Birth Management

There are several important points to remember about managing the woman with asthma during labor. The woman may fear that the stress of labor will exacerbate asthma symptoms. This is not generally the case. In fact, symptoms tend to diminish during labor. The woman should continue to receive her regularly scheduled asthma medications throughout labor (Cunningham et al., 2005). Adequate hydration and analgesia minimize the risk of bronchospasm. Fentanyl or butorphanol are the pain relievers of choice during labor because they do not cause histamine release, which could lead to bronchospasm. Epidural analgesia is the ideal method of pain control for the laboring woman with asthma (Schatz & Weinberger, 2007).

If there are indications for a surgical delivery, epidural or spinal anesthesia is preferred over general anesthesia. If a general is required, the anesthesiologist may order atropine and glycopyrrolate (Robinul) preoperatively to induce bronchodilation.

Nursing Care

Teaching is a major role when providing nursing care for the pregnant woman with asthma. Be sure that the woman does a return demonstration on the use of her inhaler. Do not assume that she knows how to use it. She should also do a return demonstration for use of the peak flow meter. Remind her of the importance of monitoring fetal activity and kick counts during the second and third trimesters.

Smoking cessation and control of the environment are critical aspects of care. Explain that smoking can increase the frequency and severity of attacks, as well as increase the risk of harm to the fetus. Instruct the woman to avoid exposure to substances to which she is allergic. She should also avoid dust, passive tobacco smoke, and other environmental pollutants (Schatz & Weinberger, 2007). Family Teaching Tips: Managing Asthma During Pregnancy outlines the major points to make when educating the pregnant woman with asthma.

EPILEPSY

Epilepsy is a group of neurologic disorders that involve a long-term tendency to have recurrent unprovoked seizures. Approximately 20,000 women with epilepsy give birth each year in the United States (Caughey, 2005). The vast majority of these women have healthy pregnancy outcomes.

Family Teaching Tips

MANAGING ASTHMA DURING PREGNANCY

- Do not stop taking your asthma medications. The risk to you and your baby is much higher from uncontrolled asthma than it is from taking your medications. Remember, you are "breathing for two."
- Check with your doctor before taking any over-the-counter medications. Some of these medications have been shown to cause harm to your developing baby.
- Protect yourself from asthma triggers.
  - Keep a symptom diary to identify your unique triggers.
  - Avoid cigarette smoke, exposure to animals, and dusty, damp environments.
  - Stay inside in air-conditioned surroundings during pollen seasons and when the pollution or mold index is high.
  - Wear a mask or scarf over your mouth on excessively cold days to help warm the air.
  - Protect yourself from colds and flu because respiratory infections can trigger acute asthma attacks.
    - ○ Avoid crowds where viruses may be prevalent.
    - ○ Wash your hands frequently.
    - ○ Take the flu shot if you have moderate or severe asthma. The flu shot is based on a killed virus, so it is safe to use during pregnancy.
  - Avoid foods or chemicals that might have caused a reaction in the past, such as sulfites or MSG.

- Continue your allergy shots as long as you are not having reactions to the shots. If you are not currently taking allergy shots, it is usually not advised to begin doing so during pregnancy because of the risk of reactions.
- Monitor your peak expiratory flow rate (PEFR) regularly, as recommended by your doctor. If you have severe asthma, you will need to measure your PEFR at least twice daily. A decrease in the PEFR usually precedes an acute asthma attack hours to days before physical symptoms begin.
- Develop a crisis management plan in consultation with your physician. The plan should include how to recognize warning signs and what to do when early signs of worsening status occur. Go immediately to the nearest emergency department if any of the following occur after rescue drugs are taken.
  - Rapid improvement does not result.
  - Improvement is not sustained.
  - Condition worsens.
  - The episode is severe.
  - Fetal movement decreases.

At the very first sign of breathing difficulties, use your peak flow meter to measure your PEFR. If it is low or has decreased from your last reading, call the doctor immediately. Other warning signs of an impending attack may include a headache, itchy throat, sneezing, coughing, or feeling tired.

Clinical Manifestations

Pregnancy presents several difficulties that relate to the condition of epilepsy. Drug metabolism changes during pregnancy, making it more difficult to establish therapeutic antiepileptic drug (AED) levels. Seventeen percent to 33% of women with epilepsy experience an increase in seizure frequency during pregnancy, whereas others experience a decrease or no change in seizure frequency (Tettenborn, 2006). The major risk to the pregnancy during a seizure results from blunt trauma. Trauma can lead to miscarriage, premature rupture of membranes, and placental abruption.

In the past, authorities believed that epilepsy itself increased the risk for birth defects in children born to women with epilepsy. However, the latest research indicates that AEDs used to treat epilepsy are the major cause of fetal defects (Caughey, 2005). Cleft lip and palate and cardiac, urinary tract, and neural tube defects comprise the majority of malformations noted in the fetus born to a woman taking AEDs (Schachter, 2007b).

Treatment

Preconception care is highly recommended for the woman with epilepsy who wishes to become pregnant. A thorough history and physical examination establishes the diagnosis of epilepsy and the efficacy of the current treatment regimen in controlling seizures. If the woman has been seizure free for several years while receiving low-dose therapy, the physician may try to wean the woman from the AED.

If AEDs are necessary, the physician will try to get control of the seizures with the fewest number of drugs at the lowest possible doses. Current recommendations are for the woman to remain on the drug that most effectively controls her seizures. The physician advises the woman to wait at least 6 months after seizures are under control before trying to become pregnant (Schachter, 2006). Her obstetrician in consultation with a neurologist should follow the woman with epilepsy.

The woman should receive high-dose (4–5 mg daily) folate supplementation in the 1 to 3 months preceding and throughout pregnancy because AEDs increase the risk for neural tube defects. The physician may order a high-resolution transvaginal ultrasound at 11 to 13 weeks' gestation to detect neural tube defects (Tettenborn, 2006). At 14 to 16 weeks' gestation, the woman should have maternal serum alpha-fetoprotein levels drawn to screen for neural tube defects. A high-resolution sonogram at 18 to 20 weeks' gestation screens for structural defects. Beginning at 36 weeks, many physicians prescribe additional vitamin K supplementation because AED therapy can lead to vitamin K-deficient hemorrhage of the newborn (Schachter, 2006).

Epilepsy is not usually an indication for cesarean delivery. Most women can expect a normal vaginal delivery. One percent to 2% of women experience seizures either during labor or after delivery. IV AEDs are usually sufficient to control the seizure (Schachter, 2006). If the seizure is severe, the woman may need an emergency cesarean delivery.

Status epilepticus is an emergency complication of epilepsy whereby seizure activity continues for 5 to 30 minutes or more after treatment is initiated or when three or more seizures occur without full recovery between seizures. The health care team takes immediate measures to protect the woman from injury while protecting the airway. Emergency intubation with mechanical ventilation is sometimes required. Blood work includes glucose, electrolytes, CBC, AED levels, and blood and urine toxicology screens. The practitioner starts at least two IV lines to allow for IV administration of benzodiazepines, such as diazepam or lorazepam (Stecker, 2007).

Nursing Care

Teach the woman the importance of carefully following her treatment regimen and of maintaining regular prenatal care. Emphasize the importance of eating a diet high in folic acid and of taking folic acid supplementation. Advise the woman to get plenty of rest and sleep and to exercise regularly. Assist her to schedule lab work at regular intervals. Provide emotional support during prenatal testing for fetal anomalies.

INFECTIOUS DISEASES

Infectious diseases are a threat to the pregnant woman in several ways. The disease may cause illness in the woman that requires treatment. Unfortunately, the best treatment for the woman is not always good for the developing fetus. The infection itself can be harmful to the fetus leading to birth defects or active infection of the newborn. Prevention is the best treatment. Table 16-2 defines terminology associated with infectious diseases.

Table 16-2 ▊ **DEFINITIONS OF TERMS ASSOCIATED WITH INFECTIOUS DISEASES DURING PREGNANCY**

Term(s)	Definition
ART	Antiretroviral therapy used in the treatment of HIV/AIDS
CD4-positive T-cell (CD4) counts	CD-4 positive T-cell counts refer to the number of Helper T-cells found in the blood. Helper T-cells are special kinds of lymphocytes that coordinate the actions of the cells of the immune system. CD-4 is a protein on the Helper T-cell to which HIV attaches. The virus then enters the cell, replicates (multiplies), kills the Helper T-cell, and moves on to other Helper T-cells. Low CD-4 counts correlate with increased symptoms and increasing severity of illness.
HAART	HAART—Highly active antiretroviral therapy that involves administration of triple-drug therapy. The CDC recommends this regimen for its effectiveness at suppressing HIV and preventing drug resistance.
Immunoprophylaxis	Prevention of disease by the production of active or passive immunity. The individual acquires passive immunity when he receives antibodies from his mother across the placenta, or when he receives an injection of antibodies to a particular infection, such as hepatitis B. Active immunity occurs when the individual's immune system produces antibodies that fight against a particular disease, such as chickenpox. Active immunity develops when a person becomes ill with certain pathogens or when she receives a vaccination.
Monotherapy	The use of a single drug to treat a particular disease or infection.
Perinatal or vertical transmission	Transmission of the infectious agent from mother to child during pregnancy, childbirth, or breast-feeding.
Seroconversion	The development of antibodies to a particular infectious agent. The person has seroconverted when lab tests can detect the antibodies in the blood.
Suppressive therapy	Treatment that suppresses the infectious agent but does not cure the individual.
Viral load	The amount of virus in the blood. High viral loads are associated with increased illness symptoms.

TORCH

TORCH is an acronym for a special group of infections that can be acquired during pregnancy and transmitted through the placenta to the fetus (Box 16-6). The "T" stands for toxoplasmosis, the "O" for other infections (hepatitis B, syphilis, varicella, and herpes zoster), the "R"

Box 16-6 ▌ TORCH INFECTIONS

TORCH (an acronym for the infections)

Toxoplasmosis
Other: hepatitis B, syphilis, varicella and herpes zoster
Rubella
Cytomegalovirus (CMV)
Herpes simplex virus (HSV)
All are teratogenic. All cross the placenta. Fetal effect is determined by gestational age at exposure. TORCH syndrome is characterized by IUGR, microcephaly, hepatosplenomegaly, rash, thrombocytopenia, and CNS findings, such as ventricular calcifications and hydrocephaly.

Assessment
1. History: flulike symptoms, fatigue, cat exposure, genital lesions, rash, exposure to sick children
2. Physical exam: lymphadenopathy, headache, malaise, jaundice, N/V, low-grade temperature, rash, ulcerated and painful lesions of the genitals
3. Psychosocial: fear, anxiety, apprehension

Diagnostics
1. Serologic tests
   - TORCH screen
   - CBC
   - HBsAg and HBeAg
   - Liver function tests
2. Cultures
   - CMV
   - HSV
3. Pap smear
4. Serial ultrasounds (monitor for IUGR and other defects throughout pregnancy)

Interventions
1. Instruct the woman regarding specifics of
   a. the infection
   b. transmission
   c. medication and medical management
2. Reinforce importance of hand washing
3. Encourage questions
4. Suggest a multidisciplinary conference with family members, if anxiety and fear levels are high
5. Encourage breast-feeding. These mothers may be afraid to breast-feed their babies.

---

is for rubella, the "C" is for cytomegalovirus (CMV), and the "H" stands for herpes simplex virus (HSV).

Each infection is teratogenic, and the effects are different, depending upon when during the pregnancy infection occurs. Fetal infection may lead to TORCH syndrome characterized by central nervous system dysfunction. Mental retardation, microcephaly, hydrocephalus, central nervous system lesions, jaundice, hepatosplenomegaly, hearing deficits, and chorioretinitis are examples of sequelae for the newborn infected with one of the TORCH agents. Fetal infection may also lead to spontaneous abortion, IUGR, stillbirth, and premature delivery. Prevention is the focus of interventions because many of the TORCH infections do not have effective treatment regimens.

The only TORCH infections that the practitioner routinely screens for during pregnancy are hepatitis B, syphilis, and rubella (Lockwood, 2007). If the practitioner has reason to believe the woman might have one of the other TORCH infections, he or she may perform a TORCH screen. Serial antibody titers confirm the diagnosis. If the woman is seronegative (no antibodies in the blood) after two titers (taken 10–20 days apart), infection is ruled out. If the woman is seropositive (antibodies in the blood) for the first titer, but the titers do not rise by the second draw, she has a latent ("old") infection. This is important because it is very rare that the fetus will acquire a latent infection. However, if the woman's antibody titers have risen by the second draw, she has an acute infection.

Toxoplasmosis

Toxoplasmosis is an infection caused by the protozoan *Toxoplasma gondii*, also referred to as "*T. gondii*." Transmission is via undercooked meat and through cat feces. Toxoplasmosis is a common infection in humans and usually produces no symptoms. However, when the infection passes from the woman through the placenta to the fetus, a condition called congenital toxoplasmosis can occur. Approximately 400 to 4,000 cases of congenital toxoplasmosis occur per year in the United States (Williams, 2007). The classic triad of symptoms for congenital toxoplasmosis is chorioretinitis, intracranial calcification, and hydrocephalus in the newborn (Williams, 2007).

Toxoplasmosis is difficult to diagnose because it rarely produces symptoms in the woman. This infection is particularly harmful if the fetus contracts the parasite between 10 and 24 weeks of pregnancy. The woman receives treatment to help prevent transmission to the fetus. Treatment is with one or all of the following medications: spiramycin (Rovamycine, an investigational drug in the United States), pyrimethamine (Daraprim), and sulfadiazine. If pyrimethamine and sulfadiazine are prescribed, the woman also takes folinic acid (Leucovorin) to prevent bone marrow suppression (Williams, 2007).

The woman can decrease the risk for infection through several common sense approaches. Advise the pregnant woman to have someone else clean the cat litter box daily. If there is no one else to perform this duty, she should wear gloves and wash her hands thoroughly before and after cleaning the box. The woman should wear gloves when working in the garden or when doing yard work. She should wash her hands thoroughly before and after handling raw meat, and she should eat only meats that have been completely cooked to 152°F or higher (i.e., no rare or medium rare meats). Instruct the woman to thoroughly clean in hot, soapy water any surface or item that is touched by raw meat. All fruits and vegetables need to be washed carefully before being served.

Other Infections: Hepatitis B, Syphilis, Varicella, and Herpes Zoster

Hepatitis B

Hepatitis B virus (HBV) is transmitted sexually or through contact with blood or body fluids. Transmission to the fetus can occur across the placenta or by contact with vaginal secretions and blood during delivery. Fortunately, due to routine vaccination of infants, the incidence of HBV infection has decreased in the United States (Teo & Lok, 2007).

The adult who becomes acutely infected may develop immunity to HBV or become a chronic carrier. Only 5% of adults who have a history of acute HBV infection convert to the chronic state of the disease. Unfortunately, infants are not so lucky. Ninety percent of infants who acquire the infection will become chronic carriers (Teo & Lok, 2007). This is an important statistic because chronic carriers are at high risk for developing cirrhosis and liver cancer. In fact, 25% of chronic carriers will die from complications of the disease (O'Donovan, 2007).

Obstetricians screen their pregnant patients for hepatitis B surface antigen (HBsAg) early in the pregnancy, and then again at delivery. A woman who has an acute HBV infection or who is chronically infected has elevated HBsAG titers. If the newborn that is born to a woman who is positive for HBsAG is not treated, the infant is highly likely to develop HBV infection. Neonatal immunoprophylaxis (see Table 16-2) can prevent as many as 90% of neonatal infections. If the mother is HBsAG positive, the neonate should receive hepatitis B immunoglobulin (HBIg) and the hepatitis B vaccine within 12 hours of birth. The immunoglobulin provides immediate protection, and the vaccine provides long-term protection from infection. Regardless of the woman's HBV status, all infants need vaccination against hepatitis B at birth, at 1 to 2 months of life, and again at approximately 12 months of age (CDC, 2007).

Syphilis

Syphilis is a sexually transmitted infection (STI) with the bacterium (spirochete) *Treponema pallidum* (*T. pallidum*). The bacteria spread via sexual contact or through broken skin. The main symptom of primary syphilis is a painless red pustule, which usually appears within 2 to 6 weeks after exposure. The pustule quickly erodes and develops a painless, bloodless ulcer called a chancre. Because it is painless, the newly infected person may not notice the chancre. The chancre, which sheds infectious fluid, usually appears on the body part that served as the portal of entry for the bacteria.

If the pregnant woman acquires a syphilis infection, the bacteria readily cross the placenta, causing infection in the developing fetus. Up to 40% of women who contract syphilis early in pregnancy and do not seek treatment have a spontaneous abortion (miscarriage). Other consequences of active syphilis infection include fetal demise, IUGR, hydrops fetalis, preterm birth, congenital infection, and neonatal death (Norwitz, 2006).

The infected infant may be born with birth defects such as blindness, deafness, or other deformities. Hutchinson's triad is characteristic and includes inflammation of the cornea, deafness, and notched teeth. Another characteristic of early congenital syphilis is snuffles, a nasal discharge that can be bloody. The newborn may have a vesicular or bullous rash that is contagious. The fluid in the bullae is highly infectious. On the other hand, the syphilis-infected infant may not immediately exhibit symptoms at birth. Symptoms can develop as long as weeks to months or years later. Swollen lymph glands, spleen and liver enlargement, jaundice, anemia, bone deformities, and vesicular rash may occur (Schelonka, Freij, & McCracken, 2005).

Screening for syphilis with the RPR or VDRL is one of the routine blood tests performed for every pregnant woman in the early part of pregnancy and repeated when she goes into labor. A positive screen requires further testing that is more specific to *T. pallidum*. Syphilis is curable, if properly treated. The treatment of choice for syphilis is benzathine penicillin B (Bicillin) administered intramuscularly as a single dose. Some authorities advocate that the woman should receive a second dose 1 week after the first dose (Norwitz, 2006). Penicillin may be given during pregnancy and is safe to use while breast-feeding. Individuals who are sensitive to penicillin receive erythromycin. Penicillin is the treatment of choice for newborns with congenital syphilis (Schelonka, Freij, & McCracken, 2005).

Varicella and Herpes Zoster

Varicella zoster is the virus that causes chickenpox. Herpes zoster is the recurrent form of the virus that lies dormant in the dorsal root ganglia of the spinal cord. Reactivation of herpes zoster results in shingles. Contact with shingles by persons who are nonimmune to chickenpox leads to the development of chickenpox in that individual. Varicella zoster and herpes zoster are members of the herpesvirus family.

Varicella zoster is spread by respiratory droplets and is highly contagious. The virus incubates for approximately 2 weeks and is contagious 2 days before onset of the skin lesions until the lesions crust over, generally 5 days after the initial onset. Herpes zoster (shingles) is characterized by a localized rash within a **dermatome**, an area on the body surface supplied by a particular sensory nerve. The rash is very painful. Occasionally pain precedes the rash. Anyone who has had chickenpox is at risk for developing shingles.

The incidence of varicella zoster during pregnancy is low, occurring in 1 to 5 of 10,000 pregnancies. Transmission of varicella zoster by the pregnant woman to her unborn child is very rare, occurring in 0.4% to 2% of cases. The highest risk (2%) occurs if the woman contracts varicella in the second trimester, between 13 and 20 weeks' gestation. Transmission of herpes zoster is even more unlikely (Riley, 2006b). However, the severity of fetal varicella syndrome gives cause to treat this infection during pregnancy with great care.

Fetal varicella syndrome is associated with low birth weight, scar-producing skin lesions, limb hypoplasia, and contractures. The syndrome can also result in damage to the ears, eyes, and central nervous system, leading to mental retardation, paralysis, and seizures. Prognosis for the neonate is poor (Riley, 2006b). The newborn is at risk for neonatal varicella, a severe form of chickenpox with a 20% to 30% mortality rate, if the woman contracts varicella from 5 days before to 2 days after delivery. Another danger of varicella during pregnancy is the risk to the woman of developing varicella pneumonitis. This form of pneumonia can be severe, with a mortality rate as high as 40% (Freij & Sever, 2005). Even if the woman survives, the severity of the pneumonia could result in death of the fetus.

Any pregnant woman who reports a possible exposure to chickenpox or shingles should have a serologic test performed to detect varicella antibodies. Varicella zoster immunoglobulin (VZIG) administered within 96 hours of exposure helps prevent the development of chickenpox. However, VZIG is no longer readily available because the sole manufacturer stopped producing the drug. VariZIG, an investigational VZIG product is available as a substitute. The neonate may be treated with VariZIG (within 96 hours of exposure), if the woman develops chickenpox 5 days before, or within 48 hours after, delivery (Riley, 2006b). Treatment of the neonate does not decrease the rate of infection, but it does decrease the severity of the disease (Freij & Sever, 2005).

The best treatment is prevention. A woman of childbearing age who has not had chickenpox should be vaccinated. She should avoid pregnancy for at least 1 month after vaccination. Vaccination is not appropriate for pregnant women (Riley, 2006b); however, susceptible individuals in the household of a pregnant woman who is susceptible to chickenpox should receive the vaccine. This is the most effective way to prevent transmission to the pregnant woman. The nonimmune woman should receive one dose of varicella vaccine immediately after delivering her baby and a second dose at the 6-week postpartum visit.

Rubella

Rubella is a virus that caused periodic epidemics in the United States. The worst epidemic occurred from 1964 to 1965. The infection caused approximately 20,000 newborns to have serious birth defects at a total estimated cost of $840 million. The Centers for Disease Control and Prevention (CDC) launched an aggressive rubella vaccination campaign. As a result, the CDC declared in 2004 that rubella was no longer endemic to the United States. This means that the rare cases of rubella infection occur in people who live or were born in countries that do not routinely administer rubella vaccine (CDC, 2007c).

Rubella is usually a mild illness when it occurs in adults and children. Twenty-five percent to 50% of rubella infections are "silent"; that is, there are no symptoms. When symptoms occur, they are generally mild and include low-grade fever, rash, lymphadenopathy, general malaise, and conjunctivitis (Riley, 2006a). Complications are not common.

The problem occurs when a woman contracts rubella while she is pregnant. Congenital rubella infection can result, which is anything but mild. Consequences of congenital rubella include spontaneous abortion, stillbirth, preterm delivery, and congenital anomalies of varying severity. Hearing impairment is the single most common defect associated with congenital rubella infection, followed by eye disorders, heart defects, and neurologic abnormalities (up to and including mental retardation). The greatest risk occurs if the woman develops rubella in the first trimester. Rubella contracted during the period of organogenesis (in the first 11 weeks of pregnancy) can result in multiple anomalies. Maternal rubella infection contracted after 20 weeks of pregnancy rarely results in birth defects (Riley, 2006a).

There is no cure for congenital rubella infection. Treatments are supportive and directed toward control of symptoms and complications. The best treatment for congenital rubella infection is prevention. Ideally, all women of childbearing age should obtain preconception care, which includes testing for immunity to rubella. Nonimmune women should be vaccinated before becoming pregnant and should wait at least 28 days after vaccination before attempting pregnancy. Routine prenatal care includes testing for immunity to rubella in early pregnancy and again before delivery. Authorities do not recommend giving rubella vaccine during pregnancy due to the small risk of congenital rubella syndrome. The nonimmune woman should carefully avoid anyone with flulike symptoms or rash while she is pregnant. The woman receives the vaccine in the early postpartum period before discharge from the hospital or birthing center. Breast-feeding is not a contraindication to rubella vaccination. Currently, the CDC (2007d) recommends that the combination measles, mumps, and rubella vaccine be given to children at 12 to 15 months of age and a second dose at age 4 to 6 years before starting school. Routine vaccination of all children decreases spread of rubella and decreases the risk that a nonimmune pregnant woman will contract the infection.

Cytomegalovirus

CMV is the silent menace because most individuals who contract the virus have no symptoms or only mild flulike symptoms. The virus will infect up to 80% of people in the United States by the time they reach the age of 40 (CDC, 2006). A virus in the herpes family causes CMV. Transmission is by contact with infected bodily fluids, such as saliva, blood, breast milk, urine, and semen. A common source of infection is young children. Once a person is infected, he or she will have the virus for life. A woman with dormant CMV who becomes pregnant can pass the virus to her fetus.

Congenital CMV infection is the most common congenital viral infection and is as common a cause of serious disability as Down's syndrome, fetal alcohol syndrome, and neural tube defects. About one third of the women who contract CMV for the first time during pregnancy will pass the infection to the fetus (CDC, 2006). The risk to the fetus from CMV infection is greatest during the first 20 weeks of pregnancy. Most affected newborns (approximately 90%) do not demonstrate symptoms at birth. However, as many as 15% of these infants develop progressive hearing loss that is usually unilateral, but may affect both ears. Signs that are likely to be present in the 10% of newborns who are symptomatic at birth include microcephaly, seizures, IUGR, hepatosplenomegaly, jaundice, and rash (Demmler, 2006). The antiviral drug ganciclovir (Cytovene), which is used to treat adult AIDS patients with CMV-related eye infections, is currently being investigated for its efficacy in treating newborns with congenital CMV infection.

Because there is no cure for congenital CMV, prevention is extremely important. Pregnant women who have contact with small children should practice meticulous hygiene. Although CMV is present in breast milk, the woman usually may breast-feed because CMV infection contracted while breast-feeding rarely causes serious problems. Family Teaching Tips: Preventing CMV Transmission During Pregnancy lists important teaching points to decrease the woman's chance she will develop CMV infection.

Herpes Simplex Virus

HSV is a STI caused by herpes simplex virus 1 (HSV-1) and herpes simplex virus 2 (HSV-2). The virus spreads by direct contact. In general, HSV-1 causes oral herpes, also known as cold sores, and HSV-2 causes genital herpes. However, both types can be transmitted to the mouth and/or genital region through kissing, oral–genital sex, and other sexual contact, and both types can cause serious illness in a newborn. Fortunately, neonatal herpes is rare, occurring in less than 0.1% of newborns (Wenner & Nashelsky, 2005); however, numbers may rise as overall rates of HSV infection are rising.

Family Teaching Tips

PREVENTING CMV TRANSMISSION DURING PREGNANCY

- Throughout the pregnancy, practice good personal hygiene, especially hand washing with soap and water, after contact with saliva and urine.
- Carefully dispose of all soiled diapers, tissues, or other potentially infected items.
- Avoid direct contact with the saliva of young children. Suggestions are to not participate in the following behaviors with young children (particularly those in day care).
  - Kissing on the lips
  - Sharing food
  - Sharing drinks or utensils
- If you develop a mononucleosislike illness (sore throat, low-grade fever, swollen lymph glands, body aches, and fatigue) during pregnancy, call your doctor to be evaluated for CMV infection.
- If you are concerned about congenital CMV, laboratory testing for antibody to CMV can be performed to determine if you already have CMV infection. If you do not have CMV antibodies, you should be especially attentive to good hygiene.
- In most cases, the demonstrated benefits of breast-feeding outweigh the minimal risk of the baby acquiring CMV from the breast milk. Talk with your doctor about your concerns so that you can make an informed decision.

Adapted from CDC recommendations found in the following reference.
Centers for Disease Control and Prevention (CDC). (2005). Information about CMV for clinicians and others in healthcare settings. Retrieved August 13, 2007, from http://www.cdc.gov/cmv/clinicians.htm

Symptoms of genital herpes usually develop within 2 to 14 days after exposure to the virus. Without antiviral treatment, the lesions may last for as long as 20 days. The first attack is generally the most severe, although approximately 80% of individuals with primary HSV infections have no symptoms. Painful lesions develop in the area exposed to the virus, usually the genital or anal regions. The lesions eventually completely heal and do not cause scarring. However, the virus lies dormant in the nervous system and can cause recurrent attacks. Flulike symptoms, such as lymphadenopathy, headache, muscle aches, and low-grade fever, sometimes occur a day or two before an outbreak (Lutwick & Seenivasan, 2006).

The majority of cases of neonatal herpes are contracted by contact with active virus in the birth canal, although small percentages (5%) of fetuses contract the infection in utero (Fischer, 2006). Most infants of women who

Table 16-3 ▌ **FORMS OF NEONATAL HSV INFECTION**

Manifestation of Neonatal Infection	Percentage of Cases
Skin, eye, or mouth disease with localized involvement	45%
Central nervous system disease with encephalitis. May or may not have the localized manifestations (above).	30%
Disseminated disease with multiple major organ involvement	25%

Note: The manifestations are listed in increasing order of severity.
Source: Cunningham, F. G., Leveno, K. J., Bloom, S. L., Hauth, J. C., Gilstrap, L. C. III, & Wenstrom, K. D. (Eds.). (2005). *Williams obstetrics* (22nd ed., pp. 1310). New York: McGraw-Hill Medical Publishing Division.

have longstanding herpes do not develop neonatal herpes. Authorities think this happens because maternal antibodies to herpes virus cross the placenta and protect the fetus. Preterm infants are more likely to contract herpes because antibodies do not begin to cross the placenta until approximately 28 weeks of gestation, so preterm infants do not have the same protection as full-term infants. The highest risk for neonatal herpes occurs in infants of women who develop herpes for the first time during the last trimester of pregnancy and who have active lesions in the birth canal at the time of delivery. In fact, the risk can be as high as 50% (Alter, 2007). Table 16-3 lists the three forms of newborn infection and the percentage at which each type occurs.

Treatment during pregnancy often includes a 1- to 2-week course of therapy with acyclovir for a first episode of HSV. Many practitioners prescribe suppressive therapy (see Table 16-2) beginning at 36 weeks' gestation because this seems to reduce the risk of an active outbreak at the time of delivery (Riley, 2007).

If the woman has a lesion at delivery, the safest alternative is cesarean delivery to prevent the baby from coming in contact with the virus in the birth canal. Vaginal examinations are withheld if there are active lesions. If there are no lesions present when the woman goes into labor, the American College of Obstetricians and Gynecologists recommends a vaginal delivery. Internal monitoring with a fetal scalp electrode is not recommended during labor in the woman with a history of genital herpes; the electrode can cause a small break in the fetal scalp and can serve as a portal of entry for the virus (Riley, 2007).

Sexually Transmitted Infections

An STI is an infection transmitted primarily by sexual contact or through contact with blood or bodily fluids. (STIs are also referred to as sexually transmitted diseases [STDs].) Many of the TORCH infections are STIs, including hepatitis B, syphilis, and herpes simplex. Other STIs of importance to the pregnant woman include chlamydia, gonorrhea, genital warts, trichomoniasis, and human immunodeficiency virus/acquired immunodeficiency syndrome (HIV/AIDS).

Many STIs are reportable diseases tracked by the CDC. Reportable infections include syphilis, chlamydia, gonorrhea, and HIV/AIDS. Some states require additional STIs to be reported. One increasing concern is that many STIs increase the risk for the individual to contract HIV/AIDS. If symptoms of the infection include a break in the integrity of the skin or mucous membranes, these sites can provide a portal of entry for HIV.

Chlamydia

Chlamydia is the most common STI in the United States, occurring in an estimated 4,000,000 cases per year (Zenilman, 2007). Infection with the bacterium *Chlamydia trachomatis* causes chlamydia. Participation in oral, vaginal, and anal sex increases the risk of contracting chlamydia.

Approximately 60% to 70% of women who have chlamydia have no symptoms (AHRQ, 2005), a fact that makes identification of the infection problematic. It also underscores the reality that although chlamydia is the most prevalent STI, it probably is grossly underreported. If the woman experiences symptoms, these may include vaginal discharge, abnormal vaginal bleeding, and abdominal or pelvic pain. Of several methods of diagnostic testing that are available, amplified DNA tests are the most sensitive. Acceptable specimens include urine and cervical secretions (Lazaro, 2006).

Untreated chlamydia increases the risk of contracting HIV/AIDS (Zenilman, 2007). The most frequent sequela of untreated chlamydia is pelvic inflammatory disease (PID), a serious infection of the reproductive tract that can lead to infertility and chronic pelvic pain. Inflammation of the fallopian tubes that occurs with PID often results in scarring, which increases the risk of ectopic pregnancy and subsequent infertility. A pregnant woman who contracts chlamydia is at increased risk for spontaneous abortion (miscarriage), preterm rupture of membranes, and preterm labor. The postpartum woman is at higher risk for endometritis (Fletcher & Ball, 2006). The fetus can encounter bacteria in the vagina during the birth process. If this happens, the newborn can develop pneumonia or conjunctivitis that can lead to blindness (Venkatesh & Hammerschlag, 2006).

Fortunately, chlamydia is easily curable with antibiotics. Treatment for the pregnant woman is with oral erythromycin or amoxicillin. As with other STIs, the sexual partners of the individual also require treatment.

Gonorrhea

Gonorrhea is an STI caused by the bacterium *Neisseria gonorrhoeae* (*N. gonorrhoeae*). Incidence rates have been declining or holding steady since 1996; however, in 2005, the rate increased for the first time since 1999. Gonorrhea is second in prevalence only to chlamydia (CDC, 2007b). Transmission of the bacteria occurs during sexual contact. The primary site of infection for the woman is the cervix, although infection can occur anywhere along the genital tract, in the urethra and rectum, and in the throat (Swygard, Seña, & Cohen, 2007).

Initial symptoms, which usually develop within 2 to 10 days of exposure to the bacteria, are mild and may go unnoticed. The woman who contracts gonorrhea may have vaginal bleeding during sexual intercourse, pain and burning while urinating, and a yellow or bloody vaginal discharge. A discharge from the rectum, itching around the anus, and painful bowel movements are signs of rectal infection, although the majority of rectal infections are asymptomatic (Swygard, Seña, & Cohen, 2007).

There are several methods used to diagnose gonorrhea. The most sensitive test for gonococcal infection is nucleic acid amplification. Urine, cervical, and vaginal specimens are appropriate for nucleic acid amplification testing. A culture taken from the cervix, rectum, or throat is often the diagnostic method of choice because it positively identifies *N. gonorrhea*, provides bacterial susceptibility information, and is widely available. In addition, culture is the only method approved for diagnosis of throat or rectal gonococcal infection (Workowski & Berman, 2006).

Treatment is usually with a combination of two antibiotics that treat both gonorrhea and chlamydia because these infections often occur together. One problem that has arisen recently is strains of *N. gonorrhoeae* that are resistant to antibiotics. Because of emerging resistant organisms, the CDC issued new treatment guidelines in 2007. One intramuscular dose of ceftriaxone, a cephalosporin, is the recommended treatment (Barclay, 2007). This treatment is appropriate for pregnant women. The CDC publishes guidelines for physicians to help prevent and treat antimicrobial resistance. Efforts are under way to develop a vaccine against gonorrhea.

Untreated gonorrhea can lead to PID, which can leave the woman infertile or susceptible to ectopic pregnancy because of scarring in the reproductive tract. The bacteria can also spread through the bloodstream and infect joints, heart valves, or the brain. Infection with gonorrhea greatly increases the risk of acquiring HIV infection.

Risk to pregnancy from gonococcal infection includes increased risk for chorioamnionitis, premature rupture of membranes, and preterm delivery (U.S. Preventive Services Task Force, 2005). Infection of the fetal eyes through contact with vaginal secretions during birth causes a condition known as ophthalmia neonatorum. Newborn blindness can result from this infection; however, cases are rare because all newborns receive prophylactic treatment with ocular antibiotic ointment within 1 hour after birth.

Human Papillomavirus

Human papillomavirus (HPV) is the most common viral STI in the United States. HPV spreads by skin-to-skin contact, usually during sexual activity. This mode of transmission differs from that of other STIs that only spread by contact with bodily fluids (Moscicki, Dempsey, & Humiston, 2006). This virus can cause condylomata acuminata (genital warts) and cervical cancer. An individual with asymptomatic HPV infection can unknowingly pass the virus on to sexual partners.

Condylomata acuminata develop in clusters on the vulva, within the vagina, on the cervix, or around the anus. The lesions may remain small, or they can develop into large clusters of warts that resemble cauliflower. An abnormal Papanicolaou (Pap) smear may be the first indication of HPV infection and should lead to further inspection for the virus. The practitioner makes the diagnosis by visualization of the warts or by applying a solution of acetic acid to areas of suspected infection. Acetic acid causes infected areas to turn white. The practitioner can take a biopsy of tissue and examine it microscopically for evidence of infection.

Genital warts can disappear without treatment. The type of treatment chosen depends on many factors, including age of the patient; duration, location, extent, and type of warts; the patient's immune status; risk of scarring; and pregnancy status. Several medical treatments are available, most of which consist of topical applications. Many of these treatments involve the use of teratogenic substances that are not for use during pregnancy. Surgical removal of the warts through a variety of techniques, including blunt dissection, laser, and cryosurgery, is a treatment option available to the pregnant woman (Fox & Tung, 2005).

Genital warts have a tendency to increase in size during pregnancy. This may result in heavy bleeding during vaginal delivery. The pregnant woman can pass HPV to her fetus during the birth process. In rare instances, neonatal HPV infection can result in life-threatening laryngeal papillomas. HPV infection transmitted to the infant may not appear for as long as 10 years after birth (Reichman, 2006a).

A vaccine for HPV became available in 2006. The FDA approved the vaccine for use in females 9 to 26 years of age. The practitioner administers the vaccine in a series of three shots over the course of 6 months. The vaccine protects against cervical cancer and genital warts.

Trichomoniasis

Trichomoniasis, or infection with Trichomonas, is an STI caused by one-celled protozoa. It can infect the urethra, vagina, cervix, and structures of the vulva. Unprotected sexual contact with someone who has the infection is the usual mode of transmission for Trichomonas. It is possible for the woman to transmit trichomoniasis to the fetus during vaginal delivery, although this is a rare occurrence.

Symptoms of trichomoniasis include large amounts of foamy, yellow-green vaginal discharge, vaginal itching, unusual vaginal odor, painful sex, and dysuria. Many women with trichomoniasis have no symptoms. The most common diagnostic test is the "wet mount." The practitioner takes a swab of vaginal secretions and examines the sample under the microscope. Unique movements of the organism allow for accurate diagnosis in 50% to 70% of cases. A culture is more sensitive than a wet mount, but results are not available for several days (Sobel, 2007).

The CDC recommends that the practitioner individualize treatment for the pregnant woman. If there are indications for treatment, the agent of choice is metronidazole (Flagyl). Although metronidazole is available in vaginal suppository and cream formats, the CDC recommends oral dosing because of its increased effectiveness in treating Trichomonas infection. The woman takes a single 2-g dose of oral metronidazole (Workowski & Berman, 2006). Expected side effects of treatment with oral metronidazole are metallic taste and dark urine. Nausea and vomiting can occur with high doses or when the woman drinks alcohol during treatment.

Trichomoniasis is associated with adverse pregnancy outcomes, in particular premature rupture of membranes, preterm delivery, and low birth weight. However, treatment with metronidazole does not reduce the incidence of these outcomes.

HIV/AIDS

In 1981, health care providers first encountered AIDS caused by HIV. HIV attacks the protective cells of the immune system, leaving the body unprotected against pathogens that normally do not cause illness in humans. Individuals who die of AIDS usually succumb to these opportunistic infections.

In 2005, there were between 4.3 and 6.6 million new cases of HIV infection in the United States, and approximately 17,000 people died of AIDS that year (Schuklenk & Kleinsmidt, 2007). African Americans are disproportionately affected. This group accounted for 49% of AIDS cases in 2005; however, African Americans only composed 13% of the population (CDC, 2007a). Women are at a higher risk than men for heterosexual transmission of the virus because the vaginal rugae are perfect for harboring the virus over time. Pregnant women are at even higher risk than are nonpregnant women for contracting HIV due to pregnancy-related physiological changes (Gray et al., 2005).

Transmission of HIV most often takes place during unprotected sexual activity with an infected partner. The virus can enter the body through the mucous membranes of the genitals, rectum, or mouth. People infected with HIV often do not look or feel sick and may transmit the virus to others before they know they are infected.

Contact with infected blood is another way to contract HIV. The risk of becoming HIV positive through receiving a blood transmission is very small because of screening and treatment of donated blood. However, exposure to HIV-infected blood by sharing needles for IV drug use, intramuscular injections of anabolic steroids, or tattooing can result in HIV infection.

A woman who has HIV during pregnancy is at risk for transmitting the infection to the fetus during pregnancy or childbirth and to the newborn while breast-feeding. Receiving appropriate antiretroviral treatment during pregnancy and childbirth and refraining from breast-feeding substantially reduce the risk of perinatal transmission.

Clinical Manifestations

There are several ways to stage HIV disease. This text describes four stages of HIV infection:

- Stage 1: Primary HIV infection
- Stage 2: Clinically asymptomatic HIV infection
- Stage 3: Symptomatic HIV infection
- Stage 4: Progression from HIV to AIDS

These stages correspond to viral loads (amounts of virus in the blood) and CD4-positive T-cell (CD4) counts (see Table 16-2).

In stage 1, the viral load is very high; the individual is highly infectious and may be asymptomatic or may have flulike symptoms. Unfortunately, the person is usually not aware of the HIV infection and continues to engage in risky behaviors, such as unprotected sexual intercourse and needle sharing. CD4 counts usually fall precipitously in stage 1 and then rebound to normal levels, above 500/mL of blood, over several weeks (Bartlett, 2007b). During this stage, the process of seroconversion (see Table 16-2) takes place. Seroconversion is complete when the individual has measurable levels of HIV antibodies. If the individual has an HIV test before seroconversion is complete, the test may show a false negative result.

In stage 2, the viral load is usually very low and sometimes undetectable; however, HIV antibodies are present, so traditional HIV tests are positive at this point. Although the viral blood count is low, the virus is busy replicating in lymphatic tissue, and the person continues to be infectious. CD4 counts are variable in stage 2, with lower counts associated with faster and more severe progression of the disease. The person is asymptomatic with the possible exception of enlarged lymph nodes (Bartlett, 2006).

In stage 3, symptomatic HIV infection, the individual has non-HIV specific symptoms. It is unknown why some HIV-positive individuals move rapidly into acute HIV disease in as little as 1 year, whereas others do not develop symptoms for 20 years or more. The average length of time from infection until onset of symptoms is 8 to 10 years. Once symptoms appear, the individual may seek treatment. Typical symptoms of acute HIV disease (Box 16-7) include swollen lymph nodes, feeling tired, weight loss, night sweats, fever, persistent oral or vaginal yeast infections, severe oral or genital herpes

Box 16-7 ▌ TYPICAL SYMPTOMS OF ACUTE HIV DISEASE

Acute HIV disease describes the symptoms that appear during Stage 3 of HIV infection. CD4 cell counts remain above 200/mL of blood during this phase. Typical symptoms include:

- Persistent generalized lymphadenopathy
- Generalized malaise
- Weight loss
- Night sweats
- Fever
- Thrush (oral yeast infection)
- Candidiasis (vaginal yeast infection)
- Oral hairy leukoplakia (lesion characterized by white plaque on the lateral aspects of the tongue)
- Aphthous ulcers (painful, shallow ulcers of the oral mucosa)
- Herpes simplex virus (outbreaks are often severe)
- Shingles (herpes zoster)
- Anemia with associated pallor
- Thrombocytopenia
- Aseptic meningitis
- Peripheral neuropathies
- Short-term memory loss

infections, shingles, skin rashes or scaly skin, and short-term memory loss. Women may develop severe PID that is not responsive to treatment.

When the individual moves into stage 4 of HIV infection, she has AIDS. The CDC defines AIDS as an HIV-positive individual who has less than 200 CD4 cells per milliliter of blood (Bartlett, 2006). Immunosuppression at this stage makes the person susceptible to opportunistic infections. Symptoms of opportunistic infections vary depending on the causative organism (bacteria, viruses, fungi, parasites, etc.). Symptoms may include extreme fatigue, dysphagia, coughing, dyspnea, nausea, vomiting, persistent diarrhea, severe weight loss, fever, confusion, ataxia, seizures, blindness, and even coma. The individual is also susceptible to various rare cancers that are difficult to treat.

Diagnosis

HIV may infect the pregnant woman during pregnancy, or she may enter pregnancy with HIV. It is very important for the practitioner to know the pregnant woman's HIV status. The CDC recommends that practitioners offer confi-

Be alert!

The HIV-positive woman may be at higher risk for domestic violence and homelessness (Lachat & Relf, 2006). Carefully assess the woman's emotional status and levels of social support.

dential HIV testing at the beginning of pregnancy and again during labor. The woman may refuse testing, but the practitioner is encouraged to counsel with the woman and explore reasons for refusal.

At present, there are several methods to test for HIV infection: the traditional enzyme-linked immunosorbent assay (ELISA) and the Western blot analysis; and newer tests that detect viral RNA. Both the ELISA and Western blot test for antibodies to the virus versus the virus itself. Antibodies to HIV usually develop within 6 to 12 weeks after exposure; however, it can take as long as 6 months for antibodies to appear. The newer tests measure viral load. At least one test is able to detect HIV, even at low levels of the virus. If levels are low at the first test, the practitioner will often test again later. Rising levels are diagnostic (Colson & Sax, 2007).

Rapid diagnostic testing of the newborn is important in order to initiate HAART quickly for the HIV-positive newborn and to allow discontinuation of therapy with concomitant side effects for the HIV-negative newborn. Unfortunately, all infants born to HIV-infected women have antibodies to HIV because the woman's antibodies cross the placenta. Therefore, an infant must be at least 18 months of age before traditional testing methods can detect HIV infection. In addition, measures of viral load are usually not accurate because the woman has been on antiretroviral therapy, which also suppresses viral load in the fetus and newborn. The standard diagnostic test for infants younger than 18 months of age is the HIV DNA polymerase chain reaction test. The practitioner orders the test at birth, and then repeats testing at 4 to 6 weeks of age, and approximately 2 months after the second test. If the results are positive at any time, the practitioner immediately orders a confirmation test. If the results of the initial tests are negative, the infant is tested at 12 months of age (Schwartzwald, 2007).

Treatment

The two main goals of treatment for the pregnant woman infected with HIV are to prevent progression of the disease in the woman and to prevent perinatal transmission of the virus to the fetus.[1] The best way to prevent perinatal transmission is to prevent HIV infection in the woman or to identify HIV infection before pregnancy or as early as possible during pregnancy. Therefore, early prenatal care for all women, regardless of risk, is imperative.

In general, therapy for the pregnant woman is the same as that recommended for the nonpregnant woman. Currently available data from the Antiretroviral Pregnancy Registry demonstrates a birth defect rate that is equal to that of the general population for infants born to women on antiretroviral therapy during the first trimester of pregnancy. For the pregnant woman with

---

[1] In depth discussion of treatment for HIV for non-pregnant individuals is outside the scope of this textbook.

HIV, therapy is composed of, at the very least, oral zidovudine (ZDV) prophylaxis, beginning as early as 14 weeks' gestation and continuing throughout pregnancy. The practitioner may withhold ZDV in the first trimester of pregnancy to avoid possible teratogenic effects, although to date the data do not demonstrate adverse fetal effects of ZDV administration in early pregnancy. The Perinatal HIV Guidelines Working Group (2006) views monotherapy (see Table 16-2) with ZDV to be suboptimal treatment for the pregnant woman, and currently recommends aggressive treatment with HAART. The Perinatal HIV Guidelines Working Group 2006 report, "Recommendations for use of antiretroviral drugs in pregnant HIV-1-infected women for maternal health and interventions to reduce perinatal HIV-1 transmission in the United States," outlines specific recommendations and precautions.

In addition, there are new therapies in development. One newly discovered medication that improves pregnancy outcomes in women with very low (<200/μL) CD4 counts is cotrimoxazole. Antepartum treatment with this medication reduces the incidence of low birth weight, preterm delivery, chorioamnionitis, and neonatal mortality (Watts & Mofenson, 2006).

The practitioner counsels the HIV-positive woman regarding the advisability of cesarean delivery scheduled at 38 weeks' gestation to further reduce the risk of perinatal transmission. Several studies have shown that women who take antiretroviral medication during pregnancy and experience vaginal delivery have an increased risk of transmitting the virus to their babies; whereas, women who take ZDV and/or HAART throughout pregnancy and have a cesarean delivery before the membranes rupture have a very low (<1%) chance of perinatal transmission. If the woman elects for a vaginal delivery, the woman receives IV ZDV during labor and birth. The infant receives oral ZDV for the first 6 weeks of life followed by prophylaxis for *P. carinii* pneumonia, a rare pneumonia associated with HIV infection. Breast-feeding by HIV-infected women is not recommended in the United States due to the risk of HIV transmission to the infant (Public Health Task Force, 2006). If these recommendations for prophylaxis are followed, the risk for perinatal transmission decreases from 25% to 35% for the untreated woman to as low as 1% to 2% for the treated woman (Simpson, 2006).

Nursing Care

Reassure the client that her care providers will protect her confidentiality. Provide information concerning HIV infection and AIDS in an open, nonjudgmental manner. Explain the benefits of knowing HIV status early in pregnancy. Encourage the woman to be tested. Be certain that the woman knows how to protect herself from HIV infection by avoiding high-risk behaviors.

If the woman is HIV-positive, ensure that she understands the risk to her sexual partners and the importance of condom use. Counsel her regarding expected treatments. Explain the risks of perinatal transmission of HIV and the benefits of therapy. Explore her understanding of the treatment regimen.

Nursing Process for the Pregnant Woman With an STI

Although different organisms cause STIs, avoiding high-risk behaviors can prevent them all. As the nurse, you can help identify women who are at risk for STIs and facilitate testing. For women who are negative for an STI, provide education regarding safe behaviors to prevent contracting an STI in the future. For women who are positive, provide nonjudgmental, compassionate care and assist the woman to cope with the diagnosis and treatment.

Assessment

Assessment begins with a thorough history. Current CDC guidelines encourage health care providers, including nurses, to routinely obtain sexual histories from all patients (Workowski & Berman, 2006). Inquire regarding risk factors for STIs in a way that makes the woman feel safe to answer honestly. Box 16-8 outlines key techniques you can use to develop rapport and elicit information that will identify risk factors for STIs.

Tact and understanding are in order! It is best not to pressure the woman to reveal risky behaviors. Instead, you can make her aware of behaviors that increase her risk of contracting an STI.

The history should include questions regarding symptoms of STI. Does she have a vaginal discharge? If so, have her describe the discharge. Is sex painful? Does she bleed during or after sex? Has she noticed swollen lymph nodes? Has she been running low-grade fevers? Has she noticed any rashes or skin lesions? Has she experienced night sweats or lost weight without trying to do so?

Take note of signs of emotional distress, anxiety, or low self-esteem. Does she practice good personal hygiene? Self-esteem issues can express themselves by self-neglect and poor grooming. Does she make appropriate eye contact? Inquire regarding her social support. Does she have friends? Does she live with anyone? Does she have a partner? Is he or she supportive of her? Notice nonverbal behaviors such as fidgeting, hand wringing, or inattention.

Psychosocial issues to consider that affect the woman's compliance with the treatment plan include the following:

■ *Substance abuse* contributes to a chaotic lifestyle and increased risk for missing medication doses and participation in high-risk behaviors.

Box 16-8 ▮ TECHNIQUES FOR TAKING A SEXUAL HISTORY

Setting the Stage

- Create an environment conducive to talking about sensitive issues.
- Appear relaxed and pursue the history as you would for any other medical problem.
- Make certain the patient is in a private location, free from distractions.
- The patient should be dressed (not in an exam gown).
- In almost all circumstances, it should just be you and the patient.

Introducing the Topic of Sexual Activity

- Explain why you are taking a sexual history and acknowledge the sensitive nature of the questions.
- Explain that you take a sexual history on every patient so the person does not feel singled-out.
- Reinforce confidentiality and convey permission to be frank.
- Integrate the sexual history into the lifestyle assessment (smoking, alcohol, caffeine intake, etc.) or into the genitourinary system review.
- Say, for example, "I take a sexual history on all patients as part as their health assessment. I know some questions may be sensitive, but the answers are important for me to know so I can provide adequate care. I need to understand if you are at risk for STIs. Any information you give me is strictly confidential and will stay between us."

Asking the Questions

- Begin with open-ended questions such as "Tell me about . . . ." This technique encourages a more complete sexual history.
- Avoid leading questions.
- Use words appropriate for the level of understanding and be clear.
- Be nonjudgmental and sensitive.
- Nonverbal communication should convey comfort and responsiveness.
- Introduce questions by a generalizing statement, such as "people have sex in many different ways." This is less threatening for the patient. She will not feel like she is the only one engaging in these activities and may feel more comfortable describing her behavior.
- Think of the "Five Ps" to cover all the topics involved in a sexual history: Partners, Prevention of Pregnancy, Protection from STIs, Practices, and Past History of STIs.

Partners

- "Do you have sex with men, women, or both?"
- "In the past 2 months, how many new partners have you had sex with?"
- "In the past 12 months, how many sexual partners have you had?"

Prevention of Pregnancy

- "Are you or your partner trying to get pregnant?"
- If no, "What are you doing to prevent pregnancy?"

Protection from STIs

- "What do you do to protect yourself from STIs and HIV?"

Practices

- "To understand your risks for STIs, I need to understand the kind of sex you have had recently."
- "Have you had vaginal sex, meaning 'penis in the vagina' sex?" If yes, "Do you use condoms: never, sometimes, or always?"
- "Have you had anal sex, meaning 'penis in the rectum/anus' sex?" If yes, "Do you use condoms: never, sometimes, or always?"
- "Have you had oral sex, meaning 'mouth on penis/vagina'?"

For condom answers

- If "never," "Why don't you use condoms?"
- If "sometimes," "In what situations or with whom do you not use condoms?"

Past History of and Risk for STIs

- "Have you ever had an STI?"
- "Have any of your partners had an STI?"
- "Have you or any of your partners ever injected drugs?"
- "Have any of your partners exchanged money or drugs for sex?"
- "Is there anything else about your sexual practices that I need to know about?"

It is always helpful to leave the door open for concerns the patient may have (e.g., "*Do you have any sexual concerns you would like to discuss?*").

Responding to the Answers

- Do not act surprised, shocked, or embarrassed by the answers you get.
- Do not be judgmental.
- Clarify the answer by asking about specific sexual behaviors (e.g., "*By sexual activity, I mean to ask if you are having any oral, vaginal, or anal sex.*"). Patients may interpret the language "sexual activity" differently than you do.

(continues on page 370)

Box 16-8 ■ TECHNIQUES FOR TAKING A SEXUAL HISTORY *(continued)*

■ Clarify the time frame (e.g., *"When was the last time you had sex?"*).

■ Ask follow-up questions (e.g., *"You told me that the last time you had sex was 1 month ago and it was oral sex. Can you tell me more about this encounter?"*).

Accepting Differences
Gender

■ Assess the gender of sexual partners (e.g., *"Do you have sex with men, women, or both?" "Tell me about your sexual partner(s) . . ."*) before asking any questions that are gender specific, such as the method of birth control, male condom use, or penile penetration.

■ The patient should feel comfortable that revealing their sexual orientation will not result in poor care, a negative reaction, or abandonment. Convey this by your comfortable and nonjudgmental attitude.

Culture

■ When seeing patients from another country, assess the degree of acculturation to the United States. Consider the following factors that may mean a lesser degree of acculturation:

• Recent immigration to the United States at an older age
• Frequent returns to the country of origin
• Emigration from a rural area
• Lack of or limited formal education
• Lower socioeconomic status
• Inexperience with Western health care systems
• Major differences in language, dress, and diet

■ For language barriers, consider obtaining the services of an interpreter.
■ Avoid jargon.
■ Speak clearly with words that the patient can easily understand. For example, use the word "sore" or "scab" versus "lesion" or "breakdown."
■ Be careful not to talk down to the patient.
■ Try to understand as much about the person and her culture as you can.

Adapted from information in the following references:
Workowski, K. A., & Berman, S. M. (2006). Sexually transmitted diseases treatment guidelines, 2006. *MMWR Recommendations and Reports, 55*(RR11), 1–94.
New England STD/HIV Prevention Training Center, (Eds.). (Undated). Sexual history taking: A case-based module of the. Retrieved August 18, 2007, from http://www.mass.gov/dph/cdc/stdtcmai/section1.pdf

---

■ *Psychiatric disorders*, such as depression or bipolar disorder, may interfere with the person's ability or desire to follow the treatment plan and avoid high-risk behaviors.

■ *Inadequate housing* can contribute to poor compliance with the treatment plan because the individual can forget to take medications or may have trouble storing medications.

■ *Support* from a friend or family member can go a long way to increase adherence to the treatment plan. If the woman is trying to hide evidence of an STI, she may miss medication doses.

■ *Work conditions*, such as irregular schedules or very rigid conditions that do not allow for appropriate breaks, including access to restrooms, can interfere with the person's ability to manage medications.

■ *Ability to pay for medications* is essential; if the individual has to choose between food and medication, there is little doubt she will choose food (Bartlett, 2007a).

Perform a physical assessment. Measure her weight. Compare her current weight to her previous or normal weight. Note any recent weight loss. Record her temperature and other vital signs. Some STIs cause a low-grade fever. Palpate the lymph nodes in the neck and groin regions. Report any swollen or nonmobile nodes. Inspect the oral mucosa and tongue for lesions. Inspect the skin thoroughly for rashes or lesions.

Selected Nursing Diagnoses

■ Risk for Infection (STI) related to unsafe sexual practices, IV drug use, or needle sharing.
■ Ineffective Protection related to altered immune status or broken skin barrier.
■ Deficient Knowledge of STI and treatment regimen.
■ Risk for Situational Low Self-Esteem related to the stigma associated with STIs.
■ Anxiety related to pregnancy outcome and fetal safety.

Outcome Identification and Planning

Goals for a pregnant woman with an STI include risk control, prevention of the spread of infection, adequate knowledge, maintaining positive self-esteem, anxiety control, and safe delivery of a healthy, infection-free infant. Individualize goals and interventions according to the needs of the woman and her fetus throughout pregnancy, birth, and the postpartum period.

Implementation
Controlling Risks for STIs

Explain the risks of contact with infected bodily fluids and blood. Clarify that women are at higher risk than are men for contracting an STI during heterosexual intercourse. Make clear that the highest risk of STI transmission during sexual activity is engaging in anal intercourse without a condom. Emphasize the importance of using a latex condom for every act of sexual intercourse and a latex barrier for oral sex. Inform the woman to avoid sexual intercourse when there are open lesions or discharge on the genitals. She should also avoid oral sex when lesions or discharge are present on the mouth or genitals.

Instruct the woman regarding proper hand-washing techniques and the importance of frequent hand washing. If the woman is an IV drug user, assist her to find a needle exchange program, if one is available in the area. Help her devise a plan to avoid needle sharing. Assist her to enter a treatment program, if this is feasible and acceptable to the woman.

Maintaining Immune Status and Protection From Additional Infections

Teach the woman that infection with one STI puts her at higher risk for contracting another STI. This is particularly true for STIs that cause lesions or skin breakdown. Explain the importance of having all sexual partners treated for the infection. She should take her medication as directed.

Give instructions specific to the STI. If the woman is HIV positive, ensure that she understands the importance of diligently taking her antiretroviral medications daily. Explain that these medications control the viral load (amount of virus in the blood) and help maintain CD4 counts in the protective range.

Ensuring Knowledge of STI and Treatment Regimen

Teach the woman the specifics of the STI she is experiencing. Be sure that she can explain how the infection is transmitted, what the symptoms of infection are, how to avoid spreading the infection to her sexual partners, how to decrease the risk of transmitting the infection to her fetus, and what the treatment plan and goals are.

Verify understanding of the treatment regimen by asking the woman to describe the medications she is taking and when and how she is to take them. Have her explain the expected action of each medication, as well as expected side effects. Teach her to immediately report side effects she may find intolerable so that the physician can adjust her medications without jeopardizing her treatment. Explain the importance of completing the full course of treatment, even after symptoms subside, to prevent the development of resistant strains of the organism.

Enhancing Self-Esteem

Maintain an open, accepting demeanor when interacting with the woman. Ensure she is in a comfortable, private place before interviewing her. Avoid asking potentially embarrassing questions in the presence of others. Avoid negative criticisms and judgmental questions such as "Why didn't you?" or "You should have . . . ." Encourage the woman to identify personal strengths. Convey confidence in the woman's ability to take care of her unborn child.

Reducing Anxiety

Use a calm, reassuring approach. Seek to understand the woman's perception of the risk to herself and to her fetus. Encourage the woman to verbalize her feelings. Use active listening. Ask for clarification when you do not understand.

Give factual information. Correct any misperceptions or misinformation the woman may have. Reassure the woman regarding the probable outcome of her pregnancy. Use up-to-date facts from reliable sources to avoid false reassurances. Help her understand the risks without causing unnecessary fear. For instance, you can explain that with treatment the risk of an HIV-positive woman transmitting HIV to her unborn child is less than 1% to 2%. Put another way, more than 98% of babies born to women with HIV disease who receive appropriate treatment will be born free of infection and will remain so.

Evaluation: Goals and Expected Outcomes

Goal: The woman will control risks for STIs.
Expected Outcomes: The woman

- verbalizes ways she will reduce her risk for contracting or transmitting STIs.
- maintains a monogamous sexual relationship with one partner who is also monogamous or partner uses a latex condom for every act of sexual intercourse.
- avoids anal sex.
- avoids IV drug use or participates in a needle exchange program.

Goal: The woman will not spread infection.
Expected Outcomes: The woman

- remains free of additional infections.
- maintains a plasma CD4 cell count above 200/mL (if HIV positive).

Goal: The woman will have adequate knowledge of the STI and its treatment.
Expected Outcomes: The woman

- explains how the STI is transmitted.
- describes how to prevent transmission to sexual partners and decrease the risk of transmission to the fetus.
- explains her treatment regimen.
- verbalizes the goals of her treatment plan.

Goal: The woman will maintain positive self-esteem.
Expected Outcomes: The woman

- demonstrates positive self-regard.
- makes positive statements about herself.
- maintains adequate personal hygiene.
- voices confidence in her ability to take care of her unborn child.

Goal: The woman will have decreased anxiety.
Expected Outcomes: The woman

- expresses reasonable expectations regarding the outcome of the pregnancy.
- verbalizes decreased anxiety.

Test Yourself

✔ Which infection is best prevented by instructing the pregnant woman to avoid changing the cat litter box?

✔ Which STI is most frequently diagnosed with a "wet mount?"

✔ What is the purpose of antiretroviral medications for the pregnant woman who is HIV positive?

PREGNANCY COMPLICATED BY INTIMATE PARTNER VIOLENCE

Intimate partner violence (IPV) is abuse perpetrated by an individual against an intimate partner. The goal of the abusive behavior is to exert and maintain power and control over the partner. Abuse refers to any type of injury committed against a person, including physical, emotional, psychological, and sexual maltreatment (Box 16-9). An intimate partner is any person who is now or who ever has been in an intimate relationship with the victim. This definition includes present and former spouses, boyfriends, girlfriends, and dating partners. IPV occurs in relationships without regard to sexual preference. In other words, IPV occurs between same sex partners, as well as between heterosexual partners. IPV crosses social, cultural, religious, and economic boundaries. Other terms used to describe IPV are domestic violence, spouse abuse, domestic abuse, and battering.

It is difficult to determine the extent of IPV, partly because it is unknown how many cases of IPV go unreported. Varied definitions used to collect and report these data contribute to the confusion. The CDC is attempting to correct this problem by developing standardized terminology and definitions. Although men can be the victims of IPV, more women report abuse. Every year in the United States, at least 2.1 million women are raped or physically assaulted. Intimate partners perpetrate an astonishing 75% of these assaults (Koenig et al., 2006).

Pregnancy is a vulnerable time for a woman. IPV may begin or escalate during pregnancy, particularly if the pregnancy is unplanned. Researchers estimate that 4% to 8% of all pregnant women experience abuse during the pregnancy. Some studies show that women who experience IPV during pregnancy are at much higher risk to be the victim of homicide (Lutz, 2005).

The pregnant woman is at risk for certain complications associated with abuse. According to Cunningham et al. (2005), a pregnant woman who is a victim of domestic violence has a three-fold increased risk of

---

Box 16-9 ■ EXAMPLES OF ABUSIVE ACTS

The terms "abuse" or "abused" are often misunderstood to refer only to egregious acts of violence that result in serious physical injury. Therefore, it is important for the health care professional to give specific examples of abuse when screening for intimate partner violence (IPV).

Physical Acts of Abuse
- Punching
- Hitting
- Kicking
- Slapping
- Shoving
- Biting
- Scratching
- Grabbing
- Choking
- Poking
- Shaking
- Hair pulling
- Burning

Emotional Acts of Abuse
- Threats of harm to self, the intimate partner, or others
- Refusing to interact with the intimate partner without explanation ("silent treatment")
- Name calling
- Put downs
- Derogatory comments
- Any act of control
  - Financial (controlling all the money)
  - Decision making (without consulting the partner)
  - Isolation from family or friends
  - Prohibiting access to transportation or telephone
- Threatening or completing acts of violence against pets or children
- Destroying property the intimate partner cares about
- Blaming the intimate partner for his or her violent outbursts

Sexual Acts of Abuse
- Forcing the partner to watch or perform any sexual act against the partner's will.

---

antepartum hemorrhage and fetal growth restriction and an eight-fold increase in fetal death. She is also at increased risk for preterm labor, chorioamnionitis, and delivering by cesarean section, and her infant is more likely to have a low birth weight.

Clinical Manifestations and Diagnosis

Abuse may begin slowly and escalate with time, or abusive episodes may begin early in a relationship. The Cycle

■ Figure 16-3 The cycle of violence.

of Violence (Fig. 16-3) is a generally accepted model that explains the pathophysiology of IPV. Abusive episodes usually progress in three identifiable phases:

1. Tension building phase
2. Explosion phase
3. Absence of tension or the "honeymoon phase"

Although it is not always possible to identify IPV during interactions with the victim or abuser, there are warning signs. The perpetrator of IPV often exhibits an overly protective attitude toward the victim. The abuser may accompany the victim to all office visits and may answer questions for the victim. It is important to remember that he may seem pleasant and congenial. Conversely, he may make degrading remarks about the victim in front of health care providers or others. If the partner refuses to leave the room so that the practitioner cannot interview the patient alone, the practitioner should be highly suspicious and look closer for other signs of abuse (Sillman, 2005).

The victim may appear quiet and passive. She may avoid eye contact. She may have an unkempt appearance and may appear depressed. She may exhibit anxiety, nervousness, and suicidal tendencies. She may abuse alcohol or drugs in response to the abuse. Box 16-10 lists clues that should raise the suspicion of abuse.

Treatment

Because every woman is at risk for IPV, routine screening of all women is the key to assisting those who are

ready to report abuse and receive help. Routine screening and direct questioning about abuse increases the likelihood that the woman will disclose that she is abused (Sillman, 2005). In particular, the prenatal period presents an excellent opportunity for screening for IPV. Prenatal visits offer opportunities for the health care provider to develop rapport and trust with the woman. The perinatal period is also a unique time of opportunity because the woman may be motivated to think about the future and the safety of her unborn child.

Although screening is a powerful tool, common barriers may get in the way. The health care provider may feel that she does not have enough time to ask about IPV. Often, providers feel uncomfortable addressing the issue. The provider may be afraid of embarrassing or offending the woman. Many times, providers avoid screening because he or she feels helpless to do anything to change the situation (Furniss et al., 2007). Because screening is a critical intervention for the victim of IPV, ACOG and the CDC recommend provider training to overcome these barriers.

Interventions for the victim of IPV are directed toward safety assessment and planning. Danger signals include statements from the woman that she or her children are in danger, that the violence has recently escalated, the partner has threatened to kill, or that there are lethal weapons (particularly guns) in the home. If the likelihood of danger exists, the health care provider assists the woman to develop a safety plan (Box 16-11).

Trained health care providers discuss options with the woman. The woman has three options:

Box 16-10 ■ CLUES THAT MAY INDICATE THE WOMAN IS BEING ABUSED

Any of the following signs should raise the suspicion of possible intimate partner violence (IPV). It is important to remember that a woman who is being abused may not show obvious signs of abuse.

- History of
  - Repeated assaults
  - Drug or alcohol abuse
  - Depression
  - Suicide attempts
- Injury* to the head, face, or neck
- Loose or broken teeth
- Injury to the breasts or abdomen
- Types of injury to include
  - Injury inflicted by a weapon
  - Cigarette and rope burns
  - Bite marks
  - Bruises and welts
- Pattern and distribution of injury to include
  - Areas normally covered by clothes
  - Occurring on both sides of the body (often on extremities)
  - Defensive posture injuries (such as to the hands or feet that occur when the victim tries to ward off the attacker)
- Injuries in various stages of healing
- Injuries that do not match the cause of trauma described by the woman or her partner

Signs unique to the pregnant woman may include

- Presents for late prenatal care or has no prenatal care
- Attends prenatal visits sporadically
- High gravidity and parity rates
- Poor weight gain during pregnancy
- History of
  - Spontaneous abortion(s)
  - STIs
  - Previous fetal death

---

*Injury can be evidenced by bruises, scrapes, scratches, or cuts, as well as burns, broken bones, etc.

(Adapted from Anderson, C. (2002). Battered and pregnant: A nursing challenge. *AWHONN Lifelines*, 6[2], 95–99; Wadman, M. C., & Foral, J. [2003]. Domestic violence. In J. A. Salomone, F. Talavera, D. E. Houry, J. Adler, & J. S. Cohen [Eds.], *eMedicine*. Last updated March 18, 2003.

Box 16-11 ■ COMPONENTS OF A SAFETY PLAN

Whether or not the woman elects to stay in the abusive relationship, she should have a safety plan. The health care provider instructs her to

- Memorize the National Domestic Violence Hotline: 1-800-799-SAFE (7233) or 1-800-787-3224 (for hearing-impaired or deaf victims).
- Pack a bag in advance with cash, credit cards, and clothes for herself and children. The bag should remain at a trusted friend or family member's house.
- Have important personal documents readily accessible. These include
  - Birth certificates
  - Driver's license
  - Bank account information
  - Important telephone numbers
  - Insurance information and cards
  - Court documents or orders
  - Copies of utility bills
- Establish a code word with family and friends to indicate when violence is escalating and help is needed.
- Identify a safe place to go. This may be a women's shelter or other safe place. Each community has unique resources that should be identified for the woman.

Nursing Care

There are many reasons that it is difficult to discuss domestic violence with patients. Myths abound, such as IPV happens in only certain socioeconomic or ethnic groups or the woman could just leave if she were not so weak or codependent. Often a nurse's own discomfort leads to avoidance of the subject. You may feel powerless to do anything about the situation, and therefore do not bring up the subject. Or, you may lack knowledge about how to screen for abuse. Whatever the barrier, you can learn to screen pregnant women for IPV.

Assist the RN to assess for abuse. Always screen the woman alone, away from children and the abuser. Provide privacy. Ask simple, direct, open-ended questions in a nonjudgmental way to show the victim that

Sometimes it is better to err on the side of caution!

You may not be the best person to screen for IPV. If you have not been trained, it is better to report your suspicions of abuse to an RN or other health care provider with training to deal with victims of abuse. However, do not allow your discomfort with the subject to hinder you from learning how to screen for violence.

- Stay with the abuser.
- Remove the abuser through arrest or with protective orders.
- Leave the relationship temporarily or permanently.

It is important for the provider to keep in mind that the woman is the only one who can truly determine which option is best for her.

you are a safe person when she is ready to disclose. Avoid questions that imply that the woman is responsible for the violence or that it is easy to walk away from a violent relationship. Questions to avoid include, "Why do you not just leave? What did you do to make your partner so angry? Why do you go back to your partner?" Remember, determining whether a woman should leave an abusive relationship is always only her decision to make.

Always document the woman's responses to questioning about IPV. If the woman denies being in an abusive relationship, document her denial. It is important to quote the woman directly. Do not use terms such as "alleges" when you are documenting the woman's replies. This terminology may cast doubt on the veracity of the woman's answers if the medical record becomes evidence in a court of law.

If the woman discloses IPV, be careful to respond with supportive statements. One of the most important things you can communicate to the victim of abuse is the fact that the abuse is not her fault! You can say, "This is not your fault. No one deserves to be treated this way." Examples of other helpful statements include, "I'm sorry that you've been hurt. Do you want to talk about it? I am concerned for your safety. You have options. Help is available."

Document your assessment objectively. If there are physical indications of abuse, draw these on a body map, then use measurable terminology to describe each lesion or observation. Photographs can be invaluable aids in a courtroom. You must get the woman's written consent before photographing her, however.

Be knowledgeable about local resources that are available for the victim of IPV. Resources include office and hospital personnel with specialized training, IPV advocacy groups, women's shelters, hotlines, child protective services, and law enforcement resources. Many cities have city-wide plans to respond to IPV. Be familiar with your city's plan.

By showing compassion and developing the trust of the abused woman, you can help turn the tide of abuse. Recovery from IPV does not happen in only one or two interventions; rather, it is a consistent atmosphere of encouragement and esteem building that may assist the victim to become a survivor.

PREGNANCY COMPLICATED BY AGE-RELATED CONCERNS

The typical childbearing years include the ages of 15 through 44 years; however, females can, and sometimes do, become pregnant anywhere from ages 9 through 56 years of age. At either end of the age spectrum, pregnancy carries higher risk for morbidity and mortality for the woman and her fetus. Although age-related concerns warrant special "at-risk" considerations, they are not in the pathophysiologic category, as are the medical conditions discussed earlier in the chapter. Instead, they are a natural part of the reproductive process requiring additional accommodations throughout the perinatal period.

Adolescent Pregnancy

Adolescent, or teen, pregnancy is pregnancy occurring at 19 years of age or younger. The consequences of teenage pregnancy are well documented. According to the CDC (2007e), teenage mothers have many roadblocks to current and future success. The major roadblocks include lower education levels and higher levels of poverty. In addition, adolescent mothers are more likely to participate in behaviors that increase the risk for poor birth outcomes, such as smoking; late, sporadic, or no prenatal care; and failure to gain sufficient weight. The pregnant adolescent is more likely to experience pregnancy complications, such as anemia, preeclampsia-eclampsia, and STIs (Malamitsi-Puchner & Boutsikou, 2006). There are also considerable consequences for the infants of adolescent mothers. Infants of teen mothers are more likely to be below normal birth weight and to be born prematurely. Infants of adolescent mothers have three times higher neonatal mortality rate than do infants of older mothers (Bryant, 2006).

Adolescent pregnancy and birth rates steadily declined from 61.8 births per 1,000 females aged 15 to 19 years in 1991, to a low of 40.5 births per 1,000 in 2005 (Hamilton, Martin, & Ventura, 2007). Unfortunately, adolescent pregnancy and birth rates significantly increased in 2006 (Hamilton, Martin, & Ventura, 2007). Nevertheless, the current rate of 41.9 births per 1,000 surpasses the *Healthy People 2010* goal of decreasing teen pregnancy to 43 pregnancies per 1,000 females. The challenges include huge racial disparities that still exist in teen pregnancy and birth rates with African American and Hispanic teenagers disproportionately affected. In addition, there is a wide range of adolescent birth rates among the states. In 2005 (the latest year for which data is available), teen birth rates ranged from a high of 61.6 in Texas and New Mexico to a low of 17.9 in New Hampshire (Martin et al., 2007). The two foremost explanations for the overall decrease in teen pregnancy and birth rates are an increased use of contraception that accounts for 77% of the decline, and increased rates of abstinence that accounts for 23% of the decline (Santelli et al., 2007).

Clinical Manifestations

Many pregnant teens seek late prenatal care, often in the third trimester, or they return sporadically for prenatal visits. Sometimes they get no prenatal care. Many factors contribute to poor prenatal care and subsequent complications of pregnancy. Recent research points to the social situation of the adolescent as the root cause of increased pregnancy risk, rather than age itself. The pregnant teen is more likely than her older counterpart is to be unmarried, have less education, be a member of an ethnic minority, and to live in poverty (Garofalo, 2006).

The adolescent faces many barriers to receiving adequate prenatal care. The pregnant teen may be fearful of disclosing her pregnancy to her parents or caregivers, so she may attempt to hide the pregnancy by wearing loose clothing, and avoiding prolonged interaction with adults.

Or she may lack family support or transportation to attend prenatal visits regularly. Because body image is extremely important to the adolescent, she may use behaviors associated with eating disorders, such as purging or self-starvation, to avoid weight gain during the pregnancy. The pregnant adolescent may not get adequate nutrition secondary to poor food choices. There is increasing evidence that pregnant teens are at increased risk for domestic violence. This situation can also lead to sporadic attendance to prenatal visits. Whatever the reason for not receiving good prenatal care, the pregnant adolescent is at increased risk for complications, such as inadequate weight gain, anemia, and preeclampsia-eclampsia. All of these conditions can result in fetal complications, such as IUGR, low birth weight, and preterm birth.

Diagnosis of adolescent pregnancy is made with the same tests used for older women. However, the diagnosis can be easily missed if the practitioner does not keep in mind the prospect of pregnancy when performing a history and physical. Adolescents often deny the possibility of pregnancy (even to themselves), making diagnosis even more challenging. The practitioner should test for pregnancy if the adolescent reports irregular periods, nausea and vomiting, or fatigue.

Treatment

The best treatment for teenage pregnancy is prevention. Many physicians and advanced practice nurses are actively involved in programs designed to prevent adolescent pregnancy. Others are involved in research studies attempting to discover which methods work and which do not. Much of the literature on adolescent pregnancy concentrates on prevention.

The challenge of managing an adolescent pregnancy is considerable. Although obtaining information about the woman's physical and psychological response to pregnancy and the social support available to her is important for any pregnant woman's care, this part of the history is particularly valuable for the pregnant teen. If the adolescent does not have adequate social support, she is more likely to experience adverse outcomes. Other areas of the history to which the practitioner pays close attention include determining the teen's perception of options available to her, HIV and other STI risk factors, and school status. Because perinatal and postpartum depression and IPV are associated with adolescent pregnancy, it is particularly important for the practitioner to screen for signs of depression and domestic violence (Nelson, Sherin, & Garland, 2006; Secco et al., 2007).

The informed practitioner does several things to assist the pregnant teen. Advocacy for the pregnant adolescent includes giving information in an open, nonjudgmental way and supporting the adolescent's choices. This approach requires that the practitioner treat the adolescent with dignity and respect by providing and protecting the right to privacy and confidentiality. Advocacy includes assisting the teen to freely make choices without coercion.

One crucial part of management includes helping the teen to develop an adequate support network. Parents, teachers, friends, and the father of the baby are all potential resources for the pregnant adolescent. These individuals may benefit from guidance on ways they can effectively help.

Nursing Care

Caring for Developmental Needs

Keep in mind the developmental needs of the pregnant adolescent. Pregnancy does not change the developmental tasks, although it may complicate the issues. According to Erikson (1963), developing an identity is an essential developmental task of the adolescent. It is important to help the pregnant teen to work on identity issues while she also begins to adopt the role of motherhood.

As with other teens, the pregnant adolescent's normal priorities include acceptance by her peer group and focusing on appearance. In addition, the adolescent, particularly the very young adolescent, is typically self-centered, a characteristic that can make it difficult for her to consider the needs of others. Take into account these priorities and characteristics as you plan your nursing care.

Caring for Physical Needs

Adequate nutrition is essential to the health of the pregnant teen. However, nutritional considerations may not have a high priority from the adolescent's viewpoint. Assist the teen to identify healthful foods that are appealing and easy to prepare. It may help to determine what foods the teen normally eats and then suggest more healthful alternatives. For instance, rather than forbidding desserts, help the teen to choose desserts that have nutritional value, such as fresh fruits or frozen yogurt. You might suggest that the teen try low-salt tortilla chips, baked potato chips, or whole-grain crackers, rather than regular potato chips.

Cultural sensitivity is in order.

Do not forget that culture influences food choices. Be sure that you understand the teen's cultural context when you counsel her regarding prenatal nutrition.

Pregnant teens are at higher risk for delivering prematurely, particularly if they experience a repeat pregnancy during their teen years. Twenty-five percent of adolescent mothers have a repeat pregnancy within 2 years of the first (Chacko, 2006). One way to help decrease the risk of a repeat pregnancy is to counsel the teen regarding birth control methods. STIs are another potential problem. Encourage the use of barrier methods of birth control (particularly male use of latex condoms) that supply protection from STIs.

Caring for Emotional and Psychological Needs

The emotional and psychological needs of the adolescent are complex. With the added emotional demands of pregnancy, the strain can be tremendous. It is frequently helpful to include significant support persons in the care planning. It is easier for them to provide meaningful support if they know how pregnancy might affect emotional functioning.

Be knowledgeable regarding community resources for the pregnant teen. If you or the primary practitioner refers the teen to another entity, follow up to make certain the adolescent receives the services for which she was referred. If she does not, try to determine the barriers that prevent her from following through with treatment. Assist her to work through the barriers to obtain needed services.

Remain nonjudgmental and open minded when dealing with pregnant teens. There are many factors working against the teen. Scolding and punishment are not helpful interventions. They tend to push the adolescent away and do little to resolve the real issues with which the teen must contend.

Pregnancy in Later Life

Although adolescent birth rates have declined over time, births for women in their late 30s and early 40s have risen. From 1990 to 2003, the birth rates for age categories experienced the following changes: the 20 to 24 year age group decreased by 12%; the 35 to 39 year age group increased by 38%; and the 40 to 44 year age group increased by 58% (Finegold, 2006). Women as old as 66 have achieved pregnancy using assisted reproductive techniques, and the oldest women to naturally conceive a pregnancy was 57 years old (Fretts, 2007).

There are risk factors that are associated with delayed childbearing. For women, fertility declines with age. Although assisted reproductive technology is much more effective than it was in the past, there is a higher incidence of multiple fetal pregnancies (i.e., twins, triplets) when these technologies are used to help a woman get pregnant. A woman older than 35 years is more likely to conceive a child with chromosomal abnormalities, such as Down's syndrome. She is also at higher risk for spontaneous abortion (miscarriage), preeclampsia-eclampsia, gestational diabetes, preterm delivery, bleeding and placental abnormalities, and other intrapartum complications. She has almost twice the risk of a younger woman of having a fetal demise; she is more likely to have cesarean delivery; and she is more likely to deliver a low-birth-weight baby (Montan, 2007; Reddy, & Co. Willinger,

2006; Tough et al., 2006). As ominous as these statistics sound, it is helpful to remember that the majority of pregnancies to women older than 35 years end with healthy babies and healthy moms.

Clinical Manifestations

In general, the woman who waits to have her first baby until she is in her late 30s or early 40s has more education than her younger counterparts do. Frequently, she has chosen to postpone childbearing to pursue career choices. She is most likely to be married, to have financial resources, and to have planned the pregnancy. She is also more likely to have a chronic condition, such as diabetes or hypertension.

Some older women report more aches and pains during pregnancy, whereas others do not. If the older woman is physically fit, it is less likely that pregnancy will cause excessive tiredness and distress. The hormonal changes of pregnancy are often a cause of facial skin breakouts, even for the older woman.

Treatment

A preconception visit is recommended for any woman who wishes to become pregnant. For the older woman it is especially important that she have a complete physical before becoming pregnant, particularly if she has a chronic medical condition. Because it may be more difficult for the older woman to conceive, fertility experts recommend that she seek medical help if she is not pregnant within 6 months of trying.

Once the woman over the age of 35 achieves pregnancy, the practitioner offers genetic testing and counseling. The miscarriage rate is higher as the woman ages, most likely because of chromosomal abnormalities of the conceptus. Trisomy 21 (Down's syndrome), trisomy 18 (Edward's syndrome), and trisomy 13 (Patau's syndrome) all occur with greater frequency as the woman ages. Therefore, the practitioner offers chorionic villus sampling or early amniocentesis. In addition, the practitioner may suggest a high-level ultrasound in the second trimester to screen for structural defects in the fetus (Fretts, 2007).

Nursing Care

Approach the older pregnant woman with an open mind. Be ready to answer questions and to suggest pregnancy and parenting resources. A woman who chooses to delay childbearing until she is past 35 years of age usually does not appreciate the label "older" pregnant woman. Neither does she want constant reminders of the increased risks associated with late childbearing. If the woman complains of receiving "rude" remarks from strangers about her age, suggest that it is OK to ignore such remarks. If she has a good sense of humor, she may be able to make a joke out of the situation. For example, when one woman was asked if she had planned to have a child at her age, she replied that she was "certainly old enough to know better."

A Personal Glimpse

My husband and I married in our late 20s. We decided to wait until we were both in our 30s to have children because we had lots of school loans to pay off and wanted to be financially secure before raising a family. I got pregnant with my daughter when I was 33. It was a normal pregnancy; I felt great, and the baby and I were completely healthy throughout. When Libby was 3 years old, we decided to try and have another baby. I conceived easily and eagerly made my first doctor appointment to officially confirm the pregnancy. I assumed that this pregnancy would be as uncomplicated as my first. Imagine my surprise when I sat down with the nurse and she started grilling me about the potential for genetic problems and health problems in my baby because I was over 35 years old. She started talking about the need for me to have special blood tests and an amniocentesis. It was all rather overwhelming and scary. I was shocked. How could 3 years make such a difference in the way that my pregnancies would be managed?

Julia

Learning Opportunity: How can the nurse present information to the woman at risk without increasing her anxiety level? Does the risk level dramatically increase at the age of 35? Why or why not?

Suggest a good skin care routine to combat facial breakouts. The older pregnant woman may benefit from a trip to a spa for a facial. It will give her a chance to relax, and she can obtain advice from a skin expert. Caution her not to begin a vigorous exercise routine during pregnancy. If she enters pregnancy already physically fit, she may continue her exercise pattern as long as she does not experience a complication of pregnancy.

Another nursing consideration highlighted by a recent study (Carolan, 2007) is that women over 35 years old may feel they have "too much" medical information and feel overwhelmed. Help by providing teaching tailored to the needs of the woman. Encourage her to discuss her concerns and questions at each visit. It is also helpful to review the sources of her information and help her decide if these sources are credible.

Test Yourself

- ✔ True or false: IPV occurs only in heterosexual relationships.
- ✔ List three components of a safety plan for a victim of IPV.
- ✔ Name two dysfunctional behaviors the pregnant adolescent might use to keep from gaining weight during pregnancy.

Key Points

- ➤ Tight glycemic control for the pregnant woman with diabetes dramatically decreases the incidence of complications. Glucose levels over time are determined by measuring glycosylated hemoglobin (HbA$_1$C).
- ➤ The pancreas of the woman with type 1 diabetes does not produce insulin, so she must receive exogenous insulin. The woman who requires insulin can self-inject insulin or use an insulin pump, which allows for more physiologic concentrations of the hormone. The cornerstone of therapy for gestational diabetes is diet therapy.
- ➤ Fetal surveillance is critical for the pregnant woman with diabetes. Fetal activity counts and NST is done to determine fetal well-being. Amniocentesis to determine fetal lung maturity in the third trimester may help determine the optimum time for delivery.
- ➤ Typical nursing concerns for the pregnant woman with DM include management of the therapeutic regimen, risk for maternal and fetal injury, risk for infection, and fetal macrosomia.
- ➤ The main goal of treatment for the pregnant woman with heart disease is prevention and early detection of cardiac decompensation. Interventions

include monitoring activity levels, managing stress, diet modification, and medication therapy.
- ➤ Iron-deficiency anemia requires iron supplementation and a diet high in iron-rich foods. Because iron supplements predispose to constipation, teach the woman to maintain adequate hydration, exercise regularly, and get plenty of fiber in the diet.
- ➤ Preventing a crisis is the goal of treatment for the woman with sickle cell anemia. Interventions involve maintaining adequate hydration, avoiding infection, getting adequate rest, and eating a well-balanced diet.
- ➤ Teaching is an important part of asthma management. The woman should continue taking her asthma medications during pregnancy. She should avoid over-the-counter medications and protect herself from asthma triggers and infection.
- ➤ Preconceptual care for the woman with epilepsy allows for stabilization on AEDs that cause lower risk to the fetus. The woman takes high-dose folic acid supplements before and throughout pregnancy to help prevent neural tube defects. Vitamin K supplementation during the last weeks of pregnancy helps to prevent neonatal hemorrhage.

➤ TORCH stands for toxoplasmosis, other (hepatitis B, syphilis, varicella, and herpes zoster), rubella, CMV, and HSV. These infections can lead to serious fetal anomalies and other complications. Prevention of infection is the best treatment strategy because many of the TORCH infections do not have effective treatment.

➤ The bacterium *Chlamydia trachomatis* causes chlamydia infection. Chlamydia spreads through sexual contact. It is frequently asymptomatic but easily treated with antibiotics.

➤ The bacterium *Neisseria gonorrhoeae* causes gonorrhea. Antibiotics treat the infection. Gonorrhea increases the risk of PID, spontaneous abortion, and preterm delivery.

➤ HPV is a virus that causes genital warts. The warts have a tendency to increase in size during pregnancy and can lead to heavy bleeding during delivery. The fetus can contract HPV through contact with vaginal secretions during birth.

➤ A protozoan causes trichomoniasis. Metronidazole (Flagyl) given orally is the treatment of choice.

➤ A pregnant woman with HIV/AIDS can pass the infection to her unborn child during pregnancy or childbirth or while breast-feeding. Disease progression and response to treatment are determined by measuring viral load and CD4 counts. Therapy during pregnancy is prophylactic administration of oral ZDV throughout pregnancy. Physicians often order combination therapies, or HAART, to keep viral loads low throughout pregnancy. Breast-feeding is contraindicated.

➤ Nursing considerations for the pregnant woman with an STI include risk for additional infection, ineffective protection, deficient knowledge, risk for low self-esteem, and anxiety. Education regarding STI prevention and treatment are important nursing functions.

➤ The Cycle of Violence describes the typical pathophysiology of IPV. Tension building is followed by the explosion phase, which leads to the honeymoon phase.

➤ Treatment of IPV includes the screening of all pregnant women to identify victims of IPV. Interventions are directed toward safety assessment and planning. Development of a safety plan is a key intervention.

➤ A pregnant teen is at high risk for poor prenatal care. Body image is an important consideration that may lead to attempts to limit weight gain during pregnancy. She is also at risk for domestic violence, anemia, and preeclampsia-eclampsia. Nutrition and social support are important areas of intervention for the pregnant adolescent.

➤ The woman who delays childbearing past 35 years of age is at increased risk for complications of pregnancy. However, she is frequently mature, has a career, is financially stable, and married. Most pregnancies to older women end successfully with a healthy mother and a healthy baby. Preconception care is ideal.

INTERNET RESOURCES

Asthma and Pregnancy

www.aaaai.org/patients/publicedmat/tips/
  asthmaandpregnancy.stm
www.nhlbi.nih.gov/health/prof/lung/index.htm
www.njc.org/disease-info/diseases/asthma/living/
  pregnancy/index.aspx

TORCH Infections and STIs

www3.niaid.nih.gov/healthscience/healthtopics/sti
www.cdc.gov/vaccines/spec-grps/default.htm#preg
www.bcm.tmc.edu/pedi/infect/cmv

Intimate Partner Violence

www.ndvh.org

Workbook

■ NCLEX-STYLE REVIEW QUESTIONS

1. A woman presents to the prenatal clinic for her 28-week prenatal visit. She has gestational diabetes mellitus (GDM). Which type of diabetes does GDM *most* closely resemble?

   a. Type 1
   b. Type 2
   c. Undetermined
   d. Uncontrolled

2. A woman with Class III heart disease is in for a prenatal visit. If she is in early heart failure, which sign is the nurse *most* likely to discover during physical assessment?

   a. Audible wheezes
   b. Persistent rales in the bases of the lungs
   c. Elevated blood pressure
   d. Low blood pressure

3. A 30-year-old gravida 1 has sickle cell anemia. She is not currently in crisis. Providing education on which topic is the highest nursing priority?

   a. avoidance of infection
   b. constipation prevention
   c. control of pain
   d. iron-rich foods

4. A 25-year-old woman is in for her first prenatal visit at 28 weeks' gestation. Which assessment finding would cause the nurse to investigate further the possibility of intimate partner violence?

   a. A calm demeanor
   b. Bilateral pedal edema
   c. A small bruise on her upper thigh
   d. Multiple bruises in varying stages of healing

■ STUDY ACTIVITIES

1. Use the following table to list and compare differences between gestational diabetes and type 1 diabetes during pregnancy.

	Gestational DM	Type I DM
Clinical presentation		
Treatment		
Nursing care		

2. Research the Internet to find at least five reliable Web sites that give patient education information regarding sickle cell anemia.

3. Investigate your community for resources to help adolescents during pregnancy and parenting. Share your findings with your clinical group.

■ CRITICAL THINKING: WHAT WOULD YOU DO?

Apply your knowledge of medical conditions during pregnancy to the following situation.

1. Elizabeth, a 32-year-old gravida 2, has just received a diagnosis of gestational diabetes.

   a. What test diagnoses the condition? What were the results of the test?
   b. What risk factors for gestational diabetes may be present in Elizabeth's history?
   c. Explain the priorities of care for Elizabeth during her pregnancy.

2. Tanya is 29 years old and has asthma. She is pregnant with her first child.

   a. What will pregnancy likely do to Tanya's asthma severity?
   b. Outline a teaching plan for Tanya.

3. Rachel is pregnant with her third child. Her HIV test just came back positive. Rachel says she does not know how she contracted HIV. She thinks it could have been from a blood transfusion she received after her last delivery.

   a. What are the most common methods of HIV transmission? Name three risk factors for HIV.
   b. What are the priorities of care for Rachel?
   c. What medication will the physician likely prescribe for her?
   d. Rachel wants to know how best to protect her unborn child from the infection. How will you respond?
   e. Rachel asks if her other children should be tested. How do you respond? Why or why not?

17 Pregnancy at Risk: Pregnancy-Related Complications

LEARNING OBJECTIVES

On completion of this chapter, you should be able to:

1. Choose appropriate nursing interventions for the woman with hyperemesis gravidarum.
2. Describe clinical manifestations of ectopic pregnancy.
3. Compare and contrast the six types of spontaneous abortion.
4. Discuss the treatment for cervical insufficiency.
5. Explain treatment and nursing care for the woman experiencing a hydatidiform mole.
6. Compare and contrast placenta previa and abruptio placentae according to characteristics of bleeding and other clinical manifestations.
7. Apply the nursing process to the care of a pregnant woman with a bleeding disorder.
8. Differentiate four categories of hypertensive disorders in pregnancy.
9. Discuss treatment and nursing interventions for the woman with preeclampsia-eclampsia.
10. Contrast the management of a multiple gestation pregnancy with that of a singleton gestation.
11. Explain the threat to pregnancy posed by ABO and Rh incompatibilities.

CHAPTER 16 examined the effect of pre-existing and acquired medical conditions on pregnancy. This chapter focuses on pregnancy-related conditions that place the woman and/or fetus at risk. The licensed practical or vocational nurse's (LPN's) role includes identification of risk factors for pregnancy-related complications through patient interview and data collection. Although the registered nurse (RN) must oversee the care for a woman with a complicated pregnancy, as the LPN, you must be able to identify signs of complications and know what problems need prompt intervention. An understanding of the basic pathology and clinical manifestations of these conditions will allow you to intervene appropriately, to teach the patient about her condition and care, and to answer questions confidently.

Do not forget or ignore the tremendous psychological and emotional impact of a complicated pregnancy. A complication that results in loss of the fetus can be devastating. The woman and her family will need support and guidance to help them cope with the loss. Sometimes the pregnancy complication puts the woman's life in danger, leaving the family to face difficult treatment choices. Often the risk to the mother of continuing the pregnancy must be weighed against the risk to the fetus if he or she is delivered early. This chapter highlights information you will need to provide basic physiologic and emotional care for the woman with an obstetric-related complication of pregnancy.

HYPEREMESIS GRAVIDARUM

Hyperemesis gravidarum is a disorder of early pregnancy that is characterized by severe nausea and vomiting that results in weight loss, nutritional deficiencies, and/or electrolyte and acid-base imbalance. Hyperemesis occurs in 0.5% to 2% of pregnancies, with a higher incidence among underweight and younger women. The disorder most often appears between 8 and 12 weeks' gestation and usually resolves by week 20. The exact cause is unclear, although there is an association between hyperemesis and high levels of human chorionic gonadotropin (hCG). Some researchers have identified a connection between pyridoxine deficiency and hyperemesis. The risk of hyperemesis is increased with a multiple gestation (pregnancy with more than one fetus), molar pregnancy, or when there is a history of hyperemesis gravidarum. Stress and psychological factors can contribute to the condition.

Clinical Manifestations

This disorder is distinguished from "morning sickness" because the nausea and vomiting are severe and result in dehydration, weight loss, and electrolyte imbalances, particularly hypokalemia. Acid-base imbalances may occur. Before the primary care provider diagnoses hyperemesis gravidarum, he or she excludes other causes of nausea and vomiting, such as hepatitis, hyperthyroidism, and disorders of the liver, gallbladder, and pancreas. An ultrasound is helpful to rule out a molar pregnancy.

Clinical features of the disorder include symptoms of dehydration, such as poor skin turgor, postural hypotension, and elevated hematocrit. Although rare, esophageal tears or perforation can occur with unremitting vomiting. Prolonged starvation from severe or untreated hyperemesis can lead to thiamine deficiency and Wernicke's encephalopathy, a severe neurologic disorder marked by inflammation and hemorrhage in the brain.

Treatment

Emergency treatment is directed toward correcting fluid, electrolyte, and acid-base imbalances. Hospitalization becomes necessary when severe dehydration is present. Normal saline or Lactated Ringers solutions are typical intravenous (IV) solutions used to treat the dehydration. Additives may include glucose to give the woman an energy source so that the body does not break down protein and fat for energy. Potassium is added if the woman's potassium is low because untreated hypokalemia can lead to cardiac disturbances. Other electrolytes or multivitamins may be added to the IV fluids as indicated to correct imbalances.

The woman takes nothing by mouth (NPO) for the first 24 hours or until the vomiting stops. Pyridoxine (vitamin B6) with or without doxylamine is the recommended first-line therapy (Wilcox, Edelman, & Logan, 2006). Often the combination of rehydration and pyridoxine is enough to control the vomiting. If not, then antiemetics may be added to the regimine. None of the antiemetics are approved by the U.S. Food and Drug Administration for treatment of nausea and vomiting during pregnancy. Because many of these medications are in pregnancy Category C (see Box 7-7 in Chapter 7), the primary care provider must carefully weigh the benefit of using the drug against the possible harmful effects to the fetus.

Antiemetics, if prescribed, are usually more effective when given on a regular, around-the-clock schedule versus as-needed (PRN) dosing. These medications are given by parenteral injection or via rectal suppository until the vomiting is under control. Once the vomiting

Cultural Snapshot

- Ginger is an herbal remedy commonly used to treat nausea. Some cultures consider ginger to be a "hot" herb that treats "cold" conditions. Although there is no information regarding possible adverse fetal effects during pregnancy, recent research demonstrates that ginger can reduce nausea significantly.
- Acupuncture/acupressure, specifically stimulation of the "P6 Neiguan point," located on the palmar aspect of the forearm above the wrist, has been shown to reduce nausea and vomiting by at least 50%. Some researchers recommend this traditional therapy as a first-line treatment before prescribing antiemetic medications.

has subsided, the woman can take antiemetics by mouth. Recent research highlights the benefits of several alternative therapies (see Cultural Snapshot). In severe cases that do not respond to conventional treatment, the primary care provider must consider additional measures. Steroid therapy is sometimes helpful for intractable (hard to treat) cases, or the woman may require enteral feeding or parenteral nutrition.

Once the vomiting has stopped, the treatment plan addresses nutrition. A clear liquid diet is given and then advanced, as tolerated, to a bland diet. A dietitian assists in determining caloric requirements. Many primary care providers order thiamine supplements to prevent Wernicke's encephalopathy.

Nursing Care

Assess the woman for nausea and administer pyridoxine/antiemetics, as ordered. It also is important to assess the amount and character of emesis. Record intake and output and weigh the woman daily. Assess for signs of dehydration, such as poor skin turgor and weight loss. Monitor laboratory values. An elevated hematocrit is associated with dehydration. Observe potassium levels, as ordered. Hypokalemia may result from severe vomiting, or hyperkalemia can occur with potassium supplementation. Monitor the fetal heart rate (FHR) at least once per shift.

After the vomiting has stopped, implement measures to promote intake. A relaxed, pleasant atmosphere is conducive to eating. The area for eating should be well ventilated and free of unpleasant odors. In addition, eating with others can promote intake. Instruct the woman to eat before or as soon as she

Did you know?

A small amount of food taken at frequent intervals is easier to tolerate than one large meal, particularly for someone who is experiencing nausea.

notices that she is hungry, because an empty stomach aggravates nausea (Funai, 2006). Make every effort to provide foods that the woman enjoys. Carbohydrates, such as breads, cereals, and grains, are sometimes easier to tolerate than other food types. She should avoid foods high in fat because such foods may exacerbate nausea.

Provide mouth care before and after meals. This reduces unpleasant tastes in the mouth, thereby encouraging intake and retention of food. In addition, it is a good idea to restrict oral fluids at mealtime to avoid early satisfaction of hunger before she consumes sufficient nutrients.

Observe family dynamics. Because psychological factors can contribute to this disorder, the woman may benefit from a psychiatric or social worker consult. Check with the RN regarding this possibility. It may be therapeutic to allow the woman to ventilate her feelings regarding the pregnancy, her condition, and the hospitalization.

BLEEDING DISORDERS

Bleeding disorders can occur during early, mid, or late pregnancy. Bleeding disorders that occur during early pregnancy include ectopic pregnancy and spontaneous abortion. Although cervical insufficiency is not technically a bleeding disorder, it is discussed in this section because it is a cause of recurrent pregnancy loss in mid-pregnancy. Diagnosis of a molar pregnancy occurs most commonly in early pregnancy, but occasionally the condition is not identified until mid-pregnancy. Placenta previa and abruptio placentae are bleeding disorders that become apparent during late pregnancy. Bleeding disorders can lead to hemorrhage during pregnancy and the birth process. You must be alert to signs and symptoms of a bleeding disorder and notify the RN and/or primary care provider if you suspect one. A prompt diagnosis may prevent hypovolemic shock from a bleeding episode.

Ectopic Pregnancy

The term "ectopic" refers to an object that is located away from the expected site or position. An **ectopic pregnancy** is a pregnancy that occurs outside of the uterus. The fertilized ovum does not find its way to the uterus, so it implants in another location. Approximately 1% of fertilized ova become ectopic pregnancies, with the vast majority implanting in a fallopian tube (Hajenius et al., 2007). The common term for this condition is "tubal" pregnancy. Other sites, such as the abdomen, ovary, or cervix, can serve as implantation sites (Fig. 17-1), although this occurs rarely. The estimated incidence is 1.3% to 2%, or 1 in 50 pregnancies (Stevens & Gilbert-Cohen, 2007). Ectopic pregnancy is the leading cause of pregnancy-related death in the first trimester.

Ectopic pregnancy occurs because some factor or condition prevents the fertilized egg from traveling down the fallopian tube, so it implants before it reaches the uterus. Adhesions, scarring, and narrowing of the tubal lumen may block the zygote's progress to the uterus. Any condition or surgical procedure that can injure a fallopian

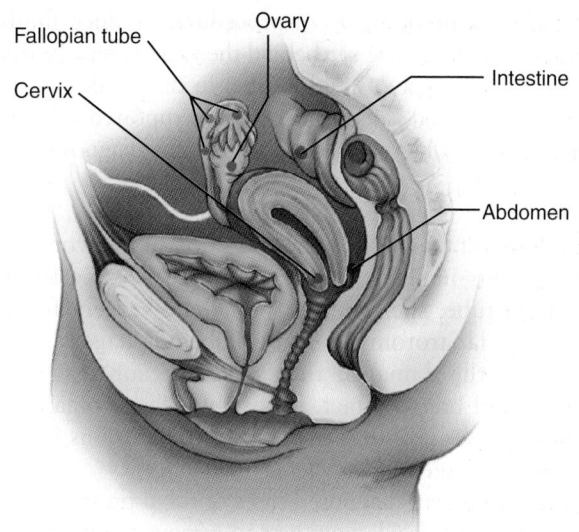

■ **Figure 17-1** Possible implantation sites for an ectopic pregnancy.

tube increases the risk. Examples include **salpingitis,** infection of the fallopian tube, endometriosis, history of prior ectopic pregnancy, any type of tubal surgery, congenital malformation of the tube, or multiple elective abortions. Conditions that inhibit peristalsis of the tube can result in tubal pregnancy. Hormonal factors may play a role because tubal pregnancy occurs more frequently in women who take fertility drugs or who use progesterone intrauterine contraceptive devices.

Clinical Manifestations

Symptoms usually appear 4 to 8 weeks after the last menstrual period, although the woman may not seek medical treatment until 8 to 12 weeks. The most commonly reported symptoms are pelvic pain and/or vaginal spotting. Other symptoms of early pregnancy, such as breast tenderness, nausea, and vomiting, also may be present.

Rarely, a woman may present with late signs, such as shoulder pain or hypovolemic shock. These signs are associated with tubal rupture, which occurs when the pregnancy expands beyond the tube's ability to stretch. The risk of tubal rupture increases with advancing gestation. Therefore, prompt diagnosis is critical to preventing rupture. If the tube ruptures, hemorrhage occurs into the abdominal cavity, which can lead to hypovolemic shock. Manifestations of shock include rapid, thready pulse; rising respiratory rate; shallow, irregular respirations; falling blood pressure; decreased or absent urine output; pale, cold, clammy skin; faintness; and thirst.

The diagnosis is not always immediately apparent because many women present with complaints of diffuse abdominal pain and minimal to no vaginal bleeding. Steps are taken to diagnose the disorder and to rule out other causes of abdominal pain. A serum or urine pregnancy test is done to detect the presence of hCG. Transvaginal ultrasound is used to locate the gestational sac and is often diagnostic. Culdocentesis (a procedure in which fluid is drawn from the cul-de-sac behind the vagina) may be done to identify the type of fluid located in the cul-de-sac. The presence of blood is associated with a ruptured tube. Laparoscopy may be required to confirm the diagnosis.

Treatment

Management depends on the condition of the woman. If she presents in shock with abdominal bleeding from a ruptured tube, she requires immediate surgery for exploratory laparotomy, control of hemorrhage, and removal of the damaged tube. The surgeon leaves the ovaries and uterus intact, if possible. The woman may need volume expanders and blood transfusions if massive hemorrhage occurs.

In nonemergent diagnosed cases of tubal pregnancy, the physician must decide how best to remove the pregnancy. Laparoscopic surgery is the most common method of removing an ectopic pregnancy. If the woman desires to have children in the future, the physician makes every attempt to save the tube by using microsurgical techniques and minimally invasive surgery. A **salpingectomy,** removal of the fallopian tube, is performed when the tube is not salvageable or if the woman has finished childbearing. A newer method of treating a small, unruptured ectopic pregnancy is intramuscular injections of methotrexate, an antineoplastic (anticancer) drug. The medication works by interfering with DNA synthesis, which disrupts cell multiplication. Because the cells of the zygote are rapidly multiplying, methotrexate targets the pregnancy for destruction. Sometimes a single dose is sufficient; or the physician may order multiple injections. The advantage to this approach is avoidance of surgery on the tube. Regardless of the treatment method, the Rh-negative, nonsensitized woman requires anti-D immunoglobulin (RhoGam).

> **Think about this.**
> Because surgery on a fallopian tube is a risk factor for ectopic pregnancy, treating an ectopic pregnancy with the anticancer drug methotrexate instead of with surgery can help prevent future ectopic pregnancies.

Nursing Care

Suspect ectopic pregnancy if the woman presents to the emergency department with abdominal pain and absence of menstrual periods for 1 to 2 months. Measure and record vital signs. Monitor the amount and appearance of vaginal bleeding. Report immediately heavy bleeding or signs and symptoms of shock to the physician or RN.

If the physician decides that surgery is necessary, assist the RN to prepare the patient. An IV line is started and laboratory testing done. At a minimum, a complete blood count and blood type and cross-match are ordered. Check to see that the woman signs a written surgical consent and that the surgical preparatory checklist is complete.

Once the patient is in stable condition, emotional issues become the focus of nursing care. Be available for emotional support of the woman and her family. It is important to remember that the woman is grieving a loss, and each individual has her own way of expressing grief. Suggest outside sources of support, such as pastoral care or grief counseling.

Before discharge, instruct the woman regarding danger signs she should report. Danger signs include fever, severe abdominal pain, or a vaginal discharge with bad odor. Explain that weekly follow-up care with her physician is necessary to measure hCG levels. Discuss contraceptive options and advise the woman that she should not attempt pregnancy until her hCG levels have returned to nonpregnant levels. If the woman desires more children, explain the possibility of another ectopic pregnancy and review the symptoms of ectopic pregnancy. Encourage her to seek grief counseling or attend a support group after discharge.

Early Pregnancy Loss

Early pregnancy loss is the most common complication of pregnancy. A more specific term used to describe early pregnancy loss is **spontaneous abortion,** loss of a pregnancy before the age of viability (<20 weeks of gestation or fetal size of <350–500 g). The common name for early pregnancy loss is *miscarriage.*

The rate of early pregnancy loss is difficult to determine because as many as 50% of losses occur before the woman realizes she is pregnant. The rate of recognized early pregnancy loss is 15% to 20%; therefore, the overall rate may be as high as 60% to 70%. Approximately 80% of spontaneous abortions occur during the first trimester (Puscheck & Pradhan, 2006). Factors that increase the risk for spontaneous abortion include advancing maternal age, history of previous spontaneous abortion, smoking, alcohol and substance abuse, increasing gravidity, uterine defects and tumors, active maternal infection, and chronic maternal health factors, such as diabetes mellitus, and renal disease.

It is difficult to determine the exact cause of miscarriage. Frequently, multiple factors contribute, and many times the cause cannot be determined. There are three overall categories of causation: fetal, maternal, and environmental. Fetal factors are usually genetic in nature. In fact, the most common cause of spontaneous abortion in the first trimester is chromosomal defects in the fetus. Faulty implantation and defects in the sperm or ovum are other fetal-related causes. There are multiple maternal-related causes. Some examples are advanced maternal age, autoimmune diseases, uterine anatomic abnormalities and fibroids, cervical in-

> **Here's a tip for you.**
> It is best to use the term "miscarriage" when talking to patients about spontaneous abortion because the term "abortion" carries negative connotations for many people.

competence, infection, endocrine dysfunction, and coagulation disorders. Environmental factors include poor nutrition; exposure to tobacco, chemicals, or radiation; and use of alcohol, street drugs, or certain prescription drugs.

Some authorities classify spontaneous abortion according to the timing of the loss. Early abortion occurs before 12 weeks and late abortion occurs between 12 and 20 weeks. Fetal factors typically cause early abortion, whereas maternal factors tend to cause late abortion.

Clinical Manifestations

Typical symptoms of spontaneous abortion include cramping and spotting or frank bleeding, which can be severe.

The woman may expel blood clots or tissue. Abdominal and suprapubic pain are common and may radiate to the lower back, buttocks, and perineum. Fever and chills are associated with sepsis.

Spontaneous abortion occurs along a continuum: threatened, inevitable, incomplete, complete, and missed (Table 17-1). The definition

This is a good rule of thumb.

Always consider any woman of childbearing age with vaginal bleeding to be pregnant until proven otherwise.

Table 17-1 ▌ COMPARISON OF SPONTANEOUS ABORTION TYPES

Abortion Type	Clinical Manifestations	Treatment
Threatened abortion	Vaginal bleeding or spotting; possibly cramping; no cervical dilatation. Symptoms may resolve and the pregnancy may progress to term, or threatened abortion can lead to one of the other types.	Vaginal rest (e.g., no sexual intercourse or douches); bed rest or light activity precautions. The woman is to report bleeding heavier than a normal menstrual period, accompanied by cramping or fever. She is to save expelled tissue for examination by the physician.
Inevitable abortion	Cramping and spotting or vaginal bleeding with cervical dilation; amniotic fluid may leak.	There are three treatment options: • Expectant management (wait for the miscarriage to occur on its own) • Misoprostol (Cytotec) orally to induce contractions • Surgical removal of the pregnancy; the type of procedure performed depends largely on the gestational age. Dilatation and curettage (D&C) is the procedure of choice for pregnancies <14 weeks. (Refer to "Induced Abortion" in Chapter 4 for a discussion of specific techniques.)
Incomplete abortion	Some, but not all, of the products of conception are expelled. Most commonly, the fetus delivers and the placenta and membranes are retained.	Treatment is similar to that used for inevitable abortion.
Complete abortion	All of the products of conception (fetus, membranes, and placenta) are expelled.	Surgical procedures are usually unnecessary. The woman goes home with instructions to monitor for complications such as heavy or increased bleeding or fever.
Missed abortion	The fetus dies, but remains in utero. Signs of pregnancy (e.g., nausea, breast tenderness) decrease, and the fundus does not grow as expected in a normal pregnancy and may regress (get smaller). No fetal heart tones are present.	Ultrasound confirms the diagnosis. If the woman carries the dead fetus for longer than 4 weeks, the risk of hemorrhage is high; therefore, a coagulation profile is drawn. The uterus is evacuated surgically by D&C, or medically by inducing labor with oxytocin or prostaglandin.
Habitual (recurrent) abortion	The loss of three or more consecutive pregnancies before the fetus is viable.	Attempts are made to determine and treat the cause. For example, cervical insufficiency is often a cause of habitual abortion.

of each category is related to whether or not the uterus is emptied, or for how long the products of conception are retained.

To make the diagnosis of spontaneous abortion the primary care provider often orders laboratory and imaging studies. An hCG level is drawn to confirm that the woman is pregnant. A complete blood count can identify anemia associated with blood loss and can provide evidence of infection. Blood typing is important to determine if the woman is Rh_o (D) negative. Blood crossmatching and coagulation studies may be ordered in cases of severe blood loss. Urinalysis rules out a urinary tract infection. Transvaginal ultrasound is the diagnostic procedure of choice to visualize the uterine cavity and determine if any products of conception are present and whether or not the embryo or fetus is alive.

Treatment

Treatment depends on which type of early pregnancy loss is occurring (see Table 17-1). Treatment for a threatened abortion is conservative because currently there is no specific therapy that can reliably prevent threatened abortion from progressing to spontaneous abortion. The primary care provider often uses a "wait-and-see" approach. Usually he or she orders bed rest and pelvic rest during which the woman does not place anything into the vagina. Pelvic rest involves no sexual intercourse, douches, or tampons. The woman should report heavy bleeding, cramping, or fever. Most other types of spontaneous abortion require some type of intervention, unless all the products of conception are expelled (complete abortion). The prostaglandin misoprostol (Cytotec) may be given by mouth to induce uterine contractions. Vacuum aspiration or dilatation and curettage (D&C) are the most common surgical methods used to clear the uterus of the products of conception (see Chapter 4). After uterine evacuation, the primary care provider often orders IV oxytocin (Pitocin) or oral methylergonovine maleate (Methergine) to help prevent bleeding. Ibuprofen controls discomfort associated with uterine cramping.

Nursing Care

Assess the woman's vital signs, amount and appearance of vaginal bleeding, and pain level. Count the number of perineal pads used or weigh perineal pads to assess the amount of bleeding. Document whether or not the pad is saturated and note if clots are present. Report a falling blood pressure and rising pulse, or other symptoms of shock, and an elevated temperature, which is associated with infection. If the pregnancy is greater than 10 to 12 weeks, evaluate the FHR with a Doppler device. Save all expelled tissue for evaluation by the physician. Administer anti-D immunoglobulin (RhoGam) if the woman is Rh_o (D) negative.

After the products of conception deliver, either spontaneously or through surgical intervention, continue to monitor vital signs and bleeding. Administer oxytocin

Family Teaching Tips

SELF-CARE AFTER SPONTANEOUS ABORTION

- Return for follow-up care if you experience any of the following danger symptoms:
  - Large amount of vaginal bleeding (soaking more than one pad in 1 hour)
  - Foul-smelling discharge
  - Severe pelvic pain
  - Temperature >38°C (100.4°F)
- Do not place anything in the vagina for approximately 2 weeks. Do not use tampons or douche and refrain from sexual intercourse.
- Return for weekly physician visits to monitor hCG levels, if ordered.
- Avoid sexual intercourse or use contraception until hCG levels become negative.
- You will likely experience intermittent menstrual-like flow and cramps during the week after miscarriage. Ibuprofen helps to control painful cramping.
- Resume regular activities when you feel well.
- Grief counseling is beneficial.

or methylergonovine maleate as ordered to control bleeding. Provide analgesics as ordered and comfort measures to treat pain. Usually the woman may go home a few hours after vacuum aspiration or D&C, if she is in stable condition. Family Teaching Tips: Self-Care After Spontaneous Abortion explains self-care at home.

Grief reactions are to be expected. Allow the woman and her partner or support person privacy to discuss their feelings with each other. Offer parents the opportunity to view the fetus. It is important to acknowledge the

This is important!

If a woman is Rh_o(D) negative, she should receive Rh_o(D) immunoglobulin (RhoGAM) any time a pregnancy is terminated for any reason. The length or type of pregnancy does not change this need.

loss and resist the temptation to reassure the woman that she "can always have more babies." The woman must work through her feelings and come to terms with the current loss before it is helpful or appropriate to focus on future pregnancies.

The intensity and range of emotional responses of the woman experiencing a spontaneous abortion vary greatly. The woman may feel overwhelmed by grief. She may feel guilty that she might have done something to cause the pregnancy loss. She may express anger with a divine power for allowing her to lose the baby. Accept

A Personal Glimpse

I was shocked when I found out I was pregnant with our fourth child. I was almost 40 years old and had a teenager and two school-aged kids. At first, my husband and I were not eager to return to the days of sleepless nights and changing diapers. However, the idea of a sweet, new baby in our family grew on my husband and me, and our three kids were thrilled and excited. During the 10th week of my pregnancy, I started to have cramping and slight bleeding. I called my OB's office and the nurse said to come to the office immediately. I called my husband at work and asked him to come home and take me to the doctor. While I was waiting for him to arrive, the cramping grew stronger and the bleeding grew heavier. I started to cry because I knew I was losing my baby. After examining me, my doctor confirmed my fear; I had experienced a miscarriage. I was told that the miscarriage wasn't complete and that they would have to do a procedure to remove what remained in my uterus. No one really explained the procedure to us, and I felt so lonely lying on the table. After the procedure, the nurse gave me some medicine for pain and made sure I was comfortable; she told me that I could probably go home in a few hours. Before leaving the room, the nurse turned to my husband and me and said, "I know this has been difficult for you, but you and your husband are very fortunate to have three children at home." Although she may have meant no harm, this nurse made me feel guilty for grieving the loss of this unexpected, but wanted pregnancy.

Elisabeth

Learning Opportunity: In what ways can the nurse acknowledge that the loss of a pregnancy is a unique and deeply personal experience for the woman and her family? Describe helpful things the nurse can say when a woman loses a pregnancy. Describe unhelpful responses.

Cultural Snapshot

Expressions of grief are influenced culturally. Some cultures discourage displays of emotion, whereas others encourage dramatic expression of grief. You cannot determine the degree of grief by the presence or absence of emotional expression.

the second trimester. Pregnancy loss is frequently inevitable. Cervical insufficiency is a leading cause of mid-pregnancy habitual, or recurrent, abortion.

The exact cause of cervical insufficiency is unknown, but there are several risk factors. Congenital defects in the reproductive tract, such as a short cervix or abnormalities related to in utero diethylstilbestrol (DES) exposure increase the risk. History of trauma to the cervix is another risk factor. Examples include surgical trauma (e.g., dilatation and curettage, conization or cauterization of the cervix) and childbirth-related injury, such as cervical lacerations and prolonged second stage of labor.

Standard treatment is cervical **cerclage,** placement of a purse-string type suture in the cervix to keep it from dilating. Generally, cerclage is done between 14 and 26 weeks of gestation following a diagnosis of cervical insufficiency in a previous pregnancy. Sometimes emergent cerclage (procedure performed when the cervix is dilated and effaced) can maintain the pregnancy long enough for corticosteroids to enhance fetal lung maturity or to allow the fetus to mature to viability. The practitioner removes the suture when the pregnancy is at term or the woman goes into labor.

Gestational Trophoblastic Disease

Gestational trophoblastic disease encompasses two related diseases of trophoblastic tissue (the tissue that develops to form the placenta). These two conditions are **hydatidiform mole** or *molar pregnancy,* characterized by benign growth of placental tissue, and **gestational trophoblastic neoplasia,** malignancy of the uterine lining.

There are two types of molar pregnancies: partial and complete. Both types involve errors in chromosomal duplication during fertilization. The consequence is grape-like (hydatidiform) swelling of the chorionic villi and trophoblastic hyperplasia; there may be no fetus (complete mole) or fetal tissue with chromosomal abnormalities (incomplete mole). A molar pregnancy has some features of a malignancy in that the trophoblastic tissue proliferates (multiplies) out of control. In fact, approximately 20% of women who experience a complete molar pregnancy develop gestational trophoblastic neoplasia within 6 months to 1 year after molar pregnancy (Chiang & Berek, 2007).

Fortunately, molar pregnancy rarely occurs. In Western countries, the rate is 1 per 1,200 pregnancies. A history

and support the woman's emotions. The woman needs ongoing grief support after discharge; be sure to refer the woman for this service.

Test Yourself

✔ An elevation in what hormone is associated with hyperemesis gravidarum?

✔ List two conditions that increase the risk for ectopic pregnancy.

✔ Name two types of abortion in which the cervix dilates.

Cervical Insufficiency

Cervical insufficiency (formerly known as incompetent cervix) results in painless cervical dilatation with bulging of fetal membranes and parts through the external os in of previous gestational trophoblastic disease increases the risk for a complete mole. Risk factors also include extremes of age; young women in their early teens and older women who are near the end of their reproductive lives are at highest risk. Women older than 40 years have a five- to 10-fold increase in risk compared with younger women (Moore & Hernandez, 2008).

Clinical Manifestations

Before the widespread use of ultrasound, diagnosis of molar pregnancy occurred most frequently in the second trimester. Now the condition is diagnosed most often in the first trimester, before classic symptoms are evident. Thus, the most common presenting sign for both partial and complete moles is vaginal bleeding. Typically, the woman presents between 8 and 16 weeks' gestation with complaints of painless (usually) brown to bright red vaginal bleeding. The bleeding may be intermittent or continuous and can be severe. The hCG level is usually higher than expected for gestational age. Transvaginal ultrasound reveals an intrauterine mass made up of many small cysts caused by grapelike vesicles that fill the uterus. (Note: older, low-resolution ultrasound equipment showed a characteristic snowstorm pattern.)

If a complete molar pregnancy continues into the second trimester undetected, other signs and symptoms appear. The woman often presents with complaints of dark to bright red vaginal bleeding and pelvic pain. Infrequently, she will report passage of grapelike vesicles. The physical examination may reveal a uterus that measures larger than expected for dates. Fetal heart tones are absent, and the examiner cannot detect fetal parts. Abdominal ultrasound reveals the characteristic tumor, and in 50% of the cases, there are giant ovarian cysts, which are the source of pelvic pain. Other less common findings include preeclampsia before the 24th week, hyperemesis gravidarum, and hyperthyroidism (Chiang & Berek, 2007).

Treatment

If the woman is hemorrhaging when she presents, the clinical team must move quickly to stabilize her condition. She requires IV volume expanders and blood transfusions. Clotting studies detect coagulation disorders that can develop as a complication of hemorrhage. Antihypertensives treat elevated blood pressure, if present.

Once the woman is in stable condition, preparation for surgery begins. A chest x-ray is used to assess the lungs, as this is the most common site of metastasis. Blood samples are drawn to establish the baseline hCG level and to type and cross-match the blood, if this has not been previously accomplished.

Surgical treatment options include evacuation of the uterus by suction curettage, if the woman wishes to have children in the future. Abdominal hysterectomy is the treatment of choice if the woman does not desire continued fertility. Labor induction techniques are not used because of the danger of hemorrhage. After the uterus is evacuated, RhoGAM is given to the woman who is $Rh_o(D)$ negative.

Continued follow-up for 1 year is extremely important. The woman returns to the doctor's office every 1 to 2 weeks to have hCG levels drawn. This monitoring is necessary to detect malignancy, which is highly treatable if caught early. If the woman cannot comply with follow-up visits, the surgeon may recommend prophylactic chemotherapy, since one in five women with hydatidiform mole will develop cancer. The woman should avoid pregnancy for at least 6 months after a molar pregnancy by using a highly reliable form of birth control, such as oral contraception.

Nursing Care

The woman is at risk for several complications; therefore, it is important to watch her closely during the postpartum period. Monitor frequently for vaginal bleeding and check the condition of the uterine fundus. Observe vital signs and the woman's level of consciousness because shock can result from hemorrhage caused by uterine atony or accidental perforation of the uterus during surgery. Administer oxytocin as ordered to control uterine atony. Methylergonovine maleate or carboprost tromethamine (Hemabate) are other medications that may be ordered to stimulate the uterine muscle to contract.

Disseminated intravascular coagulation (DIC), a bleeding disorder related to lack of clotting factors, is another possible complication. Molar tissue releases substances that break down clotting factors, increasing the woman's risk for DIC. Review clotting studies for abnormal values and monitor IV and injection sites for bleeding. Immediately report continual oozing from these sites.

Trophoblastic embolus or pulmonary edema secondary to fluid overload is a possibly fatal condition; therefore, every nursing assessment should include a thorough evaluation of respiratory status and auscultation of the lung fields. Report immediately to the RN or physician respiratory distress or crackles in the lungs.

In addition to nursing measures directed at preventing hemorrhage (see "Nursing Process for the Woman With a Bleeding Disorder") and detecting respiratory distress, emotional support is an important nursing function. The woman has to cope with a complication of pregnancy that can cause severe illness, but a baby will not result from her ordeal. Family Teaching Tips: Follow-up Care After Molar Pregnancy lists important aspects of patient education for a woman being discharged after treatment for a molar pregnancy.

Test Yourself

✔ What procedure is used to treat cervical insufficiency?

✔ How is hydatidiform mole diagnosed?

✔ Name three important discharge teaching points for the woman who has experienced a molar pregnancy.

Family Teaching Tips

FOLLOW-UP CARE AFTER MOLAR PREGNANCY

- You will need to see your primary care provider at frequent intervals for 1 year after termination of a molar pregnancy to check for cancer.
- Blood samples will be drawn at every visit to monitor serum hCG levels. Because rising hCG levels are associated with cancer, additional testing is necessary if your levels rise.
- Do not get pregnant for at least 6 months after a molar pregnancy. This is important because hCG levels rise during pregnancy making it difficult to detect cancer, if it develops.
- Immediately report unexpected or irregular vaginal bleeding because this could be a sign of developing cancer.
- Report severe persistent headaches, cough, or bloody sputum. These are symptoms of metastasis, which requires immediate, aggressive treatment.
- If you become pregnant in the future, be sure to tell your primary care provider about the history of molar pregnancy. Although the overall risk is very small, you are at a higher than average risk to experience another molar pregnancy. A sonogram done early in the pregnancy allows for immediate treatment, if needed.

Placenta Previa

Placenta previa is a condition in which the placenta is implanted close to or covers the cervical os. Normally, the placenta implants in the upper uterine segment. In placenta previa, the placenta implants in the lower part of the uterus. As the pregnancy progresses, blood vessels in the part of the placenta that covers the cervix rupture and cause vaginal bleeding.

The exact cause is not known. Any condition that could potentially scar or damage the uterus increases the risk. If scarring is present, the embryo may implant in a site that is more favorable for placental development. Conditions that increase the risk for placenta previa include history of elective abortions, multiparity, advanced maternal age (older than 35 years), previous cesarean birth or uterine incisions, maternal smoking, and prior placenta previa. The condition occurs approximately five times for every 1,000 deliveries (Ko & Yoon, 2007).

Placenta previa is classified according to the degree to which the placenta covers the cervix. Total placenta previa occurs when the placenta completely covers the cervix. If the placenta covers part of the cervix, the term partial placenta previa is used. Sometimes the placenta does not cover the cervix but is located on the border of the cervix; this condition is marginal placenta previa. Figure 17-2 compares three classifications of placenta previa. Sometimes a marginal or partial previa diagnosed early in the pregnancy becomes a normal implantation as the uterus enlarges. However, a complete placenta previa diagnosed in the second trimester rarely resolves to a normal implantation at delivery.

Clinical Manifestations

Painless, bright red bleeding that begins with no warning is a strong indicator of placenta previa. Bleeding may be light to severe and usually stops spontaneously. However, bleeding will recur, and each subsequent episode usually produces heavier bleeding than the previous one. The first bleeding episode occurs on average between 27 and 32 weeks' gestation (Ko & Yoon, 2007).

For any pregnant woman who presents with painless bleeding, a digital examination of the cervix is deferred until placenta previa has been excluded. This precaution is necessary because digital manipulation of placental

■ **Figure 17-2** Three classifications of placenta previa: **(A)** marginal, **(B)** partial, and **(C)** complete.

Placenta near OS

A   Marginal   B   Partial   C   Complete

tissue through the cervical os can cause uncontrollable bleeding. The diagnostic test of choice is transvaginal ultrasound because it is 100% predictive of placenta previa. Abdominal ultrasound is sometimes ordered; it is 95% accurate in making the diagnosis. Magnetic resonance imaging is a third method that is sometimes used (Joy & Lyon, 2008).

Usually the first bleeding episode does not harm the fetus, unless it is unusually severe. The FHR should be within normal limits. Total placenta previa is associated with atypical fetal presentations, such as breech and transverse lie. It is thought that the abnormally located placenta prevents the fetus from assuming the expected head-down presentation. In severe bleeding episodes, the fetus can become anemic, hypoxic, or develop hypovolemic shock due to blood loss and decreased oxygen transport across the placenta.

Be careful!

Never assist with a vaginal examination on a pregnant woman who is bleeding until the practitioner is sure that there is no placenta previa. During the exam, the fingers could penetrate the placenta, causing massive hemorrhage.

Treatment

If the initial bleeding episode does not stop or is massive, an immediate cesarean delivery is a life-saving measure for the woman and her fetus. If the initial bleeding episode stops and the fetus is still immature, hospitalization with bed rest is indicated. IV access is maintained, and at least 2 U of blood are placed on hold for immediate transfusion, if necessary.

If the woman is $Rh_o(D)$ negative, a Kleihauer-Betke test is performed to determine if fetal blood cells are in the maternal circulation, which indicates fetal–maternal hemorrhage. This test helps to determine the appropriate dosage of anti-D immunoglobulin (RhoGam). RhoGam is injected for each bleeding episode to prevent isoimmunization, development of antibodies against $Rh_o(D)$ positive blood in the pregnant woman. (See discussion later in this chapter.)

Serial nonstress tests (NSTs) monitor fetal well-being. Continuous electronic fetal monitoring (EFM) is required during acute bleeding episodes. In some instances, the woman is allowed to go home after the bleeding stops, but she must have someone with her at all times who can transport her immediately to the hospital if bleeding begins again.

A cesarean delivery is necessary in all cases of total placenta previa. If allowed to labor, the woman with total placenta previa would incur massive hemorrhage because placental blood vessels would break open and bleed as the cervix dilated. The physician often schedules the delivery as soon as it is reasonably certain that the fetal lungs are mature. The woman and fetus fare better when the delivery takes place in a planned fashion, as opposed to rushing to the operating room during an acute bleeding episode. Occasionally, a woman with a marginal placenta previa can deliver vaginally, as long as heavy bleeding does not occur during labor.

Nursing Care

The woman with placenta previa requires careful nursing observation. Maintain IV access at all times. Institute a perineal pad count to quantify bleeding. Monitor the vital signs at regular intervals, and assess for signs of shock. Assist with NSTs as ordered, and listen to the FHR at least every 4 hours. Instruct the woman to perform and record kick counts (see Chapter 7). If the woman is discharged home before she delivers, give her instructions for self-care (Family Teaching Tips: Home Care for the Woman With Placenta Previa).

Postpartum care of the woman with placenta previa is the same as for other women. However, it is important to observe her closely for signs and symptoms of infection and postpartum hemorrhage. She is at higher risk for both of these complications because of the proximity of the open, bleeding vessels at the former placenta site to the opening of the uterus. Also, the lower segment of the uterus cannot contract as effectively as can the upper segment; therefore, sometimes not enough pressure is exerted on the blood vessels to stop the bleeding.

Abruptio Placentae

Abruptio placentae, or placental abruption, is the premature separation of a normally implanted placenta. The incidence of abruptio placentae is 1% (Deering, 2007). Although the placenta is located in the normal place, it pulls away from the uterine wall before the end

---

Family Teaching Tips

HOME CARE FOR THE WOMAN WITH PLACENTA PREVIA

- Arrange for a dependable person with transportation to be available immediately to transport you to the hospital should a bleeding episode occur.
- Perform fetal kick counts at least daily. If your baby moves <10 times in 2 hours, or if your baby is not moving at all, immediately call your physician.
- Stay in bed at home. You may get up to use the bathroom. Do no housework or lifting. Moderate-to-vigorous activity could bring about a bleeding episode.
- Vaginal rest is essential. Do not insert anything into the vagina (e.g., no sexual intercourse, no douching, no tampons). These activities could stimulate bleeding.

of labor. The cause of abruptio placentae is unknown; however, there are associated risk factors. Conditions characterized by elevated blood pressure put the woman at risk for abruption. Preeclampsia and pre-existing chronic hypertension fall into this category. Advanced maternal age (older than 35 years) and multiparity increase the risk for placental abruption. Trauma (e.g., motor vehicle collisions or domestic violence), cigarette smoking, alcohol consumption, cocaine use, and preterm prema- ture rupture of the membranes are ad- ditional risk factors for abruption. His- tory of cesarean de- livery significantly increases the risk for placenta previa and abruption (Yang et al., 2007).

Spread the good news.
New research indicates that folic acid supple- mentation before or during pregnancy reduces the risk of placental abruption (Nilsen et al., 2008).

A placental abruption is classified in several ways. The bleeding is either concealed (hidden) or apparent, and the degree of abruption is either partial or complete (Fig. 17-3). If the middle portion of the placenta separates but the edges remain attached, massive hemorrhage can occur behind the placenta but the bleeding may remain concealed. Alternatively, a small edge of the placenta may pull away from the uterine wall and the bleeding might be readily apparent.

Maternal complications of abruptio placentae include hemorrhagic shock, DIC, uterine rupture, renal failure, and death. Sometimes the emergency requires a classic cesarean incision, in which case all future pregnancies must deliver by cesarean birth. Severity and type of fetal complications relate to the degree of placental separa- tion and maturity of the fetus. Hypoxia, anemia, growth retardation, and even fetal death may occur. When preterm delivery is indicated, the neonate is at risk be- cause of prematurity.

Clinical Manifestations

The physician often makes the preliminary diagnosis based on signs and symptoms of the patient. The diag- nosis is confirmed after delivery upon manual inspec- tion of the placenta. The classic signs are pain, dark red vaginal bleeding, a rigid, boardlike abdomen, hypertonic labor, and fetal distress. Pain has a sudden onset and is constant. Bleeding is apparent in most (approximately 80%) cases. The uterus may not relax well between con- tractions, the amniotic fluid often is bloody, and signs of maternal shock and fetal distress may be present. The fundal height may increase with severe intrauterine bleeding.

Ultrasound may assist with the diagnosis, but a nega- tive sonogram does not rule out the possibility of abrup- tion. A biophysical profile (BPP) gives additional in- formation regarding fetal status. As with other bleeding disor- ders, DIC is a poten- tial complication of placental abruption. The physician care- fully monitors fib- rinogen levels and other clotting studies to detect the devel- opment of DIC.

Maybe this will jog your memory on the exam!
You can tell the difference between placenta previa and abruptio placen- tae because the bleeding with previa is bright red and *pain- less,* whereas the bleed- ing with an abruption is usually darker red and *painful.* No pain = previa. Lots of pain = abruption.

Treatment

For cases of abruptio placentae with severe bleeding, IV fluids are infused via a large-bore IV until cryoprecipi- tate, fresh frozen plasma, or whole blood is available for transfusion. Four units of packed red blood cells are cross-matched and are readily available from the labora- tory. Oxygen is administered via face mask. The physi- cian may perform an amniotomy to decrease intrauterine pressure. If the condition of either the woman or her

▮ **Figure 17-3** Types of placen- tal abruption.

| Partial abruption, concealed hemorrhage | Partial abruption, apparent hemorrhage | Complete abruption, concealed hemorrhage |

fetus becomes unstable, the woman is delivered by emergency cesarean birth. After delivery of the fetus, if the physician is unable to control the bleeding, a hysterectomy may be required to save the woman's life.

Vaginal delivery is preferred to cesarean birth for small abruptions in which the woman and fetus remain hemodynamically stable or when the fetus has died. Contraindications for a vaginal birth include fetal distress, bleeding severe enough to threaten the life of the mother and fetus, or unsatisfactory progress of labor. The physician may rupture the membranes artificially to induce or augment labor, and oxytocin may be used. The benefits of vaginal delivery outweigh the risk of oxytocin induction in most cases (Cunningham et al., 2005).

Nursing Care

The woman with a suspected or diagnosed placental abruption requires careful monitoring. She must have nothing by mouth until her condition is stable. Assess for signs of shock. Watch for bleeding from the gums, nose, and venipuncture sites, which may indicate DIC. Insert a large-bore IV line and infuse IV fluid and blood products as ordered. Continuous EFM is necessary. The RN should evaluate the strip frequently. Immediately notify the RN if any signs of fetal distress become evident. Be prepared for an emergency cesarean birth if ordered.

After delivery, the woman requires close monitoring for postpartum hemorrhage because she is at risk for uterine atony. Continue to observe for signs of DIC. This complication may develop after delivery. Place the woman on strict intake and output. Pay particular attention to the urinary output. Acute renal failure can occur.

Nursing Process for the Woman With a Bleeding Disorder

Assessment

Take a thorough obstetric history, unless the severity of the bleeding necessitates immediate intervention. It is important to ask about the chief complaint and history of the current condition and to note any risk factors for antepartum hemorrhage (e.g., grand multiparity, advanced maternal age, or previous history of a bleeding disorder).

During an acute bleeding episode, determine the characteristics of bleeding. How much is the woman bleeding? What is the color and consistency? Is pain present? If so, where and to what degree? In some conditions, bleeding can be hidden, such as a ruptured ectopic pregnancy and some placental abruptions. Ask yourself, "Is the fundal height increasing?" Take vital signs to determine if shock is present. Initial symptoms of shock include cool, clammy skin, restlessness, apprehension, and confusion. Late signs of shock include tachycardia and, when blood loss is severe, hypotension.

Obtain the FHR and apply the EFM if the fetus is more than 20 weeks' gestation. Assess and record the baseline FHR and review the monitor strip for indications of fetal distress. Fetal tachycardia that progresses to bradycardia or decreased variability with late decelerations are ominous signs that must be reported to the charge RN or physician at once. Absence of the FHR is associated with fetal death or hydatidiform mole.

Palpate the uterus to determine if the resting tone is soft and to evaluate the characteristics of contractions, if present. Measure fundal height and compare it to previous measurements; concealed bleeding can cause increasing uterine distention.

Evaluate the woman's pain. Pelvic or shoulder pain in very early pregnancy is associated with ectopic pregnancy. Pain is generally not associated with placenta previa, unless the woman is also experiencing labor in which case the pain will subside with each contraction. Cramping and abdominal pain may accompany spontaneous abortion and abruptio placentae.

Selected Nursing Diagnoses

- Ineffective Tissue Perfusion: Placental related to hypovolemia from excessive blood loss
- Deficient Fluid Volume related to fluid volume loss from bleeding
- Risk for Injury (fetal) related to hypoxia and complications of prematurity
- Risk for Injury (maternal) related to fetal–maternal blood incompatibilities and complications of the bleeding disorder
- Risk for Infection related to open, bleeding vessels
- Acute Pain related to separation of placenta from the uterine wall or contractions associated with pregnancy loss
- Anxiety related to threat of harm and/or death to self and fetus

Outcome Identification and Planning

Maintaining the safety of the pregnant woman and her fetus is the primary goal when planning care. Goals and interventions are planned according to the individual needs and situation of the woman. Appropriate goals may include that the woman's placental perfusion and fluid volume will be maintained; fetal injury from chronic or acute hypoxia will be avoided; maternal injury and Rh isoimmunization will be avoided; the woman will remain free of signs and symptoms of infection; she will express the ability to cope with her pain; and her anxiety will be reduced.

Implementation

Maintaining Placental Perfusion and Fluid Volume

The priority of care for any woman who is bleeding is to prevent and treat shock. For acute bleeding episodes, or when the potential for hemorrhage exists, start an IV line with a large-bore catheter per physician order and state scope of practice. Infuse fluids, as ordered, to maintain blood volume. Collect blood specimens for type and cross-matching, and make certain that blood is available at all times for possible transfusion (2–4 U). If there is severe bleeding, administer blood and blood products as ordered.

It is important to monitor vital signs closely for signs of shock. Maintain strict intake and output monitoring with special attention to the urine output, which should remain above 30 mL/hr. In addition, maintain the woman in a lateral position to promote placental perfusion. Give oxygen by face mask if bleeding is heavy or if there are signs of fetal distress.

Sometimes you will need to prepare the woman for surgery, either emergently to control the bleeding, or on a planned basis to prevent hemorrhage. In a planned situation, obtain informed consent, carry out preoperative orders, and complete the preoperative checklist. When the woman must be prepared for surgery emergently, move quickly and efficiently to get her ready.

If active bleeding is not occurring, but the potential for hemorrhage exists (e.g., placenta previa), assist the woman to remain on bed rest with bathroom privileges, as ordered. It is important to maintain an ongoing perineal pad count to monitor for increased bleeding. Evaluate fundal height for sudden size increase, a condition that may occur when there is concealed hemorrhage.

Avoiding Fetal Injury

When the pregnancy has reached the point of viability (usually considered ≥20 weeks), monitor the fetus continuously during bleeding episodes until the woman is in stable condition. Watch the fetal monitoring, tracing closely for signs of fetal distress such as loss of variability, a gradually increasing or decreasing baseline, and late decelerations. If any of these signs are present, administer oxygen to the mother, reposition her to a side-lying position, and increase the rate of IV fluids. Notify the RN or physician immediately.

If the woman's condition is stable and there are no signs of fetal distress, the woman may remain hospitalized for observation. Assist her to maintain bed rest, as ordered, and institute preterm labor precautions (see Chapter 18). Administer betamethasone as ordered to increase fetal lung maturity in the event delivery must occur before term.

Preventing Maternal Injury

Maternal injury can occur from complications, such as DIC, which are sometimes the sequelae of a bleeding disorder. Obtain specimens for laboratory studies as ordered. Typical blood work includes a complete blood count to detect the presence of anemia and infection. Often, coagulation studies are necessary because some disorders (such as abruptio placentae) are associated with a high risk of clotting dysfunction. Coagulation studies include platelet and fibrinogen levels, fibrin/fibrinogen degradation products, and prothrombin time/activated partial thromboplastin time.

In addition to close monitoring of laboratory results, observe for and report signs of DIC (e.g., bleeding from the nose, gums, and venipuncture sites). Watch for cough, dyspnea, fever, confusion, and disorientation, symptoms that are also associated with DIC. Monitor the blood urea nitrogen and creatinine levels. Levels may be elevated secondary to renal failure. Assess the skin carefully for petechiae and purpura.

Injury can result from bleeding that causes fetal blood to mix with maternal blood (see Blood Incompatibilities, later in this chapter). This is why blood typing is so important with any bleeding disorder of pregnancy. The woman who is $Rh_o(D)$ negative may need a Kleihauer-Betke test to determine if any fetal blood has entered her circulation. This test can help the physician determine how much anti-D immunoglobulin (RhoGam) is needed. Every woman who is $Rh_o(D)$ negative should receive anti-D immunoglobulin (RhoGam) if there is risk of fetal–maternal hemorrhage. All bleeding episodes and evacuation of the products of conception from the uterus increase this risk.

Preventing Infection

Take measures to prevent infection. Use aseptic technique as indicated. In addition, teach the woman to wash her hands before and after eating, using the restroom, and performing perineal care. Monitor the temperature and white blood cell count. Report elevations in either parameter. Instruct the woman to report vaginal discharge with a foul odor.

Managing Pain

Assess carefully regarding the woman's pain. It is important to ask the following questions regarding pain. Where is it? What is it like? When did it start? How often does it occur? What makes it worse? What makes it better? Evaluate intensity using a pain scale. You may ask the woman to rate the pain on a scale of zero to 10. Zero represents no pain at all, and 10 represents the worst pain imaginable. If you use a pain scale, you can more effectively evaluate the success of your interventions.

Give the woman information about what is causing the pain (if you have that information) and how long she can expect it to last. Explain to her the medications the physician has ordered to help decrease her pain and tell her how frequently she can have them. For acute pain, it is often better to schedule the pain medications, rather than waiting for the woman to ask for them. Explain that it is easier to treat pain before it becomes severe. Be sure that the room temperature, lighting, and noise level are at a comfortable level for the woman. It is also helpful to try to eliminate any factors that might be interfering with her ability to cope with the pain (e.g., if the woman is overly fatigued or bored, it will be more difficult for her to deal with the pain sensation). Consult with the RN regarding nonpharmacologic methods of pain relief, such as warm or cold applications, massage, or relaxation techniques. Be sure to inform the RN or the physician right away if measures to reduce pain are ineffective.

Reducing Anxiety

Take care to attend to the woman's emotional needs. It can be frightening when there is active bleeding and health care providers are moving quickly to intervene. Use a calm and confident manner. Explain all procedures and treatments as they are being performed, using language the woman and her family can understand. Promote expression of feelings and encourage the presence of supportive family members and friends, as appropriate. If the fetus dies because of complications of the bleeding disorder, or if the woman requires an unplanned, emergency hysterectomy, she will need additional support to deal with these losses. Request a social service consult if support is inadequate.

Evaluation: Goals and Expected Outcomes

Goal: The woman and her fetus maintain adequate fluid volume and placental perfusion.

Expected Outcomes:

■ The woman's skin and mucous membranes remain hydrated.
■ The woman's hematocrit, serum electrolytes, and urine specific gravity remain within normal limits.
■ The fetus shows signs of tolerating labor.

Goal: The woman and her fetus remain free from injury.

Expected Outcomes: The woman

■ maintains coagulation studies within expected limits.
■ does not experience active bleeding.
■ does not become isoimmunized if she is Rh$_o$(D) negative.

The fetus shows signs of well-being. The fetal tracing shows

■ variability and reactivity
■ without late decelerations

Goal: The woman shows no signs of infection.

Expected Outcomes:

■ Vital signs remain within expected limits.
■ Temperature stays less than 100.4°F.
■ The white blood cell count remains within the normal range.

Goal: The woman's pain is manageable.

Expected Outcomes: The woman

■ expresses the ability to cope with her pain.
■ reports reduced pain (measured on a pain scale) after interventions.
■ reports she is able to carry on with the activities of daily living and get enough sleep and rest despite the pain.

Goal: The woman's anxiety is reduced.

Expected Outcomes: The woman

■ uses available social supports.
■ uses effective coping strategies.
■ reports decreased levels of anxiety.

Test Yourself

✔ Name two characteristics that are different between abruptio placentae and placenta previa.
✔ Name three early symptoms of shock.
✔ Name one way to evaluate the extent of concealed hemorrhage.

HYPERTENSIVE DISORDERS IN PREGNANCY

Hypertension during pregnancy is the second leading cause of maternal morbidity and mortality in the United States, complicating 6% to 8% of all pregnancies (Stella & Sibai, 2006), and is responsible for almost 15% of maternal deaths. These disorders are not only dangerous for the pregnant woman, but they also significantly increase the risk for the fetus. There are four basic categories of elevated blood pressure during pregnancy:

1. Gestational hypertension
2. Preeclampsia/eclampsia
3. Chronic hypertension
4. Preeclampsia superimposed on chronic hypertension

Gestational Hypertension

Gestational hypertension is the current term used to describe elevated blood pressure (≥140/90 mm Hg) that develops for the first time during pregnancy, without the presence of protein in the urine. Gestational hypertension may resolve spontaneously after the baby is born, in which case the condition is classified transient hypertension. If the blood pressure remains elevated after delivery, the diagnosis becomes chronic hypertension. The concern is that gestational hypertension may develop into the more serious preeclampsia-eclampsia syndrome; therefore, at each physician visit, the urine is checked for protein and the blood pressure is monitored closely. If the blood pressure increases to a level that might endanger the woman or her fetus, the physician may prescribe antihypertensives.

Preeclampsia-Eclampsia

Preeclampsia is a serious condition of pregnancy, in which the blood pressure rises to 140/90 mm Hg or higher accompanied by **proteinuria,** the presence of protein in the urine. The condition may develop into **eclampsia,** the presence of seizure activity or coma in a woman with preeclampsia. Signs and symptoms of preeclampsia usually appear after the 20th week of

Box 17-1 ▌ RISK FACTORS FOR PREECLAMPSIA-ECLAMPSIA

- Family history of preeclampsia-eclampsia
- African American descent
- Nulliparity
- Pre-existing medical conditions such as
  - Chronic hypertension
  - Systemic lupus erythematosus
  - Renal disease
  - Diabetes
- Obstetric complications including
  - Multiple gestation
  - Hydatidiform mole (molar pregnancy)
  - Carrying a fetus that develops erythroblastosis fetalis
- Extremes of age
  - Younger than 20 years (increased risk probably due in large part to nulliparity)
  - Older than 35 years (increased risk most likely related to presence of chronic diseases)

gestation and resolve when the pregnancy terminates. The syndrome may develop gradually, or it may appear suddenly without warning. The underlying cause of this disorder is unknown. Exposure to trophoblastic tissue appears to be the triggering factor, but it is not known what causes some pregnant women to develop sensitivity to the tissue, while others do not. Box 17-1 lists risk factors for preeclampsia-eclampsia.

Medical researchers want to find ways to prevent and predict preeclampsia-eclampsia because of the severe effects this condition can have on the woman and her fetus (Table 17-2). Various methods have been tried to prevent the condition, including high-protein, low-salt diets; low-dose aspirin therapy; and calcium supplementation. However, none of these therapies has been preventive to date.

Because there are no diagnostic tests available that can predict which woman will develop preeclampsia, early detection through regular prenatal care is the best alternative. Early prenatal care reduces morbidity and mortality associated with preeclampsia-eclampsia. However, recent research indicates that there are differences in outcomes between ethnic groups.

Preeclampsia occurs in approximately 5% of all pregnancies and is the third leading cause of pregnancy-related death in the United States (Jung & Erogul, 2007). Women who receive no prenatal care are more likely to die of complications of preeclampsia and eclampsia than women who receive any prenatal care. African American women are more likely to develop preeclampsia and are two to three times more likely to die of preeclampsia or eclampsia than are white women (Jung & Erogul, 2007). Although black and white women who received prenatal care had a lower risk of death, there is a far greater reduction for white women than for black women.

In a normal pregnancy, a woman's blood pressure does not rise significantly above her baseline. In fact, during the second trimester the blood pressure decreases. However, in a pregnancy complicated by preeclampsia, the blood pressure rises. The elevated blood pressure occurs because the woman's blood vessels become more sensitive to substances that cause vasoconstriction, a condition that increases peripheral resistance and blood pressure. The kidneys reinforce this rise in pressure when they respond to decreased blood flow by releasing substances that further raise the blood pressure.

The primary problem underlying the development of preeclampsia is generalized **vasospasm,** spasm of the

Table 17-2 ▌ COMPLICATIONS OF PREECLAMPSIA-ECLAMPSIA THAT CAN CAUSE MATERNAL AND/OR FETAL INJURY OR DEATH

Effects of Preeclampsia-Eclampsia	Potential Complications
Maternal Effects of Preeclampsia-Eclampsia	
Seizure activity	Bodily injury (especially the tongue), aspiration, placental abruption, or cerebral hemorrhage
Endothelial damage to pulmonary capillaries	Pulmonary edema
Severely elevated blood pressure and cerebral edema	Cerebral bleeding and complications associated with cerebral vascular accident (CVA or stroke). This complication is rare.
Edema and reduced blood flow to the liver	HELLP syndrome and/or rupture of the liver
Platelet aggregation and consumption of clotting factors	Thrombocytopenia and disseminated intravascular coagulopathy (DIC)
Fetal Effects of Preeclampsia-Eclampsia	
Reduced blood flow to the placenta	Intrauterine growth restriction (IUGR), oligohydramnios, and placental abruption
Preterm delivery to save mother or baby	Respiratory distress syndrome and other complications of prematurity

arteries, which affects every organ in the body. Vasospasm causes generalized vasoconstriction, which leads to hypertension. The elevated blood pressure adversely affects the central nervous system and decreases blood flow to the kidneys, liver, and placenta. Vasospasm also leads to endothelial damage, which causes abnormal clotting. Tiny clots (microemboli) cause damage to internal organs, especially the liver and kidneys. Edema of the tissues, body organs, or both may result from this process (Fig. 17-4).

Clinical Manifestations

Preeclampsia is diagnosed when blood pressures of greater than 140 mm Hg systolic or 90 mm Hg diastolic develop after the 20th week of gestation. The hypertension must be documented on at least two different occasions and be accompanied by proteinuria (measured initially by dipstick of a clean-catch or catheterized urine specimen followed by a 24-hour urine collection). The presence of edema or weight gain is no longer a criterion for diagnosis of this disorder because edema occurs commonly in pregnancy and is not specific to preeclampsia. However, edema is significant if it is nondependent or if it involves the face and hands.

Depending on symptoms, preeclampsia is categorized as mild or severe (Table 17-3). Symptoms of mild preeclampsia are limited to slightly elevated blood pressure and small amounts of protein in the urine. Severe preeclampsia manifests with blood pressure above 160/110 mm Hg, greater than 2+ protein in the urine, and symptoms related to edema of body organs and decreased blood flow to tissues. The central nervous system (CNS), especially the brain, is sensitive to small changes in fluid volume. Nervous system irritability occurs, resulting in hyperactive deep tendon reflexes and clonus (Fig. 17-5). A severe headache may indicate the presence of cerebral edema. If the retina of the eye becomes edematous, the woman will report blurred or double vision and spots before her eyes. Visual changes and a severe headache indicate that a seizure is likely to occur. Liver involvement results in elevation of liver enzymes. Severe edema of the liver causes nausea and pain in the epigastric region. In addition, a low platelet count may result in prolonged bleeding time, and pulmonary edema may occur when the disease process affects the lungs.

If the woman with severe preeclampsia experiences a convulsion or a coma, she has progressed from preeclampsia to eclampsia. Typically, seizures are generalized tonic-clonic in nature and only

Be careful!
Don't let the term "mild" (when applied to preeclampsia) fool you. Mild preeclampsia can progress rapidly to severe preeclampsia or eclampsia with seizures or coma. Monitor closely all pregnant women with elevated blood pressures.

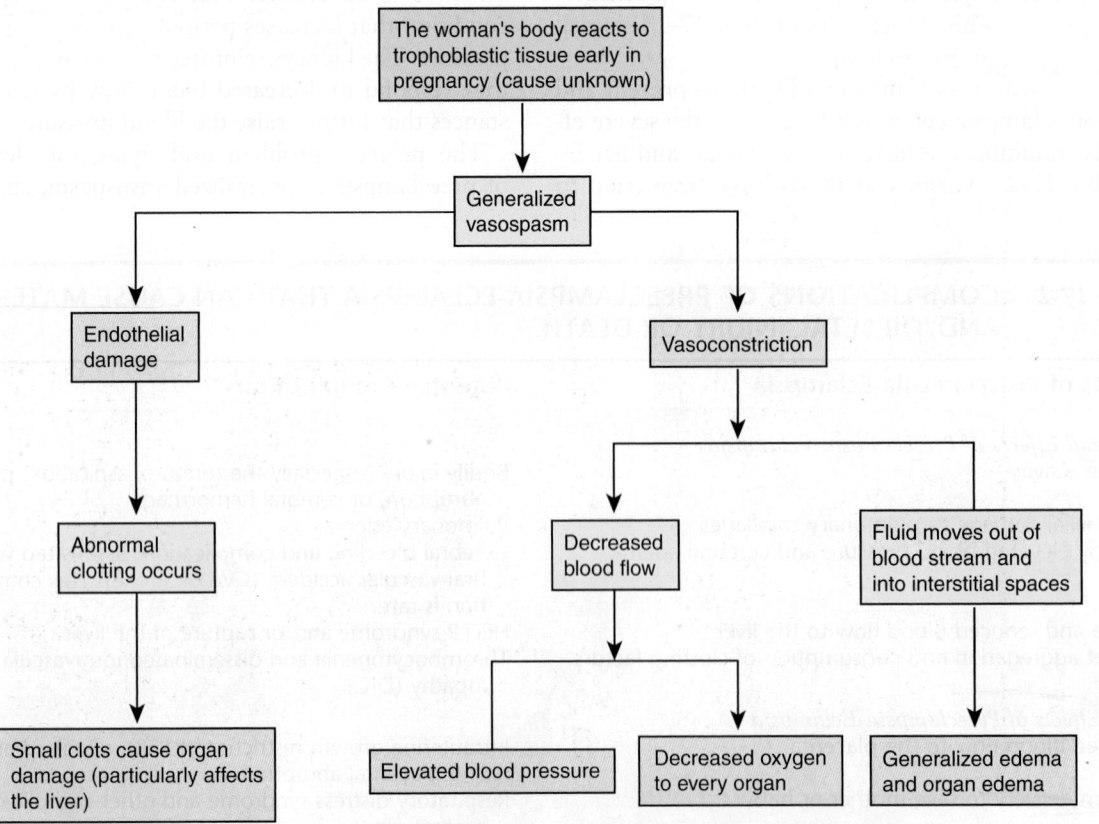

■ Figure 17-4 Pathophysiology of preeclampsia. Every body organ is affected.

Table 17-3 ▪ COMPARISON OF MILD AND SEVERE PREECLAMPSIA AND ECLAMPSIA

	Mild Preeclampsia	Severe Preeclampsia	Eclampsia
Blood pressure	140/90 mm Hg or higher; diastolic pressure remains below 100 mm Hg	160/110 mm Hg or higher	Same as for severe preeclampsia
Proteinuria	Trace to 1+ in a random specimen; 300 mg or greater in 24-hour specimen	Persistent 2+ or more; 500 mg or greater in 24-hour specimen	Same as for severe preeclampsia
Serum creatinine	Normal	Elevated	Elevated
Platelet count	Normal	Low (thrombocytopenia)	Same as for severe preeclampsia; may develop HELLP syndrome
Liver enzymes	Normal to minimally elevated	Markedly elevated	Same as for severe preeclampsia
Headache, visual disturbances, epigastric (abdominal) pain	Absent	Present	Present; epigastric pain is an important warning of an impending seizure
Fetal growth	Normal (not restricted)	May be restricted, unless there is a sudden onset near term and the baby is delivered promptly	Same as for severe preeclampsia
Edema	Trace to 1+ pedal, if present	May or may not be present; edema of the face or hands is significant	May or may not be present
Pulmonary edema	Absent	May be present	May be present
Seizure activity or coma	Absent	Absent	Present

rarely progress to status epilepticus. Potential complications of eclamptic seizure activity include aspiration, cerebral hemorrhage, stroke, hepatic rupture, abruptio placentae, fetal compromise, and death of the woman or fetus. The woman with preeclampsia remains at risk for seizure activity throughout pregnancy, labor, and in the first few days of the postpartum period. In fact, the signs of preeclampsia-eclampsia may occur suddenly in the postpartum period even if they were not noticeable before delivery.

A   B

▪ Figure 17-5 **(A)** The nurse checks the patellar reflexes. **(B)** The nurse checks for clonus.

HELLP syndrome is a severe form of preeclampsia-eclampsia. HELLP is an acronym for *h*emolysis, *e*levated *l*iver enzymes, and *l*ow *p*latelets, which are the laboratory findings in a woman with this complication of preeclampsia-eclampsia. The presence of HELLP syndrome or eclampsia greatly increases the mortality associated with preeclampsia.

Treatment

The primary goals of therapy are to deliver a healthy baby and restore the woman to a healthy state. To accomplish these goals the physician must consider several issues. The most important decision regarding management of preeclampsia involves the timing of delivery because the only cure for preeclampsia is to end the pregnancy. If the fetus is at term (>37 weeks), the physician will usually induce labor because a vaginal birth is preferred to a cesarean delivery. If the fetus is preterm, management depends on the severity of the disease and determination of fetal lung maturity. The benefits and risks of conservative management (bed rest and observation) are weighed against the benefits and risks of a preterm delivery. If the woman's condition deteriorates rapidly or the intrauterine environment becomes hostile, the physician delivers the baby promptly to save the life of the woman, the baby, or both.

Conservative management may be appropriate for the woman with mild preeclampsia. If she is compliant with the treatment plan and understands the danger signals, she may receive care at home. Otherwise, hospitalization is required with activity restriction that usually involves bed rest in a lateral position with bathroom privileges. The woman should stay in a minimally stimulating environment; therefore, visitors are usually restricted to one or two support persons.

If the physician plans conservative management to allow a preterm fetus to mature, closely observe fetal well-being. Instruct the woman to perform fetal kick counts after every meal. NSTs are done at least twice weekly. A BPP (see Chapter 7) and serial sonograms help monitor fetal status and growth. The physician may perform an amniocentesis to determine lung maturity using the lecithin/sphingomyelin (L/S) ratio. A ratio of 2:1 is indicative of lung maturity. If imminent delivery seems necessary and the baby is preterm, the woman may receive glucocorticoids (usually betamethasone) in an attempt to hasten maturity of the fetal lungs.

Preventing maternal seizures is another important goal of therapy. If severe preeclampsia ensues, institute bed rest in a darkened, quiet room and restrict visitors. The most effective medication to prevent and treat eclamptic seizures is magnesium sulfate, usually administered intravenously (Box 17-2). This medication is reserved for the woman with severe disease. The drug works by directly relaxing skeletal muscles and raising the seizure threshold. IV magnesium sulfate is the drug of choice to treat eclamptic seizures, but other anticon-

---

Box 17-2 ▮ PREVENTION AND TREATMENT OF ECLAMPTIC SEIZURES: MAGNESIUM SULFATE

Method of Action
Magnesium sulfate prevents seizures by relaxing muscles and through direct action on the central nervous system (CNS).

Usual Dosage and Administration
IV route: Loading dose of 4 to 6 g diluted in 100 mL fluid infused over 15 to 20 minutes, followed by maintenance dose of 2 g/hr.
Antidote: Calcium gluconate 1 g IV push over 2 minutes

Nursing Interventions
1. Carefully prepare and administer magnesium sulfate exactly as ordered.
2. Use a pump to regulate flow when administering via IV route.
3. Monitor vital signs per facility protocol every 15 to 30 minutes.
4. Perform hourly assessments of the following parameters
   a. Urinary output and protein levels
   b. Deep tendon reflexes
   c. Edema
5. Request serum magnesium levels every 4 to 6 hours, as ordered.
6. Discontinue magnesium sulfate and notify the physician if deep tendon reflexes are absent, respirations are <14 per minute, or urinary output is <30 mL/hr.
7. Therapeutic levels of magnesium sulfate are between 4 and 7 mEq/L. Patellar reflexes disappear at 10 mEq/L; respiratory arrest occurs at 12 mEq/L.

Note: The RN administers this medication. However, the LPN may assist with monitoring of the patient who is receiving IV magnesium.

---

vulsants, such as phenytoin (Dilantin) or diazepam (Valium), are sometimes ordered.

The therapeutic level of magnesium sulfate is 4 to 8 mg/dL. This level is effective to prevent seizures without causing toxicity. Magnesium toxicity begins when serum magnesium levels approach 9 mg/dL. First, the reflexes disappear, then as the levels increase, respiratory depression and cardiac arrest can follow. For this reason, monitor the reflexes and respiratory rate of the woman receiving magnesium sulfate at frequent intervals. Draw serum magnesium levels at prescribed intervals. Calcium gluconate is the antidote to magnesium sulfate. The RN gives this medication by IV push to treat magnesium overdose.

Magnesium sulfate leaves the body via the kidneys. If the kidneys do not function well, blood magnesium levels rise, which can lead to toxicity. Because preeclampsia can damage the kidneys, pay close attention to urinary output by measuring it hourly. Report hourly outputs of less than 30 mL.

Because magnesium sulfate causes muscular relaxation, it inhibits uterine contractions. Therefore, if delivery is indicated, the woman usually requires oxytocin induction of labor. She is also at risk for postpartum hemorrhage because the uterine muscle may be unable to contract effectively. Carefully monitor for this complication after delivery.

The treatment of hypertension is controversial. Generally, the physician orders antihypertensives only in the presence of severely elevated blood pressure (>160/105 mm Hg) because a rapid drop in the blood pressure can lead to decreased placental perfusion, resulting in fetal distress. Hydralazine (Apresoline) is the antihypertensive of choice during pregnancy. Nifedipine (Procardia) is another antihypertensive that may be ordered.

Nursing Care

Care of the woman with preeclampsia or eclampsia is challenging. The woman and fetus require frequent monitoring for symptoms of worsening condition. The experienced RN is responsible for assessment and care of the woman with preeclampsia, although you may assist.

In the hospital, monitor blood pressure at least every 4 hours for mild preeclampsia and more frequently for severe disease (Nursing Procedure 17-1). In addition, it is important to auscultate the lungs every 2 hours. Adventitious

Nursing Procedure 17-1
MEASURING BLOOD PRESSURE IN PREECLAMPSIA

EQUIPMENT

Blood pressure cuff appropriate to the size of the woman (see notes below)
Sphygmomanometer
Stethoscope

PROCEDURE

1. Wash hands.
2. Assist the woman to the same position for each reading; preferably, she should be sitting (see notes below).
3. Apply the blood pressure cuff to the arm in the usual fashion and support the arm at heart level.
4. Auscultate carefully. Note the systolic pressure; use phase 1 Korotkoff (the reading where the first clear, rhythmic sound becomes audible).
5. Note diastolic pressure at phase 5 Korotkoff (the number at which the sound completely disappears).
6. If the pressure is greater than 140/90 mm Hg, reposition the woman to her left side, wait 5 minutes, and then repeat the reading with the woman in the sitting position.
7. If the pressure continues to be elevated, determine if the woman is experiencing headache, blurred vision, or epigastric pain.
8. Reposition the woman comfortably on her left side, supported by pillows.
9. Replace equipment appropriately and wash hands.
10. Report immediately to the RN blood pressures greater than 140/90 mm Hg and/or abnormal symptoms.
11. Record the blood pressure per facility protocol. If you took the pressure more than once, record each reading, noting the time and maternal position for each.

Notes:
- Take care to choose a cuff that fits the woman correctly. If the woman is large and you use a small cuff, the reading may be elevated falsely. Conversely, if the woman is very thin and you use a large cuff, the reading may be lowered falsely.
- Measuring blood pressure with the arm at heart level is best accomplished with the woman in a sitting position. If she cannot sit up, be sure to take the pressure with the arm at heart level. If the arm is higher than the heart, the pressure reading will likely be lower than the actual pressure. Likewise, a lower than actual reading will likely result if you take the pressure with the woman in the supine position.
- Most facilities use automated blood pressure equipment, such as a Dinamap blood pressure device. These devices tend to underestimate the blood pressure in women with preeclampsia; therefore, manual blood pressures are the standard. If you use an automated device, first verify accuracy of the machine readings by comparing them with manual measurements.

Sources: (1) Gibson, P., & Carson, M. P. (2007). Hypertension and pregnancy. In G. S. Letterie, F. Talavera, F. B. Gaupp, & C. V. Smith, *eMedicine*. Last updated December 13, 2007. Retrieved January 29, 2009, from http://www.emedicine.com/med/topic3250.htm. (2) Peters, R. M. (2008). High blood pressure in pregnancy. *Nursing for Women's Health, 12*(5), 410–422.

sounds may indicate developing pulmonary edema. Weigh the woman daily on the same scale at the same time of day while she is wearing the same amount of clothing. Report any sudden increase in weight.

Teach the woman to report headache, visual changes, and epigastric pain, which are warning signs of an impending seizure. Assess deep tendon reflexes and determine if clonus is present at least once per shift. It is important to keep the environment quiet and nonstimulating because bright lights and loud noises could precipitate a seizure. Implement seizure precautions, which include padding the side rails and keeping suction equipment, an oral airway, supplemental oxygen, and medications readily available for use at the bedside. If a seizure does occur, follow proper procedure (Nursing Procedure 17-2).

The woman should remain on bed rest in the left lateral position, although some women with mild preeclampsia may have bathroom privileges. Maintain strict monitoring of intake and output. IV fluids may be ordered. It is important to control the infusion carefully with an IV pump to maintain adequate hydration without causing overload. Report urinary output of less than 30 mL/hr.

Adequate nutrition is important to promote fetal growth and maternal well-being. There is no special diet

for preeclampsia, but careful attention is needed so that nutrients are consumed in adequate amounts (see Chapter 6). Salt restriction below normal levels is not necessary, but the woman should take care to avoid excessive salt intake. See Nursing Care Plan 17-1.

Remember to care for the psychosocial needs of the woman hospitalized for preeclampsia. Boredom may be an issue because of prolonged bed rest. Encourage the woman to read, keep a journal, or do crafts. The woman may be anxious about the well-being of her fetus or because she had to leave older children at home. Keep the woman informed of the results of NSTs and other tests of fetal well-being. Reassure her that she can monitor fetal well-being by doing kick counts regularly. Allow her to ventilate her feelings of fear or frustration. Short daily visits by older children or telephone calls may also help alleviate anxiety.

Postpartum care of the woman varies depending on whether the woman received magnesium sulfate during the intrapartum period. If so, the woman receives care in the labor and delivery unit or a high-risk antepartum unit for the first 24 to 48 hours after delivery. During at time, magnesium sulfate administration continues se monitoring of respirations, deep tendon re- nus, and urinary output as before delivery. erve for postpartum hemorrhage.

Nursing Procedure 17-2
INTERVENING FOR AN ECLAMPTIC SEIZURE

EQUIPMENT

Suction equipment
Equipment to deliver oxygen
Magnesium sulfate
IV access materials
Fetal monitor

PROCEDURE

When the seizure begins:

1. If you are in the room when a seizure begins, summon help with the call bell and note the time the seizure began.
2. Gently attempt to place the woman on her side, if possible. Do not force her to this position if injury will result.
3. Provide oxygen by face mask.

During the seizure:

4. The RN will prepare and administer IV magnesium sulfate loading dose per orders or standing protocol to stop the seizure.
5. If IV access is not in place, establish access as soon as it is safe to do so.
6. Suction PRN, if it is safe to do so, because aspiration is a real threat. Do not force the

suction catheter into the mouth, particularly if you are using a hard plastic suction tip.
7. Watch for signs of spontaneous birth of the baby. Sometimes a seizure will precipitate birth.
8. Note the characteristics of the seizure so that you may accurately record a description after the emergency is over.

After the seizure:

9. Continue to suction PRN.
10. Continue administering oxygen to prevent/treat maternal–fetal hypoxia.
11. Begin continuous monitoring of the fetal heart rate, if a continuous monitor is not already in place.
12. Notify the physician of the seizure, if another nurse has not already completed this task.
13. Document the following parameters.
    a. Time the seizure began
    b. Characteristics of the seizure: tonic-clonic activity, fecal or urinary incontinence, cyanosis, etc.
    c. All nursing actions completed and medications administered
    d. Response of the woman to interventions
    e. Evaluation of the electronic fetal monitor tracing

Nursing Care Plan 17-1

THE WOMAN WITH PREECLAMPSIA

CASE SCENARIO

Hilda Rodriguez is a 35-year-old gravida 1, para 0 at 33 weeks' gestation. She was admitted to the hospital with the diagnosis of mild preeclampsia. Admitting vital signs are BP 150/98 mm Hg, T 98.7°F, P 70 bpm, R 20/min. She denies contractions, headache, blurred vision, or epigastric pain. Her deep tendon reflexes are 2+ (normal), and she does not have clonus (also a normal finding). Proteinuria of 1+ is found in a random voided specimen. Fetal heart rate is in the 150s, and a nonstress test at the physician's office today was reactive.

NURSING DIAGNOSIS

Ineffective Tissue Perfusion (maternal vital organs, peripheral tissues, and placenta) related to constriction of blood vessels (vasospasms).

GOAL: Maintenance of adequate arterial blood supply to major organs, peripheral tissues, and placenta.

EXPECTED OUTCOMES
- The woman remains alert, awake, and responsive
- Blood pressure remains 140/90 mm/Hg or lower
- Urinary output is at least 30 mL/hr
- Extremities remain warm to touch
- Peripheral edema +1 or less
- No facial edema or ascites
- Weight remains stable without sudden increases

Nursing Interventions	*Rationale*
Maintain bed rest in side-lying position, as ordered (strict or with bathroom privileges).	Bed rest in a side-lying position improves blood flow to the kidneys and other vital organs.
Monitor neurologic status (level of responsiveness) as per facility protocol.	Lowered levels of consciousness may indicate the presence of cerebral edema.
Monitor vital signs q4h or more frequently as ordered; report blood pressure >140/90 mm Hg or as ordered.	A highly elevated blood pressure can interfere with blood flow to major body organs and extremities.
Perform strict intake and output measurements.	Vasospasms associated with preeclampsia can lead to hypovolemia, a condition that decreases blood flow to vital organs.
Monitor urinary output q4h or as ordered; report outputs totaling less than 30 mL/hr, or 120 mL per 4-hour time period.	Reduced urinary output can indicate decreased blood flow to the kidneys, which should be treated promptly to prevent kidney damage.
Measure daily weights. a. Use the same scale at the same time each day with the same amount of clothing. b. Report sudden weight gain. c. Monitor for edema.	Sudden weight gain and edema indicates that fluid is being retained. Although the woman has more overall body water, the fluid is trapped in tissues so that less fluid is in the blood, a condition that leads to decreased perfusion.

NURSING DIAGNOSIS

Risk for Injury (maternal) related to cerebral irritability and possible progression of preeclampsia to eclampsia.

GOAL: Freedom from injury related to seizure activity.

EXPECTED OUTCOMES: The woman will
- Not experience injury from seizure activity
- Maintain a clear airway

(continues on page 402)

Nursing Care Plan 17-1 (continued)

THE WOMAN WITH PREECLAMPSIA

Nursing Interventions	*Rationale*
Monitor vital signs as ordered; assess for increasing blood pressure.	Increasing blood pressure indicates a worsening of status. The woman is then at risk for seizure activity.
Institute seizure precautions	A noisy, stimulating environment increases the risk for a seizure. If the woman does have a seizure, padded side rails, airway, suction equipment, and oxygen will all be needed to prevent serious injury from the seizure (e.g., aspiration).
a. Side rails up and padded	
b. Airway, suction, and oxygen equipment set up at bedside.	
c. Quiet, minimally stimulating environment (low lights, sound, etc.)	
Monitor for signs of impending seizure.	All listed signs are indicators that seizure activity will likely occur unless there is intervention.
d. Headache	
e. Blurred vision	
f. Epigastric pain	
g. Hyperactive reflexes: 4+	
h. Presence of clonus	
Assist the RN to administer magnesium sulfate, as ordered.	Magnesium sulfate is a muscle relaxant and a central nervous system depressant that can prevent eclamptic seizures.

NURSING DIAGNOSIS

Risk for Injury (fetal) related to chronic hypoxia secondary to ineffective tissue perfusion of the placenta and episodes of acute hypoxia during maternal seizure activity.

GOAL: Maintenance of adequate fetal oxygenation.

EXPECTED OUTCOMES: The fetus will
- Maintain a heart rate between 120 and 160 bpm
- Remain active with normal kick counts
- Demonstrate well-being with reactive nonstress tests

Nursing Interventions	*Rationale*
Maintain in side-lying position, or with a wedge under one hip.	A side-lying position increases perfusion to the placenta.
Monitor fetal heart tones and reactivity, as ordered.	Monitoring is done to determine fetal status.
Instruct the client to monitor fetal kick counts after each meal. (Chapter 7 outlines the procedure for performing fetal kick counts.)	If the fetus is moving as often as expected, there is reassurance the fetus is doing well. A decrease in fetal movement is an ominous sign.
Assist the RN to perform nonstress tests (NST), as ordered.	Serial NSTs will be ordered to closely monitor fetal status. A nonreactive NST indicates the fetus may be in distress.

If magnesium sulfate was not administered, the woman may be transferred to a postpartum unit. In addition to normal postpartum care, closely observe the blood pressure and monitor for other signs of worsening preeclampsia because a seizure can occur several days after delivery. Observe the woman closely because she is at increased risk for postpartum hemorrhage. Monitor the platelet count, as ordered, and watch for development of complications, such as bleeding from the mouth, gums, nose, or injection sites. If the neonate is in the neonatal intensive care unit, assist the woman to visit as soon as she is able. If she cannot visit, provide pictures of the infant and provide a daily update on the baby's condition.

Chronic Hypertension and Preeclampsia Superimposed on Chronic Hypertension

Chronic hypertension is high blood pressure that is present before the woman becomes pregnant. When a woman with pre-existing hypertension becomes pregnant, the pregnancy is already at risk. Sustained high blood pressure can be damaging to blood vessels and eventually can decrease placental perfusion, leading to fetal growth restriction. In addition, the woman with chronic hypertension is at a much higher risk of developing superimposed preeclampsia. Box 17-3 lists complications associated with chronic hypertension in the pregnant woman.

Clinical Manifestations

The definition of chronic hypertension is blood pressure that is elevated consistently above 140/90 mm Hg when the woman is not pregnant. If hypertension develops before the 20th week of gestation, chronic hypertension is suspected but is not confirmed until after pregnancy. If the blood pressure remains elevated after the pregnancy, the woman has chronic hypertension. Some women with pre-existing hypertension may begin the pregnancy with mild disease, but then experience severe disease after the 24th week.

The woman with chronic hypertension has superimposed preeclampsia when she experiences proteinuria. Preeclampsia superimposed on chronic hypertension is a particularly lethal combination. In these cases, the preeclampsia tends to develop earlier in the pregnancy and runs a more severe course. The risk of placental abruption and incidence of fetal growth restriction rises significantly.

Treatment and Nursing Care

Ideally, the woman with chronic hypertension meets with the physician before becoming pregnant to modify her treatment regimen. If she is taking a hypertensive medication that may be teratogenic, the primary care provider may change her medication to one more appropriate for pregnancy. The provider often recommends a sodium-restricted diet, explains work and exercise limitations, and recommends weight loss, if the woman is overweight. During pregnancy, prenatal visits occur at more frequent intervals, usually every 2 weeks during the first half of pregnancy, and weekly thereafter. Fetal surveillance is an area of intense focus with serial ultrasound tests, frequent NSTs, and BPPs.

Mild, uncomplicated cases of chronic hypertension tend to fare well without significant increases in perinatal mortality. In fact, the woman with mild disease may not require medication. However, in cases of severe hypertension (i.e., if the diastolic blood pressure exceeds 110 mm Hg) the woman will likely need antihypertensive therapy.

Methyldopa (Aldomet) is the antihypertensive of choice for maintenance therapy. Beta blockers and calcium channel blockers may be added to the regimen if methyldopa alone is insufficient to control the blood pressure. The benefit of treatment with one of these agents generally outweighs the risk of fetal effects when hypertension is severe. Angiotensin-converting enzyme inhibitors and angiotensin II receptor antagonists/blockers are contraindicated, and thiazide diuretics are not recommended for use during pregnancy because of adverse fetal effects.

Test Yourself

✔ List four categories of high blood pressure during pregnancy.
✔ What is the underlying process that causes most of the problems associated with preeclampsia?
✔ HELLP is an acronym for _____.

MULTIPLE GESTATION

A multiple gestation refers to a pregnancy in which the woman is carrying more than one fetus. (Singleton gestation is the term used for a pregnancy with one fetus.) Twins are the most common manifestation of multiple gestation. In the general population, twins (two fetuses) occur once in 83 deliveries, triplets (three fetuses) occur once in 6,900 deliveries, and quadruplets (four fetuses) occur once in 575,000 pregnancies (Montgomery et al., 2005). Most pregnancies resulting in more than two fetuses are the result of fertility treatments. The incidence of twins also increases with fertility techniques.

Twins can be identical (monozygotic), resulting from one ovum fertilized by one sperm, or fraternal (dizygotic), the result of two ova fertilized by two sperm (see Chapter 5 for review). A woman has an increased chance of conceiving dizygotic twins if she has one or more of the following risk factors: older maternal age, multiparity, or family history of dizygotic twins. Monozygotic twins may have one or two placentas and one or two amniotic sacs.

Box 17-3 ▎ COMPLICATIONS ASSOCIATED WITH CHRONIC HYPERTENSION IN PREGNANCY

Medical Complications
- Ventricular hypertrophy
- Heart failure
- Cerebrovascular accident (CVA; stroke)
- Chronic renal damage

Complications of Pregnancy
- Superimposed preeclampsia
- Placental abruption
- Fetal growth restriction

The best situation occurs when monozygotic twins each have their own placenta and amniotic sac.

When twins share a placenta, a serious condition called twin-to-twin transfusion syndrome can occur. In this situation, one twin (called the recipient) receives more blood from the placenta than his or her sibling. The recipient twin gets too much blood, which can overload the cardiovascular system and result in polycythemia and heart failure. The other twin, called the donor, does not get enough blood from the placenta. This twin can become severely anemic and experience intrauterine growth restriction.

A multifetal pregnancy is at risk. The woman with multifetal pregnancy is at increased risk for hyperemesis gravidarum, pyelonephritis, preterm labor, placenta previa, and preeclampsia-eclampsia. The fetuses are at risk, as well. They may be conjoined, experience growth restriction, or be born prematurely. During labor, there is a higher risk for umbilical cord prolapse. During the postpartum period, the woman is at risk for postpartum hemorrhage.

A multifetal pregnancy also increases fetal nutrient demands. The woman carrying a multifetal pregnancy requires more calories, protein, and other nutrients (Montgomery et al., 2005). This situation can easily lead to maternal anemia. Insufficient iron leads to iron-deficiency anemia, whereas insufficient folic acid may result in megaloblastic anemia.

Clinical Manifestations

The woman carrying multiple fetuses usually presents with a uterus that is large for dates. She is more likely than a woman carrying one fetus to experience anemia, fatigue, severe nausea and vomiting, and hyperemesis gravidarum. The practitioner performs an ultrasound examination to date the pregnancy and to rule out polyhydramnios, fibroid tumors, and molar pregnancy.

Treatment

Management of a multifetal pregnancy often includes consultation with a perinatologist. There is increased emphasis on the woman's diet, multivitamin and iron supplements, and rest. Obstetric ultrasounds are done every 4 to 6 weeks after diagnosis to assess fetal growth, presentation, and placental location. After 24 weeks' gestation, prenatal visits increase in frequency to every 2 weeks. The practitioner checks the cervix at every visit. Weekly NSTs begin after 32 weeks.

The practitioner must choose (or recommend) a mode of delivery. In general, a cesarean delivery is indicated if twin A (the first twin) is not in a vertex presentation. If twin A is vertex, the practitioner may opt to try a vaginal delivery. This method has a higher chance of success if both twins are vertex. If twin B (the second twin) is breech, the practitioner may schedule a cesarean delivery, or attempt a vaginal delivery but only if twin B is not larger than twin A. If a vaginal delivery is attempted, the practitioner may perform podalic version to turn twin B after twin A delivers. Alternately, the practitioner may attempt a breech delivery for twin B. If twin B experiences fetal distress or if there is difficulty delivering twin B vaginally, a cesarean delivery may be performed for twin B.

Nursing Care

Assist the physician to perform assessments to detect complications throughout the pregnancy. Instruct the woman regarding symptoms of preterm labor (Chapter 18). Teach the woman to perform fetal movement counts daily after 32 weeks gestation. Encourage the woman to get adequate rest and a well-balanced diet.

BLOOD INCOMPATIBILITIES

Incompatibilities between the woman's blood and the fetus' blood can cause problems for the fetus. Normally the two bloodstreams never meet, but occasionally some type of trauma occurs that allows intermingling of the two bloodstreams. This situation is more likely to occur during invasive procedures, such as amniocentesis. The risk also increases during active labor or a spontaneous abortion, or when the placenta separates at birth. Two types of blood incompatibilities are Rh incompatibility and ABO incompatibility.

Rh Incompatibility

The $Rh_o(D)$ factor is an antigen (protein) that is found on the surface of blood cells. When this factor is present on the blood cells, the individual is Rh positive, and when the factor is lacking, the person is Rh negative. If a woman who is Rh negative is exposed to Rh-positive blood, such as through an incorrectly cross-matched blood transfusion, her immune system produces antibodies to fight the $Rh_o(D)$ antigen. Once her body has produced antibodies to the $Rh_o(D)$ factor, she is sensitized to Rh-positive blood, a condition referred to as *isoimmunization*.

The problem arises when a woman who is Rh negative carries a fetus with Rh-positive blood. If the pregnant woman has been sensitized, the antibodies to the $Rh_o(D)$ factor readily cross the placenta and attack the fetus' blood cells. The fetus develops hemolytic anemia and often requires exchange transfusions in utero or shortly after birth. In years past, a woman who was Rh negative often became sensitized while carrying her first child. Sensitization most often occurred during childbirth, when fetal blood can leak into the woman's bloodstream during delivery. Thereafter, with each subsequent pregnancy, the fetus with Rh-positive blood would develop hemolytic anemia, with the disease becoming increasingly severe with each subsequent pregnancy. Now, sensitization rarely occurs because the Rh-negative woman receives anti-D immunoglobulin (RhoGam) within 72 hours of delivering an Rh-positive baby.

Clinical Manifestations

Routine blood and Rh typing during the first prenatal visit identify the woman at risk for Rh incompatibility. Antibody screening determines whether the woman is already sensitized. If sensitization has occurred (i.e., the antibody screen is positive), the woman will have no symptoms at all; however, the fetus may be severely affected. The physician often performs amniocentesis or cordocentesis to diagnose and assess hemolytic disease in the fetus. If sensitization has not occurred (i.e., the antibody screen is negative), the woman will be instructed about treatment and prophylaxis with RhoGam.

Treatment

RhoGam is a product derived from blood that prevents the Rh-negative woman from developing antibodies to the $Rh_0(D)$ factor. It is critical for a woman who is Rh-negative to receive RhoGam after any invasive procedure (e.g., amniocentesis or chorionic villus sampling), trauma of any kind (e.g., motor vehicle collision or physical trauma), and delivery, whether it be by abortion, miscarriage, removal of ectopic pregnancy, or vaginal or cesarean birth. It is during these times that fetal blood is most likely to contact maternal blood. Most physicians also administer a prophylactic minidose of RhoGam at 28 weeks of pregnancy.

If the woman is sensitized, she is not a candidate for RhoGam, and the fetus requires close observation. As the pregnancy progresses, fetal well-being is assessed with amniocentesis, cordocentesis, BPP, NSTs, or contraction stress tests. If hemolytic disease is severe, the fetus may require exchange transfusions, or the physician may opt to deliver the fetus prematurely (see Chapter 20 for discussion of hemolytic disease of the newborn).

It is important to note that Rh incompatibility does not occur if the woman is Rh positive. It does not matter what the fetus' Rh factor is; if the woman is Rh positive, she is not a candidate for RhoGam. An Rh-negative woman who delivers an Rh-negative child is also not a candidate for RhoGam. Because the gene for Rh-negative blood is autosomal recessive, if the woman's partner is Rh negative and she is Rh negative, the fetus will be Rh negative, and RhoGam will be unnecessary. The newborn is never a candidate for RhoGam.

> **Think of it this way.**
> A problem with Rh incompatibility can only exist if the woman is Rh negative. First, determine the woman's blood type. If she is Rh positive, then there is no problem. If she is Rh negative, a problem exists only if the fetus is Rh positive.

Nursing Care

Before discharging a woman after any invasive procedure, abdominal trauma, abortion, ectopic pregnancy, or childbirth, check her blood type. If there is a discrepancy between laboratory reports and the prenatal record, consult with the primary care provider before proceeding. If the woman is Rh negative, determine whether she is a candidate for RhoGam. The criteria for giving RhoGAM are as follows:

- The woman must be Rho(D) negative.
- The woman must not have anti-D antibodies (i.e., must not be sensitized).
- The infant must be Rho(D) positive (the fetus' blood type is not checked after an abortion).
- A direct Coombs' test (a test for antibodies performed on cord blood at delivery) must be weakly reactive or negative.

If the woman is a candidate, obtain orders and administer the RhoGam. Instruct her regarding the purpose and importance of RhoGam to subsequent pregnancies. Make certain that she understands under what circumstances she is to receive RhoGam in the future.

ABO Incompatibility

ABO incompatibility is another cause of hemolytic disease of the newborn (see Chapter 20). The problem most frequently arises when the woman's blood type is O and the fetus' blood type is A, B, or AB. Type O blood has naturally occurring antibodies against types A, B, and AB. These antibodies are large and generally do not cross the placenta. However, occasionally during pregnancy fetal blood may leak into the maternal circulation, causing the woman's immune system to produce antibodies to fetal blood. These antibodies are smaller than the naturally occurring antibodies and readily cross the placenta, where they work to destroy fetal blood. Fortunately, this type of blood incompatibility usually results in a much less severe form of hemolytic disease than does Rh incompatibility. The neonate rarely requires exchange transfusions, although he or she will likely require treatment for jaundice.

> ### Test Yourself
> ✔ List three complications for which a multiple gestation is at risk.
> ✔ Name two situations that place the fetus at increased risk for blood incompatibilities.
> ✔ What product is administered to an Rh-negative woman after she has delivered an Rh-positive fetus?

Key Points

➤ Nursing care of hyperemesis gravidarum focuses on assisting the woman to regain fluid balance and to obtain nutrition needed for healthy fetal development.

➤ Signs and symptoms of ectopic pregnancy include missed menstrual period, nausea and vomiting, abdominal pain, shoulder pain, and vaginal spotting or bleeding. If the tube ruptures, the woman experiences hemorrhage into the abdominal cavity and may develop hypovolemic shock.

➤ Spontaneous abortion is loss of a pregnancy before the fetus is able to survive outside the uterus on his or her own (before viability). Abortions are classified according to whether or not the uterus is emptied, or for how long the products of conception are retained. The six types of spontaneous abortion are threatened, inevitable, incomplete, complete, missed, and habitual (recurrent).

➤ Cerclage is the surgical procedure used to treat cervical insufficiency. A suture closes the cervix with the goal that the woman will be able to carry the pregnancy to term.

➤ For the woman with a molar pregnancy, provide patient education regarding follow-up care, including the importance of frequent physician visits, monitoring of serum hCG levels, avoiding pregnancy for at least 1 year, and reporting any symptoms of metastasis (e.g., severe persistent headache, cough or bloody sputum, or unexpected vaginal bleeding).

➤ Placenta previa causes painless, bright red bleeding during pregnancy due to an abnormally implanted placenta that is too close to or covers the cervix. Abruptio placentae is associated with dark red, painful bleeding caused by the premature separation of the placenta from the wall of the uterus at any time before the end of labor.

➤ The nursing process is used to develop the plan of care for a woman with a bleeding disorder. The focus of the care plan is maintaining placental perfusion and fluid volume, avoiding fetal injury (dealing with hypoxia), preventing maternal injury (dealing with isoimmunization), preventing infection, and reducing anxiety and pain.

➤ Hypertensive disorders are classified according to when in relation to the pregnancy the high blood pressure is first diagnosed, the presence or absence of proteinuria, and whether or not the condition resolves spontaneously after delivery. The four categories of hypertension are gestational hypertension, preeclampsia/eclampsia, chronic hypertension, and preeclampsia superimposed on chronic hypertension.

➤ Priority nursing interventions for the woman with preeclampsia-eclampsia include maintaining bed rest in a side-lying position; monitoring neurologic status, blood pressure, urinary output, and daily weights; instituting seizure precautions; observing for signs of an impending seizure (headache, blurred vision, epigastric pain, hyperactive reflexes, and presence of clonus); assisting the RN to administer magnesium sulfate; and monitoring the fetus (fetal kick counts, fetal heart rate, and NSTs).

➤ A multiple gestation (multifetal pregnancy) is at risk. The woman is more likely to experience hyperemesis gravidarum, pyelonephritis, preterm labor, placenta previa, preeclampsia-eclampsia, and postpartum hemorrhage. Close observation of the pregnancy with special attention to diet and fetal well-being is recommended. The mode of delivery is dependent on several factors, the most important of which is the presentation of each twin.

➤ Rh and ABO incompatibilities can cause hemolytic disease of the fetus/newborn. The goal of therapy for Rh incompatibility is to prevent isoimmunization of the woman. This is done by administering RhoGam to the Rh-negative woman within 72 hours of spontaneous abortion, birth, or invasive procedures, such as amniocentesis. If the woman is isoimmunized, the focus of assessment and care becomes the fetus, who may require exchange transfusions.

INTERNET RESOURCES

Hyperemesis Gravidarum
www.hyperemesis.org

Early Pregnancy Loss
www.nationalshareoffice.com
www.babycenter.com/0_understanding-miscarriage_252.bc

Ectopic and Molar Pregnancy
www.isstd.org/home.html
www.marchofdimes.com/professionals – Click on Medical References, then Quick Reference and Fact Sheets; scroll down to "Pregnancy loss and other concerns"

Preeclampsia
www.preeclampsia.org

Workbook

■ NCLEX-STYLE REVIEW QUESTIONS

1. A 28-year-old gravida 4, para 0 is at the prenatal clinic for complaints of lower abdominal cramping and spotting at 12 weeks' gestation. The nurse mid-wife performs a pelvic examination and finds that the cervix is closed. What does the nurse suspect is the cause of the cramps and spotting?

   a. Ectopic pregnancy
   b. Habitual abortion
   c. Cervical insufficiency
   d. Threatened abortion

2. A 32-year-old gravida 1, para 0 at 36 weeks' gestation comes to the obstetric department reporting abdominal pain. Her blood pressure is 164/90 mm Hg, her pulse is 100 beats per minute, and her respirations are 24 per minute. She is restless and slightly diaphoretic with a small amount of dark red vaginal bleeding. What assessment should the nurse make next?

   a. Check deep tendon reflexes.
   b. Measure fundal height.
   c. Palpate the fundus and check fetal heart rate.
   d. Obtain a voided urine specimen and determine blood type.

3. Which assessment finding best correlates with a diagnosis of hydatidiform mole?

   a. Bright red, painless vaginal bleeding
   b. Brisk deep tendon reflexes and shoulder pain
   c. Dark red, "clumpy" vaginal discharge
   d. Painful uterine contractions and nausea

4. Which instruction is appropriate to give to a woman with hyperemesis gravidarum?

   a. Eat mainly high-fat foods to supply sufficient calories.
   b. Limit fluids with meals to increase retention of food.
   c. Do all your own cooking so you will build up a tolerance for food odors.
   d. Take your antinausea medicine after meals to help control the nausea.

■ STUDY ACTIVITIES

1. Fill in the table to indicate how ectopic pregnancy, threatened abortion, inevitable abortion, and cervical insufficiency are alike and how they are different according to the signs and symptoms listed.

	Pain	Bleeding	Nausea and Vomiting	Cervical Dilation
Ectopic pregnancy				
Threatened abortion				
Inevitable abortion				
Cervical insufficiency				

2. Think of an experience you, a relative, or a friend has had that involved a miscarriage. Be ready to share your story with your clinical group. Discuss interventions the nurse can use to help the parents to cope after a miscarriage.

■ CRITICAL THINKING: WHAT WOULD YOU DO?

Apply your knowledge of hypertensive disorders of pregnancy to the following situation.

1. Maria, a 38-year-old primigravida, presents to the doctor's office for a scheduled prenatal visit at 28 weeks' gestation. During the assessment, Maria comments that she must be eating more than she thought because she gained 5 lb during the course of 2 days. Her blood pressure is 150/92 mm Hg while sitting.

   a. What should the nurse ask next? Why?
   b. What additional assessments should be done?
   c. Based on these data, what management plan is the physician likely to implement?

2. Maria is admitted to the hospital to rule out preeclampsia. The doctor's orders include bed rest with bathroom privileges, regular diet, private room, limit visitors, 24-hour urine specimen for protein and creatinine clearance, complete blood count, blood urea nitrogen and creatinine levels, liver profile, and coagulation studies.

   a. How should the nurse prepare the room for Maria? What supplies are needed? Why?
   b. If Maria has preeclampsia, what results does the nurse anticipate to see on the laboratory report for each test?
   c. Why did the doctor write an order for a private room and to limit visitors?

3. Maria receives a diagnosis of mild preeclampsia. She is to remain in the hospital on bed rest.

   a. What fetal assessment tests should be done? How frequently?

   b. What special instructions and recurring assessments should be included on the care plan?

   c. Maria asks the nurse, "Since my condition is mild, why can't I just go home? I could stay in bed there and I'd be so much more comfortable." How should the nurse reply?

4. The nurse is doing the morning assessment. Maria says, "I woke up with a terrible headache, and I can't seem to wake up enough to see well this morning. Everything looks blurry." Maria's blood pressure is 164/110 mm Hg.

   a. How is Maria's condition classified now?

   b. What other assessments should the nurse make? What should be done next after the assessment is completed?

   c. How does the nurse expect the treatment plan will change?

18 *Labor at Risk*

KEY TERMS

amnioinfusion
chorioamnionitis
external version
labor dystocia
pelvic rest
precipitous labor
tocolytic

LEARNING OBJECTIVES

On completion of this chapter, you should be able to:

1. Explain labor dystocia and describe appropriate nursing interventions.
2. Discuss treatment and nursing management of fetal malpresentation.
3. Compare and contrast premature rupture of membranes (PROM) with preterm PROM.
4. Describe clinical manifestations of preterm labor.
5. Discuss treatment options for preterm labor.
6. Apply the nursing process to the care of a woman in preterm labor.
7. Discuss potential complications, medical management, and nursing care for the woman with a postterm pregnancy.
8. Describe nursing interventions for the woman experiencing fetal demise.
9. Compare and contrast obstetric emergencies according to clinical manifestations, treatment, and nursing care.

SOMETIMES situations arise that put the laboring woman and her fetus at risk. It is for this reason that many women prefer to deliver in a hospital setting. However, a well-trained practitioner who monitors the laboring woman closely can often catch signs of developing complications so that intervention can prevent harm no matter what the treatment setting. The following discussion describes complications that the woman sometimes encounters during labor. Although you may not be directly responsible for the laboring woman, it is helpful to know the signs of labor complications to be able to summon help when needed.

DYSFUNCTIONAL LABOR (DYSTOCIA)

Labor dystocia is an abnormally slow progression of labor. Dystocia occurs because of a malfunction in one or more of the "four Ps" of labor that was discussed in Chapter 8: passageway, passenger, powers, or psyche. The pelvis may be small or contracted because of disease or injury. The fetus may be malpositioned, excessively large (macrosomic), or have an anomaly, such as hydrocephalus or omphalocele, which may not allow him to fit through the birth canal. Uterine contractions may be of insufficient quality or quantity. The woman may be unable to push effectively during the second stage of labor because of exhaustion. The woman may "fight" the contractions because of fear or pain. Frequently a combination of factors results in dysfunctional labor.

Complications

Difficult labor is associated with increased maternal and fetal morbidity and mortality. The risk for infection increases during prolonged labor, particularly in association with ruptured membranes. Bacteria can ascend the birth canal, resulting in fetal or maternal bacteremia and sepsis. Neonatal pneumonia can result from the fetus aspirating infected amniotic fluid. Uterine rupture can result from obstructed labor. This complication can be lethal for the woman and her fetus. Labor dystocia is the most common reason cited for performing a primary cesarean delivery, which carries increased risk for mother and baby. The American College of Obstetricians and Gynecologists attributes approximately 60% of cesarean deliveries to labor dystocia (Cunningham et al., 2005).

Some complications of labor dystocia relate only to the woman. Fistula formation is more common in prolonged labor because the presenting part exerts pressure for prolonged periods on maternal soft tissue, a situation that can result in tissue necrosis and subsequent fistula development. Pelvic floor injury is more common for the woman who experiences a difficult labor or delivery.

Clinical Manifestations and Diagnosis

Before the clinician can diagnose abnormal labor, he or she must first be aware of what constitutes normal labor. Table 18-1 compares expected rates of labor progress for the primipara and multipara. For additional review of normal labor, refer to Chapters 8 and 10.

Table 18-1 ▌ EXPECTED LABOR PROGRESS

	Primipara	Multipara
Expected length of the latent phase of labor	<20 hour	<14 hours
Expected rate of dilation during active labor	At least 1.2 cm/hr	At least 1.5 cm/hr
Expected rate of fetal descent during active labor	At least 1 cm/hr	At least 2 cm/hr

Labor dystocia can occur in any stage of labor, although it occurs most commonly once the woman is in active labor or when she reaches the second stage of labor. There are two types of labor dystocia: disorders of protraction and arrest. A protraction disorder occurs when there is abnormally slow progression of labor. An arrest disorder refers to total lack of progress (Satin, 2007). A primipara in active labor receives a diagnosis of protraction of dilation if cervical dilation progresses at less than 1.2 cm/hr. She has a diagnosis of protraction of descent if the fetal head descends at less than 1 cm/hr. If a multipara in active labor experiences less than 1.5 cm/hr cervical dilation or fetal descent of less than 2 cm/hr, the diagnosis is a protraction disorder. Traditionally, the practitioner diagnoses a disorder of arrest when there is no change in cervical dilation or fetal descent for a period of 2 hours, provided the woman is in adequate labor. Recently, some experts are proposing a more conservative waiting period of 4 hours before making a diagnosis of an arrest disorder (Cunningham et al., 2005).

Causes of Labor Dysfunction

Labor dysfunction can occur because of problems with the uterus or problems with the fetus.

Uterine Dysfunction

There are two types of uterine dysfunction: hypotonic and hypertonic. The most common is hypotonic dysfunction. This labor pattern manifests by uterine contractions that may or may not be regular, but the quantity or strength is insufficient to dilate the cervix.

Hypertonic dysfunction presents in two ways. The most common is frequent ineffective contractions. Some clinicians refer to this syndrome as uterine "irritability." The underlying problem with this disorder is that the uterine muscle cells do not contract in a coordinated fashion. The result is an elevated resting uterine tone with small, short, but frequent contractions.

The other type of hypertonic dysfunction manifests as increased frequency and intensity of uterine contractions. This type of hypertonic dysfunction often results in **precipitous labor**—labor that lasts less than 3 hours from the start of uterine contractions to birth. The complication that most frequently results from a precipitous labor is maternal soft tissue damage, such as lacerations of the cervix, vaginal wall, and perineum; and bruising or other trauma to the infant from rapid descent through the birth canal.

Be careful!

Don't confuse precipitous labor with precipitous delivery. Precipitous labor is an abnormally fast labor (lasting < 3 hours); whereas, a precipitous delivery refers to a delivery that is unattended by the physician or nurse midwife.

Cephalopelvic Disproportion

Practitioners sometimes refer to labor arrest as "failure to progress." If hypotonic labor is not the cause of failure to progress, the practitioner may suspect cephalopelvic disproportion (CPD). In this situation, the diameters of the fetal head are too large to pass through the birth canal. CPD can be due to a condition that causes an enlarged fetal head, such as fetal macrosomia or hydrocephalus. CPD can also result from a small maternal pelvis. In the past, maternal rickets frequently was the cause of a contracted pelvis. Improved nutrition has decreased the incidence of rickets, so today most cases of CPD are due to other causes. Nongynecoid pelvic types, such as android, anthropoid, or platypelloid, may result in CPD.

Fetal Malposition

Fetal malposition (discussed next) can cause prolonged labor. When the back of the fetal head is toward the posterior portion of the maternal pelvis, the position is occiput posterior (see Chapter 8 for a review of fetal positions). A labor complicated by occiput posterior position is usually prolonged and characterized by maternal perception of increased intensity of back discomfort. The lay term for this type of labor is "back labor." Face presentation is another cause of prolonged labor. When the fetal face presents, the largest diameters of the fetal head present to the maternal pelvis, and labor is generally prolonged. Breech presentation, transverse lie, and compound presentations may also cause labor dystocia. Any of these fetal positions may result in the need for cesarean delivery, although vaginal delivery may be possible.

Treatment

Treatment depends on the cause of labor dystocia. However, because the cause is not always readily apparent, practitioners usually give a "trial of labor." If uterine hypofunction is the cause of inadequate progress, augmentation of labor with artificial rupture of membranes or intravenous (IV) oxytocin infusion or both is usually the treatment of choice (Satin, 2007). (The augmentation orders require the same process as that for labor induction; see Chapter 11.) Oxytocin augmentation is the treatment of choice for uterine irritability in the absence of placental abruption. In this situation, oxytocin assists the uterus to contract more effectively so that the pattern spaces out, but individual contractions become stronger and more effective.

Hypertonic labor may result from an increased sensitivity of uterine muscle to oxytocin induction or augmentation. Treatment for this iatrogenic cause of hypertonic labor is to decrease or shut off the oxytocin infusion. If the hypertonic pattern causes the fetal heart rate to drop precipitously, the practitioner may order administration of a **tocolytic**, a substance that relaxes the uterine muscle, to slow the labor.

If the cause of labor dystocia is fetal malposition, the practitioner may attempt to manipulate the fetus to a more favorable position. For occiput posterior position, the fetus may rotate unaided to an anterior position, although this process generally prolongs labor because the fetus must rotate 180 degrees, as compared with 90 degrees when the fetal head begins descent in a transverse position. If the woman completes the first stage of labor and the fetal head has not rotated, the practitioner may use the vacuum extractor or forceps to attempt to rotate the head to an anterior position. This requires that the fetal head be at +2 station, or lower. It is possible for the fetus to deliver from an occiput posterior position. In this situation, the baby is born face up.

Nursing Care

Carefully assess fetal lie, presentation, and position when the woman presents to the labor and delivery area. During the active phase, assess the contraction pattern every 30 minutes. Check for uterine contractions of adequate frequency and intensity. Assess fetal response to uterine contractions. Perform a thorough pain assessment every hour to include a pain scale to rate intensity. Ask the woman to describe her pain. Inquire regarding the presence of intense back pain.

Plot cervical changes and fetal descent on a labor graph (Joy & Lyon, 2005). Observe for slow progression or arrest of labor. Identify slow progression if a primipara in active labor dilates more slowly than 1.2 cm/hr or the fetal head descends at less than 1 cm/hr; or if a multipara in active labor dilates more slowly than 1.5 cm/hr or the fetal head descends at less than 1.5 cm/hr, over a period of several hours. Identify arrest of dilation if no cervical change occurs during a 2-hour period and arrest of descent if no descent occurs during a 2-hour period.

If a disorder of dilation or descent is noted, notify the physician. However, make several assessments before calling. Check to see if the woman has a full bladder. Remember that a full bladder can interfere with the progress of labor. Next, determine if the contraction pattern is adequate. Contractions should occur every 2 to 3 minutes apart, last 60 to 90 seconds, and be of moderate to strong intensity during the active phase of labor.

If the bladder is empty and the contraction pattern is adequate, try to determine if the fetus is in an occiput posterior position. Inquire regarding the character of the woman's pain. Suspect occiput posterior position if the woman complains of severe lower back pain. Current nursing literature (Ridley, 2007) indicates that the most effective noninvasive intervention for labor complicated by occiput posterior position is to place the mother in Sims' on the same side as the fetal spine. This positioning helps the fetus rotate from occiput posterior to occiput anterior, which decreases the chance of a cesarean delivery.

Determine if the woman might benefit from pain relief measures. IV sedation or epidural anesthesia might be helpful. If the woman is "fighting" the contractions, pain control might help her relax and allow the cervix to dilate.

> **Don't underestimate the value of comfort measures.**
>
> Counter pressure applied to the lower back with a fisted hand sometimes helps the woman to cope with the "back labor" that is characteristic of occiput posterior positioning.

Call a full report of your labor assessments to the physician. Carefully note any orders for sedation, anesthesia, or oxytocin augmentation. After carrying out the ordered interventions, continue to evaluate for adequate labor progress. Notify the physician if interventions do not result in progression of labor or if signs of fetal distress occur.

FETAL MALPRESENTATION

In the majority of pregnancies at term, the fetus presents head down. Two diversions from vertex presentation are breech and shoulder presentation, more commonly known as transverse lie.

In a breech presentation, the fetal buttocks and/or the feet present to the birth canal (refer to Chapter 8 for pictures of breech presentation). Frequently the preterm fetus is breech because there is room to turn and maneuver in the uterus. At term, approximately 3% to 4% of fetuses are breech (Jenis, 2006). Breech presentation can cause several birth problems. Labor progress can be slow because the soft buttocks do not provide as much pressure on the cervix as does the head in a vertex presentation. There is an increased risk for umbilical cord prolapse (refer to discussion later in this chapter) and cervical spine injury, and the head can become trapped during delivery.

Transverse lie (shoulder presentation) occurs once in approximately 300 deliveries (Bowes, 2006). As with breech presentation, transverse lie is more common early in pregnancy with most fetuses turning to cephalic presentation before term. Factors that predispose to fetal malpresentation include multiparity, placenta previa, hydramnios, contracted pelvis, and uterine anomalies.

Clinical Manifestations and Diagnosis

There are three types of breech presentation: (1) frank (hips flexed, knees extended; also known as pike position), (2) complete (hips and knees flexed; also know as tailor position), and (3) footling or incomplete (one or both hips extended with the foot or feet presenting). Frank breech is the preferred breech position for vaginal delivery (Fischer, 2006). If a transverse lie persists, the fetus cannot deliver vaginally.

The most common method the practitioner uses to diagnose fetal malpresentation is Leopold's maneuvers (Chapter 10) followed by ultrasound. Sometimes the practitioner notes transverse lie by looking at the contour of the abdomen, which tends to be in the shape of a football, wider side to side than top to bottom.

Treatment

There are three basic options for a breech presentation. The practitioner may use **external version**, a process of manipulating the position of the fetus while in utero, to try to turn the fetus to a cephalic presentation (Fig. 18-1). Approximately 60% of the time this procedure is effective; however, sometimes the fetus turns back to a breech presentation before labor ensues (Cunningham et al., 2005). Some practitioners allow the woman to labor with the fetus in a breech presentation and attempt a vaginal delivery, although this practice has become less common because of success-

ful version techniques and malpractice concerns. A cesarean delivery is the third option for delivering a breech presentation.

For a transverse lie (shoulder presentation), there are two options. Either the practitioner will use external version to try to turn the fetus to a cephalic presentation, or he or she will deliver by cesarean.

This is a good review tip.

When you prepare a table in anticipation of a vaginal breech delivery, be sure to include a set of piper forceps. These special forceps can help deliver the head after the rest of the body has been born in a breech presentation.

Nursing Care

You may need to assist with the external version procedure, which is done only in facilities that have the capability to do an emergency cesarean delivery. The RN performs a nonstress test (NST) before and immediately after the procedure. Assist the woman to empty her bladder just before the procedure. Position her supine with a pillow or wedge under the right hip. If ordered, the RN administers tocolytics to relax the uterus. Take and record vital signs before and after the procedure. The procedure is uncomfortable and occasionally has to be stopped because of the woman's discomfort. Administer Rho(D) immunoglobulin (RhoGAM) to the Rh-negative woman, as ordered after the procedure.

If the fetus in breech presentation is to deliver vaginally, expect to see passage of thick meconium. This normally occurs as the buttocks are squeezed during labor, and does not usually cause a problem because the meconium does not mix with the amniotic fluid. Assist the RN to prepare for a difficult delivery. Check that all neonatal resuscitation supplies are available and in working order. Have piper forceps available on the delivery table and be prepared to assist the delivery attendant. You may need to don sterile gloves and hold the infant's body while the attendant applies piper forceps to help deliver the head. A specialist, such as a pediatrician, neonatal nurse practitioner, or neonatologist, should be present at all vaginal breech deliveries.

■ Figure 18-1 External version. One or two physicians manipulate the fetus through the abdominal wall to coax the fetus to turn to a vertex presentation.

Test Yourself

✔ Name four complications associated with labor dystocia.

✔ What is the usual medical treatment for uterine hypofunction?

✔ What nursing assessments must be done before notifying the physician of a disorder of dilation or descent? Name three.

PREMATURE RUPTURE OF MEMBRANES

Premature (or prelabor) rupture of membranes (PROM) refers to spontaneous rupture of the amniotic sac before the onset of labor. PROM occurs in approximately 10% of pregnancies at term (Jazayeri & Galan, 2006). This condition is different from preterm labor, which is the onset of labor before the end of 37 weeks' gestation. PROM is also different from preterm PROM, which refers to rupture of the amniotic sac before the onset of labor in a woman who is less than 37 weeks' gestation. Complications include maternal and neonatal infection, abruptio placentae, umbilical cord compression or prolapse, fetal pulmonary hypoplasia, and fetal/neonatal death.

Preterm PROM occurs in approximately 3% of all pregnancies and is a leading cause of preterm delivery (Medina & Hill, 2006). Infection is the most common cause of preterm PROM (Duff, 2006). Risk factors for preterm PROM include African American ethnicity, cigarette smoking, previous preterm delivery, vaginal bleeding, low-socioeconomic conditions, sexually transmitted infections, and conditions causing uterine distension (e.g., polyhydramnios, multifetal pregnancy). Some procedures, such as cerclage and amniocentesis, can result in preterm PROM. The farther along in the pregnancy that PROM occurs, the better the chance for a healthy outcome. Most women with preterm PROM deliver within 1 week after the amniotic sac ruptures. PROM before the age of viability rarely results in a good outcome.

Clinical Manifestations and Diagnosis

The woman with PROM usually presents to the delivery suite with reports of a large gush or continuous, uncontrollable leaking of fluid from the vagina. She may report vaginal discharge or bleeding and pelvic pressure. However, she does not present with regular uterine contractions because she is not in labor.

Sometimes the diagnosis is obvious when large amounts of amniotic fluid are visible. The practitioner performs a speculum exam, looks for pooling of amniotic fluid, and then tests the fluid with nitrazine paper, which turns blue in the presence of amniotic fluid. The practitioner may perform a fern test if the nitrazine test is equivocal (uncertain). For the fern test, the practitioner collects a specimen of fluid from the vagina on a sterile cotton swab and then smears the specimen on a slide. When the practitioner views the specimen under the microscope, a ferning pattern indicates that amniotic fluid is present.

Treatment

The major problem for the woman with PROM at term is increased risk for infection, specifically **chorioamnionitis**, bacterial or viral infection of the amniotic fluid and membranes. With each hour that passes after PROM that delivery does not occur, the risk for infection increases. Fortunately, most women go into spontaneous labor within 24 hours of PROM. However, many practitioners prefer to induce labor with oxytocin rather than wait for nature to take its course. Current research indicates that induction of labor for term PROM results in fewer maternal infections and fewer neonatal intensive care admissions (Dare et al., 2006). Hospitalization is required for both treatment options: expectant management (wait and see) and induction of labor.

Management of preterm PROM is more complicated. If there are signs of infection, such as elevated maternal temperature; maternal tachycardia; cloudy, foul-smelling amniotic fluid; and uterine tenderness, the practitioner obtains cultures, starts antibiotics, and facilitates delivery, regardless of gestational age. However, if there is no infection, the practitioner may choose expectant management. The goal is to allow the fetus time to mature and achieve delivery before the woman or her fetus becomes infected.

The practitioner often orders a course of IV antibiotics (usually ampicillin and erythromycin) for 48 hours, followed by oral antibiotics for 5 days to treat preterm PROM. The usual practice is to administer 7 days of antibiotic therapy. The National Institutes of Health does not recommend antibiotic therapy for longer than 7 days because this practice does not improve outcomes and increases the risk for development of resistant strains of bacteria.

For preterm PROM between 24 and 34 weeks, intramuscular corticosteroids given to the mother reduce the risk of neonatal respiratory distress syndrome, intraventricular hemorrhage, and necrotizing enterocolitis (Medina & Hill, 2006). Some practitioners administer a tocolytic to prolong the pregnancy long enough for the corticosteroid injections to work. The presence of infection is a contraindication for tocolytic administration.

The practitioner may order strict bed rest or bed rest with bathroom privileges. **Pelvic rest**, a situation in which nothing is placed in the vagina (including tampons and the practitioner's fingers to perform a cervical examination), is instituted because the risk for infection increases whenever the cervix is manipulated. The practitioner may elect to perform periodic sterile speculum examinations to check for cervical changes. A digital examination is not necessary unless signs of labor, such as pelvic pressure, cramping, regular contractions, or bloody show, are present.

The practitioner orders fetal surveillance at least daily. Generally, the woman performs kick counts after every meal. Daily NSTs may also be ordered. The practitioner performs frequent ultrasound examinations to measure the amount of amniotic fluid and fetal growth.

Nursing Care

Assess the woman who presents with reports of PROM. Ask the woman to describe the sequence of events that occurred in association with the rupture of the amniotic sac. Check for visible signs of PROM—pooling of fluid and positive nitrazine or fern test.

Once the diagnosis is established, follow the practitioner's orders for management of PROM. If the woman is at term, expect continuous fetal heart rate monitoring. Watch for the sudden onset of deep variable decelerations, which may indicate umbilical cord prolapse. Take her temperature at least every 2 hours. Promptly report temperature elevation, prolonged maternal or fetal tachycardia, and cloudy or foul-smelling amniotic fluid. Watch for the natural onset of labor or administer oxytocin induction, if ordered.

Always give a thorough report!

The length of time from when the membranes rupture until delivery is an important part of the report to the pediatrician and to the newborn's nurse. They will monitor the newborn closely for signs of sepsis in the event of prolonged rupture of membranes.

PRETERM LABOR

Preterm labor (PTL) is labor that occurs after 19 weeks' and before the end of 37 weeks' gestation. PTL often leads to preterm birth, which accounts for 70% of neonatal morbidity and mortality (Giarratano, 2006). Despite years of research, the incidence of preterm birth has actually increased from approximately 8% to 9% in the 1980s to 12.5% in 2004 (Institute of Medicine, 2006), which represents a greater than 30% increase since 1981 (Lyndon, 2006). The current rate is much higher than the *Healthy People 2010* goal of 7.6%. It is widely accepted that the development of effective treatments for PTL would greatly reduce the health care burden of sick neonates.

Often the cause of PTL is not readily apparent. In fact, there is no associated risk factor in one-half of woman presenting with PTL (Gray, 2006). The top three risk factors are history of previous preterm birth, current multiple gestation pregnancy (twins, triplets, or more), and uterine or cervical abnormalities. Although history of previous preterm birth is one of the better predictors, this association is not helpful for predicting PTL for the primigravida. Box 18-1 lists selected risk factors for PTL.

Clinical Manifestations and Diagnosis

It is not always easy to diagnose PTL. The presence of painful uterine contractions does not by itself indicate that the woman is in PTL, because pain is a subjective phenomenon affected by many variables. The definitive diagnosis of PTL is made when uterine contractions result in cervical change. The earlier the diagnosis is made, the greater the likelihood that treatment will be effective. If the practitioner makes the diagnosis after the cervix

---

Box 18-1 ▌ RISK FACTORS FOR PRETERM LABOR AND BIRTH

Obstetric and Gynecologic Risk Factors
- Multifetal pregnancy (twins, triplets)
- History of preterm birth
- Uterine or cervical abnormalities:
  - Fibroid tumors
  - Bicornuate uterus
  - Cervical insufficiency
- Preterm premature rupture of membranes
- Placenta previa
- Retained intrauterine device
- Short time period (<6–9 months) between pregnancies
- Poor pregnancy weight gain
- In Vitro fertilization

Demographic and Lifestyle Risk Factors
- Extremes of maternal age (<17 years of age or >35 years of age)
- Member of an ethnic minority
- Low socioeconomic status
- Late or no prenatal care
- Smoking
- Alcohol or illicit drug use
- Intimate partner violence
- Lack of social support
- High levels of stress
- Long working hours with long periods of standing

Medical Risk Factors
- Infection
  - Chorioamnionitis
  - Bacterial vaginosis
  - Bacteriuria
  - Acute pyelonephritis
  - Sexually transmitted infections
- High blood pressure
- Diabetes
- Clotting disorders
- Entering the pregnancy underweight
- Obesity

Fetal-Related Risk Factors
- Intrauterine growth restriction
- Congenital anomalies

---

has dilated to greater than 3 cm, it is unlikely that labor will stop, and it is highly likely that the baby will be born prematurely.

The woman in PTL often presents with signs that include uterine contractions, which may be painless; pelvic pressure; menstrual-like cramps; vaginal pain; and low, dull backache accompanied by vaginal discharge and bleeding. The membranes may be intact or ruptured. The most frequent examinations used to diagnose PTL include assessment of contraction frequency, fetal fibronectin test (Box 18-2), and measurement of cervical length. No change in cervical length in the presence of a negative fetal fibronectin test indicates that the woman has a very low chance of delivering prematurely in the next 2 weeks (Rideout, 2005).

Treatment

Standard obstetric care includes evaluation of risk factors for preterm delivery as early as the first office visit. If there are risk factors for PTL, the practitioner examines the cervix for evidence of injury and performs a workup to detect asymptomatic bacteriuria, sexually transmitted infections, and bacterial vaginosis. The practitioner may prescribe antibiotics to treat these infections, if present. At 20 and 26 weeks' gestation, cervical length may be measured using transvaginal ultrasound. A cervical length of less than 2.5 cm is abnormal (Gray, 2006). The woman receives education regarding signs and symptoms of PTL. Weekly telephone contact with a nurse and regular prenatal visits are encouraged.

Once PTL is diagnosed, the practitioner must determine how best to treat it. The traditional treatments, bed rest and hydration, are no longer recommended due to numerous potentially dangerous side effects (Gray, 2006). The practitioner must decide if tocolytics (Table 18-2) are appropriate. A fetus less than 23 weeks' gestation has almost no chance of surviving outside of the womb, so tocolytics generally are not used below this gestational age. Likewise, practitioners do not often pre-

scribe tocolytics after 34 weeks' gestation because the risk of prolonging the pregnancy at this point is often greater than the risk of neonatal morbidity and mortality if the fetus delivers. Therefore, administration of tocolytics usually occurs between 24 and 33 weeks' gestation. Although the medication may not prevent preterm birth, tocolytics often buy enough time to allow for corticosteroid injections to help mature the fetal lungs, treatment of group B streptococcal infections, if present, or to allow transfer to a facility with a higher level of neonatal intensive care. All of these interventions have consistently improved perinatal outcomes (Wyatt & Rhoads, 2006).

One particularly promising new treatment is for the practitioner to administer weekly injections of progesterone to the pregnant woman with a history of preterm delivery. This treatment option may prevent preterm birth in up to one third of the women who are candidates for this therapy (American College of Obstetricians and Gynecologists, 2005; Cypher, 2007).

Nursing Process for the Woman With Preterm Labor

Assessment

Collect a thorough history, including history of previous preterm birth, multifetal pregnancy, infections, cigarette smoking, and other risk factors for PTL (see Box 18-1). Inquire if the woman is experiencing symptoms of PTL, such as uterine contractions; uncontrollable leaking of fluid from the vagina; backache; menstrual-like cramps; and vaginal pain, discharge, or bleeding.

The physical assessment includes nitrazine testing. If the nitrazine test results are uncertain, prepare to assist the RN or practitioner to perform a speculum exam to check for pooling of fluid and to obtain a fern test. Place the woman on the fetal monitor. Observe for uterine irritability or contractions. Palpate the uterus carefully. A hard, boardlike uterine rigidity and pain that does not relent may indicate placental abruption.

Assess the woman's emotional response. The threat of PTL may cause apprehension, fear, and anxiety. The woman and her partner may be concerned for the well-being of the fetus. Once the diagnosis is established, the woman may be concerned about the side effects of tocolytic therapy.

Selected Nursing Diagnoses

- Risk for Imbalanced Fluid Volume related to dehydration, infusion of high volumes of IV fluid, and/or side effects of tocolytic therapy
- Risk for Injury related to side effects of tocolytic therapy
- Acute Pain related to labor contractions
- Anxiety related to threat of harm to or death of self and fetus

---

Box 18-2 ▌ FETAL FIBRONECTIN TEST

Fetal fibronectin is a protein that acts as a cellular adhesive (glue) to help the placenta and fetal membranes adhere to the uterus during pregnancy. It is normally absent between weeks 22 and 37 of gestation.

Testing

The practitioner uses a cotton swab to collect a sample of cervical secretions and sends the sample to a laboratory for analysis. It takes approximately 6 to 36 hours to get the results.

Interpreting Results

A negative result (absence of fetal fibronectin) is a reliable indicator that delivery is unlikely to occur within the 2 weeks following the test. A positive test (presence of fetal fibronectin) is a less reliable indicator. A positive test may or may not mean that the woman is in preterm labor.

Table 18-2 ■ **TOCOLYTIC AGENTS**

Medication	Route of Administration	Maternal Side Effects	Fetal/Neonatal Side Effects
terbutaline (Bricanyl)	Subcutaneous	Tachycardia, palpitations, anxiety, hypokalemia, hyperglycemia, hypotension, shortness of breath, headache, nausea or vomiting, chest pain, pulmonary edema, cardiac ischemia, cardiac insufficiency	Tachycardia, elevated serum glucose
magnesium sulfate	IV	*At therapeutic levels:* Flushing, feelings of warmth, lethargy, pulmonary edema *At toxic levels:* Respiratory depression, tetany, paralysis, profound hypotension, cardiac arrest	*At therapeutic levels:* Nonreactive nonstress test; decreased to no fetal breathing movements
indomethacin	*Loading dose:* Rectal suppository *Maintenance dose:* Oral	Nausea, heartburn, renal failure, hepatitis, gastrointestinal bleeding	Premature closure of the ductus arteriosus, oligohydramnios, neonatal necrotizing enterocolitis, intraventricular hemorrhage, pulmonary hypertension, hyperbilirubinemia
nifedipine (Procardia)	Oral	Flushing, headache, dizziness, nausea, transient hypotension	None known

Note: Ritodrine (Yutopar), an older tocolytic, is no longer available in the United States. The use of magnesium sulfate as a tocolytic has fallen out of favor with many researchers because it does not prolong pregnancy and it increases the risk of fetal/neonatal death (Simhan & Caritis, 2007). A new investigational drug, atosiban, was developed specifically to treat preterm labor. Atosiban is showing promise as a tocolytic with fewer maternal and fetal side effects (Husslein et al., 2007; Lyndrup & Lamont, 2007; Shim et al., 2006).

Planning and Goals

Maintaining the safety of the pregnant woman and her fetus is the primary goal when planning care. Appropriate goals may include that the woman will maintain a balanced fluid volume with clear lung fields; she will not experience injury from tocolytic therapy; she will report a tolerable pain level; and she will report a reduction in anxiety. Additional goals and interventions are planned according to the individual needs and situation of the woman. (Nursing care for the preterm newborn is discussed in Chapter 20.)

Implementation

Maintaining a Balanced Fluid Volume

Monitoring fluid status is an important nursing function for the woman in PTL. Monitor the IV site and the rate of infusion. Administer a fluid bolus of 500 to 1,000 mL only if ordered, and then reduce to the ordered maintenance rate.

Monitor vital signs. A normal blood pressure in conjunction with a rising pulse upon moving from a recumbent to a sitting or standing position is associated with low fluid volume. Hypotension is associated with severe dehydration. Monitor urinary output. Record urine characteristics. Concentrated urine with a high specific gravity may indicate dehydration.

Watch for signs of fluid overload. Normally a healthy pregnant woman can withstand high fluid volumes; however, if she is receiving tocolytics, watch closely for signs of developing pulmonary edema, such as dyspnea, tachycardia, productive cough, and adventitious breath sounds.

Preventing Injury

If the woman is receiving magnesium sulfate therapy to stop PTL, assess her at least once per hour. Report dyspnea, tachycardia, productive cough, or adventitious breath sounds to the RN or practitioner. Monitor respiratory rate. Report bradypnea or periods of apnea. Check deep tendon reflexes at least hourly. Report decreased or absent reflexes immediately. Refer to Chapter 17 for other nursing actions necessary for magnesium infusion.

Monitor serum potassium and glucose levels, as ordered, if the woman is receiving terbutaline, a Beta₂-

adrenergic receptor agonist. Report low potassium or elevated glucose levels to the RN or practitioner.

Monitor for and report any significant changes in the vital signs, in particular tachycardia or hypotension. The practitioner usually leaves orders detailing the pulse and blood pressure levels that require reporting. Assess for shortness of breath, anxiety, and palpitations. Immediately report any complaints of chest pain. Monitor for signs of pulmonary edema.

Managing Pain

Assess the woman's pain using a pain scale at the frequency ordered by the RN. Ask the woman at what level the pain is tolerable. Be sure to assess and record location, characteristics, and intensity. Administer pain medication as ordered by the practitioner. Keep in mind that a sudden increase in pain intensity or pain that does not relent may be the sign of a developing complication. Report any changes in the character or intensity of pain.

Reducing Anxiety

Encourage the woman and her partner to verbalize their fears and concerns. Answer questions honestly and to the best of your ability. If you do not know the answer, say so, and explain that you will find the answer as soon as possible. Make certain that the woman and her partner know the treatment plan. Explain procedures before performing them. Allow the woman to ventilate regarding her feelings. Explore with the RN coping strategies that the woman is using. Assist the woman to use positive coping strategies whenever possible. If she is alone without a support system, ask for a social services or pastoral care consult.

Evaluation: Goals and Expected Outcomes

Goal: The woman maintains fluid volume balance.
Expected Outcomes:

- Skin and mucous membranes remain hydrated.
- Lung fields remain clear to auscultation.
- Hematocrit, serum electrolytes, and urine specific gravity remain within normal limits.

Goal: The woman remains injury free.
Expected Outcomes: The woman

- reports onset of respiratory distress immediately, such as dyspnea or productive cough.
- reports cardiac signs immediately, such as chest pain, heart palpitations, or racing pulse.

Goal: The woman expresses the ability to cope with her pain.
Expected Outcomes: The woman

- reports reduced pain (measured on a pain scale) after interventions.
- reports she is able to get sufficient sleep and rest despite the pain.

Goal: The woman verbalizes that she is coping with her anxiety.
Expected Outcomes: The woman

- uses available social supports.
- uses effective coping strategies.
- reports decreased levels of anxiety.

Test Yourself

- ✔ What is the difference between PROM and preterm PROM?
- ✔ Describe four nursing interventions appropriate for the woman with PROM.
- ✔ List three treatment options that reduce neonatal morbidity and mortality for the woman in PTL.

POSTTERM PREGNANCY AND LABOR

A postterm pregnancy is one that lasts longer than 2 weeks after the due date, (i.e., 42 weeks). The incidence of postterm pregnancy is 3% to 12% (Butler & Wilkes, 2006). Miscalculation of gestational age can lead to an incorrect diagnosis of postterm pregnancy. When the woman seeks late prenatal care and is unsure of her last menstrual period, miscalculation of gestational age occurs more frequently. This is true because early sonograms are the most accurate tool to determine gestational age.

A postterm pregnancy is at risk for increased perinatal mortality, particularly during labor. Oligohydramnios and meconium staining of the amniotic fluid are common complications of postterm pregnancy. Oligohydramnios increases the incidence of cord compression, which can lead to fetal distress during labor. Thick meconium-stained fluid increases the risk for meconium aspiration syndrome (discussed in Chapter 20). The risk for birth of an unusually large infant increases as the gestation advances. The woman in labor with a large infant is at higher risk for shoulder dystocia. A postterm pregnancy that is also complicated by intrauterine fetal growth restriction is particularly at risk for perinatal mortality (Cunningham et al., 2005).

Clinical Manifestations and Diagnosis

The woman presents with an intrauterine pregnancy that has been determined to be at or past 42 completed weeks. Usually the practitioner will attempt to use several methods to determine fetal age, such as when the practitioner could first hear the fetal heart rate by Doppler and by fetoscope, early ultrasound measurements, and recorded fundal height measurements. Decreased amniotic fluid volume may be present, as measured by ultrasound. The practitioner should suspect fetal macrosomia (birth weight >4,500 g). Meconium stain-ing of the amniotic fluid frequently is noted.

Treatment

There are two basic treatment plans for the woman who is carrying a postterm pregnancy. One plan is ex-pectant management. This treatment protocol involves frequent testing for fetal well-being. The practitioner instructs the woman to report decreased fetal move-ment immediately. The woman must have NSTs and ul-trasounds to measure amniotic fluid volume at least twice weekly. Other testing may include biophysical profiles. The second strategy for managing a postterm pregnancy is induction of labor at 41 to 42 weeks' ges-tation. (Chapter 11 discusses labor induction.) Clinical research has shown that similar outcomes occur using either strategy (Butler & Wilkes, 2006; Gülmezoglu, Crowther, & Middleton, 2006).

One intrapartum treatment that the practitioner might order for the postterm pregnancy is **amnioinfusion**, infu-sion of sterile fluid into the uterine cavity during labor. In the postterm pregnancy, amnioinfusion may be done to relieve persistent deep variable decelerations associated with cord compression from oligohydramnios (Hofmeyr, 2007). Some practitioners order amnioinfusion to dilute thick meconium-stained amniotic fluid in an effort to decrease morbidity and mortality from meconium as-piration syndrome; however, current evidence is that amnioinfusion for thick meconium is not helpful (Fraser et al., 2005; Spong & Ross, 2006). Possible complica-tions of this procedure include polyhydramnios from trapped amniotic fluid, high intrauterine pressures, pla-cental abruption, and chorioamnionitis.

Nursing Care

Teach the woman who is postterm to monitor fetal movements daily. (Refer to Chapter 7 for description of fetal kick counts.) Explain the importance of reporting decreased fetal movement to her practitioner immedi-ately. She may be anxious regarding the well-being of her fetus. Provide realistic reassurances. Be certain that the practitioner has answered all her questions and concerns adequately. If you identify a knowledge deficit, instruct her appropriately or refer her to the RN or practitioner for clarification.

During labor, observe the fetal monitor strip closely for signs of fetal distress. Report these immediately to the RN in charge. Carefully note and record the color and amount of amniotic fluid when the water bag breaks. No fluid is worrisome because it may indicate oligohydramnios with thick meconium staining. If you assisted with the amniotomy, be sure to inform the RN of this finding.

The RN is responsible for monitoring the woman who receives an amnioinfusion. The nurse connects the appro-priate solution to IV tubing and primes the tubing and then assists the physician or nurse midwife to insert the IUPC. After the IUPC is in place, the nurse attaches the IV tub-ing to the infusion port and administers a fluid bolus of 250 mL (or the amount ordered). The nurse then connects the tubing to an IV pump and decreases the rate to approxi-mately 150 mL/hr, or as ordered.

Exercise caution! Don't ever place IV fluids or solutions for amnioin-fusion in a baby blan-ket warmer or in the microwave. This prac-tice could result in serious burns.

The RN monitors the resting tone of the uterus at least every 30 minutes. The resting tone should not exceed 25 mm Hg. You may help monitor the resting tone and as-sist the woman with perineal care. Assess and record the amount, color, and odor of the fluid expelled onto the under-buttocks pad. If no fluid is returning at all, notify the RN immediately.

INTRAUTERINE FETAL DEATH

Fetal death is death of the fetus in utero (lack of car-diac activity) at 20 weeks' or greater gestation or a weight of 500 g (some states use 350 g) or more. This definition distinguishes fetal death from early preg-nancy loss, such as occurs with spontaneous abortion (miscarriage).

Causes of fetal death fall into four general types: fetal, placental, maternal, and unknown. Approximately 25% to 40% of fetal deaths can be attributed to fetal causes, 25% to 35% placental causes, 25% to 35% unknown causes, and 5% to 10% maternal causes (Cunningham et al., 2005). Examples of fetal causes include genetic or congenital abnormalities and infection. The most com-mon cause of fetal demise is placental abruption, which is usually categorized under placental causes; however, preeclampsia and other maternal disorders can increase the risk for placental abruption. Cord accidents (such as prolapse or true knot), premature rupture of the mem-branes, and twin-to-twin transfusion syndrome are other placental causes. Maternal causes include advanced ma-ternal age; medical disorders, such as diabetes mellitus and hypertension; and pregnancy-related complications such as preeclampsia-eclampsia, Rh disease, uterine rup-ture, and infection.

Clinical Manifestations and Diagnosis

Often the woman presents for treatment when she can no longer detect fetal movements. Inability to find the fe-tal heart rate leads the practitioner to suspect fetal death. Ultrasound confirms death (Lindsey & Azad, 2007).

Treatment

The current recommendation is to induce labor as soon as possible after diagnosis of fetal death to avoid the rare complication of a coagulopathy (Lindsey & Azad, 2007). The physician induces labor, as described in Chapter 11, for fetal demise at or near term. When the gestational age is less than 28 weeks, the cervix is rarely favorable for induction. In these cases, the practitioner may prescribe prostaglandin E_2 vaginal suppositories or oral or intravaginal misoprostol to induce labor.

Nursing Care

Physical care of the woman is similar to that for other women having labor induced. Pay careful attention to the history because the woman with a uterine scar from previous surgery is at risk for rupture. For the woman at term, use the tocodynamometer to monitor uterine contractions during labor. Postpartum care is the same as for other women.

Emotional care of the woman is more complex. She may experience shock, denial, anger, and depression. Remember that grief responses vary from individual to individual (Callister, 2006). Allow the woman and her family space to comfort one another, but do not avoid her. Offer to call a pastor or other spiritual leader she may desire. Be sure to determine if the woman would like any religious sacraments or rituals. Most institutions provide postpartum care in a unit or room away from the nursery.

> **Don't forget the golden rule!**
> A woman who has just received a diagnosis of fetal demise is experiencing a terrific loss. Be available to her without intruding. Answer her questions honestly. Encourage her to hold and name her baby, if she is able.

Be sure that mementos are collected. Take pictures as dictated by institutional policy. Pictures are usually taken even if the woman refuses them. The chaplain or social worker may keep the pictures on file for a year or more. Inform the woman that she can change her mind and come get the pictures at any time. Collect a lock of hair, footprints, and other reminders of the baby (Capitulo, 2005). Refer to Chapter 19 for further discussion of how to care for the grieving woman.

Test Yourself

✔ Name five complications for which the postterm pregnancy is at risk.

✔ List four categories of causes of fetal death.

✔ Describe at least three ways you can provide support for the woman with a fetal demise.

EMERGENCIES ASSOCIATED WITH LABOR AND BIRTH

Although most births occur without major complications, true emergencies can develop rapidly. The two goals of treatment in any obstetric emergency are prompt recognition of the problem and timely team in-

tervention. Good communication skills are essential for team functioning. It is important for you to recognize risk factors for obstetric emergencies in order to anticipate possible complications. You must also be knowledgeable and skillful in responding to emergent situations.

Amniotic Fluid Embolism

Amniotic fluid embolism (AFE) is a rare obstetric emergency that frequently results in death or severe neurologic impairment of the woman and her fetus. Anaphylactoid syndrome of pregnancy is another name for AFE because research indicates that AFE more resembles anaphylaxis and septic shock than it does pulmonary embolism.

AFE is a rare complication of pregnancy with a maternal mortality rate as high as 80% (Schoening, 2007). Very few women survive AFE without neurologic damage (Moore & Ware, 2005). AFE occurs in two major phases: respiratory distress, followed by hemodynamic instability, which includes pulmonary edema and hemorrhage. The woman may become comatose, and if she survives, may remain in a vegetative state.

Clinical Manifestations and Diagnosis

In most cases, symptoms of AFE occur suddenly during or immediately after labor. The woman usually develops symptoms of acute respiratory distress, cyanosis, and hypotension. If she is in labor, the fetus typically demonstrates signs of fetal distress, with bradycardia occurring in most cases.

The physician bases the diagnosis on the clinical symptoms and laboratory studies. Arterial blood gases demonstrate acidosis and hypoxemia. Bleeding times are usually prolonged. The chest x-ray may show evidence of pulmonary edema (Moore & Ware, 2005).

Treatment

Unfortunately, there is currently no curative therapy; therefore, treatment aims to support vital functions. An immediate response to the woman's initial complaint of respiratory distress is necessary to increase the woman's chances of survival. The woman often progresses quickly to full cardiopulmonary arrest and requires advanced cardiac life support, including mechanical intubation and ventilation. Authorities recommend delivery of the infant by cesarean within 5 minutes after the start of cardiopulmonary resuscitation (CPR) if the mother does not respond (Moore & Ware, 2005). Typically, the physician treats disseminated intravascular coagulopathy with massive fluid resuscitation and blood product replacement therapy. Once the woman is in stable condition, she requires care in an adult intensive care unit.

Nursing Care

Respond promptly and summon for immediate assistance if a laboring or postpartum woman reports dyspnea.

Administer oxygen via face mask. Measure the vital signs, particularly the blood pressure and pulse. Hypotension, tachycardia, and other signs of shock are usually evident. Initiate CPR, if needed, and be prepared to assist with a cesarean delivery at the bedside, if needed. Be prepared to assist the RN during fluid resuscitation and blood product administration. Anticipate transfer to the intensive care unit as soon as the woman is stable enough to transfer.

Shoulder Dystocia

Shoulder dystocia is an obstetric emergency dreaded by all obstetric practitioners. The fetal head delivers, but the shoulders become stuck in the bony pelvis, preventing delivery of the body. The fetus can suffer permanent brain damage because his chest cannot expand, and he cannot take his first breath. Although macrosomia (fetal weight >4,500 g) and maternal diabetes are the two risk factors known to be associated with shoulder dystocia, many cases occur in fetuses of normal weight (Camune

& Brucker, 2007; Rodis, 2006a). Therefore, nurses and practitioners should anticipate this complication at every delivery.

Shoulder dystocia puts the woman and the fetus at risk. Even if correct maneuvers are used, injury and fetal death can still result. The woman is at increased risk for postpartum hemorrhage due to cervical or vaginal lacerations or uterine atony (failure of the uterus to contract effectively to stop bleeding). The fetus is at increased risk for brachial plexus injuries and fractures of the humerus and clavicle (Cunningham et al., 2005).

Clinical Manifestations and Diagnosis

The "turtle sign" is the classic sign that alerts the practitioner to the probability of shoulder dystocia. The fetal head delivers, but then retracts similar to a turtle. The fetal head may wiggle from side to side and fail to rotate (Camune & Brucker, 2007). The practitioner tries gentle downward pressure on the fetal head in an attempt to deliver the anterior shoulder, but is unable to do so using normal maneuvers (Rodis, 2006b).

Treatment

Several maneuvers are available to the practitioner that may relieve shoulder dystocia. Two of them require the direct assistance of the nurse:

- *McRoberts maneuver* (Fig. 18-2A). This intervention is frequently successful and is often tried first. McRoberts requires the assistance of two individuals. Two nurses are ideal; however, a support person or a technician can serve as the second assistant. With the woman in lithotomy position, each nurse holds one leg and sharply flexes the leg toward the woman's shoulders. This opens the pelvis to its widest diameters and allows the anterior shoulder to deliver in almost half of the cases (Rodis, 2006b).
- *Suprapubic pressure* (see Fig. 18-2B). In addition to McRoberts maneuver, one nurse can use a fist to apply suprapubic pressure. This will sometimes dislodge the impacted shoulder.

The practitioner can try other maneuvers, such as placing a hand in the vagina and attempting to push one of the shoulders in a clockwise or counter-clockwise motion. Intentionally fracturing a clavicle may help dislodge the fetus. In some cases, the practitioner may push the fetal head back in the birth canal and perform an emergency cesarean delivery. This maneuver, called Zavanelli maneuver, has been successful, but is associated with increased risk of trauma.

Nursing Care

Because shoulder dystocia often cannot be predicted, be prepared at every delivery for this emergency. Ensure that the woman's bladder is empty before every delivery. If she cannot void, you may need to use an in-and-out

A Personal Glimpse

My wife, Sally, had just delivered our daughter. We had waited to have a child until we were in our 30s, and then it had taken us 2 years to get pregnant. I was so awed by the whole birth experience. I was taking pictures of my daughter when I heard Sally say to the nurse, "I can't breathe!" I looked over and saw that she was very pale, almost gray. In the blink of an eye, she stopped breathing and one of the nurses started helping her breathe. The other nurse took the baby and me to the nursery. The nursery nurse was very kind. She let me stay with the baby as long as I wanted; however, I couldn't concentrate on the baby because I was so worried about my wife. I went to the waiting room and I was pacing up and down. After what seemed like an eternity, the doctor came to talk to me. He said that he thought Sally had an embolism. He told me that she had a breathing tube and was connected to a machine that was helping her breathe. The nurse came out and took me to the ICU. I felt so frightened by all the tubes and machines that were connected to my wife. I felt very helpless. I also felt guilty for putting my wife through this. I didn't know if I could forgive myself if she didn't make it. Slowly, over the next week, Sally started to get better. I have never felt more thankful in my life than on the day I was able to take Sally home. She was very weak, but she was alive. It was such a joy to see her finally able to hold our little Jessica.

Bill

Learning Opportunity: What could the nurses in this situation have done to help the husband cope with his wife's severe illness? What interventions could the nurse use to help promote attachment between the newborn and the woman when the woman who has been critically ill begins to get better?

■ **Figure 18-2** Maneuvers to relieve shoulder dystocia. **(A)** McRoberts maneuver. **(B)** Suprapubic pressure.

A

B

catheter to drain the bladder. Make sure that a hard surface is available, such as a CPR backboard, to place under the mattress or bed linens beneath the woman's hips when shoulder dystocia is diagnosed (Camune & Brucker, 2007). Make certain that all neonatal resuscitation supplies are present and working before every delivery. Call for the neonatology team and extra nurses to attend the delivery as soon as the diagnosis is made.

Assist the birth attendant with maneuvers, as described above. Be prepared to go for a stat cesarean delivery if the body does not deliver. If maneuvers are successful and a vaginal delivery is accomplished, perform a careful assessment of the newborn. Check for crepitus in the area of the clavicle, which might indicate the bone is broken. Check for spontaneous movements of both arms. Sometimes the newborn will move only one arm, which may indicate Erb's palsy. This injury involves nerve damage (usually temporary) and inability to move the arm. When edema subsides, full function normally returns, although injury can persist.

> **This is important!**
> Don't EVER apply pressure to the fundus (fundal pressure). The shoulder can become more impacted, and the woman has an increased chance of uterine or bladder rupture when fundal pressure is applied with shoulder dystocia.

Umbilical Cord Prolapse

Umbilical cord prolapse occurs when the umbilical cord slips down in front of the presenting part. It occurs rarely in vertex presentations. Factors that increase the risk include fetal malpresentation, multiple gestation, multiparity, prematurity, polyhydramnios, and rupture of the membranes (Belogolovkin, Bush, & Eddleman, 2005) with the fetus at a high station.

Clinical Manifestations and Diagnosis

Prolapse of the umbilical cord can occur at any time (Fig. 18-3). Infrequently, the condition happens before the membranes rupture. Sometimes the woman presents with a cord prolapse. The cord may be visible at the introitus, or it may be palpable in the vaginal vault. An occult prolapse results in cord compression, but the cord is not easily palpable. The woman may report feeling "something coming out" when the membranes rupture. The majority of cases of cord prolapse happen immediately after spontaneous or artificial rupture of the membranes. The fetal heart rate drops precipitously. Vaginal examination typically confirms the diagnosis.

Treatment

When the fetal presenting part compresses the umbilical cord against the bony pelvis, it can compromise fetal circulation and result in fetal death unless the health care team intervenes quickly. Immediate cesarean delivery is the treatment of choice to save the fetus' life. The examiner who discovers the condition should push upward on the presenting part with the fingers to move the fetus away from the cord. Bladder filling with a Foley catheter is another method that can temporarily relieve cord compression while the woman is prepared for delivery.

Nursing Care

Always check fetal heart tones after spontaneous or artificial rupture of the membranes. If the fetal heart rate drops, perform a vaginal examination (or call the RN to

A   B

■ **Figure 18-3** Prolapsed cord. **(A)** Prolapse within the uterus (occult prolapse). **(B)** Prolapse with the cord visible at the vulva.

do one), and palpate for the umbilical cord. If the woman presents with a visible prolapse, quickly place her in bed and gently palpate the cord for pulsations to verify fetal viability. Then use your fingers to press upward on the presenting part. Continue to hold the presenting part off the cord until delivery of the infant. (You will be transported with the woman to the operating room. The sterile drapes will be placed over you.) If you discover the condition and are unable to call for help, place the patient in knee–chest position, call for help, and then continue to intervene as previously described. If another nurse is holding the presenting part off the cord, move quickly to prepare the woman for emergency cesarean delivery.

Uterine Rupture

Uterine rupture occurs when the uterus tears open, leaving the fetus and other uterine contents exposed to the peritoneal cavity. Rarely is this a spontaneous occurrence. It is usually associated with a uterine scar from previous uterine surgery. Often the scar results from a prior cesarean delivery; however, any surgery that requires an incision into the uterus can place the woman at risk for uterine rupture. Traumatic rupture can occur in connection with blunt trauma, such as occurs in an automobile collision or intimate partner violence.

Clinical Manifestations and Diagnosis

Abrupt change in the fetal heart rate pattern is often the most significant sign associated with uterine rupture (Cunningham et al., 2005). Other signs are complaints of pain in the abdomen, shoulder, or back in a laboring woman who had previous good pain relief from epidural anesthesia. Falling blood pressure and rising pulse may be associated with hypovolemia caused by occult bleeding. A vaginal examination may demonstrate a higher fetal station than was present previously. There may or may not be changes in the contraction pattern (Nahum & Pham, 2006).

Treatment

As soon as uterine rupture is recognized, the treatment is immediate cesarean delivery. This action is necessary to save the woman's life and, it is hoped, that of the fetus as well, although uterine rupture is associated with a high incidence of fetal death. This is true because the fetus can withstand only approximately 20 minutes in utero after uterine rupture. This time can be even shorter if the cord prolapses through the tear in the uterine wall and becomes compressed.

Nursing Care

Recognizing the signs of uterine rupture is critical for the obstetric nurse because the complication requires quick recognition and action to avoid fetal and maternal death. In cases of trial-of-labor-after-cesarean, the RN should monitor the woman during labor, particularly if oxytocin is infusing to induce or augment the labor. If signs of rupture occur, immediately prepare the woman for cesarean delivery and institute interventions to treat hypovolemic shock.

Placental and Umbilical Cord Abnormalities

Although, technically, abnormalities of the placenta and umbilical cord are not obstetric emergencies, they can lead to emergencies and can have dire outcomes for the woman and her fetus. Table 18-3 lists selected conditions that can result in maternal and fetal complications.

Test Yourself

✔ Describe three clinical manifestations of amniotic fluid embolism.

✔ Describe two maneuvers with which the nurse can assist when shoulder dystocia complicates delivery.

✔ Define vasa previa.

Table 18-3 ▌ PLACENTAL ABNORMALITIES

Condition	Description	Risk Factors	Maternal and Fetal Implications
Placenta accreta	Abnormal adherence of the placenta to the uterine wall. Variations of penetration occur, including • Placenta increta—the placenta invades the uterine muscle. • Placenta percreta—the placenta penetrates through the uterine muscle, sometimes invading the bladder and other pelvic structures.	History of previous uterine surgery; such as • Cesarean delivery (risk increases with each subsequent C section) • Myomectomy • Dilation and curettage • Induced abortion Other risk factors include • Age older than 35 • Placenta previa	*Maternal implications:* Interferes with normal placental separation in the third stage of labor, resulting in hemorrhage, which may require hysterectomy to control. May also cause uterine rupture during pregnancy or labor. *Fetal implications:* Fetal death may occur if the condition results in uterine rupture.
Velamentous insertion of the umbilical cord	The umbilical cord is attached to the side (versus the center) of the placenta, and the fetal vessels separate in the membranes before reaching the placenta. Vasa previa is a variation in which the fetal vessels are in the part of the membrane that is in front of the presenting part.	Low-lying placenta, antepartum hemorrhage, in vitro fertilization (IVF) pregnancy	*Fetal implications:* Exsanguination (the fetus may bleed out) resulting in fetal death may occur when the membranes rupture.
Succenturiate placenta	An "accessory" placenta that develops at a distance from the main placenta. Vasa previa can occur in this situation when the fetal vessels traverse the membranes between the two placentas.	Same as for velamentous placenta	*Maternal implications:* May result in hemorrhage when the accessory placenta is retained. Hemorrhage may require blood transfusions and/or hysterectomy to control. *Fetal implications:* The same as for vasa previa.
Nuchal cord	The umbilical cord is wrapped once (or more) around the fetus' neck.	This condition occurs frequently in normal pregnancies with no identifiable risk factors.	*Fetal implications:* Moderate-to-deep variable decelerations may occur during labor. Rarely, a tight nuchal cord can lead to fetal death.
True knot	A true knot occurs when the umbilical cord is tied in a knot.	This condition can occur in an active fetus with a long cord.	*Fetal implications:* A true knot sometimes results in fetal death.

Key Points

➤ Labor dystocia is an abnormally slow progression of labor. Nursing interventions include carefully assessing the fetal lie, presentation, and position and the woman's labor pattern throughout labor. Compare the woman's progress with expected norms, and notify the practitioner when progress deviates from the expected. Assist the woman to keep her bladder empty, frequently assess adequacy of the contraction pattern, and administer pain relief interventions.

➤ Two types of fetal malpresentation are breech and transverse lie (shoulder presentation). For breech presentation, the practitioner may use external version, allow the woman to attempt vaginal delivery, or perform a cesarean delivery. For transverse lie, external version or cesarean delivery is needed.

➤ PROM is spontaneous rupture of the amniotic sac before the onset of labor in a full-term fetus; preterm PROM is PROM in a pregnancy that is less than 37 weeks' gestation. In both cases, the woman presents to the delivery suite with uncontrollable leaking of fluid from the vagina. Monitor the woman's temperature frequently to detect early signs of infection.

➤ Clinical manifestations of PTL include uterine contractions, with or without pain; pelvic pressure; cramping; backache; and vaginal discharge and bleeding.

➤ PTL is not easy to treat. If the membranes are not ruptured and cervical dilation is less than 3 cm, the practitioner may prescribe tocolytics and injectable steroids to stop the labor long enough to allow the fetal lungs to mature.

➤ Nursing interventions for the woman in PTL include maintaining a balanced fluid volume, preventing injury, managing the woman's pain, and reducing anxiety.

➤ Complications associated with postterm pregnancy include oligohydramnios with resultant cord compress, meconium staining of the amniotic fluid that can lead to meconium aspiration syndrome, macrosomia, and fetal death.

➤ Patient teaching for the woman carrying a postterm pregnancy includes discussing the plan of care. Frequently labor is induced. Sometimes the practitioner orders expectant management, which involves frequent fetal kick counts and NSTs to monitor fetal well-being. Instruct the woman to report decreased fetal movement immediately.

➤ During labor induction of a woman with fetal demise, monitor the contraction pattern to avoid uterine hyperstimulation. Monitor the woman for signs of disseminated intravascular coagulopathy. Provide emotional care for the woman and her family.

➤ AFE occurs suddenly during labor or in the immediate postpartum period. The woman becomes acutely dyspneic, apprehensive, hypotensive, and cyanotic. Treatment is supportive, and the woman requires care in the intensive care unit.

➤ Shoulder dystocia occurs when the fetal head is born but the shoulders fail to deliver. McRoberts maneuver and suprapubic pressure are two interventions that require the active involvement of the nurse. Carefully observe the newborn for signs of birth injury.

➤ Umbilical cord prolapse occurs when the umbilical cord slips down in front of the presenting part. Unless pressure is immediately relieved, the fetus will die or will experience permanent brain damage from lack of oxygen. An immediate cesarean delivery is required.

➤ History of a previous uterine scar increases the risk of uterine rupture during labor. Ominous fetal heart rate patterns on the fetal monitor are usually the most significant sign of rupture. Prompt cesarean delivery is necessary to save the fetus and the woman.

INTERNET RESOURCES

http://pregnancy.about.com/od/laborcomplications
www.childbirth.org/articles/labor/laborcomp.html

www.merck.com/mmhe/sec22/ch261/ch261a.html
www.moonlily.com/obc/complications.html

Workbook

▮ NCLEX-STYLE REVIEW QUESTIONS

1. A 35-year-old gravida 1 delivered after 24 hours of labor. Her membranes ruptured 4 hours after she started labor. Two hours before she delivered, she spiked a temperature of 101°F. For which of the following complications is her newborn most at risk?

   a. ABO incompatibility
   b. Fistula formation
   c. Pelvic floor injury
   d. Pneumonia

2. A 26-year-old primigravida is attempting natural childbirth. Her doula has been supporting her through the past 16 hours of labor. The laboring woman is now 6 cm dilated. She continues to report severe pain in her back with each contraction. She finds it comforting when her doula uses the ball of her hand to put counterpressure on her lower back. What is the likely cause of the woman's back pain?

   a. Breech presentation
   b. Fetal macrosomia
   c. Occiput posterior position
   d. Nongynecoid pelvis

3. A 31-year-old gravida 3, para 1 calls the clinic. She is at 29 weeks' gestation. She says that she has been having uterine contractions every 10 minutes for the past 2 hours. She also feels "heaviness" in her vaginal area. Her first baby was born prematurely at 28 weeks' gestation. What advice by the nurse is best for this woman?

   a. "Come into the hospital immediately. These signs strongly indicate that you may be in premature labor."
   b. "Drink two large glasses of water. Lie down on your left side. If the contractions don't stop in an hour, come in to the hospital."
   c. "Monitor your contractions for 1 more hour. If they increase in frequency, or get stronger, come in right away."
   d. "It is not likely that you will deliver a second baby prematurely. Don't panic. If you continue to have contractions, come in to be checked."

4. The nurse is assisting in a delivery that is complicated by shoulder dystocia. Which nursing action is indicated?

   a. Give fundal pressure.
   b. Start rescue breathing.
   c. Assist the RN to flex the woman's thighs.
   d. Watch the fetal monitor for signs of fetal distress.

▮ STUDY ACTIVITIES

1. Use the table provided to compare fetal and maternal causes of labor arrest.

Fetal Causes of Labor Arrest	Maternal Causes of Labor Arrest

2. Interview your local March of Dimes representative to see what is being done in your community to learn more about and prevent preterm labor. Share your findings with your clinical group.

3. Develop a teaching plan for a woman with a postterm pregnancy that is being managed expectantly.

▮ CRITICAL THINKING: WHAT WOULD YOU DO?

Apply your knowledge of labor at risk to the following situations.

1. Julia, a gravida 2, para 0, just found out that her fetus is in a breech position at 36 weeks' gestation. Julia is afraid that she will have to have a cesarean delivery. What options does Julia have in this situation?

2. Julia's pregnancy proceeds to 39 weeks' gestation. She presents to labor and delivery because her "water bag broke." After the midwife confirms that the membranes have ruptured, she explains to Julia that the plan is for Julia and her husband to wait in the hospital until labor begins. Julia wants to know why she and her husband can't just go home to wait for contractions to begin.

   a. How do you reply to Julia?
   b. What nursing interventions will you plan for Julia during the wait before labor begins?
   c. How would your care be different if Julia were at 30 weeks' gestation with ruptured membranes versus 39 weeks?

3. Kimberly has been receiving tocolytic terbutaline for the past 12 hours. You are taking Kimberly's vital signs at the beginning of your shift. You notice that Kimberly's pulse is 130 and her blood pressure is 88/50 mm Hg. When you ask her how she is feeling, she replies, "I feel out of breath, and I have a feeling of pressure in my chest." What should you do?

19 Postpartum Woman at Risk

KEY TERMS

deep vein thrombosis (DVT)
endometritis
exudate
hematoma
hypovolemic shock
malattachment
mastitis
pulmonary embolism
uterine atony
uterine subinvolution
venous thromboembolism (VTE)

LEARNING OBJECTIVES

On completion of this chapter, you should be able to:

1. Identify major conditions that place a woman at risk during the postpartal period.
2. Differentiate between early and late postpartum hemorrhage.
3. Describe nursing interventions for the woman with postpartum hemorrhage, appropriate to the cause.
4. Compare and contrast four types of infection that may occur in the postpartum period.
5. Identify factors that place a postpartum woman at risk for venous thromboembolism.
6. Explain treatment and nursing care for the postpartum woman experiencing venous thromboembolism (deep vein thrombosis and/or pulmonary embolism).
7. Describe two major psychiatric problems that can complicate the postpartum period.
8. Discuss the nurse's role when caring for a postpartal woman who is grieving.
9. Identify behaviors that would suggest malattachment.

OFTEN CONSIDERED the "fourth trimester of pregnancy," the postpartum period encompasses the first 6 weeks after childbirth. After delivery, the woman begins to experience physiologic and psychological changes that return her body to the prepregnancy state. These changes usually occur without difficulty. However, factors such as blood loss, trauma during delivery, infection, or fatigue can place the postpartum woman at risk. As the practical/vocational nurse, you play a key role in identifying the woman at risk for complications to ensure early detection and prompt intervention. You may be the person who identifies the problem and alerts the registered nurse (RN) or primary medical provider of the pressing need for intervention. Interventions for the postpartum woman at risk focus on treating the complication, thereby minimizing the effects on the woman's return to her pre-pregnant state; promoting adaptation to her role as mother of a new infant; and supporting and enhancing maternal–infant bonding.

This chapter addresses major complications associated with the postpartum period, including hemorrhage, infection, venous thromboembolism, and psychiatric disorders. The chapter emphasizes priority aspects of care for each complication. The chapter also describes special postpartum situations, such as postpartal grieving and malattachment.

POSTPARTUM HEMORRHAGE

Postpartum hemorrhage is one of the leading causes of maternal deaths, accounting for approximately 30% of all pregnancy-related deaths. It can occur early, within the first 24 hours after delivery, or late, anytime after the first 24 hours through the 6-week postpartum period. The woman is most vulnerable to hemorrhage during the first 24 hours after delivery, with the greatest risk occurring in the first hour after delivery.

Traditionally, postpartum hemorrhage was defined as any blood loss in an amount greater than 500 mL after a vaginal delivery or greater than 1,000 mL after a cesarean birth. However, because blood loss estimates during delivery are often inaccurate and the amount of blood loss that can be tolerated varies from woman to woman, the definition has been broadened. Most authorities accept the definition of postpartum hemorrhage as blood loss resulting in hemodynamic changes (e.g., change in the quality or rate of the pulse or blood pressure), blood loss of greater than 1,000 mL, or a decrease in the hematocrit of 10% or greater after delivery when compared with that before delivery (Wainscott, 2006).

There are four major causes of postpartum hemorrhage: **uterine atony**, inability of the uterus to contract effectively; lacerations to the uterus, cervix, vagina, or perineum; retained placenta; and disruption in maternal

---

Box 19-1 ▐ **RISK FACTORS FOR POSTPARTUM HEMORRHAGE**

Risk factors are listed by cause.

Uterine Atony
- Multiparity
- Intrauterine infection
- Previous uterine surgery
- Prolonged or difficult labor
- History of postpartum hemorrhage
- Placenta previa or abruptio placentae
- Use of oxytocin for labor stimulation or augmentation
- Use of agents during labor that relax the uterus (tocolytics), such as
  - magnesium sulfate
  - terbutaline
  - certain anesthetics
  - nitroglycerin
- Overdistention of the uterus, such as occurs with
  - multiple gestation
  - polyhydramnios
  - fetal macrosomia

Lacerations and Hematomas
- Episiotomy
- Macrosomia
- Precipitous labor
- Traumatic delivery
- Use of forceps or vacuum extraction for delivery

Retained Placenta
- Abruptio placentae
- Placenta accreta
- Prolonged third stage of labor

Disruption in Maternal Clotting Abilities
- Fetal demise
- Thrombocytopenia
- Preeclampsia

---

clotting mechanisms. It is important to monitor all postpartum women for excessive bleeding because two-thirds of the women who experience postpartum hemorrhage have no risk factors. However, there are factors known to increase the risk for postpartum hemorrhage (Box 19-1). Early detection and prompt intervention are necessary to control the hemorrhage. Otherwise, the woman can progress to shock, renal failure, and ultimately death from the loss of blood.

Early Postpartum Hemorrhage

Early postpartum hemorrhage refers to blood loss (>500 mL) within the first 24 hours after delivery. Early

postpartum hemorrhage usually results from one of the three following conditions:

- Uterine atony
- Lacerations
- Hematoma

Most cases of early postpartum hemorrhage result from uterine atony. With this condition, the uterus does not contract as it should. Thus, the muscles of the uterus remain relaxed and exert no compression on the open uterine blood vessels at the former placenta site. As a result, the vessels continue to bleed. This blood loss can be extensive and rapid. Lacerations can occur as small tears or cuts in the perineal tissue, vaginal sidewall, or cervix. A **hematoma** is a collection of blood within tissues that can lead to concealed blood loss.

Regardless of the cause, the woman is at risk for developing hypovolemia, a system-wide decrease in blood volume from too much blood loss. If the blood loss continues, the woman may develop **hypovolemic shock**, which is characterized by a weak, thready, rapid pulse; drop in blood pressure; cool, clammy skin; and changes in level of consciousness. These findings may occur abruptly and be dramatic if the blood loss is large and occurs quickly. However, with bleeding of a more gradual onset, these signs and symptoms may be extremely subtle because of the body's ability to compensate for the blood loss over time. With continued bleeding, the woman's body eventually is overwhelmed and is no longer able to compensate for the loss. At that point, she exhibits the typical signs and symptoms of shock.

The woman who experiences postpartum hemorrhage is also at risk for developing anemia from the blood loss. The woman may require emergency surgical intervention, which may include hysterectomy with loss of childbearing capability, or blood transfusions. Other complications associated with postpartum hemorrhage include further bleeding, which may occur if clotting factors are used up or if disseminated intravascular coagulation (DIC) develops, and multiple organ failure.

Clinical Manifestations

Clinical manifestations of early postpartum hemorrhage differ according the cause of the hemorrhage.

Hemorrhage Caused by Uterine Atony

If the underlying cause of hemorrhage is uterine atony, the woman's fundus usually will be difficult to palpate. When the fundus is identified on palpation, it is soft (boggy), relaxed, and located above the level of the umbilicus. If the woman has a distended bladder, this condition further interferes with uterine contraction. A full bladder may cause the uterus to deviate to one side, rather than being at the midline. Vaginal bleeding (lochia) typically is moderate to heavy, possibly with numerous large clots.

■ **Figure 19-1** Perineal hematoma. Note the bulging, swollen mass.

Hemorrhage Caused by Lacerations

When lacerations are the cause of bleeding, the fundus is firm on palpation. However, the bleeding continues in a steady trickle. Characteristically, the bleeding is bright red in color, in contrast to the dark red color of lochia.

Hemorrhage Caused by Hematoma

Unlike uterine atony and lacerations, the bleeding associated with hematoma formation may not be apparent. A blood vessel ruptures and leaks into the surrounding tissue. This causes pressure, pain, swelling (edema), and dark red or purple discoloration, most commonly on one side of the perineum (Fig. 19-1). Initially, the area may feel soft. However, as leakage into the tissues continues, the area becomes firm to the touch. The area is tender on palpation.

A hematoma also can form deep in the pelvis, where it is much more difficult to identify. The primary symptom is deep pain unrelieved by comfort measures or medication and accompanied by vital sign instability. Regardless of where the hematoma occurs, the woman's lochia usually is within expected parameters. However, if the hematoma is large, she may experience a significant loss of blood into the tissues, leading to signs and symptoms of hypovolemic shock.

Diagnosis

Clinical signs and changes in laboratory values point to the diagnosis. Because of blood loss, the woman's hemoglobin and hematocrit levels are decreased from her prelabor (baseline) levels, approximately 1 to 1.5 g/dL and 2% to 4%, respectively. An underlying coagulation defect manifests with increased clotting times and decreased platelet and prothrombin levels.

Treatment

The goals of treatment for postpartal hemorrhage are to correct the underlying cause while attempting to control the hemorrhage and reduce its effects. If the woman is exhibiting signs and symptoms of hypovolemic shock, emergency measures are instituted to support vital functions. These include rapid intravenous (IV) fluid replacement, blood transfusions, oxygen administration, and frequent close monitoring of all vital functions. Insertion of an indwelling urinary catheter may be necessary to monitor the urine output hourly.

Treatment for Uterine Atony

If uterine atony is present, fundal massage is initiated. Massage may help the uterus to contract, thereby compressing the blood vessels and ultimately decreasing the bleeding. Once the uterus contracts firmly, steady, gentle fundal pressure is applied to help express any clots that may have collected in the uterus. The woman's bladder must be empty; otherwise, the uterus will not remain contracted once the massage stops.

Drug therapy may be necessary if fundal massage fails to maintain the uterus in a contracted state. Typical medications include oxytocic agents, such as oxytocin (Pitocin), ergonovine (Ergotrate), methylergonovine (Methergine), carboprost (Hemabate), and misoprostol (Cytotec) administered parenterally. If drug therapy is ineffective, the primary care provider may need to intervene. Bimanual compression of the uterus is frequently the first method attempted. Exploration of the uterine cavity may be the next option when other treatment measures fail. Uterine packing may be required to control hemorrhage. Another option is uterine artery embolization or ligation to control bleeding. When postpartum hemorrhage due to uterine atony continues despite all efforts to control it, a hysterectomy may be done, usually only as a last resort.

Treatment for Lacerations and Hematomas

Postpartal hemorrhage caused by lacerations requires surgical repair of the lacerations. Small hematomas usually require no additional treatment other than application of ice and analgesics to control pain. In most instances, small hematomas absorb spontaneously, usually during a period of 4 to 6 weeks. Surgical incision with drainage and evacuation of clots and ligation of the bleeding vessel may be required if the hematoma is large.

Nursing Process for the Woman with Early Postpartum Hemorrhage

You play an important role in monitoring the woman's status, assisting with measures to control bleeding, providing support to the woman and her family, and educating the woman about her condition. Maintaining the woman's safety is paramount.

Assessment

As with any patient, thorough, frequent assessment is necessary to allow for early detection and prompt intervention should hemorrhage occur. Be aware of the woman's history, labor progress, and risk factors for postpartum hemorrhage. Note the use of any analgesia or anesthesia during labor and delivery or the use of oxytocin for labor induction or augmentation. This information helps to identify potential factors that would place the woman at risk for hemorrhage.

Ask the woman about the onset of the bleeding, if appropriate. For example, "Did the bleeding seem to increase suddenly or have you noticed a constant trickling?" Ask about any associated symptoms, such as "Do you have any pain or pressure?" These types of questions help to provide information about the possible cause of the hemorrhage. Ask the woman how frequently she is changing her perineal pads, how saturated they appear, and when she changed the pad last. The bleeding of a woman who has changed her perineal pads twice in the last hour with each pad containing approximately a half-dollar–sized amount of lochia is far different from that of a woman who has changed her perineal pads twice in the last hour because they were saturated. Additional evaluation of the second woman is necessary. In this case, notify the RN and the primary care provider.

Assess the fundus for consistency, shape, and location. Remember that the uterus should be firm, in the midline, and decrease 1 cm each postpartum day. Inability to locate the fundus suggests that it is not firm and contracting. Displacement to one side suggests that the woman has a distended bladder.

Observe lochia for color, amount, odor, and character, including evidence of any clots. When evaluating the lochia, turn the woman to her side and look under the buttocks for any pooling of blood that may occur while she is in bed. Note amount and characteristics of the bleeding. Dark red is the normal color of lochia in the first few postpartum days. A bright red color is associated with fresh bleeding, such as that from a laceration. Note whether bleeding decreases with fundal massage.

Determine when the woman last urinated. Remember that a full bladder can impede uterine contraction, predisposing her to hemorrhage. Inspect the woman's perineal area closely for evidence of lacerations or hematomas. Do not mistake an episiotomy for a laceration. Typically, an episiotomy is approximately 1 to 2 inches in length and has clean, regular sutured edges, whereas a laceration varies in length, and its edges appear irregular and somewhat jagged. Evaluate pain and other associated symptoms. Severe pain and pressure that are unrelieved by ordinary pain control measures may indicate the presence of a hematoma.

Assess the woman's vital signs to obtain a baseline and then monitor vital signs as ordered, noting any changes suggesting hypovolemic shock. Note the color and temperature of the woman's skin and her level of consciousness. Recall that cool, clammy skin and decreasing level of consciousness may indicate hypovolemic shock. Table 19-1 highlights assessment findings for the major causes of postpartum hemorrhage.

Cultural Snapshot

For people of color (e.g., African American, Hispanic, and Asian), assess skin "color" (pale, red, cyanotic, jaundiced) by looking at the mucous membranes of the mouth, tongue, and gums. The unpainted nail bed also gives a clear, nonpigmented view of color.

Selected Nursing Diagnoses

- Deficient Fluid Volume related to excessive blood loss
- Risk for Injury related to hemorrhage and possible development of hypovolemic shock
- Ineffective Tissue Perfusion related to decreased circulating blood volume subsequent to postpartum hemorrhage and development of hypovolemic shock

Outcome Identification and Planning

Appropriate goals for the woman experiencing postpartum hemorrhage include the following: The woman will demonstrate signs and symptoms of restored fluid balance, she will remain free of any injury, and she will exhibit signs of adequate tissue perfusion.

Implementation

Nursing care for the woman experiencing postpartum hemorrhage focuses on stopping the bleeding, restoring fluid balance, preventing injury, and promoting adequate tissue perfusion. As with any postpartal complication, be sure to provide emotional support to the woman and her family, explaining all events and procedures to minimize anxiety and fear. Keep the family informed of the situation, explaining laboratory tests, procedures, and signs of improvement. Allow the partner and family to discuss feelings, which may be very intense. Frustration, anger, blame, disbelief, and sorrow are common emotions. Listen, be patient, be present, and acknowledge that this is a difficult time.

Controlling and Restoring Fluid Balance

Key to restoring fluid balance is stopping the bleeding. First, try fundal massage to contract the uterus and stop the bleeding (see Nursing Procedure 12-1 in Chapter 12). Make sure the woman's bladder is empty before beginning massage. Be aware that the uterus may relax quickly when massage stops, placing the woman at risk for continued hemorrhage.

Don't do it!

Never attempt uterine massage without first placing one hand over the symphysis pubis. Doing so could cause the uterus to turn inside out (inversion) and lead to massive hemorrhage that can quickly lead to death.

Table 19-1 ▮ ASSESSING THE SOURCE OF POSTPARTUM HEMORRHAGE

| | Sources of Early Postpartum Hemorrhage | | | Sources of Late Postpartum Hemorrhage | |
	Uterine Atony	Lacerations	Hematoma	Retained Placental Fragments	Subinvolution of the Uterus
Occurrence	Early	Early	Early	Early or late	Late
Condition/ placement of uterus	Fundus is boggy and high. If bladder is full, fundus is displaced to one side.	Normal	Normal	Fundus is slightly boggy but often becomes firm when massaged.	Fundus may be firm when palpated but boggy a short time later.
Characteristics of lochia	Moderate to heavy lochia (i.e., a perineal pad fills up with blood in <1 hour)	Bleeding is heavy, bright red, and continues in a steady trickle or flow.	Normal	Lochia contains intermittent clots.	Initially, lochia flow is normal. Then lochia increases over what is expected and/or reverts to an earlier type of flow (e.g., the lochia becomes rubra after it has changed to serosa, etc.).
Characteristics of pain	May be absent.	May be constant.	Pressure and severe pain at the site (perineal hematoma). Deep pain unrelieved by comfort measures or medication (deep pelvic hematoma).	May be intermittent or heavier than normal cramping.	May be absent or there may be constant cramping. Backache may be present.
Other signs and symptoms	Tachycardia, hypotension, and other signs of hypovolemic shock if blood loss is severe.	Bruising may be apparent.	Swelling (edema) and dark red or purple discoloration (perineal hematoma). Accompanied by unstable blood pressure, pulse, and hemoglobin and hematocrit (deep pelvic hematoma).	Portions of maternal surface of placenta are missing at birth.	Dizziness, lightheadedness, and fatigue when changing positions or doing simple self-care tasks. Fever and other signs of infection may be present.

Administer oxytocics, as ordered. If an IV line with oxytocin is present, increase the rate of flow to a fast drip. Prepare the woman for surgical intervention if less drastic measures do not control bleeding. If the woman is going to surgery, withhold all food and fluids, unless allowed by the physician. If the woman continues to hemorrhage, anticipate transfer to the intensive care unit for closer, more frequent monitoring.

When a woman experiences postpartum hemorrhage, fluid is lost. Encourage her to increase her oral fluid intake, if allowed. If the woman is not able to drink oral fluids, or if fluid loss is significant, expect to administer IV fluids. Expect an isotonic IV solution, such as normal saline or lactated Ringer's solution, to be ordered for replacement therapy. Assist with IV catheter insertion if the woman does not have one already inserted, and administer fluids as ordered. Use care in administering fluids to avoid circulatory overload from too rapid or too great an infusion.

Continue to monitor the woman's fundus and lochia frequently for changes indicating continuation or resolution of the hemorrhage. If uterine atony is causing the bleeding and the woman received IV oxytocin, fundal assessment is crucial. Although oxytocin helps to contract the uterus, and this effect is immediate, the drug has a short duration of action, placing the woman at risk for hemorrhage secondary to recurrence of atony once the IV rate of administration slows or stops.

Inspect the perineum closely for evidence and amount of bleeding. Monitor pad count to help determine the amount of blood lost. Be sure to turn the woman on her side and inspect the area under the buttocks because blood can pool, presenting a misleading picture.

Monitor the woman's intake and output closely, possibly every hour if necessary, to determine the effectiveness of therapy and progression or resolution of the fluid imbalance. Urine output should be at least 30 mL/hr, indicating adequate renal function. Encourage the woman to void frequently to prevent bladder distention from interfering with uterine contraction. If the woman has difficulty voiding, try measures such as running warm water over the perineum, placing the woman's hand in a basin or sink of warm water, or having the woman hear running water at the sink. If all else fails and the woman is unable to void, anticipate the need for insertion of an indwelling urinary catheter.

Expect to assist with obtaining blood specimens for laboratory testing, such as complete blood count (CBC), electrolyte levels, coagulation studies, and type and cross-matching for blood. If ordered, administer blood component therapy to aid in replacing fluid and blood loss.

Continue to monitor the woman's vital signs frequently for changes. Be alert for a rising pulse rate, changing pulse characteristics to rapid and thready, or decreasing blood pressure, which may indicate hypovolemic shock.

Preventing Injury

A postpartum woman who is hemorrhaging is at risk for injury. Reduction in blood supply to the brain can lead to changes in the woman's level of consciousness, placing her at risk for injury from confusion, disorientation, and falls. Therefore, safety measures are necessary.

Keep the call light close by and urge the woman to remain in bed. Check on her frequently, and encourage a family member to stay with her, if necessary. If the woman has bathroom privileges, instruct her to sit at the side of the bed for a short time before rising to prevent orthostatic hypotension, and then assist her to ambulate and stay nearby in the event that she complains of light-headedness or dizziness.

Continue to monitor the woman's vital signs for changes. If she reports dizziness or light-headedness when getting up, obtain her blood pressure while lying, sitting, and standing, noting any change of 10 mm Hg or more. Should the woman's blood pressure drop with position changes, notify the RN and/or primary care provider.

Promoting Adequate Tissue Perfusion

A decrease in circulating blood volume secondary to hemorrhage affects tissue perfusion because the blood does not transport oxygen to the required areas in adequate amounts. Therefore, the woman needs oxygen supplementation. Administer oxygen therapy via nasal cannula or face mask, as ordered. Evaluate oxygen saturation levels with continuous pulse oximetry. Notify the RN or primary care provider if the oxygen saturation falls below 95%.

Arterial blood gas studies may be performed to evaluate the woman's acid-base balance and provide a more definitive evaluation of the woman's status. Be prepared to adjust the oxygen flow rate based on the arterial blood gas findings.

Continue to assess the woman's skin color and temperature for changes. Cold, clammy skin may indicate constriction of the peripheral vessels, suggesting that the woman is developing hypovolemic shock or that her condition is worsening. Check nail beds for color and capillary refill. Keep in mind that a capillary refill greater than 3 seconds suggests impaired blood flow.

Monitor the woman's level of consciousness for changes. A woman who is alert and oriented is exhibiting adequate cerebral perfusion. However, confusion, disorientation, or deteriorating levels of consciousness suggest diminished blood flow and inadequate cerebral perfusion.

When adequately perfused, the kidneys function to produce urine. Urine output of at least 30 mL/hr demonstrates adequate renal function. Therefore, monitor the woman's urine output for changes. Report decreased urine output immediately.

Evaluation: Goals and Expected Outcomes

Goal: The woman will maintain fluid balance.
Expected Outcomes: The woman's

- intake and output are within acceptable parameters.
- output is at least 30 mL/hr.
- vital signs are within normal limits.
- lochia is moderate in amount, without clots.
- laboratory test results, including hemoglobin and hematocrit levels, return to acceptable levels.

Goal: The woman will remain free of injury.
Expected Outcomes: The woman

- maintains vital signs within acceptable parameters.
- demonstrates no signs and symptoms of hypovolemic shock.
- maintains a well-contracted uterus.
- remains alert and oriented.
- remains free of falls.

Goal: The woman will exhibit signs of adequate tissue perfusion.
Expected Outcomes: The woman

- is alert and oriented to person, place, and time.
- has pink, warm, and dry skin with quick capillary refill.
- maintains vital signs within acceptable parameters.
- maintains an oxygen saturation above 95%.
- has urine output of at least 30 mL/hr.

Late Postpartum Hemorrhage

Late postpartum hemorrhage refers to blood loss (>500 mL) occurring after the first 24 hours after delivery, and at any time throughout the 6-week postpartum period. Most cases of late postpartum hemorrhage result from retained placental fragments or **uterine subinvolution**, a condition in which the uterus returns to its prepregnancy shape and size at a rate that is slower than expected (usually the result of retained placental fragments or an infection). The woman who has had uterine surgery, including a previous cesarean birth or an abortion, is at high risk for retained placental fragments along the site of the surgical scar.

Clinical Manifestations

As with early postpartum hemorrhage, the woman with late postpartal hemorrhage notices an increase in bleeding. This increase usually occurs abruptly several days after discharge. Along with an abrupt onset of bleeding, the woman's uterus is not well contracted. On palpation, the uterus is not descending at the usual rate of 1 cm or fingerbreadth per postpartum day. Lochia is heavier than expected. The woman may report episodes of intermittent, irregular, or excessive vaginal bleeding. In addition, the woman may report backache, fatigue, and general malaise. She may also report pelvic pain or heaviness. Her temperature may be elevated slightly and lochia may be foul smelling if an infection is present. (See Table 19-1 for assessment findings for specific causes of postpartum hemorrhage.)

Diagnosis

Similar to the findings of early postpartum hemorrhage, the woman's hemoglobin and hematocrit levels are low. If retained placental fragments are the cause, the woman's serum human chorionic gonadotropin levels remain elevated. Ultrasound may reveal evidence of placental fragments. An elevated white blood cell (WBC) count may indicate infection. However, this result may not be conclusive because a postpartal woman's WBC count typically is elevated in the early postpartum period.

Treatment

Treatment of late postpartum hemorrhage focuses on correcting the underlying cause of the hemorrhage. Oxytocic therapy, similar to that used for uterine atony, may assist the uterus to contract. Often, uterine contraction aids in removing any fragments from the uterus. If necessary, surgery, specifically dilation and curettage, may be done to remove the fragments from the myometrium. Surgical intervention is a last resort when other treatment measures have been ineffective because it can traumatize the uterus further, leading to additional bleeding. Antibiotic therapy treats an infection, if present.

Nursing Care

Most cases of late postpartum hemorrhage occur after the woman leaves the health care or birthing facility. Therefore, patient education before discharge about expected changes and danger signs and symptoms is crucial. Instruct the woman to call her primary care provider if she experiences any signs of infection, such as fever greater than 100.4°F (38°C), chills, or foul-smelling lochia. She should also report lochia that increases (versus decreasing) in amount, or reversal of the pattern of lochia (i.e., moves from serosa back to rubra).

Test Yourself

- ✔ What is the definition of postpartum hemorrhage?
- ✔ Name the most common cause of early postpartum hemorrhage.
- ✔ Name three nursing actions appropriate for the woman who is bleeding due to uterine atony.

POSTPARTUM INFECTION

Postpartum infection, also called puerperal infection, refers to any infection that occurs after delivery. Most commonly, the infection involves the reproductive tract, but it also can involve other areas, such as the breast, wound, or urinary tract. Currently, approximately 1% to 8% of all postpartum women experience puerperal infection, with the maternal mortality rate for infection ranging from 4% to 8% (Kennedy, 2007).

A postpartum infection is suspected when the woman develops a fever of 100.4°F (38°C) or greater on two consecutive occasions at least 6 hours apart during the first 10 days postpartum, but not including the first 24 hours (Chen, 2007). Various organisms are associated with postpartum infections, including but not limited to staphylococcus, streptococcus, *Escherichia coli*, and Chlamydia.

The major risk factor for postpartum infection is a nonelective cesarean birth. Antepartum risk factors include history of infection; history of chronic conditions, such as diabetes, anemia, or poor nutrition; infections of the genital tract; smoking; and obesity. Intrapartal risk factors include:

- Urinary catheterization
- Episiotomy or lacerations
- Frequent vaginal examinations
- Retained placenta or one requiring manual removal
- Prolonged rupture of membranes (usually >24 hours)
- Chorioamnionitis (infection/inflammation of the fetal membranes)
- Traumatic birth, including the use of instruments, such as forceps or vacuum extractor
- Use of invasive procedures, such as internal fetal monitoring, fetal scalp sampling, and amnioinfusion

Use of poor aseptic technique and inadequate hand washing by health care personnel or the woman increase the risk. A woman who experiences postpartum hemorrhage has a greater risk for postpartal infection because of her weakened state and reduced ability to fight off the infection.

Although postpartal infection usually remains localized, it can progress and spread to nearby structures such as the peritoneum, causing peritonitis, or to the blood, causing septicemia and posing a significant risk to the woman's well-being. Most postpartal infections occur once the woman goes home from the health care facility. Therefore, patient teaching about possible signs and symptoms is crucial to ensure early detection and prompt intervention.

Endometritis

Endometritis refers to an infection of the uterine lining. It is the most common postpartal infection, occurring in approximately 3% of women who deliver vaginally and up to 30% of women who had a cesarean birth (Chen, 2007). Bacteria, frequently normal vaginal flora, gain entrance to the uterus during birth or the immediate postpartum period.

Endometritis is a serious complication because the infection can spread to nearby organs, such as the fallopian tubes (causing salpingitis), ovaries (causing oophoritis), connective tissues and ligaments (causing parametritis), and the peritoneum (causing peritonitis).

Clinical Manifestations

The woman with endometritis typically looks ill and commonly develops a fever of 100.4°F (38°C) or higher (more commonly 101°F [38.4°C], possibly as high as 104°F [40°C]) on the third to fourth postpartum day. The rise in temperature at this specific time is the most significant finding. The woman exhibits tachycardia, typically a rise in pulse rate of 10 beats per minute for each rise in temperature of 1°F. In addition, the woman may report chills, anorexia, and general malaise. She also may report abdominal cramping and pain, including strong afterpains. Fundal assessment reveals uterine subinvolution and tenderness. Lochia typically increases in amount, and is dark, purulent, and foul smelling. However, with certain microorganisms, her lochia may be scant or absent.

Diagnosis

A CBC reveals an elevated WBC count with increased eosinophiles or polymorphonuclear leukocytes. Urine culture to rule out urinary tract infection is negative. Vaginal cultures confirm the diagnosis and reveal the offending organisms. Pelvic ultrasound may reveal an abscess or possible retained placental fragments.

Pay close attention!
The WBC count of a postpartal woman is normally elevated, ranging up to 20,000 to 30,000/mm³. Before you report a high WBC count, assess for other signs of infection. This will help the provider make an accurate diagnosis.

Treatment

The mainstay of treatment is antibiotic therapy. Typically, the woman is admitted to the health care facility for IV therapy. Until culture and sensitivity reports are available, broad-spectrum IV antibiotic therapy commences and continues until the woman has been afebrile longer than 24 hours. The woman typically does not need oral antibiotics (Simmons, 2007).

The primary care provider may prescribe oxytocic agents to aid in uterine involution and promote uterine drainage. Analgesics are appropriate for strong afterpains or abdominal discomfort. Hydration with IV and oral fluids and adequate nutrition also are important treatment measures.

Nursing Care

The woman with endometritis is visibly ill. Therefore, nursing care focuses on administering drug therapy to combat the infection, promoting physical and emotional comfort, alleviating anxiety, and teaching the woman about measures used to treat the infection and to prevent a recurrence, including proper perineal care and hand washing.

Managing Antibiotic Therapy

Administer prescribed broad-spectrum IV antibiotics, and assess the woman for changes indicating an improvement. Monitor the woman's vital signs every 2 to 4 hours, or more often if indicated. Expect to see a reduction in temperature and a return of the pulse rate to preinfection levels as the infection resolves. Monitor for a decrease in abdominal pain and tenderness and a change in the woman's lochia to normal color (based on the postpartum day) and amount. Palpate the fundus to evaluate for uterine contraction. Expect to administer oxytocic agents, as ordered, to promote uterine involution. As with any medication, check with the primary care provider or lactation consultant to determine whether the woman can continue to breast-feed. In the rare instance that antibiotic therapy precludes breast-feeding, encourage the woman to pump her breasts to maintain the milk supply.

Keep in mind

Many antibiotics are nephrotoxic (damaging to the kidneys). Encourage a liberal fluid intake preferably to 3,000 mL/day. Report urine output less than 30 mL/hr.

Semi-Fowler's position promotes uterine drainage and prevents the infection from spreading. Encourage frequent ambulation to promote drainage, unless contraindicated. Be alert for signs and symptoms of peritonitis, such as pronounced abdominal pain with distention, a rigid, boardlike abdomen, and absent bowel sounds. Assess for tachycardia, tachypnea, hypotension, changes in sensorium, and decreased urine output. These suggest septic shock, a rare, but serious and possibly fatal complication.

Encourage frequent changing of perineal pads to remove infected drainage. Remind the woman to remove the pad using a front-to-back motion to avoid contaminating the perineal area. Reinforce the need to wash her hands after each change. Offer perineal care every 2 hours or as necessary. Be sure to wear gloves when handling soiled perineal pads to prevent infection transmission.

Providing Comfort Measures

The woman needs comfort care during this time. Provide cool washcloths and frequent linen changes, especially if she is febrile and diaphoretic. If she reports chills, add extra blankets to keep her warm; however, be careful that she does not become overheated. Keep the room calm and quiet to promote rest.

Administer analgesics, as ordered, for reports of abdominal pain. Encourage frequent position changes. Keep the head of the bed elevated. Fatigue is common during an infection. Allow for frequent rest periods so that she does not overtax herself. Assist with personal hygiene measures, including perineal care.

Alleviating Anxiety

The woman with endometritis typically develops symptoms after discharge home. She may become anxious and upset when readmission is necessary because this entails separation from her newborn. Allow her to verbalize her feelings. Provide support and guidance as necessary. Enlist the aid of the woman's spouse or significant other and family to help in alleviating her anxiety.

If breast-feeding is allowed, encourage the woman to pump her breasts for feedings. Arrangements with the facility and/or the primary care provider may allow the woman and her baby to be together for feedings. If not, encourage the family to bring in pictures of the baby for the woman to keep in her room.

Providing Patient Teaching

Patient teaching is a major focus of nursing care. One key area of teaching is medication therapy, especially if the woman is to continue medications at home. Other areas to address include proper hand-washing techniques, perineal care, expected changes in lochia, signs and symptoms of a recurrent infection, and danger signs to notify the physician. Family Teaching Tips: Endometritis outlines the major discharge teaching points.

Wound Infection

Postpartal wound infections typically involve infections of the perineum that develop at the site of an episiotomy or laceration. Wound infection also can occur at the site of the abdominal incision after a cesarean birth. Perineal wound infections, although rare, commonly develop on the third or fourth postpartum day. Factors increasing the risk of perineal wound infections include infected lochia, fecal contamination of the wound, and inadequate hygiene measures.

Risk Factors

Risk factors for a postpartum wound infection include:

- History of a chronic medical disorder, such as diabetes or hypertension
- Anemia or malnutrition
- Obesity
- Chorioamnionitis
- Immunosuppression, including treatment with corticosteroids
- Development of a hematoma
- Prolonged labor, rupture of membranes, or operative time
- Hemorrhage

Clinical Manifestations

The woman with a perineal wound infection most likely will report pain out of proportion to what is expected. Inspection of the perineum reveals redness of the area and edema of the surrounding tissue. The wound edges may be separated (Fig. 19-2A). Often there is a foul-smelling, possibly purulent, vaginal drainage. The area is tender on palpation. Fever and general malaise also may be present.

The woman with an infected incision after a cesarean birth frequently has endometritis before the wound

ENDOMETRITIS

- Be sure to complete all of your antibiotics, even though you are feeling better.
- Call your care provider if you have any of the following symptoms of recurrent infection:
  - Temperature >100.4°F (38°C)
  - Chills
  - Abdominal pain that does not go away with pain medication
  - Vaginal discharge that smells bad (like rotten meat)
- You should do the following things to prevent additional infection:
  - Wash your hands thoroughly before and after eating, using the restroom, or touching your vaginal area.
  - Wipe from front to back after using the restroom.
  - Remove soiled sanitary pads from front to back. Fold the pad so that the discharge is contained in the middle section of the pad, and then wrap it in toilet paper, or preferably a plastic bag. Dispose in the trash.
  - Wash hands before applying a new pad. Apply the pad from front to back. Do not touch the middle section of the pad. This part should remain very clean because it will be touching your vaginal area.
- You will heal faster and be less likely to get sick again if you do the following things:
  - Get at least 8 hours of sleep every night.
  - Rest frequently. Take a nap when the baby is napping.
  - Eat a nutritious diet.
  - Gradually increase your activity as you are able to tolerate it.
  - Drink plenty (1–2 L) of fluids each day.
- Be sure to attend your scheduled follow-up visits with your primary care provider.

becomes infected. When this happens, she continues to be febrile, even with antibiotic treatment. Inspection of the abdominal wound reveals erythema and induration (area of hardened tissue). In addition, the wound edges may be separated (Fig. 19-2B). **Exudate** (drainage) may be present and may be purulent. The area surrounding the wound typically is warm and tender on palpation, and the woman reports pain.

Diagnosis

A CBC with differential may reveal an elevation in WBC count. A culture of the area reveals the causative organism and guides treatment. If the primary care provider suspects sepsis, blood cultures may be drawn. Ultrasound can locate abscesses that may require draining.

Treatment

Antibiotic therapy is used to treat the infection, regardless of location. Supportive therapy is appropriate for perineal infections to include analgesics, local anesthetic sprays, warm compresses, and sitz baths. An infected incision requires regular cleansing and often a wound dressing. Surgical intervention may become necessary. This involves opening the wound for drainage, irrigation, debridement, and possibly packing. The goal of debridement is to clean the wound and promote granulation.

▮ **Figure 19-2** Postpartum wound infections. **(A)** Infected episiotomy site. **(B)** Infected cesarean birth incision.

A

B

Nursing Care

For the woman with a perineal infection, place warm compresses to the wound site several times each day, as ordered. Assist with sitz baths to provide comfort. These measures aid the healing process by increasing circulation to the area.

Keeping the perineal area clean is important. Encourage the woman to change her perineal pads and to perform perineal care frequently. She should use a front-to-back motion when removing perineal pads and when cleaning the perineum after elimination. Remind her to wash her hands after performing any perineal care and using the bathroom. Although always important, thorough hand washing is essential when the woman cares for an infected wound at home to prevent transmitting the infection to the newborn.

For the woman with an incisional infection, perform wound care, as ordered. This may include dressing changes, irrigations, debridement, or possibly wound packing. Always use aseptic technique when performing wound care. With each dressing change or procedure, inspect the wound for signs and symptoms indicating resolution of the infection and evidence of healing. If necessary, record measurements of the wound to aid in evaluating progress. If wound care will continue after discharge, teach the woman or another family member how to perform the care. The woman or family member should be able to detect signs and symptoms of increasing infection and know the signs that indicate the wound is healing. Have the person perform a return demonstration of any procedure.

Mastitis

Mastitis refers to an infection of the mammary gland (breast). Typically, only one breast is affected. Although the infection can occur at any time when the woman is breast-feeding, it is most common during the second and third weeks after delivery.

Mastitis occurs when organisms are transferred from the woman's hands, staff's hands, or newborn's mouth to the breast and enter the breast tissue through a small, often microscopic, crack, fissure, or injured area on the nipple or breast tissue. Certain risk factors contribute to the development of mastitis. These include

- Inadequate or incomplete breast emptying during feeding or lack of frequent feeding leading to milk stasis
- Engorgement
- Clogged milk ducts
- Cracked or bleeding nipples
- Nipple piercing
- Use of plastic-backed breast pads

If left untreated, mastitis can progress to an abscess, which may require surgical drainage.

Clinical Manifestations

The woman usually develops mastitis after discharge. Common complaints include general flulike symptoms

■ **Figure 19-3** Mastitis. The woman with mastitis usually has a reddened, painful area on one breast that is warm to palpation.

that occur suddenly, such as fever, malaise, and possibly chills. In addition, the woman reports tenderness, pain, and heaviness in her breast. Inspection reveals erythema and edema in an area localized to one breast (Fig. 19-3). The area is hard, warm, and tender on palpation. Purulent drainage may be present.

Diagnosis

No specific test confirms the diagnosis of mastitis. Typically, signs and symptoms form the basis for diagnosis.

Treatment

Supportive care in conjunction with antibiotic therapy is the treatment for mastitis. Penicillinase-resistant agents effective against *Staphylococcus aureus*, such as dicloxacillin (Dynapen) or cephalexin (Keflex), are the drugs of choice. Therapy usually continues for 10 days. The woman may need analgesics for comfort.

Did you know?

Antibiotic resistant organisms are increasingly the cause of mastitis. This infection passes from the hands of nursery personnel to the baby who then passes it to his or her mother during breast-feeding. Meticulous hand washing is the best prevention.

Nursing Care

Nursing care focuses on supporting continued breast-feeding, preventing milk stasis, and administering ordered antibiotics. Milk stasis is an important cause of discomfort and extension of the infection with possible

A Personal Glimpse

Breast-feeding my daughter was a challenge from the very beginning. She didn't want to latch on, she arched her back and cried, and she fussed at the breast. It took us several months to finally get a good pattern down. When she was about 6 months old, she and I were visiting my grandmother at the beach. One morning I woke up and felt awful. I had a hard, red spot on my breast and I felt hot and cold and exhausted. I took my temperature and it was 103°F. The only option I had was to go to the emergency room. I knew it had to be mastitis, and the emergency room doctor verified this. All I wanted was the prescription for antibiotics so that I could get back to my daughter. While writing the prescription, the doctor said to me, "You know you should really stop breast-feeding." I must have looked at him rather strangely because he said, "The infection and the antibiotics aren't good for the baby." I did not want to stop nursing my daughter after all we had been through. As soon as I got home, I called a friend who is a nurse. I told her what antibiotic I was taking, and she assured me that it was perfectly fine for me to continue breast-feeding my daughter. In fact, she told me that I should breast-feed frequently to help unclog the blocked milk duct in my breast. I was very relieved.

Jill

Learning Opportunity: Why is it important for breast-feeding to continue while the woman is being treated for mastitis? What can the nurse do to help a woman with mastitis continue breast-feeding?

abscess formation. Encourage the woman to breast-feed every 1.5 to 2 hours. Frequent feeding enhances complete emptying of the breast. If the woman is unable to breast-feed, for example because the affected breast is too sore or antibiotic therapy contraindicates breast-feeding, encourage the woman to manually express breast milk or use a breast pump to empty her breasts.

Recommend the use of warm compresses or a warm shower before feeding to promote the let-down reflex and stimulate the flow of milk. Warm compresses also are soothing and increase blood flow to the area to stimulate healing. Suggest that the woman begin breast-feeding on the affected breast first, if possible, so that the breast completely empties. If this is too painful, suggest that she start on the unaffected breast until after the let-down reflex, then switch to the affected breast. This strategy should result in less pain when the baby latches. Explain that massaging the affected area during feeding helps to ensure complete emptying.

Provide support and encouragement for continuing breast-feeding. Encourage liberal fluid intake to ensure adequate milk formation. Review proper techniques for breast-feeding and proper infant positioning (refer to Chapter 15). A lactation consultant is a valuable resource

for the woman with mastitis. Nursing Care Plan 19-1 discusses the care of a woman with mastitis.

Urinary Tract Infection

Urinary tract infection (UTI) involves an infection of the bladder (cystitis) or the kidneys (pyelonephritis). Trauma during birth and inadequate bladder emptying during labor or postpartum may lead to urinary stasis, which increases the risk for developing a UTI. Frequent vaginal examinations during labor, urinary catheterizations, and delivery involving instrumentation further compound the risk.

Clinical Manifestations

The signs and symptoms of cystitis differ from those of pyelonephritis. Typically, those associated with pyelonephritis are more dramatic and severe. The woman with cystitis characteristically reports burning and pain on urination. She reports urgency and frequency and voids only small amounts at a time. The woman usually has a low-grade fever and possibly suprapubic pain.

In addition to burning, pain, urgency, and frequency, the woman with pyelonephritis presents with a high, spiking fever that rises and falls abruptly. Often she has shaking chills and reports nausea and vomiting. Flank pain and tenderness are common. Tenderness at the costovertebral angle (the area on the back just above the waistline) is present on palpation.

Diagnosis

A urinalysis and clean catch urine for culture and sensitivity provide evidence of an infection. The urinalysis typically reveals WBCs, protein, blood, and presence of bacteria. The clean catch urine specimen, considered diagnostic for UTI, reveals greater than 10^5 colony-forming units. A CBC may reveal an elevated WBC count.

Treatment

Antibiotic therapy is the treatment of choice based on the urine culture and sensitivity results. For the woman with cystitis, oral antibiotics are appropriate. For the woman with pyelonephritis, IV antibiotic therapy is the treatment of choice. Typically, therapy begins with a broad-spectrum antibiotic and is later adjusted based on the urine culture and sensitivity reports.

In addition to antibiotic therapy, antipyretics and analgesics, such as acetaminophen (Tylenol); antispasmodics; urinary analgesics, such as phenazopyridine hydrochloride (Pyridium); and antiemetics may be ordered. Hydration and good perineal hygiene also are important.

Nursing Care

Nursing care focuses on promoting comfort, ensuring adequate hydration, and providing patient teaching. The woman with cystitis typically does not require admission to a health care facility for treatment. However, the

Nursing Care Plan 19-1

THE WOMAN WITH MASTITIS

CASE SCENARIO

Jessica Thompson is a 22-year-old gravida 1 para 1, who delivered her baby vaginally 2 weeks ago. She is breast-feeding. She is readmitted to the hospital with a diagnosis of mastitis in the right breast. Her admitting vital signs are BP 128/70, T 101.2°F, P 106 bpm, R 22/min. She is tired all the time, and her body aches all over. Assessment of her breast-feeding techniques indicates that the baby feeds better from the left breast, so Jessica usually starts with the left breast. Since her right breast began hurting 2 days ago, she has avoided using that breast to feed the baby because she says, "It just hurts too much." She also reports that sometimes the baby uses a pacifier between feedings. Jessica says that she isn't sure that she should keep breast-feeding because she is afraid that "the infection might hurt my baby." The physician has ordered clindamycin (Cleocin) 900 mg IV every 8 hours; acetaminophen (Tylenol) 1,000 mg PO every 4 hours PRN temperature >100.4°F; ibuprofen (Motrin) 800 mg PO every 8 hours PRN pain.

NURSING DIAGNOSIS

Hyperthermia related to inflammation secondary to infectious process as evidenced by T 101.2°F.

GOAL: Temperature regulation

EXPECTED OUTCOMES
- Temperature will decrease to <100.4°F.
- Pulse rate will decrease to <100 bpm.
- Muscle aches will resolve.

Nursing Interventions	*Rationale*
Monitor vital signs, including temperature every 4 hours until it has been <100.4°F for at least 24 hours. Monitor WBC, as ordered.	Monitoring the vital signs will allow tracking of temperature spikes and overall response to therapy. White blood cell count will begin decreasing as the infection resolves.
Administer the antipyretic, acetaminophen, as ordered. Administer antibiotic, clindamycin, as ordered.	Antipyretics control body temperature. Antibiotics will treat the infection that is causing the fever.
Place a pitcher of ice water at the bedside and refill it frequently, as needed. Offer juices, popsicles, and other liquids every 1 to 2 hours.	Temperature elevation can result in fluid loss. In addition, adequate hydration is needed so that the body can effectively fight infection.

NURSING DIAGNOSIS

Ineffective Breast-feeding Pattern related to incomplete emptying of the right breast and pacifier use.

GOAL: Maintenance of effective breast-feeding.

EXPECTED OUTCOMES
- Initiates breast-feeding on demand at least every 1.5 to 2 hours.
- Infant exhibits proper latch during breast-feeding.
- Empties both breasts regularly.

Nursing Interventions	*Rationale*
Encourage Jessica to continue breast-feeding.	Breast-feeding with mastitis is safe for the baby. Stopping breast-feeding increases the risk for abscess formation.
Request a consult with a lactation specialist.	A lactation specialist can evaluate for subtle factors that may be interfering with the breast-feeding process and can help the baby to latch on well.

(continued)

Nursing Care Plan 19-1 (continued)

THE WOMAN WITH MASTITIS

Assist Jessica to breast-feed every 1.5 to 2 hours until symptoms begin to resolve.	Regular emptying of the breasts improves milk flow and decreases stasis, which can lead to blocked milk ducts and further infection.
Instruct Jessica to start on the right breast first, if she is able. If not, it may help to assist her to use a breast pump on the right breast while she is feeding on the left breast.	It is important to completely empty the affected breast at every feeding to increase milk flow and circulation to the area.
Instruct Jessica to gently massage the affected area (the lump that is warm and tender) as the breast is emptied (i.e., during breast-feeding or pumping).	Gentle massage helps relieve the obstruction in the clogged duct to promote milk flow.
Encourage rooming in with the infant, if allowed by the facility, as long as a friend or family member can stay in the room with Jessica.	Rooming in allows for breast-feeding on demand, which is ideal. A competent adult must remain at the bedside to take responsibility for the baby, because the baby is not a patient. It is not appropriate for the patient to have responsibility for the infant until she is well enough to go home.
If the baby is unavailable to breast-feed, assist Jessica to pump her breasts every 2 hours. Refrigerate the milk for later consumption by the baby.	Pumping the breasts stimulates milk production, increased blood flow, and increased milk flow, all of which help decrease the symptoms of mastitis.
Discourage pacifier use.	Sucking on a pacifier or artificial nipple can decrease the amount that the infant suckles, thereby increasing the risk for milk stasis.

NURSING DIAGNOSIS

Acute Pain related to mastitis (particularly associated with breast-feeding).

GOAL: Tolerable pain levels

EXPECTED OUTCOMES
- Verbalizes adequate relief from pain after interventions.
- Empties affected breast without undue pain.

Nursing Interventions	*Rationale*
Administer ibuprofen, as ordered. In the first 24 to 48 hours, administer the medication around the clock versus PRN.	Ibuprofen usually provides excellent pain relief for the pain associated with mastitis. It also has anti-inflammatory properties, which further help reduce pain. Around-the-clock dosing prevents acute pain from becoming severe. Once pain becomes severe, it is more difficult to treat.
Assist Jessica to apply warm compresses or a heating pad to the affected breast. Alternatively, or additionally, encourage her to take warm showers.	Warmth helps to decrease pain and increases blood flow to the area, which increases milk flow.

NURSING DIAGNOSIS

Fatigue related to infectious process.

GOAL: Ability to perform self- and baby-care functions.

EXPECTED OUTCOMES
- Verbalizes feeling rested.
- Reports increased energy levels.
- Performs self- and baby-care without complaints of fatigue.

(continues on page 440)

Nursing Care Plan 19-1 (continued)

THE WOMAN WITH MASTITIS

Nursing Interventions	Rationale
Encourage frequent rest periods.	Promotes healing.
Limit visitors, as appropriate.	Reduces stimuli and allows for rest.
Encourage adequate nutrition.	Promotes healing and provides energy source.
Encourage wakefulness during the early evening hours. Discourage late afternoon naps.	Promotes sleep during the night, which provides the most restful sleep.
Encourage the use of bedtime rituals, preferably ones she uses at home, and reduce light and noise stimuli at bedtime.	These interventions promote sleep.
Encourage significant other to care for the baby (other than feedings) during the night.	Promotes periods of uninterrupted sleep.
Group nursing interventions and care activities.	Avoids unnecessary interruptions and promotes rest.

NURSING DIAGNOSIS
Deficient Knowledge: Self-care after discharge

GOAL: Demonstrates ability to care for self at home.

EXPECTED OUTCOMES
• Washes hands before and after using the restroom, eating, touching the breasts.
• Answers questions accurately regarding self-care.
• Breast-feeds infant every 2 to 3 hours without prompting.

Nursing Interventions	Rationale
Teach importance of hand washing. Encourage frequent hand washing at appropriate times.	Helps prevent the spread and recurrence of infection.
Encourage Jessica to continue breast-feeding as instructed (refer to breast-feeding guidelines above).	Proper breast-feeding techniques decrease the likelihood that mastitis will recur.
Instruct regarding early warning signs, which include	If the woman initiates intervention at the first warning sign, she may be able to prevent a recurrence of mastitis.
• Breast engorgement	
• Nipple soreness or cracking	
• A painful lump in one breast, which is a sign of a plutted duct.	
If she has any of the warning symptoms, she should do the following	These measures encourage the flow of milk, help prevent milk stasis, and prevent early mastitis from becoming more severe.
• Rest in bed, if possible.	
• Breast-feed frequently from the affected breast.	
• Put a warm compress on the affected breast.	
• Gently massage lumpy areas while the infant is feeding.	
• Call her physician if she develops a fever ≥100.4°F or if she does not get better within 24 hours.	

woman with pyelonephritis usually requires hospitalization for IV hydration and antibiotic therapy.

Providing Comfort

The woman with a UTI typically has pain and burning on urination, which can make voiding difficult. The dis-

comfort can prevent the woman from emptying her bladder completely, resulting in urinary stasis. Urinary stasis provides a good medium for organism growth, further compounding her risk for infection, and possibly increasing her risk for extension of the infection, for example, from the bladder to the kidneys. Therefore, assist the woman with comfort measures, such as running warm water over the perineum or using a sitz bath when attempting to urinate. Administer analgesics such as acetaminophen (Tylenol), as ordered. A urinary analgesic (e.g., phenazopyridine hydrochloride [Pyridium]) is comforting, if ordered.

Consider this.

The woman with a UTI may not drink enough fluid, fearing that she will need to void more frequently and thus increase her pain. Explain that a high-urinary output often decreases the pain associated with UTI.

Promoting Adequate Hydration

Adequate hydration is necessary to dilute the bacterial concentration in the urine and aid in clearing the organisms from the urinary tract. Encourage the woman to drink at least 3,000 mL of fluid a day. Suggest she drink one glass per hour to ensure adequate intake. Be sure to keep a record of her intake.

Advise the woman to drink fluids that make the urine acidic, deterring organism growth. Fluids such as cranberry, plum, prune, or apricot juices are examples. Tell the woman to avoid carbonated beverages because they increase the alkalinity of urine, which promotes organism growth. If the woman has pyelonephritis, expect to administer IV fluids in addition to oral fluid to ensure adequate hydration.

Providing Patient Teaching

Patient teaching is essential for ensuring compliance with therapy and preventing a recurrence of cystitis or pyelonephritis. Instruct the woman to complete the full drug regimen, which can range from 5 to 10 days. The woman with pyelonephritis receives IV antibiotic therapy initially. The primary care provider may order oral antibiotics for the woman to continue after discharge (depending on her length of stay in the health care facility). If the woman is breast-feeding, provide instruction concerning the safety of continued breast-feeding based on the particular antibiotic she is taking. Other important patient teaching topics include hydration measures, comfort measures, perineal care, and preventive measures, including signs and symptoms of a recurrence.

Test Yourself

✔ List five risk factors for postpartum infection.
✔ Name five signs and symptoms of endometritis.
✔ Describe four clinical manifestations of postpartum wound infection.

VENOUS THROMBOEMBOLISM

Venous thromboembolism (VTE) is the umbrella term for deep vein thrombosis (DVT) and pulmonary embolism. VTE is the leading cause of maternal mortality in the United States (Dresang et al., 2008). Most deaths occur due to the more serious manifestation of VTE, pulmonary embolism.

Risk Factors

The pregnant and postpartal woman is at risk for VTE for three reasons:

1. Clotting factors increase during pregnancy and remain elevated in the early postpartum to promote blood clotting.
2. Pressure of the pregnant uterus on lower extremity veins leads to venous dilation and pooling of blood (venous stasis), which increase the risk for clots to form.
3. Vascular trauma during childbirth (particularly during forceps-assisted or cesarean delivery) and/or prolonged periods in lithotomy position also cause venous stasis, resulting in risk for clot formation.

Box 19-2 lists factors that further increase the postpartum woman's risk for VTE.

Deep Vein Thrombosis

Deep vein thrombosis (DVT) is formation of a blood clot (thrombus) in the deeper veins of the calf, thigh, or pelvis. These deep veins carry the majority of venous return from the legs to the heart, increasing the likelihood that all or part of the clot will break off and travel to the lungs, resulting in pulmonary embolism (discussed below).

Clinical Manifestations

The woman with DVT may have no symptoms. If she does exhibit signs, these typically include swelling and calf pain or tenderness in the affected leg. The area may

---

Box 19-2 ▌ RISK FACTORS FOR POSTPARTUM VENOUS THROMBOEMBOLISM

Medical Risk Factors
- Thrombophilia
- Personal history of venous thromboembolism
- Family history of venous thromboembolism
- Obesity
- Smoking
- Age >35 years
- Severe varicose veins
- Bedrest or immobility >3 days

Obstetrical Risk Factors
- History of three or more pregnancies
- Prolonged labor
- Use of forceps
- Cesarean birth

be warm, tender, and red. Homans' sign (pain on dorsiflexion of the foot) may be positive. Historically, a positive Homans' sign was indicative of DVT. However, this is not a reliable sign because the pain may be attributable to other conditions, such as muscle strain or contusion. The leg may appear visibly pale or white with diminished pedal pulses due to arterial spasm, which decreases circulation to the area.

Diagnosis

The primary care provider may order several diagnostic tests, such as venous compression ultrasonography or venography with a contrast medium. These tests reveal altered blood flow, confirming the presence of blood clots. Other tests may include computed tomography and magnetic resonance imaging (Cunningham et al., 2005c).

Treatment

The primary goals of medical therapy for DVT are to prevent further thrombus formation and to prevent pulmonary embolism, a potentially fatal complication. Anticoagulation therapy is the treatment of choice. Supportive therapy involves analgesics, heat, bed rest, application of compression stockings, and elevation of the affected leg. Anticoagulation therapy may start with subcutaneous enoxaparin (Lovenox) every 12 hours or heparin administered subcutaneously or intravenously. IV heparin requires a loading dose followed by a maintenance infusion, both of which require a continuous infusion pump. After several days of, or in conjunction with, heparin or enoxaparin therapy, the woman begins oral anticoagulant therapy with warfarin (Coumadin). Parenteral anticoagulants continue until laboratory values are in the therapeutic range. The woman continues on oral warfarin for approximately 6 weeks.

Nursing Care

Nursing care for the woman with DVT includes instituting bed rest; applying compression stockings, as ordered; and elevating the affected extremity to promote venous return. Inspect the lower extremities for changes in color, temperature, and size and palpate pedal pulses. Measure the circumference of each lower extremity and compare the results bilaterally to determine the degree of edema. Assist the woman to remove the compression stockings for an hour every 8 to 12 hours.

Apply warm compresses, as ordered. When applying the compresses, ensure that they are at the proper temperature. Altered blood flow may diminish the woman's ability to sense temperature extremes, placing her at risk for a burn injury. Make sure that the weight of the compresses does not rest on the leg, compromising blood flow. Check the woman's bed linens and change them as necessary because the linens may become damp or wet from the moist heat applications. If possible, use a waterproof pad to protect the linens. Warm moist compresses can cool quickly. Provide the woman with extra blankets if necessary to prevent chilling. Use chemical heat packs or a pad such as an Aquathermia pad to help keep the compresses warm.

It is important to monitor the woman's vital signs closely for slight elevations in temperature, possibly to 101°F (38.3°C), and report this finding. Because the woman with DVT is at risk for developing a pulmonary embolism, be alert for, and immediately report, any sudden onset of breathing difficulties.

Administer anticoagulant therapy, as ordered. When giving heparin, always have the antidote, protamine sulfate, readily available. Place the woman on bleeding precautions, which includes monitoring for evidence of bleeding, applying 5 to 10 minutes of pressure to injection or venipuncture sites, and avoiding unnecessary injections. Teach the woman to report any increase in vaginal bleeding, saturation of perineal pads or evidence of bruising, oozing at IV sites, or gingival bleeding.

The woman typically goes home on oral anticoagulant therapy. Therefore, teach her about the drug and signs and symptoms to report immediately (Family Teaching Tips: Anticoagulant Therapy).

Family Teaching Tips

ANTICOAGULANT THERAPY

While you are on anticoagulant therapy, you are at risk for bleeding. Look for the following signs of bleeding:
- Bruising
- Bleeding gums
- Nosebleed
- Oozing from scratches and scrapes
- Blood in the urine
- Black or tarry stools
- Increased vaginal bleeding
- Notify the primary care provider of any change in level of consciousness, decreased ability to follow commands, or decreased sensation or ability to move extremities. These signs may indicate a cerebral bleed. This emergency requires immediate intervention.

The following precautions will help prevent excessive bleeding:
- Use a soft toothbrush.
- Avoid using razor blades (use an electric razor to shave).
- Avoid aspirin-containing products.
- Check with the primary care provider before taking any over-the-counter medications.
- Notify your dentist and any other health care provider that you are on anticoagulant therapy.
- Apply pressure for 5 to 10 minutes after any injections or after blood is drawn or if you accidentally cut or scrape yourself.

Pulmonary Embolism

Pulmonary embolism occurs when a clot (thrombus) breaks free from the vessel wall (most commonly from the pelvic vein), travels to the heart, and then through the pulmonary circulation, where it lodges and interrupts the blood flow to the lungs. (The clot that migrates and creates a blockage is called a *pulmonary embolus*.) If a large area of lung tissue is deprived of blood flow, cardiovascular collapse ultimately occurs, which can be fatal.

Clinical Manifestations

The postpartum woman who develops a pulmonary embolism typically exhibits a sudden onset of dyspnea, pleuritic chest pain, and an impending sense of severe apprehension or doom. If the woman experiences any of these, report them immediately. In addition, the woman may be tachypneic, tachycardic, and hypotensive. She may have a cough with bloody sputum (hemoptysis) and report abdominal pain. Cyanosis and changes in level of consciousness also may occur.

Diagnosis

Arterial blood gases reveal a decrease in the partial pressure of oxygen and partial pressure of carbon dioxide. Ventilation/perfusion scan demonstrates a mismatching between lung tissue perfusion and ventilation, that is, a decrease in or absence of perfusion in parts of the lung to which ventilation is normal. Pulmonary angiography reveals filling defects or abrupt cessation of blood flow at the location of the embolus. A chest radiograph may show atelectasis, infiltrates, or pleural effusions, all of which suggest a pulmonary embolism.

Treatment

Pulmonary embolism is a life-threatening emergency requiring immediate treatment. Treatment is supportive therapy and includes oxygen via face mask and medications to treat the symptoms. For example, if the woman is hypotensive, the primary care provider may order dopamine to raise her blood pressure. Heparin therapy prevents further clot formation. The primary care provider may consider thrombolytic agents to dissolve the existing clot; however, this therapy is not used routinely in the postpartum period. Continuous monitoring via pulmonary artery catheterization and continuous electrocardiogram monitoring often are necessary. Because of the woman's critical status, she usually receives care in the intensive care unit.

Nursing Care

Immediate action is crucial for the woman who develops a pulmonary embolism. Immediately raise the head of the bed to at least 45 degrees to facilitate breathing. Begin oxygen therapy at 8 to 10 L/min via face mask, and notify the physician. Assist with obtaining specimens for arterial blood gas analysis, and prepare the woman for diagnostic testing. Monitor vital signs closely. Provide emotional support and explain all procedures and treatments to the woman, who is most likely apprehensive about what is happening. Prepare the woman for transfer to the intensive care unit.

Test Yourself

✔ What three factors put the postpartum woman at risk for thrombus formation?

✔ Name four nursing interventions appropriate for the woman with DVT.

✔ What symptoms are associated with pulmonary embolism?

POSTPARTUM PSYCHIATRIC DISORDERS

Three psychiatric conditions manifest themselves during the postpartum period. These include: postpartum blues (also known as "baby blues" or "maternity blues"), postpartum depression, and postpartum psychosis. Of these three conditions, postpartum blues is the most common and least serious. Research reveals that at least 50% of all postpartum women experience this transitory phase of sadness and crying. (See Chapter 12 for more discussion of this condition.)

Postpartum depression and postpartum psychosis are distinct disorders. Depression affects the woman's ability to function; however, her perception of reality remains intact. Conversely, the woman with postpartum psychosis experiences a severe distortion in her view of reality, often accompanied by hallucinations and delusions. Both disorders respond well to treatment, if caught early.

The exact cause of these disorders is unknown. Researchers believe that multiple factors are responsible for their development. These factors may include:

- Stress arising from the pregnancy and responsibilities associated with child rearing
- Sudden decrease in endorphins with labor and abrupt changes in hormonal levels (estrogen and progesterone) after delivery
- Low serum levels of free tryptophan (also associated with the psychiatric diagnosis of major depression)
- Possible thyroid gland dysfunction

Regardless of the cause, you may play a key role in teaching the woman about the signs and symptoms of each disorder and in early detection to facilitate prompt treatment.

Postpartum Depression

Postpartum depression is a nonpsychotic depressive disorder that appears within the first 6 months postpartum, or symptoms may develop during pregnancy but persist after the birth. This disorder is the most common complication of childbirth, occurring in up to 19.2% of women in the first 3 months postpartum (Beck, 2008a). Box 19-3 lists risk factors for postpartum depression.

Consequences of untreated postpartum depression include difficulty with normal maternal–infant attachment, altered family dynamics, cognitive and behavioral problems in the offspring, and maternal suicide (Driscoll, 2006a). Postpartum depression may also adversely affect the father's mental health (Horowitz & Goodman, 2005).

Clinical Manifestations

The woman with postpartum depression commonly demonstrates strong feelings of sadness, irritability, and anxiety. She is frequently tearful. She may have a lack of interest in her surroundings and have trouble motivating herself to do normal activities. She may show disinterest in others and a lack of enjoyment with life. Intense feelings of inadequacy, inability to cope, ambivalence, guilt, and unworthiness are often noted. The woman often reports problems sleeping, loss of libido, decreased appetite, inability to concentrate, overwhelming fatigue, and obsessive thinking. She may contemplate harming herself (suicide) or the infant.

Diagnosis

Signs and symptoms are the basis for diagnosis. Depressive symptoms must be present on most days for at least 2 weeks for the diagnosis to apply. The primary care provider usually screens the woman for medical conditions such as hypothyroidism and anemia that can cause symptoms of depression.

Treatment

Usually treatment for postpartum depression occurs on an outpatient basis, although severe cases may require hospitalization in a psychiatric facility. A trained mental health professional guides the treatment plan, which includes the woman's family.

Antidepressant therapy is the mainstay of treatment. Agents such as selective serotonin reuptake inhibitors, including paroxetine (Paxil), fluoxetine (Prozac), and sertraline (Zoloft), are first-line drugs in the treatment of postpartum depression. Current research indicates that these agents are safe for use in women who are breast-feeding; however, the woman should know that all of these medications are found in breast milk.

Electroconvulsive treatment is effective for women with severe postpartum depression, especially if the woman has thoughts of suicide (Nonacs, 2007).

Nursing Care

Early detection and treatment are critical because the disorder can disrupt the woman's life and frequently interferes with interpersonal relationships. Therefore, all postpartum women and their families need information regarding the warning signs and symptoms. This teaching should be part of routine postpartum discharge instructions. In fact, some states mandate that every pregnant woman receive written information about postpartum depression along with a list of local resources as a part of prenatal care and again before discharge from the hospital after giving birth.

It is normal for the postpartum woman to be reluctant to verbalize any feelings of sadness or lack of enthusiasm about motherhood or child caring and rearing because of fear of rejection or feelings of guilt. As the nurse, you play a key role in dispelling the myth that happiness automatically occurs after the birth of a child.

Instruct the woman and her family that postpartum depression can occur at any time after delivery. Therefore, the family needs to keep a listening ear to the woman's concerns. Instruct the family to be especially alert for complaints about problems sleeping, lack of energy or lack of interest in daily activities, or fatigue out of proportion to the woman's status. It is especially important the woman understand that she should seek help immediately if she has thoughts of harming herself or her baby.

Explain the importance of the treatment plan. If the woman is hesitant to take antidepressants because she is breast-feeding, help her understand the possible consequences of not taking the medication (e.g., adverse effects on bonding with the baby and long-term negative effects on the baby's cognitive, emotional, and behavioral growth and development, etc.).

Acknowledge any feelings that the woman with postpartum depression expresses. Avoid statements that provide false reassurance or that discount the woman's feelings, such as, "Don't worry, you'll feel better soon," or "Your baby is so cute. You shouldn't feel so sad!" Assist the woman in obtaining support as necessary. Contact with others in a support group can help to alleviate feelings of isolation.

A Personal Glimpse

When I gave birth to our oldest daughter, my husband and I were living away from our families and friends. I remember bringing our daughter home from the hospital and feeling completely overwhelmed and anxious. Our daughter was fussy and didn't nurse well. I had no mother, sister, or girl-friend nearby to talk with or get advice from. My husband was calm and very supportive, but he worked full-time shift work. I remember feeling so lonely and depressed. I kept thinking that these feelings would go away after a few weeks. But they didn't. I wasn't eating or sleeping well, and I know I was miserable to be around. I felt completely inadequate as a mother. Finally, after 8 weeks of this, my husband suggested we go see the doctor. Reluctantly, I made an appointment. When we first got to the doctor's office, the nurse sat down with us to ask us questions. When she asked why we were there, I started crying but managed to explain what I had been feeling since the birth of our daughter. She handed me some tissues and put her hand on my arm. She assured me that she and the doctor would work with me to help me feel better and return to my normal emotional state.

I am so glad that my husband suggested I get help. The doctor gave me a prescription for Paxil, and the nurse gave me all sorts of great suggestions, like joining a new mom support group and making sure that I got daily exercise. In just a few weeks, I felt so much better and now have much more confidence in my ability to be a mother to our daughter.

Lynne

Learning Opportunity: What clues did this woman give that indicate she was suffering from postpartum depression versus the "baby blues?" What specific actions can the nurse take to quickly recognize and provide support for the woman who has postpartum depression?

Postpartum Psychosis

Postpartum psychosis is a rare psychiatric disorder with severe consequences for the woman, the newborn, and family, if left untreated. The disorder mimics severe bipolar disorder in that the woman exhibits symptoms of mania, depression, and psychosis. Symptoms appear abruptly sometime during the first few months postpartum. The disorder may have its onset as early as 48 hours after delivery, although the typical onset is within the first 2 to 3 weeks after delivery. Postpartum psychosis is an emergency that requires inpatient treatment in a psychiatric facility.

Clinical Manifestations

The onset of psychotic symptoms is abrupt and associated with a stressful life situation. Symptoms of postpartum psychosis include the following:

- Delusions (she may express the belief that the infant is dead or defective)
- Hallucinations (she may hear voices telling her to kill herself or her child)
- Severe agitation, restlessness, or irritability
- Hyperactivity, euphoria, or little concern for self or infant (manic phase of bipolar disorder)
- Depression including preoccupation with guilt, feelings of worthlessness and isolation, extreme overconcern for the infant's health, and sleep disturbances
- Poor judgment and confusion

Because of the woman's misperception of reality, suicide and infanticide are possible.

Treatment

Postpartum psychosis is a psychiatric emergency, requiring immediate psychiatric hospitalization. Antipsychotic agents are the treatment of choice, although the treatment plan may also include antidepressants. The psychiatric care provider may consider electroconvulsive therapy, especially if the woman is suicidal (Engqvist et al., 2007).

Nursing Care

Caring for the woman with postpartum psychosis requires specialized psychiatric training beyond the scope of practice for the obstetric nurse. However, you need to be aware of the signs and symptoms of postpartum psychosis so that early detection and prompt intervention can occur.

SPECIAL POSTPARTUM SITUATIONS

In addition to complications that can occur in the postpartum period, two other situations may require nursing intervention. These include grief and malattachment.

Grief in the Postpartal Period

Typically, the postpartum period is a happy time of celebrating the birth of a newborn. However, not all pregnancies conclude in a happy family taking home a healthy newborn. These situations may include the woman who is placing her newborn for adoption, the family faced with a newborn with congenital anomalies, and the family dealing with the death of the fetus or newborn.

Grief is a universal process that each individual experiences uniquely. Grief is a natural response to a loss, whether the loss is the result of a choice, such as occurs with adoption, or when the situation is completely out of the individual's control, such as when the newborn has a congenital anomaly or dies. Shock and disbelief are often the first feelings expressed. This feeling of numbness or unreality may last hours, days, or weeks. Anger, even to the point of rage, bargaining, and depression are natural expressions of the grieving process. It is normal for individuals to demonstrate many emotions as they work through their feelings.

Men and women may differ in their responses to grief. These differences can cause a rift between the woman and her spouse unless the couple receives intervention to help them work through the differences. Sometimes the woman responds to feelings of sadness and guilt with tearfulness and isolation. The man may respond to these same feelings by throwing himself into his work. The woman may misperceive that her spouse "doesn't care" or that he "isn't grieving." Counseling can be beneficial.

The Woman Placing the Newborn for Adoption

Giving the newborn up for adoption is a complicated and difficult choice some women face. Each woman's circumstances are unique, and responses to this challenge are individualized. The woman often enters into a very somber period of grief and detachment. She may express intense emotions and need to discuss the dreams and hopes that she is releasing with this decision, or she may be withdrawn and quiet. In all cases, the woman requires support, personal care, and comfort through the early postpartum period.

The woman placing her newborn for adoption requires nonjudgmental support. It is critical for you to be aware of your own attitudes and avoid the temptation to influence the outcome toward your beliefs. Your role is to be an advocate for the woman, which involves keeping her informed of her rights and options and supporting her in whatever decision that she makes. It is important for you to recognize that each state has laws that govern the rights of each party in the adoption process. Be knowledgeable of your institution's policies regarding handling of the adoption process.

The Family Whose Newborn Has Congenital Anomalies

Helping parents adjust to a newborn with congenital anomalies is a challenge for the postpartum nurse. The woman and her family must grieve the loss of the "dream" child and learn to accept one that is not as they had imagined (see Chapters 20 and 21).

Encourage frequent interaction with the newborn. Point out positive features. Role model healthy behaviors by talking and playing with the baby as you would with any newborn. When the family goes home, they may benefit by participation in a parent support group.

The Family Whose Fetus or Newborn Has Died

Death often forces individuals to face core issues and personal values; it leaves emotions raw, while people struggle for meaning. When a newborn or fetus dies, the parents are often unprepared to deal with their new reality. They frequently voice questions to which there are no good answers.

Coping with death of the fetus or newborn can be stressful for you as well as the family. You may feel inadequate to help and be tempted to withdraw from the situation. It is important to recognize your feelings so that you do not let your feelings interfere with your ability to care for the woman and her family. It may be helpful to talk through your feelings with a friend or co-worker. Do not let personal beliefs and values overshadow the family's beliefs and values. Allow the family to experience their own grief process; provide assistance and support in ways that are meaningful and helpful to them.

Several measures can help provide meaning to the family during this difficult time. The baby who died is a part of a family and has a place with them. Encourage the family to name their newborn, even if it was stillborn. Memory items, such as footprints and handprints, a name record, blessing, and souvenir birth record, identify this baby as a member of a particular family. Parents have identified photos of the newborn as a precious memory. Keep in mind that the photos must be comforting photos, that is, ones with the baby clothed, washed, and positioned comfortably. Allow the family or mother to assist with clothes, bathing, animal toys, or blankets.

Malattachment in the Postpartal Period

Attachment is an enduring emotional bond between the baby and primary caregiver. The relationship of attachment begins when a women first finds out that she is pregnant. Through the prenatal visits, information about the well-being of her baby reinforces this attachment. As she hears the heart beat, sees the baby's movements on ultrasound, and feels the movement inside her uterus, the woman begins to perceive this something inside her body as a "someone" other than herself. Preparations of the nursery and choosing names continue this bonding process. A stable relationship, good prenatal course, and positive anticipation of a healthy infant help a woman to begin an internal relationship with her baby before he or she is born.

Many things influence the degree of attachment. A stable relationship, good prenatal course, and positive anticipation of a healthy infant help a woman to begin an internal relationship with her baby before he or she is born. However, difficulties during the pregnancy, immaturity on the part of the woman, or an unreliable support system puts the family at risk for malattachment, emotional distancing in the maternal–infant relationship. Pregnancy complications or difficult relationships with the father of the baby can also adversely affect attachment. In addition, alcohol and drug abuse can contribute to malattachment and infant neglect.

Key signs of malattachment include lack of eye contact, lack of verbal stimulation, and a lack of response to the newborn's cries or cues. Table 19-2 lists behaviors that may indicate malattachment. If you observe any of these

Table 19-2 ▮ COMPARING ATTACHMENT AND MALATTACHMENT

Attachment	Malattachment
Uses endearments and pet names	Speaks of the newborn as an object; "it"
Speaks softly and uses "baby talk"	Makes no eye contact with the newborn
Calls newborn by name, often	Does not use the newborn's name
Becomes involved in routine care of diapering, bathing, and feeding	Shows disinterest in daily care and feeding of the newborn
Holds newborn close to body or in direct face-to-face contact	Places newborn in crib or lays newborn on lap facing away from mother
Responds to crying, smiling, feeding, and elimination with positive reinforcement	Ignores crying and newborn cue behaviors; reacts negatively to elimination needs
Easily calms upset newborn	Does not perceive newborn's needs; newborn is frustrated and nervous

signs, report them to the RN. Lack of bonding between the mother and her newborn can be very serious if the woman goes home without proper support. Therefore, interventions include involving the whole family in the bonding process. Discharge planning includes a predischarge consult with a clinical psychologist or clinical social worker to assess support systems available for the mother. A referral for home care may be appropriate.

Test Yourself

✔ What signs indicate that the woman may be experiencing postpartum depression versus the "baby blues"?

✔ List three things you can do to help a family cope with the birth of a newborn with a congenital anomaly.

✔ Name three ways you can create memories for parents whose newborn has died.

Cultural Snapshot

In the United States, fathers take a more active role in the direct care of their newborns shortly after birth. Families from different cultures may incorporate other relatives in newborn care. Be careful not to misinterpret lack of the father's involvement as malattachment. Family cultural beliefs may prescribe that only female members, such as the woman's sisters, mother, or mother-in-law, are allowed to handle the baby until the child is older. In some cultures, the woman is expected to remain secluded at home for approximately 4 to 6 weeks after delivery. Ask the family directly about who will be attending to the needs of the woman and infant once they go home.

Key Points

➤ Hemorrhage, infection, venous thromboembolism, and psychiatric disorders are conditions that put the postpartum woman at risk.

➤ Early postpartum hemorrhage occurs in the first 24 hours after birth and is most frequently caused by uterine atony. Late postpartum hemorrhage can occur anytime after the first 24 hours. Frequent causes are infection, subinvolution, and retained placental fragments.

➤ Nursing interventions for the woman with postpartum hemorrhage are focused on identifying the cause and stopping the bleeding. Establishing an IV line, if not already in place, and frequent monitoring of vital signs and urinary output are critical actions. For uterine atony, massage the uterus and administer ordered oxytocics. For lacerations and hematomas, notify the physician.

➤ Endometritis, infection of the uterine lining, is the most common postpartal infection. IV antibiotics are necessary for serious infections.

➤ Wound infection can involve the episiotomy, laceration, or cesarean incision. Risk factors include chronic medical conditions, obesity, and any factor that decreases a woman's resistance. Antibiotic therapy and drainage of the wound may be required.

➤ Mastitis is a localized infection of breast tissue caused by stasis in a milk duct and infection with organisms that enter the breast through a crack or fissure in the nipple. Treatment involves antibiotics, emptying the breasts (preferably by breast-feeding), and warm compresses.

➤ UTI symptoms include frequency, urgency, and burning upon urination. Pyelonephritis (kidney infection) is a more serious infection than cystitis (bladder infection). High, intermittent fever with flank tenderness accompanies pyelonephritis. Antibiotics are the therapy of choice.

➤ All postpartum women are at risk for thromboembolic disorders because of increased clotting factors that remain elevated after birth, pressure of the gravid uterus on the veins of the lower extremities during pregnancy, and the length of time in labor and delivery of being inactive or placed in stirrups, which can lead to stasis and pooling of blood in the extremities.

➤ The two major psychiatric disorders that can affect the woman in the postpartum period include postpartum depression and postpartum psychosis. Postpartum depression is a major mood disorder that interferes with the woman's ability to function in daily life. Postpartum psychosis is an emergency that requires inpatient psychiatric care. Both disorders require treatment by a mental health professional.

➤ The nurse's role is to support the woman who is grieving. Listen and be accepting of her feelings. Encourage the use of a support group and counseling for the couple. If the newborn dies, help the family make memories by encouraging them to hold the baby and say goodbye, by taking pictures, and by giving them a memento box with clothes the baby wore or blankets, etc.

➤ Assess for malattachment if the woman does not interact with or hold her baby, or if she turns away or does not talk to the baby or call him by name. Notify the RN if you notice any of these symptoms.

INTERNET RESOURCES

Postpartum Hemorrhage
www.pphprevention.org

Postpartum Depression
www.nimh.nih.gov/publicat/depwomenknows.cfm
www.4woman.gov/faq/postpartum.pdf

Workbook

■ NCLEX-STYLE REVIEW QUESTIONS

1. A woman is in for her postpartum checkup. She has a fever of 101°F and reports abdominal pain and a "bad smell" to her lochia. The nurse recognizes that these symptoms are associated with which condition?

   a. Mastitis
   b. Endometritis
   c. Subinvolution
   d. Episiotomy infection

2. The nurse enters the room of a woman who delivered 12 hours ago. The woman is leaning forward in bed and is obviously having difficulty breathing. The area around her mouth is blue. What should the nurse do first?

   a. Administer oxygen by nasal cannula.
   b. Obtain arterial blood for blood gas analysis.
   c. Raise the head of the bed.
   d. Tell the woman that she doesn't need to worry.

3. A woman delivered a healthy baby girl 2 days ago. Which observation by the nurse indicates the need for additional assessment and follow-up?

   a. The woman actively participates in the care of her baby.
   b. The woman comments that her baby has red hair like her grandmother.
   c. The woman reports that she will be happy to get home because she does not like hospital food.
   d. The woman tells a friend, referring to her baby, "it just cries all the time."

4. When caring for a postpartum woman who exhibits a large amount of bleeding, which areas would the nurse need to assess before the woman ambulates?

   a. Attachment, lochia color, complete blood cell count
   b. Blood pressure, pulse, complaints of dizziness
   c. Degree of responsiveness, respiratory rate, fundus location
   d. Height, level of orientation, support systems

■ STUDY ACTIVITIES

1. Use the following table to compare deep vein thrombosis and pulmonary embolism.

	Deep Vein Thrombosis	Pulmonary Embolism
Clinical manifestations		
Diagnosis		
Treatment		
Nursing care		

2. Research the resources in your community for postpartum depression. How many of these are available at no charge to the woman? How can the woman find out about these resources? Share your findings with your clinical group.

3. Develop a teaching plan for young teenage mothers to help them decrease their chances for developing a postpartum infection.

■ CRITICAL THINKING: WHAT WOULD YOU DO?

Apply your knowledge of postpartum complications to the following situation.

1. Josie is an outgoing 15-year-old girl who delivered a baby girl 24 hours ago. You walk in because you hear the newborn crying. Josie is talking to a friend on the telephone about the football game next week. When you check on the baby in the crib beside Josie's bed, the baby is jittery and red in the face.

   a. What is your impression of this situation? What ongoing assessments will you do to evaluate this situation?
   b. What do you need to do for the baby? Which individuals do you need to involve in the discharge planning process?

2. You just received Tiffany from the labor and delivery (L&D) unit after a normal delivery of a little girl. Her fundus is slightly firm, above the umbilicus, and positioned to the right. Her sanitary pad is full, but the L&D nurse reported that she received perineal care just before transport.

   a. What is the likely source of the heavy lochia? What nursing interventions should be done?
   b. If the fundus remains firm and in the midline, but a steady flow of lochia is noted despite fundal massage, what do you suspect is causing the problem? What nursing interventions should be done in this instance?

3. A woman who had a cesarean birth 3 days ago asks you to look at her incision, which is red and warm to touch with a small amount of yellow drainage along the edges.

   a. What conclusions do you reach as a result of your assessment? What additional assessments should be made? What interventions are appropriate in this situation?
   b. What if the woman reported hardness in an area of one of her breasts? How would you assess her breasts? What instructions would you give her?

20 The Newborn at Risk: Gestational and Acquired Disorders

KEY TERMS

apnea

appropriate for gestational age (AGA)

Erb palsy

extremely low birth weight (ELBW)

gestational age

intrauterine growth restriction (IUGR)

intraventricular hemorrhage

kernicterus

large for gestational age (LGA)

low birth weight (LBW)

macroglossia

meconium aspiration syndrome

necrotizing enterocolitis (NEC)

polycythemia

postterm

preterm

respiratory distress syndrome (RDS)

retinopathy of prematurity

small for gestational age (SGA)

very low birth weight (VLBW)

LEARNING OBJECTIVES

On completion of this chapter, you should be able to:

1. Define the classifications used to describe newborns based on their size, gestational age, or weight.

2. Explain the various components of the gestational age assessment.

3. Describe the most common underlying condition that causes a newborn to be SGA, and explain the reason this condition occurs.

4. Differentiate between symmetric and asymmetric growth restriction in infants.

5. List factors that contribute to a newborn being large for gestational age (LGA).

6. List possible contributing factors for preterm birth.

7. Compare characteristics of the preterm newborn with those of the term newborn.

8. Identify complications commonly associated with preterm newborns.

9. Describe the goals of care for the preterm newborn.

10. Describe major aspects of nursing care for the postterm newborn.

11. Give details of care for three acquired respiratory disorders associated with newborns.

12. Describe hemolytic disease of the newborn.

13. Explain important features of treatment, clinical manifestations, and nursing considerations for the newborn of a diabetic mother.

14. Discuss the clinical manifestations of and nursing care for a newborn of a chemically dependent mother.

15. Differentiate causes of and care for newborns with congenitally acquired infections.

DESPITE ALL that can go wrong, it is a wonder that the majority of babies are born healthy. However, for the 10% that are born ill or that develop health problems shortly after birth, the beginning of life can be a struggle. These fragile newborns need specialized care in the neonatal intensive care unit (NICU). Many Level III NICUs do not hire licensed practical/vocational nurses because the care of sick newborns can be complex and fall outside the scope of practical nursing. However, licensed practical/vocational nurses often work in Level II NICUs because these babies are more stable and have predictable needs. It is important for you to understand the major disorders and principles of care for sick newborns. If you work in a newborn nursery, you must be able to identify when the newborn's condition is deteriorating so that you can get help quickly.

This chapter focuses on newborn conditions that result when the newborn differs in size from the norm or is born earlier or later than expected. It also discusses disorders that the newborn acquires as a result of factors present during the pregnancy or birth.

VARIATIONS IN SIZE AND GESTATIONAL AGE

The majority of newborns are born around 40 weeks' gestation, weighing from 5.5 to 10 lb (2.5–4.6 kg) and measuring 18 in to 23 in (45–55 cm) in length. However, there are variations in birth size and **gestational age**, the length of time between fertilization of the egg and birth, that increase the newborn's risk for perinatal problems.

Terminology that describes newborns based on their size or gestational age is useful to facilitate communication. Size classifications consider the newborn's weight, length, and head circumference; these classifications include the following:

- **small for gestational age (SGA)** describes a newborn whose weight, length, and/or head circumference falls below the 10th percentile for gestational age
- **appropriate for gestational age (AGA)** describes a newborn whose weight, length, and/or head circumference falls between the 10th and 90th percentiles for gestational age
- **large for gestational age (LGA)** describes a newborn whose weight, length, and/or head circumference is above the 90th percentile for gestational age

There are three classifications that describe a newborn's size based on weight: **low birth weight (LBW)**, weight less than 2,500 g; **very low birth weight (VLBW)**, weight less than 1,500 g; and **extremely low birth weight (ELBW)**, weight less than 1,000 g.

Newborn classification based on gestational age includes:

- **preterm**, or premature, a newborn born at less than 37 weeks' gestation
- **postterm**, or postmature, a newborn born at greater than 42 weeks' gestation
- **term**, a newborn born between 37 and 42 weeks' gestation.

GESTATIONAL AGE ASSESSMENT

Assessment of gestational age is a critical evaluation. The registered nurse (RN) is ultimately responsible for performing the gestational age assessment. However, you should be familiar with the instruments used and be able to differentiate characteristics of the full-term newborn from those of the premature or postterm newborn. Although prenatal estimates of gestational age, particularly the sonogram, yield reliable information, the most precise way to assess gestational age is through direct evaluation of the newborn in the first few hours after birth.

The Ballard scoring system (Fig. 20-1) is a common gestational age assessment tool used in newborn nurseries. Gestational age assessment involves evaluation of two main categories of maturity: neuromuscular and physical maturity. The RN rates each category on a scale of –1 to 5, with 5 being the highest or most completed development. Table 20-1 compares gestational assessment findings in a term, preterm, and postterm newborn.

Neuromuscular Maturity

Six categories determine neuromuscular maturity:

1. Posture
2. Square window (measurement of wrist angle with flexion toward forearm until resistance is met)
3. Arm recoil (extension and release of arm after arm is completely flexed and held in position for approximately 5 seconds)
4. Popliteal angle (measurement of knee angle on flexion of thigh with extension of lower leg until resistance is met)
5. Scarf sign (arm pulled gently in front of and across top portion of body until resistance is met)
6. Heel to ear (movement of foot to near the head as possible)

Physical Maturity

Six categories determine physical maturity:

1. Skin
2. Lanugo
3. Plantar creases
4. Breast buds
5. Ears
6. Genitals

THE SMALL-FOR-GESTATIONAL AGE (GROWTH-RESTRICTED) NEWBORN

Small for gestational age (SGA) describes an infant who is born smaller than the average size (in weight, length, and/or head circumference) for the number of weeks' gestation at the time of delivery. The criteria are that the SGA newborn's weight falls below the 10th percentile of that expected for his or her gestational age, or that two of the three categories (weight, length, and head circumference) fall below the 10th percentile. Early identification of the SGA fetus with ultrasound is ideal.

Although some SGA babies are small because their parents are small (genetics), most are small because of circumstances that occurred during the pregnancy, causing limited fetal growth. This condition is **intrauterine growth restriction (IUGR)** or fetal growth restriction. It occurs when the fetus does not receive adequate amounts of oxygen and nutrients necessary for the proper growth and development of organs and tissues. IUGR can begin at any time during the pregnancy. The discussion for the remainder of this section focuses on the newborn who is SGA because of IUGR.

Contributing Factors

IUGR, the most common underlying condition leading to SGA newborns, results from interference in the supply of nutrients to the fetus. Inadequate maternal nutrition

NEUROMUSCULAR MATURITY

NEUROMUSCULAR MATURITY SIGN	SCORE							RECORD SCORE HERE
	−1	0	1	2	3	4	5	
POSTURE								
SQUARE WINDOW (Wrist)	>90°	90°	60°	45°	30°	0°		
ARM RECOIL		180°	140°–180°	110°–140°	90°–110°	<90°		
POPLITEAL ANGLE	180°	160°	140°	120°	100°	90°	<90°	
SCARF SIGN								
HEEL TO EAR								
					TOTAL NEUROMUSCULAR MATURITY SCORE			

SCORE

Neuromuscular ____
Physical ____
Total ____

MATURITY RATING

Score	Weeks
−10	20
−5	22
0	24
5	26
10	28
15	30
20	32
25	34
30	36
35	38
40	40
45	42
50	44

PHYSICAL MATURITY

PHYSICAL MATURITY SIGN	SCORE							RECORD SCORE HERE
	−1	0	1	2	3	4	5	
SKIN	sticky, friable, transparent	gelatinous, red, translucent	smooth, pink, visible veins	superficial peeling and/or rash, few veins	cracking pale areas, rare veins	parchment, deep cracking, no vessels	leathery, cracked, wrinkled	
LANUGO	none	sparse	abundant	thinning	bald areas	mostly bald		
PLANTAR SURFACE	heel-toe 40–50 mm:−1 <40 mm:−2	>50 mm no crease	faint red marks	anterior transverse crease only	creases ant. 2/3	creases over entire sole		
BREAST	impercep-tible	barely perceptible	flat areola no bud	stippled areola 1–2 mm bud	raised areola 3–4 mm bud	full areola 5–10 mm bud		
EYE-EAR	lids fused loosely: −1 tightly: −2	lids open pinna flat stays folded	sl. curved pinna; soft; slow recoil	well-curved pinna; soft but ready recoil	formed and firm instant recoil	thick cartilage, ear stiff		
GENITALS (Male)	scrotum flat, smooth	scrotum empty, faint rugae	testes in upper canal, rare rugae	testes descending, few rugae	testes down, good rugae	testes pendulous, deep rugae		
GENITALS (Female)	clitoris prominent and labia flat	prominent clitoris and small labia minora	prominent clitoris and enlarging minora	majora and minora equally prominent	majora large, minora small	majora cover clitoris and minora		
					TOTAL PHYSICAL MATURITY SCORE			

▮ Figure 20-1 Ballard's gestational age assessment tool, including neuromuscular and physical assessment criteria. (From Ballard, J. L. [1991]. New Ballard score expanded to include extremely premature infants. *Journal of Pediatrics*, 119, 417–423.)

may be a contributing factor. If the mother is unable to meet the increased nutritional demands of pregnancy, the fetus does not receive the necessary nutrients for growth. Another factor may involve an abnormality in the placenta or its function. Placental damage, such as when the placenta separates prematurely, or a decrease in blood flow to the placenta reduces its ability to trans-port nutrients. Maternal conditions that interfere with adequate blood flow to the placenta, such as preeclamp-sia/eclampsia or uncontrolled diabetes, contribute to placental malfunction. Maternal smoking interferes with placental blood flow and is the most common preventa-ble cause of IUGR. In some situations, placental func-tioning may be normal, but the fetus is unable to use the

Table 20-1 ▌ COMPARING GESTATIONAL AGE ASSESSMENT FINDINGS

Assessment Parameter	Term Newborn	Preterm Newborn	Postterm Newborn
Neuromuscular Maturity			
Posture	Flexed position with good muscle tone	Hypotonic with extension of the extremities	Full flexion of arms and legs
Square window	Flexible wrists with a small angle, usually ranging from 0 to 30 degrees	Angle greater than 45 degrees	Similar to that for term newborn
Arm recoil	Quick recoil with angle at elbow less than 90 degrees	Slowed recoil time with angle greater than 90 degrees	Similar to that for term newborn
Popliteal angle	Resistance to extension with knee angle 90 degrees or less	Decreased resistance to extension with large angle at knee	Similar to that for term newborn
Scarf sign	Increased resistance to movement with elbow unable to reach midline	Increased flexibility with elbow extending past midline	Similar to that for term newborn
Heel to ear	Moderate resistance to movement	Little to no resistance to movement	Similar to that for term newborn
Physical Maturity			
Skin	Cracking of the skin and few visible veins	Very thin with little subcutaneous fat and easily visible veins	Leathery, cracked, and wrinkled
Lanugo	Thinning of lanugo with balding areas	Abundance of fine-downy hair up to 34 weeks	Almost absent lanugo with many balding areas
Plantar creases	Creases covering at least the anterior 2/3 of foot	Smooth feet with few creases	Creases covering entire foot
Breast buds	Raised areola with 3- to 4-mm breast bud	Flat areola with little to no breast bud	Full areola with 5- to 10-mm breast bud
Ear	Cartilage present within pinna with ability for natural recoil when folded	Little cartilage, allowing shape to be maintained when folded	Cartilage thick; pinna stiff
Genitals	Male with pendulous scrotum covered with rugae; testicles descended Female with large labia majora covering minora	Male with smooth scrotum and undescended testicles Female with prominent clitoris; labia minora not covered by majora	Male with pendulous scrotum with deep rugae Female with clitoris and labia minora completely covered by labia majora

supplied nutrients, such as when the fetus develops an intrauterine infection. Box 20-1 lists factors that contribute to IUGR.

Clinical Manifestations

The two classification of IUGR are symmetrical growth restriction and asymmetrical growth restriction. Approximately 20% to 30% of newborns with IUGR have symmetrical growth restriction (Divon & Ferber, 2007). These newborns have not grown at the expected rate for gestational age on standard growth charts, but the growth pattern is symmetrical. In other words, both head and body parts are in proportion but are below normal size for gestational age. Generally, all three growth measurements (weight, length, and

head circumference) fall below the 10th percentile when plotted on a standard growth chart. Symmetrical growth restriction is the more serious of the two types because it begins earlier in the pregnancy, frequently has a genetic cause, and the condition is generally chronic.

The majority (70%–80%) of newborns with IUGR have asymmetric growth restriction. The asymmetrically growth-restricted newborn's head is large in comparison with the body. For this reason, asymmetric growth restriction is described as "head sparing." When the three growth measurements (weight, length, and head circumference) are plotted on a standard growth chart, one or two of the measurements falls below the 10th percentile. These newborns typically have normal measurements for

Box 20-1 ▌ CONTRIBUTING FACTORS TO IUGR AND PRETERM BIRTH

Maternal Factors

Lifestyle
- Smoking
- Alcohol use
- Substance abuse (e.g., narcotics, heroin, cocaine)
- Severe malnutrition during pregnancy

Chronic Diseases
- Heart disease
- Chronic hypertension
- Diabetes
- Anemia
- Connective tissue disorders (e.g., lupus)

Genetics and Demographics
- Race/Ethnicity (African Americans have higher incidence; Latino Americans have lower incidence when compared to whites)
- Extremes of age (under 16 or over 40)
- Short stature

Pregnancy-Related
- Prior history of IUGR or other poor pregnancy outcomes (e.g., stillbirth or preterm delivery)
- Multiple pregnancy (e.g., twins, triplets)
- Preeclampsia/eclampsia
- Intrauterine infections
- Umbilical cord defects
- Placenta previa
- Abruptio placentae

Fetal Factors
- Chromosomal abnormalities
- Congenital defects
- Congenital infections (TORCH)
- Hemolytic disease

head circumference and length but demonstrate a comparatively LBW.

The IUGR newborn typically appears pale, thin, and wasted. The skin is loose and peeling with very little vernix. The face has a shrunken or "wizened" appearance. Skull sutures may overlap or be too wide, and the abdomen may be sunken. The umbilical cord appears thin and dull, compared with the shiny, plump cord of a normal newborn. Meconium staining is a frequent finding. Compared with the AGA newborn, breast buds are smaller, ear cartilage is less developed, and female genitalia appear less mature.

The IUGR newborn may have neurologic involvement. The cry may be shrill. The infant may have a wide-eyed expression and appear hyperalert. He or she may be irritable, jittery, and difficult to soothe with an exaggerated Moro reflex. The newborn may have difficulty sleeping and startle easily.

Complications

Harsh conditions in utero can lead to a decrease in oxygen available to the fetus (hypoxia), causing the fetus to experience chronic fetal distress. Unable to meet the demands of normal labor and birth, the fetus may gasp in utero or with the first breaths at delivery, resulting in aspiration (breathing foreign matter into the lungs) of amniotic fluid. If the aspirated fluid contains meconium (the first stool), the newborn can develop meconium aspiration syndrome (see Meconium Aspiration Syndrome section later in this chapter).

The growth-restricted fetus is at increased risk for cesarean delivery because of fetal distress. He or she may be born prematurely with all the complications that accompany preterm birth. The newborn may have a difficult cardiopulmonary transition.

The IUGR newborn has difficulty with thermoregulation for several reasons. This newborn has very little subcutaneous tissue and brown fat because he or she consumed stores in utero. Compared to the AGA infant, the IUGR newborn has a large ratio of body surface area to weight. As a result, the newborn may develop hypothermia. In addition, the IUGR newborn typically experiences hypoglycemia (low blood sugar) because of a high metabolic rate in response to heat loss and low glycogen stores. Hypothermia and hypoglycemia can each lead to respiratory distress.

In response to chronic hypoxia in utero, the fetus increases red blood cell (RBC) production, leading to **polycythemia** (excess number of RBCs) and hyperviscosity of the blood. This newborn often has impaired immune function that continues throughout childhood. The IUGR newborn has a much higher mortality rate compared to the AGA infant. Symmetrically growth-restricted newborns have the highest mortality rate.

Nursing Care

The RN is responsible for assessing gestational age, identifying potential complications, and initiating the plan of care. As the licensed practical/vocational nurse, you play an important role in carrying out interventions identified in the plan of care.

Review the maternal history and note any factors that might contribute to SGA or IUGR. Be alert for potential complications and risk factors related to respiratory distress, hypothermia, hypoglycemia, polycythemia, and altered parental interaction with the newborn. Conduct and document routine nursing care with special emphasis on the following:

- Monitor respiratory status, including respiratory rate and pattern and observe for signs and symptoms of respiratory distress, such as cyanosis, nasal flaring, and expiratory grunting.

- Maintain a neutral thermal environment so that the skin temperature remains between 97.7°F and 99.5°F (36.5°C and 37.5°C).
- Monitor blood glucose levels, as ordered and more frequently if symptoms develop. Maintain levels greater than or equal to 50 mg/dL.
- Monitor results of other blood studies, such as hematocrit (<65%), hemoglobin (<22 g/dL), and bilirubin (<12 mg/dL).
- Observe feeding tolerance, including amounts taken and any difficulties or problems encountered, such as inability to suck at breast, fatigue, excessive spitting up, or diarrhea.
- Monitor intake and output and daily weights.
- Observe for jaundice.
- Encourage parents to visit frequently and care for their infant.

THE LARGE-FOR-GESTATIONAL AGE NEWBORN

A large-for-gestational age (LGA) newborn is one whose size (weight, length, and/or head circumference) is above the 90th percentile when plotted on a standard growth chart. The full term LGA newborn weighs more than 4,000 g, or two of the three categories (weight, length, and head circumference) lie above the 10th percentile for gestational age. Generally, the newborn's overall body size is proportional, but both head and weight fall in the upper limits of growth charts. Most LGA infants are genetically and nutritionally adequate. The newborn could receive an incorrect designation of LGA due to miscalculation of the due date. A postbirth gestational age assessment is essential.

Size can be misleading!
An LGA newborn may look mature because of his size. However, he could be developmentally immature because of gestational age.

Contributing Factors

In the majority of cases, the underlying cause of LGA is unknown. However, certain factors contribute. Maternal diabetes, particularly if it is poorly controlled, is the strongest known contributing factor. Genetic makeup may be a factor. For example, parents of large stature (height and/or weight) have an increased tendency to reproduce a LGA newborn. Obesity is a strong contributing factor. Latino women have a higher incidence of LGA newborns. Male newborns also are typically larger than female newborns. In addition, multiparous women have two to three times the number of LGA newborns than do primiparous women.

Congenital disorders play a role in LGA. Beckwith-Wiedemann syndrome, a rare genetic disorder, causes hormonally induced excessive weight gain and **macroglossia** (abnormally large tongue), which can cause feeding difficulties. Transposition of the great vessels, a congenital heart disease (see Chapter 21), is associated with LGA newborns. Other factors include umbilical abnormalities such as omphalocele, hypoglycemia, and hyperinsulinemia of the newborn.

Potential Complications

Most commonly, LGA newborns develop complications associated with the large body size. This newborn is more than twice as likely to deliver by cesarean section as his or her AGA counterpart is. The increased size is a leading cause of breech presentation and shoulder dystocia, which results in an increased incidence of birth injuries and trauma from a difficult extraction. Subsequent problems include fractured skull or clavicles, cervical or brachial plexus injury, and **Erb palsy** (a facial paralysis resulting from injury to the cervical nerves).

Nursing Care

Identifying the newborn at risk for LGA is important for anticipating the plan of care. Carefully review the maternal history for any risk factors that would contribute to an LGA newborn. Note any prenatal ultrasound reports, such as fetal skull size measurement. Assist the RN to perform a gestational age assessment. Conduct and document routine nursing care with a special emphasis on the following:

- Monitor vital signs frequently, especially respiratory status for changes indicating respiratory distress.
- Observe for signs and symptoms of hypoglycemia, including monitoring results of blood glucose levels.
- Document and report any signs of birth trauma or injury.
- Help parents verbalize feelings about any bruising or trauma they notice, including their fears of causing their newborn more pain.
- Encourage parent–newborn bonding by providing interaction and support, such as showing how to arouse a sleepy newborn, console a fussy newborn, and offer feedings.

Test Yourself

✔ What two major areas does a gestational age assessment evaluate?

✔ What is the underlying factor commonly associated with most SGA newborns?

✔ LGA newborns are at an increased risk for what complications associated with their size?

THE PRETERM NEWBORN

The preterm (premature) newborn is any infant born at less than 37 weeks' gestation. The preterm newborn's needs and care differs with the level of prematurity. Micro-premies are the tiniest newborns, weighing less than 1,000 g. The late preterm newborn is at the more mature end of the spectrum, born between 34 and 37 weeks' gestation. Determining the gestational age of the preterm newborn is crucial (see earlier discussion of gestational age assessment and Figure 20-1).

The preterm infant's untimely departure from the uterus may mean that various organs and systems are not sufficiently mature to adjust to extrauterine life. Often, small community hospitals or birthing centers are not equipped to care adequately for the preterm infant. When preterm delivery is expected, transport of the pregnant woman to a facility with a NICU is ideal. However, if delivery occurs before transport, then transportation of the newborn may be necessary. A team of specially trained personnel may come from the NICU to transport the neonate by ambulance, van, or helicopter. The newborn travels in a self-contained, battery-powered unit that provides warmth and oxygen. Intravenous (IV) fluids, monitors, and other emergency equipment are available during the transport.

Preparation is vital! Because so many things can go wrong during a preterm birth, make sure that neonatal care providers know about the impending birth so that equipment for resuscitation and emergency care is ready.

Contributing Factors

The underlying cause of preterm birth, in most cases, is unknown. The discovery and use of tocolytics (medications that relax the uterus) brought hope that the incidence of preterm delivery would decrease; however, the number of preterm births is actually on the rise. Tocolytics have brought about better outcomes because they delay the delivery long enough for corticosteroids to enhance lung maturity, but they have had a negligible effect on the rate of occurrence of preterm births. Prematurity remains the leading cause of perinatal death and disability (Mandy, 2006).

The main cause of the continued increase in the incidence of preterm birth is advances in fertility treatments resulting in multiple births. Multiple births are often preterm because of polyhydramnios (excessive amniotic fluid), a larger than average intrauterine mass, and/or early cervical dilation. Another of the most common contributing factors is preterm premature rupture of membranes. This may occur due to various underlying conditions, particularly infection of the membranes, which is an indication for immediate delivery. The increased numbers of pregnant women with diabetes is

another major contributor. All of the contributing factors to IUGR also increase the risk of preterm birth (see Box 20-1).

Characteristics of the Preterm Newborn

Compared with the term infant, the preterm infant is tiny, scrawny, and red. The extremities are thin, with little muscle or subcutaneous fat. The head and abdomen are disproportionately large, and the skin is thin, relatively translucent, and usually wrinkled. Veins of the abdomen and scalp are more visible. Lanugo is plentiful over the extremities, back, and shoulders. The ears have soft, minimal cartilage and thus are extremely pliable. The soft bones of the skull tend to flatten on the sides, and the ribs yield with each labored breath. Testes are undescended in the male; the labia and clitoris are prominent in the female. The soles of the feet and the palms of the hands have few creases. Many of the typical newborn reflexes are weak or absent. Figure 20-2 shows several typical physical characteristics of the preterm newborn.

The preterm newborn's physiologic immaturity causes many difficulties involving virtually all body systems, the most critical of which is the respiratory system. Typically, respirations are shallow, rapid, and irregular with periods of **apnea**, absence of breathing that lasts for at least 20 seconds or that causes cyanosis and/or bradycardia. Retractions of the chest wall and sternum indicate labored respirations.

Thermoregulation and maintaining fluid and electrolyte balance are major problems for the preterm newborn because he or she loses heat and fluids more quickly and has fewer compensatory mechanisms than does the term newborn. Rapid heat and water loss occur because the preterm newborn does not have the insulation provided by subcutaneous and brown fat that is available to the term newborn, water and heat can escape through the thin skin, and this newborn has an increased surface area to body mass. The preterm newborn cannot shiver to produce heat and cannot assume a flexed posture to conserve heat and water. Immaturity of the CNS and the lack of integrated reflex control of peripheral blood vessels (to cause vasodilation or vasoconstriction) also affect the preterm newborn's ability to maintain body temperature.

The preterm newborn has high caloric needs, but has a digestive system that may be unprepared to receive and digest food. The stomach is small, with a capacity that may be less than 1 to 2 oz. The sphincters at either end of the stomach are immature, causing regurgitation or vomiting if feedings distend the stomach. The immature liver cannot manage all the bilirubin produced by hemolysis (destruction of RBCs with the release of hemoglobin), making the infant prone to jaundice and high blood bilirubin levels (hyperbilirubinemia) that may result in brain damage.

■ **Figure 20-2** Characteristics of a preterm newborn. **(A)** Few plantar creases. **(B)** Soft, pliable ear cartilage, matted hair, and fused eyelids. **(C)** Lax posture with poor muscle development. **(D)** Breast and nipple area barely noticeable. **(E)** Male genitalia. Note the minimal rugae on the scrotum. **(F)** Female genitalia. Note the prominent labia and clitoris.

The preterm infant does not receive enough antibodies from the mother and cannot produce them. This characteristic makes the infant particularly vulnerable to infection.

Muscle weakness in the premature infant contributes to nutritional and respiratory problems and to a posture distinct from that of the term infant (Fig. 20-3). The infant may not be able to change positions and is prone to fatigue and exhaustion, even from eating and breathing. Skilled, gentle intensive care is needed for the newborn to survive and develop. The parents also need supportive, intensive care.

■ Figure 20-3 Typical resting posture of preterm newborn. Note the lax position and immature muscular development.

Treatment of Complications

The preterm newborn is at risk for a variety of complications. The most vulnerable body systems are respiratory, gastrointestinal, and central nervous systems. The most frequent complications include hypothermia, hypoglycemia, respiratory disorders, patent ductus arteriosus, intracranial hemorrhage, necrotizing enterocolitis, jaundice, infection, and retinopathy of prematurity (ROP). Treatment of the preterm newborn and his or her complications is individualized because each newborn responds to the challenge of preterm transition to extrauterine life in his or her unique way. This section discusses treatment and special considerations of some of the most common conditions associated with prematurity.

Respiratory Distress Syndrome

Respiratory distress syndrome (RDS), also known as hyaline membrane disease, occurs in about 20,000 to 30,000 premature infants born in the United States each year. The risk of RDS is higher the lower the gestational age. In fact, almost half of the neonates at 26 to 28 weeks' gestation develop RDS compared to less than 30% of neonates born at 30 to 31 weeks' gestation (Pramanik, 2006).

RDS occurs in the preterm newborn because the lungs are too immature. Normally, the lungs remain partially expanded after each breath because of surfactant, a biochemical compound that reduces surface tension inside the air sacs. The premature infant's lungs are deficient in surfactant and thus collapse after each breath, greatly increasing the work of breathing. The complex interplay of disease process and treatments (in particular oxygen therapy) causes damage to the lung cells. These damaged cells combine with other substances present in the lungs to form a hyaline membrane. This fibrous membrane lines the alveoli and blocks gas exchange.

The preterm newborn with RDS may exhibit problems breathing immediately or a few hours after birth. Typically, respirations increase to greater than 60 breaths per minute. Nasal flaring and retractions may be noted. Mucous membranes may appear cyanotic. As respiratory distress progresses, the newborn exhibits seesawlike respirations in which the chest wall retracts and the abdomen protrudes on inspiration and then the sternum rises on expiration. Breathing is labored, the respiratory rate continues to increase, and expiratory grunting occurs. Breath sounds usually diminish, and the newborn may develop periods of apnea.

Surfactant replacement therapy was the treatment breakthrough in the 1970s that dramatically increased survival rates. More recent therapy advances include the use of antenatal steroids, appropriate resuscitation techniques, immediate use of continuous positive airway pressure (CPAP), and gentle (versus aggressive) ventilation procedures (Pramanik, 2006).

Treatment begins shortly after birth with synthetic or naturally occurring surfactant, obtained from animal sources or extracted from human amniotic fluid. The newborn receives surfactant as an inhalant through a catheter inserted into an endotracheal tube. The therapy may be preventive ("rescue") treatment to avoid the development of RDS in the newborn at risk. Newborns with RDS usually receive additional oxygen through continuous positive airway pressure, using intubation or a plastic hood. This helps the lungs to remain partially expanded until they begin producing surfactant, usually within the first 5 days of life. The preterm newborn that develops RDS requires supportive care to promote adequate oxygenation and prevent complications.

> **Did you know?**
>
> Too much oxygen is toxic to tiny lungs and eyes. Research demonstrates that newborns with RDS have decreased incidence of chronic lung and eye conditions when oxygen saturation levels remain between 85% and 94% versus the 95% to 98% levels targeted in times past.

Intraventricular Hemorrhage

Intraventricular hemorrhage (IVH), bleeding into the brain's ventricles, is a complication of preterm birth that occurs more often in the newborn of less than 32 weeks' gestation. In addition to early gestational age, other factors commonly associated with IVH include birth asphyxia, LBW, respiratory distress, and hypotension. Ultrasonography, computed tomography, and magnetic resonance imaging screen for and provide the basis to diagnose the condition.

Two factors place the extremely premature infant at risk for IVH. First, the developing brain has a fragile capillary network that ruptures easily with cerebral pressure changes. Second, the preterm newborn may be unable to autoregulate cerebral pressure, which leaves the newborn with little protection from pressure fluctuations. In addition, too much stimulation and abrupt movements during care increase the risk.

Most infants who develop IVH are asymptomatic or have subtle symptoms, such as a sudden drop in hematocrit levels, pallor, and poor perfusion. Therefore, the primary care provider orders screening exams to identify bleeding. Signs that may accompany IVH include hypotonia, apnea, bradycardia, a full (or bulging) fontanelle, cyanosis, and increased head circumference. Neurologic signs such as twitching, convulsions, and stupor may be noted.

Supportive care is the foundation for medical intervention. The focus is on preventing, diagnosing, and correcting acid-base imbalances, fluid and electrolyte imbalances, respiratory compromise, and cardiovascular disturbances. Nursing intervention focuses on prevention (see the nursing care section that follows for further discussion of preventative interventions).

Retinopathy of Prematurity

Retinopathy of prematurity (ROP) is a form of retinopathy (degenerative disease of the retina) commonly associated with the preterm newborn, particularly infants born at less than 28 weeks' gestation. Immature retinal blood vessels grow abnormally, often resulting in retinal scarring and/or detachment. These events lead to varying degrees of blindness. Wide fluctuations in oxygen levels and oxygen saturation limits maintained above 94% are major causes.

Prevention is the best treatment. The nursing process section that follows discusses prevention strategies. It is not always possible to prevent ROP, so treatment begins with early identification. An ophthalmologist with special training performs a screening exam at 31 weeks' corrected age[1] to detect the changes associated with developing ROP. Laser surgery is the current treatment of choice. This therapy has proved more effective and less damaging to surrounding eye tissues than cryosurgery.

Necrotizing Enterocolitis

Necrotizing enterocolitis (NEC) is an acute inflammatory necrotic disease of the intestine. This devastating condition has a mortality rate of 25%, and surviving newborns often face life-long health challenges and disability (Yeo, 2006). The incidence is highest in small preterm newborns. The cause is unknown; however, the key risk factor is prematurity. Precipitating factors include formula feeding, bowel ischemia, and bacterial invasion of the intestine.

Initial clinical manifestations may be subtle and are not specific to NEC. The newborn feeds poorly, and may experience lethargy, temperature instability, and vomiting of bile. Other findings include abdominal distention and occult blood in the stool. Abdominal radiographs (x-rays) confirm the diagnosis. Abdominal ultrasound is a useful diagnostic tool when performed by a skilled practitioner.

Initially, oral feedings are discontinued and nasogastric suction is applied to rest the bowel. IV fluids, including total parenteral nutrition, and antibiotics are given. Bowel perforation or necrosis necessitates surgical intervention to repair, bypass, or remove parts of the intestine.

Because NEC can lead to devastating outcomes, prevention is the focus of much research. The most promising medical therapy at present is the use of probiotics. These oral supplements provide microbes that are normally present in the intestine of older children and adults. These microbes enhance the gut's ability to form a protective barrier against insults that could lead to NEC (Thompson & Bizzarro, 2008).

> **Nurses definitely make a difference.**
> Your observation skills are critical to detecting early and subtle changes associated with NEC. The sooner the newborn receives treatment for NEC, the better the outcomes.

> ### Test Yourself
> ✔ Describe three characteristics of a preterm newborn.
> ✔ Which complication associated with preterm newborns is due to a surfactant deficiency?
> ✔ What factors increase the risk for ROP?

Nursing Process for the Preterm Newborn

The complex needs of a preterm newborn require skilled nursing care. Priorities of care include maintenance of adequate oxygenation, continuous electronic cardiac and respiratory monitoring, frequent manual monitoring of vital signs, thermoregulation, infection control, hydration, provision of adequate nutrition and developmental care for the newborn, and emotional support for the parents.

Assessment

Assessment of the preterm newborn is similar to that for any newborn, but the initial assessment focuses on the status of the respiratory, circulatory, and neurologic systems to determine the immediate needs of the infant. Although monitoring equipment provides a continual reading of the heart rate, take apical pulses periodically, listening to the heart through the chest using a stetho-

> **Don't check out!**
> Although sophisticated monitoring equipment is available in the modern NICU, do not rely on monitors in place of careful assessment. Observe the equipment, make sure it is functioning properly, and systematically assess the infant.

---

[1]Calculate the corrected age by adding the weeks since birth to the gestational age at birth. For example, if the birth occurred at 26 weeks' gestation, then the newborn would be 31 weeks' corrected age at the chronological age of 5 weeks.

scope for 1 full minute so as not to miss an irregularity in rhythm. Note the pulse rate, rhythm, and strength. The pulse rate is normally rapid (120–140 beats per minute [bpm]) and unstable. Premature newborns are subject to dangerous periods of bradycardia (as low as 60–80 bpm) and tachycardia (as high as 160–200 bpm). Your observations of the pulse rate, rhythm, and strength are essential to determining how the infant is tolerating treatments, activity, feedings, and the temperature and oxygen concentration of the environment.

Selected Nursing Diagnoses

Based on the initial assessment, nursing diagnoses that may be appropriate include the following:

- Ineffective Breathing Pattern related to an immature respiratory system
- Ineffective Thermoregulation related to immaturity and transition to extrauterine life
- Risk for Infection related to an immature immune system and environmental factors
- Risk for Injury related to cerebral bleeding secondary to premature status
- Risk for Fluid Volume Deficit related to increased insensitive water loss secondary to premature skin that favors evaporation, and therapies, such as overhead warmers and phototherapy, that also promote fluid loss
- Risk for Imbalanced Nutrition, Less Than Body Requirements related to an inability to suck
- Risk for Impaired Skin Integrity related to prematurity and exposure to phototherapy light
- Activity Intolerance related to poor oxygenation and weakness
- Risk for Disorganized Infant Behavior related to prematurity and excess environmental stimuli
- Parental Anxiety related to a seriously ill newborn with an unpredictable prognosis
- Risk for Impaired Parenting related to separation from the newborn and difficulty accepting loss of ideal newborn
- Interrupted Family Processes related to the effect of prolonged hospitalization on the family

Outcome Identification and Planning

The major goals for the preterm newborn include improving respiratory function, maintaining body temperature, preventing infection, protecting neurologic status, maintaining fluid and electrolyte balance, maintaining adequate nutrition, preserving skin integrity, conserving energy, and supporting growth and development. Goals for the family include reducing anxiety and improving parenting skills and family functioning.

Implementation
Improving Respiratory Function

Not all preterm newborns need extra oxygen, but many do. Isolettes have oxygen inlets and humidifiers for raising the oxygen concentration inside from 20% to 21% (room air) to a higher percentage. An oxyhood, a clear plastic hood placed over the infant's head, is another way to supply humidified oxygen for infants with mild respiratory distress. For newborns that require a little more help, CPAP is the preferred modality. This therapy does not allow the alveoli to collapse at the end of respiration, which greatly reduces the work of breathing and improves oxygenation. There several ways to administer CPAP including nasal prongs, face masks, and nasopharyngeal or endotracheal tubes. The preterm newborn with severe RDS will likely need mechanical ventilation.

Pulse oximetry continuously monitors blood oxygen saturation. The RN programs the pulse oximeter to alarm when oxygen saturation levels fall below 85% or rise higher than 94%. If the alarm rings, respond immediately and adjust the oxygen concentration, as ordered, to maintain the oxygen saturation within the prescribed limits. Teach the parents, other caregivers, and all staff (e.g., unit secretaries, housekeepers) to report alarms immediately. These actions are neuroprotective and can limit the occurrence of ROP and NEC.

Observe the preterm newborn's respirations carefully. Observe for changes in respiratory effort, rate, depth, breath sounds, and regularity of respirations. Note any expiratory grunting or chest retractions (substernal, suprasternal, intercostal, subcostal), including severity, and nasal flaring to determine the newborn's ability to maintain respirations. Assist the RN to ensure that oxygen support or ventilator settings and endotracheal tube placement, if present, are as prescribed to ensure adequacy of ventilation and respiratory assistance.

Reposition the newborn every 2 hours to reduce the risk for pneumonia and atelectasis. Frequent suctioning may be necessary to prevent airway obstruction, hypoxia, and asphyxiation. If not contraindicated, elevate the head of the bed as needed to maintain a patent airway. Promote rest times between procedures because organized care helps to conserve the newborn's energy and reduce oxygen consumption.

One of the most hazardous characteristics of the preterm newborn is the tendency to stop breathing periodically (apnea). The hypoxia caused by apnea and general respiratory difficulty may lead to long-term neurologic disability, such as cerebral palsy or mental retardation. Monitors with apnea alarms alert the caregiver when an episode of apnea occurs. Electrodes positioned on the infant's chest with leads to the apnea monitor provide a continuous reading

Don't succumb to temptation.

You may want to lower the sound when false alarms occur frequently. This highly unsafe practice can lead to tragedy if you miss a newborn's distress because the alarms are off. Instead, troubleshoot and fix the problem causing the false alarms.

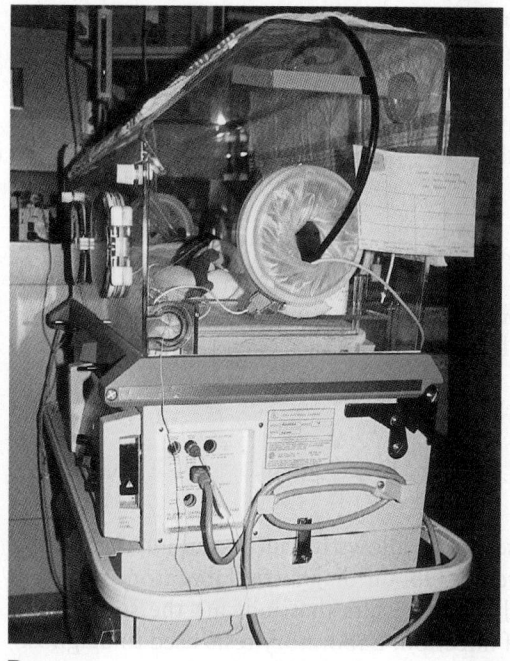

A   **B**

■ **Figure 20-4** Maintenance of thermoregulation. **(A)** Newborn under a radiant warmer. **(B)** Newborn in an isolette.

of the respiratory rate. Visual and audio alarms go off when the rate goes too high or too low or if the infant waits too long to take a breath.

It is a nursing responsibility to place, check, and replace the leads on the newborn. Each day, remove electrodes and reapply them in a slightly different location to protect the infant's sensitive skin from damage by the electrode paste and adhesive. Cleanse the skin carefully between applications of the electrodes. When an episode of apnea occurs, first try gentle tactile stimulation, such as wiggling a foot. Sometimes this is enough to remind the newborn to breathe. If not, the newborn may require respiratory assistance with a bag and mask.

Maintaining Body Temperature

Monitor the preterm newborn's body temperature closely. Observe for signs of cold stress such as low temperature, body cold to touch, pallor, and lethargy.

Protect the newborn from heat loss. If the newborn becomes wet, be sure to dry him or her quickly and remove wet linen to avoid heat loss via evaporation. Avoid positioning the preterm newborn on cold surfaces or placing cold objects (e.g., a cold stethoscope) on the newborn. Protect the infant from drafts. Be sure to expose as little of the newborn's skin as possible during procedures to minimize heat loss. Conversely, the preterm newborn must not be overheated because this causes increased consumption of oxygen and calories, possibly jeopardizing the newborn's status.

An isolette or a radiant warmer prevents heat loss and helps control other aspects of the premature infant's envi-

ronment (Fig. 20-4). A heat-sensing probe attached to the newborn's skin controls the temperature of the isolette or the radiant warmer. The isolette has a clear Plexiglas top that allows a full view of the newborn from all aspects. The isolette maintains ideal temperature, humidity, and oxygen concentrations and isolates the infant from infection. Portholes at the side allow access to the newborn with minimal temperature and oxygen loss. Open units with overhead radiant warmers allow maximum access to the infant when sophisticated equipment or frequent manipulation for treatment and assessment is necessary.

Preventing Infection

Infection control is an urgent concern in the care of the preterm newborn. The preterm infant cannot resist bacterial invasions, so caregivers must provide an atmosphere that protects him or her from such attacks. The primary means of preventing infection is hand washing. All persons must practice good hand washing immediately before touching the newborn and when moving from one newborn to another.

Other important aspects of good housekeeping include regular cleaning or changing of humidifier water; IV tubing; and suction, respiratory, and monitoring equipment. The NICU is separate from the normal newborn nursery and usually has its own staff. This separation helps eliminate sources of infection. Personnel in this area usually wear scrub suits or gowns. Personnel from other departments (radiology, respiratory therapy, or laboratory) put a cover gown over their uniforms while working with these newborns.

Signs of infection are nonspecific and subtle. Report these signs and symptoms of infection including:

- Temperature instability (decrease or increase)
- Glucose instability and metabolic acidosis
- Poor sucking
- Vomiting
- Diarrhea
- Abdominal distention
- Apnea
- Respiratory distress and cyanosis
- Hepatosplenomegaly
- Jaundice
- Skin mottling
- Lethargy
- Hypotonia
- Seizures

Close observation allows for successful intervention if infection occurs. Obtain diagnostic laboratory work as ordered and report results that indicate the source and treatment of infection. Laboratory tests used to diagnose and treat infections include blood cultures, cerebral spinal fluid analysis, urinalysis and urine cultures, tracheal aspirate culture, and superficial cultures. Expect antibiotics to be ordered to treat suspected or confirmed bacterial infections.

Protecting Neurologic Status

Because the preterm newborn is at risk for IVH, protecting neurologic status is critical. Neuroprotection involves avoiding activities that could cause wide fluctuations of cerebral blood pressures. Assist the RN to assess fluid volume status and prevent fluid overload. Ensure that the head and body remain in alignment when moving and turning the newborn (i.e., avoid twisting the head at the neck). Minimal stimulation is a necessary precaution to minimize pain and stress. Reduce procedures that cause crying, such as routine suctioning. Avoid painful procedures and disturbances when possible. Use narcotics, as ordered, to treat pain when avoidance is not possible. Control noise level in the environment. Provide developmental care and positioning.

Little things make a big difference.

Because excessive noise can overstimulate and increase the risk for IVH, speak gently and softly around the preterm newborn. Don't tap on the sides of the isolette, and avoid frequent opening and closing of portholes.

Maintaining Fluid and Electrolyte Balance

Maintaining fluid and electrolyte balance is a major challenge for the preterm newborn. In many instances, an IV "life line" is necessary immediately after delivery. Fluids infuse through a catheter placed in the umbilical vein in the stump of the umbilical cord. Intravenous fluids may infuse through other veins, particularly the peripheral veins of the hands, feet, or scalp. Extremely small amounts of fluid are needed, perhaps as little as 5 to 10 mL/hr or even less. An infusion pump is critical to measure accurately and administer fluids at a steady rate. Keep accurate, complete records of IV fluids and observe frequently for signs of infiltration or overhydration.

Monitor lab values, as ordered. Serum electrolytes, blood urea nitrogen, creatinine, and plasma osmolarity levels are the most common tests. Report abnormal values. Ensure that the appropriate IV fluids are infusing and that the proper amounts of supplemental sodium, potassium, chloride and other additives are included, as ordered.

Observe and record the number of voidings, the color of the urine, and note any edema. Keep strict intake and output records. Measure and record all urinary output by weighing the diapers before and after they are used. Urinary output should be at least 1 mL/kg/hr.

This is how it's done.
One gram equals approximately 1 mL. Weigh the wet diaper, and then subtract the weight of the dry diaper. The difference in grams is the output in mL.

Maintaining Adequate Nutrition

At birth, a preterm newborn may be too weak or sick to suck. Commonly, the preterm newborn has difficulty coordinating sucking, swallowing, and breathing so that he or she can breast- or bottle-feed. Other problems that may inhibit oral feedings include limited stomach capacity, contributing to distention and inadequate intake; poor muscle tone of the cardiac sphincter, leading to regurgitation with secondary apnea and bradycardia; and muscle weakness, which leads to exhaustion. Premature newborns are likely to have problems with aspiration because the gag reflex does not develop until about the 32nd to 34th week of gestation, which predisposes them to distention and regurgitation. As a result, alternative feeding methods may be needed.

At first, some preterm newborns receive all their fluid, electrolyte, vitamin, and calorie needs by the IV route (usually with total parenteral nutrition); others can start with a nipple and bottle. However, many require gavage-feeding (feeding by a tube passed from the mouth or nose to the stomach). It is important for the preterm newborn to receive enteral-feedings as soon as possible after birth. Enteral feedings keep the gastrointestinal system functioning and healthy. Lack of food in the gut leads to atrophy of the mucosa. It then becomes more difficult to initiate feedings.

There are other feeding methods available if the preterm newborn cannot tolerate either gavage or nipple-feeding, and if IV fluids are inadequate. Some preterm newborns do better if fed with a rubber-tipped medicine dropper. Others may require gastrostomy-feedings (feeding by a tube passed through the skin to the stomach; see Chapter 30). Whatever the alternate method used, the preterm newborn who is not receiving nipple-feedings should receive nonnutritive sucking opportunities, such as with a pacifier.

It is important to assess nutritional health of the preterm newborn. Perform daily weights. Weight gain or loss patterns give an indication of overall health and indicate whether the newborn is consuming enough calories. Weigh the newborn with the same clothing, using the same scale, and at the same time each day to help ensure accurate, comparable data. Other indicators of nutritional health include skin condition, hair growth, and achievement of adequate growth patterns and developmental milestones.

Sources of Nutrition. Breast milk, the preferred source of nutrition for the preterm newborn, offers many benefits. Breast milk stimulates the newborn's immune system and provides immunoglobulins from the woman. Human milk protects from NEC, infections, cancers, metabolic disorders, and certain childhood disorders. Mothers can pump their breast milk and freeze it to use for bottle or gavage-feedings until the preterm newborn is strong enough to breast-feed. Providing food, which only she can supply, to nourish her newborn provides a tremendous boost to the emotional satisfaction of the mother.

If the woman chooses not to breast-feed, human donor breast milk is a satisfactory substitute. A centralized milk bank collects pumped breast milk for distribution to NICU newborns, as needed. Before accepting and storing the donated milk, the milk bank screens the lactating donor for communicable diseases and other conditions that could adversely affect milk composition.

If the newborn is to receive formula, then a preterm formula with 20 calories/oz is the typical type chosen. Preterm formula has a different nutrient mix than formula for term newborns. This is because the preterm newborn has specialized nutritional needs. For example, if the formula is too rich (too high in carbohydrates and fats), vomiting and diarrhea may occur. Some preterm newborns require higher-density caloric formula. These formulas provide 22 or 24 calories/oz.

Gavage-Feeding. When the preterm newborn is not able to receive oral feedings, gavage-feedings through an orogastric or nasogastric tube may be necessary. The frequency and quantity of gavage-feedings are individualized. Usually, feeding frequency is every 2 hours to allow for small amounts at frequent intervals. Preterm infants have a difficult time tolerating large amounts at one time due to limited stomach capacity, and if the feeding takes too long, the infant may tire. Figure 20-5 shows a nurse assisting a mother to gavage-feed her newborn.

Check prefeed gastric residuals (aspiration of gastric contents before a feeding). If the stomach is not empty by the next feeding, allow more time between feedings or give smaller feedings. The newborn's tolerance level dictates the quantity. Increase the amount of formula or

■ Figure 20-5 The nurse helps the caregiver administer a gavage-feeding to her premature infant.

breast milk slowly (milliliter by milliliter) as quickly as tolerated. The feeding is too large if the newborn's stomach distends so that it causes respiratory difficulty, vomiting, or regurgitation and if there is formula left in the stomach by the next feeding. See Chapter 30 for more information on gavage-feeding.

Pay attention.
Report immediately gradually increasing residuals and abdominal girth, or return of more than 2 mL of undigested formula. These signs indicate feeding intolerance and could herald the onset of NEC.

Nipple- (Bottle-) Feeding. When a preterm newborn who is being gavage-fed begins to suck vigorously on the fingers, hands, pacifier, or gavage tubing and demonstrates evidence of a gag reflex, it is time to introduce bottle-feeding, and in some cases, breast-feeding. The infant who can take the same quantity of formula or breast milk by bottle that he or she took by gavage-feeding without becoming too tired is ready for oral feeding. Alternating gavage- and nipple-feedings may be necessary in some cases to assist the preterm newborn in making the transition. Special nipples and smaller bottles prevent too much liquid from flowing into the newborn's mouth. The nipple for a preterm newborn usually is made of softer rubber than is a regular nipple. It is also smaller, but no shorter, than the regular nipple.

To nipple-feed, hold the newborn in your arms or on your lap at a 45-degree angle. Be careful to prevent aspiration throughout the feeding. Make sure that oxygen is available, as needed. Burp the preterm newborn often during and after feedings. Sometimes simply changing the infant's position is enough assistance; at other times, it may help to gently rub or pat the infant's back.

Preserving Skin Integrity

Assess skin integrity frequently (at least every shift) for changes in color, turgor, texture, vascularity, and signs of irritation or infection. Pay special attention to areas in which equipment is attached or inserted. Frequent skin assessment allows for early detection and prompt intervention.

A preterm newborn's skin is extremely fragile and injures easily, so handle the infant gently. Reposition the preterm newborn every 2 to 4 hours and as needed. Preterm infants have a knack for wriggling into corners and cracks from which they cannot extract themselves, so close observation is necessary.

Keep the skin clean and dry, but avoid excessive bathing, which further dries the skin. Use water only or mild soaps when bathing twice weekly. Change the diaper as soon as possible after soiling to help prevent breakdown in the perineal area. Pad pressure-prone areas by using sheepskin blankets, waterbeds, pillows, or egg crate mattresses to help prevent additional skin breakdown to these areas. Monitor intake and output and avoid dehydration and over hydration. Box 20-2 outlines interventions to prevent preterm skin breakdown.

Promoting Energy Conservation

The preterm newborn uses most of his or her energy to breathe and maintain vital functions. Plan ahead and cluster care activities to avoid exhaustion from constant handling and movement. Energy conservation does not include ignoring or avoiding the newborn or discouraging the contact essential to establishing a normal relationship. Gentle touch and newborn massage are therapeutic.

Box 20-2 ▪ INTERVENTIONS TO PROTECT PRETERM SKIN

- Keep the infant's skin clean with water.
- Modify typical newborn bathing:
  - Schedule twice weekly.
  - Between baths, clean visibly soiled areas, face, and perineum as needed with water.
  - Use water only for infants less than 32 weeks' gestation.
  - For infants greater than 32 weeks' gestation, mild nonalkaline soap may be used at bath time only.
- Avoid alcohol on the skin.
- Avoid creams and ointments, unless specifically ordered.
- Use water or mineral oil to help remove adhesives. Avoid adhesive remover.
- Use iodine or benzoin with caution because the newborn's skin readily absorbs these products.
- Use transparent dressings such as Tegaderm or OpSite to protect IV sites and over bony prominences, as needed, to prevent breakdown.

Supporting Growth and Development

All NICU newborns need developmental care, including preterm newborns. Interventions include decreasing environmental noise and stress, maintaining flexed positioning, and clustering care to conserve energy. Providing opportunities for nonnutritive sucking helps develop feeding skills. Kangaroo (skin-to-skin) care assists with keeping the newborn warm and promotes parental bonding (Beal, 2005).

As the preterm infant grows, he or she increasingly needs sensory stimulation. Mobiles hung over the isolette and toys placed in or on the infant unit may provide visual stimulation. A radio with the volume turned low, a music box, or a wind-up toy in the isolette may provide auditory stimulation. An excellent form of auditory stimulation comes from the voices of the infant's family, physicians, and nurses talking and singing. Being bathed, held, cuddled, and fondled provides needed tactile stimulation. Contact is essential to the infant and the family. Some NICUs have "foster grandparents" who regularly visit long-term NICU infants and provide them with sensory stimulation, cuddling, loving, crooning, and talking. These programs have proven beneficial to both the infants and the volunteer grandparents.

Reducing Parental Anxiety

Birth of a preterm newborn creates a crisis for the family caregivers. Often their long-awaited baby is whisked away from them, sometimes to a distant neonatal center, and hooked up to a maze of machines. They cannot share the early, sensitive attachment period. It may take weeks to establish touch and eye contact, ordinarily achieved in 10 minutes with a term infant. Sometimes the woman's condition inhibits early contact with the preterm newborn. If the birth was by cesarean, or if the labor was difficult or prolonged, she may not have the strength to go to the NICU and to become involved with the baby. Parents often leave the hospital empty-handed, without the perfect, healthy infant of their dreams. How can they learn to know and love the strange, scrawny creature that now lives in that plastic box?

Parents feel anxiety, guilt, fear, depression, and perhaps anger. These feelings are normal. Accept and encourage the parent(s) to express their feelings. If the parent(s) ignore these feelings, long-term damage to the parental–child relationship can result. Unfortunately, unresolved negative feelings can even lead to child neglect or abuse.

Nurses who work with high-risk infants can do much to help families cope with the crisis of prematurity and early separation. To ease some of the apprehension of the family caregivers, transport teams prepare the newborn for transportation, then take the newborn in the transport incubator into the mother's room so that the parents may see (and touch, if possible) the newborn before the child is whisked away. In many cases, instant photos provide the family some concrete reminder of the newborn until they can visit in person.

A Personal Glimpse

My son was born 8.5 weeks before his expected due date. I was unable to hold him until 12 hours after his birth. I was discharged from the hospital with a Polaroid snapshot of him and the phone number of the hospital's neonatal intensive care unit.

For 2 weeks I visited him, learning new medical terms and gaining an understanding of all the obstacles he would have to overcome before being released. These days were an emotional roller coaster filled with feelings of joy over being blessed with a son; enormous concern over his condition; and a great deal of guilt. The thing I wanted most in the world was to take him home, healthy and without the IVs, equipment, monitors, and the hard hospital chairs. When I left him each day, I was leaving a part of myself, and I felt as though I would not be whole until he was home with me.

Looking back, I so appreciated that the staff was optimistic when informing me of things, but not overly so. Unmet expectations can be devastating! There is not a moment that I am not thankful for my son and his health and not a night that I don't sleep better after I have checked on him sleeping in bed.

Kerry

Learning Opportunity: Give specific examples of what the nurse could do to support this mother and help decrease her fears and anxieties.

■ Figure 20-6 Encouraging sibling interaction with the preterm newborn.

Explain what is happening to the newborn in the NICU and periodically report on his or her condition (by phone if the NICU is not in the same hospital) to reassure the family that the child is receiving excellent care and to keep them informed. Listen to the family and encourage them to express their feelings and support one another. As soon as possible, the family should see, touch, and help care for the newborn. Most NICUs do not restrict visiting hours for parents or support persons, and they encourage families to visit often, whenever it is convenient for them. Many hospitals offer 24-hour phone privileges to families so that they are never out of touch with their newborn's caregivers.

Improving Parenting Skills and Family Functioning

Ideally, before the woman goes home from the hospital, she is able to visit the preterm newborn and to begin participating in the infant's care. The parents need to feel that the newborn belongs to them, not to the hospital. To help foster this feeling and strengthen the attachment, encourage activities that help them take on the parenting role. Pumping her milk to feed the newborn is an excellent way to promote assumption of the maternal role. Encouraging the father to provide kangaroo care is one way to help him feel like he is being a father.

Siblings should be included in the visits to see the preterm newborn (Fig. 20-6). The monitors, warmers, ventilators, and other equipment may be frightening to

siblings and family caregivers. Make the family feel welcome and comfortable when they visit. A primary nurse assigned to care for the infant gives the family a constant person to contact, increasing their feelings of confidence in the care the newborn is receiving.

Support groups for families who have experienced the crisis of a preterm newborn are of great value. Members of these support groups can visit the families in the hospital and at home, helping the parents and other family members to deal with their feelings and solve the problems that may arise when the infant is ready to come home or if the infant does not survive.

As the time for discharge of the infant nears, the family is understandably apprehensive. The NICU nurses must teach the parents and support persons the skills they need to care for the infant. This knowledge gives them confidence that they can take care of the infant. Some hospitals allow caregivers to stay overnight before the infant's discharge so that they can participate in around-the-clock care. The knowledge that they can telephone the physician and nurse at any time after discharge to have questions answered is reassuring.

In addition to feeding, bathing, and general care of the infant, many families of premature newborns need to learn infant cardiopulmonary resuscitation and the use of an apnea monitor, before the infant is discharged. Some preterm infants go home with oxygen, gastrostomy feeding tubes, and many other kinds of sophisticated equipment. This helps place the infant in the home much earlier, but it requires intensive training and support of the family members who care for the infant. Support from a home health nurse may be required in this situation.

After the baby goes home, a nurse, usually a community health nurse, visits the family to check on the health of the mother and the baby. The nurse provides additional support and teaching about the infant's care, if necessary, and answers any questions the family might have.

Evaluation: Goals and Expected Outcomes

Evaluation of the preterm newborn is an ongoing process that demands continual readjustment of the nursing diagnoses, planning, and implementation. Goals and expected outcomes include:

Goal: The preterm newborn's respiratory function will improve.

Expected Outcomes: The newborn

- maintains a respiratory rate less than 60 breaths per minute with symmetrical chest expansion.
- does not grunt or retract with breathing.
- has clear breath sounds.
- maintains oxygen saturation levels between 85% and 94%.
- remains free of episodes of apnea.

Goal: The preterm newborn's temperature will remain stable.

Expected Outcome: The newborn maintains temperature between 97.7°F and 99.5°F (36.5°C and 37.5°C).

Goal: The infant remains free of infection.

Expected Outcomes: The newborn

- maintains vital signs within normal limits.
- has clear breath sounds.
- maintains intact skin.

Goal: The preterm newborn's nutritional status will remain adequate.

Expected Outcomes: The infant

- ingests increased amounts of oral nutrition.
- gains weight daily.
- maintains adequate skin turgor.

Goal: The preterm newborn will remain free of skin breakdown.

Expected Outcome: The newborn's skin remains intact and free of redness, rashes, and irritation.

Goal: The preterm newborn will show improved tolerance to activity.

Expected Outcomes: The newborn

- has stable vital signs.
- maintains pink skin color during activity.
- requires supplemental oxygen in decreasing amounts until oxygen is no longer necessary.

Goal: The preterm newborn will demonstrate appropriate development.

Expected Outcome: The newborn

- responds appropriately to stimuli.
- achieves developmental milestones.
- increasingly interacts with the environment and caregivers.
- demonstrates appropriate behavior states with integrated responses.

Goal: The parents will demonstrate a reduction in anxiety level.

Expected Outcomes: Parents and family caregivers

- express feelings and anxieties concerning the newborn's condition.
- visit and establish a relationship with the newborn.
- demonstrate interaction with the newborn, holding and helping to provide care.

Goal: Parents will demonstrate appropriate parenting skills.

Expected Outcomes: Parents and family caregivers

- learn how to care for the newborn in the hospital and at home.
- hold, cuddle, talk to, and feed the preterm newborn.
- demonstrate knowledge of appropriate infant care.

Goal: The family will adapt to the crisis and begins functioning at an appropriate level.

Expected Outcomes: The family

- has an adequate support system and uses it.
- contacts a support group for families of high-risk infants.

THE POSTTERM NEWBORN

When pregnancy lasts longer than 42 weeks, the infant is postterm (postmature), regardless of birth weight.

Contributing Factors

About 12% of all infants are postterm. The causes of delayed birth are unknown. However, some predisposing factors include first pregnancies between the ages of 15 and 19 years, the woman older than 35 years with multiple pregnancies, and certain fetal anomalies.

Characteristics of the Postterm Newborn

Some postterm newborns have an appearance similar to term infants, but others look like infants 1 to 3 weeks old. He or she has a wide-eyed, hyper-alert expression. Little lanugo or vernix remains, scalp hair is abundant, and fingernails are long. The skin is dry, cracked, wrinkled, peeling, and whiter than that of the normal newborn. The infant has little subcutaneous fat and appears long and thin.

These infants are at risk for intrauterine hypoxia during labor and delivery due to failing placental function. Thus, it is customary for the physician or nurse–midwife to induce labor or perform a cesarean delivery before the baby is markedly overdue. Many physicians do not allow a pregnancy to continue beyond the end of 42 weeks' gestation.

Potential Complications

In the last weeks of gestation, the infant relies on glycogen for nutrition. This depletes the liver glycogen stores and may lead to neonatal hypoglycemia. Polycythemia may develop in response to intrauterine hypoxia. Polycythemia puts the infant at risk for cerebral ischemia, hypoglycemia, thrombus formation, and respiratory distress because of hyperviscosity of the blood. Often, the postterm infant expels meconium in utero. At birth, he or she may aspirate meconium into the lungs, obstructing the respiratory passages and irritating the lungs, resulting in meconium aspiration syndrome (see later discussion).

Treatment

Prevention of postterm birth is the mainstay of treatment in modern obstetrical practice. Early ultrasounds are done routinely because these establish the most accurate dating of the pregnancy. Later in the pregnancy (after 42 weeks), ultrasound is used to evaluate fetal development, weight, the amount of amniotic fluid, and the placenta for signs of aging. This information allows the physician to make an informed decision regarding the safest form and timing of delivery.

Nursing Care

Typically, postterm newborns are ravenous eaters at birth. If the newborn is free from respiratory distress, offer feedings at 1 or 2 hours of age, and remain observant for potential aspiration and possible asphyxia. Monitor serial blood glucose levels. The newborn may require intravenous glucose infusions to stabilize the glucose level.

Provide a thermoneutral environment to promote thermoregulation. A radiant heat warmer or isolette may be helpful. Use measures to minimize heat loss, such as reducing drafts and drying the skin thoroughly after bathing.

Draw venous and arterial hematocrit levels, as ordered, to evaluate for polycythemia. If polycythemia is present, a partial exchange transfusion may be done to prevent or treat hyperviscosity.

Anticipate that the stressed postterm newborn will not tolerate the labor and delivery process well. Observe and monitor the newborn's cardiopulmonary status closely. Administer supplemental oxygen therapy, as ordered for respiratory distress.

Postterm newborns can appear very different from what parents expect. Help facilitate a positive parent–newborn bond by explaining the newborn's condition and reasons for treatments and procedures. Point out positive features. Encourage them to express their feelings and to participate in their newborn's care, if possible, to alleviate their stresses and fears about the newborn's condition.

Test Yourself

✔ Name three alternatives to breast- or bottle-feeding for a preterm newborn who cannot tolerate oral feedings.

✔ List three ways you can encourage the parents to take on the parental role.

✔ Name three potential complications associated with the postterm newborn.

ACQUIRED DISORDERS
RESPIRATORY DISORDERS

A newborn is at risk for developing respiratory disorders after birth as the newborn adapts to the extrauterine environment. The risk for these disorders increases when the newborn experiences a gestational age variation.

Transient Tachypnea of the Newborn

Transient tachypnea of the newborn (TTN) involves the development of mild respiratory distress. It typically occurs within a few hours after birth, with the greatest degree of distress occurring at approximately 36 hours of life. TTN commonly disappears spontaneously around the third day.

TTN results from a delay in absorption of fetal lung fluid after birth. In utero the lungs are filled with fluid. As the fetus passes through the birth canal during delivery, some of the fluid squeezes out as the thoracic area is compressed. After birth, the newborn breathes and fills the lungs with air, thus expelling additional lung fluid. The newborn typically absorbs any remaining fluid into the bloodstream or expels it by coughing. However, this process is incomplete for newborns that develop TTN.

Contributing Factors

TTN commonly occurs in newborns born by cesarean delivery. The newborn does not experience the compression of the thoracic cavity that occurs with passage through the birth canal, so he or she retains some fluid in the lungs. Other contributing factors include prematurity, SGA, maternal diabetes, and maternal smoking during pregnancy.

Clinical Manifestations and Diagnosis

A newborn who develops TTN typically exhibits mild respiratory distress, with a respiratory rate greater than 60 breaths per minute. Mild retractions, nasal flaring, and some expiratory grunting may be noted. However, cyanosis usually does not occur. Often the newborn has difficulty feeding because he or she is breathing at such a rapid rate and is, therefore, unable to suck and breathe at the same time.

Arterial blood gases may reveal hypoxemia and decreased carbon dioxide levels. A chest x-ray usually indicates some fluid in the central portion of the lungs with adequate aeration.

Treatment

Treatment depends on the newborn's gestational age, overall status, history, and extent of respiratory distress. Unless an infection is suspected, medication therapy is not typically required. IV fluids and gavage-feedings may meet the newborn's fluid and nutritional requirements until the condition resolves. Supplemental oxygen often is ordered.

Nursing Care

Care for the newborn with TTN is supportive. Monitor the newborn's vital signs and oxygen saturation levels closely. Remain alert for changes that would indicate that the newborn is becoming fatigued from the rapid breathing. Administer IV fluids and supplemental oxygen as ordered. Assist the parents to understand what their newborn is experiencing. Help allay any fears or anxieties that they may have by explaining that the condition typically resolves without long-term consequences.

Meconium Aspiration Syndrome

Meconium aspiration syndrome (MAS) refers to a condition in which the fetus or newborn develops respiratory distress after inhaling meconium mixed with amniotic fluid. Meconium is a thick, pasty, greenish black substance that is present in the fetal bowel as early as 10 weeks' gestation. Meconium staining of amniotic fluid usually occurs as a reflex response that allows the rectal sphincter to relax. Subsequently, the fetus expels meconium into the amniotic fluid. The fetus may aspirate meconium while in utero or with his or her first breath after birth. The meconium can block the airway partially or completely and can irritate the newborn's airway, causing respiratory distress.

Contributing Factors

Typically, MAS is associated with fetal distress during labor. The fetus may experience hypoxia, causing peristalsis to increase and the anal sphincter to relax. The fetus then gasps or inhales the meconium-stained amniotic fluid. Other factors that contribute to the development of MAS include a maternal history of diabetes or hypertension, difficult delivery, advanced gestational age, and poor intrauterine growth.

Clinical Manifestations and Diagnosis

MAS is suspected whenever amniotic fluid is stained green to greenish black. Other manifestations include:

- Difficulty initiating respirations after birth
- Low Apgar score
- Tachypnea or apnea
- Retractions
- Hypothermia
- Hypoglycemia
- Cyanosis

The physician suspects the diagnosis when the newborn develops respiratory distress after a delivery in which the amniotic fluid is meconium-stained. Typically, a chest x-ray confirms the diagnosis.

Treatment

If the amniotic fluid is meconium-stained, a pediatrician, neonatologist, or caregiver with expertise intubating newborns attends the delivery. If the newborn does not breathe immediately after birth, the attendant intubates the newborn and attempts to suction below the vocal cords. The hope is that any meconium present below the cords will be suctioned out before the newborn takes his first breath. If the newborn breathes immediately, intubation is not done. After delivery, gastric lavage may be performed to remove any meconium swallowed and to prevent aspiration of vomitus.

The physician may order tracheal and bronchial suctioning to remove meconium plugs from the respiratory tract. Oxygen therapy and assisted ventilation may be necessary to support the newborn's respiratory status. In some cases, extracorporeal membrane oxygenation supports the newborn's oxygen requirements. Prophylactic antibiotics may prevent development of pneumonia. The physician may order chest physiotherapy with clapping and vibration to help remove any remaining meconium from the lungs.

Nursing Care

Newborns with MAS are extremely ill and require care in the NICU. Nursing care focuses on observing the neonate's respiratory status closely and ensuring adequate oxygenation. Measures to maintain thermoregulation are key factors to reducing the body's metabolic demands for oxygen. Be prepared to administer respiratory support and medication therapy, as ordered.

Sudden Infant Death Syndrome

Sudden infant death syndrome (SIDS) has caused much grief and anxiety among families for centuries. One of the leading causes of infant mortality worldwide, SIDS claims an estimated 2,500 lives annually in the United States alone. Although there has been a dramatic drop in the incidence of deaths during the past 20 years, SIDS is still the leading cause of death in infants between 7 and 365 days of age (Carroll & Laughlin, 2006).

Commonly called "crib death," SIDS is the sudden and unexpected death of an apparently healthy infant in whom the postmortem examination fails to reveal an adequate cause. The term SIDS is not a diagnosis but rather a description of the syndrome. Varying theories have been suggested about the cause of SIDS. Despite much research over the years, no single cause has been identified.

Contributing Factors

Infants who die of SIDS are usually 2 to 4 months old, although some deaths have occurred during the first and second week of life. Few infants older than 6 months of age die of SIDS. It is a greater threat to LBW infants than to term infants. It occurs more often in winter and affects more male infants than female infants, as well as more infants from minority and lower socioeconomic groups. Infants born to mothers younger than 20 years of age, infants who are not first born, and infants whose mothers smoked during pregnancy are also at greater risk. Research has revealed that a greater number of

■ Figure 20-7 An apnea monitor for home monitoring.

infants with SIDS have been sleeping in a prone (face down) position than in a supine (lying on the back with the face up) position. Because of these studies, the American Academy of Pediatrics recommends avoiding the prone position for sleep until the infant is 6 months old.

Clinical Manifestations

SIDS is rapid and silent and occurs at any time of the day. There is no evidence of a struggle. People who have been nearby claim that they heard no unusual sounds before the death was discovered. The infant frequently is to all appearances in excellent health before the death. The autopsy often reveals a mild respiratory disorder but nothing considered serious enough to have caused the death.

A closely related syndrome is an apparent life-threatening event. The infant is found in distress but responds immediately to stimulation. This infant recovers with no lasting problems. The physician orders a home apnea monitor for this infant (Fig. 20-7). The apnea monitor is set to sound an alarm if the infant does not take a breath within a given number of seconds. Family caregivers learn infant cardiopulmonary resuscitation so that they can respond quickly if the alarm sounds. Infants who have had an episode of an apparent life-threatening event are at risk for additional episodes and may be at risk for SIDS. The infant stays on home apnea monitoring until he or she is 1 year old.

Nursing Care

The effects of SIDS on caregivers and families are devastating. Grief coupled with guilt is a frequent response. Disbelief, hostility, and anger are common reactions. Even though the family caregivers are told that they are not to blame, it is difficult for most not to keep search-

ing for evidence of some possible neglect on their part. Prolonged depression usually follows the initial shock and anguish over the infant's death.

The immediate response of the emergency department staff should be to allow the family to express their grief, encouraging them to say good-bye to their infant and providing a quiet, private place for them to do so. Compassionate care of the family caregivers includes helping to find someone to accompany them home or to meet them there. Immediately refer the family to the local chapter of the National SIDS Foundation. Sudden Infant Death Alliance is another resource for help. In some states, specially trained community health nurses who are knowledgeable about SIDS are available. These nurses are prepared to help families and can provide written materials, as well as information, guidance, and support in the family's home. They maintain contact with the family as long as necessary and provide support in a subsequent pregnancy.

Caregivers are particularly concerned about subsequent infants. Recent studies have indicated that the risk for these infants is no greater than that for the general population. Many care providers, however, continue to recommend monitoring these infants for the first few months of life to help reduce the family's stress. Monitoring continues until the new infant is past the age of the SIDS infant's death.

HEMOLYTIC DISEASE OF THE NEWBORN

Hemolytic disease of the newborn, also known as *erythroblastosis fetalis*, is a condition in which the infant's RBCs are broken down (hemolyzed) and destroyed, producing severe anemia and hyperbilirubinemia. In severe cases, heart failure, brain damage, and death can result.

Causes

There are two main causes of hemolytic disease of the newborn. Before the mid-1960s, hemolytic disease was largely the result of Rh incompatibility. The introduction of immune globulin, or RhoGAM, in the mid-1960s has markedly reduced the incidence of this disorder (see Chapter 17 for administration criteria). Today, hemolytic disease is principally the result of ABO incompatibility, which is generally much less severe than the Rh-induced disorder.

Rh Incompatibility

Rh factor is a protein substance (antigen) found on the surface of RBCs of individuals who are Rho(D) positive. Individuals whose blood cells do not carry the Rh antigen are Rho(D) negative. If an individual who is Rho(D) negative encounters Rho(D)-positive blood, that individual's immune system views the Rh factor as foreign and produces anti-D antibodies that attack and destroy the antigen. This becomes a problem for the Rho(D)-positive fetus whose mother has developed the anti-D antibodies. The antibodies easily cross the placenta, enter the fetal circulation, and attack the fetus' RBCs. The result is hemolysis (destruction) of the fetal RBCs, which leads to severe fetal anemia. The Rho(D)-positive fetus is vulnerable to hemolytic disease only if his mother is Rho(D) negative and has been sensitized to Rho(D)-positive blood (i.e., she has anti-D antibodies).

> **Think about this.**
>
> If the fetus is Rho(D) negative, his RBCs do not carry the antigen. Therefore, even if his or her mother is sensitized, the fetus will not experience hemolysis because the anti-D antibodies do not have anything to attack.

The first-born child does not usually develop hemolytic disease for two reasons. First, in response to the initial exposure to the Rho(D) antigen, the woman's body produces a large antibody that does not cross the placenta. Subsequent exposures induce production of the small anti-D antibody that crosses the placenta. Second, most sensitization occurs at birth when fetal blood cells escape into the woman's blood stream as the placenta separates from the uterine wall. This puts subsequent pregnancies at risk.

With the next pregnancy, the small maternal antibodies enter the fetal circulation and begin to hemolyze (destroy) the fetus' RBCs. The fetus makes a valiant attempt to replace the destroyed RBCs by releasing large amounts of immature RBCs (erythroblasts) into the bloodstream (thus the name erythroblastosis fetalis). As the rapid destruction of the fetus' RBCs continues, anemia develops. If the anemia is severe enough, the fetus develops heart failure and hydrops fetalis (extensive fetal edema), which can lead to fetal death.

Rapid destruction of the fetus' RBCs releases bilirubin, which is not usually a problem in utero because the woman's body processes and excretes the excess bilirubin (Salem & Singer, 2008). After birth, the newborn's immature liver cannot handle the high levels of bilirubin and he or she develops pathologic jaundice. This condition can lead to **kernicterus**, a disorder in which excess bilirubin stains neurons in the brain and spinal cord leading to irreversible injury or death.

ABO Incompatibility

The major blood groups are A, B, AB, and O, and each has antigens that may be incompatible with those of another group. The most common incompatibility in the newborn occurs between a woman with type O blood and an infant with type A or B blood. The reactions are usually less severe than in Rh incompatibility.

Diagnosis

When titers show the presence of anti-D antibodies, the provider monitors fetal well-being. Because direct sampling of fetal blood increases the risk of fetal loss, the provider usually uses indirect means to measure disease severity.

Traditionally, amniocentesis established the diagnosis (see Chapter 7 for discussion of amniocentesis). Analysis of a sample of amniotic fluid shows the amount of bile pigments (bilirubin) present. Thus, it can be determined if the fetus is mildly, moderately, or severely affected. Now, Doppler velocimetry is the diagnostic method of choice. It has the advantage of being noninvasive and yields more sensitive data about the fetal condition.

After birth, the following tests help determine presence of disease and severity:

- Direct Coombs' test detects the presence of maternal antibodies
- Rh and ABO typing help identify the cause
- Hemoglobin levels and RBC counts determine severity of anemia
- Plasma bilirubin levels help determine disease severity

A positive direct Coombs' test indicates that maternal anti-D antibodies are present on the surface of the infant's RBCs. Conversely, a negative direct Coombs' test indicates that there are no antibodies on the infant's RBCs.

Clinical Manifestations

The initial exam for infants with known incompatibility (either Rh or ABO) includes evaluation for pallor, edema, jaundice, and an enlarged spleen and liver. If prenatal care was inadequate or absent, a severely affected infant may be stillborn or have hydrops fetalis, a condition marked by extensive edema, marked anemia and jaundice, and enlargement of the liver and spleen. If untreated, infants with hydrops are at risk for severe brain damage from kernicterus. Death occurs in about 75% of infants with kernicterus; those who survive may be mentally retarded or develop spastic paralysis or nerve deafness.

Treatment

Because ABO incompatibilities are typically milder than are Rh incompatibilities, treatment during pregnancy is not required. For the severely affected fetus with an Rh incompatibility, the provider (usually an obstetrician or maternal–fetal medicine specialist) may perform an intrauterine transfusion of Rho(D)-negative blood. If the fetus is beyond 32 weeks' gestation, delivery by labor induction or cesarean is the best treatment option.

After delivery, a positive Coombs' test indicates the presence of the disease but not the degree of severity. If bilirubin and hemoglobin levels are within normal limits, the provider orders close observation and frequent laboratory tests. A newborn that has mild-to-moderate disease usually receives hydration and phototherapy after birth. Phototherapy involves the use of special lights to help reduce bilirubin levels. The lights work by converting fat-soluble unconjugated bilirubin, which the

■ **Figure 20-8** A newborn receiving phototherapy.

serum bilirubin levels routinely when the infant is receiving phototherapy.

Phototherapy may also be administered using a fiberoptic blanket consisting of a pad attached to a halogen light source with illuminating plastic fibers. A disposable protective cover protects the blanket that wraps about the infant to disperse therapeutic light. These blankets are appropriate for home use, which can cut hospitalization costs and reduce the family separation time. The neonate's eyes do not require protection when the fiberoptic blanket is used. The blanket can stay on all the time without interfering with newborn care.

Infants whose bilirubin levels return to normal may leave the hospital for routine home care. Remain sensitive to the parents' feelings of guilt and anxiety. Give them the opportunity to ventilate their feelings.

Here's what you can do!

Turn off the phototherapy lights whenever you draw a blood sample to measure bilirubin levels. If you leave the lights on, the sample may read falsely low.

body cannot expel, to water-soluble conjugated bilirubin that the body excretes via the gastrointestinal and renal routes. A severely affected newborn requires care in a NICU and usually receives an exchange transfusion immediately after birth.

Nursing Care

Nursing care for the newborn with risk factors for hemolytic disease involves initial and ongoing assessment for jaundice. Always report jaundice to the RN. Jaundice found within the first 24 hours after birth is always pathologic. Report this finding immediately.

For the newborn receiving phototherapy, place the lights above and outside the isolette at the appropriate height (Fig. 20-8). If the lights are too far away from the newborn, the therapy will not work. If they are too close, the newborn may receive burns. The infant is nude (except for possibly a diaper under the perineal area to collect urine and feces) to maximize the skin surface area exposed to the light. Turn the newborn every 3 to 4 hours to rotate the area of exposure. Do not turn off the lights except to feed and to change the diaper.

Always shield the newborn's eyes from the ultraviolet light. Carefully apply eye patches to avoid eye irritation. If the eye patch is too loose, it can slip down and obstruct the nares or lead to retinal damage from the light. Remove the patches every 4 hours to cleanse the eyes and examine for irritation, inflammation, and/or dryness. Clean and change the patches daily.

The light may cause the infant to have skin rashes; "sunburn" or tanning; loose, greenish stools; hyperthermia; an increased metabolic rate; increased evaporative water loss; and priapism (a prolonged erection of the penis). Infants undergoing phototherapy need as much as 25% more fluids to prevent dehydration. Monitor the

NEWBORN OF A DIABETIC MOTHER

Maternal diabetes places the fetus and newborn at risk for serious complications. Perinatal outcome has a direct relationship with the severity and control of the mother's diabetes (see Chapter 16). The diabetic woman who closely controls her blood glucose level before conception and throughout pregnancy, particularly in the early months, decreases her risk of having an infant with congenital anomalies. Fetal death is less likely with excellent control.

Clinical Manifestations

Infants of mothers with poorly controlled type 2 or gestational diabetes have a distinctive appearance. They are LGA, plump and full-faced with bulky shoulders, and coated with vernix caseosa. Both the placenta and the umbilical cord are oversized. In contrast, infants of mothers with poorly controlled, long-term, or severe type 1 diabetes actually may suffer from IUGR.

Consistently elevated fetal insulin levels cause the distinctive growth pattern. Because maternal glucose levels are elevated and glucose readily crosses the placenta, the fetus responds by increasing insulin production. Because insulin acts as a fetal growth hormone, consistently high levels cause fetal *macrosomia*, birth weight of greater than 4,500 g (9 lb, 14 oz). Insulin also causes disproportionate fat buildup to the shoulders and upper body, increasing the risk for shoulder dystocia and birth trauma.

Newborns of diabetic mothers are at risk for hypoglycemia in the first few hours after birth. In utero, the fetal pancreas adapts to the high blood glucose levels by producing and secreting more insulin. After birth, the glucose source is abruptly cut off when the umbilical cord is cut. The newborn's pancreas cannot readjust quickly enough, so it continues to produce insulin, leading to neonatal hypoglycemia. This condition may cause permanent brain damage or death unless care providers detect it quickly and treat the newborn with oral or IV glucose. See Chapter 13 for in-depth discussion of neonatal hypoglycemia.

High insulin levels can also delay fetal lung maturity; therefore, newborns of diabetic mothers have a higher incidence of respiratory distress syndrome and other respiratory difficulties. These infants are subject to many other hazards, including congenital anomalies, preterm delivery, difficult cardiopulmonary transition at birth, and enlarged heart. Other issues include hypocalcemia, hypomagnesemia, polycythemia with hyperviscosity, and hyperbilirubinemia. This infant is at increased risk for developing early onset diabetes in adolescence or early adulthood.

Nursing Care

Newborns of diabetic mothers require especially careful observation. Perform early (as soon as possible after birth) and frequent blood glucose checks. Administer early feedings or if the newborn has respiratory distress or is otherwise ill give IV glucose, as ordered. Hypoglycemia can return after treatment, so watch for signs and symptoms. Watch for signs of respiratory distress. Anticipate supplemental oxygen and surfactant therapy. Some infants need ventilator support. Monitor electrolyte levels, especially magnesium and calcium, as ordered. Assist the RN to perform a gestational age assessment, as these infants can be deceptively large and still be preterm. Watch for and report any heart murmurs or other signs of cardiac dysfunction. Check carefully for signs of birth trauma.

Test Yourself

✔ What respiratory disorder is associated with a delay in the absorption of fetal lung fluid after birth?

✔ List three signs that may indicate the infant is suffering from meconium aspiration.

✔ What medication has dramatically reduced the incidence of hemolytic disease of the newborn?

NEWBORN OF A MOTHER WITH SUBSTANCE ABUSE

Alcohol and illicit drug use by the mother during pregnancy can lead to many problems in the newborn. The newborn of a woman who uses alcohol is at risk for fetal alcohol syndrome (FAS). The newborn of a chemically dependent woman may be SGA and/or experience withdrawal symptoms.

Unfortunately, identifying the pregnant woman who abuses alcohol or drugs is often difficult. Many of these women have no prenatal care or only infrequent care. They may not keep appointments because of apathy or simply because they are not awake during the day. As a result, many of these infants suffer prenatal insults that result in intrauterine growth retardation, congenital abnormalities, and premature birth.

Fetal Alcohol Syndrome

Alcohol is one of the many teratogenic substances that readily cross the placenta to the fetus. Many newborns exposed to alcohol in utero exhibit withdrawal symptoms during the first few hours after delivery. FAS is often apparent in newborns of mothers with chronic alcoholism and sometimes appears in newborns whose mothers are low to moderate consumers of alcohol. Binge drinking appears to be more harmful to the developing fetus than does drinking small amounts every day. Because we do not know exactly how much alcohol is safe, the woman should stop drinking at least 3 months before she plans to become pregnant.

Clinical Manifestations

The newborn that is withdrawing from alcohol typically is hyperactive, irritable, has trouble sleeping, and may have tremors or seizures. Characteristics of FAS include LBW, small height and head circumference, short palpebral fissures (eyelid folds), reduced ocular growth, and a flattened nasal bridge. This newborn is prone to respiratory difficulties, hypoglycemia, hypocalcemia, and hyperbilirubinemia. Growth during infancy and childhood continues to fall below average growth rates. Unfortunately, the brain damage that occurs during fetal development is permanent, resulting in mental retardation.

Nursing Care

FAS is highly preventable. Societal interventions, of which nurses can be a part, include increasing the public's awareness of the detrimental effects of alcohol use during pregnancy. Other helpful interventions include screening women of reproductive age for alcohol problems and encouraging women to obtain adequate prenatal care and use appropriate resources for decreasing alcohol use.

Nursing care for the newborn that is withdrawing from alcohol includes the supportive interventions of swaddling, decreasing sensory stimulation, and ensuring adequate nutrition. Keep the newborn's environment quiet and dark during the first few days of withdrawal. Administer benzodiazepine or other anticonvulsants, as ordered, to prevent or treat seizure activity. Adequate nutrition is key to supporting weight gain. The newborn's sucking reflex may be weak, and he or she may be too irritable to feed. Give small amounts of formula or breast milk frequently. Monitor the newborn's daily weight, intake, and output. Encourage the parents to feed the newborn. This measure also helps to promote bonding.

Neonatal Substance Withdrawal

The newborn of the woman addicted to cocaine, heroin, methadone, or other drugs is born dependent upon these substances. Newborns may also be born dependent on a certain class of antidepressants, serotonin reuptake inhibitors. Many of these infants suffer withdrawal symptoms during the early neonatal period. However, the time of onset varies widely. For example, the newborn experiencing withdrawal from opioids typically experiences withdrawal symptoms within 24 to 48 hours after birth. However, it may take up to 2 weeks before the newborn exhibits any symptoms.

Clinical Manifestations

Withdrawal symptoms commonly include tremors, restlessness, hyperactivity, disorganized or hyperactive reflexes, increased muscle tone, sneezing, tachypnea, vomiting, diarrhea, disturbed sleep patterns, and a shrill high-pitched cry (Fig. 20-9). Ineffective sucking and

Irritability
Disturbed sleep patterns
Frequent sneezing
Shrill, high-pitched cry
Vomiting
Constant movement
Tremors
Tachypnea
Diarrhea
Hyperreflexia, clonus

■ **Figure 20-9** Manifestations of a newborn with substance withdrawal.

swallowing reflexes create feeding problems, and regurgitation and vomiting occur often after feeding.

Nursing Care

Care of the newborn experiencing substance withdrawal focuses on providing physical and emotional support. Medications such as chlorpromazine, clonidine, diazepam, methadone, morphine, paregoric, or phenobarbital may ease the withdrawal and prevent complications, such as seizures.

Because of neuromuscular irritability, many of these newborns respond favorably to gentle rocking movements while in close bodily contact with their caregivers. Therefore, some nurseries place the newborns in special carriers that hold them close to the nurse's chest while the nurse moves about the nursery. Swaddling the infant (wrapping securely in a small blanket) with arms across the chest also is a method of quieting the agitated newborn. Keep the newborn's environment dimly lit to minimize stimulation. Maintain the airway and monitor respiratory status closely. Provide small frequent feedings. Keep the newborn's head elevated to promote effective sucking and reduce the risk of aspiration. Vomiting and diarrhea may lead to fluid and electrolyte imbalances. Monitor intake and output closely and give supplemental fluids as ordered. Use a nonjudgmental approach when interacting with the newborn and his or her mother.

NEWBORN WITH A CONGENITALLY ACQUIRED INFECTION

All newborns are at increased risk for infections because their immune systems are immature and they cannot localize infection. At-risk newborns are even more susceptible than are normal newborns. The newborn may acquire an infection prenatally from the mother (through the placenta), during the intrapartum period (during labor and delivery) from maternal vaginal infection or inhalation of contaminated amniotic fluid and after birth from cross-contamination with other infants, health care personnel, or contaminated equipment.

A variety of organisms can cause newborn infection. Table 20-2 summarizes several prominent neonatal infections. (See Chapter 16 for a detailed discussion of congenitally acquired infections.) The newborn that develops an infection often does not have any specific signs of illness. The clue that alerts you to a possible problem may be signs such as cyanosis, pallor, thermal instability (difficulty keeping temperature within normal range), convulsions, lethargy, apnea, jaundice, or just "not looking right." Blood, urine, cerebrospinal fluid cultures, and other laboratory and radiographic tests necessary to isolate the specific organism confirm the diagnosis. Treatment consists of intensive antibiotic therapy, IV fluids, respiratory therapy, and other supportive measures.

Table 20-2 ■ NEONATAL INFECTIONS

Infectious Agent	Mode of Transmission to Fetus or Neonate	Onset	Clinical Manifestations/ Complications	Prevention/ Treatment	Notes
Chlamydia trachomatis (chlamydia) or *Neisseria gonorrhoeae* (gonorrhea)	Birth canal during a vaginal birth	Variable	Ophthalmia neonatorum, a serious form of conjunctivitis that can lead to blindness	Prevention: Routine ophthalmic administration of erythromycin ointment after birth	
Group B streptococcus (GBS)	In utero or via the birth canal during vaginal delivery	Early onset is within the first 24 hours of life. Late onset is up to 7 days of life	Septicemia (blood infection) and meningitis	Prevention: Antibiotics to GBS positive women during labor	The woman does not have an infection; GBS colonizes the vagina and gastrointestinal tracts of healthy women. GBS is the most common cause of neonatal sepsis; however, neonatal GBS infection is a rare event.
Hepatitis B virus	Contact with infected blood during birth	Variable	Most infants with hepatitis B become chronic carriers, which puts them at risk for cirrhosis and liver cancer	Prevention: Newborns of mothers with hepatitis B receive hepatitis B immune globulin within 12 hours of birth. All newborns receive the first in a series of hepatitis B vaccines before discharge from the hospital	Incidence has decreased dramatically since newborns began receiving the vaccine.
Herpes simplex virus type 1 or 2	Contact with vaginal secretions during birth (mother with active lesions is the most common mode) or in utero infection when virus crosses the placenta to the fetus.	At about 1 week of age	Initial signs and symptoms are nonspecific, such as irritability, lethargy, fever, or failure to feed. Later manifestations: Skin, eye, or mouth disease; central nervous system disease with encephalitis; or disseminated disease with multiple major organ involvement	Prevention: Suppressive therapy for the mother with acyclovir beginning at 36 weeks' gestation; Cesarean delivery for women with active lesions at term.	Neonatal herpes infection is rare
Human immunodeficiency virus (HIV)	In utero across the placenta; contact with infected blood in the birth canal; and breast-feeding	Commonly between 4 months and 1 year of age.	Bacterial infections, such as pneumonia, meningitis, and bacteremia; thrush, mouth sores, and severe diaper rash	Prevention: Antiretroviral therapy during pregnancy to suppress maternal viral load; and sometimes antiretroviral therapy to the newborn during the first 6 weeks of life	Very poor prognosis for infants who develop symptoms before 1 year of age.

(continued)

Table 20-2 ▌ NEONATAL INFECTIONS *(continued)*

Infectious Agent	Mode of Transmission to Fetus or Neonate	Onset	Clinical Manifestations/ Complications	Prevention/ Treatment	Notes
Methicillin-resistant *S aureus* (MRSA)	In NICUs due to over-crowding, lack of adequate cleaning procedures, poorly trained staff, or cross-contamination from a parent or family member visiting an infant; can also be transmitted during breast-feeding	Variable	Symptoms range from pustules or eye discharge to septicemia, pneumonia, and infant death	Prevention: Screening at-risk pregnant women on admission to the hospital; careful adherence to infection control measures, such as hand washing and environmental cleanliness.	
Rubella virus	In utero across the placenta	In utero	Spontaneous abortion, stillbirth, preterm delivery, and congenital anomalies; hearing impairment is the single most common defect followed by eye disorders, heart defects, and neurologic abnormalities, including mental retardation	Prevention: Rubella vaccine. There is no cure; treatment is supportive.	
Treponema pallidum (*T. pallidum*) causes syphilis	In utero across the placenta	In utero, at birth, or months later	Intrauterine growth restriction, hydrops fetalis, fetal death, preterm birth, congenital infection, and neonatal death, blindness, deafness, or other deformities; Hutchinson's Triad and snuffles (bloody discharge) are characteristic symptoms.	Prevention: Treat maternal infection during pregnancy. Treatment: Penicillin for the infected newborn.	

Key Points

➤ Newborns are classified by size as SGA, AGA, and LGA. Based on weight, newborns may be classified as LBW, very low birth weight, or extremely low birth weight. Classifications by gestational age are preterm, postterm, or term.

➤ A gestational age assessment evaluates two major categories of maturity: neuromuscular maturity and physical maturity.

➤ IUGR is the most common underlying condition leading to SGA newborns. It occurs when the fetus does not receive adequate amounts of oxygen and nutrients necessary for the proper growth and development of organs and tissues.

➤ Neither the symmetrically growth-restricted newborn nor the asymmetrically growth-restricted newborn has grown at the expected rate for gestational age on standard growth charts. When plotted on a standard growth chart, the symmetrically growth-restricted newborn's weight, length, and head circumference fall below the 10th percentile; whereas, the asymmetrically growth-restricted newborn's falls below the 10th percentile on one or sometimes two of the measurements. For the asymmetrically growth-restricted infants the birth weight is most commonly affected.

➤ The underlying cause of a newborn being LGA is unknown. Contributing factors may include maternal diabetes; genetic factors, such as parent size and male sex of the newborn; congenital disorders; or the number of pregnancies the mother has had, with multiparous women having two to three times the number of LGA newborns.

➤ Preterm births may result from maternal lifestyle conditions related to health, diet, living conditions, overwork, low income, frequent pregnancies, and maternal age extremes. One of the most common factors is preterm premature rupture of membranes. Multiple births, the need for an earlier delivery to ensure maternal or fetal well-being, emotional or physical trauma to the woman, fetal infection, and fetal malformations are also often causes for preterm deliveries.

➤ Characteristics of the preterm newborn as compared to the term newborn include little muscle or subcutaneous fat; thin, translucent skin; visible veins on abdomen and scalp; plentiful lanugo; extremely pliable ears, due to minimal cartilage; undescended testes in the male and prominent labia minor and clitoris in the female; very few creases in the soles of the feet or palms of the hands; and weak or absent newborn reflexes.

➤ Common complications associated with preterm newborns include hypothermia, hypoglycemia, respiratory disorders, patent ductus arteriosus, intracranial hemorrhage, necrotizing enterocolitis, jaundice, infection, and ROP.

➤ Care of the preterm newborn focuses on improving respiratory function, maintaining body temperature, preventing infection, protecting neurologic status, maintaining fluid and electrolyte status, maintaining adequate nutrition, preserving skin integrity, conserving energy, and supporting growth and development. Goals for the family include reducing anxiety and improving parenting skills and family functioning.

➤ Potential complications seen in the postterm newborn are meconium aspiration; hypoglycemia;

and polycythemia, due to intrauterine hypoxia. Polycythemia puts the infant at risk for cerebral ischemia, hypoglycemia, thrombus formation, and respiratory distress because of hyperviscosity of the blood. These are focus areas for nursing care.

➤ Common acquired respiratory disorders of the newborn include TTN, MAS, and sudden SIDS. TTN occurs in the first few hours of life and is caused by retained lung fluid. MAS occurs when the newborn inhales meconium into the respiratory passages, often with the first breath; this leads to pneumonia. The incidence of SIDS has decreased since newborns have been put on their backs to sleep.

➤ Hemolytic disease of the newborn, a condition in which the infant's RBCs are broken down and destroyed, may be the result of Rh or ABO incompatibility. Hyperbilirubinemia occurs and may be treated by exchange transfusions or phototherapy.

➤ Newborns of diabetic mothers are at risk for hypoglycemia, delayed fetal lung maturity resulting in respiratory disorders, shoulder dystocia, and birth trauma. Characteristic appearance includes LGA, plump with bulky shoulders, and coated with vernix caseosa.

➤ The newborn of a mother who is chemically dependent on alcohol may develop FAS. The newborn is prone to respiratory difficulties, hypoglycemia, hypocalcemia, hyperbilirubinemia, slowed growth, and retarded mental development. Nursing care for the newborn with FAS is supportive and focuses on preventing complications, such as seizures.

➤ The newborn of a mother who is dependent on illicit drugs may experience withdrawal symptoms. These include tremors, restlessness, hyperactivity, disorganized or hyperactive reflexes, increased muscle tone, sneezing, tachypnea, vomiting, diarrhea, disturbed sleep patterns, and a shrill high-pitched cry. Ineffective sucking and swallowing reflexes create feeding problems. Nursing care for the newborn focuses on providing physical and emotional support.

➤ Group B beta-hemolytic streptococcus is the major cause of congenitally acquired infections in the newborn. Other causes include rubella virus, *Chlamydia trachomatis* or *Neisseria gonorrhoeae* (leading to ophthalmia neonatorum), hepatitis B, herpes virus types 1 and 2, *Treponema pallidum* (*T. pallidum*) that causes syphilis, and human immunodeficiency virus. A newer infection concern is methicillin-resistant *S. aureus*.

INTERNET RESOURCES

Human Milk Bank
www.hmbana.org

Prematurity
www.marchofdimes.com/prematurity

SIDS
www.sids.org
www.sidsfamilies.com

Workbook

▪ NCLEX-STYLE REVIEW QUESTIONS

1. The nurse is assisting in a newborn assessment of gestational age using the Newborn Maturity Rating and Classification (Ballard) scoring system. Of the following physical characteristics, which is associated with a newborn with the oldest gestational age?

   a. abundant lanugo, flat areola, and pinna flat.
   b. anterior transverse plantar crease, ear recoil, and few scrotal rugae.
   c. transparent skin, no lanugo, and prominent clitoris.
   d. bald areas, plantar creases cover sole, and 3- to 4-mm breast bud.

2. A newborn is considered large for gestational age (LGA) when the newborn is larger than the average baby is. Which of the following is most likely to be a contributing factor in a newborn that is LGA?

   a. The mother of the newborn has no other children.
   b. The mother of the newborn has gained little weight during pregnancy.
   c. The mother of the newborn has a diagnosis of diabetes.
   d. The mother of the newborn has a history of smoking during pregnancy.

3. The nurse is caring for a preterm newborn. When developing a plan of care for the preterm newborn, which of the following nursing interventions would be the most important to include?

   a. Repositioning at least every 2 hours
   b. Monitoring body temperature
   c. Promoting rest periods between procedures
   d. Recording urinary output

4. The nurse is caring for the newborn of a mother who abused cocaine during her pregnancy. Which of the following characteristics would the nurse likely see in this newborn?

   a. The newborn weighs above average when born.
   b. The newborn sleeps for long periods of time.
   c. The newborn cries when touched.
   d. The newborn has facial deformities.

5. The preterm newborn has specific characteristics that differ from those of the term newborn. Which of the following are preterm characteristics? Select all that apply.

   a. Extremities are thin, with little muscle or subcutaneous fat.
   b. Skin is thickened and without wrinkles.
   c. Head and abdomen are disproportionately large.
   d. Veins of the abdomen and scalp are visible.
   e. Lanugo is not evident on the back and shoulders.
   f. Ears have soft, minimal cartilage and are pliable.

▪ STUDY ACTIVITIES

1. Research your community to find sources of help for families who have lost children to sudden infant death syndrome (SIDS). What support groups and organizations are available that you might recommend to families who have lost a child because of SIDS? Discuss with your peers what you found and make a list of resources to share.

2. Go to the following Internet site: http:/www.kidshealth.org. Click on "Parents Site." Type "premature" in the search box. Click on "A Primer on Preemies."

   a. What are the two basic needs of a premature infant discussed on this site?
   b. What are the common health problems often seen in premature infants?
   c. What suggestions does this site offer to families of children who have a premature infant?

▪ CRITICAL THINKING: WHAT WOULD YOU DO?

1. The physician just told Andrea, the mother of Andrew, a newborn, that her son's bilirubin level is elevated and he is going to be given phototherapy. Andrea appears concerned and anxious and looks as if she is about to cry.

   a. What is the first thing you would do and say to Andrea?
   b. What would you explain to Andrea regarding the purpose of the phototherapy for Andrew?
   c. What will you teach this mother in regards to what she might expect while Andrew is under the light?

2. You are teaching a nutrition class to a group of pregnant women. One of the women says that she heard it was not a problem to drink a little alcohol while she was pregnant. Another member of the group says she has heard about something called fetal alcohol syndrome.

   a. What will you teach this group regarding the use of alcohol during pregnancy?
   b. What is fetal alcohol syndrome?
   c. What are the characteristics of infants with fetal alcohol syndrome?
   d. What are the possible long-term complications of fetal alcohol syndrome?

21 *The Newborn at Risk: Congenital Disorders*

KEY TERMS

atresia
atrial septal defect
bilateral
brachycephaly
chordee
coarctation of the aorta
congestive heart failure (CHF)
cyanotic heart disease
epispadias
galactosemia
hernia
hip dysplasia
hypospadias
hypothermia
imperforate anus
overriding aorta
phenylketonuria (PKU)
pulmonary stenosis
right ventricular hypertrophy
spina bifida
supernumerary
talipes equinovarus
tetralogy of Fallot
transposition of the great arteries
unilateral
ventricular septal defect
ventriculoatrial shunting
ventriculoperitoneal shunting

LEARNING OBJECTIVES

On completion of this chapter, you should be able to:

1. Differentiate the three types of spina bifida.
2. Discuss the two types of hydrocephalus, including the symptoms, treatment, and nursing care.
3. Describe five common types of congenital heart defects, tracing the blood flow in each defect and discussing the treatment and nursing care.
4. Differentiate between cleft lip and cleft palate, including treatment and nursing care.
5. Discuss esophageal atresia and tracheoesophageal fistula.
6. Explain what occurs when an infant has an imperforate anus.
7. List and describe the five types of hernias that newborns may have.
8. Describe hypospadias, epispadias, exstrophy of the bladder, and ambiguous genitalia.
9. Discuss congenital talipes equinovarus.
10. Explain congenital dislocation of the hip, including signs and symptoms, treatment, and nursing care.
11. Compare phenylketonuria, congenital hypothyroidism, galactosemia, and maple syrup urine disease.
12. Discuss Down syndrome including common characteristics, treatment, and nursing care.
13. Differentiate Turner and Klinefelter syndromes.

CHAPTER 20 discussed variations in size and gestational age as well as acquired disorders of the newborn. This chapter discusses congenital disorders, which are problems that occur during fetal development and are present in the infant at birth. Congenital disorders include malformations, or *congenital anomalies*, which can often be corrected during the first months or years of life. Other congenital disorders result from inborn errors of metabolism, which are hereditary disorders, or chromosomal abnormalities.

The birth of a newborn with a congenital defect (anomaly) is a crisis for parents and caregivers. Depending on the defect, immediate or early surgery may be necessary. Early, continuous, skilled observation and highly skilled nursing care are required. Rehabilitation of the newborn and education of the family caregivers in the newborn's care are essential. The emotional needs of the newborn and the family must be integrated into nursing care plans. Many of these newborns have a brighter future today as a result of increased diagnostic and medical knowledge and advances in surgical techniques.

Family caregivers experience a grief response whether the newborn's defect is a result of abnormal intrauterine

A   B   C   D

▪ Figure 21-1 Degrees of spinal cord anomalies. **(A)** The normal spinal closure. **(B)** Spina bifida occulta. **(C)** Spina bifida with meningocele. **(D)** Spina bifida with myelomeningocele, clearly showing the spinal cord involvement.

development or a chromosomal abnormality. They mourn the loss of the perfect child of their dreams, question why it happened, and may wonder how they will show the newborn to family and friends without shame or embarrassment. This grief may interfere with the process of parent–newborn attachment. Parents need to understand that their response is normal and that they are entitled to honest answers to their questions about the newborn's condition. Other children in the family should be informed gently but honestly about the newborn and should be allowed to visit the newborn when accompanied by adult family members. Sufficient time and attention must be devoted to the older siblings to avoid jealousy toward the newborn.

CONGENITAL MALFORMATIONS

Congenital anomalies or malformations may be caused by genetic or environmental factors. Approximately 2% of all infants born have a major malformation (Holmes, 2006). These anomalies include defects of the central nervous, cardiovascular, gastrointestinal, genitourinary, and skeletal systems. Defects such as cleft lip and severe neural tube defects are apparent at birth, but others may be discovered only after a complete physical examination. Congenital anomalies account for a large percentage of the health problems seen in newborns and children.

CENTRAL NERVOUS SYSTEM DEFECTS

Central nervous system defects include disorders caused by an imbalance of cerebrospinal fluid (CSF) (as in hydrocephalus) and a range of disorders resulting from malformations of the neural tube during embryonic development (often called "neural tube defects"). These defects vary from mild to severely disabling.

Spina Bifida

Caused by a defect in the neural arch, generally in the lumbosacral region, **spina bifida** is a failure of the poste-

rior laminae of the vertebrae to close; this leaves an opening through which the spinal meninges and spinal cord may protrude (Fig. 21-1).

Clinical Manifestations

A bony defect that occurs without soft-tissue involvement is called *spina bifida occulta*. In most instances, it is asymptomatic and presents no problems. A dimple in the skin or a tuft of hair over the site may cause one to suspect its presence, or it may be overlooked entirely.

When part of the spinal meninges protrudes through the bony defect and forms a cystic sac, the condition is termed *spina bifida with meningocele*. No nerve roots are involved, so no paralysis or sensory loss below the lesion appears. However, the sac may rupture or perforate, introducing infection into the spinal fluid and causing meningitis. For this reason, as well as for cosmetic purposes, surgical removal of the sac with closure of the skin is indicated.

In *spina bifida with myelomeningocele*, there is a protrusion of the spinal cord and the meninges, with nerve roots embedded in the wall of the cyst (Fig. 21-2). The effects of this defect vary in severity from sensory loss or

▪ Figure 21-2 A newborn with a myelomeningocele and hydrocephalus.

partial paralysis below the lesion to complete flaccid paralysis of all muscles below the lesion. Complete paralysis involves the lower trunk and legs, as well as bowel and bladder sphincters.

Making a clear-cut differentiation in diagnosis between a meningocele and a myelomeningocele on the basis of symptoms alone is not always possible. Myelomeningocele may also be termed *meningomyelocele*; the associated "spina bifida" is always implied but not necessarily named. *Spina bifida cystica* is the term used to designate either of these protrusions.

Diagnosis

Elevated maternal alpha-fetoprotein (AFP) levels followed by ultrasonographic examination of the fetus may show an incomplete neural tube. An elevated AFP level in the maternal serum or amniotic fluid indicates the probability of central nervous system abnormalities. Additional examination may confirm this and allow the pregnant woman the opportunity to consider terminating the pregnancy. The best time to perform these tests is between 13 and 15 weeks' gestation, when peak levels are reached. Most obstetricians perform AFP testing.

Diagnosis of the newborn with spina bifida is made from clinical observation and examination. Additional evaluation of the defect may include magnetic resonance imaging (MRI), ultrasonography, computed tomography, and myelography. The newborn needs to be examined carefully for other associated defects, particularly hydrocephalus, genitourinary defects, and orthopedic anomalies.

Treatment

Many specialists are involved in the treatment of these newborns, especially in the case of myelomeningocele. These specialists may include neurologists, neurosurgeons, orthopedic specialists, pediatricians, urologists, and physical therapists. After a thorough evaluation of the newborn, a plan of surgical repair and treatment is developed.

Highly skilled nursing care is necessary in all aspects of the newborn's care. The child requires years of ongoing follow-up and therapy. Surgery is required to close the open defect but may not be performed immediately, depending on the surgeon's decision. Waiting several days does not seem to cause additional problems, and this period gives the family an opportunity to adjust to the initial shock and become involved in making the necessary decisions.

Nursing Process for the Newborn With Myelomeningocele

Assessment

A routine newborn examination is conducted with emphasis on neurologic impairment. When collecting data during the examination, observe the movement and response to stimuli of the lower extremities. Carefully measure the head circumference and examine the fontanelles. Thoroughly document the observations made. When handling the newborn, take great care to prevent injury to the sac.

The family needs support and understanding during the newborn's initial care and for the many years of care during the child's life. Determine the family's knowledge and understanding of the defect as well as their attitude concerning the birth of a newborn with such serious problems.

Selected Nursing Diagnoses

- Risk for Infection related to vulnerability of the myelomeningocele sac
- Risk for Impaired Skin Integrity related to exposure to urine and feces
- Risk for Injury related to neuromuscular impairment
- Compromised Family Coping related to the perceived loss of the perfect newborn
- Deficient Knowledge of the family caregivers related to the complexities of caring for a newborn with serious neurologic and musculoskeletal defects

Outcome Identification and Planning: Preoperative Care

The preoperative goals for care of the newborn with myelomeningocele include preventing infection, maintaining skin integrity, preventing trauma related to disuse, increasing family coping skills, education about the condition, and support.

Implementation

Preventing Infection

Monitor the newborn's vital signs, neurologic signs, and behavior frequently to observe for any deviations from normal that may indicate an infection. Prophylactic antibiotics may be ordered. Carry out routine aseptic technique with conscientious hand washing, gloving, and gowning, as appropriate. Until surgery is performed, the sac must be covered with a sterile dressing moistened in a warm sterile solution (often sterile saline). Change this dressing every 2 hours; do not allow it to dry to avoid damage to the covering of the sac. The dressings may be covered with a plastic protective covering. Maintain the newborn in a prone position so that no pressure is placed on the sac. After surgery, continue this positioning until the surgical site is well healed.

Diapering is not advisable with a low defect, but the sac must be protected from contamination with fecal material. Placing a protective barrier between the anus and the sac may prevent this contamination. If the anal sphincter muscles are involved, the newborn may have continual loose stools, which adds to the challenge of keeping the sac free from infection.

Promoting Skin Integrity

The nursing interventions discussed in the previous section on infection also are necessary to promote skin integrity around the area of the defect and the diaper area. As mentioned, leakage of stool and urine may be continual. This leakage causes skin irritation and breakdown if the newborn is not kept clean and the diaper area is not free of stool and urine. Scrupulous perineal care is necessary.

Preventing Contractures of Lower Extremities

Newborns with spina bifida often have **talipes equinovarus** (clubfoot) and congenital **hip dysplasia** (dislocation of the hips), both of which are discussed later in this chapter. If there is loss of motion in the lower limbs because of the defect, conduct range-of-motion exercises to prevent contractures. Position the newborn so that the hips are abducted and the feet are in a neutral position. Massage the knees and other bony prominences with lotion regularly, then pad them, and protect them from irritation. As stated, avoid putting pressure on the sac during care activities.

Promoting Family Coping

The family of a newborn with such a major anomaly is in a state of shock on first learning of the problems. Be especially sensitive to their needs and emotions. Encourage family members to express their feelings and emotions as openly as possible. Recognize that some families express emotions much more freely than others do, and adjust your responses to the family with this in mind. Provide privacy, as needed, for the family to mourn together over their loss, but do not avoid the family because this only exaggerates their feelings of loss and depression. If possible, encourage the family members to cuddle or touch the newborn using proper precautions for the safety of the defect. With the permission of the physician, the newborn may be held in a chest-to-chest position to provide closer contact.

Providing Family Teaching

Give family members information about the defect, and encourage them to discuss their concerns and ask questions. Provide information about the newborn's present state, the proposed surgery, and follow-up care. Remember that anxiety may block understanding and processing knowledge, so information may need to be repeated. Provide information in small segments to facilitate learning.

After surgery, the family needs to be prepared to care for the newborn at home. Teach the family to hold the newborn's head, neck, and chest slightly raised in one hand during feeding. Also, teach them that stroking the newborn's cheek helps stimulate sucking. Showing the family how to care for the newborn, allowing them to participate in the care, and guiding them in performing return demonstrations are all methods to use in family teaching.

For long-term care and support, refer the family to the Spina Bifida Association of America (www.sbaa.org). Give them materials concerning spina bifida. These children need long-term care involving many aspects of medicine and surgery, as well as education and vocational training. Although children with spina bifida have many long-term problems, their intelligence is not affected; many of these children grow into productive young adults who may live independently.

Evaluation: Goals and Expected Outcomes

Goal: The newborn will be free from signs and symptoms of infection.

Expected Outcomes: The newborn

- has vital signs and neurologic signs that are within normal limits.
- shows no signs of irritability or lethargy.

Goal: The newborn will have no evidence of skin breakdown.

Expected Outcome: The newborn's skin

- remains clean, dry, and intact.
- has no areas of reddening or signs of irritation.

Goal: The newborn will remain free from injury.

Expected Outcome:

- The newborn's lower limbs show no evidence of contractures.

Goal: The family caregivers will show positive signs of beginning coping.

Expected Outcomes: The family members

- verbalize their anxieties and needs.
- hold, cuddle, and soothe the newborn as appropriate.

Goal: The family caregivers will learn to care for the newborn.

Expected Outcomes: The family

- demonstrates competence in performing care for the newborn.
- verbalizes understanding of the signs and symptoms that should be reported.
- has information about support agencies.

Hydrocephalus

Hydrocephalus is a condition characterized by an excess of CSF within the ventricular and subarachnoid spaces of the cranial cavity. Normally, a delicate balance exists between the rate of formation and absorption of CSF; the entire volume is absorbed and replaced every 12 to 24 hours. In hydrocephalus, this balance is disturbed.

CSF is formed mainly in the lateral ventricles by the choroid plexus and is absorbed into the venous system through the arachnoid villi. CSF circulates within the ventricles and the subarachnoid space. It is a colorless fluid consisting of water with traces of protein, glucose, and lymphocytes.

In the *noncommunicating* type of congenital hydrocephalus, an obstruction occurs and CSF is not able to pass between the ventricles and the spinal cord. The blockage causes increased pressure on the brain or spinal cord. One of the most common causes of noncommunicating hydrocephalus occurs when there is a narrowing in the aqueduct of Sylvius (Fig. 21-3). In the *communicating* type of hydrocephalus, no obstruction of the free flow of CSF exists between the ventricles and the spinal theca; rather the condition is caused by defective absorption of CSF, which increases pressure on the brain or spinal cord. Congenital hydrocephalus is most often the obstructive or noncommunicating type.

Hydrocephalus may be recognized at birth, or it may not be evident until after a few weeks or months of life. The condition may not be congenital but instead may occur during later infancy or during childhood as the result of a neoplasm, a head injury, or an infection such as meningitis.

When hydrocephalus occurs early in life before the skull sutures close, the soft, pliable bones separate to allow head expansion. This condition is manifested by a rapid increase in head circumference. The fact that the soft bones can yield to pressure in this manner may partially explain why many of these newborns fail to show the usual symptoms of brain pressure and may exhibit little or no damage in mental function until later in life. Other newborns show severe brain damage, which has often occurred before birth.

Clinical Manifestations

An excessively large head at birth is suggestive of hydrocephalus. Rapid head growth with widening cranial sutures is also strongly suggestive and may be the first manifestation of this condition. An apparently large head in itself is not necessarily significant. Normally, every newborn's head is measured at birth, and the rate of growth is checked at subsequent examinations. If a newborn's head appears to be abnormally large at birth or appears to be enlarging, it should be measured frequently.

As the head enlarges, the suture lines separate and the spaces may be felt through the scalp. The anterior fontanelle becomes tense and bulging, the skull enlarges in all diameters, and the scalp becomes shiny and its veins dilate (Fig. 21-4). If pressure continues to increase without intervention, the eyes appear to be pushed downward slightly with the sclera visible above the iris—the so-called setting sun sign.

If the condition progresses without adequate drainage of excessive fluid, the head becomes increasingly heavy, the neck muscles fail to develop sufficiently, and the newborn has difficulty raising or turning the head. Unless hydrocephalus is arrested, the newborn becomes increasingly helpless and symptoms of increased intracranial pressure

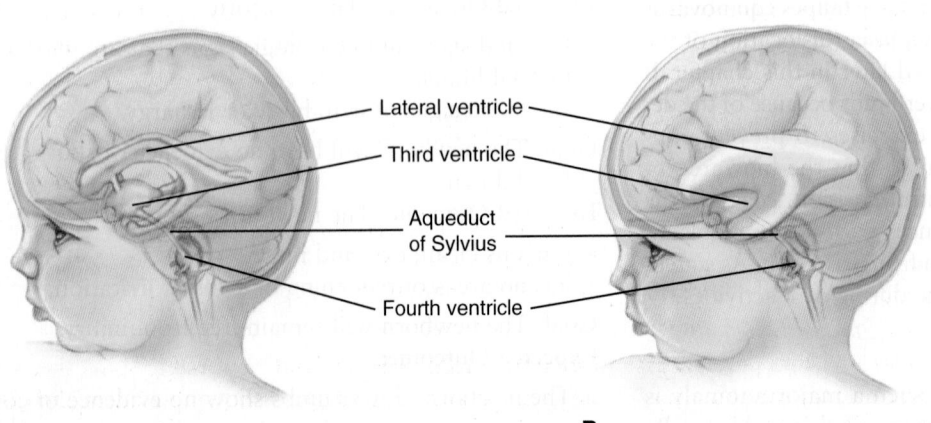

A   B

■ **Figure 21-3 (A)** Infant *without* hydrocephalus. Note the ventricles of the brain and channels for the normal flow of cerebrospinal fluid. **(B)** Infant *with* hydrocephalus. Note broadening of the forehead and large head size.

Lateral ventricle
Third ventricle
Aqueduct of Sylvius
Fourth ventricle

■ **Figure 21-4** A newborn with hydrocephalus. Note the pull on the eyes giving the "setting sun" appearance.

(IICP) develop. These symptoms may include irritability, restlessness, personality change, high-pitched cry, ataxia, projectile vomiting, failure to thrive, seizures, severe headache, changes in level of consciousness, and papilledema.

Diagnosis

Positive diagnosis of hydrocephalus is made with computed tomography and magnetic resonance imaging. Echoencephalography and ventriculography also may be performed for further definition of the condition.

Treatment

Surgical intervention is the only effective means of relieving brain pressure and preventing additional damage to the brain tissue. If minimal brain damage has occurred, the child may be able to function within a normal mental range. Motor function is usually retarded. In some instances, surgical intervention may remove the cause of the obstruction, such as a neoplasm, a cyst, or a hematoma, but most children require placement of a shunting device that bypasses the point of obstruction, draining the excess CSF into a body cavity. This procedure arrests excessive head growth and prevents additional brain damage.

Many shunt procedures use a silicone rubber catheter that is radiopaque so that its position may be checked by radiographic examination. The silicone rubber catheter reduces the problem of tissue reaction. A valve or regulator is an essential part of each catheter that prevents excessive build-up of fluid or too-rapid decompression of the ventricle. The most common procedure, particularly for newborns and small children, is **ventriculoperitoneal shunting** (VP shunt). In this procedure, the CSF is drained from a lateral ventricle in the brain; the CSF runs through the subcutaneous catheter and empties into the peritoneal cavity (Fig. 21-5). This procedure allows the insertion of some excess tubing to accommodate growth. As the

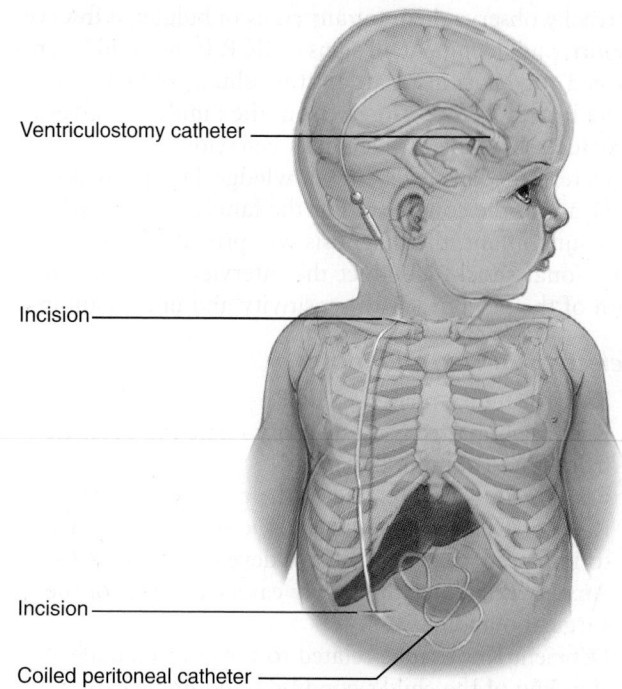

Ventriculostomy catheter

Incision

Incision

Coiled peritoneal catheter

■ **Figure 21-5** Ventriculoperitoneal shunting to drain excess cerebrospinal fluid in hydrocephalus.

child grows, the catheter needs to be revised and lengthened.

In **ventriculoatrial shunting,** CSF drains into the right atrium of the heart. This procedure cannot be used in children with pathologic changes in the heart. The CSF drained from the ventricle is absorbed into the bloodstream.

Other pathways of drainage have been used with varying degrees of success. All types of shunts may have problems with kinking, blocking, moving, or shifting of tubing. The danger of infection in the tubing is a constant concern. Children with shunts must be observed constantly for signs of malfunction or infection.

The long-term outcome for a child with hydrocephalus depends on several factors. If untreated, the outcome is very poor, often leading to death. With shunting, the outcome depends on the initial cause of the increased fluid, the treatment of the cause, the brain damage sustained before shunting, complications with the shunting system, and continued long-term follow-up. Some of these children can lead relatively normal lives if they have follow-up and revisions as they grow.

Nursing Process for the Postoperative Newborn With Hydrocephalus

Assessment

Obtaining accurate vital and neurologic signs is necessary before and after surgery. Measurement of the newborn's head is essential. If the fontanelles are not closed, carefully observe them for any signs of bulging. Observe, report, and document all signs of IICP. If the child has returned for revision of an existing shunt, obtain a complete history before surgery from the family caregiver to provide a baseline of the child's behavior.

Determine the level of knowledge family members have about the condition. For the family of the newborn or young infant, the diagnosis will probably come as an emotional shock. Conduct the interview and examination of the newborn with sensitivity and understanding.

Selected Nursing Diagnoses

- Risk for Injury related to IICP
- Risk for Impaired Skin Integrity related to pressure from physical immobility
- Risk for Infection related to the presence of a shunt
- Risk for Delayed Growth and Development related to impaired ability to achieve developmental tasks
- Anxiety related to the family caregiver's fear of the surgical outcome
- Deficient Knowledge related to the family's understanding of the child's condition and home care

Outcome Identification and Planning

The goals for the postoperative care of the newborn with shunt placement for hydrocephalus include preventing injury, maintaining skin integrity, preventing infection, maintaining growth and development, and reducing family anxiety. Family goals include increasing knowledge about the condition and providing loving, supportive care to the newborn.

Implementation

Preventing Injury

At least every 2 to 4 hours, monitor the newborn's level of consciousness. Check the pupils for equality and reaction, monitor the neurologic status, and observe for a shrill cry, lethargy, or irritability. Measure and record the head circumference daily. Carry out appropriate procedures to care for the shunt as directed. To prevent a rapid decrease in ICP, keep the newborn flat. Observe for signs of seizure, and initiate seizure precautions. Keep suction and oxygen equipment convenient at the bedside.

Promoting Skin Integrity

After a shunting procedure, keep the newborn's head turned away from the operative site until the physician allows a change in position. If the newborn's head is enlarged, prevent pressure sores from forming on the side where the child rests. Reposition the newborn at least every 2 hours, as permitted. Inspect the dressings over the shunt site immediately after the surgery, every hour for the first 3 to 4 hours, and then at least every 4 hours.

Preventing Infection

Infection is the primary threat after surgery. Closely observe for and promptly report any signs of infection, which include redness, heat, or swelling along the surgical site; fever; and signs of lethargy. Perform wound care thoroughly as ordered. Administer antibiotics as prescribed.

Promoting Growth and Development

Every newborn has the need to be picked up and held, cuddled, and comforted. An uncomfortable or painful experience increases the need for emotional support. A newborn perceives such support principally through physical contact made in a soothing, loving manner.

The newborn needs social interaction and needs to be talked to, played with, and given the opportunity for activity. Provide toys appropriate for his or her physical and mental capacity. If the child has difficulty moving about the crib, place toys within easy reach and vision; a cradle gym, for example, may be tied close enough for the newborn to maneuver its parts.

> **This is important!**
> Always support the head of a newborn with hydrocephalus when picking up, moving, or positioning. Using egg-crate pads, lamb's wool, or a special mattress can prevent pressure and breakdown of the scalp.

Unless the newborn's nervous system is so impaired that all activity increases irritability, the newborn needs stimulation just as any child does. If repositioning from side to side means turning the newborn away from the sight of activity, the crib may be turned around so that vision is not obstructed.

A newborn who is given the contact and support that all newborns require develops a pleasing personality because he or she is nourished by emotional stimulation. Use the time spent on physical care as a time for social interaction. Talking, laughing, and playing with the newborn are important aspects of the newborn's care. Make frequent contacts, and do not limit them to the times when physical care is being performed.

Reducing Family Anxiety

Explain to the family the condition and the anatomy of the surgical procedure in terms they can understand. Discuss the overall prognosis for the child. Encourage family members to express their anxieties and ask questions. Giving accurate, nontechnical answers is extremely helpful. Give the family information about support groups, such as the National Hydrocephalus Foundation (www.nhfonline.org), and encourage them to contact the groups.

Providing Family Teaching

Demonstrate care of the shunt to the family caregivers and have them perform a return demonstration. Provide them with a list of signs and symptoms that should be reported. Review these with the family members and make sure they understand them. Discuss appropriate growth and developmental expectations for the child, and stress realistic goals.

Evaluation: Goals and Expected Outcomes

Goal: The newborn will be free from injury related to complications of excessive CSF.

Expected Outcomes: The newborn

- has no signs of IICP, such as lethargy, irritability, and seizure activity.
- has a stable level of consciousness.

Goal: The newborn's skin will remain intact.

Expected Outcome:

- The newborn's skin shows no evidence of pressure sores, redness, or other signs of skin breakdown.

Goal: The newborn will remain free of infection.

Expected Outcomes: The newborn

- shows no signs of infection.
- has stable vital signs.
- has no redness, drainage, or swelling at the surgical site.

Goal: The newborn will have age-appropriate growth and development.

Expected Outcomes: The newborn

- has his or her social and developmental needs met.
- interacts and plays appropriately with toys and surroundings.

Goal: The family caregiver's anxiety will be reduced.

Expected Outcomes: The family

- expresses fears and concerns.
- interacts appropriately with the newborn.

Goal: The family will learn care of the child.

Expected Outcomes: The family

- participates in the care of the newborn.
- asks appropriate questions.
- lists signs and symptoms to report.

CARDIOVASCULAR SYSTEM DEFECTS: CONGENITAL HEART DISEASE

Cardiovascular system defects range from mild to severe. They may be detected immediately at birth or may not be detected for several months. When a newborn is suspected of having a heart abnormality, the family is understandably upset. The heart is *the* vital organ; a person can live without a number of other organs and appendages, but life itself depends on the heart. The family caregivers will have many questions. The nurse may answer some; the care provider must answer others. Many answers will not be available until after various evaluation procedures have been conducted.

Technological advances have progressed rapidly in this field, making earlier detection and successful repair much more likely. However, heart defects are still the leading cause of death from congenital anomalies in the first year of life. A brief review of the development and function of the embryonic heart is useful to understanding the malformations that occur.

Development of the Heart

The heart begins beating early in the third to eighth week of intrauterine life. When first formed, the heart is a simple tube receiving blood from the placenta and pumping it out into its developing body. During this period, the heart rapidly develops into its normal, but complex, four-chambered structure.

Fetal circulation is unique. The fetal lungs are inactive, requiring only a small amount of blood to nourish their tissues. Blood is circulated through the umbilical arteries to the placenta, where waste products and carbon dioxide are exchanged for oxygen and nutrients. The blood is then returned to the fetus through the umbilical vein.

At birth, the umbilical cord is cut, and the newborn's own independent circulatory system is established. Certain circulatory bypasses, such as the *ductus arteriosus*, the *foramen ovale*, and the *ductus venosus*, are no longer necessary (see Chapter 5). They close during the first several weeks after birth. In addition, the pressure in the heart, which has been higher on the right side during fetal life, now changes so that the left side of the heart has the higher pressure (Fig. 21-6).

During this period of complex development, any error in formation may cause serious circulatory difficulty. The incidence of cardiovascular malformations is about 8 in 1,000 live births. Some abnormalities are slight and

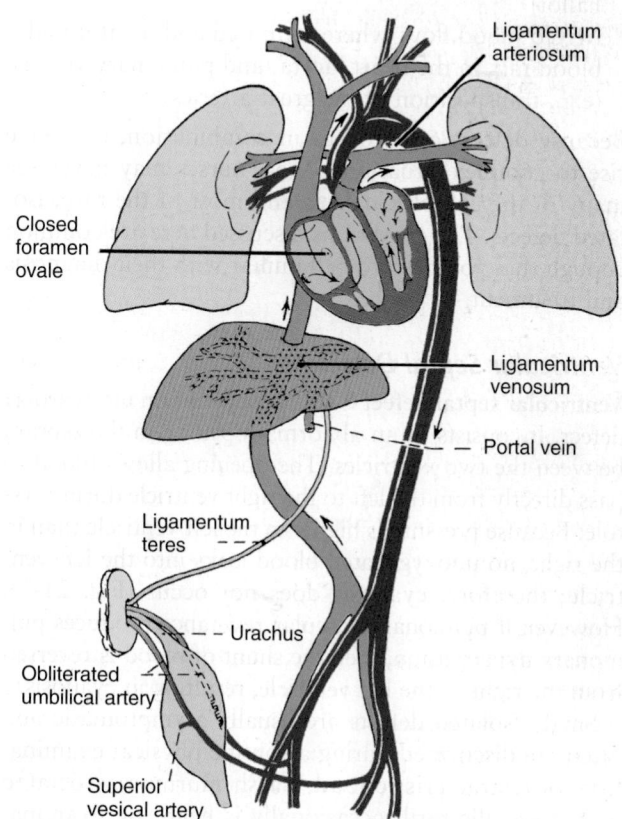

■ **Figure 21-6** Normal blood circulation in the newborn. Highlighted ligaments indicate pathways that should close at or soon after birth. Arrows indicate normal flow of blood.

allow the person to lead a normal life without correction. Others cause little apparent difficulty but need correction to improve the chance for a longer life and for optimal health. Some severe anomalies are incompatible with life for more than a short time; others may be helped but not cured by surgery.

Common Types of Congenital Heart Defects

Traditionally, congenital heart defects have been described as cyanotic or acyanotic conditions. **Cyanotic heart disease** implies an oxygen saturation of the peripheral arterial blood of 85% or less. This condition occurs when a heart defect allows any appreciable amount of oxygen-poor blood in the right side of the heart to mix with the oxygenated blood in the left side of the heart (*right-to-left shunting*). Defects that permit right-to-left shunting may occur at the atrial, ventricular, or aortic level. However, because defects are often complex and occur in various combinations, this is an inadequate means of classification. A more clear-cut classification system is based on blood flow characteristics:

- Increased pulmonary blood flow (e.g., ventricular septal, atrial septal, and patent ductus arteriosus)
- Obstruction of blood flow out of the heart (e.g., coarctation of the aorta)
- Decreased pulmonary blood flow (e.g., tetralogy of Fallot)
- Mixed blood flow, where saturated and desaturated blood mix in the heart, aorta, and pulmonary vessels (e.g., transposition of the great arteries)

Because defects often occur in combination, they give rise to complex situations. Most nurses may never see many of the complex defects and most of the rare, isolated defects. The conditions discussed here are common enough that you need to be familiar with their diagnosis and treatment.

Ventricular Septal Defect

Ventricular septal defect is the most common intracardiac defect. It consists of an abnormal opening in the septum between the two ventricles. The opening allows blood to pass directly from the left to the right ventricle during systole. Because pressure is higher in the left ventricle than in the right, no unoxygenated blood leaks into the left ventricle; therefore, cyanosis does not occur (Fig. 21-7). However, if pulmonary vascular resistance produces pulmonary hypertension, then the shunt of blood is reversed from the right to the left ventricle, resulting in cyanosis.

Small, isolated defects are usually asymptomatic and often are discovered during a routine physical examination. A characteristic loud, harsh murmur associated with a systolic thrill occasionally is heard on examination. A history of frequent respiratory infections may occur during infancy, but growth and development are unaffected. The child leads a normal life.

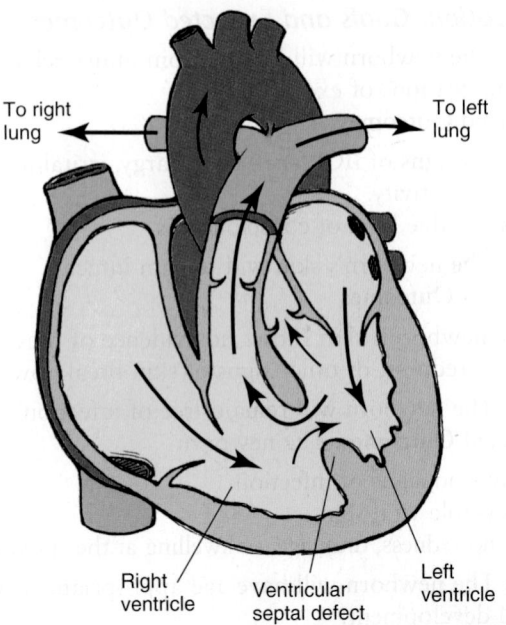

To right lung   To left lung

Right ventricle   Ventricular septal defect   Left ventricle

■ **Figure 21-7** A ventricular septal defect is an abnormal opening between the right and left ventricle. Ventricular septal defects vary in size and may occur in the membranous or muscular portion of the ventricular septum.

Corrective surgery may be postponed until the age of 18 months to 2 years, when the surgical risk is less than that for newborns. However, improved surgical techniques enable the repair to be made in the first year of life with high rates of success. The child is observed closely and may be prescribed a regimen of prophylactic antibiotics to prevent frequent respiratory infections. If pulmonary involvement becomes a problem, the repair is done without further delay. Repairs in children who are at high risk are done by the use of cardiac catheterization procedures.

Atrial Septal Defects

An **atrial septal defect** is an abnormal opening between the right and left atria. The opening may be the result of an incompetent foramen ovale or incorrect development of the atrial septum (Fig. 21-8). In general, left-to-right shunting occurs in all true atrial septal defects. However, many healthy people have a patent foramen ovale that normally causes no problems because its valve is anatomically structured to withstand left chamber pressure, rendering it functionally closed.

True atrial septal defects are common heart anomalies and may occur as isolated defects or in combination with other heart anomalies. Atrial septal defects are amenable to surgery with a low surgical mortality risk. The surgical repair may be performed in a dry field using a heart–lung bypass machine. The opening is closed with sutures or a Dacron patch.

Patent Ductus Arteriosus

In fetal circulation, the ductus arteriosus is a vascular channel between the left main pulmonary artery and the

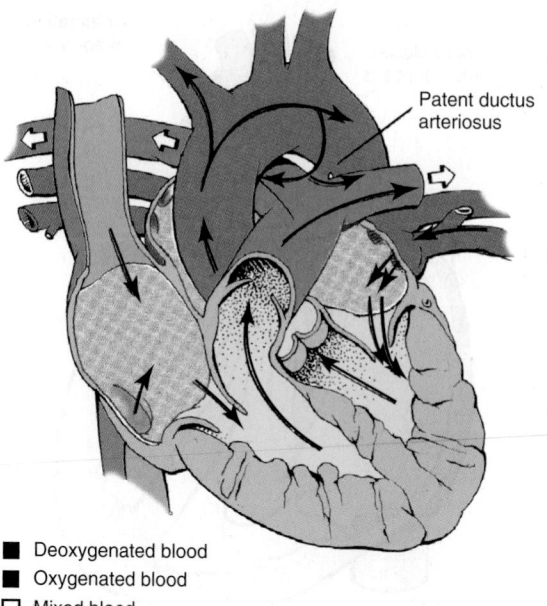

■ Deoxygenated blood
■ Oxygenated blood
□ Mixed blood

■ **Figure 21-8** An atrial septal defect is an abnormal opening between the right and left atria that allows left-to-right shunting of blood. The opening can result from three types of abnormalities: (1) An incompetent foramen ovale, the most common defect. (2) An ostium secundum defect, an opening in the middle of the septum that results from abnormal development of the septum secundum. (3) An ostium primum defect, an opening at the lower end of the septum that results from improper development of the septum primum; the defect frequently involves the atrioventricular valves.

■ **Figure 21-9** Patent ductus arteriosus occurs when the ductus arterious fails to close soon after birth. If the ductus fails to close, the blood is shunted from the aorta to the pulmonary artery, rather than going into the systemic circulation.

descending aorta. It allows blood to bypass the non-functioning lungs and go directly from the pulmonary artery to the aorta and into the systemic circuit. After birth, the duct normally closes, eventually becoming obliterated and forming the ligamentum arteriosum. However, if the ductus arteriosus remains patent after birth, the higher pressure in the aorta reverses the direction of blood flow in the ductus. Blood is then shunted from the aorta into the pulmonary artery. This situation results in a flooding of the lungs and an overloading of the left heart chambers (Fig. 21-9).

Normally, the ductus arteriosus is nonpatent after the first or second week of life and should be obliterated by the fourth month. Why it fails to close is unknown. Patent ductus arteriosus is common in newborns who exhibit the rubella syndrome, but most newborns with this anomaly have no history of exposure to rubella during fetal life. It is also common in preterm newborns weighing less than 1,200 g and in newborns with Down syndrome.

Symptoms of patent ductus arteriosus are often absent during childhood. Growth and development may be retarded in some children, with an easy fatigability and dyspnea on exertion. The diagnosis may be based on a characteristic machinerylike murmur over the pulmonary area, a wide pulse pressure, and a bounding pulse. Cardiac catheterization is diagnostic but is not required in the presence of classic clinical features.

Indomethacin (Indocin), a prostaglandin inhibitor, may be administered with some success to premature newborns to promote closure of the ductus arteriosus. If this fails to close the ductus, surgery is indicated in all diagnosed cases, even if they are asymptomatic. Some persons live a normal life span without correction, but the risks of the defect far outweigh the surgical risks. Surgical correction consists of closure of the defect by ligation or by division of the ductus. Division is the method of choice if the child's condition permits because the ductus occasionally reopens after ligation. The optimal age for surgery is before the age of 2 years, with earlier surgery for severely affected newborns. Prognosis is excellent after a successful repair.

Coarctation of the Aorta

Coarctation of the aorta is a constriction or narrowing of the aortic arch or the descending aorta usually adjacent to the ligamentum arteriosum (Fig. 21-10). The constriction obstructs blood flow through the aorta, increasing left ventricular pressure and workload.

Most children with this congenital condition have no symptoms until later childhood or young adulthood. This delay of symptoms occurs because, in the average child, blood is able to bypass the constricted portion of the aorta by way of collateral circulation (chiefly through the branches of the subclavian and carotid arteries that arise from the arch of the aorta). Eventually, however, the enlarged collateral arteries erode the rib margins, and the rib notching may be visualized by radiographic examination. A few newborns do have severe symptoms in their first year of life; they show dyspnea, tachycardia, and cyanosis, which are all signs of developing **congestive heart failure (CHF)**.

■ **Figure 21-10** Coarctation of the aorta is characterized by a narrowed aortic lumen. It exists as a preductal or postductal obstruction, depending on the position of the obstruction in relation to the ductus arteriosus. The defect obstructs blood flow through the aorta, causing an increased left ventricular pressure and workload.

In older children, the condition is easily diagnosed based on hypertension in the upper extremities and hypotension in the lower extremities. The radial pulse is readily palpable, but the femoral pulses are weak or even impalpable. Blood pressure is normal or elevated in the arms and is low or undetectable in the legs. A high-pitched systolic murmur is usually present and heard over the base of the heart and over the interscapular area of the back. The diagnosis may be confirmed by aortography.

Uncorrected coarctation may cause hypertension and cardiac failure later in life. The optimal age for elective surgery is before the age of 2 years. Early surgery may be necessary for a gravely ill newborn who presents with severe CHF. In early infancy, the mortality rate depends on the presence of other congenital heart problems.

Surgery consists of resection of the coarcted area with an end-to-end anastomosis of the proximal and distal ends of the aorta. Occasionally a long defect may necessitate an end-to-end graft using tubes of Dacron or similar material. Prognosis is excellent for the restoration of normal function after surgery.

Tetralogy of Fallot

Tetralogy of Fallot is a fairly common congenital heart defect involved in 50% to 70% of all cyanotic congenital heart diseases. It consists of a grouping of heart defects (tetralogy denotes four abnormal conditions): (1) **pulmonary stenosis,** (2) ventricular septal defect, (3) **overriding aorta,** and (4) **right ventricular hypertrophy.** The pulmonary stenosis is usually seen as a narrowing of

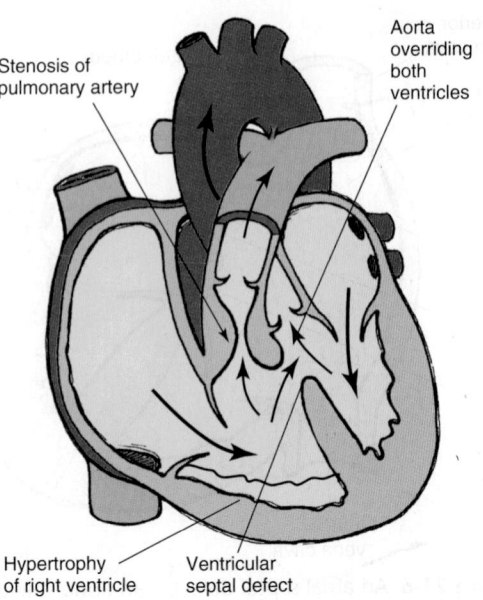

■ **Figure 21-11** Tetralogy of Fallot is characterized by the combination of four defects: (1) pulmonary stenosis, (2) ventricular septal defect, (3) overriding aorta, and (4) hypertrophy of the right ventricle.

the upper portion of the right ventricle and may include stenosis of the valve cusps. Pulmonary stenosis results, in turn, in right ventricular hypertrophy (increase in size). The aorta appears to straddle the ventricular septum, overriding the ventricular septal defect. This defect allows a shunt of unsaturated blood from the right ventricle into the aorta or into the left ventricle (Fig. 21-11).

Tetralogy of Fallot is the most common defect causing cyanosis in patients surviving beyond 2 years of age. The child with this defect may be precyanotic in early infancy, with the cyanotic phase starting at 4 to 6 months of age. However, some severely affected newborns may show cyanosis earlier. As long as the ductus arteriosus remains open, enough blood apparently passes through the lungs to prevent cyanosis.

The severity of symptoms depends on the degree of pulmonary stenosis, the size of the ventricular septal defect, and the degree to which the aorta overrides the septal defect. The infant presents with feeding difficulties and poor weight gain, resulting in retarded growth and development. Dyspnea and easy fatigability become evident. Exercise tolerance depends in part on the severity of the disease; some children become fatigued after little exertion. In the past, on experiencing fatigue, breathlessness, and increased cyanosis, the child was described as assuming a squatting posture for relief. Squatting apparently increased the systemic oxygen saturation. However, squatting rarely is seen today because these newborns' defects usually are repaired by the time they are 2 years old.

Attacks of paroxysmal dyspnea are common during infancy and early childhood. An anoxic spell is heralded by sudden restlessness, gasping respiration, and increased cyanosis that lead to a loss of consciousness and, possibly, convulsions. These attacks, called "tet spells," last from a few minutes to several hours and appear to be unpredictable, although stress does seem to trigger some episodes.

The history and clinical manifestations are usually sufficient to make a diagnosis. However, cardiac catheterization, electrocardiography, chest radiography, and laboratory tests to determine polycythemia and arterial oxygen saturation may be performed for additional definition.

The preferred repair of these defects is total surgical correction. This procedure requires the use of a cardiopulmonary bypass machine. The heart is opened, and extensive resection is done. The repair relieves the pulmonary stenosis, and the septal defect is closed by use of a patch. Successful total correction transforms a grossly abnormal heart into a functionally normal one. However, most of these children are left without a pulmonary valve.

In infants who cannot withstand the total surgical correction until they are older, the Blalock-Taussig procedure is performed. This procedure is an end-to-end anastomosis of a vessel arising from the aorta, usually the subclavian artery, to the corresponding right or left pulmonary artery. These shunts are now seen only occasionally because total surgical repair has much greater success and lower mortality rates.

Transposition of the Great Arteries

In **transposition of the great arteries**, the aorta arises from the right ventricle instead of the left, and the pulmonary artery arises from the left ventricle instead of the right. These newborns are usually cyanotic from birth. This severe defect was once almost always fatal. However, advancements in diagnosis and treatment have increased the survival rate.

Test Yourself

✔ What is the difference between spina bifida with meningocele and spina bifida with myelomeningocele?

✔ What does the newborn have an excess of in the condition of hydrocephalus? How is hydrocephalus treated?

✔ List the five common types of congenital heart defects.

Risk Factors

Maternal alcoholism, maternal irradiation, ingestion of certain drugs during pregnancy, maternal diabetes, and advanced maternal age (older than 40 years) increase the incidence of heart defects in newborns. Rubella in the expectant mother during the first trimester can also cause cardiac malformations. Maternal malnutrition and heredity may be contributing factors. Recent studies have shown that the offspring of mothers who had congenital heart anomalies have a much higher risk of having congenital heart anomalies. If one child in the family has a congenital heart abnormality, later siblings have a very high risk for such a defect.

Clinical Manifestations

The newborn with a severe cardiovascular abnormality, such as a transposition of the great vessels, is cyanotic from birth and requires oxygen and special treatment. A less seriously affected child, whose heart can compensate to some degree for the impaired circulation, may not have symptoms severe enough to call attention to the difficulty until he or she is a few months older and more active. Others may live a fairly normal life and not be aware of any heart trouble until a murmur or an enlarged heart is discovered during physical examination in later childhood.

A cardiac murmur discovered early in life necessitates frequent physical examinations. This murmur may be a functional, "innocent" murmur that may disappear as the child grows older, or it may be the chief manifestation of an abnormal heart or an abnormal circulatory system. The most common parental concern is that of feeding difficulties. Newborns with cardiac anomalies severe enough to cause circulatory difficulties have a history of being poor eaters, tiring easily from the effort to suck, and failing to grow or thrive normally. These manifestations of CHF may appear during the first year of life in newborns with conditions such as large ventricular septal defects, coarctation of the aorta, and other defects that place an increased workload on the ventricles.

Treatment and Nursing Care

Advances in medical technology have enabled heart repairs to be performed in newborns as young as less than 1 day old. Miniaturization of instruments, earlier diagnosis through the use of improved diagnostic techniques, pediatric intensive care facilities staffed with highly skilled nurse specialists, and more sophisticated monitoring techniques have all contributed to these advances.

Most physicians now think it is important to operate as early as possible to repair defective hearts. Inadequate circulation may prevent adequate growth and development and cause permanent, irreparable physical, mental, and emotional damage. If the child receives a diagnosis early and correction or repair is possible, CHF may be avoided.

In cases where the child has CHF, it is important that the CHF be treated. The primary goals in the treatment of CHF are to reduce the workload of the heart and to improve the cardiac functioning, thus increasing oxygenation of the tissues. This is done by removing excess sodium and fluids, slowing the heart rate, and decreasing the demands on the heart. See Chapter 37 for a complete discussion of CHF and its treatment.

Care at Home Before Surgery

A child with congenital heart disease may show easy fatigability and retarded growth. If the child has a cyanotic type of heart disease with clubbing of the fingers or toes, periods of cyanosis and reduced exercise tolerance are evident. This young child may assume a squatting position, which reduces the return flow to the heart, thus temporarily reducing the workload of the heart.

Such a child should be allowed to lead as normal a life as possible. Families are naturally apprehensive and find it difficult not to overprotect the child. They often increase the child's anxiety and cause fear in the child about participating in normal activities. Children are rather sensible about finding their own limitations and usually limit their activities to their capacity if they are not made unduly apprehensive.

Some families can adjust well and provide guidance and security for the sick child. Others may become confused and frightened and show hostility, disinterest, or neglect; these families need guidance and counseling. As the nurse, you have a great responsibility to support the family. The primary nursing goal is to reduce anxiety in the child and family. This goal may be accomplished through open communication and ongoing contact.

Routine visits to a clinic or a physician's office become a way of life, and the child may come to feel different from other people. Physicians and nurses have a responsibility both to the family caregivers and the child to give clear explanations of the defect, using readily understandable terms and diagrams, pictures, or models. A child who knows what is happening can accept a great deal and can continue with the business of living.

Cardiac Catheterization

Cardiac catheterization may be performed before heart surgery to obtain more accurate information about the child's condition. The child or newborn is sedated or anesthetized for this process, and a radiopaque catheter is inserted through a vein into the right atrium. In the newborn or young child, the femoral vein often is used. Close observation of the child after the procedure is essential. Carefully monitor the site used and check the extremity for pulses, edema, skin temperature and color, and any other signs of poor circulation or infection. A pressure dressing is used over the catheterization site and left in place until the day after the procedure. The dressing should be snug and intact and monitored closely for any signs of bleeding from the site. The child is kept flat in bed with the extremity straight for as long as 6 hours after the procedure. Monitor vital signs closely.

Preoperative Preparation

When a child enters the hospital for cardiac surgery, it is seldom a first admission; generally, it has been preceded by cardiac catheterization or perhaps other hospitalizations. The child may be admitted a few days before surgery to allow time for adequate preparation, or preoperative procedures may be done on an outpatient basis. Preoperative teaching should be intensive for the family and the child at an age-appropriate level. They should understand that blood might be obtained for typing and cross-matching and for other determinations as ordered. Additional x-ray studies may be done.

The equipment to be used after surgery should be described with drawings and pictures. If possible, the family caregivers and the child should have the opportunity to visit a cardiac recovery room and see chest tubes and an oxygen tent. They should meet the nursing personnel and see the general appearance of the unit. Of course, use good judgment about the timing and the extent of such preparation; nothing is gained by arousing additional anxiety with premature or excessively graphic descriptions. A young child may become familiar with the surgical clothing worn by personnel and with the oxygen tent and can perhaps listen to a heartbeat. The child should learn how to cough and should practice coughing. He or she should understand that coughing is important after surgery and must be done regularly, even though it may hurt.

Cardiac Surgery

Open-heart surgery using the heart–lung machine has made extensive heart correction possible for many children who otherwise would have been disabled and lived limited lives. Machines have been refined for use with newborns and small children. Heart transplants may be performed when no other treatment is possible.

Inducing **hypothermia**—reducing the body temperature to 68°F to 78.8°F (20°C–26°C)—is a useful technique that helps to make early surgery possible. A reduced body temperature increases the time that the circulation may be stopped without causing brain damage. The blood temperature is reduced by the use of cooling agents in the heart–lung machine. This also provides a dry, bloodless, motionless field for the surgeon.

Postoperative Care

At the end of surgery, the child is taken to the pediatric intensive care unit for skillful nursing by specially trained personnel for as long as necessary. Children who have had closed-chest surgery need the same careful nursing management as those who have had open-heart surgery.

By the time the child returns to the regular pediatric unit, chest drainage tubes usually have been removed and the child has started taking oral fluids and is ready to sit up in bed or in a chair. The child probably feels weak and helpless after such an experience and needs encouragement and reassurance. However, with recovery a child is usually ready for activity. Family caregivers usually need to reorient themselves and to accept their child's new status. This attitude is not easy to acquire after what seemed like a long period of anxious watching. The surgeon and the surgical staff evaluate the results of the surgery and make any necessary recommendations regarding resumption of the child's activities. Plans should be made for follow-up and supervision, as well as counseling and guidance.

GASTROINTESTINAL SYSTEM DEFECTS

Most gastrointestinal system anomalies are apparent at birth or shortly thereafter. The anomalies are often the result of interruption of embryonic growth at a crucial stage. Many of these anomalies interfere with the normal nutrition and digestion essential to the newborn's normal growth and development. Many anomalies require immediate surgical intervention.

Cleft Lip and Cleft Palate

Cleft lip and cleft palate are the most common facial malformations. Cleft lip occurs in about 1 in 1,000 live births and is more common in males. Cleft palate occurs in 1 newborn in 2,500 live births, more often in females. Their causes are not entirely clear; they appear to be genetically influenced, but they sometimes occur in isolated instances with no genetic history. Although a cleft lip and a cleft palate often appear together, either defect may appear alone.

The cleft lip and cleft palate defects result from failure of the primary and secondary palates to fuse. If the maxillary processes do not fuse during the fifth to eighth week of intrauterine life, a cleft (fissure) occurs, resulting in a cleft lip. The secondary palate closes later in embryonic development, and the failure to close occurs for different reasons. In an 8-week-old embryo, there is still no roof to the mouth; the tissues that are to become the palate are two shelves running from the front to the back of the mouth and projecting vertically downward on either side of the tongue. The shelves move from a vertical position to a horizontal position; their free edges meet and fuse in midline. Later, bone forms within this tissue to form the hard palate, normally by the 10th to 12th week of fetal life. Exactly what happens to prevent this closure is not known for sure. The incidence of cleft palate is higher in the close relatives of people with the defect than it is in the general population, and some evidence indicates that environmental and hereditary factors play a part in this defect.

Clinical Manifestations

The cleft lip may be a simple notch in the vermilion line, or it may extend up into the floor of the nose (Fig. 21-12). It may be either **unilateral** (one side of the lip) or **bilateral** (both sides). The cleft palate may be a small opening or it may involve the entire palate (Fig. 21-13). Cleft palate occurs with a cleft lip about 50% of the time, most often with bilateral cleft lip. The child born with a cleft palate but with an intact lip does not have the external disfigurement that may be distressing to the new parent. However, the problems are more serious. Cleft palate is often accompanied by nasal deformity and dental disorders, such as deformed, missing, or **supernumerary** (excessive in number) teeth.

Diagnosis

The physical appearance of the newborn confirms the diagnosis of cleft lip. Diagnosis of cleft palate is made at

■ **Figure 21-12** A cleft lip may extend up into the floor of the nose.

birth with the close inspection of the newborn's palate. To be certain that a cleft palate is not missed, the examiner must insert a gloved finger into the newborn's mouth to feel the palate to determine that it is intact. If a cleft is found, consultation is set up with a clinic specializing in cleft palate repair.

Treatment

Surgery, usually performed by a plastic surgeon, is a major part of the treatment of a newborn with a cleft lip, palate, or both. Total care involves many other specialists, including pediatricians, nurses, orthodontists, prosthodontists, otolaryngologists, speech therapists, and occasionally psychiatrists. Long-term, intensive, multidisciplinary care is needed for newborns with major defects.

Plastic surgeons' opinions differ as to the best time for repair of the cleft lip. Some surgeons favor early repair, before the newborn is discharged from the hospital.

■ **Figure 21-13** The cleft lip may be **(A)** a simple notch, **(B)** unilateral, or **(C)** bilateral. The cleft palate may **(D)** be a small opening or **(E)** involve the entire palate.

They believe that early repair can alleviate some of the family's feelings of rejection of the newborn. Other surgeons prefer to wait until the newborn is 1 or 2 months old, weighs about 10 lb, and is gaining weight steadily. Newborns who are not born in large medical centers with specialists on the staff are discharged from the birth hospital and referred to a center or physician specializing in cleft lip and palate repair.

If early surgery is contemplated, the newborn should be healthy and of average or above-average weight. The newborn must be observed constantly because a newborn has a higher likelihood of aspiration than does an older infant. These newborns must be cared for by competent plastic surgeons and experienced nurses.

The goal in repairing the cleft palate is to give the child a union of the cleft parts to allow intelligible and pleasant speech and to avoid injury to the maxillary development. The timing of cleft palate repair is individualized according to the size, placement, and degree of deformity. The surgery may need to be done in stages over a period of several years to achieve the best results. The optimal time for surgical repair of the cleft palate is considered to be between 6 months and 5 years of age. Because the child cannot make certain sounds when starting to talk, undesirable speech habits are formed that are difficult to correct. If surgery must be delayed beyond the third year, a dental speech appliance may help the child develop intelligible speech.

Nursing Process for the Newborn With Cleft Lip and Cleft Palate

The birth of a newborn with a facial deformity may change the atmosphere of the delivery from one of joyous anticipation to one of awkward tension. Parents and family are naturally eager to see and hold their newborn and must be prepared for the shock of seeing the facial disfigurement of a cleft lip. Their emotional reaction to such an obvious malformation is usually much stronger than to a "hidden" defect, such as congenital heart defect. They need encouragement and support, as well as considerable instruction about the newborn's feeding and care.

Assessment

One primary concern in the nursing care of the newborn with a cleft lip with or without a cleft palate is the emotional care of the newborn's family. In interviewing the family and collecting data, explore the family's acceptance of the newborn. Practice active listening with reflective responses, accept the family's emotional responses, and demonstrate complete acceptance of the newborn.

The family caregivers who return to the hospital with their infant for the beginning repair of a cleft palate have already faced the challenges of feeding their infant. Conduct a thorough interview with the caregiver that includes a question about the methods they found to be most effective in feeding the infant.

Physical examination of the infant includes temperature, apical pulse, and respirations. Listen to breath sounds to detect any pulmonary congestion. Observe skin turgor and color, noting any deviations from normal. In addition, observe the infant's neurologic status, noting alertness and responsiveness. Document a complete description of the cleft.

Selected Nursing Diagnoses

Nursing diagnoses for the newborn before surgery may include:

- Imbalanced Nutrition: Less than Body Requirements related to inability to suck secondary to cleft lip
- Compromised Family Coping related to visible physical defect
- Anxiety of family caregivers related to the child's condition and surgical outcome
- Deficient Knowledge of family caregivers related to the care of the child before surgery and the surgical procedure

Nursing diagnoses applicable to the newborn after the surgical repairs are:

- Risk for Aspiration related to a reduced level of consciousness after surgery
- Ineffective Breathing Pattern related to anatomical changes
- Risk for Deficient Fluid Volume related to NPO status after surgery
- Imbalanced Nutrition: Less than Body Requirements related to difficulty in feeding after surgery
- Acute Pain related to surgical procedure
- Risk of Injury to the operative site related to newborn's desire to suck thumb or fingers and anatomical changes
- Risk for Infection related to surgical incision
- Risk for Delayed Growth and Development related to hospitalizations and surgery
- Deficient Knowledge of family caregivers related to long-term aspects of cleft palate

Outcome Identification and Planning: Preoperative Care

Goal setting and planning must be modified to adapt to the surgical plans. If the newborn is to be discharged from the birth hospital to have surgery 1 to 2 months later, nursing care may focus on preparing the family to care for the newborn at home and helping them cope with their emotions. The major goals include maintaining adequate nutrition, increasing family coping, reducing the parents' anxiety and guilt regarding the newborn's physical defect, and preparing parents for the future repair of the cleft lip and palate.

Implementation
Maintaining Adequate Nutrition

The newborn must be in good nutritional condition before surgery can be scheduled. However, feeding the

A

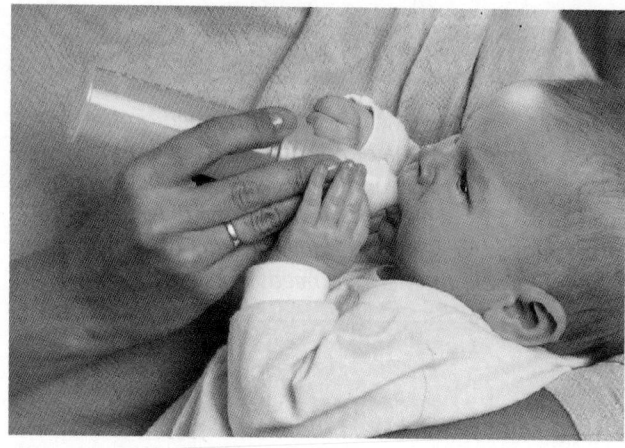
B

■ **Figure 21-14** Specialty feeding devices used for the newborn with a cleft lip or palate include **(A)** special nipples and devices and **(B)** a special feeder.

newborn with a cleft lip or palate before repair is a challenge. Feeding may be time consuming and tedious because the newborn's ability to suck is inadequate. Breast-feeding may be successful because the breast tissue may mold to close the gap. If the newborn cannot breast-feed, the mother's breast milk may be expressed and used instead of formula until after the surgical repair heals. Various nipples and feeding devices may be tried to find the method that works best. A soft nipple with a crosscut made to promote easy flow of milk or formula may work well. A large nipple with holes that allow the milk to drip freely makes sucking easier. If the cleft lip is unilateral, the nipple should be aimed at the unaffected side. The infant should be kept in an upright position during feeding (Fig. 21-14).

If the infant does not have a cleft lip or if the lip has had an early repair, sucking may be learned more easily, even though the suction generated is not as good as in the infant with an intact palate. Lamb's nipples (extra-long nipples) and special cleft palate nipples molded to fit into the open palate area to close the gap have been used with success.

One of the simplest and most effective methods may be the use of an eyedropper or an Asepto syringe with a short piece of rubber tubing on the tip (Breck feeder). The dropper or syringe is used carefully to drip formula into the newborn's mouth at a rate slow enough to allow the newborn to swallow. As the newborn learns to eat, coughing, sputtering, and choking may occur. Be alert for signs of aspiration when feeding the newborn, and teach family caregivers to be alert as well.

Whatever feeding method is used, the experience may be frustrating for both the feeder and the newborn. Have family caregivers practice the feeding techniques under supervision. During the teaching process, give them ample opportunity to ask questions so they feel able to care for the newborn (see Family Teaching Tips: Cleft Lip/Cleft Palate).

Promoting Family Coping

Encourage family members to verbalize their feelings regarding the defect and their disappointment. Convey to the family that their feelings are acceptable and normal. While caring for the newborn, demonstrate behavior that clearly displays acceptance of the newborn. Serve as a model for the family caregivers' attitudes toward the child.

Family Teaching Tips

CLEFT LIP/CLEFT PALATE

- Sucking is important to speech development.
- Holding the baby upright while feeding helps avoid choking.
- Burp the baby frequently because a large amount of air is swallowed during feeding.
- Don't tire the baby. Limit feeding times to 20–30 minutes maximum. If necessary, feed the baby more often.
- Feed strained foods slowly from the side of the spoon in small amounts.
- Don't be alarmed if food seeps through the cleft and out the nose.
- Have baby's ears checked any time he or she has a cold or upper respiratory infection.
- Talk normally to baby (no "baby talk"). Talk often; repeat baby's babbling and cooing. This helps in speech development.
- Try to understand early talking without trying to correct baby.
- Good mouth care is very important.
- Early dental care is essential to observe teething and prevent caries.

Cultural Snapshot

In some cultures, genetic defects are blamed on the mother—something she did or ate, stress or trauma that occurred during pregnancy, viewing a child with a defect caused her child to have the same defect. The mother may have feelings of guilt or fears of being an unacceptable mother and needs nursing support.

Reducing Family Anxiety

Give the family caregivers information about cleft repairs. Pamphlets are available that present photographs of before and after corrections that will answer some of their questions. Encourage them to ask questions and reassure them that any question is valid.

Providing Family Teaching

By the time the infant is actually admitted for the repair, the family will have received a great amount of information, but all families need additional support throughout the procedure. Explain the usual routine of preoperative, intraoperative, and postoperative care. Written information is helpful, but be certain the parents understand the information. Simple things are important; show families where they may wait during surgery, inform them how long the surgery should last, tell them about the postanesthesia care unit procedure, and let them know where the surgeon will expect to find them to report on the surgery.

Outcome Identification and Planning: Postoperative Care

Major goals for the postoperative care of the infant who is hospitalized for surgical repair of cleft lip or palate include preventing aspiration, improving respiration, maintaining adequate fluid volume and nutritional requirements, relieving pain, preventing injury and infection to the surgical site, promoting normal growth and development, and increasing the family caregivers' knowledge about the child's long-term care.

Implementation
Preventing Aspiration and Improving Respiration

To facilitate drainage of mucus and secretions, position the infant on the side, never on the abdomen, after a cleft lip repair. The infant may be placed on the side or the abdomen after a cleft palate repair. Watch the infant closely in the immediate postoperative period. Do not put anything in the infant's mouth to clear mucus because of the danger of damaging the surgical site, particularly with a palate repair.

Immediately after a palate repair, the infant must change from a mouth-breathing pattern to nasal breathing. This change may frustrate the infant, but the infant positioned to ease breathing and given encouragement should be able to adjust quickly.

Monitoring Fluid Volume

In the immediate postoperative period, the infant needs parenteral fluids. Follow all the usual precautions: check placement, discoloration of the site, swelling, and flow rate every 2 hours. Document intake and output accurately. Parenteral fluids are continued until the infant can take oral fluids without vomiting.

Maintaining Adequate Nutrition

As soon as the infant is no longer nauseated (vomiting should be avoided if possible), the surgeon usually permits clear liquids. After the cleft lip repair, no tension should be placed on the suture line, to prevent the sutures from pulling apart and leaving a scar. A specialized feeder may need to be used because bottle or breast-feeding may increase the tension on the suture line.

For an infant who has had a palate repair, no nipples, spoons, or straws are permitted; only a drinking glass or a cup is recommended. A favorite cup from home may be reassuring to the older infant. Offer clear liquids such as flavored gelatin water, apple juice, and synthetic fruit-flavored drinks. Red juices should not be given because they may conceal bleeding. Infants do not usually like broth. The diet is increased to full liquid, and the infant is usually discharged on a soft diet. When permitted, foods such as cooked infant cereals, ice cream, and flavored gelatin are often favorites. The surgeon determines the progression of the diet. Nothing hard or sharp should be placed in the infant's mouth. After each feeding, clear water is used to rinse the mouth and suture line.

Relieving Pain

Observe the infant for signs of pain or discomfort from the surgery. Administer ordered analgesics as needed. Relieving pain not only comforts the infant, but may also prevent crying, which is important because of the danger of disrupting the suture line. Make every effort to prevent the infant with a lip repair from crying to prevent excessive tension on the suture line.

Preventing Postoperative Injury

Continuous, skilled observation is essential. Swollen mouth tissues cause excessive secretion of mucus that is handled poorly by a small infant. For the first few postoperative hours, never leave the infant alone because aspiration of mucus occurs quickly and easily. Because nothing is permitted in the infant's mouth, particularly the thumb or finger, elbow restraints are necessary. The thumb, although comforting, may quickly undo the repair or cause undesirable scarring along the suture line. The infant's ultimate happiness and well-being must take precedence over immediate satisfaction. Accustoming the infant to elbow restraints gradually before admission is helpful.

Elbow restraints must be applied properly and checked frequently (see Fig, 30-2 in Chapter 30). Place the restraints firmly around the arm and pin to the infant's shirt or gown to prevent them from sliding down below the elbow. The infant's arms can move freely but cannot bend at the elbows to reach the face. Apply the restraint snugly, but do not allow the circulation to be hindered. The older infant may need to be placed in a jacket restraint. The use of restraints must be documented.

Remove restraints at least every 2 hours; remove them only one at a time, and control the released arm so that the thumb or fingers do not pop into the mouth. Explore various means of comforting the infant. Talk to the infant continuously while providing care. Inspect and massage the skin, apply lotion, and perform range-of-motion exercises. Replace restraints when they become soiled.

Preventing Infection

Aseptic technique is important while caring for the infant undergoing lip or palate repair. Good hand-washing technique is essential. Instruct the family caregivers about the importance of preventing anyone with an upper respiratory infection from visiting the infant. Observe for signs of otitis media that may occur from drainage into the eustachian tube.

Care of Lip Suture Line

The lip suture line is left uncovered after surgery and must be kept clean and dry to prevent infection and subsequent scarring. A wire bow called a Logan bar or a butterfly closure is applied across the upper lip and attached to the cheeks with adhesive tape to prevent tension on the sutures caused by crying or other facial movement (Fig. 21-15). Gently clean the infant's mouth with tepid water or clear liquid after feeding to clear the suture area of any food or liquids. Carefully clean the sutures after feeding and as often as necessary to prevent

Some nurses find this approach helpful.
Playing "Peek-a-Boo" and other infant games will help to comfort and entertain the infant in restraints; however "Patty Cake" does not work well with an infant in elbow restraints.

collection of dried formula or serum. Clean the sutures gently with sterile cotton swabs and saline or the solution of the surgeon's choice. Application of an ointment, such as bacitracin, may also be ordered. Care of the suture line is extremely important because it has a direct effect on the cosmetic appearance of the repair. Frequent cleaning is essential as long as the sutures are in place. Teach the family how to care for the suture line because the infant will probably be discharged before the sutures are removed (7–10 days after surgery). The infant probably will be allowed to suck on a soft nipple at this time.

Promoting Sensory Stimulation

The infant needs stimulating, safe toys in the crib. Nurses and family caregivers must use every opportunity to provide sensory stimulation. Talking to the infant, cuddling and holding him or her, and responding to cries are important interventions. Provide freedom from restraints within the limitations of safety as much as possible. One caregiver should be assigned to provide stability and consistency of care. Family caregivers and health care personnel must encourage the older child to use speech and help enhance the child's self-esteem. A baby experiences emotional frustration because of restraints, so satisfaction must be provided in other ways. Rocking, cuddling, and other soothing techniques are an important part of nursing care and family caregiving.

Providing Family Teaching

After effective surgery and skilled, careful nursing care, the appearance of the baby's face should be improved greatly. The scar fades in time. Family caregivers need to know that the baby will probably need a slight adjustment of the vermilion line in later childhood, but they can expect a repair that is barely, if at all, noticeable.

Cleft lip and cleft palate centers have teams of specialists who can provide the services that these children and their families need through infancy, preschool, and the school years. Explain to the caregivers the services offered by the pediatrician, plastic surgeon, orthodontist, speech therapist, nutritionist, and public or home health nurse. These professionals can give explanations and counseling about the child's diet, speech training, immunizations, and general health. Encourage family caregivers to ask them any questions they may have. Be alert for any evidence that the caregivers need additional information and arrange appropriate meetings.

Dental care for the deciduous teeth is even more important than usual. The incidence of dental caries is high in children with a cleft palate, but preservation of the deciduous teeth is important for the best results in speech and appearance.

Evaluation: Goals and Expected Outcomes
Preoperative

Goal: The newborn will show appropriate weight gain.

■ **Figure 21-15** Logan bar for easing strain on sutures.

Expected Outcome:

- The newborn's weight increases at a predetermined goal of 1 oz or more per day.

Goal: The family will demonstrate acceptance of the newborn.

Expected Outcomes: Family caregivers

- verbalize their feelings about the newborn.
- cuddle and talk to the newborn.

Goal: The family caregiver's anxiety will be reduced.

Expected Outcomes: Family caregivers

- ask appropriate questions about surgery and openly discuss their concerns.
- voice reasonable expectations.

Goal: The family will learn how to care for the newborn and will have an understanding of surgical procedures.

Expected Outcomes: Family caregivers

- ask appropriate questions.
- demonstrate how to feed the newborn before surgery.
- describe the surgical procedures.

Postoperative

Goal: The infant's respiratory tract will remain clear, the infant will breathe easily, and the respiratory rate will be within normal limits.

Expected Outcomes: The infant

- has clear lung sounds with no aspiration.
- has a respiratory rate that stays within normal range.

Goal: The infant will adjust his or her breathing pattern.

Expected Outcomes: The infant

- breathes nasally with little stress.
- maintains normal respirations.

Goal: The infant will show signs of adequate hydration during NPO period.

Expected Outcomes: The newborn

- has good skin turgor and moist mucous membranes.
- has adequate urine output.
- shows no evidence of parenteral fluid infiltration.

Goal: The infant will have adequate caloric intake and retain and tolerate oral nutrition.

Expected Outcomes: The infant

- gains 0.75 to 1 oz/day (22–30 g/day) if younger than 6 months of age or 0.5 to 0.75 oz/day (13–22 g/day) if older than 6 months.
- does not experience nausea or vomiting.

Goal: The infant's pain and discomfort will be minimized.

Expected Outcome: The infant

- rests quietly, does not cry, and is not fretful.

Goal: The surgical site will remain free of injury.

Expected Outcomes: The infant

- has an intact surgical site.

- puts nothing into the mouth such as straws, sharp objects, thumb, or fingers.

Goal: The infant's incision site will remain free of signs and symptoms of infection.

Expected Outcomes:

- The incisional site is clean with no redness or drainage.
- The infant's temperature is within normal limits.
- The caregivers and family members practice good hand-washing and aseptic techniques.

Goal: The infant will show evidence of normal growth and development.

Expected Outcomes: The infant

- is content most of the time and responds appropriately to the caregiver and family.
- engages in age- and development-appropriate activities within the limits of restraints.

Goal: The family will learn how to care for the infant's long-term needs.

Expected Outcomes: The family caregivers

- ask appropriate questions and respond appropriately to staff queries.
- describe services available for the child's long-term care.

Esophageal Atresia and Tracheoesophageal Fistula

Atresia is the absence of a normal body opening or the abnormal closure of a body passage. Esophageal atresia (EA) with or without fistula into the trachea is a serious congenital anomaly and is among the most common anomalies causing respiratory distress. This condition occurs in about 1 in 2,500 live births. Several types of EA occur; in more than 90% of affected newborns, the upper, or proximal, end of the esophagus ends in a blind pouch, and the lower, or distal, segment from the stomach is connected to the trachea by a fistulous tract (Fig. 21-16). This is referred to as a tracheoesophageal fistula.

Clinical Manifestations

Any mucus or fluid that a newborn swallows enters the blind pouch of the esophagus. This pouch soon fills and overflows, usually resulting in aspiration into the trachea. Few other conditions depend so greatly on careful nursing observation for early diagnosis and, therefore, improved chances of survival. The newborn with this disorder has frothing and excessive drooling and periods of respiratory distress with choking and cyanosis. Many newborns have difficulty with mucus, but be alert to the possibility of an anomaly and report such difficulties immediately. No feeding should be given until the newborn has been examined.

If early signs are overlooked and feeding is attempted, the newborn chokes, coughs, and regurgitates as the food

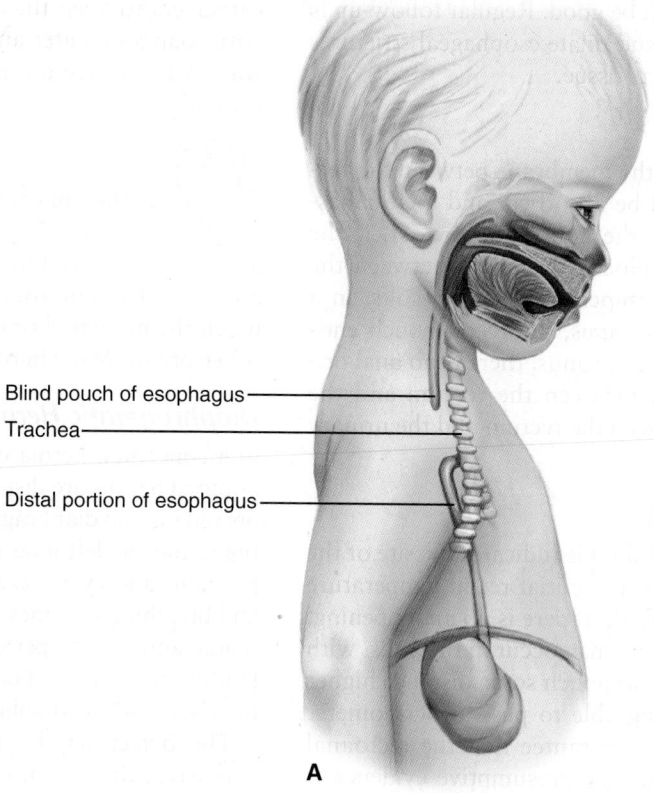

Blind pouch of esophagus———
Trachea———

Distal portion of esophagus———

A

■ **Figure 21-16** Types of esophageal atresia. **(A)** In the most common form of esophageal atresia, the esophagus ends in a blind pouch, and a fistula connects the trachea with the distal portion of the esophagus. **(B)** Both segments of the esophagus are blind pouches. **(C)** The esophagus is continuous but with a narrowed segment. **(D)** The upper segment of the esophagus opens into trachea via a fistula.

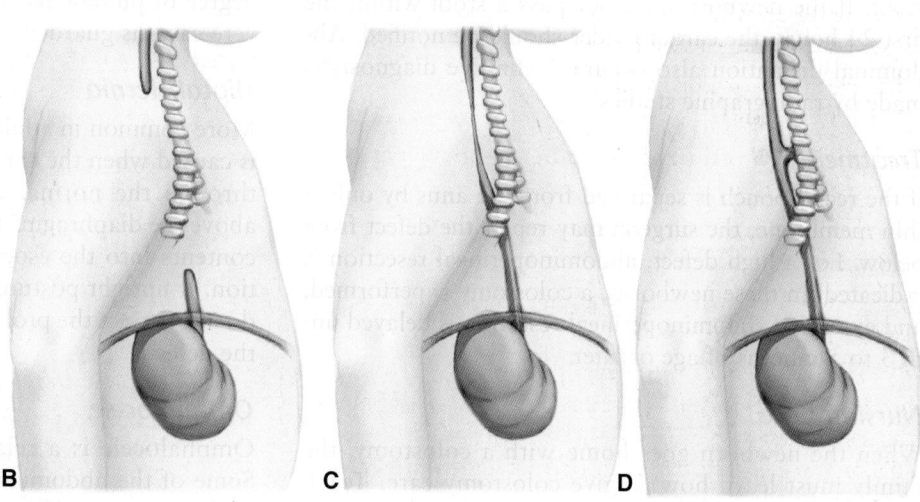

B   **C**   **D**

enters the blind pouch. The newborn becomes deeply cyanotic and appears to be in severe respiratory distress. During this process, some of the formula may be aspirated, resulting in pneumonitis, increasing the risk of surgery. This newborn's life may depend on your careful observation. If there is a fistula of the distal portion of the esophagus into the trachea, the gastric contents may reflux into the lungs and cause a chemical pneumonitis.

Treatment and Nursing Care

Surgical intervention is necessary to correct the defect. Timing of the surgery depends on the surgeon's prefer-

ence, the anomaly, and the newborn's condition. Aspiration of mucus must be prevented, and continuous, gentle suction may be used. The newborn needs intravenous fluids to maintain optimal hydration. The first stage of surgery may involve a gastrostomy and a method of draining the proximal esophageal pouch. A chest tube is inserted to drain chest fluids. An end-to-end anastomosis is sometimes possible. If the repair is complex, surgery may need to be done in stages.

Often these defects occur in premature newborns, so additional factors may complicate the surgical repair and prognosis. If there are no other major problems, the long-term outcome should be good. Regular follow-up is necessary to observe for and dilate esophageal strictures that may be caused by scar tissue.

Imperforate Anus

Early in intrauterine life, the membrane between the rectum and the anus should be absorbed, and a clear passage from the rectum to the anus should exist. If the membrane remains and blocks the union between the rectum and the anus, an **imperforate anus** results. In a newborn with imperforate anus, the rectal pouch ends blindly at a distance above the anus; there is no anal orifice. A fistula may exist between the rectum and the vagina in females or between the rectum and the urinary tract in males.

Clinical Manifestations

In some newborns, only a dimple indicates the site of the anus (Fig. 21-17A). When the initial rectal temperature is attempted, it is apparent that there is no anal opening. However, a shallow opening may occur in the anus, with the rectum ending in a blind pouch some distance higher (Fig. 21-17B). Thus, being able to pass a thermometer into the rectum does not guarantee that the rectoanal canal is normal. More reliable presumptive evidence is obtained by watching carefully for the first meconium stool. If the newborn does not pass a stool within the first 24 hours, the care provider should be notified. Abdominal distention also occurs. Definitive diagnosis is made by radiographic studies.

Treatment

If the rectal pouch is separated from the anus by only a thin membrane, the surgeon may repair the defect from below. For a high defect, abdominoperineal resection is indicated. In these newborns, a colostomy is performed, and extensive abdominoperineal resection is delayed until 3 to 5 months of age or later.

Nursing Care

When the newborn goes home with a colostomy, the family must learn how to give colostomy care. Teach caregivers to keep the area around the colostomy clean with soap and water and to diaper the baby in the usual way. A protective ointment is useful to protect the skin around the colostomy.

Hernias

A **hernia** is the abnormal protrusion of a part of an organ through a weak spot or other abnormal opening in a body wall. Complications occur depending on the amount of circulatory impairment involved and how much the herniated organ impairs the functioning of another organ. Most hernias can be repaired surgically.

Diaphragmatic Hernia

In a congenital hernia of the diaphragm, some of the abdominal organs are displaced into the left chest through an opening in the diaphragm. The heart is pushed toward the right, and the left lung is compressed. Rapid, labored respirations and cyanosis are present on the first day of life, and breathing becomes increasingly difficult. Surgery is essential and may be performed as an emergency procedure. During surgery, the abdominal viscera are withdrawn from the chest and the diaphragmatic defect is closed.

This defect may be minimal and repaired easily, or so extensive, that pulmonary tissue has failed to develop normally. The outcome of surgical repair depends on the degree of pulmonary development. The prognosis in severe cases is guarded.

Hiatal Hernia

More common in adults than in newborns, hiatal hernia is caused when the cardiac portion of the stomach slides through the normal esophageal hiatus into the area above the diaphragm. This action causes reflux of gastric contents into the esophagus and subsequent regurgitation. If upright posture and modified feeding techniques do not correct the problem, surgery is necessary to repair the defect.

Omphalocele

Omphalocele is a relatively rare congenital anomaly. Some of the abdominal contents protrude through into

■ **Figure 21-17** Imperforate anus (anal atresia). **(A)** Membrane between anus and rectum. **(B)** Rectum ending in a blind pouch at a distance above the perineum.

A

B

■ **Figure 21-18** Omphalocele with membrane sac covering the organs.

■ **Figure 21-19** Small umbilical hernia in newborn.

the root of the umbilical cord and form a sac lying on the abdomen. This sac may be small, with only a loop of bowel, or large and containing much of the intestine and the liver (Fig. 21-18). The sac is covered with peritoneal membrane instead of skin.

These defects may be detected during prenatal ultrasonography so that prompt repair may be anticipated. At birth, the defect should be covered immediately with gauze moistened in sterile saline, which then may be covered with plastic wrap to prevent heat loss. Surgical replacement of the organs into the abdomen may be difficult with a large omphalocele because there may not be enough space in the abdominal cavity. Other congenital defects often are present.

With large omphaloceles, surgery may be postponed and the surgeon will suture skin over the defect, creating a large hernia. As the child grows, the abdomen may enlarge enough to allow replacement.

Umbilical Hernia

Normally the ring that encircled the fetal end of the umbilical cord closes gradually and spontaneously after birth. When this closure is incomplete, portions of omentum and intestine protrude through the opening. More common in preterm and African-American newborns, umbilical hernia is largely a cosmetic problem (Fig. 21-19). Although upsetting to parents, umbilical hernia is associated with little or no morbidity. In rare instances, the bowel may strangulate in the sac and require immediate surgery. Almost all of these hernias close spontaneously by the age of 3 years; hernias that do not close, should be corrected surgically before the child enters school.

Did you know?

Some people believe that taping a coin on an umbilical hernia will help reduce the hernia. This can actually result in a serious problem for the newborn and should not be done.

Inguinal Hernia

Primarily seen in males, inguinal hernias occur when the small sac of peritoneum surrounding the testes fails to close off after the testes descend from the abdominal sac into the scrotum. This failure allows the intestine to slip into the inguinal canal, with resultant swelling (Fig. 21-20). If the intestine becomes trapped (incarcerated) and the circulation to the trapped intestine is impaired (strangulated), surgery is necessary to prevent intestinal obstruction and gangrene of the bowel. As a preventive measure, inguinal hernias normally are repaired as soon as they are diagnosed.

Test Yourself

✔ What are two major concerns for the newborn with a cleft lip or cleft palate?

✔ What is a potential complication for the newborn who has EA?

✔ How are hernias most often treated?

■ **Figure 21-20** Inguinal hernia: note the bulge in the groin area.

A   B

▮ Figure 21-21 Exstrophy of the bladder. **(A)** Prior to surgery, note the bright-red color of the bladder. **(B)** Following surgical repair.

GENITOURINARY TRACT DEFECTS

Most congenital anomalies of the genitourinary tract are not life threatening, but may present social problems with lifelong implications for the child and family. Thus, early recognition and supportive, understanding care are essential.

Hypospadias and Epispadias

Hypospadias is a congenital condition affecting males in which the urethra terminates on the ventral (underside) surface of the penis, instead of at the tip. A cord-like anomaly (a **chordee**) extends from the scrotum to the penis, pulling the penis downward in an arc. Urination is not affected, but the boy cannot void while standing in the normal male fashion. Surgical repair is desirable between the ages of 6 and 18 months, before body image and castration anxiety become problems. Microscopic surgery makes early repair possible. Surgical repair is often accomplished in one stage and is often done as outpatient surgery. These newborns should not be circumcised because the foreskin is used in the repair. Severe hypospadias may require additional surgical procedures.

In **epispadias,** the opening is on the dorsal (top) surface of the penis. This condition often occurs with exstrophy of the bladder. Surgical repair is indicated.

Exstrophy of the Bladder

Exstrophy of the bladder is a urinary tract malformation that occurs in 1 in 30,000 live births in the United States. It is usually accompanied by other anomalies, such as epispadias, cleft scrotum, cryptorchidism (undescended testes), a shortened penis, and cleft clitoris. It also is associated with malformed pelvic musculature, resulting in a prolapsed rectum and inguinal hernias. Children with this defect have a widely split symphysis pubis and posterolaterally rotated hip sockets, causing a waddling gait.

In this condition, the anterior surface of the urinary bladder lies open on the lower abdomen (Fig. 21-21). The exposed mucosa is red and sensitive to touch and allows direct passage of urine to the outside. This condition makes the area vulnerable to infection and trauma. Surgical closure of the bladder is preferred within the first 48 hours of life. Final surgical correction is completed before the child goes to school. If bladder repair is not done early in the child's life, the family caregivers must be taught how to care for this condition and how to deal with their feelings toward this less-than-perfect child. Their emotional reaction may be further complicated if the malformation is so severe that the sex of the child may be determined only by a chromosome test (see the following section on ambiguous genitalia).

Nursing care of the newborn with exstrophy of the bladder should be directed toward preventing infection, preventing skin irritation around the seeping mucosa, meeting the newborn's need for touch and cuddling, and educating and supporting the family during this crisis.

Ambiguous Genitalia

If a child's external sex organs did not follow a normal development in utero, at birth it may not be possible to determine by observation if the child is a male or female. The external sexual organs are either incompletely or abnormally formed. This condition is called ambiguous genitalia. Although rare, the birth of a newborn with ambiguous genitalia presents a highly charged emotional climate and has possible long-range social implications.

Regardless of the cause, it is important to establish the genetic sex and the sex of rearing as early as possible so that surgical correction of anomalies may occur before the child begins to function in a sex-related social role. Authorities believe that the newborn's anatomical structure, rather than the genetic sex, should determine the sex of rearing. It is possible to construct a functional vagina surgically and to administer hormones to offer an anatomically incomplete female a somewhat normal life. Currently, it is impossible to offer comparable surgical reconstruction to males with an inadequate penis. Parents may feel guilt, anxiety, and confusion about their child's condition and need understanding and support to help them cope with this emergency.

SKELETAL SYSTEM DEFECTS

Skeletal system defects in the newborn may be noted and treatment begun soon after birth. Some skeletal system defects may not be evident until later in the child's life. Two common skeletal defects are congenital talipes equinovarus (clubfoot) and hip dysplasia (dislocation of the hip). Children with these conditions and their parents often face long periods of exhausting, costly treatment; therefore, they need continuing support, encouragement, and education.

Congenital Talipes Equinovarus

Congenital clubfoot is a deformity in which the entire foot is inverted, the heel is drawn up, and the forefoot is adducted. The Latin word *talus,* meaning ankle, and *pes,* meaning foot, make up the word *talipes,* which is used in connection with many foot deformities. *Equinus,* or plantar flexion, and *varus,* or inversion, denotes the kind of foot deformity present in this condition. The equinovarus foot has a clublike appearance, thus the term "clubfoot" (Fig. 21-22*A*). This defect is usually evident at birth.

Congenital talipes equinovarus is the most common congenital foot deformity, occurring in about 1 in 1,000 births. It appears as a single anomaly or in connection with other defects, such as myelomeningocele. It may be bilateral (both feet) or unilateral (one foot). The cause is unclear, although a hereditary factor is observed occasionally. One hypothesis is that it results from an arrested embryonic growth of the foot during the first trimester of pregnancy.

Clinical Manifestations

Talipes equinovarus is detected easily in a newborn but must be differentiated from a persisting "position of comfort" assumed in utero. The positional deformity may be corrected easily by the use of passive exercise, but the true clubfoot deformity is fixed. The positional deformity should be explained to the parents immediately to prevent anxiety.

Treatment

Nonsurgical Treatment

If treatment is started during the neonatal period, correction can usually be accomplished by manipulation and bandaging or by application of a cast. The cast often is applied while the newborn is still in the neonatal nursery. While the cast is applied, the foot is first moved gently into as nearly normal a position as possible. Force should not be used. If the family caregiver can be pres-

▮ **Figure 21-22** **(A)** Bilateral clubfoot. **(B)** Casting for clubfoot in typical overcorrected position.

ent to help hold the newborn while the cast is applied, the caregiver will have the opportunity to understand what is being done. The very-young newborn gets satisfaction from sucking, so a pacifier helps prevent squirming while the cast is applied.

The cast is applied over the foot and ankle (and usually to midthigh) to hold the knee in right-angle flexion (Fig. 21-22*B*). Casts are changed frequently to provide gradual, atraumatic correction—every few days for the first several weeks, then every week or two. Treatment is usually continued for a matter of months until radiograph and clinical observation confirm complete correction.

Any cast applied to a child's body should have some type of waterproof material protecting the skin from the cast's sharp plaster edges. One method is to apply strips of adhesive vertically around the edges of the cast in a manner called "petaling." To petal a cast, strips of adhesive are cut 2 or 3 in long and 1 in wide. One end is notched, and the other end is cut pointed to aid in smooth application. Family caregivers must be taught cast care.

After correction with a cast, a Denis Browne splint with shoes attached may be used to maintain the correction for another 6 months or longer (Fig. 21-23). After overcorrection has been attained, the child should wear a special clubfoot shoe, which is a laced

■ **Figure 21-23** A Denis Browne splint with shoes attached is used to correct clubfoot.

shoe whose turning out makes it appear that the shoe is being worn on the wrong foot. The Denis Browne splint still may be worn at night, and the caregivers should carry out passive exercises of the foot. The older infant may resist wearing the splint, so family caregivers must be taught the importance of gentle, but firm, insistence that the splint be worn.

Surgical Treatment

Children who do not respond to nonsurgical measures, especially older children, need surgical correction. This approach involves several procedures, depending on the age of the child and the degree of the deformity. It may involve lengthening the Achilles tendon and operating on the bony structure for the child older than 10 years. Prolonged observation after correction by either means should be carried out, at least until adolescence; any recurrence is treated promptly.

Congenital Hip Dysplasia

Congenital hip dysplasia results from defective development of the acetabulum, with or without dislocation.

The malformed acetabulum permits dislocation, with the head of the femur becoming displaced upward and backward. The condition is difficult to recognize during early infancy. When there is a family history of the defect, increased observation of the young newborn is indicated. The condition is often bilateral and about six times more common in girls than in boys.

Clinical Manifestations

Early recognition and treatment before an infant starts to stand or walk are extremely important for successful correction. The first examination should be part of the newborn examination. Experienced examiners may detect an audible click when examining the newborn using the Barlow's sign and Ortolani's maneuver (see Chapter 13, Nursing Procedure 13-2). These tests, used together on one hip at a time, show a tendency for dislocation of the hip in adduction and abduction and should be conducted only by an experienced practitioner. The tests are effective only for the first month; after this time, the clicks disappear. Signs that are useful after this include:

■ Asymmetry of the gluteal skin folds (higher on the affected side) (Fig. 21-24*A*).
■ Limited abduction of the affected hip (Fig. 21-24*B*). This is tested by placing the infant in a dorsal recumbent position with the knees flexed, then abducting both knees passively until they reach the examination table without resistance. If dislocation is present, the affected side cannot be abducted more than 45 degrees.
■ Apparent shortening of the femur (Fig. 21-24*C*).

After the child has started walking, later signs include lordosis, swayback, protruding abdomen, shortened extremity, duck-waddle gait, and a positive Trendelenburg sign. To elicit this sign, the child stands on the affected leg and raises the normal leg. The pelvis tilts down, rather than up toward the unaffected side. X-ray studies usually

A   **B**   **C**

■ **Figure 21-24** Signs of congenital hip dysplasia. **(A)** Asymmetry of the gluteal folds of the thighs. **(B)** Limited abduction of the affected hip. **(C)** Apparent shortening of the femur.

■ **Figure 21-25** A Pavlik harness for treatment of congenital hip dysplasia. The harness is composed of shoulder straps, stirrups, and a chest strap. It is placed on both legs, even if only one hip is dislocated.

are made to confirm the diagnosis in the older newborn. Uncorrected dislocation causes limping, easy fatigue, hip and low back discomfort, and postural deformities.

Treatment

Correction may be started in the newborn period by placing two or three diapers on the infant to hold the legs abducted, in a froglike position. Cloth diapers work best for this purpose. Another treatment option, when the dislocation is discovered during the first few months, consists of manipulation of the femur into position and the application of a brace. The most common type of brace used is the Pavlik harness (Fig. 21-25). The primary care provider assesses the infant weekly while the infant is in the harness and adjusts the harness to align the femur gradually. Sometimes, no additional treatment is needed.

If treatment is delayed until after the child has started to walk or if earlier treatment is ineffective, open reduction followed by application of a spica cast usually is needed. A spica or "hip spica cast," as it is often called, covers the lower part of the body, from the waist down and either one or both legs, usually leaving the feet open. The cast maintains the legs in a frog-like position, with the hips abducted. There may be a bar placed between the legs to help support the cast. After the cast is removed, a metal or plastic brace is applied to keep the legs in wide abduction.

Nursing Process for the Newborn in an Orthopedic Device or Cast

Although the actual hospitalization of the infant is relatively short (if no other abnormalities require hospitalization), it is important to teach the family about cast

care or care of the infant in an orthopedic device, such as a Pavlik harness. Determine the family caregiver's ability to understand and cooperate in the infant's care. Emotional support of the family is important.

Assessment

The observation of the infant varies depending on the orthopedic device or cast used. Immediately after the application of a cast, observe for signs that the cast is drying evenly. Check the toes for circulation and movement. Check the skin at the edges of the cast for signs of pressure or irritation. If an open reduction has been performed, observe the child for signs of shock and bleeding in the immediate postoperative period.

Selected Nursing Diagnoses

- Acute Pain related to discomfort of orthopedic device or cast
- Risk for Impaired Skin Integrity related to pressure of the cast on the skin surface
- Risk for Delayed Growth and Development related to restricted mobility secondary to orthopedic device or cast
- Deficient Knowledge of family caregivers related to home care of the infant in the orthopedic device or cast

Outcome Identification and Planning

Goals include relieving pain and discomfort, maintaining skin integrity, promoting growth and development, and increasing family knowledge about the infant's home care. Goals for the family focus on the desire for correction of the defect with minimal disruption to the infant's growth and development and care of the infant at home.

Implementation
Providing Comfort Measures

The infant may be irritable and fussy because of the restricted movement caused by the device or cast. Useful methods of soothing the infant include nonnutritive sucking, stroking, cuddling, and talking. If irritability seems excessive, check the infant for signs of irritation from the device or cast. The infant in a cast may be held after the cast is completely dry. Do not remove the harness

Cultural Snapshot

Cradleboards are devices used as baby carriers and to provide security for newborns in some cultures. Using a cradleboard can sometimes aggravate hip dysplasia. Encourage the caregivers to use thick diapers, sometimes more than one, to help in keeping the hips in a slightly abducted position when the child is carried on a cradleboard. Cloth diapers work better than disposable diapers for this purpose.

unless specific permission for bathing is granted by the provider. Teach the family caregivers how to reapply the harness correctly. The infant in a Pavlik harness is not as difficult to handle as the infant in a cast.

Promoting Skin Integrity

For the first 24 to 48 hours after application of a cast, place the infant on a firm mattress and support position changes with firm pillows. When handling the cast, use the palms of the hands to avoid excessive pressure on the cast. Carefully inspect the skin around the cast edges for signs of irritation, redness, or edema. Petal the edges of the cast around the waist and toes and protect the cast with plastic covering around the perineal area. If the covering becomes soiled, remove it, wash and dry thoroughly, then reapply or replace it. With the Pavlik harness, monitor the skin under the straps frequently and massage it gently to promote circulation. To relieve pressure under the shoulder straps, place extra padding in the area.

Diapering can be a challenge for the infant in a cast. Take great care to protect the diaper area from becoming soiled and moist. Disposable diapers are usually the most effective way to provide good protection of the cast and prevent leakage.

Avoid using powders and lotions because caking of the powder or lotion can cause areas of irritation. Daily sponge baths are important and must include close attention to the skin under the straps of the device or around the edge of the cast.

Observe the infant in a cast carefully for any restriction of breathing caused by tightness over the abdomen and lower chest area. Vomiting after a feeding may be an indication that the cast is too tight over the stomach. In either case, the cast may have to be removed and reapplied.

Prevent the older infant or child from pushing any small particles of food or toys down into the cast.

Providing Sensory Stimulation

Because the infant will be in the device or cast for an extended period when much growth and development occur, provide him or her with stimulation of a tactile nature. Provide mobiles, musical toys, and stuffed toys. Do not permit the infant to cry for long periods. Keep feeding times relaxed. Hold the infant if possible and encourage interaction. Provide a pacifier if the infant desires it. Encourage activities that use the infant's free hands. The older infant may enjoy looking at picture books and interacting with siblings. Diversionary activities should include transporting the infant to other areas in the home or in the car. Strollers and car seats may be adapted to allow safe transportation.

Here's an idea.
For older infants or toddlers in a hip spica cast, a wagon may provide a convenient and fun way to explore the environment, encourage stimulation, and promote independence.

Providing Family Teaching

Determine the family caregiver's knowledge and design a thorough teaching plan because the infant will be cared for at home for most of the time. Use complete explanations, written guidelines, demonstrations, and return demonstrations. Provide the family with a resource person who may be called when a question arises and encourage them to feel free to call that person. Make definite plans for return visits to have the device or cast checked. The caregiver needs to understand the importance of keeping these appointments. Provide a public or home health nurse referral when appropriate (see Nursing Care Plan 21-1: The Infant With an Orthopedic Cast).

Evaluation: Goals and Expected Outcomes

Goal: The infant will show signs of being comfortable.
Expected Outcomes: The infant

- is alert and content with no long periods of fussiness.
- interacts with caregivers with cooing, smiling, and eye contact.

Goal: The infant's skin will remain intact.
Expected Outcomes:

- The infant's skin around the edges of the cast shows no signs of redness or irritation.
- The diaper area is clean, dry and intact, and protected from soiling.

Goal: The infant will attain appropriate developmental milestones.
Expected Outcomes: The infant

- responds positively to audio, visual, and diversionary activities.
- shows age-appropriate development.

Goal: The family caregivers will learn home care of the infant.
Expected Outcome:

- The family demonstrates care of the infant in the orthopedic device or cast, asks pertinent questions, and identifies a resource person to call.

Test Yourself

✔ How is congenital clubfoot treated?
✔ What three signs are seen in the infant with a congenital hip dysplasia?
✔ List five nursing interventions used to promote skin integrity for an infant in a cast.

INBORN ERRORS OF METABOLISM

Inborn errors of metabolism are hereditary disorders that affect metabolism. These disorders include phenylketonuria, galactosemia, congenital hypothyroidism, and maple syrup urine disease. Nursing care for the newborn

Nursing Care Plan 21-1

THE INFANT WITH AN ORTHOPEDIC CAST

Six-month-old Melissa Davis has right congenital hip dysplasia. After a trial with a Pavlik harness, she has been placed in a hip spica cast. The cast has just been applied. This is a new experience for her and her caregiver.

NURSING DIAGNOSIS
Acute Pain related to discomfort of hip spica cast

GOAL: The infant will show signs of being comfortable.

OUTCOME CRITERIA
- The infant is alert and contended.
- The infant has no long periods of fussiness.
- The infant interacts with caregivers by cooing, smiling, and eye contact.

Nursing Interventions	*Rationale*
Check edges of cast for smoothness; petal edges of cast.	Rough edges can cause irritation and discomfort.
Soothe by stroking, cuddling, and talking to infant.	These comfort measures help the infant feel safe, secure, and loved and provide distraction from discomfort and restriction of cast.
Provide infant with a pacifier.	Nonnutritive sucking is a means of self-comfort.

NURSING DIAGNOSIS
Risk for Impaired Skin Integrity related to pressure of the cast on the skin surface

GOAL: The infant's skin will remain intact.

OUTCOME CRITERIA
- The infant's skin around the cast shows no signs of redness or irritation.
- The infant's skin in the diaper area is clean, dry, and intact with no signs of perineal redness of irritation.

Nursing Interventions	*Rationale*
Place infant on firm mattress for 24 to 48 hours until cast is dry.	The cast is still pliable until dry. Undue pressure on any point must be avoided.
Use palms when handling damp cast.	Using palms instead of fingers prevents excessive pressure in any one area.
Petal all edges of cast.	Petalling provides a smooth edge along cast to avoid irritation.
Inspect skin around the cast edges for redness and irritation during each shift.	Early signs of irritation indicate areas that may need added protection.
Protect perineal area of cast with waterproof covering.	Urine and feces can easily cause irritation, skin breakdown, or a softened and malodorous cast.
Remove, wash, and thoroughly dry perineal covering if wet or soiled.	A clean, dry perineal cast protective covering decreases the problem of breakdown.

NURSING DIAGNOSIS
Risk for Delayed Growth and Development related to restricted mobility secondary to hip spica cast

GOAL: The infant will attain appropriate developmental milestones.

OUTCOME CRITERIA
- The infant responds positively to audio, visual, and diversional activities.
- The infant smiles, coos, and squeals in response to family caregivers.
- The infant shows age-appropriate development.

(continues on page 506)

Nursing Care Plan 21-1 *(continued)*

THE INFANT WITH AN ORTHOPEDIC CAST

Nursing Interventions	Rationale
Provide mobiles, musical toys, stuffed toys, and toys infant can manipulate. Encourage caregiver to interact with infant during feeding. Plan activities that include changes of environment, such as moving to the playroom in the hospital or to a different room in the home.	Visual, tactile, and auditory stimulation are important for infant development. Interacting (babbling, cooing) with others in her or his environment encourages development. Environmental variety provides increased visual, auditory, and tactile stimulation.

NURSING DIAGNOSIS
Deficient Knowledge of family caregivers related to the home care of the infant in a cast

GOAL: The family caregivers will learn home care of the infant.

OUTCOME CRITERIA
* The family caregivers demonstrate care of the infant in the hip spica cast.
* The family caregivers ask pertinent questions.
* The family caregiver identifies a resource person to call.

Nursing Interventions	Rationale
Determine the family caregivers' knowledge level and design a teaching plan. Choose teaching methods most suited to family caregivers' recognized needs and learning style.	An effective teaching plan is tailored to begin with the knowledge base of the family. The family's ability to read, understand, and follow directions and their cognitive abilities affect the results.
Before discharge, schedule follow-up appointment for return visit to have the cast checked.	Scheduling the follow-up appointment emphasizes to family caregivers the importance of close follow-up.

involves accurate observation of manifestations to aid in prompt diagnosis and initiation of treatment. Family teaching might include dietary guidelines, information about the disorder, and genetic counseling. The family also needs support and information to prepare for the long-term care of a chronically ill child (see Chapter 32).

Phenylketonuria

Phenylketonuria (PKU) is a recessive hereditary defect of metabolism that, if untreated, causes severe mental retardation in most but not all affected children. It is an uncommon defect, appearing in about 1 in 12,000 births. Children with this condition lack the enzyme that normally changes the essential amino acid phenylalanine into tyrosine.

As soon as the newborn with this defect begins to take milk (either breast or cow's milk), phenylalanine is absorbed in the normal manner. However, because the affected newborn cannot metabolize this amino acid, phenylalanine builds up in the blood serum to as much as 20 times the normal level. This build-up

occurs so quickly that increased levels of phenylalanine appear in the blood after only 1 or 2 days of ingestion of milk. Phenylpyruvic acid appears in the urine of these newborns between the second and the sixth week of life.

Most untreated children with this condition develop severe and progressive mental deficiency. The high levels of phenylalanine in the bloodstream and tissues cause permanent damage to brain tissues. The newborn appears normal at birth but begins to show signs of mental arrest within a few weeks. Therefore, this disorder must be diagnosed as early as possible, and the child must be placed immediately on a low-phenylalanine formula.

Clinical Manifestations

Untreated newborns may experience frequent vomiting and have aggressive and hyperactive traits. Severe, progressive retardation is characteristic. Convulsions may occur, and eczema is common, particularly in the perineal area. There is a characteristic musty smell to the urine.

Diagnosis

Most states require newborns to undergo a blood test to detect the phenylalanine level. This screening procedure, the Guthrie inhibition assay test, uses blood from a simple heel prick. The test is most reliable after the newborn has ingested some form of protein. The accepted practice is to perform the test on the second or third day of life. If the newborn leaves the hospital before this time, the newborn is brought back to have the test performed. The test may be repeated in the third week of life if the first test was done before the newborn was 24 hours old. Health practitioners caring for newborns not born in a hospital are responsible for screening these newborns. When screening indicates an increased level of phenylalanine, additional testing is done to make a firm diagnosis.

Treatment and Nursing Care

Dietary treatment is required. A formula low in phenylalanine (e.g., Lofenalac or Phenyl-free) should be started as soon as the condition is detected. Best results are obtained if the special formula is started before the newborn is 3 weeks of age. A low-phenylalanine diet is a very restricted one; foods to be omitted include breads, meat, fish, dairy products, nuts, and legumes. A nutritionist should supervise the diet carefully. The child remains on the diet at least into early adulthood, and it may even be recommended indefinitely.

Maintaining the newborn on the restricted diet is relatively simple compared with the problems that arise as the child grows and becomes more independent. As the child ventures into the world beyond home, more and more dietary temptations are available, and dietary compliance is difficult. The family and child need support and counseling throughout the child's developmental years.

If a woman who has PKU decides to have a child and is not following a diet low in phenylalanine, she should return to following the dietary treatment for at least 3 months before becoming pregnant. The diet is continued through the pregnancy to help in preventing the child from being born with a mental impairment. Routine blood testing is done to maintain the serum phenylalanine level at 2 to 8 mg/dL.

Galactosemia

Galactosemia is a recessive hereditary metabolic disorder in which the enzyme necessary to convert galactose into glucose is missing. Galactose is one of the component monosaccharides of milk. The newborns generally appear normal at birth but experience difficulties after ingesting milk (breast, cow's, or goat's).

Clinical Manifestations

Early feeding difficulties with vomiting and diarrhea severe enough to produce dehydration and weight loss and jaundice are primary manifestations. Unless milk is withheld early, other difficulties include cataracts, liver and spleen damage, and mental retardation, with a high mortality rate early in life. A screening test (Beutler test) can be used to test for the disorder.

Treatment and Nursing Care

Galactose must be omitted from the diet, which in the young newborn means a substitution for milk. Nutramigen and Pregestimil are formulas that provide galactose-free nutrition for the newborn. The diet must continue to be free of lactose when the child moves on to table foods, but the diet allows more variety than does the phenylalanine-free diet.

Congenital Hypothyroidism

At one time referred to by the now unacceptable term "cretinism," congenital hypothyroidism is associated with either the congenital absence of a thyroid gland or the inability of the thyroid gland to secrete thyroid hormone. The incidence of congenital hypothyroidism is about 1 in 4,000 births.

Clinical Manifestations

The newborn appears normal at birth, but clinical signs and symptoms begin to be noticeable at about 6 weeks of life. The facial features are typical and include depressed nasal bridge, large tongue, and puffy eyes. The neck is short and thick. The voice (cry) is hoarse, the skin is dry and cold, and the newborn has slow bone development. Two common features are chronic constipation and abdomen enlargement caused by poor muscle tone (Fig. 21-26). The newborn is a poor feeder and often characterized as a "good" baby by the parent or caretaker because he or she cries very little and sleeps for long periods.

Diagnosis

Most states require a routine test for triiodothyronine (T_3) and thyroxine (T_4) levels to determine thyroid function in all newborns before discharge for early diagnosis of congenital hypothyroidism. This test is done as part of the heel-stick screening, which includes the Guthrie screening test for PKU.

▊ **Figure 21-26** A newborn with congenital hypothyroidism; note the short, thick neck and enlarged abdomen.

Treatment and Nursing Care

The thyroid hormone must be replaced as soon as the diagnosis is made. Levothyroxine sodium, a synthetic thyroid replacement, is the drug most commonly used. Blood levels of T_3 and T_4 are monitored to prevent overdosage. Unless therapy is started in early infancy, mental retardation and slow growth occur. The later that therapy is started, the more severe the mental retardation. Therapy must be continued for life.

> ### Test Yourself
>
> ✔ Why is it desirable for genitourinary tract defects such as hypospadias to be corrected by the time the child is 18 months old?
> ✔ What is a serious outcome that can occur if phenylketonuria, congenital hypothyroidism, and galactosemia are not treated?

Maple Syrup Urine Disease

Maple syrup urine disease (MSUD) is an inborn error of metabolism of the branched chain amino acids. It is autosomal recessive in inheritance. It is rapidly progressive and often fatal.

Clinical Manifestations

The onset of MSUD occurs very early in infancy. In the first week of life, these newborns often have feeding problems and neurologic signs such as seizures, spasticity, and opisthotonos. The urine has a distinctive odor of maple syrup. Diagnosis is made through a blood test for the amino acids leucine, isoleucine, and valine. This is easily done at the same time the heel stick for PKU is performed.

Treatment and Nursing Care

Treatment of MSUD is dietary and must be initiated within 12 days of birth to be successful. The special formula is low in the branched chain amino acids. The special diet must be continued indefinitely.

CHROMOSOMAL ABNORMALITIES

Chromosomal abnormalities are often evident at birth and frequently cause physical and cognitive challenges for the child throughout life. There are various forms of chromosomal abnormalities, including nondisjunction, deletion, translocation, mosaicism, and isochromosome abnormalities.

The most common abnormalities are nondisjunction abnormalities, which occur when the chromosomal division is uneven. Normally during cell division of the cells of reproduction, the 46 chromosomes divide in half, with 23 chromosomes in each new cell. Nondisjunction abnormalities occur when a new cell has an extra chromosome (e.g., 24) or not enough chromosomes (e.g., 22). When

■ **Figure 21-27** Karotype showing trisomy 21. Note three chromosomes in the 21 position.

this defective chromosome joins with a normal reproductive cell having 23 chromosomes, an abnormality occurs. Down syndrome, the most common chromosomal abnormality, most often is a result of chromosomal nondisjunction with an extra chromosome on chromosome 21. Two other common chromosomal abnormalities are the Turner and Klinefelter syndromes, which are nondisjunction abnormalities occurring on the sex chromosomes.

Down Syndrome

Down syndrome is the most common chromosomal anomaly, occurring in about 1 in 700 to 800 births. Langdon Down first described the condition in 1866, but its cause was a mystery for many years. In 1932, it was suggested that a chromosomal anomaly might be the cause, but the anomaly was not demonstrated until 1959.

Down syndrome has been observed in nearly all countries and races. Most people with Down syndrome have trisomy 21 (Fig. 21-27); a few have partial dislocation of chromosomes 15 and 21. A woman older than 35 years of age is at a greater risk of bearing a child with Down syndrome than is a younger woman, but children with Down syndrome are born to women of all ages. Older women and increasing numbers of younger women are choosing to undergo screening at 15 weeks' gestation for low maternal serum AFP levels and high chorionic gonadotropin levels, which indicates the possibility of Down syndrome in the fetus. Amniocentesis and chorionic villus sampling are more accurate and will confirm the blood test results. These screening tests give women the option of aborting the fetus or continuing with the pregnancy and preparing themselves for the birth of a disabled child.

Clinical Manifestations

All forms of the condition show a variety of abnormal characteristics. Mental status is usually within the moderate to severe range of retardation, with most children being moderately retarded. The most common anomalies include:

- **Brachycephaly** (shortness of head)
- Retarded body growth

- Upward and outward slanted eyes (almond-shaped) with an epicanthic fold at the inner angle
- Short, flattened bridge of the nose
- Thick, fissured tongue
- Dry, cracked, fissured skin that may be mottled
- Dry and coarse hair
- Short hands with an incurved fifth finger
- A single horizontal palm crease (simian line)
- Wide space between the first and second toes
- Lax muscle tone (often referred to as "double jointed" by others)
- Heart and eye anomalies
- Greater susceptibility to leukemia than that of the general population

Not all these physical signs are present in all people with Down syndrome. Some may have only one or two characteristics; others may show nearly all the characteristics (Fig. 21-28).

Treatment and Nursing Care

The physical characteristics of the child with Down syndrome determine the medical and nursing management. Lax muscles, congenital heart defects, and dry skin contribute to a large variety of problems. The child's relaxed muscle tone may contribute to respiratory complications as a result of decreased respiratory expansion. The relaxed skeletal muscles contribute to late motor development. Gastric motility is also decreased, leading to problems with constipation. Congenital heart defects and vision or hearing problems add to the complexities of the child's care.

In infancy, the child's large tongue and poor muscle tone may contribute to difficulty breast-feeding or ingesting formula and can cause great problems when the time comes to introduce solid foods. The family caregivers need support during these trying times. As the child gets older, concern about excessive weight gain becomes a primary consideration.

The family caregivers of the child with Down syndrome need strong support and guidance from the time the child is born. Early intervention programs have yielded some encouraging results, but depending on the level of cognitive impairment, the family may have to decide if they can care for the child at home, or if other living arrangements need to be considered for the child. A cognitively impaired child who is undisciplined or improperly supervised may threaten the safety of others in the home and the neighborhood. Caring for the child may demand so much sacrifice from other family members that the family structure may be significantly affected. However, with consistent care, patience, and guidelines, families of children with Down syndrome often find joy and pleasure in the gentle and loving nature of the child.

Turner Syndrome

The newborn with Turner syndrome has one less X chromosome than normal. Characteristics of Turner syndrome include short stature, low-set ears, a broad-based neck that appears webbed and short, a low-set hairline at the nap of the neck, broad chest, an increased angle of the arms, and edema of the hands and feet. These children frequently have congenital heart defects as well. Females are most often affected by Turner syndrome and, with the exception of pubic hair, do not develop secondary sex characteristics.

Children with Turner syndrome have normal intelligence but may have visual-spatial concerns, learning

Figure 21-28 Typical features of a child with Down syndrome: **(A)** facial features; **(B)** horizontal palm crease (simian line).

A

B

disabilities, problems with social interaction, and may lack physical coordination. Growth hormones are given to increase the height, as well as the hormonal levels, but females with Turner syndrome rarely can become pregnant.

Klinefelter Syndrome

The presence of an extra X chromosome causes Klinefelter syndrome. The syndrome is most commonly seen in males. Characteristics are not often evident until puberty, when the child does not develop secondary sex characteristics. The testes are usually small and do not produce mature sperm. Increased breast size and a risk of developing breast cancer are frequently seen.

Boys with Klinefelter syndrome often have normal intelligence but frequently have behavior problems, show signs of immaturity and insecurity, and have difficulty with memory and processing. Hormone replacements of testosterone may be started in the early teens to promote normal adult development.

Key Points

➤ Spina bifida is caused when the spinal vertebrae fail to close and an opening is left where the spinal cord or meninges may protrude. In spina bifida occulta, soft tissue is not involved and only a dimple in the skin may be seen. In spina bifida with meningocele, the spinal meninges protrude through and form a sac, and in spina bifida with myelomeningocele, both the spinal cord and meninges protrude. Myelomeningocele is the most difficult type to treat because of the concern of complete paralysis below the lesion.

➤ Noncommunicating hydrocephalus occurs when there is an obstruction in the circulation of CSF. With communicating hydrocephalus, absorption of CSF is defective. The most obvious symptom of hydrocephalus is the rapid increase in head circumference. Ventriculoperitoneal shunting (VP shunt) drains CSF from the brain into the peritoneal cavity. Ventriculoatrial shunting drains the CSF into the heart. Nursing care focuses on preventing injury, maintaining skin integrity, preventing infection, and maintaining growth and development.

➤ Ventricular septal defects allow the blood to pass from the left to the right ventricle; in the atrial septal defect the blood flows from the left to the right atria. With a patent ductus arteriosus, blood is shunted from the aorta into the pulmonary artery. When coarctation of the aorta occurs, there is a narrowing of the aortic arch and an obstruction of blood flow.

➤ Tetralogy of Fallot is a group of heart defects including pulmonary stenosis, ventricular septal defect, overriding aorta, and right ventricular hypertrophy. The child with tetralogy of Fallot has cyanosis and low oxygen saturation. The severe and usually fatal defect, transposition of the great arteries, causes cyanosis and occurs because the aorta arises from the right ventricle, instead of the left, and the pulmonary artery arises from the left ventricle, instead of the right.

➤ A failure of the maxillary and premaxillary processes to fuse during fetal development can cause a cleft lip on one or both sides of the lip or a cleft palate, in which the tissue in the roof of the mouth does not fuse properly. Surgery is a major part of the treatment of either condition. Nursing care focuses on maintaining adequate nutrition, increasing family coping, and reducing the parents' anxiety and guilt. After surgery, nursing care focuses on preventing aspiration, improving respiration, maintaining adequate fluid volume and nutritional requirements, relieving pain, preventing injury and infection to the surgical site, and promoting normal growth and development.

➤ EA is the absence of a normal opening in or the abnormal closure of the esophagus. A tracheoesophageal fistula occurs when the upper, or proximal, end of the esophagus ends in a blind pouch and the lower, or distal, segment from the stomach is connected to the trachea by a fistulous tract. Early signs of EA include frothing and excessive drooling and periods of respiratory distress with choking and cyanosis. The newborn with tracheoesophageal fistula is at risk for aspiration, pneumonitis, and respiratory distress. Surgical correction of the defect is necessary.

➤ If the membrane between the rectum and the anus remains after birth and blocks the union between the rectum and the anus, an imperforate anus results. If the newborn does not pass a stool within the first 24 hours, the care provider should be notified. The infant requires surgery and may have a colostomy placed.

➤ A diaphragmatic hernia occurs when abdominal organs are displaced into the left chest through an opening in the diaphragm. A hiatal hernia occurs if the cardiac portion of the stomach slides into the area above the diaphragm. A rare occurrence, an omphalocele is seen when the abdominal contents protrude through the umbilical cord and form a sac lying on the abdomen. If the end of the umbilical cord does not close completely and a portion of the intestine protrudes through the opening, an umbilical hernia forms. Inguinal hernias occur mostly in males when a part of the intestine slips into the inguinal canal.

➤ Hypospadias is a congenital condition in which the urethra terminates on the ventral (underside) surface of the penis, instead of at the tip. Epispadias occurs when the opening of the urethra is on the dorsal (top) surface of the penis. In the child with exstrophy of the bladder, the anterior surface of the urinary bladder lies open on the lower abdomen; surgical closure of the bladder is preferred within the first 48 hours of life. Ambiguous genitalia is a condition in which the external sexual organs are either incompletely or abnormally formed, and it may not be possible to determine by observation at birth if the child is a male or female.

➤ Talipes equinovarus (clubfoot) and congenital hip dysplasia are the most common skeletal deformities in the newborn. Clubfoot is treated by manipulation and bandaging or by application of a cast. Children who do not respond to nonsurgical measures need surgical correction. Signs and symptoms of congenital hip dysplasia include asymmetry of the gluteal skin folds, limited abduction of the affected hip, and apparent shortening of the femur. To treat hip dislocation, the femur is manipulated and a brace applied. A hip spica cast may be used after an open reduction, if necessary. Nursing care focuses on relieving pain and discomfort, maintaining skin integrity, promoting growth and development, and increasing family knowledge.

➤ PKU is a recessive hereditary defect of metabolism that, if untreated, causes severe mental retardation.

PKU is detected by the Guthrie inhibition assay test to detect phenylalanine levels in the blood. Dietary treatment using a formula and diet low in phenylalanine is started and continued as the child gets older. Galactosemia is a hereditary metabolic disorder in which the enzyme necessary to convert galactose into glucose is missing. Galactose is omitted from the diet to treat the disorder. Congenital hypothyroidism is detected by performing tests for triiodothyronine (T_3) and thyroxine (T_4) levels to determine thyroid function. The thyroid hormone must be replaced to treat the disorder. MSUD is an inborn error of metabolism, which is autosomal recessive in inheritance. It is rapidly progressive and often fatal.

➤ If phenylketonuria, congenital hypothyroidism, and galactosemia are not treated, the newborn often has severe mental retardation.

➤ Down syndrome is sometimes called trisomy 21 because of the three-chromosome pattern seen on the 21st pair of chromosomes. Signs and symptoms seen in children include brachycephaly (shortness of head); slowed growth; slanted (almond shaped) eyes; short, flattened nose; thick tongue; dry, cracked, fissured skin; dry and coarse hair; short hands with an incurved fifth finger; single horizontal palm crease (simian line); wide space between the first and second toes; lax muscle tone; heart and eye anomalies; and a greater susceptibility to leukemia.

➤ The newborn with Turner syndrome has one less X chromosome than normal. The presence of an extra X chromosome causes Klinefelter syndrome.

INTERNET RESOURCES

Spina Bifida
www.sbaa.org

Cleft Lip and Cleft Palate
www.cleft.org

Congenital Heart Defects
www.congenitalheartdefects.com
www.americanheart.org

Workbook

■ NCLEX-STYLE REVIEW QUESTIONS

1. The nurse is doing an admission examination on a newborn with a diagnosis of hydrocephalus. If the following data were collected, which might indicate a common symptom of this diagnosis?

    a. Sac protruding on the lower back
    b. Respiratory rate of 30 breaths a minute
    c. Gluteal folds higher on one side than the other
    d. Head circumference of 18 in

2. When collecting data during an admission interview and examination on a newborn, the nurse finds the newborn has cyanosis, dyspnea, tachycardia, and feeding difficulties. These symptoms might indicate the newborn has which of the following conditions?

    a. Spina bifida
    b. Tetralogy of Fallot
    c. Congenital rubella
    d. Hip dysplasia

3. In caring for a newborn who has had a cleft lip/cleft palate repair, which nursing action is the *highest* priority?

    a. Document the time period the restraints are on and off.
    b. Observe the incision for redness or drainage.
    c. Teach the caregivers about dental care and hygiene.
    d. Provide sensory stimulation and age-appropriate toys.

4. In planning care for an infant who had a spica cast applied to treat a congenital hip dysplasia, which of the following nursing interventions would be included in this newborn's plan of care?

    a. Inspect skin for redness and irritation.
    b. Change bedding and clothing every 4 hours.
    c. Weigh every morning and evening using same scale.
    d. Monitor temperature and pulse every 2 hours.

5. The nurse is caring for a newborn who has a myelomeningocele and has not yet had surgery to repair the defect. Which of the following measures will be used to prevent the site from becoming infected? (Select all that apply.)

    a. Give antibiotics as a prophylactic measure.
    b. Cover the sac with a saline-soaked sterile dressing.
    c. Maintain the newborn in a supine position.
    d. Place a plastic protective covering over the dressing.
    e. Change the dressing every 8 hours.

■ STUDY ACTIVITIES

1. Using a table like the one below, list the common types of congenital heart defects. Include the description of the defect (chambers and parts of the heart involved), the blood flow characteristics, symptoms, and treatment.

Defect	Description of Defect	Blood Flow Characteristics	Symptoms	Treatment

2. Make a list of the maternal risk factors that may cause congenital heart defects. For each of these risk factors, state what could be done to decrease the occurrence of these risks.

3. Develop a teaching project by creating a mobile or gathering a collection of appropriate toys and activities that could be used for sensory stimulation with a newborn who is in an orthopedic cast. Present your project to your classmates and explain why and how these items would be appropriate to use for developmental stimulation.

4. Go to the following Internet site: www.pediheart.org

    a. Click on "Parent's Place."
    b. Click on "Prepare for Surgery."
    c. Read the section "Preparing Your Child for Surgery."
    d. Read the section "Helpful Parent Tips."

5. List eight tips to share with parents whose child is having heart surgery.

6. List three books that parents could use with the child who is having heart surgery.

■ CRITICAL THINKING: WHAT WOULD YOU DO?

1. Diane's baby was born with a bilateral cleft lip and cleft palate. When you bring the baby to her for feeding, she breaks down and sobs uncontrollably.

    a. Describe what your immediate response would be.
    b. What feelings and emotions do you think Diane is experiencing?

c. Write out an example of a therapeutic response you could make.

2. Cody was born with hydrocephalus and has been admitted to the pediatric unit to have a ventriculoperitoneal (VP) shunt placed. You walk into Cody's room after the pediatrician has discussed the procedure with Cody's parents. They seem anxious and begin asking you questions. How will you answer the following questions?

   a. What is hydrocephalus and what caused Cody to have the disorder?
   b. Why does Cody need to have a shunt and how does it work?
   c. What long-term problems will Cody have because of the disorder?

3. *Dosage calculation:* The nurse is preparing the preoperative medication of Demerol (meperidine) for an infant who is having a surgical procedure to correct a congenital heart defect. The infant weighs 9.9 lbs (9 lbs, 14.4 oz). The usual dosage range of this medication is 1 to 2.2 mg/kg. Answer the following:

   a. How many kilograms does the infant weigh?
   b. What is the low dose of Demerol (in milligrams) that this infant could be given?
   c. What is the high dose of Demerol (in milligrams) that this infant could be given?

HEALTH PROMOTION FOR NORMAL GROWTH AND DEVELOPMENT

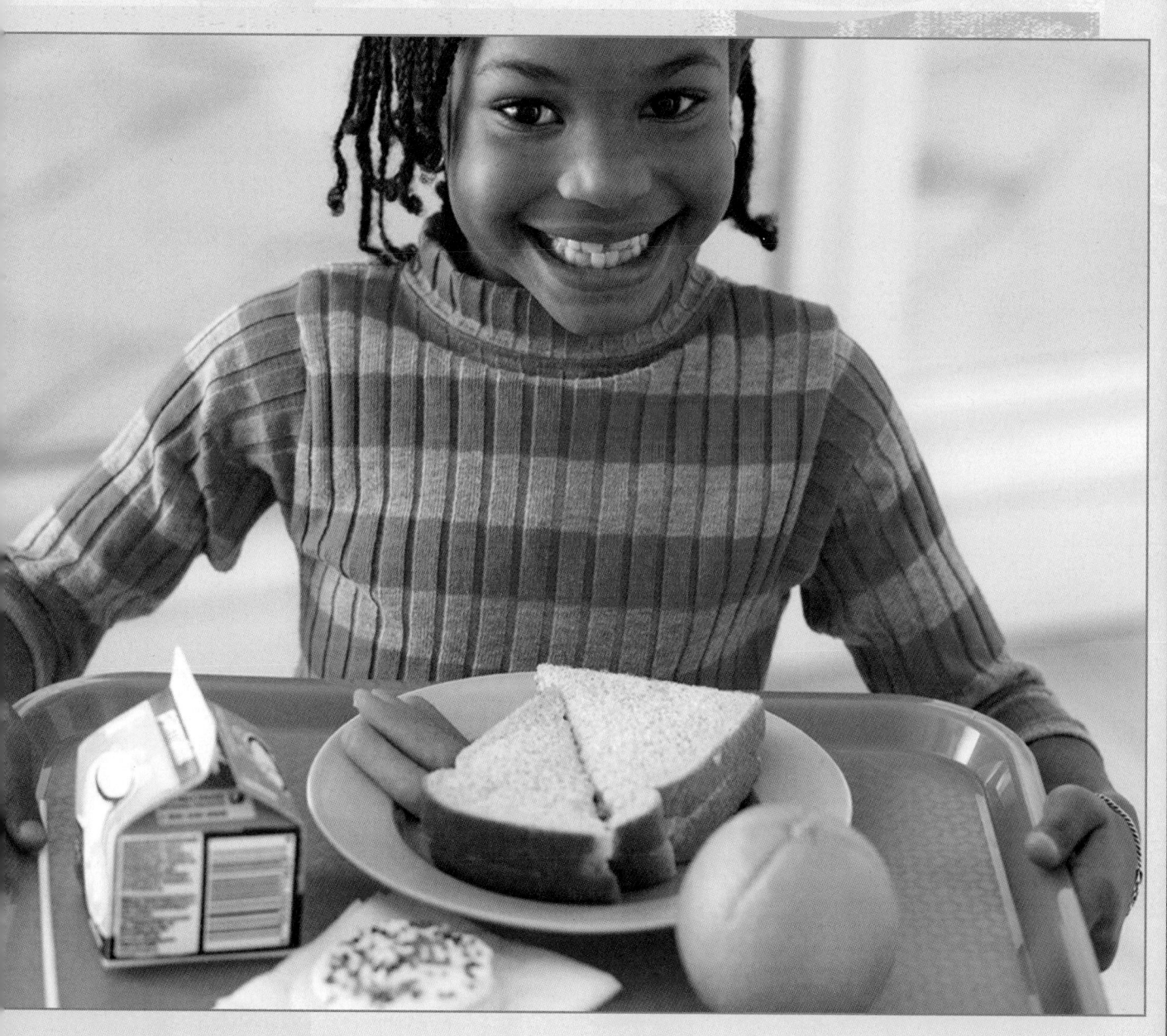

22 Principles of Growth and Development

KEY TERMS

archetypes
cephalocaudal
cognitive development
development
developmental tasks
ego
egocentric
growth
id
latchkey child
libido
maturation
proximodistal
sublimation
superego
temperament

LEARNING OBJECTIVES

On completion of this chapter, you should be able to:

1. Explain growth, development, and maturation.
2. Describe cephalocaudal and proximodistal patterns of growth.
3. Explain how height and weight are used to monitor growth and development.
4. Discuss how tools for measuring standards of growth and development are used.
5. Describe genetic, nutritional, and environmental factors that can influence a child's growth and development.
6. List and discuss the six stages of psychosexual development according to Freud.
7. Identify and describe the eight stages of Erikson's theory of psychosocial development and the developmental tasks in each stage.
8. Identify and describe the four stages of Piaget's theory of cognitive development.
9. Discuss the ideas included in Kohlberg's theory of the development of moral reasoning.
10. Discuss the important aspects of communicating with children of various ages and family caregivers.
11. Discuss the role of the nurse in understanding growth and development.

THE PROCESS of growth and development continues from conception all the way to death. There are periods of time when growth is more rapid than others and times when development is slowed. Growth and development is influenced by many factors. Some basic foundations of growth and development are important to understand when working and communicating with infants, children, and adolescents.

FOUNDATIONS OF GROWTH AND DEVELOPMENT

"Growth and development" refers to the total growth of the child from birth toward maturity. **Growth** is the physical increase in the body's size and appearance caused by increasing numbers of new cells. **Development** is the progressive change in the child toward maturity or **maturation**, completed growth and development. As children develop, their capacity to learn and think increases.

Growth of the child follows an orderly pattern starting with the head and moving downward. This pattern is referred to as **cephalocaudal**. The child is able to control the head and neck before being able to control the arms and legs. Growth also proceeds in a pattern referred to as **proximodistal**, in which growth starts in the center and progresses toward the periphery or outside (Fig. 22-1). Following this pattern, the child can control movement of the arms before being able to control movement of the hands. Another example of proximodistal growth is the ability to hold something in the hand before being able to use the fingers to pick up an object. The process of growth moves from the simple to complex.

Developmental tasks or milestones are basic achievements associated with each stage of development. These tasks must be mastered to move successfully to the next developmental stage. Developmental tasks must be completed successfully at each stage for a person to achieve maturity.

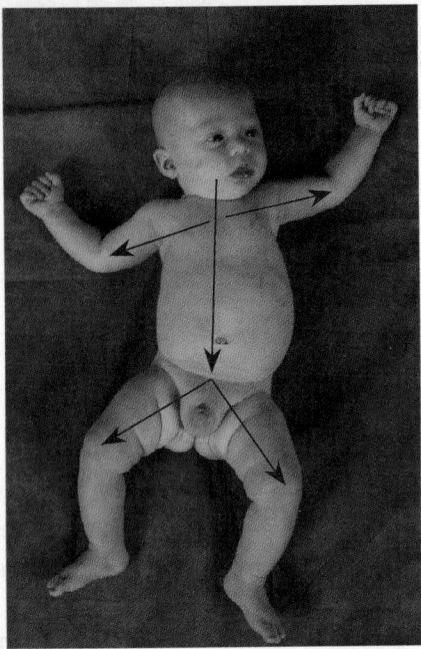

■ **Figure 22-1** The pattern of growth starting with the head and moving downward is cephalocaudal. Proximodistal growth starts in the center and progresses outward.

Patterns of Growth

Each child has a unique pattern of growth. These patterns are related to height and weight. Monitoring these patterns and recognizing deviations from the child's normal pattern can be helpful in discovering medical issues and concerns.

Height

As the child grows, the height, or distance from the head to the feet, increases in a predictable pattern. The changes in a child's height provide a concrete measurement of the child's growth. Although predictable, the increases in height are not uniform but often are seen in growth spurts, or time periods when there is rapid growth, and

other periods of time when growth is slowed. The length of the infant and the increasing height of the child are measured routinely (see Chapter 28), and the patterns are monitored and plotted on a growth chart. The increase in height seen in children and adolescents results from the skeletal growth that is taking place.

Weight

The weight gain of the child also progresses in a predictable pattern. Although for many different reasons there are variations in the weight of children the same age, the weight gain of each individual child is an important factor in the growth of the child. Patterns of weight increases are monitored and plotted on growth charts.

Body Proportions

From fetal life through adulthood body proportions vary and change. As the fetus develops and the child grows, the development of body systems and organs affects and changes the body proportions (Fig. 22-2). In early fetal life, the head is growing faster than the rest of the body and is thus proportionately larger. During infancy, the trunk portion of the body grows significantly. The legs grow rapidly during childhood, again changing the body proportions. As the child grows into an adolescent, the trunk portion grows and the body proportions are those of an adult.

Standards of Growth

A growth chart with predictable patterns or growth curves is used to plot and monitor a child's growth through the years. These growth charts allow for comparison of children of the same age and sex. They also allow for comparison of the child's current measurements with the child's previous measurements. Standard growth charts are used to determine if the child's pattern is appropriate or if for some reason the child's growth is above or falls below a standardized normal range (see Appendix G). A growth chart is used for comparison only; if a child does not fall into the "normal" range, it does not necessarily indicate that there is something of concern for that child.

| 2-month fetus | 5-month fetus | Newborn | 2 years | 6 years | 12 years | 25 years |

■ **Figure 22-2** From fetal life through adulthood the body proportions change.

A Personal Glimpse

Every time I had to take my baby to the pediatrician's office for his well-baby checkup I would worry for days. The nurse would always weigh and measure him and look at the growth chart, then look at me with a curious look. Sometimes she would weigh him again and then just stare at me. I would ask what was wrong and she would say in an accusing voice, "Well, he is in the 95th percentile for height and in the 5th percentile for weight." She would start asking me questions like was I feeding him often enough, did he cry all the time, did he have a babysitter who took care of him while I worked, or just why was he not gaining enough weight. I would get so upset because they acted like I was starving or neglecting my baby, and I knew I wasn't. Finally when he was 11 months old, it was discovered that he had a digestive problem and couldn't drink milk or eat wheat or oatmeal—his low weight didn't have anything to do with the way I was taking care of him. I started giving him soy milk, changed his diet and right away he started gaining weight. I was so relieved that now finally he was in a higher percentile on the growth chart. I will never forget how bad I felt when I was treated as if I was a neglectful mother, that was so hard. I am glad the disorder was discovered—by the time he was 21 he was 6 ft and 3 in tall and weighed 190 lb!

Diane

Learning Opportunity: What were the benefits in this situation of plotting this child's growth on a growth chart? What do you think this mother was feeling when she was in the pediatrician's office? What could the nurse have done to support this mother?

Standards of Development

Developmental screening is done by using standardized developmental tools, such as the Denver Developmental Screening Test. Development in children occurs in a range of time rather than at an exact time. Developmental screening identifies any delays in what is considered a standard or normal pattern. Although one child might develop at a faster rate than another child within a time range, both children will have mastered developmental tasks or milestones, thus following a normal and predictable pattern.

It is important to recognize that developmental screening is used for the sake of comparison and does not automatically mean there is a concern if the child does not fit exactly into the standardized normal pattern.

A word of caution is in order.

Growth charts and developmental tools should be used only as a guide. Not every child, even though normal, follows the same growth and development pattern as other children the same age.

Test Yourself

✔ Define growth, development, and maturation.

✔ What do cephalocaudal and proximodistal mean?

✔ How do body proportions in the child differ from those in the adult?

✔ Why is the child's height and weight plotted on a growth chart?

INFLUENCES ON GROWTH AND DEVELOPMENT

There are many influences on the growth and development of a child. Prenatal factors that influence the fetus and child's growth and development include the mother's general health and nutrition, as well as her behaviors during pregnancy. These factors as well as genetic, nutritional, and environmental factors all affect the growth and development of the child.

Genetics

The science of genetics studies the ways in which normal and abnormal traits are transmitted from one generation to the next. The scientist Gregor Mendel did experiments that proved each parent's individual characteristics could reappear unchanged in later generations. Human cells contain 46 chromosomes, consisting of 23 essentially identical pairs. At conception, the union of the sperm and egg forms a single cell. This cell is made up of one member of each pair contributed by the father and one member of each pair contributed by the mother. This combination determines the sex and inherited traits of the new organism.

The genetic makeup of each child helps determine characteristics such as the child's sex, race, eye color, height, and weight. Growth and development of the child is influenced by these factors. For example, each child is genetically programmed to grow to be a certain height. With adequate nutrition and good health, most children will attain this height. Some diseases are genetically transmitted. If a child has a genetic predisposition to a certain disease, that child might not grow and develop as completely as a healthy child would. Physical and mental disorders can occur as a result of a child's genetic factors.

Cultural Snapshot

Some cultural groups are more prone to certain diseases and disorders. Many of these are genetically passed from generation to generation. Being aware of these and sensitive to the concerns, fears, and feelings of people from various cultures helps the nurse remain supportive and objective.

The child's heredity also influences personality characteristics, including **temperament**. Temperament is the combination of all of an individual's characteristics, the way the person thinks, behaves, and reacts to something that happens in his or her environment. Not all children react alike to situations. Depending on the child's temperament, one child might react to a situation with a quiet, shy response, whereas another child might react with acting out or aggressive behavior in the same situation. Children with differing temperaments might adapt in different time frames to new situations. One child might adapt quickly, whereas another child might adapt more slowly to the new situation. Characteristics that evidence a child's temperament include areas such as his or her activity level; the development of regular patterns, such as waking, eating, and elimination patterns, in daily life; and how he or she approaches and adapts to situations. Temperament also plays a part in a child's attention span and how easily he or she becomes distracted. All of these characteristics of temperament play a part in the child's development.

Nutrition

The quality of a child's nutrition during the growing years has a major effect on the overall health and development of the child. The child needs adequate amounts of food and nutrients for the body to grow. Nutrition is also a factor in the child's ability to resist infection and diseases. Motor skill development is influenced by inadequate, as well as excessive, food intake. The child establishes nutritional habits and patterns early in life; these patterns are carried into adulthood, thus influencing the individual's growth, development, and health throughout life.

The U.S. Department of Agriculture has developed MyPyramid, on which daily dietary guidelines are based. These guidelines provide a healthy, balanced diet when followed. Foods from the main food groups necessary for good nutrition are included. Figure 22-3 shows the MyPyramid for Kids with explanations of each of the food groups and food sources for each group. The U.S. Department of Agriculture also provides families with recommendations for eating right and exercising (Family Teaching Tips: Tips for Eating Right and Exercising).

Family Teaching Tips

EATING RIGHT AND EXERCISING

EATING RIGHT

- *Make half your grains whole.* Choose whole-grain foods, such as whole-wheat bread, oatmeal, brown rice, and low-fat popcorn, more often.
- *Vary your veggies.* Go dark green and orange with your vegetables—eat spinach, broccoli, carrots, and sweet potatoes.
- *Focus on fruits.* Eat them at meals and at snack time too. Choose fresh, frozen, canned, or dried, and go easy on the fruit juice.
- *Get your calcium-rich foods.* To build strong bones, serve low-fat and fat-free milk and other milk products several times a day.
- *Go lean with protein.* Eat lean or low-fat meat, chicken, turkey, and fish. Also, change your tune with more dry beans and peas. Add chickpeas, nuts, or seeds to a salad; pinto beans to a burrito; or kidney beans to soup.
- *Change your oil.* We all need oil. Get yours from fish, nuts, and liquid oils, such as corn, soybean, canola, and olive oil.
- *Don't sugarcoat it.* Choose foods and beverages that do not have sugar and caloric sweeteners as one of the first ingredients. Added sugars contribute calories with few, if any, nutrients.

EXERCISE

- *Set a good example.* Be active and get your family to join you. Have fun together. Play with the kids

or pets. Go for a walk, tumble in the leaves, or play catch.
- *Take the President's Challenge as a family.* Track your individual physical activities together and earn awards for active lifestyles at www.presidentschallenge.org.
- *Establish a routine.* Set aside time each day as activity time—walk, jog, skate, cycle, or swim. Adults need at least 30 minutes of physical activity most days of the week, and children need 60 minutes everyday or most days.
- *Have an activity party.* Make the next birthday party centered on physical activity. Try backyard Olympics or relay races. Have a bowling or skating party.
- *Set up a home gym.* Use household items, such as canned foods, as weights. Stairs can substitute for stair machines.
- *Move it!* Instead of sitting through TV commercials, get up and move. When you talk on the phone, lift weights or walk around. Remember to limit TV watching and computer time.
- *Give activity gifts.* Give gifts that encourage physical activity—active games or sporting equipment.

From United States Department of Agriculture, "Tips for Families." http://teamnutrition.usda.gov/resources/mpk_tips.pdf. Retrieved November 12, 2007.

MyPyramid For Kids

Eat Right. Exercise. Have Fun.

MyPyramid.gov

Grains
Make half your grains whole

Start smart with breakfast Look for whole-grain cereals.

Just because bread is brown doesn't mean it's whole-grain. Search the ingredients list to make sure the first word is "whole" (like "whole wheat").

1 oz. = 1 slice bread; 3–4 crackers; 1 cup dry cereal; or ½ cup cooked cereal, rice, or pasta

Vegetables
Vary your veggies

Color your plate with all kinds of great-tasting veggies.

What's green and orange and tastes good? Veggies! Go dark green with broccoli and spinach, or try orange ones like carrots and sweet potatoes.

Also try green beans, cauliflower, and squash.

Fruits
Focus on fruits

Fruits are nature's treats – sweet and delicious. Eat a variety.

Go easy on juice and make sure it's 100%.

Milk
Get your calcium-rich foods

Move to the milk group to get your calcium. Calcium builds strong bones.

Look at the carton or container to make sure your milk, yogurt, cheese, or cottage cheese is lowfat or fat-free.

Meat & Beans
Go lean with protein

Fat lean or lowfat meat, chicken, turkey, and fish. Ask for it baked, broiled, or grilled – not fried.

It's nutty, but true. Nuts*, seeds*, peas, and beans are all great sources of protein, too.

(*After age 3 because of risk of choking.)

1 oz. = 1 egg, 2 Tbsp. peanut butter, or ½ cup beans

💧 **Oils**   Oils are not a food group, but you need some for good health. Get your oils from fish, nuts, and liquid oils such as corn oil, soybean oil, and canola oil.

Find your balance between food and fun

- Move more. Aim for at least 60 minutes everyday, or most days.
- Walk, dance, bike, rollerblade – it all counts. How great is that!

Fats and sugars — know your limits

- Get your fat facts and sugar smarts from the Nutrition Facts label.
- Limit solid fats as well as foods that contain them.
- Choose food and beverages low in added sugars and other caloric sweeteners.

MyPyramid.gov
STEPS TO A HEALTHIER YOU

U.S. Department of Agriculture
Food and Nutrition Service
September 2005
FNS-381

USDA is an equal opportunity provider and employer.

■ **Figure 22-3** MyPyramid for Kids (Adapted from the U.S. Department of Agriculture Food and Nutrition Service).

Normal nutritional needs and daily requirements vary at each stage of development. In addition, eating patterns, skills, and behaviors vary at each stage. These aspects of nutrition are discussed in the chapters covering each of the stages of growth and development.

Environment

Many aspects of the child's environment affect growth and development. The family structures, including family size, sibling order, parent–child relationships, and cultural background, all affect the growth and development of the child (see Chapter 2). The socioeconomic level of the family can affect the child, especially if there are not sufficient funds to provide adequate nutrition, childcare, and health care for the growing child. Living in a household in which parents are addicted to drugs or alcohol can affect the child (see Chapter 33). Play and entertainment are important environmental aspects in the development of a child. Other environmental factors that can affect growth and development include family homelessness and divorce; a latchkey situation, in which children come home from school to an empty house each day; and running away from home.

Play and Entertainment

Throughout the stages of growth and development, the role and types of play differ. Through play, children learn about themselves, the environment around them, and relationships with others. Various aspects of play, including the roles, types, and functions of play, are discussed in each of the chapters covering the stages of growth and development.

> **"Playing" is the job of every child!**
>
> The use of movies, television, video games, computers, and the Internet can have both positive and negative influences on the child. Children who have little or no supervision may not have the ability to recognize what is appropriate and healthy for their development.

The Homeless Family

A growing number of families are homeless in the United States. Causes of homelessness include job loss, loss of housing, drug addiction, insufficient income, domestic turmoil, and separation or divorce. Single mothers with children make up an increasing number of these families. Many of these homeless single mothers and their families have multiple problems. Often there are higher rates of abuse, drug use, and mental health problems in homeless families. Many of these families lived with relatives for a time before being reduced to living in a car, an empty building, a welfare hotel, or perhaps a cardboard box. These families sometimes seek temporary housing in a shelter for the homeless. They often move from one living situation to another, living in a shelter for the time allowed and then moving elsewhere, only to return after a while to repeat the cycle.

Homelessness creates additional stresses for the family. Many homeless families have young children but have problems gaining entry into the health care system, even though these children are at high risk for developing acute and chronic conditions. Health care for these families commonly occurs as crisis intervention, instead of the more effective preventive intervention. Pregnant homeless women with their attendant problems receive little if any prenatal care, are poorly nourished, and bear low-birth-weight infants. Most of the children of homeless families do not have adequate immunizations. Homeless children often have chronic illnesses at a higher rate than that of the general population. These chronic conditions may include anemia, heart disease, peripheral vascular disease, and neurologic disorders. Many homeless children have developmental delays, perform poorly when they attend school, suffer from anxiety and depression, and exhibit behavioral problems.

Many shelters available to the homeless are overcrowded, lack privacy (the bathroom facilities are used by many people), have no personal bedding or cribs for infants, and no facilities for cooking or refrigerating food. Because of limits to the length of stay, many families must move from one shelter to another. This adds to the problems these families face by contributing to a lack of consistency in the services and programs available to them.

As a nurse, you can set the tone of the interaction between the homeless family and the health care facility. Establishing an environment in which the child's caregiver feels respected and comfortable is important. Focusing initially on the positive factors in the caregiver's relationship with the children alleviates some of the caregiver's guilt and fear of being criticized. Make every effort to offer down-to-earth suggestions and help the family in the most practical manner.

On the child's admission to the health care facility, the health care team performs a complete admission assessment. Ask the caregiver about the family's living arrangements; such information will help in the care and planning for the child. During this interview, you may become aware of problems of other family members that need attention. When giving assistance and guidance, be careful to supplement, not take over, the family's functioning. For instance, tell the family how to go about getting a particular benefit and be certain they have complete and accurate information but do not take the steps for them. These families need to feel self-reliant and in control, and they need realistic solutions to their problems.

Outreach programs for the homeless have been established in many major cities. These programs conduct screening, treat acute illnesses, and help families contact local health care services when needed. Provide information to the family about any assistance that is available.

Divorce and the Child

Divorce has increased to the point that one in two marriages ends in divorce. About 50% of children experience the separation or divorce of their parents before they complete high school. Some children may experience more than one divorce because many people who remarry divorce a second time. Divorce can be traumatic for children but may be better than the constant tension and turmoil that they have lived through in their home.

Children often feel responsible for the breakup and believe that it would not have occurred if they had just done the right thing or been good. On the other hand, children may blame one of the parents for deciding to end the marriage and causing them grief and unhappiness. Counseling can help children to acknowledge and understand their anger and their need to blame one or the other parent. This process may take a considerable amount of time to resolve. Both parents should make every effort to eliminate the child's feeling of guilt and should avoid using the child as a spy or go-between with the estranged spouse. Parents must avoid trying to buy the affection of the children. This is especially true for the noncustodial parent, who must not shower the children with special gifts, trips, and privileges when the children are visiting.

Sensitivity and understanding go a long way. Children whose parents are getting a divorce commonly feel unloved and, in a sense, feel that they too are being divorced.

Children should be encouraged to ask questions about the separation and divorce. A child who does not ask questions may be afraid to ask for fear of retaliation by one of the parents. Children should be discouraged from thinking that they might be able to do something that would get the parents back together again. They must be helped to recognize the finality of the divorce. Plans for the children should be made (e.g., where and with whom the children will live, where they will go to school) and shared with the children as soon as possible. This can give the children a sense of security in their chaotic personal world. Each child's confidence and self-esteem must be strengthened through careful handling of the transition (Fig. 22-4).

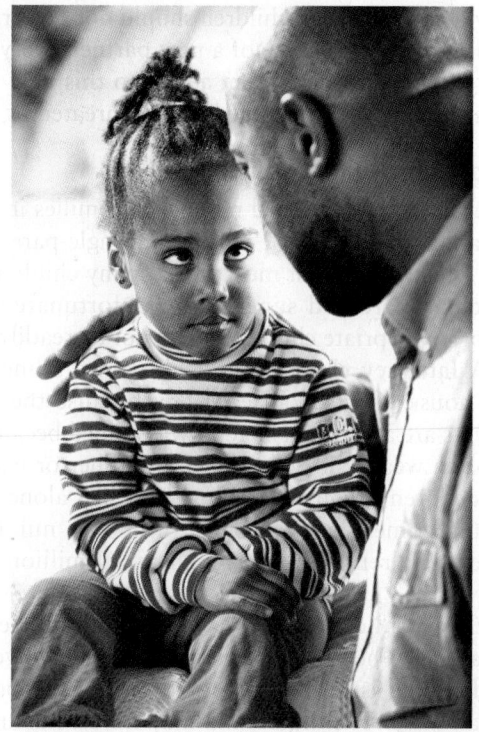

■ **Figure 22-4** This father explains to his daughter that even though he and her mother will not be married and live in the same house anymore, he loves her and will see her often.

When a child of a divorce is hospitalized, be certain to have clear information about who is the custodial parent, as well as who may visit or otherwise contact the child. The custodial parent's instructions and wishes should be honored.

Encourage the child to express feelings of fear and guilt. Help the child understand that other children have divorced parents. The school nurse may function as an advocate for a counseling program in the school setting that brings together children of divorces. During counseling, children can voice their fears and concerns and begin to work through them with the help of an objective counselor in a protected environment. One of the most important aspects of such groups is the reassurance the children get that they are not alone in this crisis.

When the custodial parent begins to date and plans to remarry, the child may again have strong emotions that must be worked through. If the remarriage brings together a blended family of children from the previous marriages of both adults, the children may need extra support in accepting the new step-parent and stepsiblings. Adults who seek preventive counseling when planning to form a step-family have greater success than do those who seek help only after problems are overwhelming.

Children react in various ways to a parent's new marriage, depending in part on age. The new marriage may introduce additional problems of a new home, a new neighborhood, and a new school that can cause anxiety for any child. Although children should not be permitted to veto the parent's choice of a new partner, every effort should be made to help them adjust to this new family member and view the change in a nonthreatening way.

The Latchkey Child

As a result of the increased number of families in which both parents work and the increase in single-parent families in which the parent must work, many children need after-school care and supervision; unfortunately, adequate or appropriate child care may not be readily available. A **latchkey child** is one who comes home to an empty house after school each day because the family caregivers are at work. The term was coined because this child often wears the house key around her or his neck. These children usually spend several hours alone before an adult comes home from work. The number of latchkey children may be as high as 10 million in the United States.

Latchkey children often have fears about being at home alone. When more than one child is involved and the older child is responsible for the younger one, conflicts can arise. The older child may have to assume responsibility that is beyond the normal expectations for the child's age. This can be a difficult situation for the caregivers and the children. The caregivers must carefully outline permissible activities and safety rules (Fig. 22-5). A plan should be in place to help the older child solve any arising problems that involve both children. The older child should not feel that the complete responsibility is on his or her shoulders, but rather that it is a shared responsibility with the caregiver. Some schools have after-school programs that provide safe activities for children. In addition, some communities have programs in which an adult telephones the child regularly every day after school, or there is a telephone hotline that the child can call (see Family Teaching Tips: Tips for Parents of Latchkey Children).

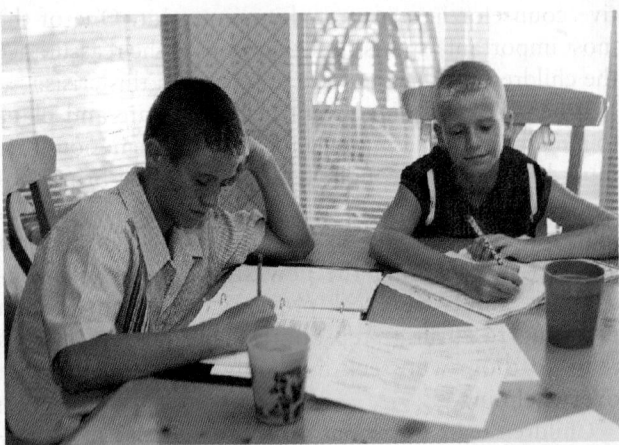

■ **Figure 22-5** "Latchkey" children come home to an empty house after school. These boys have specific rules about activities to be done as they wait the arrival of their caregiver.

Family Teaching Tips

TIPS FOR PARENTS OF LATCHKEY CHILDREN

- Teach the child to keep the key hidden and not show it to anyone.
- Plan with the child the routine to follow when arriving home; plan something special each day.
- Plan a telephone contact on the child's arrival home; either have the child call you or you call the child.
- Always let the child know if you are going to be delayed.
- Review safety rules with the child. Post them on the refrigerator as a reminder.
- Use a refrigerator chart to spell out daily responsibilities, and have the child check off tasks as they are completed.
- Let the child know how much you appreciate his or her responsible behavior.
- Have a trusted neighbor for backup if the child needs help; be sure the child knows the telephone number, and post it by the telephone.
- Post telephone emergency numbers that the child can use; practice when to use them.
- Teach the child to tell telephone callers that the caregiver is busy but never to say that the caregiver is not home.
- Teach the child not to open the door to anyone.
- Be specific about activities allowed and not allowed.
- Carefully survey your home for any hazards or dangerous temptations (e.g., guns, motorcycle, ATV, swimming pool). Eliminate them, if possible, or ensure that rules about them are clear.
- See if your community has a telephone friend program available for latchkey children.
- A pet can relieve loneliness, but give the child clear guidelines about care of the pet during your absence.

Despite concerns that latchkey children are more likely to become involved with smoking, stealing, or taking drugs, researchers have not found sufficient data to support this fear. Children who are given responsibility of this kind and who are recognized for their dependability usually live up to the expectations of the adults in their social environment.

Nurses must recognize the need for after-school services for these children and take an active role in the community to plan and support such services. Maintain a list of the facilities available to support families with latchkey children. Give caregivers guidance in planning children's after-school activities and offer support to the caregivers in their attempts to provide for their children.

The Runaway Child

In the United States, as many as 750,000 to 2 million adolescents run away from home each year. A child can be considered a runaway after being absent from home overnight or longer without permission from a family caregiver. Most children who run away from home are 10 to 17 years of age.

A child may run away from home in response to circumstances that he or she views as too difficult to tolerate. Physical or sexual abuse, alcohol or drug abuse, divorce, step-families, pregnancy, school failure, and truancy may contribute to a child's desire to escape. However, some adolescents are not runaways but rather "throwaways" who have been forced to leave home and are not wanted by the adults in the home. Often the throwaways have been forced out of the home because their behavior is unacceptable to family caregivers or because of other family stresses such as divorce, remarriage, and job loss.

Runaway or throwaway adolescents often turn to stealing, drug dealing, and prostitution to provide money for alcohol, drugs, food, and possibly shelter. Many of these adolescents live on the streets because they cannot pay for shelter; they avoid going to public shelters for fear of being found by police. They may become victims of pimps or drug dealers who use the adolescents for their own gain.

There are numerous programs to help runaways, especially in urban areas. The 24-hour-a-day National Runaway Switchboard (1-800-RUNAWAY, 1-800-786-2929) is available to give runaways information and referral (www.nrscrisisline.org). This service may help the runaway to find a safe place to stay and may provide counseling, shelter, health care, legal aid, message relay to the family, and transportation home if desired. Runaways are not forced to go home but may be encouraged to inform their families that they are all right. Other free hotline numbers are also available.

A sexually transmitted disease, pregnancy, acquired immunodeficiency syndrome, or drug overdose are the usual reasons that runaways are seen at a health care facility. When caring for such a child, be nonjudgmental. Any indication of being disturbed or disgusted by the adolescent's lifestyle may end any chance of cooperation and cause the adolescent to refuse to give any additional information. Try to build a trusting relationship with the child. Remember that the runaway viewed his or her problems as so great that escaping was the only way to resolve them. Counseling is necessary to begin to resolve the problems.

Health teaching for the runaway must be suited to his or her lifestyle and must be at a level the child can understand. Without prying excessively, try to find out the runaway's living circumstances and adjust the teaching plans accordingly. Remember that the child's problems did not come about overnight, and they will not be resolved quickly. Caring for a runaway can be frustrating, challenging, and sometimes rewarding for the health care staff.

Test Yourself

✔ What are three commonly seen responses in children whose parents divorce?

✔ What are some concerns that might be expressed by caregivers of "latchkey" children?

✔ Why is it especially important as a nurse to be nonjudgmental and to develop a trusting relationship with the runaway child?

THEORIES OF CHILD DEVELOPMENT

How a helpless infant grows and develops into a fully functioning, independent adult has fascinated scientists for years. Four pioneering researchers whose theories in this area are widely accepted are Sigmund Freud, Erik Erikson, Jean Piaget, and Lawrence Kohlberg (Table 22-1). Their theories present human development as a series of overlapping stages that occur in predictable patterns. These stages are only approximations of what is likely to happen in children at various ages, and each child's development may differ from these stages.

Sigmund Freud

Most modern psychologists base their understanding of children at least partly on the work of Sigmund Freud. His theories focus primarily on the **libido** (sexual drive or development). Although Freud did not study children, his work focused on childhood development as a cause of later conflict. Freud believed that a child who did not adequately resolve a particular stage of development would have a fixation (compulsion) that correlated with that stage. Freud described three levels of consciousness: the **id**, which controls physical need and instincts of the body; the **ego**, the conscious self, which controls the pleasure principle of the id by delaying the instincts until an appropriate time; and the **superego**, the conscience or parental value system. These consciousness levels interact to check behavior and balance each other. The psychosexual stages in Freud's theory are the oral, anal, phallic, latency, and genital stages of development.

Oral Stage (Ages 0–2 Years)

The newborn first relates almost entirely to the mother (or someone taking a motherly role), and the first experiences with body satisfaction come through the mouth. This is true not only of sucking but also of making noises, crying, and breathing. It is through the mouth

Table 22-1 ■ COMPARATIVE SUMMARY OF THEORIES OF FREUD, ERIKSON, PIAGET, AND KOHLBERG

Age (years)	Stage	Freud (Psychosexual Development)	Erikson (Psychosocial Development)	Piaget (Intellectual Development)	Kohlberg (Moral Development)
1	Infancy	Oral Stage	Trust vs. Mistrust	Sensorimotor Phase	Stage 0—Do what pleases me
2–3	Toddlerhood	Anal Stage	Autonomy vs. Shame		Preconventional Level Stage 1—Avoid punishment
4–6	Preschool (early childhood)	Phallic (infant genital) Oedipal Stage	Initiative vs. Guilt	Preoperational Phase	Preconventional Level Stage 2—Do what benefits me
7–12	School-age (middle childhood)	Latency Stage	Industry vs. Inferiority	Concrete Operational Phase	Conventional Level Stage 3 (Age 7–10)—Avoid disapproval Stage 4 (Age 10–12)—Do duty, obey laws
13–18	Adolescence	Genital Stage (puberty)	Identity vs. Role Confusion	Formal Operational Phase	Postconventional Level Stage 5 (Age 13)—Maintain respect of others Stage 6 (Age 15)—Implement personal principles

that the baby expresses needs, finds satisfaction, and begins to make sense of the world.

Anal Stage (Ages 2–3 Years)

The anal stage is the child's first encounter with the serious need to learn self-control and take responsibility. Toilet training looms large in the minds of many people as an important phase in childhood. Because elimination is one of the child's first experiences of creativity, it represents the beginnings of the desire to mold and control the environment; this is the "mud pie period" in the child's life.

The child has pride in the product created. Cleanliness and this natural pride do not always go together, so it may be necessary to help direct this pride and interest into more acceptable behaviors. Playing with such materials as modeling clay, crayons, and dough helps put the child's natural interests to good use, a process called **sublimation.**

Phallic (Infant Genital) Stage (Ages 3–6 Years)

In Freud's third stage, the child's interest moves to the genital area as a source of pride and curiosity. To the child's mind, this area constitutes the difference between boys and girls, a difference that the child is beginning to be aware of socially. The superego begins to develop during this stage.

During this stage, the child begins to understand what it means to be a boy or a girl. The child learns to identify

with the parent of the same sex (Fig. 22-6). At about this time, a boy begins to take pride in being a male and a girl in being a female. In many families, a new brother or sister also arrives, arousing the child's natural interest in human origins. The parents' reaction to the child's genital exploration may influence whether the child learns to feel satisfied with him- or herself as a sexual being, or is laden with feelings of guilt and dissatisfaction throughout life.

Freud hypothesized that this awareness of genital differences also leads to a time of conflict in the child's emotional relationships with parents. The conflict occurs

■ Figure 22-6 The preschool child learns to identify with the parent of the same sex.

between attachment to and imitation of the parent of the same sex and the appeal of the other parent. The boy who for years has depended on his mother for all his emotional and physical needs now is confronted by his desire to be a man (Oedipus complex). The girl, who has imitated her mother, now finds her father a real attraction (Electra complex). It is through contact with parents that the child learns to relate to the opposite sex. The child learns the interests, attitudes, concerns, and wishes of the opposite sex.

Latency Stage (Ages 6–10 Years)

The latency stage is the time of primary schooling, when the child is preparing for adult life but must await maturity to exercise initiative in adult living. The child's sense of moral responsibility (the superego) develops, based on what has been taught through the parents' words and actions.

During this stage, the child is involved with learning, developing cognitive skills, and actively participating in sports activities, with little thought given to sexual concerns. The child's main relationships are with peers of the same sex. Developing positive friendships at this stage helps the child learn about caring relationships.

When placed in an unfamiliar setting, children in this stage may become confused because they do not know what is expected of them. They need the sense of security that comes from approval and praise and usually respond favorably to a brief explanation of "how we do things here."

Genital Stage (Ages 11–13 Years)

Physical puberty is occurring at an increasingly early age, and social puberty occurs even earlier, largely because of the influence of sexual frankness on television, in movies, and in the print media. At puberty, all of the child's earlier learning is concentrated on the powerful biological drive of finding and relating to a mate. In earlier societies, mating and forming a family occurred at a young age. Our society delays mating for many years after puberty, creating a time of confusion and turmoil during which biological readiness must take second place to educational and economic goals. This is a sensitive period when privacy is important, and great uncertainty exists about relating to any member of the opposite sex. This development depends on a self-healing process that helps counterbalance the stresses created by natural and accidental crises. The self-healing process is delayed by any major crisis, such as hospitalization, that interrupts normal development. Interruptions may cause regression to an earlier stage, such as the older child who begins to wet the bed when hospitalized.

Erik Erikson

Building on Freud's theories, Erikson described human psychosocial development as a series of tasks or crises. According to Erikson and Senn (1958), "children 'fall apart' repeatedly, and unlike Humpty Dumpty, grow together again," if they are given time and sympathy and are not interfered with.

Erikson formulated a series of eight developmental tasks or crises; the first five pertain to children and youth. To present a complete view of Erikson's theory, all eight tasks are presented. In each task, the person must master the central problem before moving on to the next one. Each task holds positive and negative counterparts, and each of the first five implies new developmental tasks for parents (Table 22-2).

Table 22-2 ■ CHILD AND PARENT DEVELOPMENTAL TASKS ACCORDING TO ERIKSON

Developmental Level	Basic Task	Stage of Parental Development	Parental Task
Infant	Trust	Learning to recognize and interpret infant's cues	To interpret cues and respond positively to the infant's needs; hold, cuddle, and talk to infant
Toddler	Autonomy	Learning to accept child's need for self-mastery	To accept child's growing need for freedom while setting consistent, realistic limits; offer support and understanding when separation anxiety occurs
Preschooler	Initiative	Learning to allow child to explore surrounding environment	To allow independent development while modeling necessary standards; generously praise child's endeavors to build child's self-esteem
School-Age	Industry	Learning to accept rejection without deserting	To accept child's successes and defeats, assuring child of acceptance to be there when needed without intruding unnecessarily
Adolescent	Identity	Learning to build a new life, supporting the emergence of the adolescent as an individual	To be available when adolescent feels need: provide examples of positive moral values; keep communication channels open; adjust to changing family roles and relationships during and after the adolescent's struggle to establish an identify.

Trust Versus Mistrust (Ages 0–1 Year)

The infant has no way to control the world other than crying for help and hoping for rescue. During the first year, the child learns whether the world can be trusted to give love and concern or only frustration, fear, and despair. The infant who is fed on demand learns to trust that cries, communicating a need, will be answered. The baby fed according to the nurse's or caregiver's schedule does not understand the importance of routine but only that these cries may go unanswered.

This is critical to remember.

Trust has to be established and then reinforced at each stage of growth and development. Help the child build a trusting relationship by being consistent and responding appropriately to the child's needs at every age.

Autonomy Versus Doubt and Shame (Ages 1–3 Years)

Even the smallest child wants to feel in control and needs to learn to perform tasks independently, even when this takes a long time or makes a mess. The toddler gains reassurance from self-feeding, from crawling or walking alone where it is safe, and from being free to handle materials and learn about things in the environment (Fig. 22-7).

A toddler exploring the environment begins to explore and learn about his or her body too. If caregivers react appropriately to this normal behavior, the child will gain self-respect and pride. However, if caregivers shame the child for responding to this natural curiosity, the child may develop and sustain the belief that somehow the body is dirty, nasty, and bad.

Initiative Versus Guilt (Ages 3–6 Years)

During this period, the child engages in active, assertive play. Steadily improving physical coordination and expanding social skills encourage "showing off" to gain adult attention and, the child hopes, approval. The preschool child, still self-centered, plays alone, although in the company of other children; interaction comes later. These children want to know what the rules are and enjoy "being good" and the adult approval that action gains. During this time, the child develops a conscience and accepts punishment for doing wrong because it relieves feelings of guilt.

Children in this phase of development generally do not have a concept of time. The child needs a familiar frame of reference to understand when something is going to happen. For example, the parent or caregiver may say, "I will be back when your lunch comes" or "I will be back when the cartoons come on TV." Explaining that it is time for "Mommy and Daddy to go to work" might help an unhappy child realize that the parent or caregiver is not leaving because of any negative behavior of the child's.

Notice this difference.

When working with children who have not fully developed a concept of time, explaining at the end of a shift that you must go home to your own family may help the child understand and realize you are not leaving because of any negative behavior of the child's.

Industry Versus Inferiority (Ages 6–12 Years)

Children begin to seek achievement in this phase. They learn to interact with others and sometimes to compete with them. They like activities they can follow through to completion and tangible results (Fig. 22-8).

Competition is healthy as long as the standards are not so high that the child feels there is no chance of winning. Praise, not criticism, helps the child to build self-esteem and avoid feelings of inferiority. It is important to emphasize that everyone is a unique person and deserves to be appreciated for his or her own special qualities.

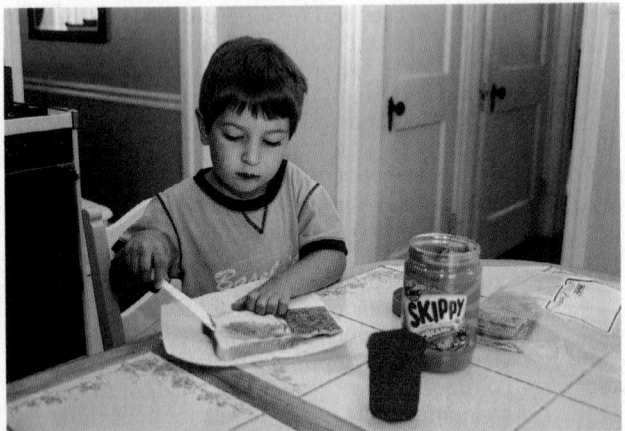

■ **Figure 22-7** This toddler has a desire to do things independently, by himself.

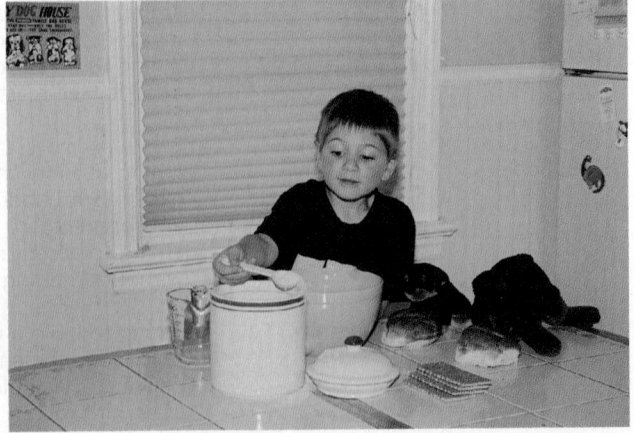

■ **Figure 22-8** The school-aged child enjoys activities that produce tangible results.

Identity Versus Role Confusion (Ages 12–18 Years)

Adolescents are confronted by marked physical and emotional changes and the knowledge that soon they will be responsible for their own lives. The adolescent develops a sense of being an independent person with unique ideals and goals and may feel that parents, caregivers, and other adults refuse to grant that independence. Adolescents may break rules just to prove that they can. Stress, anxiety, and mood swings are typical of this phase. Relationships with peers are more important than ever.

Intimacy Versus Isolation (Early Adulthood)

During early adulthood, the person tries to establish intimate personal relationships with friends and an intimate love relationship with one person. Difficulty in establishing intimacy results in feelings of isolation.

Generativity Versus Self-Absorption (Young and Middle Adulthood)

For many people, this phase means marriage and family, but for others it may mean fulfillment in some other way—a profession, a business career, or a religious vocation. The person who does not find this fulfillment becomes self-absorbed or stagnant and ceases to develop socially.

Ego Integrity Versus Despair (Old Age)

This final phase is the least understood of all, for it means finding satisfaction with oneself, one's achievements, and one's present condition without regret for the past or fear for the future.

Jean Piaget

Freud and Erikson studied psychosexual and psychosocial development; Jean Piaget brought new insight into **cognitive development** or intellectual development—how a child learns and develops that quality called intelligence. He described intellectual development as a sequence of four principal stages, each made up of several substages (Piaget, 1967). All children move through these stages in the same order, but each moves at his or her own pace.

Sensorimotor Phase (Ages 0–2 Years)

The newborn behaves at a sensorimotor level linked entirely to desires for physical satisfaction. The newborn feels, hears, sees, tastes, and smells countless new things and moves in an apparently random way. Purposeful activities are controlled by reflexive responses to the environment. For example, while nursing, the newborn gazes intently at the mother's face, grasps her finger, smells the nipple, and tastes the milk, thus involving all senses.

As the infant grows, an understanding of cause and effect develops. When random arm motions strike the string of bells stretched across the crib, the newborn

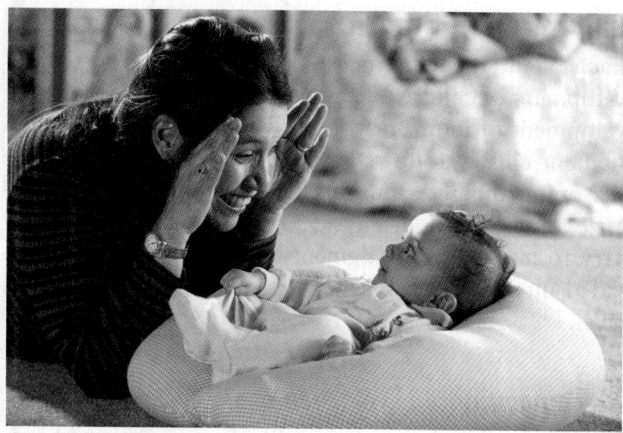

■ Figure 22-9 The infant responds to mother's voice and her facial expressions.

hears the sound made and eventually can manipulate the arms deliberately to make the bells ring.

In the same way, newborns cannot understand words or even the tone of voice; only through hearing conversation directed to them can they pick out sounds and begin to understand (Fig. 22-9). As the infant produces verbal noises, the responses of those nearby are encouraging and eventually help the infant learn to talk.

Preoperational Phase (Ages 2–7 Years)

The child in this phase of development is **egocentric**; that is, he or she cannot look at something from another's point of view. The child's interpretation of the world is from a self-centered point of view and in terms of what is seen, heard, or otherwise experienced directly.

This child has no concept of quantity; if it looks like more, it is more. Four ounces of juice poured into two glasses looks like more than 4 oz in one glass. A sense of time is not yet developed; thus, the preschooler or early school-aged child cannot always tell if something happened a day ago, a week ago, or a year ago.

Concrete Operations (Ages 7–11 Years)

During this stage, children develop the ability to begin problem solving in a concrete, systematic way. They can classify and organize information about their environment. Unlike in the preoperational stage, children begin to understand that volume or weight may remain the same even though the appearance changes. These children can consider another's point of view and can deal simultaneously with more than one aspect of a situation.

Formal Operations (Ages 12–15 Years)

The adolescent is capable of dealing with ideas, abstract concepts described only in words or symbols. The person in this stage begins to understand jokes based on double meanings and enjoys reading and discussing theories and philosophies. Adolescents can observe and then draw logical conclusions from their observations.

Lawrence Kohlberg

Each of the theorists focuses on one element in the development of children. Kohlberg's theory is about the development of moral reasoning in children. Moral development closely follows cognitive development because reasoning and abstract thinking (the ability to conceptualize an idea without physical representation) are necessary to make moral judgments. Kohlberg's theory is divided into three levels with two or three stages in each level.

Preconventional Level (Premoral Level)

During the first 2 years (stage 0), there is no moral sensitivity. This is a time of egocentricity; decisions are made with regard only to what pleases the child or makes him or her feel good and what displeases or hurts the child. The child is not aware of how his or her behavior may affect others. The child simply reacts to pleasure with love and to hurtful experiences with anger.

In stage 1, punishment and obedience orientation (ages 2–3 years), the child determines right or wrong by the physical consequence of a particular act. The child simply obeys the person in power with no understanding of the underlying moral principle.

In stage 2, naive instrumental self-indulgence (ages 4–7 years), the child views a specific act as right if it satisfies his or her needs. Children follow the rules to benefit them-selves. They think, "I'll do something for you if you'll do something for me" and, on the other hand, "If you do something bad to me, I'll do something bad to you." This is basically the attitude of "an eye for an eye."

> **Think about this.**
> When working with children who are in the process of developing a sense of right and wrong, it is important to understand that the child thinks if he or she gets punished for doing something, then it is wrong; if the child does not get punished, he or she thinks the behavior is right or acceptable.

Conventional Level

As concrete operational thought develops, children can engage in moral reasoning. School-aged children become aware of the feelings of others. Living up to expectations is a primary concern, regardless of the consequences.

In stage 3, "good-boy" orientation (ages 7–10 years), being "nice" is very important. Children want to avoid a guilty conscience. Pleasing others is very important.

In stage 4, law and order orientation (ages 10–12 years), showing respect to others, obeying the rules, and maintaining social order are the desired behaviors. "Right" is defined as something that finds favor with family, teachers, and friends. "Wrong" is symbolized by broken relationships.

Postconventional Level (Principled Level)

By adolescence, the child usually achieves Piaget's formal operational stage. To achieve the postconventional level of moral development, the adolescent must have attained the formal operational stage of cognitive development. As a result, many persons do not reach this level.

In stage 5, social contract orientation (ages 13–18 years), culturally accepted values define personal standards and personal rights. A person's rights must not be violated for the welfare of the group. The end no longer justifies the means. Laws are for mutual good, cooperation, and development.

Stage 6, personal principles, is not attained very frequently. The person who reaches this level does what he or she thinks is right without regard for legal restrictions, the cost to self, or the views of others. Because of this person's deep respect for life, he or she would not do anything that would intentionally harm him- or herself or another.

> ### Test Yourself
> ✔ What are the five stages of growth and development according to Freud?
> ✔ What are the tasks that must be mastered at each of the five stages of child development according to Erikson?
> ✔ How are Piaget and Kohlberg's theories of development similar?

Other Theorists

Freud, Erikson, Piaget, and Kohlberg are only four of the many researchers who have studied the development of children and families. During the 1940s and 1950s, Arnold Gesell studied many infants and talked with their parents concerning children's behavior. From his studies emerged a series of developmental landmarks that are still considered valid and the observation that children progress through a series of "easy" and "difficult" phases as they develop. For example, he labeled one period the "terrible twos," the time when a toddler begins to assert new mobility and coordination to gain parental attention, even if the attention is unfavorable. Knowing that these cycles are normal makes it easier for parents to cope.

Carl Jung's contribution to the study of child growth and development focused on the inner sequence of events that shape the personality. He emphasized that human development follows predetermined patterns called **archetypes**. These archetypes replace the instinctive behavior present in other animals. Interaction of the archetypes with the outside environment is evident throughout human life. For example, a normal child learns to suck, crawl, walk, and talk without any instruction, but the details of how the child does these things come from observation and imitation of others.

Jung believed that the first 3 years of a child's life are spent coordinating experiences and learning to make a conscious personality, a distinct person who is separate from the rest of the environment. In the following years, the child learns to make sense of the environment by associating new discoveries to a general approach to the world. Dreams and nightmares help express personality developments that for some reason do not find a conscious outlet.

Jung points out that what happens to a child is not so critical to the child's development as the responses to these happenings. A hospital experience may permanently scar a child's personality if the child's natural feeling of terror is overlooked. Hospitalization may be accepted and even become a point of pride, however, if carried out in an atmosphere of assurance and support of the child's emotional concern and the need for love and acceptance.

The interaction between inner development and the environment is particularly clear in studies of young children who have been deprived in some way. John Bowlby's studies of children who were not held or loved and Bruno Bettelheim's studies of children given good physical care but little or no emotional satisfaction indicate how vital psychological interaction is.

In recent years, the theories of Erikson, Piaget, and Kohlberg have been criticized for being gender specific to males and culturally specific to whites. In response, several theorists have conducted research on the growth and development of females and varying ethnic groups. Most notably, Carol Gilligan researched the moral development of males and females, and Patricia Green sought to construct a "truly universal theory of development through the empirical and theoretical understanding of cultural diversity" (Cocking & Greenfield, 1994).

DEVELOPMENTAL CONSIDERATIONS FOR COMMUNICATING WITH CHILDREN AND FAMILY CAREGIVERS

Communicating with children and family caregivers is a primary source of data collection during a well-child visit or in any health crisis situation. Communication occurs in all settings and focuses on data collection as well as information related to immunizations, developmental assessment, teaching, and anticipatory guidance. Information about the child is derived from the child, the caregivers, and observations of the child and family. Understanding the developmental level of the child and influences on the child's and caregiver's communication (e.g., family, culture, community, age, personality) are critical for communicating effectively.

Principles of Communication

Communication includes spoken and written words as well as the body language, facial expressions, voice intonations, and emotions behind the words. Listening is one of the most important aspects of communication.

When listening, think about what the person is saying and *not* about how you are going to respond. Listening includes attending (giving the other person physical signs that you are listening) and following (encouraging the speaker to fully express what it is he or she needs to say). Silence is also a form of communication; it might indicate that the person is thinking, is unclear about what is being said, is having difficulty responding, is angry, and so on.

> **Always remember.**
> Listening includes more than hearing. It includes tuning into the other person, being sensitive to the person's feelings, and concentrating on what the other person is trying to express.

Time management is an important aspect of communication. Communicate in a calm and unhurried manner, even though work demands and time constraints often make this difficult. It is important to gain skill in balancing communication needs of children and families with other nursing responsibilities.

Some nurses have difficulty accepting their own feelings while working with children. A nurse might feel anxious or inadequate when starting new relationships and beginning to communicate with children. Remember that this feeling is normal and that your communication skills will improve with experience over time.

To direct the focus of a conversation, use open-ended questions followed by guided statements. It is always important to clarify statements and feelings expressed by caregivers and children. Reflective statements help indicate what you believe was expressed. For example, you might state, "You seem worried about Maria's loss of appetite."

One of the biggest challenges when several people are present is deciding to whom you should direct questions. Although eventually you will need information from the child and caregivers, start with the child if he or she can talk. Even at age 3, some children can tell you about the specific problem. Good strategies when communicating with children include maintaining eye contact, playful engagement, and talking about what interests the child or caregiver. Play is an important form of communication for children and can be an effective technique in communicating with children.

Avoid communication blocks, which include socializing, giving unasked for advice, providing false assurances, being defensive, giving pat or clichéd responses, being judgmental or stereotyping, not allowing issues to be fully explored, interrupting, and not allowing the person to finish a response.

Sometimes it is necessary to communicate through an interpreter because of language barriers or hearing impairments. A medical interpreter trained in the language of the child is preferable but not always available. When using an interpreter, ensure that the interpreter understands the goal of the conversation. Allow the interpreter and family to become acquainted, and then communicate directly with the family and child, observing nonverbal responses. Pose questions to elicit one answer at a time, and do not interrupt the conversation between the interpreter and family. It is important not to talk about the family and child to the interpreter in English because the family might understand some information. Avoid medical jargon, and respect cultural differences. Follow up with the interpreter regarding his or her impression of the interaction and arrange for the interpreter to meet with the family on subsequent visits.

Communicating With Infants

Infants evaluate only actions and respond to only sensory cues. Infants cannot realize that a nurse who handles them abruptly and hurriedly may be rushed or insecure; they feel only that the nurse is frightening and unloving. To comfort the infant, hold, cuddle, and soothe him or her, or allow caregivers to do so. Spending time in the beginning of an interaction to calm down and connect with the infant is helpful.

It is important to establish a relationship with the caregiver up front. Begin by recognizing and praising the hard work of parenting. Allow the caregiver to hold the infant as you initiate conversation, and begin observing the infant, caregiver, and their interactions. When appropriate, ask the caregiver for permission to hold the infant yourself or to place him or her on an examination table or bed.

Sensory play activities, such as massaging the infant, stretching the arms and legs, looking at a colorful or moving object, and playing peek-a-boo and "this little piggy," can ease the child and convey a sense of safety and comfort.

Communicating With Young Children

Allow the caregiver to hold the young child as you initiate conversation, and begin observing the child, caregiver, and their interactions. When appropriate, ask the caregiver permission to hold the child yourself or to place him or her on an examination table or bed.

Remember that, according to normal stages of development, young children are egocentric. Explain to them how they will feel or what they can do. Experiences of others have no relevance. Use short sentences, positive explanations, familiar and nonthreatening terms, and concrete explanations.

Young children tend to be frightened of strangers. Sudden abrupt or noisy approaches signal danger. The child needs time to evaluate the situation while still in the arms of the caregiver. Do not rush the situation, but allow time for the child to initiate the relationship. Spending time calming down or connecting with the child is helpful. Conversation might be started through a doll, toy, or puppet. "What's doll's name?" "How does doll feel?" A casual approach with reluctant children is most effective. Games that pique the younger child's curiosity ("Which hand has the car?") might also help put him or her at ease. Children who show rejecting or aggressive behavior are putting up a defense. Ignore these behaviors unless they are harmful to the child or someone else.

Allow young children to handle or explore equipment that will come in contact with them. For example, have them touch the bell of a stethoscope, listen to their teddy bear's heart, or play a simple game with these objects (Fig. 22-10). Such activities may communicate better than words because young children cannot yet understand abstract ideas.

When speaking with young children, do not stand over and talk down to them. Instead, get down on eye level with them. Speak in a slow, clear, positive voice. Use simple words. Keep sentences short. Express statements and questions positively. Listen to the child's fears and worries and be honest in your answers. When possible, give the child choices so that he or she will feel a sense of having some control over the situation and often will be more cooperative. Choices should be simple and limited. Only offer choices if they exist. Do not ask, "Do you want medicine now?" if that is not an option. Do ask, "Would you like the red cup or the blue cup for your medicine?" Consult with the caregiver about which choices are reasonable.

Young children tend to be literal and cannot separate fantasy from reality. Do not use analogies. For example, "This will be a little bee sting." Young children visualize a bee sting, which might be traumatic.

Because verbal skills are limited, pay particular attention to nonverbal clues, such as pushing an object away, covering the eyes, crying, kicking, pointing, clinging, and exploring an object with the fingers.

Most nurses find this approach helpful. Use your knowledge of growth and development to talk to the child at his or her level of development and understanding. Doing so will enable you to quickly establish rapport and begin a trusting relationship with the child.

■ Figure 22-10 The nurse encourages the child to communicate by allowing her to play with the medical equipment.

Communicating With School-Aged Children

Remember to begin by calming down or connecting with the child. If caregivers are present, briefly acknowledge them. Then, focus on the child. Include the child in the plan of care. School-aged children are interested in knowing the "what" and "why" of things. They will ask more questions if their curiosity is not satisfied. Provide simple, concrete responses using age-appropriate vocabulary. Complex or detailed explanations are not necessary. Provide explanations that help them understand how equipment works.

Be sensitive to the child's concern about body integrity. Children are particularly concerned about anything that poses a threat of injury to their bodies. Help reduce their anxieties by allowing them to voice concerns and by providing reassurances.

Play, re-enactment, or artwork can give insight into how well a child understands a procedure or experience. These activities also can reveal the child's perception of interpersonal relationships. Subsequent play can provide clues to the child's progress or changing feelings.

Here's a helpful hint.
When working with school-aged children, explain what is going to happen and why it is being done to *them* specifically. Charts, diagrams, and metaphors might be helpful. Elicit the child's cooperation by offering reasonable and limited choices.

Communicating With Adolescents

Communicating with adolescents might be challenging. Adolescents waiver between thinking like an adult and thinking like a child. Behavior is related to their developmental stage and not necessarily to chronological age or physical maturation. Their age and appearance may fool you into assuming that they are functioning on a different level.

Adolescents respond positively to individuals who show a genuine interest in them. Show interest early and sustain a connection. Focus the interview on them rather than the problem. Build rapport by opening with informal conversation about friends, school, hobbies, and family. Once you have established rapport, return to more open-ended questions.

Adolescents might need to relate information they do not wish others to know, so they might not reveal much with caregivers present. If adolescents and caregivers are to be interviewed, it might help to first interview the adolescent alone (thereby establishing relationship), then the adolescent and caregivers together, and then the caregivers separately. A discussion about confidentiality with both parent and adolescent might set concerns at ease. Explain to the parent and adolescent that some degree of independence will improve health care. Discuss why confidentiality is important, what will not be shared with caregivers, and what must be shared with caregivers (i.e., what the adolescent states is confidential unless the adolescent indicates that he or she intends to harm him- or herself or somebody else). Adolescents and caregivers might not always agree. In this case, clearly define the problem so an agreement might be reached. Encourage adolescents to discuss sensitive issues with caregivers.

This is important.
Do not impose your values on adolescents or give unwanted advice; they will likely reject you. Adolescents need to feel they can express their own ideas and opinions.

Let adolescents know that you will listen in an open-minded, nonjudgmental way. Avoid asking prying or embarrassing questions. Phrase questions regarding sensitive information in a way that encourages the adolescent to respond without feeling embarrassed. When feeling threatened, adolescents might not respond or only respond with monosyllabic answers. Reduce anxiety by confining conversations to nonthreatening topics until the adolescent feels at ease. Be aware of clues that he or she is ready to talk.

Make contracts with adolescents so that communication can remain open and honest and the plan of care may be more closely followed.

Communicating With Caregivers

Much of the information collected about the child comes from the family. In general, family members provide most of the care and are allies in promoting the health of the child. View the caregivers as experts in the care of their child and you as their consultant. Identify the child's family caregivers (not always mom or dad) and clarify roles. When the family structure is not immediately clear, you may avoid embarrassment by asking directly about other family members. "Who else lives in the home?" "Who is Jimmy's father?" "Do you live together?" Do not assume that because parents are separated that the other parent is not actively involved in care of the child. When talking with caregivers, observe how they interact with the child and how the child interacts with the environment. Watch how caregivers set limits or fail to set limits.

Include caregivers in providing information, problem solving, and planning of care (Fig. 22-11). Keep caregivers well informed of what is going on. Explain procedures and invite caregivers to help, but do not force them to participate if they are not comfortable doing so. Make the caregiver feel welcome and important. Encourage conferences between family caregivers and members of the health care team. Such meetings help caregivers form a clearer picture of the child and his or her behavior, condition, and health needs, and give them an opportunity to consider different types of treatments and relationships.

Pay attention to the verbal and nonverbal clues a parent uses to convey concerns, worries, and anxieties

■ **Figure 22-11** The nurse teaches the child and parent together.

about the child. Worries might be conveyed in an off-handed manner or referenced frequently. Remember the chief complaint might not relate to the real reason the parent has brought the child to the health care facility. Create a trusting atmosphere that allows parents to be open about all of their concerns. Ask facilitating questions: "Do you have any other concerns about Richie that you would like to tell me about?" "What did you hope I would be able to do for you today?" "Was there anything else that you wanted to tell or ask me about today?" When a parent introduces a concern or offers information without prompting, follow up with clarifying questions. Other times, it might be necessary to direct the conversation based on observations. When communicating with the parent, provide positive reinforcement and ask open-ended questions. This approach is non-threatening and encourages description. Be supportive, not judgmental. "Why didn't you bring him sooner?" or "What did you do that for?" does not improve the relationship. Rather, acknowledge the hard work of parenting and praise successes.

To elicit information, it might be useful to compare what is actually happening with what the parent expects to be happening. If a mother says, "My 2-year-old son barely eats anything," it might be helpful to ask, "What do you think your child should be eating?" If the mother responds, "Three full meals a day, including green vegetables," you may interpret the problem differently from how the mother initially presented it to you.

Each individual in the room, including the health care provider, might have a different idea about the nature of the problem. Discover as many of these perspectives as possible. Family members who are not present may also have concerns. It is a good idea to ask about those concerns: "If Sally's father were here today, what questions or concerns would he have?" Agreement about a problem might not be mutual. Sometimes caregivers might not perceive a problem you see; other times parents might perceive a problem that you do not see. Explore what is behind the parents' perception and work toward a mutual agreement. Other members of the health care team might be needed.

Parents' concerns, anxieties, and negative attitudes might be conveyed to the child, which sometimes causes negative reactions from the child. Be alert to negative attitudes. Provide caregivers with opportunities to discuss and explore their anxieties, concerns, or problems. Demonstrate genuine care and concern to help ease these feelings. Some children might feel self-sufficient and view the caregivers' presence as being treated like a baby. However, it is often normal for the child to regress during illness, in which case the caregivers' presence may offer support.

Provide anticipatory guidance related to normal growth and development, nurturing childcare practices, and safety and injury prevention. In addition to providing information, help parents in using the information.

THE NURSE'S ROLE RELATED TO GROWTH AND DEVELOPMENT

As a pediatric nurse, it is important to have an understanding of factors and influences, as well as normal or expected patterns related to the growth and development of the infant, child, and adolescent. Knowledge of growth and development will help when working with the child in a well-child setting, during illness, or when a child is having surgery.

When interviewing the child and family caregiver, an understanding of growth and development will help you to ask appropriate questions to assess whether the child's development is within the normal range or if there are variations or abnormalities present. Knowledge of growth and development helps you to ask age-related questions, as well as answer the caregiver's questions regarding the child. In communicating with children, being aware of a child's language skills and development enables you to communicate at the child's level of understanding.

Much of your role as a pediatric nurse involves teaching and working with family caregivers. Providing them with examples of normal growth and development and helping them to anticipate safety and nutritional needs of their child is vital.

When working with a sick child or one with a disease or disorder, be aware that the child's age and stage of growth and development can affect the way the child copes with the situation or responds to treatment. In developing a plan of care for any child, use knowledge of growth and development to provide the best care for the child.

This advice could be a lifesaver.

An understanding of growth and development helps you offer suggestions to the caregivers about what behaviors to expect and what safety precautions to initiate for their child.

Key Points

- Growth is the physical increase in the body's size. Development is the progression of changes in the child toward maturity or maturation, which is completed growth and development.
- Growth following an orderly pattern from the head downward is called cephalocaudal. Proximodistal growth starts in the center and progresses outward.
- Height and weight are monitored and plotted on growth charts to provide a comparison of measurements and patterns of a child's growth.
- Growth charts and developmental assessment tools are used to compare a child's growth to other children of the same age and sex. They are also used to compare the child's current measurements with his or her previous measurements.
- Genetic factors influence a child's physical characteristics such as the child's gender, race, eye color, height, and weight, as well as the child's overall growth and development. Some diseases as well as some physical and mental disorders are genetically transmitted. Personality characteristics, including temperament, are genetically influenced.
- The quality of a child's nutrition during the growing years has a major effect on the overall health and development of the child and throughout life. Nutrition is also a factor in the child's ability to resist infection and diseases.
- A lower socioeconomic level, decreased caregiver time and involvement, media exposure, and living in a household in which parents are addicted to drugs or alcohol are environmental factors that may influence growth and development. Homelessness, divorce, latchkey situations, and running away from home are also environmental factors that influence a child's growth and development.
- According to Freud, in the oral stage of development the newborn experiences body satisfaction through the mouth. During the anal stage, the child begins to learn self-control and taking responsibility. The child finds a source of pride and develops curiosity regarding the body in the phallic stage. Moral responsibility and preparing for adult life occur in the latency stage, and in the genital stage, puberty and the drive to find and relate to a mate occurs.
- Erikson's theory of psychosocial development sets out sequential tasks that the child must successfully complete before going on to the next stage. His theory describes developmental tasks in 8 stages:
  - Trust vs. Mistrust—the infant learns that his or her needs will be met.
  - Autonomy vs. Doubt and Shame—the toddler learns to perform independent tasks.
  - Initiative vs. Guilt—the child develops a conscience and sense of right and wrong.
  - Industry vs. Inferiority—the child competes with others and enjoys accomplishing tasks.
  - Identity vs. Identity Confusion—the adolescent goes through physical and emotional changes as he or she develops as an independent person with goals and ideas.
  - Intimacy vs. Isolation—the young adult develops intimate relationships.
  - Generativity vs. Self-Absorption—the middle-aged adult finds fulfillment in life.
  - Ego Integrity vs. Despair—the older adult is satisfied with life and the achievements attained.
- Piaget's four stages of cognitive development include the sensorimotor phase, in which the infant uses the senses for physical satisfaction. The young child in the preoperational phase sees the world from an egocentric or self-centered point of view. During the concrete operations phase, the child learns to problem solve in a systematic way, and in the formal operations phase, the adolescent has his or her own ideas and can think in abstract ways.
- Kohlberg's theory relates to the development of moral reasoning in children. The child progresses from making decisions with no moral sensitivity to making decisions based on personal standards and values.
- Understanding the growth and development of the child and influences on the child and family caregivers is important for effective communication. Listening, maintaining eye contact, and playing with children can encourage communication. Infants evaluate actions and respond to sensory cues. Young children are egocentric and tend to be frightened of strangers. Use short sentences, positive explanations, familiar and nonthreatening terms, and concrete explanations. School-aged children are interested in knowing the "what" and "why" of things. Provide simple, concrete responses using age-appropriate vocabulary. Choices should be simple and limited. Let adolescents know that you will listen in an open-minded, nonjudgmental way. Phrase questions regarding sensitive information in a way that encourages the adolescent to respond without feeling embarrassed. Include caregivers in providing information, problem solving, and planning of care. Keep caregivers well informed.
- The nurse who understands normal growth and development is better able to develop an appropriate plan of care for the child, including the areas of communication, safety, and family teaching.

INTERNET RESOURCES

www.nacd.org
www.piaget.org
www.keepkidshealthy.com/growthcharts

Workbook

■ NCLEX-STYLE REVIEW QUESTIONS

1. The nurse observes that during feeding the newborn looks at the mother's face and holds her finger. According to Piaget, these observations indicate the child is in which phase of development?

   a. Sensorimotor
   b. Preoperational
   c. Concrete operations
   d. Formal operations

2. The nurse is caring for a toddler who has recently turned 2 years old. Of the following behaviors by the toddler, which would indicate the toddler is attempting to become autonomous? The toddler

   a. cries when the caregiver leaves.
   b. walks alone around the room.
   c. "shows off" to get attention.
   d. competes when playing games.

3. In working with a preschool-aged child, which of the following statements made by the child's caregiver would indicate an understanding of this child's stage of growth and development?

   a. "My child always wants her own way."
   b. "Why won't my child play with other children?"
   c. "I will tell my child I will be back after lunch."
   d. "She doesn't know when she has done something wrong."

4. In an interview, a 9-year-old child makes the following statement to the nurse: "I like to play basketball, especially when we win." This statement indicates this child is developing which basic task of child development?

   a. Trust
   b. Autonomy
   c. Initiative
   d. Industry

5. In discussing needs of adolescents with family caregivers, the nurse explains that to support the adolescent in developing his or her own identity, it would be *most* important for the adolescent caregiver to

   a. respond to physical needs.
   b. praise the child's actions.
   c. accept the child's defeats.
   d. maintain open communication.

6. Using the growth charts in Appendix G, plot the measurements of a male child who is 18 months old, 33 in tall, and weighs 26 lbs. What percentile is this child for height? Weight?

■ STUDY ACTIVITIES

1. Using the following table, compare the theories of Freud, Erikson, Piaget, and Kohlberg regarding children who are in the early elementary school years.

	Name of Theorist	Main Ideas and Similarities Between Theorists' Ideas
Latency stage		
Industry stage		
Concrete operational stage		
Conventional level		

2. Erikson identified trust as the development task for the first stage of life. Discuss why successful accomplishment of this task is essential to the person's future happiness and adjustment.

3. Go to the following Internet site: www.cdc.gov/ncbddd/child/tools.htm

   a. What is the main objective for doing developmental screening?
   b. What should be considered when selecting a screening tool?
   c. What are some myths about screening tools?

4. Do an Internet search on "safety for kids at home alone."

   a. Make a list of some of the sites you discovered.
   b. List two questions that parents should ask themselves when considering leaving a child at home alone.
   c. List six factors that a parent should consider before allowing a child to stay home alone.

■ CRITICAL THINKING: WHAT WOULD YOU DO?

1. The mother of a 4-month-old infant brings the baby to the health care clinic for her well-baby check. The baby is measured and weighed and the measurements are plotted on a growth chart. The baby is in the 75th percentile for height and the 60th percentile for weight. When the provider examines the baby, the notion of doing a developmental screening on the child is discussed.

   a. What will you explain to this mother when she asks you the purpose of the growth chart?
   b. How often will the baby's measurements be plotted on the growth charts?
   c. What will you expect to see after the child has had several measurements plotted?
   d. What is the purpose of doing a developmental screening?

2. A group of family caregivers is participating in a class discussing influences on a child's growth and development. If you were the nurse doing this teaching session, how would you answer the following questions?

   a. What influence does genetics have on growth and development?

   b. What are the effects of nutrition on a child's growth?

   c. What are some environmental factors that influence a child's development?

23

Growth and Development of the Infant: 28 Days to 1 Year

KEY TERMS

bottle mouth or nursing bottle caries
deciduous teeth
extrusion reflex
pedodontist
pincer grasp
primary circular reactions
seborrhea
secondary circular reactions

LEARNING OBJECTIVES

On completion of this chapter, you should be able to:

1. Explain the major developmental task of the infant according to Erikson.
2. Describe physical growth and development that occurs during the first year of life, including weight and height, head and skull, skeletal growth, teeth, circulatory system, respiratory rate, and neuromuscular development.
3. Describe the fear of strangers seen in the infant, including the age this usually appears and the reason it occurs.
4. Discuss a useful purpose of the game "Peek-a-Boo."
5. Discuss nutritional requirements and concerns of the infant.
6. Describe the process and challenge of adding solid foods to the infant's diet.
7. Discuss weaning: (a) the usual age when the baby becomes interested in a cup, and (b) criteria to determine the appropriate time.
8. State the cause of bottle mouth caries and discuss ways to prevent bottle mouth caries.
9. List examples of foods to offer the infant who does not drink enough milk from a cup.
10. Discuss immunization of infants including (a) communicable diseases against which children are immunized, (b) schedule of immunizations, and (c) common side effects and treatments following immunization.
11. Outline caregiver teaching to present during routine health maintenance visits for the infant.
12. Describe early dental care for the infant.
13. Discuss important safety issues for the infant.
14. Discuss the nurse's and family caregivers' role related to the hospitalization of the infant.

THE 1-MONTH-OLD infant has a busy year ahead. During this year, the infant grows and develops skills more rapidly than he or she ever will again. In the brief span of a single year, this tiny, helpless bit of humanity becomes a person with strong emotions of love, fear, jealousy, and anger and gains the ability to rise from a supine to an upright position and move about purposefully.

Erikson's psychosocial developmental task for the infant is to develop a sense of trust. The development of trust occurs when the infant has a need and that need is met consistently. The infant feels secure when the basic needs are meet. This stage creates the foundation for the developmental tasks of the next stages to be met. If the infant does not receive food, love, attention, and comfort, the infant learns to mistrust the environment and those who are responsible for caring for the child.

PHYSICAL DEVELOPMENT

Despite the many factors, such as genetic background, environment, health, gender, and race, that affect growth in the first year of life, the healthy infant progresses in a predictable pattern. By the end of the year, the dependent infant who at 1 month of age had no teeth and could not roll over, sit, or stand blossoms into an emerging toddler with teeth who can sit alone, stand, and begin to walk alone. The growth seen in the prenatal development of the fetus continues.

Weight and Height

In the first year, both weight and height increase rapidly. During the first 6 months, the infant's birth weight doubles and height increases about 6 in. Growth slows slightly during the second 6 months but is still rapid. By 1 year of age, the infant has tripled his or her birth weight and has grown 10 to 12 in.

Thinking in terms of the "average" child is misleading. To determine if an infant is reaching acceptable levels of development, birth weight and height must be the standard to which later measurements are compared. A baby weighing 6 lb at birth cannot be expected to weigh as much at 5 or 6 months of age as the baby who weighed 9 lb at birth, but each is expected to double his or her birth weight at about this time. A growth graph is helpful for charting a child's progress (Fig. 23-1).

Head and Skull

Head Circumference

At birth, an infant's head circumference averages about 13.75 in (35 cm) and is usually slightly larger than the chest circumference. The chest measures about the same as the abdomen at birth. At about 1 year of age, the head circumference has grown to about 18 in (47 cm). The chest also grows rapidly, catching up to the head circumference at about 5 to 7 months of age. From then on, the chest can be expected to exceed the head in circumference.

Fontanels and Cranial Sutures

The posterior fontanel is usually closed by the second or third month of life. The anterior fontanel may increase slightly in size during the first few months of life. After the sixth month, it begins to decrease in size, closing between the 12th and the 18th months. The sutures between the cranial bones do not ossify until later childhood.

Skeletal Growth and Maturation

During fetal life, the skeletal system is completely formed in cartilage at the end of 3 months' gestation. Bone ossification and growth occur during the remainder of fetal life and throughout childhood. The pattern of maturation is so regular that the "bone age" can be determined by radiologic examination. When the bone age matches the child's chronological age, the skeletal structure is maturing at a normal rate. To avoid unnecessary exposure to radiation, radiologic examination is performed only if a problem is suspected.

Eruption of Deciduous Teeth

Calcification of the primary or **deciduous teeth** starts early in fetal life. Shortly before birth, calcification begins in the permanent teeth that are the first to erupt in later childhood. The first deciduous teeth, usually the lower central incisors, usually erupt between 6 and 8 months of age (Fig. 23-2).

Babies in good health who show normal development may differ in the timing of tooth eruption. Some

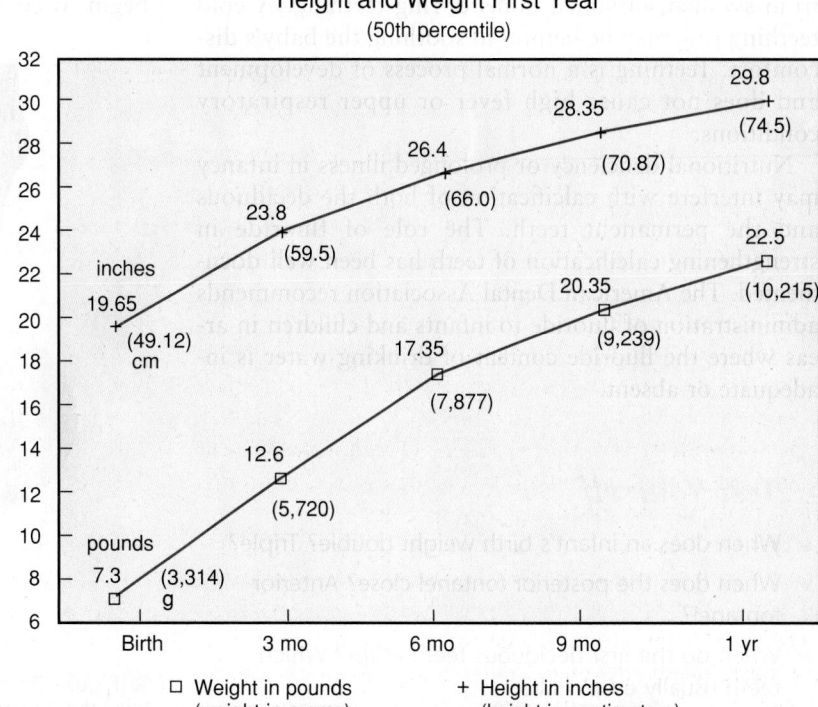

■ Figure 23-1 Chart of infant growth representing an infant in the midrange birth-weight 7.3 lb (3,314 g) and birth length 19.65 in (49.12 cm). Infants of different races vary in average size. Asian infants tend to be smaller, and African American infants tend to be larger.

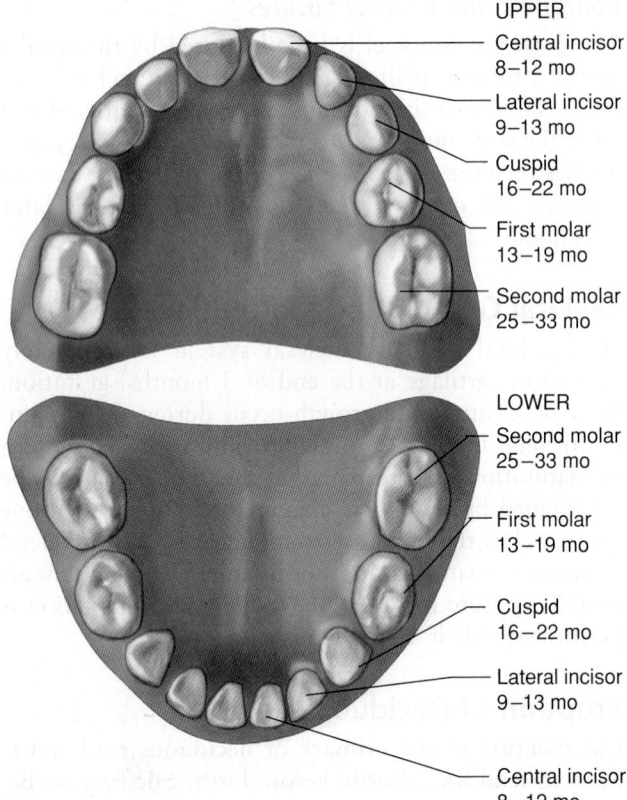

UPPER
Central incisor
8–12 mo

Lateral incisor
9–13 mo

Cuspid
16–22 mo

First molar
13–19 mo

Second molar
25–33 mo

LOWER
Second molar
25–33 mo

First molar
13–19 mo

Cuspid
16–22 mo

Lateral incisor
9–13 mo

Central incisor
8–12 mo

■ Figure 23-2 Approximate ages for the eruption of deciduous teeth.

families show a tendency toward very early or very late eruption without having other signs of early or late development. Some infants may become restless or fussy from swollen, inflamed gums during teething. A cold teething ring may be helpful in soothing the baby's discomfort. Teething is a normal process of development and does not cause high fever or upper respiratory conditions.

Nutritional deficiency or prolonged illness in infancy may interfere with calcification of both the deciduous and the permanent teeth. The role of fluoride in strengthening calcification of teeth has been well documented. The American Dental Association recommends administration of fluoride to infants and children in areas where the fluoride content of drinking water is inadequate or absent.

Test Yourself

✔ When does an infant's birth weight double? Triple?

✔ When does the posterior fontanel close? Anterior fontanel?

✔ When do the first deciduous teeth erupt? Which teeth usually erupt first?

Circulatory System

In the first year of life, the circulatory system undergoes several changes. During fetal life, high levels of hemoglobin and red blood cells are necessary for adequate oxygenation. After birth, when the respiratory system supplies oxygen, hemoglobin decreases in volume, and red blood cells gradually decrease in number until 3 months of age. Thereafter, the count gradually increases until adult levels are reached.

Obtaining an accurate blood pressure measurement in an infant is difficult. Electronic or ultrasonographic monitoring equipment is often used (see Chapter 28). The average blood pressure during the first year of life is 85/60 mm Hg. However, variability is expected among children of the same age and body build.

An accurate determination of the infant's heartbeat requires an apical pulse count. Place a pediatric stethoscope with a small-diameter diaphragm over the left side of the chest in a position where the heartbeat can be clearly heard (Fig. 23-3). Then, count the pulse for 1 full minute (see Chapter 28). During the first year of life, the average apical rate ranges from 70 (asleep) to 150 (awake) beats per minute and as high as 180 beats per minute while the infant is crying.

Body Temperature and Respiratory Rate

Body temperature follows the average normal range after the initial adjustment to postnatal living. Respirations average 30 breaths per minute, with a wide range (20–50 breaths per minute) according to the infant's activity.

Neuromuscular Development

As the infant grows, nerve cells mature and fine muscles begin to coordinate in an orderly pattern of develop-

■ Figure 23-3 A pediatric stethoscope is used to clearly hear the heartbeat of the infant.

ment. Naturally, the family caregivers are full of pride in the infant who learns to sit or stand before the neighbor's baby does, but accomplishing such milestones early means little. Each child follows a unique rhythm of progress within reasonable limits.

Average rates of growth and development are useful for purposes of making comparisons. Few landmarks call for special attention, and their absence may indicate the need for additional environmental stimulation. Do not emphasize routine developmental tables with family caregivers; a small time lag may be insignificant. A large time lag may require greater stimulation from the environment or a watchful attitude to discover how overall development is proceeding.

Table 23-1 and Figure 23-4 summarize the accepted norms in physical, psychosocial, motor, language, and cognitive growth and development in the first year of life.

PSYCHOSOCIAL DEVELOPMENT

The infant who actively seeks food to fulfill feelings of hunger experiences the give-and-take of life. The infant begins to develop a sense of trust when fed on demand. However, the infant eventually learns that not every need is met immediately on demand. Slowly the infant becomes aware that something or someone separate from oneself fulfills one's needs. Gradually, as a result of the loving care of family caregivers, the infant learns that the environment responds to desires expressed through one's own efforts and signals. The infant is now aware that the environment is separate from self.

Caregivers who expect too much too soon from the infant are not encouraging optimal development. Rather than teaching the rules of life before the infant has learned to trust the environment, the caregivers are actually teaching that nothing is gained by one's own activity and that the world does not respond to one's needs.

Conversely, caregivers who rush to anticipate every need give the infant no opportunity to test the environment. The opportunity to discover that through one's own actions the environment may be manipulated to suit one's own desires is withheld from the infant by these "smothering" caregivers. Family Teaching Tips: Infants From Birth to 1 Year suggests healthy child-rearing patterns during infancy.

No one is perfect, and every family caregiver misinterprets the infant's signals at times. The caregiver may be tired, preoccupied, or responding momentarily to his or her own needs. The caregiver may not be able to ease the infant's pain or soothe the restlessness, but this also is a learning experience for the baby.

As mentioned earlier, the infant's development depends on a mutual relationship with give and take between the infant and the environment in which the family caregivers play the most important role. Table 23-2 summarizes significant caregiver–infant interactions indicating positive behaviors.

Family Teaching Tips

INFANTS FROM BIRTH TO 1 YEAR

- *First 6 weeks:* Frequent holding of infant gives infant feeling of being loved and cared for. Rocking and soothing baby are important.
- *6 weeks to 3½ months:* Continue to give infant feeling of being loved and cared for; respond to cries; provide visual stimulation with toys, pictures, mobiles, and auditory stimulation by talking and singing to baby; and repeat sounds that infant makes to encourage vocal stimulation.
- *3½ to 5 months:* Play regularly with baby; give child variety of things to look at; talk to baby; offer a variety of items to touch—soft, fuzzy, smooth, and rough—to provide tactile stimulation; continue to respond to infant's cries; move baby around home to provide additional visual and auditory stimulation; and begin placing infant on floor to provide freedom of movement.
- *5 to 8 months:* Continue to give infant feeling of being loved and cared for by holding, cuddling, and responding to needs; talk to infant; put infant on floor more often to roll and move about; and fear of strangers is common at this age.
- *8 to 12 months:* Accident-proof the house; give the infant maximum access to living area; supply infant with toys; stay close by to support infant in difficult situations; and continue to talk to infant to provide language stimulation. The baby at this age loves surprise toys like jack-in-the-box and separation games like "Peek-a-Boo"; loves putting-in and taking-out activities. The child is developing independence, and temper tantrums may begin.

During the first few weeks of life, actions such as kicking and sucking are simple reflex activities. In the next sequential stage, reflexes are coordinated and elaborated. For example, in early infancy hand movements are random (Fig. 23-5A). The infant finds that repetition of chance movements brings interesting changes, and in the latter part of the first year, these acts become clearly intentional (Fig. 23-5B). The infant expects that certain results follow certain actions.

The infant soon connects the smiling face looking down with the pleasure of being picked up, fed, or bathed. Anyone who smiles and talks softly to the infant may make that small face light up and cause squirming of anticipation. In only a few weeks, however, the infant learns that one particular person is the main source of comfort and pleasure.

An infant cannot apply abstract reasoning but understands only through the five senses. As the infant matures enough to recognize the mother or primary caregiver, the

Table 23-1 ▪ GROWTH AND DEVELOPMENT: BIRTH TO 1 YEAR

Age	Physical	Personal-Social	Fine Motor	Gross Motor	Language	Cognition
Birth–4 wk	Weight gain of 5–7 oz (150–270 g) per wk. Height gain of 1" per mo first 6 mo. Head circumference increases 1/2" per mo. Moro, Babinski, rooting, and tonic neck reflexes present	Some smiling begins. Erikson's stage of "trust vs. mistrust."	Grasp reflex very strong. Hands flexed.	Catches and holds objects in sight that cross visual field. Can turn head from side to side when lying in a prone position (see Fig. 23-4A). When prone, body in a flexed position. When prone, moves extremities in a crawling fashion.	Cries when upset. Makes enjoyment sounds during mealtimes.	At 1 mo, sucking activity with associated pleasurable sensations.
6 wk	Tears appear	Smiling in response to familiar stimuli. Less flexion noted.	Hands open. Holds head up when prone.	Tries to raise shoulders and arms when stimulated. Smiles to familiar voices. Less flexion of entire body when prone.	Cooing predominant. Begins to repeat actions. Babbling sounds.	**Primary circular reactions** (explores objects by touching or putting in mouth; infant unaware actions are what bring pleasure).
10–12 wk	Posterior fontanel closes.	Aware of new environment. Less crying. Smiles at significant others.	No longer has grasp reflex. Pulls on clothes, blanket, but does not reach for them. Pumps arms, shoulders, and head from prone position (Fig. 23-4B).	No longer has Moro reflex. Symmetric body positioning.	Makes noises when spoken to.	Beginning of coordinated responses to different kinds of stimuli.
16 wk	Moro, rooting, and tonic neck reflexes disappear; drooling begins.	Responds to stimulus. Sees bottle, squeals, and laughs. Aware of new environment and shows interest.	Grasps objects with two hands. Eye–hand coordination beginning.	Plays with hands. Brings objects to mouth. Balances head and body for short periods in sitting position.	Laughs aloud. Sounds "n," "k," "g," and "b."	Likes social situations. Defiant, bored if unattended.

Table 23-1 ■ GROWTH AND DEVELOPMENT: BIRTH TO 1 YEAR *(continued)*

Age	Physical	Personal-Social	Fine Motor	Gross Motor	Language	Cognition
20 wk	May show signs of teething.	Smiles at self in mirror. Cries when limits are set or when objects are taken away.	Holds one object while looking for another one. Grasps objects voluntarily and brings them to mouth.	Able to sit up (Fig. 23-4C). Can roll over.	Cooing noises. Squeals with delight. Can bear weight on legs when held in a standing position. Able to control head movements.	Visually looks for an object that has fallen.
24 wk	Birth weight doubles; weight gain slows to 3–5 oz (90–150 g) per wk. Height slows to 1/2" per mo. Teething begins with lower central incisors.	Likes to be picked up. Knows family from strangers. Plays "Peek-a-Boo." Knows likes and dislikes. Fear of strangers.	Holds a bottle fairly well. Tries to retrieve a dropped article.	Tonic neck reflex disappears. Sits alone in high chair, back erect. Rolls over and back to abdomen.	Makes sounds "guh," "bah." Sounds "p," "m," "b," and "t" are pronounced. Babbling sounds.	**Secondary circular reactions** (realizes actions bring pleasure). Repeats actions that affect an object. Beginning of object permanence.
28 wk	Lower lateral incisors are followed in the next month by upper central incisors.	Imitates simple acts. Responds to "no." Shows preferences and dislikes for food.	Holds cup. Transfers objects from one hand to the other.	Reaches without visual guidance. Can lift head up when in a supine position.	Babbling decreases. Duplicates "ma-ma" and "pa-pa" sounds.	
32 wk	Teething continues.	Dislikes diaper and clothing change. Afraid of strangers. Fear of separating from mother.	Gradually palmar grasp reflex lessens and the **pincer grasp** (using thumb and index finger) develops (Fig. 23-4D). Adjusts body position to be able to reach for an object. May stand up while holding on.	Crawls around (Fig. 23-4E). Pulls toy toward self.	Combines syllables but has trouble attributing meaning to them.	
40 wk-1 yr	Birth weight tripled; has six teeth; Babinski reflex disappears. Anterior fontanel closes between now and 18 mo.	Does things to attract attention. Tries to follow when being read to. Imitates parents. Looks for objects not in sight.	Holds tools with one hand and works on it with another. Puts toy in box after demonstration. Starts blocks. Holds crayon to scribble on paper.	Stands alone; begins to walk alone (Fig. 23-4F). Can change self from prone to sitting to standing position.	Words emerge. Says "da-da" and "ma-ma" with meaning.	Coordination of secondary schemes; masters barrier to reach goal, symbolic meanings.

A

B

C

D

E   **F**

■ **Figure 23-4** Growth and development of the infant. **(A)** At 4 weeks, this infant turns head when lying in a prone position. **(B)** At 12 weeks, this infant pushes up from a prone position. **(C)** At 21 weeks, the infant sits up but tilts forward for balance. **(D)** At 32 weeks, this infant uses the pincer grasp to pick up a piece of cereal. **(E)** At 32 weeks, this infant is crawling around and on the go. **(F)** At 43 weeks, this infant is getting ready to walk.

Table 23-2 ▌ CRITERIA OF POSITIVE CAREGIVER–INFANT INTERACTIONS

Area of Interaction	Positive Caregiver Response
Feeding	Offers infant adequate amounts and proper types of food and prepares food appropriately
	Holds infant in comfortable, secure position during feeding
	Burps infant during or after feeding
	Offers food at a comfortable pace for infant
Stimulation	Provides appropriate nonaggressive verbal stimulation to infant
	Provides a variety of tactile experiences and touches infant in caring ways other than during feeding times or when moving infant away from danger
	Provides appropriate toys and interacts with infant in a way satisfying to infant
Rest and sleep	Provides a quiet, relaxed environment and a regular, scheduled sleep time for infant
	Makes certain infant is adequately fed, warm, and dry before putting down to sleep
Understanding of infant	Has realistic expectations of infant and recognizes infant's developing skills and behavior
	Has realistic view of own parenting skills
	View of infant's health condition similar to the view of medical or nursing diagnosis
Problem-solving initiative	Motivated to manage infant's problems; diligently seeks information about infant; follows through on plans involving infant
Interaction with other children	Demonstrates positive interaction with other children in home without aggression or hostility
Caregiver's recreation	Seeks positive outlets for own recreation and relaxation
Parenting role	Expresses satisfaction with parenting role; expresses positive attitudes

infant becomes fearful when this person disappears. To the infant, out of sight means out of existence, and the infant cannot tolerate this. For the infant, self-assurance is necessary to confirm that objects and people do not cease to exist when out of sight. This is a learning experience on which the infant's entire attitude toward life depends.

Think about this.

The ancient game of "Peek-a-Boo" is a universal example of how the infant learns. It is one of the joys of infancy as the child affirms the ability to control the disappearance and reappearance of self. In the same manner by which the infant affirms self-existence, he or she confirms the existence of others, even when they are temporarily out of sight.

NUTRITION

During the first year of life, the infant's rapid growth creates a need for nutrients greater than at any other time of life. The Academy of Pediatrics Committee on Nutrition endorses breast-feeding as the best method of feeding infants. (See Chapter 15 for discussion of factors that influence the choice of a feeding method.)

Most of the infant's requirements for the first 4 to 6 months of life are supplied by either breast milk or commercial infant formulas. Nutrients that may need to be supplemented are vitamins C and D, iron, and fluoride. Breast-fed infants need supplements of iron, as well as vitamin D, which can be supplied as vitamin drops. Most commercial infant formulas are enriched with vitamins C and D. Some infant formulas are fortified with iron. Infants who are fed home-prepared formulas

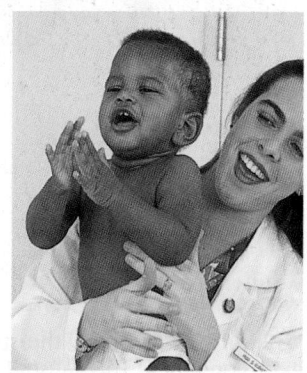

■ Figure 23-5 **(A)** In the early stages of infancy, hand movements are random. **(B)** Later in infancy, hand movements are coordinated and intentional.

A

B

(based on evaporated milk) need supplemental vitamin C and iron; however, evaporated milk has adequate amounts of vitamin D, which is unaffected by heating in the preparation of formula. Vitamin C can be supplied in orange juice or juices fortified with vitamin C.

Fluoride is needed in small amounts (0.25 mg/day) for strengthening calcification of the teeth and preventing tooth decay. A supplement is recommended for breast-fed and commercial formula-fed babies and for those whose home-prepared formulas are made with water that is deficient in fluoride. Vitamin preparations are available combined with fluoride.

Addition of Solid Foods

The time or order requirement for starting solid foods is not exact. However, at about 4 to 6 months of age, the infant's milk consumption alone is not likely to be sufficient to meet caloric, protein, mineral, and vitamin needs. In particular, the infant's iron supply becomes low, and supplements of iron-rich foods are needed. Table 23-3 provides guidelines for introducing new foods into an infant's diet.

Infant Feeding

The infant knows only one way to take food, namely to thrust the tongue forward as if to suck. This is called the **extrusion** (protrusion) **reflex** (Fig. 23-6) and has the effect of pushing solid food out of the infant's mouth. The process of transferring food from the front of the mouth to the throat for swallowing is a complicated skill that must be learned. The eager, hungry baby is puzzled over this new turn of events and is apt to become frustrated and annoyed, protesting loudly and clearly. Taking the edge off the very hungry infant's appetite by giving part of the formula is best before proceeding with this new experience. If the family caregivers understand that

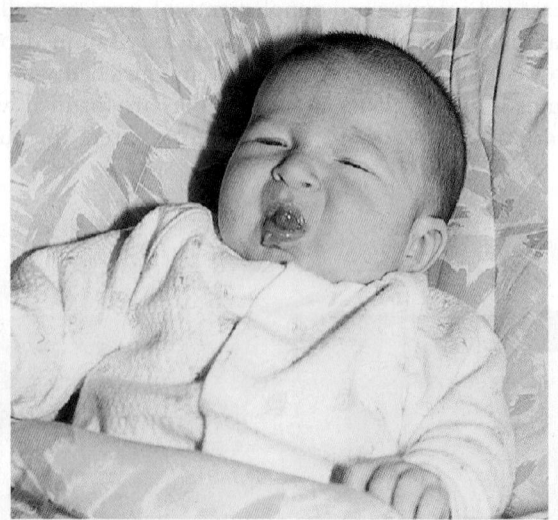

▮ **Figure 23-6** A baby thrusts the tongue forward using the extrusion reflex. This causes food to be pushed out of the mouth.

pushing food out with the tongue does not mean rejection, their patience will be rewarded.

The baby's clothing (and the caregiver's as well) needs protection when the baby is held for a feeding. A small spoon fits the infant's mouth better than a large one and makes it easier to put food further back on the tongue—but not far enough to make the baby gag. If the food is pushed out, the caregiver must catch it and offer it again. The baby soon learns to manipulate the tongue and comes to enjoy this novel way of eating. To avoid the danger of aspiration, the caregiver must quiet an upset or crying baby before proceeding with feeding.

Foods are started in small amounts, 1 or 2 tsp daily. Babies like their food smooth, thin, lukewarm, and bland. The choice of mealtime does not matter. It works best, at first, to offer one new food at a time, allowing 4 or 5 days before introducing another so that the baby becomes accustomed to it. This method also helps determine which food is responsible if the baby has a reaction to a new food.

When teeth start erupting, anytime between 4 and 7 months of age, the infant may enjoy a teething biscuit or cookie to practice chewing and to offer comfort. At about 9 or 10 months of age, after a few teeth have erupted, chopped foods can be substituted for pureed foods. Breast milk or formula gradually is replaced with whole milk as the infant learns to drink from a cup. This change takes some time because the infant continues to derive comfort from sucking at the breast or bottle. Infants need fat and should not be given reduced-fat milk (skim, 1%, or 2%).

Preparation of Foods

Various pureed baby foods, chopped junior foods, and prepared milk formulas are available on the market. These products save caregivers much preparation time, but many families cannot afford them. No matter which type of food is used, family caregivers should read food labels carefully to avoid foods that have undesirable additives, especially sugar and salt, or other unnecessary ingredients.

Point out that vegetables and fruits can be cooked and strained or pureed in a blender and are as acceptable to the baby as commercially prepared baby foods. Baby foods prepared at home should be made from freshly prepared foods, not canned, to avoid commercial additives. Caregivers should carefully check labels of frozen foods used because sugar and salt are commonly added. Excess blended food can be stored in the freezer in ice cube trays for future use. Caregivers can cook cereals and prepare formulas at home as well. Instead of purchasing junior foods, the caregiver can substitute well-cooked, unseasoned table foods that have been mashed or ground.

Preparation and storage of baby food at home require careful sanitary practices. All equipment used in the preparation of the infant's food must be carefully cleaned with hot, soapy water and rinsed thoroughly.

Table 23-3 ▌ SUGGESTED FEEDING SCHEDULE FOR THE FIRST YEAR OF LIFE

Age	Food Item	Amount*	Rationale
Birth–6 mo	Human milk or iron-fortified formula	Daily totals 0–1 mo 18–24 oz 1–2 mo 22–28 oz 2–3 mo 25–32 oz 3–4 mo 28–32 oz 4–5 mo 27–39 oz 5–6 mo 27–45 oz	Infants' well-developed sucking and rooting reflexes allow them to take in milk and formula. Infants do not accept semisolid food because their tongues protrude when a spoon is put in their mouths. They cannot transfer food to the back of the mouth. Human milk needs supplementation.
	Water	Not routinely recommended	Small amounts may be offered under special circumstances (e.g., hot weather, elevated bilirubin level, or diarrhea).
4–6 mo	*Iron-fortified infant cereal;[†] begin with rice cereal (delay adding barley, oats, and wheat until 6th mo)	4–8 tbsp after mixing	At this age, there is a decrease of the extrusion reflex, the infant can depress the tongue and transfer semisolid food from a spoon to the back of the pharynx to swallow it. Cereal adds a source of iron and B vitamins; fruit juices introduce a source of vitamin C.
	*Unsweetened fruit juices;[†‡] plain, vitamin C–fortified	2–4 oz	
	Dilute juices with equal parts of water		Delay orange, pineapple, grapefruit, or tomato juice until 6th mo.
	Human milk or iron-fortified formula	Daily totals 4–5 mo 27–39 oz 5–6 mo 27–45 oz	Do not offer water as a substitute for formula or breast milk, but rather as a source of additional fluids.
	Water	As desired	
7–8 mo	*Fruits, plain strained; avoid fruit desserts	1–2 tbsp	Teething is beginning; thus, there is an increased ability to bite and chew.
	*Yogurt[†]		
	*Vegetables,[†] plain strained; avoid combination meat and vegetable dinners	5–7 tbsp	Vegetables introduce new flavors and textures.
	*Meats,[†] plain strained; avoid combination or high-protein, dinners	1–2 tbsp	Meat provides additional iron, protein, and B vitamins.
	*Crackers, toast, zwieback[†]	1 small serving	
	Iron-fortified infant cereal or enriched cream of wheat	4–6 tbsp	
	Fruit juices[‡]	4 oz	
	Human milk or iron-fortified formula	24–32 oz	Iron-fortified formula or iron supplementation with human milk is still needed because the infant is not consuming significant amounts of meat.
	Water	As desired	May introduce a cup to the infant.
9–10 mo	*Finger foods[†]—well-cooked, mashed, soft, bite-sized pieces of meat and vegetables	In small servings	Rhythmic biting movements begin; enhance this development with foods that require chewing.
	Iron-fortified infant cereal or enriched cream of wheat	4–6 tbsp	Decrease amounts of mashed foods as amounts of finger foods increase.
	Fruit juices[‡]	4 oz	
	Fruits	6–8 tbsp	
	Vegetables	6–8 tbsp	
	Meat, fish, poultry, yogurt, cottage cheese	4–6 tbsp	Formula or breast milk consumption may begin to decrease; thus, add other sources of calcium, riboflavin, and protein (e.g., cheese, yogurt, and cottage cheese).
	Human milk or iron-fortified formula	24–32 oz	
	Water	As desired	

(continues on page 548)

Table 23-3 ▮ **SUGGESTED FEEDING SCHEDULE FOR THE FIRST YEAR OF LIFE** *(continued)*

Age	Food Item	Amount*	Rationale
11–12 mo	Soft table foods† as follows:		Motor skills are developing; enhance this development with more finger foods.
	Cereal; iron-fortified infant cereal; may introduce dry, unsweetened cereal as a finger food	4–6 tbsp	
	Breads; crackers, toast, zwieback	1 or 2 small servings	Rotary chewing motion develops; thus, child can handle whole foods that require more chewing.
	Fruit juice‡	4 oz	
	Fruit: soft, canned fruits or ripe banana, cut up, peeled raw fruit as the infant approaches 12 mo	1/2 cup	Infant is relying less on breast milk or formula for nutrients; a proper variety of solid foods (fruits, vegetables, starches, protein sources, and dairy products) will continue to meet the young child's needs.
	Vegetables: soft cooked, cut into bite-sized pieces	1/2 cup	
	Meats and other protein sources: strips of tender, lean meat, cheese strips, peanut butter	2 oz or 1/2 cup chopped	Delay peanut butter until 12th month.
	Mashed potatoes, noodles		
	Human milk or iron-fortified infant formula	24–30 oz	
	Water	As desired	

*Amounts listed are daily totals and goals to be achieved gradually. Intake varies depending on the infant's appetite.
†New food items for age group.
(Adapted from Twin Cities District Dietetic Association. *Manual of clinical nutrition,* with permission from its publisher, Chronimed Publishing, 13911 Ridgedale Dr, Minneapolis, MN 55343,1994:54–56.)
‡The Committee on Nutrition of the American Academy of Pediatrics recommends that fruit juices be introduced when infant can drink from a cup.

Some families prefer to spend more money for convenience and economize elsewhere, but no one should be made to feel that a baby's health or well-being depends on commercially prepared foods.

The healthy baby's appetite is the best index of the proper amount of food. Healthy babies enjoy eating and accept most foods, but they do not like strongly flavored or bitter foods. If the baby shows a definite dislike for any particular food, forcing it may develop into a battle of wills. A dislike for a certain food is not always permanent, and the rejected food may be offered again later. The important point is to avoid making an issue of likes or dislikes. The caregiver also should avoid introducing any personal attitudes about food preferences.

Self-feeding

The infant has an overpowering urge to investigate and to learn. At around 7 or 8 months of age, the baby may grab the spoon from the caregiver, examine it, and mouth it. The baby also sticks fingers in the food to feel the texture and to bring it to the mouth for tasting (Fig. 23-7). This is an essential, although messy, part of the learning experience.

After preliminary testing, the infant's next task is to try self-feeding. The baby soon finds that the motions involved in getting a spoon right side up into the mouth are too complex, so fingers become favored over the spoon. However, the infant returns to the spoon again until he or she eventually succeeds in getting some food from spoon to mouth, at least part of the time. Help family caregivers understand that all this is not deliberate messiness to be forbidden but rather a necessary part of the infant's learning.

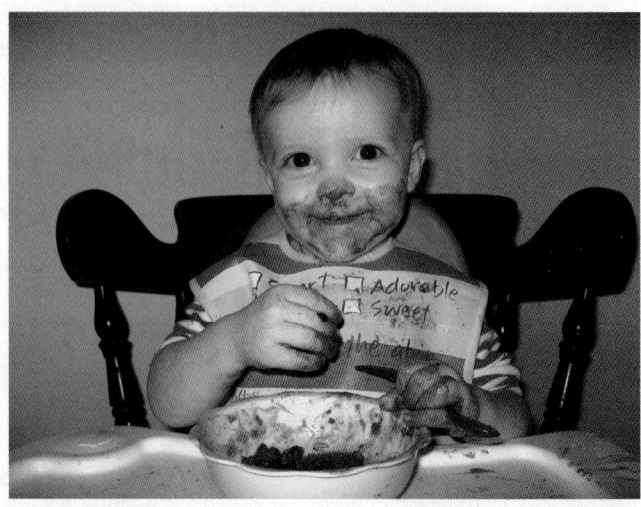

▮ Figure 23-7 Eating by yourself is a messy business but so much fun!

Weaning the Infant

Weaning, either from the breast or from the bottle, must be attempted gradually without fuss or strain. The infant is still testing the environment. The abrupt removal of a main source of satisfaction—sucking—before basic distrust of the environment has been conquered may prove detrimental to normal development. The speed with which weaning is accomplished must be suited to each infant's readiness to give up this form of pleasure for a more mature way of life.

At the age of 5 or 6 months, the infant who has watched others drink from a cup usually is ready to try a sip when it is offered. The infant seldom is ready at this point, however, to give up the pleasures of sucking altogether. Forcing the child to give up sucking creates resistance and suspicion. Letting the infant set the pace is best.

An infant who takes food from a dish and milk from a cup during the day may still be reluctant to give up a bedtime bottle. However, the infant must never be permitted to take a bottle of formula, milk, or juice to bed. **Pedodontists** (dentists who specialize in the care and treatment of children's teeth) discourage the bedtime bottle because the sugar from formula or sweetened juice coats the infant's teeth for long periods and causes erosion of the enamel on the deciduous teeth, resulting in a condition known as **bottle mouth** or **nursing bottle caries**. This condition can also occur in infants who sleep with their mother and nurse intermittently throughout the night. In addition to the caries, liquid from milk, formula, or juice can pool in the mouth and flow into the eustachian tube, causing otitis media (ear infection) if the infant falls asleep with the bottle.

Good judgment is in order.
A bottle of plain water or a pacifier can be used if the infant needs the comfort of sucking at bedtime.

A few babies resist drinking from a cup. Milk needs (calcium, vitamin D) may be met by offering yogurt, custard, cottage cheese, and other milk products until the infant becomes accustomed to the cup. The caregiver should be cautioned not to use honey or corn syrup to sweeten milk because of the danger of botulism, which the infant's system is not strong enough to combat.

Test Yourself

✔ What nutrients may need to be supplemented for the infant?
✔ Why is fluoride given to an infant?
✔ Why is one new food at a time introduced?
✔ What might occur if the infant is given a bottle of formula at bedtime?

Women, Infants, and Children Food Program

Women, Infants, and Children (WIC) is a special supplemental food program for pregnant, breast-feeding, or postpartum women, infants, and children as old as 5 years of age. This federal program provides nutritious supplemental foods, nutrition information, and health care referrals. It is available free of charge to persons who are eligible based on financial and nutritional needs and who live in a WIC service area. The family's food stamp benefits or school children's breakfast and lunch program benefits are unaffected. The foods prescribed by the program include iron-fortified infant formula and cereal, milk, dry beans, peanut butter, cheese, juice, and eggs. These foods may be purchased with vouchers or distributed through clinics. To encourage the use of WIC services, many health care facilities give WIC information to eligible mothers during prenatal visits or at the time of delivery.

HEALTH PROMOTION AND MAINTENANCE

Routine checkups, immunizations, family teaching, and education about accident prevention are important aspects of health promotion and maintenance. Immunizations and frequent well-baby visits help ensure good health. Family teaching and accident prevention help caregivers provide the best care for their rapidly growing child.

Routine Checkups

During the first year of life, at least six visits to the health care facility are recommended. These are considered well-baby visits and usually occur at 2 weeks, 2 months, 4 months, 6 months, 9 months, and 12 months. During these visits, the infant receives immunizations to guard against disease. Collect data regarding the infant's growth and development, nutrition, and sleep; the caregiver–infant relationship; and any potential problems. Document the infant's weight, height, and head circumference. Family teaching, particularly for first-time caregivers, is an integral part of health promotion and maintenance.

Immunizations

Every infant is entitled to the best possible protection against disease. Obviously, infants cannot take proper precautions, so family caregivers and health professionals must be responsible for them. This care extends beyond the daily needs for food, sleep, cleanliness, love, and security to a concern for the infant's future health and well-being. Protection is available against a number of serious or disabling diseases, such as diphtheria, tetanus, pertussis, rotavirus, hepatitis A and B, polio, measles, mumps, German measles (rubella), varicella (chickenpox), *Haemophilus influenzae* meningitis, pneumococcal diseases, and meningococcal disease, making it unnecessary to take chances with a child's health because of inadequate immunization.

The American Academy of Pediatrics, through its committee on the control of infectious diseases and the Advisory Committee on Immunization Practices for the Centers for Disease Control and Prevention (CDC), recommends a schedule of immunizations for healthy children living in normal conditions (see Appendix J). Additional recommendations are made for children who live in certain regions and areas or who have certain risk factors. Immunizations should be given within the prescribed timetable unless the child's physical condition makes this impossible. An immunization need not be postponed if the child has a cold but should be postponed if the child has an acute febrile condition or a condition causing immunosuppression or if he or she is receiving corticosteroids, radiation, or antimetabolites.

Side effects vary with the type of immunization but usually are minor in nature. The most common side effect is a low-grade fever within the first 24 to 48 hours and possibly a local reaction, such as tenderness, redness, and swelling at the injection site. These reactions are treated symptomatically with acetaminophen for the fever and cool compresses to the injection site. The child may be fussy and eat less than usual. The child is encouraged to drink fluids, and holding and cuddling is comforting to the child. Encourage the caregivers to call the provider if they are concerned, if there are any other reactions, or if these symptoms do not go away within about 48 hours.

Many children do not get their initial immunizations in infancy and may not get them until they reach school age, when immunizations are required for school entrance. Health care personnel should make every effort to encourage parents to have their children immunized in infancy to avoid the danger of possible epidemic outbreaks. For instance, measles outbreaks resulting in the deaths of children have been increasing at an alarming rate because of inadequate immunization. Serious illnesses, permanent disability, and deaths from inadequate immunizations are senseless and tragic. Answer any questions the caregiver may have about immunizations. Remember, however, that the caregiver has a right to refuse immunization if he or she has been fully informed about immunizations and any possible reactions. Maintain a nonjudgmental viewpoint throughout the discussion.

This advice could save the day.

Preparing caregivers by giving information regarding common side effects following immunizations may help decrease the caregivers' anxiety and concerns. A written information sheet gives the caregiver something to refer to at home if the child has a side effect.

Test Yourself

✔ Discuss the reasons immunizations are given.

✔ What are the diseases that children can be immunized against?

Family Teaching

Because mothers are discharged so early after giving birth, use every opportunity to perform teaching and promote healthy baby care. Well-baby visits provide an opportunity to ask the caregiver about concerns and to provide teaching. During well visits, offer guidance to help caregivers prepare for the many changes that occur with each developmental level. Discuss normal growth and development milestones but emphasize that these milestones vary from infant to infant. The infant's overall progress is the most important concern, not when he or she accomplishes a given task as compared with another infant or a developmental table. Discuss any infant sleep and activity concerns that the caregiver has. Encourage the caregiver to seek information about any other problems, worries, or anxieties he or she has. Provide ample time and opportunity for the caregivers to ask questions and gain information. It is not only wise to ask if the caregiver has concerns but also to suggest possible topics that may need to be reinforced. Some of those topics are discussed here.

Bathing the Infant

A daily bath is unnecessary but is desirable and soothing in very hot weather. Placing the baby into a small tub for a bath, rather than giving a sponge bath, may have a soothing and comforting effect as long as the baby is healthy and has no open skin areas. The small tub or large basin bath is described in the Family Teaching Tips: Giving a Small Tub Bath.

The bathing procedure is essentially the same for the older infant. When old enough to sit and move about freely, the infant may enjoy the regular bathtub, but this is often frightening to him or her. Splashing about in a small tub may be more fun, especially with a floating toy. An infant in a tub should always be held securely (Fig. 23-8). If possible, time should be scheduled so that bathing is a leisurely process, a time for the caregiver and baby to enjoy. As noted in Chapter 41, regular shampooing is important to prevent seborrheic dermatitis (cradle cap), which is caused by a collection of **seborrhea**, yellow crusty patches of lesions on the scalp.

Scented or talcum powder should not be used after the bath; powder tends to cake in creases, causing irritation, and may cause respiratory problems when inhaled by the infant. Scented powders and lotions cause allergic reactions in some babies. In any case, a clean baby has a sweet smell without the use of additional fragrances. Excessively dry skin may benefit from the application of

Family Teaching Tips

GIVING A SMALL TUB BATH

PREPARATION

Make sure room is warm and draft-free. Wash hands, put on protective covering, and assemble the following equipment:

- Large basin or small tub
- Mild soap/shampoo
- Nonsterile protective gloves
- Clean cotton balls
- Soft washcloth
- Large soft towel or small cotton blanket
- Clean diaper and clothes for infant

Fill tub with several inches of warm water (95°F–100°F [35°C–37°C]). This is comfortably warm to the elbow. Place basin or tub in crib or other protected surface.

Never turn from the baby during bathing. *Always* keep at least one hand holding the infant.

BATHING PROCEDURE

Wash the infant's face and head at the beginning of the bath. Use clear water with no soap. Wash each eye with a separate cotton ball, from the inner canthus outward. Gently wash the outer folds of the ears and behind them. Wash the rest of the face. Hold the infant with your nondominant arm using the football hold. Lather the hair with a mild shampoo, intended for use with infants, and rinse thoroughly.

After drying the head, undress the infant and examine for skin rashes or excoriations. Wearing protective gloves, remove diaper and wipe any feces from diaper area.

Place the infant in tub and soap the body while supporting the infant's head and shoulders on your arm. If the infant's skin is dry, soap may be eliminated or a prescribed soap substitute used. If the baby is enjoying the experience, make it leisurely by engaging the infant in talk, paddling in the water, and playing for a few extra minutes. When finished, lift the infant from the tub, place on a dry towel and pat dry with careful attention to folds and creases (underarms, neck, perineal area).

After the bath, gently separate the female infant's labia and cleanse with moistened cotton balls and clean water, wiping from *front to back* to avoid bacterial contamination from the anal region. Circumcised male infants need only be inspected for cleanliness. Uncircumcised males may have the foreskin gently retracted to remove smegma and accumulated debris. The foreskin is gently replaced. Do not force foreskin if not easily retracted, but document and report this occurrence.

---

lanolin or A+D Ointment, but oils are believed to block pores and cause infection. Various medicated ointments are available for excoriated skin areas.

After the bath, the baby's fingernails need to be inspected and cut, if long. Otherwise, the baby may scratch his or her face during random arm movements. The nails should be cut straight across with great care. While cutting, hold the arm securely and the hand firmly.

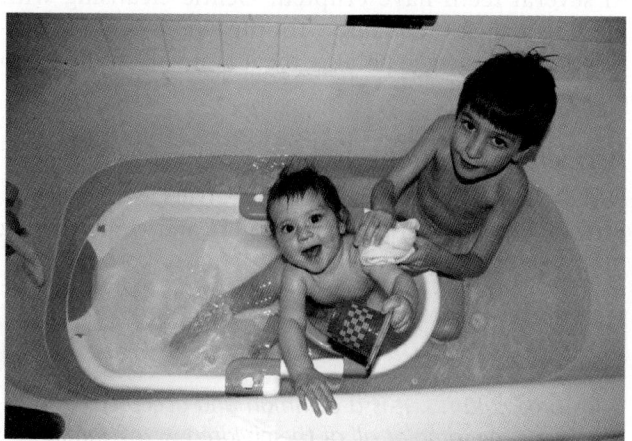

■ Figure 23-8 Bath time can be an enjoyable experience for the infant, especially when held securely in a bath seat.

Caring for the Diaper Area

To prevent diaper rash, soiled diapers should be changed frequently. The caregiver should check every 2 to 4 hours while the infant is awake to see if the diaper is soiled. Waking the baby to change the diaper is not necessary. Cleanse the diaper area with water and a mild soap if needed (see Family Teaching Tips: Preventing and Treating Diaper Rash in Chapter 41). Commercial diaper wipes also may be used, but they are an added expense (Fig. 23-9).

Diapers are available in various sizes and shapes. The choice of cloth versus disposable diapers is controversial. Disposable diapers have an environmental impact, but cloth diapers are inconvenient and associated with a higher risk of infection. Whatever the type, size, and folding method used, there should be no bunched material between the thighs. Two popular cloth diaper styles are the oblong strip pinned at the sides or the square diaper folded kite-fashion. The latter has the advantage of being useful for different ages and sizes. When folding a cloth diaper for a boy, the excess material is folded in the front, but for a girl, it is folded to the back. Safety pins must always be closed when they are used to fasten the diaper. When removed, they must be closed and placed out of the infant's reach.

■ **Figure 23-9** While the father changes his child's diaper, the nurse takes this opportunity to provide teaching on care of the diaper area.

For the older infant, the diaper must be fastened snugly at the hips and legs to prevent feces from running out of the open spaces. Cleaning a soiled crib and a smeared baby once or twice serves as an effective reminder!

Dressing the Infant

Dressing an infant can sometimes create a dilemma, especially for the first-time caregiver. Sometimes merely getting clothes on the baby is difficult. For instance, babies tend to spread their hands when the caregiver is trying to put on a top with long sleeves. The easiest way to put an infant's arm into a sleeve is to work the sleeve so that the armhole and the opening are held together, then to reach through the armhole and pull the arm through the opening. Clothing should not bind but should allow freedom of movement and be appropriate for the weather.

One rule of thumb is to dress the infant with the same amount of clothing that the adult finds comfortable. Overdressing in hot weather can cause overheating and prickly heat (miliaria rubra; see Chapter 41). In very hot weather, a diaper may be sufficient. When the infant begins to crawl, long pants help protect the knees from becoming chafed from the rug or flooring. When dressing the infant to go outdoors in cold weather, a head covering is important because infants lose a large amount of heat through their heads. In hot, sunny weather, the infant should not spend much time in the direct sun because the infant's skin is tender and burns easily.

Choosing shoes for the infant can be a problem for the new caregiver. Infants do not need hard-soled shoes; in fact, health care providers often recommend that infants be allowed to go barefoot and wear shoes only to protect them from harsh surfaces. Shoes with stiff soles actually hamper the development of the infant's foot. Sneakers made with a smooth lining with no rough surfaces to irritate the infant's foot are a good choice. They should be durable and flexible and have ample room in the toe. Properly made moccasins also are a good choice. High-topped shoes are unnecessary. Socks should provide plenty of toe room. Shoes should be replaced frequently as the infant's feet grow.

Promoting Sleep

Most infants sleep 10 to 12 hours at night and take two to three naps during the day. Each child develops his or her own sleeping patterns, and these vary from child to child. Caregivers often have concerns about their child's sleep needs and patterns. Infants should not have pillows placed in bed with them because of the possibility of suffocation. Sleep habits and patterns vary, but a consistent bedtime routine is usually helpful in establishing healthy sleeping patterns and in preventing sleep problems. Placing the child in the crib while awake and letting the child fall asleep in the crib creates good sleeping habits. In addition, this will often prevent the child from waking up when he or she is moved from the position or place he or she has fallen asleep. Using the crib for sleeping only, not for play activities, helps the child associate the bed with sleep rather than play. Sleep disturbances may be learned behaviors. Explore in depth any concern expressed by the caregiver. With the older child, bedtime rituals, consistent limits, and use of a reward system may decrease bedtime and sleep concerns and problems.

Dental Care

When teething begins in the second half of the first year, the caregiver can start practicing good dental hygiene with the infant. Initially the caregiver can rub the gums and newly erupting teeth with a clean, damp cloth while holding the infant in the lap. This time can be made pleasant by talking or singing to the infant. Brushing the teeth with a small, soft brush usually is not started until several teeth have erupted. Gentle cleansing with plain water is adequate. Toothpaste is not recommended at this stage because the infant will swallow too much of it.

Accident Prevention

Discussing safety issues with caregivers is important. Provide information about car safety and childproofing

Cultural Snapshot

In some cultures, it is a common and accepted practice for some or all of the children in the family to sleep in the bed with the parents.

Family Teaching Tips

INFANT SAFETY

Be one step ahead of child's development and prepared for the next stage.

ASPIRATION/SUFFOCATION
- Always hold bottle when feeding, **never** prop bottle.
- Crib and playpen bars should be spaced no more than 2-3/8 inches apart.
- Check toys for loose or sharp parts or small buttons.
- Keep small articles (such as buttons, marbles, safety pins, lint, balloons) off the floor and out of infant's reach.
- Store products such as baby powder out of child's reach.
- Keep plastic bags out of child's reach.
- Do not use pillows in a crib.
- Avoid giving child foods such as hot dogs, grapes, nuts, candy, and popcorn.
- Remove bibs at nap and bed times.
- Do not tie pacifier on a string around the child's neck.

FALLS
- Never leave child unattended on a high surface such as a high chair, bed, couch, or countertop.
- Place gates at the tops and bottoms of stairways.
- Raise crib rails and be sure they are securely locked.

MOTOR VEHICLE
- Place infant in an approved infant car carrier in the back seat when in a car. Follow the manufacturer's instructions regarding the age and size of the infant regarding placement of the carrier (rear or front facing)
- Never leave child unattended in a car.

DROWNING
- Never leave child alone in the bathtub, or near any water, including toilets, buckets, or swimming pools.
- Fence and use locked gates around swimming pools.

BURNS/INJURIES
- Cover unused plugs with plastic covers.
- Keep electrical cords out of sight.
- Remove tablecloths or dresser scarves that child might grasp and pull.
- Pad sharp corners of low furniture or remove them from child's living area.
- Turn household hot water to a safe temperature— 120°F (48.8°C).

POISONING
- Check toys for nontoxic material.
- Move all toxic substances (cleaning fluids, detergents, insecticides) out of reach and keep them in locked areas.
- Remove any houseplants that may be poisonous.
- Protect child from inhaling lead paint dust (from remodeling) or chewing on surfaces painted with lead paint.
- Place medicines in locked cupboards; remind family and friends (especially those with grown children or no children) to do the same.

and preventing aspiration, falls, burns, poisoning, and bathing accidents. Remind caregivers that the infant is developing rapidly and safety precautions should stay one step ahead of the infant's developmental abilities. Caregivers should teach older children in the family to be watchful for possible dangers to the infant, and they must be alert to potential dangers that the older sibling may introduce, such as unsafe toys, rough play, or jealous harmful behavior (see Family Teaching Tips: Infant Safety).

Test Yourself

✔ List the areas of family teaching that are important for the caregivers of infants.

✔ What are the areas of concern for the safety of an infant?

THE INFANT IN THE HEALTH CARE FACILITY

Hospitalization, however brief, hampers the infant's normal pattern of living. Disruption occurs even if a family caregiver stays with the infant during hospitalization. All or most of the sick infant's energies may be needed to cope with the illness. If given sufficient affection and loving care and if promptly restored to the family, however, the infant is not likely to suffer any serious psychological problems. Long-term hospitalization, though, may present serious problems, even with the best of care.

Illness itself is frustrating; it causes pain and discomfort and limits normal activity, none of which the infant can understand. If the hospital atmosphere is emotionally unresponsive and offers little if any cuddling or rocking, the infant may fail to respond to treatment, despite cleanliness and proper hygiene. Touching, rocking,

A Personal Glimpse

By the time my second son Noah was 6 months old, my husband and I were relaxed and confident parents. Perhaps too much so! Noah had just begun crawling. "We need to dig out the gates," I said to my husband, Richard. He agreed. However, we didn't do it right away, being busy with two kids and work.

Shortly afterward, Richard was working in our upstairs office. Noah was playing underfoot. I opened the door to the office and walked in to put something away. On my way out, I carelessly left the door open. I went downstairs to the kitchen and began coloring with my older son Jacob. A few minutes later, Noah crawled past my husband and out into the hallway. Richard was reading e-mail and didn't notice.

Then I heard something heavy and hard tumbling down the stairs and knocking into the walls, followed by my husband's screaming. I ran to the foyer and found Noah wailing face down on the hardwood floors. I fell to the ground, scooped him up, rocked him, and began crying. Will he be OK? Did he break anything? How could I be so careless? Why didn't we put the gates up? Why am I such a bad parent? I should have known better.

In the end, Noah was fine. His cheek was bruised, and his arm was sore. My husband and I were shaken, but we were OK too. The gates went up that afternoon!

Darlene

Learning Opportunity: What would you say to these parents to support and reassure them? What recommendations would you make to caregivers regarding safety in the home?

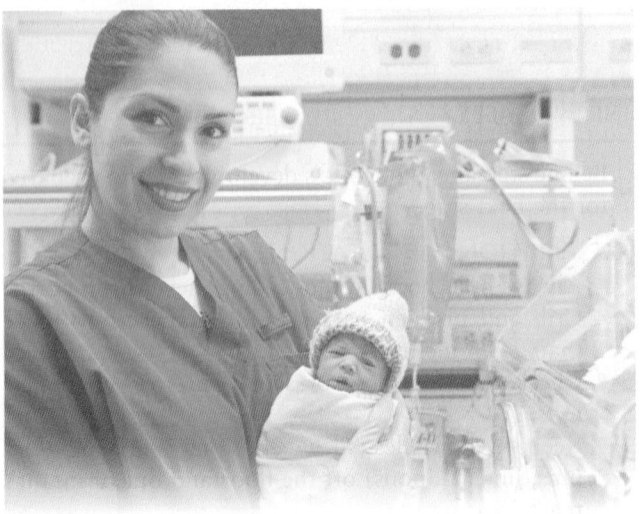

■ **Figure 23-10** Holding and cuddling can ease the discomfort of the hospital experience.

and cuddling a child are essential elements of nursing care (Fig. 23-10).

Hospitalization may have other adverse effects. The small infant matures largely as a result of physical development. If hindered from reaching out and responding to the environment, the infant becomes apathetic and ceases to learn. This situation is particularly apparent when restraints are necessary to keep the child from undoing surgical procedures or dressings or to prevent injury. The child in restraints needs an extra measure of love and attention and the use of every possible method to provide comfort.

Spending time, playing music in the room, or encouraging someone to stay with the infant might help to make the infant more comfortable. Provide age-appropriate sensory stimulation within the constraints of the infant's condition. Coo to and cuddle the infant, talk to him or her in warm and soft tones, and provide opportunities to fulfill sucking needs. Engage the infant in play. Singing songs, looking at picture books, reading stories,

reciting rhymes, playing "Peek-a-Boo," and other activities are strongly recommended. Introduce toys that are safe and age appropriate and that stimulate interest and responsiveness. Provide family caregivers with information about normal developmental activities appropriate for the infant, and encourage them to provide sensory and cognitive stimulation. This approach helps the infant build trust in the caregiver, which is a major developmental task, according to Erikson. It also helps caregivers feel needed and useful.

As the nurse, your relationship with family caregivers is extremely important. The hospitalized infant needs continued stimulation, empathetic care, and loving attention from family caregivers. Encourage caregivers to feed, hold, diaper, and participate in their infant's care as much as they can. Through conscientious use of the nursing process, collect data regarding the needs of the caregivers and the infant and plan care with these needs in mind. Identify and acknowledge the caregivers' apprehensions and develop plans to resolve or eliminate them. Make arrangements for rooming-in for the family caregiver, if possible. Family caregivers often are sensitive to changes in their infant that may help to identify discomfort, pain, or fear. Caregivers may sometimes assist during treatments and other procedures by stroking, talking to, and looking directly at the infant, thus helping to provide comfort during a time of stress. After the procedure, the infant may benefit from rocking, cuddling, singing, stroking, and other comfort measures that the family caregivers may provide. If the family caregivers are unavailable or can spend only limited time with the infant, the nursing staff must meet these emotional needs.

Key Points

➤ According to Erikson, the developmental task for the infant is to develop a sense of trust, which happens when the needs of the infant are consistently met.

➤ An infant's birth weight doubles by age 6 months and triples by 1 year.

➤ At birth, an infant's head circumference is usually slightly larger than the chest circumference. The head and chest grow rapidly and after about 5 to 7 months of age, the chest can be expected to exceed the head in circumference.

➤ The posterior fontanel closes by the second or third month and the anterior fontanel closes between the 12th and 18th months.

➤ The first tooth to erupt is usually one of the upper or lower incisors. This occurs between 6 and 8 months of age in most children. Family history, nutritional status, and prolonged illness affect the eruption of teeth. Fluoride is recommended to strengthen calcification of teeth and prevent tooth decay.

➤ The average apical rate ranges from 70 (asleep) to 150 (awake) beats per minute and as high as 180 beats per minute when the infant is crying.

➤ As the infant grows, nerve cells mature and fine muscles begin to coordinate in an orderly pattern of development.

➤ Between the ages of 6 and 7 months, most children develop a fear of strangers. As the infant matures enough to recognize the mother or primary caregiver, the infant becomes fearful when this person disappears. To the infant, out of sight means out of existence, and the infant cannot tolerate this. The game "Peek-a-Boo" is useful in affirming self-existence to the infant and that even when temporarily out of sight others still exist.

➤ The infant's nutritional requirements for the first 4 to 6 months are supplied by either breast milk or commercial infant formulas. Nutrients that may need to be supplemented are vitamins C and D, iron, and fluoride. At about 4 to 6 months of age, the infant's iron supply becomes low and supplements of iron-rich foods are needed. At around 7 or 8 months of age, the baby begins experimenting with finger foods and self-feeding.

➤ Infants have a tendency to push solid food out of their mouths with their tongue thrust forward because of the extrusion reflex.

➤ New foods are introduced one at a time to determine the food responsible if the infant has a reaction.

➤ An infant can be gradually weaned to a cup as her or his desire for sucking decreases, usually around the age of 1 year.

➤ Bottle mouth caries can occur when an infant is given a bottle at bedtime; the sugar from the formula causes erosion of the tooth enamel. To prevent bottle mouth caries, a bottle of plain water or a pacifier for sucking can be given at bedtime.

➤ If an infant resists drinking milk from a cup, calcium and vitamin D needs can be met by giving foods such as yogurt, custard, and cottage cheese.

➤ Children are immunized against hepatitis B virus, diphtheria, tetanus, pertussis, rotavirus, *Haemophilus influenzae* type b, polio, measles, mumps, rubella, varicella (chickenpox), pneumococcal disease, and meningococcal disease. In addition, they may be immunized against the hepatitis A virus. Immunizations should be given according to The American Academy of Pediatrics' recommended schedule. The most common side effect is a low-grade fever and possibly tenderness, redness, and swelling at the injection site. Acetaminophen is given for fever and cool compresses are applied to the injection site. The child may be fussy and eat less than usual. The child is encouraged to drink fluids, and holding and cuddling is comforting to the child.

➤ During routine health maintenance visits, teach caregivers information regarding normal growth and development milestones, bathing, diapering, dressing, sleep patterns, dental care, and safety.

➤ Infants' gums and teeth should be cleaned with a clean, damp cloth and plain water.

➤ Accident prevention for the infant includes closely watching the infant and monitoring the environment for safety hazards.

➤ In addition to nursing care, touching, rocking, and cuddling are essential for the hospitalized infant. Age-appropriate sensory stimulation and play within the constraints of the infant's condition are important. When an infant is hospitalized, the family caregiver can give the child stimulation, care, and attention by feeding, holding, and diapering the infant.

INTERNET RESOURCES

General Resources
www.cdc.gov
www.kidshealth.org/parent/growth
www.drspock.com

Child Passenger Safety
www.nhtsa.dot.gov

Workbook

■ NCLEX-STYLE REVIEW QUESTIONS

1. The nurse would expect an infant who weighs 7 lbs 2 oz at birth to weigh approximately how many pounds at 6 months of age?

   a. 10 lbs
   b. 14 lbs
   c. 17 lbs
   d. 21 lbs

2. In caring for a 4-month-old infant, which of the following actions by the infant would the nurse note as appropriate for a 4-month-old infant?

   a. Grasping objects with two hands.
   b. Holding a bottle well.
   c. Trying to pick up a dropped object.
   d. Transferring an object from one hand to the other.

3. When assisting with a physical exam on an infant, the nurse would expect to find the posterior fontanel closed by what age?

   a. 3 months
   b. 5 months
   c. 8 months
   d. 10 months

4. In teaching a group of parents of infants, the nurse would teach the caregiver that between 6 and 8 months of age, which of the following teeth usually erupt?

   a. First molars
   b. Upper lateral incisors
   c. Lower central incisors
   d. Cuspid

5. An infant had the following intake in the 12 hours after receiving immunizations. Calculate the 12-hour intake for this infant.

   Pedialyte, 4 oz
   Rice cereal, 4 tbsp.
   Dilute apple juice, 3 oz
   Applesauce, 1½ cup
   Iron-fortified formula, 8 oz
   Yogurt, ¼ cup
   Crackers, 4 small
   Iron-fortified formula, 5 oz
   Strained vegetables, 1 jar
   Iron-fortified formula, 7 oz
   12-hour intake _____

■ STUDY ACTIVITIES

1. List and compare the fine motor and gross motor skills in each of the following ages.

	4 Weeks Old	24 Weeks Old	32 Weeks Old
Fine motor skills			
Gross motor skills			

2. Answer the following regarding immunizations.

   a. By the time the infant is 1 year old, immunizations should have been given to prevent which diseases?
   b. How many doses of the hepatitis B vaccine are recommended?
   c. What are the two most common side effects of immunizations? How are these treated?

3. List five safety tips important in the infant stage of growth and development.

4. Go to the following Internet site: www.cdc.gov. Search for "Vaccines & Immunizations." Click on "Immunization Schedules." Open the schedules for children and adolescents and answer the following questions:

   a. What is the date of this immunization schedule?
   b. Compare the information on this site to Appendix J. Are there any changes? What changes have been made?
   c. Why do you think these changes in the immunization schedule have been made?

■ CRITICAL THINKING: WHAT WOULD YOU DO?

1. Tony Ricardo brings 6-month-old Essie for a routine checkup. You are responsible for formulating a plan for the visit.

   a. What characteristics would you observe for during the physical examination?
   b. What immunizations will the child need at this visit (assuming she is up to date)?
   c. What nutritional factors and guidelines will you observe for and teach?
   d. What other age-appropriate teaching will you do with Essie's father?

2. As you review nutrition with Mr. Ricardo, he states that Essie loves her bedtime bottle.

   a. What will you teach Mr. Ricardo regarding this practice?
   b. What suggestions will you make to help prevent the problems that often result from bedtime bottles?

3. At Nicole's 6-month checkup, her mother tells you that Nicole doesn't like the baby food and she just spits it out.

   a. What will you tell Nicole's mother to help her understand what is happening?
   b. What other information about feeding infants will you provide for this mother?

24 Growth and Development of the Toddler: 1 to 3 Years

KEY TERMS

autonomy
dawdling
discipline
negativism
parallel play
punishment
ritualism
temper tantrum

LEARNING OBJECTIVES

On completion of this chapter, you should be able to:

1. Identify characteristics of the toddler age group.
2. Explain the major developmental task of the toddler according to Erikson.
3. Describe physical growth that occurs during toddlerhood.
4. Define the following terms as they relate to the psychosocial development of the toddler: (a) negativism, (b) ritualism, (c) dawdling, and (d) temper tantrums.
5. Discuss psychosocial development of the toddler in relationship to (a) play, (b) discipline, and (c) the addition of a sibling to the toddler's home situation.
6. Discuss nutritional concerns of the toddler and the progression of the toddler's self-feeding skills.
7. Describe routine checkups as an important part of health promotion and maintenance for the toddler.
8. Identify important aspects of family teaching for the caregivers of toddlers, including (a) bathing, (b) dressing, (c) dental care, (d) toilet training, and (e) sleep.
9. State why accident prevention is a primary concern when caring for a toddler.
10. Discuss the four leading causes of accidental death of toddlers and preventive measures.
11. Discuss important aspects of nursing care for the toddler in the health care facility.

Soon after a child's first birthday, important and sometimes dramatic changes take place. Physical growth slows considerably; mobility and communication skills improve rapidly; and a determined, often stubborn little person creates a new set of challenges for the caregivers. "No" and "want" are favorite words. Temper tantrums appear.

During this transition from infancy to early childhood, the child learns many new physical and social skills. With additional teeth and better motor skills, the toddler's self-feeding abilities improve and include the addition of a new assortment of foods. Left unsupervised, the toddler also may taste many nonfood items that may be harmful, even fatal.

This transition is a time of unpredictability. One moment, the toddler insists on "me do it"; the next moment, the child reverts to dependence on the mother or other caregiver. While seeking to assert independence, the toddler develops a fear of separation. The toddler's curiosity about the world increases, as does his or her ability to explore. Family caregivers soon discover that this exploration can wreak havoc on orderly routine and a well-kept house and that the toddler requires close supervision to prevent injury to self or objects in the environment (Fig. 24-1). The toddler justly earns the title of "explorer."

Toddlerhood can be a difficult time for family caregivers. Just as parents are beginning to feel confident in their ability to care for and understand their infant, the toddler changes into a walking, talking person whose attitudes and behaviors disrupt the entire family. Accident-proofing, safety measures, and firm but gentle discipline are the primary tasks for caregivers of toddlers. Learning to discipline with patience and understanding is difficult but eventually rewarding. At the end of the toddlerhood stage, the child's behavior generally becomes more acceptable and predictable.

■ **Figure 24-1** This curious toddler explores in a kitchen drawer while mom supervises closely.

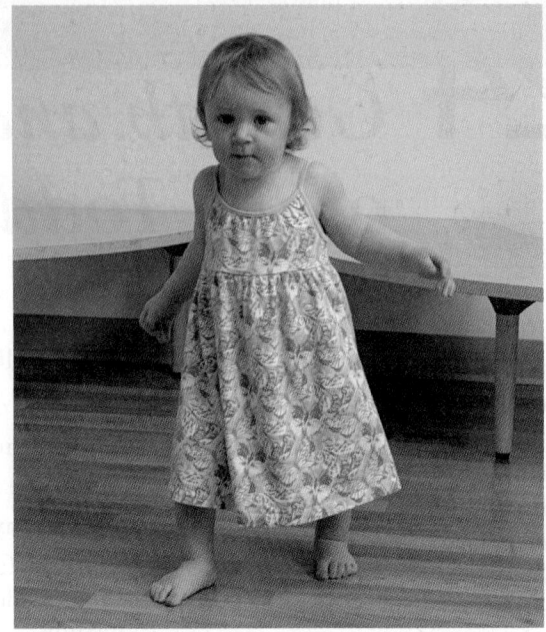

■ **Figure 24-2** The toddler is proud of her ability to walk.

Erikson's psychosocial developmental task for this age group is **autonomy** (independence) while overcoming doubt and shame. In contrast to the infant's task of building trust, the toddler seeks independence, wavers between dependence and freedom, and gains self-awareness. Stubborn behavior asserting independence is so common that the stage is commonly referred to as the "terrible twos," but it is just as often referred to as the "terrific twos" because of the toddler's exciting language development, the exuberance with which he or she greets the world, and a newfound sense of accomplishment. Both aspects of being 2 years old are essential to the child's development, and caregivers must learn to manage the fast-paced switching between anxiety and enthusiasm.

PHYSICAL DEVELOPMENT

Toddlerhood is a time of slowed growth and rapid development. Each year the toddler gains 5 to 10 lb (2.26–4.53 kg) and about 3 in (7.62 cm). Continued eruption of teeth, particularly the molars, helps the toddler learn to chew food. The toddler learns to stand alone and to walk (Fig. 24-2) between the ages of 1 and 2 years. By the end of this period, the toddler may have learned partial or total toilet training.

The rate of development varies with each child, depending on the individual personality and the opportunities available to test, explore, and learn. Table 24-1 summarizes significant landmarks in the toddler's growth and development.

PSYCHOSOCIAL DEVELOPMENT

During this time, most children say their first words and continue to improve and refine their language skills. The toddler develops a growing awareness of self as a being, separate from other people or objects. Intoxicated with newly discovered powers and lacking experience, the child tends to test personal independence to the limit.

Behavioral Characteristics

Negativism, ritualism, dawdling, and temper tantrums are characteristic behaviors seen in toddlers.

Negativism

This age has been called an age of **negativism**. Certainly, the toddler's response to nearly everything is a firm "no," but this is more an assertion of individuality than of an intention to disobey. Limiting the number of questions asked of the toddler and making a statement, rather than asking a question or giving a choice, is helpful in decreasing the number of negative responses from the child.

> **Here's a helpful hint.**
> Limiting the number of questions asked and offering a choice to the toddler will help decrease the number of "no" responses. For example, the question, "Are you ready for your bath?" might be replaced by saying, "It is bath time. Do you want to take your duck or your toy boat to the tub with you?"

Ritualism

Ritualism, employed by the young child to help develop security, involves following routines that make rituals of even simple tasks. At bedtime, all toys must be in accustomed places, and the caregiver must follow a habitual practice. This passion for a set routine is not found in

Table 24-1 ▎ GROWTH AND DEVELOPMENT: THE TODDLER

Age (months)	Personal–Social	Fine Motor	Gross Motor	Language	Cognition
12–15	Begins Erikson's stage of "autonomy versus shame and doubt" Seeks novel ways to pursue new experiences Imitations of people are more advanced	Builds with blocks; finger paints Able to reach out with hands and bring food to mouth Holds a spoon Drinks from a cup	Movements become more voluntary Postural control improves; able to stand and may take few independent steps	First words are not generally classified as true language. They are generally associated with the concrete and are usually activity-oriented.	Begins to accommodate to the environment, and the adaptive process evolves
18	Extremely curious Becomes a communicative social being Parallel play Fleeting contacts with other children "Make-believe" play begins	Better control of spoon; good control when drinking from cup Turns page of a book Places objects in holes or slots	Walks alone; gait may still be a bit unsteady Begins to walk sideways and backward	Begins to use language in a symbolic form to represent images or ideas that reflect the thinking process Uses some meaningful words such as "hi," "bye-bye," and "all gone" Comprehension is significantly greater	Demonstrates foresight and can discover solutions to problems without excessive trial-and-error procedures Can imitate without the presence of a model (deferred imitation)
24	Language facilitates autonomy Sense of power from saying "no" and "mine" Increased independence from mother	Turns pages of a book singly Adept at building a tower of six or seven cubes When drawing, attempts to enclose a space	Runs well with little falling Throws and kicks a ball Walks up and down stairs one step at a time	Begins to use words to explain past events or to discuss objects not observably present Rapidly expands vocabulary to about 300 words; uses plurals	Enters preconceptual phase of cognitive development State of continuous investigations Primary focus is egocentric
36	Basic concepts of sexuality are established Separates from mother more easily Attends to toilet needs	Copies a circle and a straight line Grasps spoon between thumb and index finger Holds cup by handle	Balances on one foot; jumps in place; pedals tricycles	Quest for information furthered by questions like "why," "when," "where," and "how" Has acquired the language that will be used in the course of simple conversation during adult years	Preconceptual phase continues; can think of only one idea at a time; cannot think of all parts in terms of the whole

every child to the same degree, but it does provide a comfortable base from which to step out into new and potentially dangerous paths. These practices often become more evident when a sitter is in the home, especially at bedtime. This gives the child some measure of security when the primary caregiver is absent.

Dawdling

Dawdling, wasting time or being idle, serves the purpose of asserting independence. The young child must decide between following the wishes and routines of the caregiver or asserting independence by following personal desires. Because he or she is incapable of making such a choice, the toddler compromises and tries both. If the task to be done is an important one, the caregiver with a firm and friendly manner should help the child to follow along the way he or she should go; otherwise, dawdling can be ignored within reasonable limits.

Temper Tantrums

Temper tantrums, aggressive displays of temper where the child reacts with rebellion to the wishes of the caregiver, spring from the many frustrations that are natural results of a child's urge to be independent. Add to this a child's reluctance to leave the scene for necessary rest, and frequently the frustrations become too great. Even the best of caregivers may lose patience and show a temporary lack of understanding. The child reacts with enthusiastic rebellion, but this, too, is a phase that the family must live through while the child works toward becoming an individual.

Reasoning, scolding, or punishing during a tantrum is useless. A trusted person who remains calm and patient needs to be nearby until the child gains self-control. After the tantrum is over, diverting attention with a toy or some other interesting distraction can help the child relax. However, do not yield the

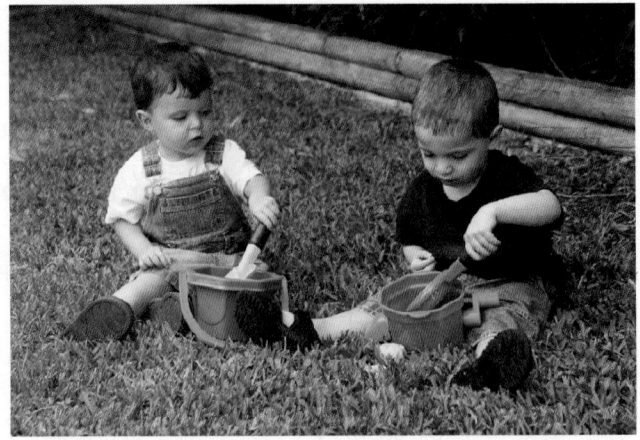

■ Figure 24-3 Toddlers engaged in parallel play.

point or give in to the child's whim. Giving in would tell the child that to get whatever he or she wants, a person need only throw oneself on the floor and scream. The child would have to learn painfully later in life that people cannot be controlled in this manner.

These tantrums can be accompanied by head banging and breath holding. Breath holding can be frightening to the caregiver, but the child will shortly lose consciousness and begin breathing. Head banging can cause injury to the child, so the caregiver needs to provide protection.

The caregiver should try to be calm when dealing with a toddler having a tantrum. The child is out of control and needs help to regain control; the adult must maintain self-control to reassure the child and provide security.

Play

The toddler's play moves from the solitary play of the infant to **parallel play**, in which the toddler plays alongside other children but not with them (Fig. 24-3). Much of the playtime involves imitation of the people the child sees as role models: adults around him or her, siblings, and other children. Toys that involve the toddler's new gross motor skills, such as push-pull toys, rocking horses, large blocks, and balls, are popular. Fine motor skills develop through use of thick crayons, play dough, finger paints, wooden puzzles with large pieces, toys that fit pieces into shaped holes, and cloth books. Toddlers enjoy talking on a play telephone and like pots, pans, and toys, such as brooms, dishes, and lawn mowers, that help them imitate the adults in their environment and promote socialization. The toddler cannot share toys until the later stage of toddlerhood, and adults should not make an issue of sharing at this early stage.

Adults should carefully check toys for loose pieces and sharp edges to ensure the toddler's safety. Toddlers still put things into their mouths; therefore, small pieces that may come loose, such as small beads and buttons, must be avoided.

For an adult, staying quietly on the sidelines and observing the toddler play can be a fascinating revelation of

---

Remaining calm is a must.

It is not easy to handle a small child who drops to the floor screaming and kicking in rage in the middle of the supermarket or to deal with comments from onlookers. The best a caregiver can do is pick up the out-of-control child as calmly as possible and carry him or her to a quiet, neutral place to regain self-control. The caregiver must ensure the child's safety by remaining near but ignoring the child's behavior.

Cultural Snapshot

A common cultural belief is that children are to respect their elders, be quiet and humble, and often to be "seen and not heard." This may create a problem for the toddler who is attempting to express his or her independence and having a "temper tantrum."

what is going on in the child's world. However, the adult must intervene if necessary to avoid injury.

Discipline

The word "discipline" has come to mean punishment to many people, but the concepts are not the same. To **discipline** means to train or instruct to produce a particular behavior pattern, especially moral or mental improvement, and self-control. **Punishment** means penalizing someone for wrongdoing. Although all small children need discipline, the need for punishment occurs much less frequently.

The toddler learns self-control gradually. The development from an egotistic being, whose world exists only to give self-satisfaction, into a person who understands and respects the rights of others is a long, involved process. The child cannot do this alone but must be taught.

Two-year-old children begin to show some signs of accepting responsibility for their own actions, but they lack inner controls because of their egocentricity. The toddler still wants the forbidden thing but may repeat "no, no, no" while reaching for a desired treasure, recognizing that the act is not approved. Although the child understands the act is not approved, the desire is too strong to resist. Even at this age, children want and need limits. When no limits are set, the child develops a feeling of insecurity and fear. With proper guidance, the child gradually absorbs the restraints and develops self-control or conscience.

Consistency and timing are important in the approach that the caregiver uses when disciplining the child. The toddler needs a lot of help during this time. People caring for the child should agree on the methods of discipline, and they should all operate by the same rules so that the child knows what is expected. This need for consistency can cause disagreement for family caregivers who have experienced different types of child-rearing themselves. The caregivers may be confused by this child who had been a sweet, loving baby and now has turned into a belligerent little being who throws tantrums at will.

This period can be challenging to adults. The child needs to learn that the adults are in control and will help the child to gain self-control while learning to be independent. When the toddler hits or bites another child, caregivers should calmly remove the offender from the situation. Negative messages such as "You are a bad boy for hitting Jamal" or "Bad girl! You don't bite people" are not helpful. Instead, messages such as "Biting hurts—be gentle" do not label the child as bad but label the act as unacceptable.

Another useful method for a child who is not cooperating or who is out of control is to send the child to a "time out" chair. This should be a place where the child can be alone but observed without other distractions. The duration of the isolation should be limited—1 minute per year of age is usually adequate. Caregivers should warn the child in advance of this possibility, but only one warning per event is necessary.

"Extinction" is another discipline technique effective with this age group. If the child has certain undesirable behaviors that occur frequently, caregivers ignore the behavior. In this technique, adults do not react to the child as long as the behavior is not harmful to the child or others. Caregivers must be consistent and never react in any way to that particular behavior. However, when the child responds acceptably in a situation in which the undesirable behavior was the usual response, it is important to compliment the child. Suppose, for example, that the child screams or makes a scene when the caregiver will not buy cookies in the grocery store. If, after the caregiver practices extinction, the child talks in a normal voice on another visit to the grocery store, caregivers should compliment the child's "grown-up" behavior.

Notice the difference. Praise children for good behavior with attention and verbal comments and, when possible, ignore negative behavior.

Spanking or other physical punishment usually does not work well because the child is merely taught that hitting or other physical violence is acceptable, and the child who is spanked frequently becomes immune to it.

Sharing With a New Baby

The first child has the caregivers' undivided attention until a new baby arrives, often when the first child is a toddler. Preparing a child just emerging from babyhood for this arrival is difficult. Although the toddler can feel the mother's abdomen and understand that this is where the new baby lives, this alone does not give adequate preparation for the baby's arrival. This real baby represents a rival for the mother's affection.

As in many stressful situations, the toddler frequently regresses to more infantile behavior. The toddler who no longer takes milk from a bottle may need or want a bottle when the new baby is being fed. Toilet training, which may have been moving along well, may regress with the toddler having episodes of soiling and wetting.

The new infant creates considerable change in the home, whether he or she is the first child or the fifth. In homes where the previous baby is displaced by the newcomer, some special preparation is necessary. Moving the older child to a larger bed some time before the new baby appears lets the toddler take pride in being "grown up" now.

■ **Figure 24-4** The toddler is meeting her new baby brother.

Preparation of the toddler for a new brother or sister is helpful but should not be intense until just before the expected birth. Many hospitals have sibling classes for new siblings-to-be that are scheduled shortly before the anticipated delivery. These classes, geared to the young child, give the child some tasks to do for the new baby and discuss both negative and positive aspects of having a new baby in the home. Many books are available to help prepare the young child for the birth and that explore sibling rivalry.

Probably the greatest help in preparing the child of any age to accept the new baby is to help the child feel that this is "our baby" not just "mommy's baby" (Fig. 24-4). Helping to care for the baby, according to the child's ability, contributes to a feeling of continuing importance and self-worth.

The displaced toddler almost certainly will feel some jealousy. With careful planning, however, the mother can reserve some time for cuddling and playing with the toddler just as before. Perhaps the toddler may profit from a little extra parental attention for a time. The toddler needs to feel that parental love is just as great as ever and that there is plenty of room in the parents' lives for both children.

The child should not be made to grow up too soon. The toddler should not be shamed or reproved for reverting to babyish behavior but should receive understanding and a bit more love and attention. Perhaps the father or other family member can occasionally take over the care of the new baby while the mother devotes herself to the toddler. The mother also may plan special times with the toddler when the new infant is sleeping and the mother has no interruptions. This approach helps the toddler feel special.

NUTRITION

The toddler needs foods from the major food groups each day. The USDA guidelines found in the MyPyramid for Kids in Figure 22-3 in Chapter 22 are appropriate for

Table 24-2 ■ DAILY NUTRITIONAL NEEDS OF THE 1- TO 3-YEAR-OLD

For a 1,000- to 1,400-calorie diet, the toddler needs the amounts below from each food group. Toddlers should be moderately active for 60 minutes every day, or most days.

Grains	Vegetables	Fruits	Milk	Meat and Beans
3–5 oz	1–1.5 cups	1–1.5 cups	2 cups	2–4 oz

children beginning at age 2. Daily nutritional needs for the toddler, including caloric requirements and the appropriate number of servings per day, are listed in Table 24-2.

Eating problems commonly appear between the ages of 1 and 3 years. These problems occur for a number of reasons, such as

- The child's growth rate has slowed; therefore, he or she may want and need less food than before. Family caregivers need to know that this is normal.
- The child's strong drive for independence and autonomy compels an assertion of will to prove his or her individuality, both to self and to others.
- A child's appetite varies according to the kind of foods offered. "Food jags," the desire for only one kind of food for a while, are common.

To minimize these eating problems and ensure that the child gets a balanced diet with all the nutrients essential for health and well-being, caregivers should plan meals with an understanding of the toddler's developing feeding skills. Family Teaching Tips: Feeding Toddlers offers guidance for toddler mealtimes. Messiness is to be expected and prepared for when learning begins; it gradually diminishes as the child gains skill in self-feeding. At 15 months, the toddler can sit through meals, prefers finger feeding, and wants to self-feed. He or she tries to use a spoon but has difficulty with scooping and spilling. The 15-month-old grasps the cup with the thumb and forefinger but tilts the cup instead of the head. By 18 months, the toddler's appetite decreases. The 18-month-old has improved control of the spoon, puts spilled food back on the spoon, holds the cup with both hands, spills less often, and may throw the cup when finished if no one is there to take it. At 24 months, the toddler's appetite is fair to moderate. The toddler at this age has clearly defined likes and dislikes and food jags. The 24-month-old grasps the spoon between the thumb and forefinger, can put food on the spoon with one hand, continues to spill, and accepts no help ("Me do!"). By 30 months, refusals and preferences are less evident. Some toddlers at this age hold the spoon like an adult, with the palm turned inward. The cup, too, may be handled in an adult manner. The 30-month-old tilts his or her head back to get the very last drop.

Family Teaching Tips

FEEDING TODDLERS

- Serve small portions, and provide a second serving when the first has been eaten. One or 2 teaspoonfuls is an adequate serving for the toddler. Too much food on the dish may overwhelm the child.
- There is no *one* food essential to health. Allow substitution for a disliked food. Food jags where toddlers prefer one food for days on end are common and not harmful. If the child refuses a particular food such as milk, use appropriate substitutes such as pudding, cheese, yogurt, and cottage cheese. Avoid a battle of wills at mealtime.
- Toddlers like simply prepared foods served warm or cool, not hot or cold.
- Provide a social atmosphere at mealtimes; allow the toddler to eat with others in the family. Toddlers learn by imitating the acceptance or rejection of foods by other family members.
- Toddlers prefer foods that they can pick up with their fingers; however, they should be allowed to use a spoon or fork when they want to try.

- Try to plan regular mealtimes with small nutritious snacks between meals. Do not attach too much importance to food by urging the child to choose what to eat.
- Dawdling at mealtime is common with this age group and can be ignored unless it stretches to unreasonable lengths or becomes a play for power. Mealtime for the toddler should not exceed 20 minutes. Calmly remove food without comment.
- Do not make desserts a reward for good eating habits. It gives unfair value to the dessert and makes vegetables or other foods seem less desirable.
- Offer regularly planned nutritious snacks such as milk, crackers and peanut butter, cheese cubes, and pieces of fruit. Plan snacks midway between meals and at bedtime.
- Remember that the total amount eaten each day is more important than the amount eaten at a specific meal.

HEALTH PROMOTION AND MAINTENANCE

Three important aspects of health promotion and maintenance for the toddler are routine checkups, family teaching, and accident prevention. Routine checkups help protect the toddler's health and ensure continuing growth and development. Use these opportunities to encourage good health through family teaching, support of positive parenting behaviors, and reinforcement of the toddler's achievements. Toddlers need a stimulating environment and the opportunity to explore it. This environment, however, must be safe to help prevent accidents and infection. Give caregivers information regarding accident prevention and home safety.

Routine Checkups

The practitioner sees the child at 15 months of age for immunization boosters and at least annually thereafter. Routine physical checkups include assessment of growth and development, oral hygiene, toilet training, daily health care, the caregiver–toddler relationship, and parenting skills. Interviews with caregivers, observations of the toddler, observations of the caregiver–toddler interaction, and communication with the toddler are all effective means to elicit this information. Remember that caregiver interpretations may not be completely accurate. Communicate with the toddler on his or her level and offer only realistic options.

The child should receive current immunizations (see Appendix J). Table 24-3 details nursing measures to ensure optimal health practices.

Family Teaching

The toddler is learning rapidly about the world in which she or he lives. As part of that process, the toddler learns about everyday care needed for healthy growth and development. The toddler's urge for independence and the caregiver's response to that urge play an important part in everyday life with the toddler. Some of these activities are included in the following discussion.

Bathing

Toddlers generally love to take a tub bath. Setting a regular time each day for the bath helps give the toddler a sense of security about what to expect. Although the toddler can sit well in the tub, he or she should never be left alone. An adult must supervise the bath continuously to prevent an accident. The toddler enjoys having tub toys to play with. Caregivers should avoid using bubble bath, especially for little girls, because it can create an environment that encourages the growth of organisms that cause bladder infections. A bath often is relaxing and may help the toddler quiet down before bedtime.

Dressing

By their second birthday, toddlers take an active interest in helping to put on their clothes. They often begin

Table 24-3 ▪ GUIDELINES FOR HEALTH PROMOTION IN THE TODDLER

Developmental Characteristics of Toddler (2–3 Yr)	Possible Deviations From Health	Nursing Measures to Ensure Optimal Health Practices
Self-feeding (foods and objects more accessible for mouthing, handling, and eating)	Inadequate nutritional intake Accidental poisoning Gastrointestinal disturbances: Instability of gastrointestinal tract Infection from parasites (pinworm)	Diet teaching Childproofing the home Careful hand washing (before meals, after toileting) Avoidance of rich foods Observe for perianal itching (Scotch tape test, administer anthelmintic)
Toilet training	Constipation (if training procedures are too rigid) Urinary tract infection (especially prevalent in girls due to anatomic structure and poor toilet habits)	Teaching toileting procedures Urinalysis when indicated (e.g., burning) Teaching hygiene (at the onset of training, instruct girls to wipe from front to back, and wash hands to prevent cross-infection)
Increased socialization	Increased prevalence of upper respiratory infections (immune levels still at immature levels)	Hygienic practices (e.g., use of tissue or handkerchief, not drinking from same glass) Immunizations for passive immunity against communicable disease
Primary dentition	Caries with resultant infection or loss of primary as well as beginning permanent teeth	Oral hygiene, regular tooth brushing, dental examination at 2.5–3 years Proper nutrition to ensure dentition
Sleep disturbances	Lack of sleep may cause irritability, lethargy, decreased resistance to infection	Teaching regarding recommended amounts of sleep (12–14 hr in first year, decreasing to 10–12 hr by age 3); need for rituals to enhance transition process to bedtime; possibility of need for nap; setting bedtime limits

around 18 months by removing their socks and shoes whenever they choose. This behavior can be frustrating to the caregiver, but if accepted as another small step in development, the caretaker may feel less frustration. Between the ages of 2 and 3 years, the toddler can begin by putting on underpants, shirts, or socks. Often the clothing ends up backward, but the important thing is that the toddler accomplished the task. Encourage the caregiver to take a relaxed attitude as the toddler learns to dress himself or herself. If clothes must be put on correctly, the caregiver should try to do it without criticizing the toddler's job. The caregiver should warmly acknowledge the toddler's accomplishment of putting on a piece of clothing that he or she may have struggled with for some time. Roomy clothing with easy buttons; large, smooth-running zippers; or Velcro is easier for the toddler to handle.

As in late infancy, shoes need to be worn primarily to protect the toddler's feet from harsh surfaces. Sneakers are still a good choice. Avoid hard-soled shoes. High-topped shoes are unnecessary.

Dental Care

Dental caries (cavities) are a major health problem in children and young adults. Sound teeth depend in part on sound nutrition. The development of dental caries is linked to the effect the diet has on the oral environment.

Bacteria that act in the presence of sugar and form a film, or dental plaque, on the teeth cause tooth decay. People who eat sweet foods frequently accumulate plaque easily and are prone to dental caries. Sugars eaten at mealtime appear to be neutralized by the presence of other foods and, therefore, are not as damaging as between-meal sweets and bedtime bottles. Foods consisting of hard or sticky sugars, such as lollipops and caramels that remain in the mouth for longer periods, tend to cause more dental caries than those eaten quickly. Sugarless gum or candies are not as harmful.

When the child is about 2 years of age, he or she should learn to brush the teeth or at least to rinse the mouth after each meal or snack. Because this is the period when the toddler likes to imitate others, the child learns best by example. Plain water should be used until the child has learned how to spit out toothpaste. An adult should also brush the toddler's teeth until the child becomes experienced (Fig. 24-5). One good method is to stand behind the child in front of a mirror and brush the child's teeth. In addition to cleaning adequately, this also helps the child learn how it feels to have the teeth thoroughly brushed. The use of fluoride toothpaste strengthens tooth enamel and helps to prevent tooth decay, particularly in communities with unfluoridated water. An adult should supervise the use of fluoride toothpaste; the child should use only a

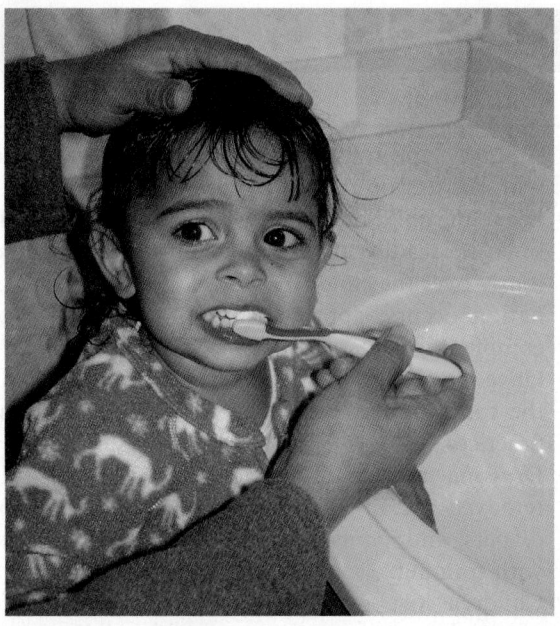

Figure 24-5 An adult helps the toddler brush her teeth.

small pea-sized amount. The physician may recommend supplemental fluoride, but families on limited incomes may find this difficult to afford. A fluoride supplement is a medication and should be treated and stored as such. Fluoride also can be applied during regular visits to the dentist, but the greatest benefit to the tooth enamel occurs before the eruption of the teeth.

The first visit to the dentist should occur at about 2 years of age so the child gets acquainted with the dentist, staff, and office. A second visit might be a good time for a preliminary examination, and subsequent visits twice a year for checkups are recommended. If there are older siblings, the toddler can go along on a visit with them to help overcome the fears of a strange setting. Some clinics are recommending earlier visits to check the child and give dietary guidance. Children of low-income families often have poor dental hygiene and care, both because of the cost of care and parental lack of knowledge about proper care and nutrition. Some caregivers may believe it is unnecessary to take proper care of baby teeth because "they fall out anyway." However, the care and condition of the baby teeth affect the normal growth of permanent teeth, which are forming in the jaw under the baby teeth.

Pay attention to the little details.

It is important to teach the caregivers the importance of proper care of the child's baby teeth.

Toilet Training

Learning bowel and bladder control is an important part of the socialization process. In Western culture, a great sense of shame and disgust has been associated with body waste products. To function successfully in this culture, one must learn to dispose of body waste products in a place considered proper by society.

The toddler has been operating on the pleasure principle by simply emptying the bowel and bladder when the urge is present without thinking of anything but personal comfort. During toilet training, the child, who is just learning about control of the personal environment, finds that some of that control must be given up to please those most important people, the caregivers. The toddler now must learn to conform not only to please those special loved ones, but also to preserve self-integrity, the toddler must persuade himself or herself that this acceptance of the dictates of society is voluntary. These new routines make little sense to the child.

Timing is an important aspect of toilet training. To be able to cooperate in toilet training, the child's anal and urethral sphincter muscles must have developed to the stage where the child can control them. Control of the anal sphincter usually develops first. The child also must be able to postpone the urge to defecate or urinate until reaching the toilet or potty and must be able to signal the need before the event. In addition, before toilet training can occur, the child must have a desire to please the caregiver by holding feces and urine, rather than satisfying his or her own immediate need for gratification. This level of maturation seldom takes place before the age of 18 to 24 months.

At the start of toilet training, the child does not understand the use of the potty chair but will sit there for a short time to please the caregiver (Fig. 24-6). If the child's bowel movements occur at about the same time every day, one day a bowel movement will occur while the child is sitting on the potty. Although there is no sense of special achievement for this event itself, the child does like the praise and approval caregivers provide.

Figure 24-6 Toddlers will sit on the potty chair to please a caregiver.

A Personal Glimpse

My husband and I decided it was time to potty train our near 3-year-old son, William. We started by "introducing" him to the potty. In the morning, my husband would casually ask William if he'd like to sit on the potty. "No," he'd assert. Before a bath, I'd ask William if he would like to sit on the Elmo chair and get a treat. "No," he'd say again, "gimme back my diaper." Taking this as a sign that he wasn't ready, we decided to delay potty training. Then, one day, William followed our 5-year-old son, Jack, into the bathroom. From the other room I heard Jack say, "See, Will, this is how I use the potty." William, ever eager to please his brother, pulled up a step stool and mimicked Jack. Nothing happened, but William was starting to show interest. I praised them and gave them both a small treat. I suggested to Jack that he ask William to sit on the little potty while he sat on the big potty to "pee," which would be easier for William. "Got it," Jack said with two thumbs up. We resumed potty training. Jack took the lead in our family effort. A week later, Jack and William came bounding out of the bathroom together. "We did it," Jack exclaimed. "We did it," William repeated. "I go pee-pee like Jack!" Upon further inspection, I found that William had in fact successfully used the little potty. "High-five," Jack begged. "High-five," William dutifully repeated. "High-five all around," I giggled. We still have a long way to go, but we are making progress—all four of us together!

Melanie (and Joe)

Learning Opportunity: What behavioral characteristics commonly seen in the toddler did this child show? What would you suggest these parents do to praise and support both of their children in the toilet training process?

Family Teaching Tips

TOILET TRAINING

- A potty chair in which a child can comfortably sit with the feet on the floor is preferable.
- Leave the child on the potty chair for only a short time. Be readily available but do not hover anxiously over the child. If a bowel movement or urination occurs, approval is in order; if not, no comment is necessary.
- Have the child wash her/his hands after sitting on the toilet or potty chair to instill good hygiene practices.
- Dressing the child in clothes that are easily removed and in training pants or "pull-up" type diapers and pants increases the child's success with training.
- Children love to copy and imitate others, and often, observing a parent or an older sibling gives the toddler a positive role model for toilet training.
- During the beginning stages of training, the child is likely to have a bowel movement or wet diaper soon after leaving the potty. This is not willful defiance and need not be mentioned.
- Empty the potty chair unobtrusively after the child has resumed playing. The child has cooperated and produced the product desired. If it is immediately thrown away, the child may be confused and not so eager to please the next time. However, some children enjoy the fun of flushing the toilet and watching as the materials disappear.
- Be careful not to flush the toilet while the child is sitting on it, as this can be frightening to the child.
- The ability to feel shame and self-doubt appears at this age. Therefore, the child should not be teased about reluctance or inability to conform. This teasing can shake the child's confidence and cause feelings of doubt in self-worth.
- Do not expect perfection; even after control has been achieved, lapses inevitably occur.

Eventually the child will connect this approval with the bowel movement in the potty, and the child will be happy that the caregiver is pleased.

Generally, the first indication of readiness for bladder training is when the child makes a connection between the puddle on the floor and something he or she did. In the next stage, the child runs to the caregiver and indicates a need to urinate, but only after it has happened. Sometimes the child who is ready for toilet training will pull on a wet or soiled diaper or even bring a clean diaper to the caregiver to indicate they need a diaper change. A serious training program will have little benefit, however, until the child is sufficiently mature to control the urethral sphincter and reach the desired place. When the child stays dry for about 2 hours at a time during the day, this may indicate sufficient maturity.

Give this a try.

Offering small rewards, such as stickers, nutritious treats, or toys, can encourage the child who is in the process of toilet training.

The caregiver should not expect perfection, even after control has been achieved. Each child follows an individual pattern of development, so no caregiver should feel embarrassed or ashamed because a child continues to have accidents. Lapses inevitably occur, perhaps because the child is completely absorbed in play or because of a temporary episode of loose stools. Occasionally a child feels aggression, frustration, or anger and may use this method to "get even." As long as the lapses are occasional, caregivers should ignore them. If the lapses are frequent and persistent, the cause should be explored.

No one should expect the child to accomplish self-training, and family caregivers should be alert to the signs of readiness. Patience and understanding by the caregivers are essential. Family Teaching Tips: Toilet Training offers suggestions for caregivers. Complete control, especially at night, may not be achieved until 4 or 5 years of age. Each child should be taught a term or phrase to use for toileting that is recognizable to others, clearly understood, and socially acceptable. This is especially true for children who are cared for outside the home.

> **Here's a tip for caregivers.**
> To help the child remember to use the toilet or potty chair, set a timer to sound at appropriate intervals. When the timer sounds, the child will be reminded to go to the bathroom.

Sleep

The toddler's sleep needs change gradually between the ages of 1 and 3 years. A total daily need for 12 to 14 hours of sleep is to be expected in the first year of toddlerhood, decreasing to 10 to 12 hours by 3 years of age. The toddler soon gives up a morning nap, but most continue to need an afternoon nap until sometime near the third birthday.

Bedtime rituals are common. A bedtime ritual provides structure and a feeling of security because the toddler knows what to expect and what is expected of him or her. The separation anxiety common in the toddler may contribute to some of the toddler's reluctance to go to bed. Family caregivers must be careful that the toddler does not use this to manipulate them and delay bedtime. Gentle, firm consistency by caregivers is ultimately reassuring to the toddler. Regular schedules with set bedtimes are important.

> **Check out this tip.**
> Bedtime routines, such as reading a story or having a quiet time, are helpful in providing a calming end to a busy day for the toddler.

> ## Test Yourself
> ✔ List the areas of family teaching that are important for the caregivers of toddlers.
> ✔ What must develop in order for the toddler to be physically ready for toilet training? By what age are most children toilet trained?

Accident Prevention

Toddlers are explorers who require constant supervision in a controlled environment to encourage autonomy and prevent injury. When supervision is inadequate or the environment is unsafe, tragedy often results; accidents are the leading cause of death for children between the ages

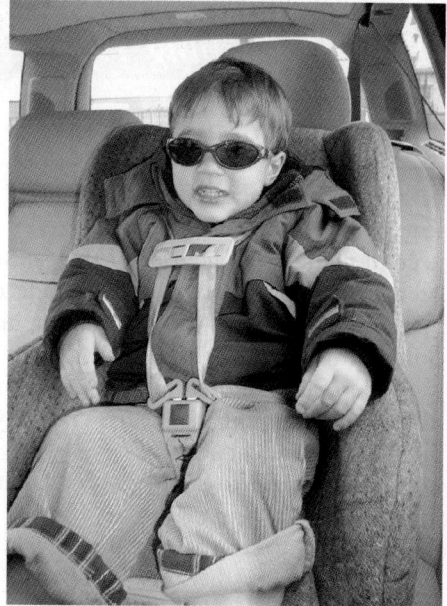

■ **Figure 24-7** Car seats are used for safety when toddlers ride in a vehicle.

of 1 and 4 years. Accidents involving motor vehicles, drowning, burns, and poisoning are the most common causes of death. The number of motor vehicle deaths in this age group is more than three times greater than the numbers of deaths caused by burns or drowning. Family teaching can help minimize the risk for accident and injury.

Motor Vehicle Accidents

Many childhood deaths or injuries resulting from motor vehicle accidents can be prevented by proper use of restraints. Federally approved child safety seats are designed to give the child maximum protection if used correctly (Fig. 24-7). Adults must be responsible for teaching the child that seat belts are required for safe car travel and that he or she must be securely fastened in the car seat before the car starts. Adults in the car with a child should set the example by also using seat belts. Many toddlers are killed or injured by moving vehicles while playing in their own driveways or garages. Caregivers need to be aware that these tragedies can occur and must take proper precautions at all times. See Family Teaching Tips: Preventing Motor Vehicle Accidents.

Drowning

Although drowning of young children is often associated with bathtubs, the increased number of home swimming pools has added significantly to the number of accidental drownings. Often, these pools are fenced on three sides to keep out nonresidents but are bordered on one side by the family home, making the pool accessible to infants and toddlers. Even small plastic wading pools hold enough water to drown an unsupervised toddler. Any family living near a body of water, no matter how small, must not leave a mobile infant or toddler

Family Teaching Tips

PREVENTING MOTOR VEHICLE ACCIDENTS

- Never start the car until the child is securely in the car seat.
- If the child manages to get out of the car seat or unfasten it, pull over to the curb or side of the road as soon as possible, turn off the car, and tell the child that the car will not go until he or she is safely in the seat. Children love to go in the car, and they will comply if they learn that they cannot go unless in the car seat.
- Never permit a child to stand in a car that is in motion.
- Teach the toddler to stop at a curb and wait for an adult escort to cross the street. An older child should be taught to look both ways for traffic. Start this as a game with toddlers, and continually reinforce it.
- Teach the child to cross only at corners.
- Begin in toddlerhood to teach awareness of traffic signals and their meanings. As soon as the child recognizes color, he or she can tell you when it is all right to cross.
- Never let a child run into the street after a ball.
- Teach a child never to walk between parked cars to cross.
- As a driver, always be on the alert for children running into the street when in a residential area.

Family Teaching Tips

PREVENTING BURNS

- Do not let electrical cords dangle over a counter or table. Repair frayed cords. Newer small appliances have shorter cords to prevent dangling.
- Cover electrical wall outlets with safety caps.
- Turn handles of pans on the stove toward the back of the stove. If possible, place pans on back burners out of the toddler's reach.
- Place cups of hot liquid out of reach. Do not use overhanging tablecloths that toddlers can pull.
- Use caution when serving foods heated in the microwave; they can be hotter than is apparent.
- Supervise small children at all times in the bathtub so they cannot turn on the hot water tap.
- Turn thermostat on home water heater down so that the water temperature is no higher than 120°F.
- Place matches in metal containers and out of reach of small children. Keep lighters out of reach of children.
- Never leave small children unattended by an adult or responsible teenager.

unattended, even for a moment. Even a small amount of water, such as that in a bucket, may be enough to drown a small child.

Burns

Burn accidents occur most often as scalds from immersions and spills and from exposure to uninsulated electrical wires or live extension cord plugs. Children also are burned while playing with matches or while left unattended in a home where a fire breaks out. Whether the fire results from a child's mischief, an adult's carelessness, or some unforeseeable event, the injuries, even if not fatal, can have long-term or permanent effects. Burns can often be prevented by following simple safety practices (Family Teaching Tips: Preventing Burns).

Ingestion of Toxic Substances

The curious toddler wants to touch and taste everything. Left unsupervised, the toddler may sample household cleaners, prescription or over-the-counter drugs, kerosene, gasoline, peeling lead-based paint chips, or dust particles. Poisoning is still the most common medical emergency

in children, with the highest incidence between the ages of 1 and 4 years.

Caregivers need continual reminders about the possibility of childhood poisoning. Even with precautionary labeling and "child-resistant" packaging of medication and household cleaners, children display amazing ingenuity in opening bottles and packages that catch their curiosity. Mr. Yuk labels are available from the nearest poison control center. The child can be taught that products are harmful if they have the Mr. Yuk label on them. However, labeling is not sufficient: All items that are in any way toxic to the child must be placed under lock and key or totally out of the child's reach.

Preventive measures that all caregivers of small children should observe are listed in Family Teaching Tips: Preventing Poisoning.

Always exercise caution.

The importance of careful, continuous supervision of toddlers and other young children cannot be overemphasized.

The following medications are most commonly involved in cases of childhood poisoning:

- Acetaminophen
- Salicylates (aspirin)
- Laxatives
- Sedatives

Family Teaching Tips

PREVENTING POISONING

- Keep medicines in their original containers with original labels in a locked cupboard. Do not rely on a high shelf being out of a child's reach.
- Never refer to medicines as candy.
- Nevel give medications to a child in the dark. Wrong medications or doses could be given.
- Discard unused medicines by a method that eliminates any possibility of access by children, other persons, or animals (e.g., flush them down the toilet).
- Replace safety caps properly, but do not depend on them to be childproof. Children can sometimes open them more easily than adults can.
- Keep the telephone number of the Poison Help Line (1-800-222-1222) posted near every telephone.
- Store household cleaning and laundry products out of children's reach.
- Never put kerosene or other household fluids in soda bottles or other drink containers.

- Tranquilizers
- Analgesics
- Antihistamines
- Cold medicines
- Birth control pills

Test Yourself

✔ What are the major causes of accidents in the toddler?

✔ List measures you can teach caregivers of toddlers to prevent accidents.

THE TODDLER IN THE HEALTH CARE FACILITY

Although hospitalization is difficult and frightening for a child of any age, the developmental stage of the toddler intensifies these problems. When providing care, keep in mind the toddler's developmental tasks and needs. The toddler, engaged in trying to establish self-control and autonomy, finds that strangers seem to have total power; this eliminates any control on the toddler's part. Add these fears to the inability to communicate well, discomfort from pain, separation from family, the presence of unfamiliar people and surroundings, physical restraint, and uncomfortable or frightening procedures, and the toddler's reaction can be clearly understood.

Maintaining Routines

Part of the child's admission procedure includes a social assessment survey conducted by interviewing the family caregiver who has accompanied the child to the facility.

Usually part of the standard pediatric nursing assessment form, the social assessment covers eating habits and food preferences, toileting habits and terms used for toileting, family members and the names the child calls them, the name the child is called by family members, pets and their names, favorite toys, sleeping or napping patterns and rituals, and other significant information that helps the staff better plan care for the toddler (Fig. 28-2 in Chapter 28). This information should become an indispensable part of the nursing care plan. The nursing care plan should provide opportunities for independence for the toddler, whenever possible.

Separation anxiety is high during the toddler age. As discussed in detail in Chapter 29, the stages of protest and despair are common. Acknowledge these stages, and communicate to the child that it is acceptable to feel angry and anxious at being separated from the primary family caregiver, the person foremost in the child's life. Never interpret the toddler's angry protest as a personal attack. Many facilities encourage family involvement in the child's care to minimize separation anxiety. The mother is often the family member who stays with the child, but in many families, other members who are close to the child may take turns staying. Having a family caregiver with the toddler can be extremely helpful. However, do not neglect caring for the toddler who has a loved one present. In many families, it is impossible for the family caregiver to stay with the child for any of a number of reasons. These children need extra attention and care. All children should be assigned a constant caregiver while in the facility, but this is especially important for the toddler who is alone (Fig. 24-8).

As the nurse assigned to the toddler, you may become a surrogate parent while caring for the child. Maintaining as much as possible the pattern, schedule, and rituals

▮ Figure 24-8 The nurse may become a surrogate parent for the hospitalized toddler.

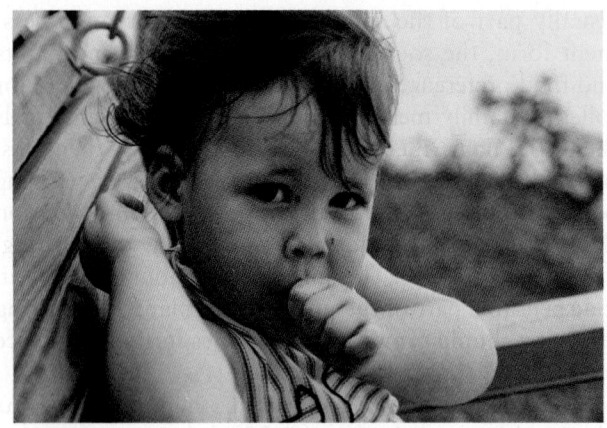

■ **Figure 24-9** The toddler finds security and comfort in her "beloved" thumb.

that the toddler is used to helps to provide some measure of security to the child. This is a time when the toddler needs the security of a beloved thumb or other "lovey," a favorite stuffed animal or blanket. It is important to recognize that the toddler uses this to provide self-comfort (Fig. 24-9). The lovey may be well worn and dirty, but the toddler finds great reassurance in having it to snuggle or cuddle. Do not ridicule the child for its unkempt appearance, and make every effort to allow the toddler to have it whenever desired.

When the family caregiver must leave the toddler, it may be helpful for the adult to give the child some personal item to keep until the adult returns. The caregiver can tell the child he or she will return "when the cartoons come on TV" or "when your lunch comes." These are concrete times that the toddler will probably understand.

Special Considerations

The busy toddler just learning to use the toilet, self-feed, and be disciplined presents a unique challenge to the staff nurse. Maintain control on the pediatric unit, promote safety, and help establish the toddler's sense of security while allowing the toddler's development to continue.

The toddler learning sphincter control is still dependent on familiar surroundings and the family caregiver's support. For this reason, some pediatric personnel automatically put toddlers back in diapers when they are admitted. This practice should be discouraged. Under the right circumstances and especially with the caregiver's help, many of these children can maintain control. They at least should be given a chance to try. Potty chairs can be provided for the child when appropriate. The nursing staff must know the method and times of accomplishing toilet training used at home and must try to comply with them as closely as possible in the hospital.

Some limits are needed for the toddler, but be careful when setting them. Toddlers, like children of any age, need to feel that someone is in control and need limits set with love and understanding. A child who has been overindulged for a long time may need firm, calm statements of limits delivered in a no-nonsense but kind manner. Explaining what is going to be done, what is expected of the toddler, and what the toddler can expect from you as the nurse may be helpful. Sometimes giving some tactful guidance to the family caregiver may help to set limits for the toddler. This is an area where nursing experience helps you to solve difficult problems. Discipline on the pediatric unit is discussed in Chapter 29.

A toddler's eating habits may loom large in your mind as a potential problem. In the hospital or clinic, as at home, food can assume an importance out of proportion to its value and create unnecessary problems. Eating concerns for the pediatric patient are fully discussed in Chapter 29. Some helpful hints to minimize potential problems are

- View mealtime as a social event.
- Encourage self-feeding.
- Do not push the child to eat.
- Allow others to eat with the child.
- Offer familiar foods.
- Provide fluids in small but frequent amounts.

Safety is a concern with all hospitalized children, but safety promotion for a toddler may be particularly challenging. The curious toddler needs to be watched with extra care, but the toddler should not be unnecessarily prohibited from exploring and moving about freely. Safety in the hospital setting is discussed in detail in Chapter 29.

Key Points

➤ The toddler tries to assert his or her independence, is curious about the world around him/her, and at times fears separation from caregivers. Because of the toddler's new-found independence, parenting can be frustrating and a challenge, especially related to creating a safe environment and disciplining the child.

➤ Erikson's developmental task for the toddler is autonomy (independence) while overcoming doubt and shame. The toddler seeks independence, wavers between dependence and freedom, and gains self-awareness.

➤ The toddler's physical growth slows while motor, social, and language development rapidly increase. Each year the toddler gains 5 to 10 lb (2.26–4.53 kg) and about 3 in (7.62 cm).

➤ Using negativism, the toddler often responds "no" to almost everything to assert individuality. To develop security, the toddler likes to follow specific sets of routines; this is referred to as "ritualism." Dawdling occurs when toddlers follow their own desires, rather than the caregiver's wishes and routines. Temper tantrums are an aggressive display of temper, in which the child reacts with rebellion to the wishes of the caregiver.

➤ The toddler's play is often parallel play, in which the toddler plays alongside other children but not with them. Playtime involves imitation of the people the child sees as role models. The toddler learns self-control gradually, and the development from an egotistic being into a person who understands and respects the rights of others is a long, involved process, which the child must be taught.

➤ Toddlers want and need limits. Consistency and timing are important in the caregivers' approach to disciplining the child.

➤ The toddler frequently regresses to more infantile behavior when a new sibling arrives. Special preparation and parental attention is necessary to show that there is room in the parents' lives for both children.

➤ Nutritional concerns and eating problems occur in the toddler because of a slower growth rate, a drive for independence, "food jags," and variations in appetite. A balanced diet should be planned with an understanding of the toddler's developing feeding skills. The toddler progresses from finger feeding and tilting the cup to being able to hold a spoon and handle a cup in an adult manner.

➤ The toddler undergoes routine checkups at 15 months of age for immunization boosters and at least annually thereafter.

➤ Family teaching includes aspects of everyday life with a toddler:

• A regular time for a bath helps give the toddler a sense of security. Caregivers should avoid using bubble bath, especially for girls, because it can create an environment that encourages the growth of organisms that cause bladder infections.

• Encourage the caregiver to take a relaxed attitude as the toddler learns to dress him- or herself.

• Bacteria forms dental plaque on teeth because of the presence of sugar in foods. By the age of

2 years, a toddler can be taught to brush his or her teeth by following the example of adults. Around this same age, the toddler should visit the dentist to be introduced to the process of a dental checkup.

• Toilet training can be started when the child's sphincter muscles have developed enough so the child can control them; this usually occurs at age 18 to 24 months. Perfection should not be expected. To aid in training, the caregiver leaves the child on the potty chair for only a short time. If the child has a bowel movement or urinates after leaving the potty, this is ignored. The child should not be teased, and the potty chair should not be emptied until the child has gone back to playing or other activities.

• A child needs a total of 12 to 14 hours of sleep daily in the first year of toddlerhood; this need decreases to 10 to 12 hours by 3 years of age. A bedtime ritual provides structure and a feeling of security.

➤ Supervision and prevention of accidents is especially important because of the exploring nature of the toddler.

➤ The leading causes of death in toddlers are accidents involving motor vehicles, drowning, burns, and poisons. Toddlers should always be secured in a car seat when in a motor vehicle. Supervision is important when toddlers are near motor vehicles, streets, bathtubs, and swimming pools. Toxic substances should be stored out of reach and in child-proofed containers. The most common medications involved in child poisonings are acetaminophen, aspirin, laxatives, sedatives, tranquilizers, analgesics, antihistamines, cold medicines, and birth control pills.

➤ Keep in mind the toddler's developmental tasks and needs. When the toddler is hospitalized, it is important to know their specific habits, terms used, patterns, and rituals. Maintaining as much as possible the pattern, schedule, and rituals that the toddler is used to helps to provide security. The curious toddler needs to be watched closely to maintain safety, but should not be unnecessarily prohibited from exploring.

INTERNET RESOURCES

Toddlers
www.babycenter.com/toddler

Poison Control
www.aapcc.org

Accident Prevention
www.childrens.com

Workbook

■ NCLEX-STYLE REVIEW QUESTIONS

1. The nurse is weighing a toddler who is 3 years old. If this child has had a typical pattern of growth and weighed 18 lb at the age of 1 year, the nurse would expect this toddler to weigh approximately how many pounds?

   a. 22 lb
   b. 30 lb
   c. 36 lb
   d. 42 lb

2. The nurse is observing a group of 2-year-old children. Which of the following actions by the toddlers would indicate a gross motor skill seen in children this age?

   a. Turns pages of a book
   b. Uses words to explain an object
   c. Drinks from a cup
   d. Runs with little falling

3. The toddler-aged child engages in "parallel play." The nurse observes the following behaviors in a room where two children are playing with dolls and stuffed animals. Which of the following is an example of parallel play?

   a. Sharing stuffed animals with each other
   b. Sitting next each other, each playing with her or his own doll
   c. Taking turns playing with the same stuffed animal
   d. Feeding the first doll, then feeding the second doll

4. In preparing snacks for a 15-month-old toddler, which of the following would be the *best* choice for this age child?

   a. Small cup of yogurt
   b. Five or six green grapes
   c. Handful of dry cereal
   d. Three or four cookies

5. The nurse is working with a group of caregivers of toddlers. The nurse explains that accident prevention and safety are very important when working with children. Which of the following statements is true regarding accidents and safety for the toddler? Select all that apply.

   a. Child car restraints are required for children.
   b. Accidents are the leading cause of death in children up to age 4 years.
   c. At least 5 to 6 in of water is necessary for drowning to occur.
   d. Touching and tasting substances in the environment is a concern.
   e. Poisonous items should be kept in a locked area.
   f. Child-resistant packaging keeps children from opening any bottle.

■ STUDY ACTIVITIES

1. List and compare the fine motor and gross motor skills in each of the following ages:

	15 Months	24 Months	36 Months
Fine motor skills			
Gross motor skills			

2. Discuss the development of language seen in toddlerhood. Compare the language development of the 15-month-old child to the language development of the 36-month-old child.

3. List the four leading causes of accidents in toddlers. For each of these causes state three prevention tips that you could share with family caregivers of toddlers.

4. Do an Internet search on the topic "Toilet training readiness checklist."

   a. What are the common physical, behavioral, and cognitive signs of toilet training readiness?
   b. After reading this information, what could you share with the caregivers of a toddler regarding toilet training?

■ CRITICAL THINKING: WHAT WOULD YOU DO?

1. You are in the supermarket with your 2-year-old niece, Lauren. She is having a loud, screaming temper tantrum because you will not buy some expensive cookies she wants. As you are trying to talk with her, she is yelling, "No, I want them."

   a. What are the reasons toddlers have temper tantrums?
   b. What is the best way to respond to a toddler who is having a temper tantrum? Why?
   c. What would you say to Lauren in this situation?
   d. What actions would you take during the temper tantrum? After the temper tantrum?

2. Marti complains to you that 2-year-old Tasha is very difficult to put to bed at night. Marti often just gives up and lets Tasha fall asleep in front of the television.

   a. What are some of the factors that might be affecting Tasha at bedtime?
   b. What would you explain to Marti regarding bedtime rituals and routines for toddlers?
   c. What would you suggest Marti do with Tasha at her bedtime?

3. Jed is a 26-month-old child whose family caregivers work outside the home. He goes to a day care center 3 days a week and is kept by his grandmother the other 2 days. Jed's mother asks you for advice in toilet training Jed.

   a. What questions would you ask Jed's mother regarding his physical readiness for toilet training?

   b. What suggestions will you offer regarding bowel training? Bladder training?

   c. How might the variety of caregivers Jed has affect his toilet training?

   d. What could Jed's mother do to provide consistency in toilet training for her child?

25 Growth and Development of the Preschool Child: 3 to 6 Years

KEY TERMS

associative play
cooperative play
dramatic play
magical thinking
noncommunicative language
onlooker play
solitary independent play
unoccupied behavior

LEARNING OBJECTIVES

On completion of this chapter, you should be able to:

1. State the major developmental task of the preschooler according to Erikson.
2. Discuss the physical development of the preschooler: (a) growth rate, (b) dentition, (c) visual development, and (d) skeletal growth.
3. Discuss the progression of language development in the preschooler, including factors that delay or enhance progress.
4. Discuss the role of magical thinking and imagination in the preschooler.
5. Discuss the nurse's role in helping parents understand their preschooler's sexual curiosity and masturbation.
6. List six types of play in which preschoolers engage; define each type.
7. Discuss aggression in the preschooler and the family caregivers' role and response.
8. Discuss the role of discipline for the preschooler and the effects of caregivers' behavior when disciplining.
9. Discuss the special needs of the disadvantaged preschooler and the value of Head Start programs.
10. Describe nutritional needs of preschoolers, including (a) daily needs, (b) appetite variations, (c) suggested snacks, and (d) television commercials and other influences.
11. Discuss the recommended health maintenance checkup schedule for the preschooler.
12. Identify important aspects of family teaching for the caregivers of preschool-aged children, including (a) bathing, (b) dressing, (c) dental care, (d) toileting, and (e) sleep.
13. List guidelines for accident prevention in the preschool-aged population.
14. Discuss infection prevention in the preschooler, describing the need for it and preventive measures to teach the child.
15. Discuss important aspects of nursing care for the preschool child in the health care facility.

PRESCHOOLERS are fascinating creatures. As their social circles enlarge to include peers and adults outside the family, preschoolers' language, play patterns, and appearance change markedly. Their curiosity about the world around them grows, as does their ability to explore that world in greater detail and see new meanings in what they find. It can be said that preschoolers soak up information "like a sponge." "Why?" and "how?" are favorite words. This curiosity also means that accidents are still a serious concern.

At 3 years of age, the child still has the chubby, baby-face look of a toddler; by age 5, a leaner, taller, better-coordinated social being emerges. The child works and plays tirelessly, "making things" and telling everyone about them. In children this age, exploring and learning go on continuously. They sometimes have problems separating fantasy from reality. According to Erikson, the developmental task of the preschool age is initiative versus guilt. Preschoolers often try to find ways to do things to help, but they may feel guilty if scolded when they fail because of inexperience or lack of skill.

PHYSICAL DEVELOPMENT

The physical development seen in the preschool child includes a slowed growth rate, changes in dentition and visual development, and skeletal growth changes, especially in the feet and legs.

Growth Rate

The preschool period is one of slow growth. The child gains about 3 to 5 lb each year (1.4 –2.3 kg) and grows about 2.5 in (6.3 cm). Because the increase in height is proportionately greater than the increase in weight, the 5-year-old child appears much thinner and less babyish than the 3-year-old child does. Boys tend to be leaner than girls are during this time. Gross and fine motor skills continue to develop rapidly (Fig. 25-1). Balance improves and confidence emerges to try new activities. By age 5, the child generally can throw and catch a ball well, climb effectively, and ride a bicycle. Table 25-1 summarizes important milestones for growth and development.

Dentition

By 6 years of age, the child's skull is 90% of its adult size. The deciduous teeth have completely emerged by the beginning of the preschool period. Toward the end of the preschool stage, these teeth begin to be replaced by permanent teeth. This is an event that most children an-

■ **Figure 25-2** The smiling 6-year-old is often seen without front teeth.

ticipate as an indication that they are "growing up." Pictures of smiling 5- and 6-year-olds typically show missing front teeth (Fig. 25-2).

The age at which permanent teeth erupt varies with individual children and with various ethnic and economic groups. Permanent teeth of African-American children erupt at least 6 months earlier than those of American children of European ancestry. The central incisors are usually the first to go, just as they were the first to erupt in infancy.

Visual Development

Although the preschooler's senses of taste and smell are acute, visual development is still immature at age 3. Eye-hand coordination is good, but judgment of distances generally is faulty, leading to many bumps and falls. During the preschool years, the child's vision should be checked to screen for amblyopia. Usually by age 6, the child achieves 20/20 vision, but mature depth perception may not develop in some children until 8 to 10 years of age.

Skeletal Growth

Between the third and sixth birthdays, the greatest amount of skeletal growth occurs in the feet and legs. This contributes to the change from the wide-gaited, potbellied look of the toddler into the slim, taller figure of the 6-year-old child. In addition, the carpals and tarsals mature in the hands and feet, which contributes to better hand and foot control.

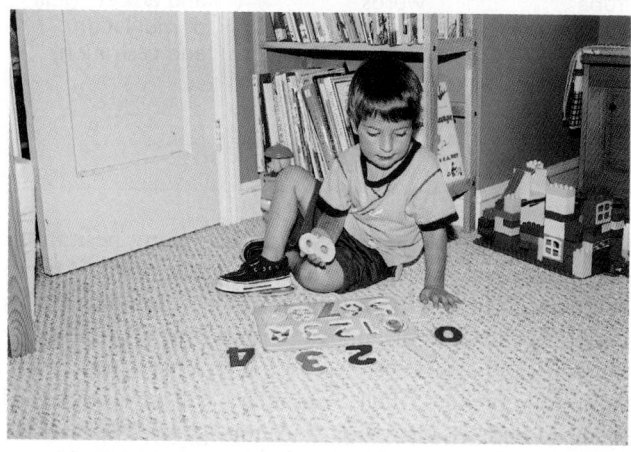

■ **Figure 25-1** This 3-year-old child is developing fine motor skills, has good hand–eye coordination, and shows preference for using his right hand in putting a puzzle together.

Test Yourself

✔ When do children start to lose their deciduous teeth?

✔ Give examples of fine motor skill development.

✔ Give examples of gross motor skill development.

Table 25-1 ▪ GROWTH AND DEVELOPMENT: THE PRESCHOOLER

Age (yr)	Personal–Social	Fine Motor	Gross Motor	Language	Cognition
3	Begins Erikson's stage of "initiative vs. guilt." Conscience develops. Shy with strangers and inept with peers. Sufficiently independent to be interested in group experiences with age mates (e.g., nursery school)	Able to button clothes Copies ○ and + Uses pencils, crayons, paints Shows preference for right or left hand (see Fig. 25-2)	Tends to watch motor activities before attempting them Can jump several feet Uses hands in broad movements Rides tricycle Negotiates stairs well	Vocabulary up to 1,000 words Articulates vowels accurately Talks a lot Sings and recites Asks many questions	Continues in preoperational state (2–7 years) characterized by: 1. *Centration,* or the inability to attend to more than one aspect of a situation 2. *Egocentricity,* or the inability to consider the perception of others 3. The static and irreversible quality of thought that makes the child unable to perceive the processes of change
4	Boisterous and inflammatory Aggressive physically and verbally but developing behaviors to become socially acceptable Becomes socially acceptable Accepts punishment for wrongdoing because it relieves guilt	Can use scissors; copies a square Adds three parts to stick figures	Has some hesitation but tends to try feats beyond ability Greater powers of balance and accuracy Hops on one foot; can control movements of hands	Vocabulary of about 1,500 words Constant questions Sentences of four or five words Uses profanity Reports fantasies as truth	Reality and fantasy are not always clear to the preschooler. Believes that words make things real—"magical thinking"
5	Initiates contacts with strangers and relates interesting little tales Interested in telling and comparing stories about self Peer relations are important ("best friends" abound) Responds to social values by assuming sex roles with rigidity	Ties shoelaces Copies a diamond and a triangle Prints a few letters or numbers May print first name Cuts food	Will not attempt feats beyond ability Throws and catches ball well Jumps rope Walks backward with heel to toe Skips and hops Adept on bicycle and climbing equipment	Vocabulary of 3,000 words Speech is intelligible Asks meanings of words Enjoys telling stories	Thinks feelings and thoughts can happen Intrusions into the body cause fear and anxiety (fear of mutilation and castration)

PSYCHOSOCIAL DEVELOPMENT

The preschool age is characteristic of rapid language development. Imagination, sexual and social development, and a variety of types of play also characterize the preschool child's psychosocial development.

Language Development

Between the ages of 3 and 5 years, language development is generally rapid. Most 3-year-old children can construct simple sentences, but their speech has many hesitations and repetitions as they search for the right word or try to make the right sound. Stuttering can develop during this period but usually disappears within 3 to 6 months. By the end of the fifth year, preschoolers use long, rather complex sentences; their vocabulary will have increased by more than 1,500 words since the age of 2.

Preschoolers' use of language changes during this period. Three-year-old children often talk to themselves or to their toys or pets without any apparent purpose other than the pleasure of using words. Piaget called this "egocentric" or **noncommunicative language.** By 4 years of age, children increase their use of communicative language, using words to transmit information other than their own needs and feelings.

Four- and 5-year-olds delight in using "naughty" words or swearing. Bathroom words become favorites, and taunts such as "you're a big doo-doo" bring heady excitement to them. Caregivers may become concerned by this turn of events, but the child simply may be trying words out to test their impact.

Table 25-2 summarizes typical development of preschoolers' verbal abilities.

Here's a helpful hint.

By using a calm, matter-of-fact response when a preschooler uses "naughty" or swear words, some of the power of using that type of language will be diffused. The child learns that this is not language to use in the company of others.

Delays or other difficulties in language development may result from one or more of the following factors:

- Hearing impairment or other physical problem
- Lack of stimulation
- Overprotection
- Lack of parental interest or rejection by parents

Good language skills develop as the child engages regularly in conversation with caregivers and others. The conversation should be on a level that the child can understand. Reading to the child is an excellent method of contributing to language development. Talking with the child about the pictures in storybooks can enhance this. Praise, approval, and encouragement are all part of supporting attempts at communication.

Family and cultural patterns also influence language development. Some children come from bilingual families and are trying to learn the rules of both languages. Others may come from geographic or social communities that have dialects different from the general population.

Development of Imagination

Preschoolers have learned to think about something without actually seeing it—to visualize or imagine. This normal development, sometimes called **magical thinking,** makes it difficult for them to separate fantasy from reality. Preschoolers believe that words or thoughts can make things real, and this belief can have either positive or negative results. For example, in a moment of anger, a child may wish that a parent or a sibling would die; if that person is hurt later, the child feels responsible and suffers guilt. The child needs reassurance that this is not so.

Imagination makes preschoolers good audiences for storytelling, simple plays, and television, as long as the characters and events are not too frightening or sad. When preschoolers see a television character die, they believe it is real and often cry. The child's television viewing should be supervised to avoid programs with negative impact or overstimulation.

During this stage, children often have imaginary playmates who are very real to them. This occurs particularly with families with one child for whom imaginary playmates fill times of loneliness. The imaginary friend often has the characteristics that the child might wish for in a real friend. Sometimes the child blames the imaginary friend for breaking a toy or engaging in another act for which the child does not want to take responsibility. Caregivers need assurance that this is normal behavior.

The preschooler's active imagination often leads to a fear of the dark or nightmares. Consequently, problems with sleep are common (see the Sleep Needs section later in this chapter).

Table 25-2 ▌ VERBAL MASTERY BY PRESCHOOLERS

Age (yr)	Characteristics of Language Usage	Vocabulary Size, Pattern, Comprehension, Rhythm
3–4	Loves to talk; talks a lot; makes up words; sings or recites own version of song; likes new words; asks many questions and wants answers. Not always logical in sentences and concepts. Uses four- or five-word phrases. Aggressive with words rather than actions.	Vocabulary of 900–1,500 words; at 3 understands up to 3,600 words, up to 5,600 words by 4. By 4 years, speech understandable even with mispronunciations. May have hesitations, repetitions, and revisions while trying to imitate adult speech. Stuttering may occur but disappears within 3–6 months; may continue up to 2 years without being permanent.
4–5	Understands out-of-context words. Speech highly emotional. Difficulty finding right word; tells function rather than name of item. Changes subject rapidly. Boasts, brags, quarrels; loves "naughty" words. Relates fanciful tales.	Vocabulary of 3,000 words; understands up to 9,600 words by 5 years. Speech completely understandable.

A Personal Glimpse

We had just returned from a weekend visit to my parent's house. My 2-year-old was sleeping quietly. I was in the laundry room doing the laundry from our weekend trip and my 5-year-old (Kayla) was playing in the family room (or so I thought). Suddenly I heard a loud crashing sound that came from the kitchen. I asked, "What was that?" "Nothing Mom." I asked again, "What WAS that?" and headed toward the kitchen. When I got to the kitchen, I discovered what the sound had been—the entire sugar canister was empty—the canister on its side, rolling on the floor with the contents all over the cabinet and kitchen floor. Clearly, SOMETHING had happened. I called to Kayla to come to the kitchen. This time I said, "Kayla, tell me how this happened." She told me, "I was playing Legos and Sandy (her imaginary friend) was making cookies just like at Gramma's house and Sandy was getting the sugar and then it was all over the floor." As I looked at the mess she continued, "Like last time Sandy got the toothpaste all over the wall, only this time it was in the kitchen." As upset as I was at having to clean the mess, I thought it was creative of Kayla to use her "imaginary friend" as the mess maker.

Ann

Learning Opportunity: What would you tell this mother regarding preschoolers and imaginary friends? What would you suggest this mother should say to respond to her child in this situation?

Sexual Development

The preschool period is the stage that Freud termed the "oedipal" or "phallic" (genital) period. During these years, children become acutely aware of their sexuality, including sexual roles and organs. They generally develop a strong emotional attachment to the parent of the opposite sex. Children's curiosity about their own genitalia and those of peers and adults may make parents uncomfortable and evoke responses that indicate to the child that sex is dirty and something to be ashamed and guilty about.

Despite today's abundance of sexually oriented literature, many families find it difficult to deal with the young child's questions and actions. You can help caregivers understand that the child's sexual curiosity is a normal, natural part of total curiosity about oneself and the surrounding world. The informed, understanding family caregiver can help children develop positive attitudes toward sexuality and toward themselves as sexual human beings.

In addition to responsible teaching of sexual information, the caregiver also should teach the child about "good touch" and "bad touch." The child needs to understand that no one should touch the child's body in a way that is unpleasant.

Exploration of the genitalia is as natural for the preschooler as thumb sucking is for the infant. It is one way the child learns to perceive the body as a possible source of pleasure and is the beginning of the acceptance of sex as natural and pleasurable.

Caregivers can be reassured that this is not uncommon behavior, and a calm, matter-of-fact response to the child found masturbating is the most effective approach. The child should be helped to understand that masturbation is not an activity that is appropriate in public. If the child seems to be masturbating excessively, counseling may be needed, especially if the child's life has been unsettled in other aspects.

Social Development

Preschoolers are outgoing, imaginative, social beings. They play vigorously and, in the process, learn about the world in which they live. As they gain control over their environment, preschoolers try to manipulate it, and this may lead to conflict with caregivers. Preschool children are delightful to watch as they go about the business of growing and learning.

Play

Play activities are one way that children learn. Normally by 3 years of age, children begin imitative play, pretending to be the mommy, the daddy, a policeman, a cowboy, an astronaut, or some well-known person or television character (Fig. 25-3). Caregivers can gain good insight into the way their child interprets family behavior by watching the child play. Listening to a preschooler scold a doll or stuffed animal for "bothering me while I'm busy talking on the phone," lets the adults hear how they sound to the child.

■ Figure 25-3 Imitative play is common; this preschooler pretends to be a "cowboy."

Preschoolers engage in various types of play: dramatic, cooperative, associative, parallel, solitary independent, onlooker, and unoccupied behavior. **Dramatic play** allows a child to

Watch out!.
Preschoolers love to imitate adults. Dressing up like Mommy or Daddy is a favorite play activity. Listening to a preschooler gives adults an idea of how they sound to the preschooler!

act out troubling situations and to control the solution to the problem. This is important to remember when teaching children who are going to be hospitalized. Using dolls and puppets to explain procedures makes the experience less threatening. In **cooperative play,** children play in an organized group with each other, as in team sports. **Associative play** occurs when children play together and are engaged in a similar activity but without organization, rules, or a leader, and each child does what she or he wishes. In parallel play, children play alongside each other but independently. Although common among toddlers, parallel play exists in all age groups; for example, in a preschool classroom where each student is working on an individual project or craft. **Solitary independent play** means playing apart from others without making an effort to be part of the group or group activity. Watching television is one form of **onlooker play** in which there is observation without participation. In **unoccupied behavior,** the child may be daydreaming or fingering clothing or a toy without apparent purpose.

Drawing is another form of play through which children learn to express themselves. During the preschool years as fine motor skills improve, children's drawings become much more complex and controlled and can be revealing about the child's self-concept and perception of the environment.

Children need all types of play to aid in their total development. Too much of one kind may signal a problem; for example, a youngster who spends most of the time unoccupied may be troubled, depressed, or not stimulated. Cooperative play helps to develop social interaction skills and often physical health.

Too much onlooker play, particularly television viewing, means that children are missing the benefits of other kinds of play and may be forming strong, highly inaccurate impressions of people and their behaviors. Caregivers should limit the amount of time that preschoolers spend watching television, and they should encourage interactive play.

Test Yourself

✔ What is magical thinking? Why do preschoolers have imaginary friends?

✔ Who do preschool children imitate when they are playing?

✔ List the types of play seen in the preschool-aged child.

Aggression

Temper tantrums are an early form of aggression. The preschooler with newly developed language skills uses words aggressively in name-calling and threats. Four-year-old children use physical aggression as well; they push, hit, and kick in an effort to manipulate the environment. The family caregivers' task during these years is to help the child understand that the anger and frustration that result in aggressive behavior are normal but need to be handled differently because aggressive behavior is not socially acceptable.

Children who come from unhappy home situations are likely to be more aggressive than children from a comfortable family situation. Their caregivers have served as role models, and their aggressive behavior toward each other has said to the child, "this is acceptable."

Discipline

Family caregivers need to remember that preschoolers are developing initiative and a sense of guilt. They want to be good and follow instructions, and they feel bad when they do not, even if they are not physically punished. Discipline during this time should strive to teach the child a sense of responsibility and inner control. All the child's caregivers must understand and agree to the limits and discipline measures for the child. If one caregiver says "no" and another one says "yes," the child soon learns to play one against the other, leading to confusion about limits. Spanking and other forms of physical punishment remove the responsibility from the child. Taking away a privilege from a child who has misbehaved until he or she can demonstrate that there has been an improvement in behavior is much more effective. Because the child's concept of time is not clear, the period should be comparatively brief (Fig. 25-4).

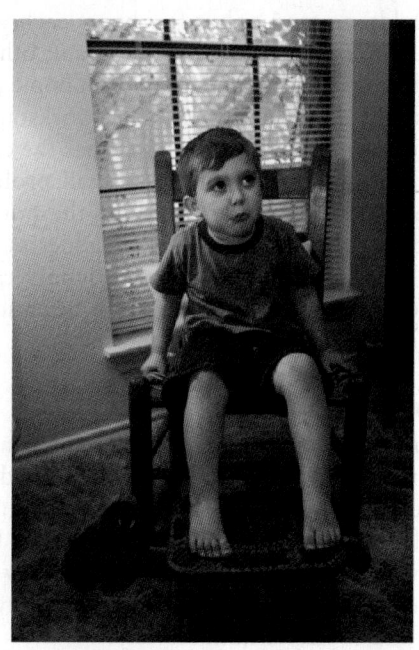

■ **Figure 25-4** Although he may not like it, quiet solitude helps the preschooler develop inner control.

Table 25-3 ■ **EFFECTS OF POSITIVE AND NEGATIVE CAREGIVER BEHAVIOR**

Behavior	Effect on Child	Effect on Adult
Attending only to desired behaviors Calm reasoning with expression of dislike of behavior Physical restraint with adult present Isolation of child for a period of time equal to 1 min per year of age Withholding of desired treats, outings, presents	Development of inner control	Feelings of adequacy as a parent
Yelling, screaming, and implying guilt and punishment Telling child that he or she is bad Physical punishment	Development of fears and compulsive behaviors	Feelings of guilt and inadequacy
Giving treats, presents, or food for lack of undesired behavior Physical punishment Threatening punishment from God or other authority figure	Development of control based on external forces	Feelings of being manipulated by child

Table 25-3 presents some examples of the effects of caregivers' positive and negative responses.

Nursery School or Day Care Experience

Group experiences with peers and adults outside the immediate family are important to a child's development. However, the transition to new experiences, new people, and new surroundings can be threatening to some preschoolers. Children vary in their willingness or ability to handle new situations; being introduced gradually according to individual readiness produces the most satisfactory adjustment.

Some children spend only a few hours each week in a nursery school or other day care program; others must spend a great deal more time away from home and family because the adult family members work outside the home. The family should understand that the child who spends more time away from home will probably demand more of their attention during the hours when they are together. As the child grows older and the attachment to peers becomes stronger, family caregivers sense a decrease in the need for adult attention and a greater sense of independence in the child.

The Disadvantaged Child

Discussions of normal growth and development assume that children come from a secure, well-adjusted home in which there is ample opportunity for social, cultural, and intellectual enrichment. Many children, however, are deprived of such a background for many reasons. This population is the one most likely to have health problems and to need health services.

Children who have not been able to achieve a sense of security and trust, for whatever reason, need special understanding, warm acceptance, and intelligent guidance to grow into self-accepting people. Society is gradually awakening to the needs of these children and is trying to provide enriched nursery school and kindergarten experiences for those whose home life cannot do this for them.

Recognition that environmental enrichment is often unavailable in families with limited social, cultural, and economic resources led to the establishment of Head Start programs. Head Start programs are funded by federal and local money and are free to the children enrolled. Children in such programs have an opportunity to broaden their horizons through varied experiences and to increase their understanding of the world in which they live. Family caregiver participation is a central component of the Head Start concept and often has a positive effect on other children in the household. In some programs, teachers go into the home to help the caregiver teach the young child motor, cognitive, self-help, and language skills. Counseling and referral services are also provided through Head Start programs. Children who have had a background of Head Start enrichment are better prepared to enter kindergarten or first grade and compete successfully with their peers.

NUTRITION

The preschool period is not a time of rapid growth, so children do not need large quantities of food. Children do need foods from the major food groups each day. Protein needs continue to remain high to provide for muscle growth. Refer to the USDA guidelines found in the MyPyramid for Kids in Figure 22-3 in Chapter 22. Daily nutritional needs including caloric requirements and the appropriate number of servings per day for the preschool child are listed in Table 25-4.

Table 25-4 ▌ DAILY NUTRITIONAL NEEDS OF THE 3- TO 6-YEAR-OLD				
For a 1,200 to 1,800-calorie diet, the preschooler needs the amounts below from each food group. Preschoolers should be moderately active for 60 minutes every day, or most days.				
Grains	Vegetables	Fruits	Milk	Meat and Beans
4–6 oz	1.5–2.5 cups	1–1.5 cups	2–3 cups	3–5 oz

The preschooler's appetite is erratic; at one sitting, the preschooler may devour everything on the plate, and at the next meal, he or she may be satisfied with just a few bites. Portions are smaller than adult-sized portions, so the child may need to have meals supplemented with nutritious snacks (Box 25-1). Note that certain snacks are recommended only for the older child to avoid any danger of choking. The preschooler generally best accepts frequent, small meals with snacks in between.

Among the preschooler's favorites are soft foods, grain and dairy products, raw vegetables, and sweets. Television commercials for sugar-coated cereals, snacks, and fast foods of questionable nutritional value exert a powerful influence on the preschooler and can make supermarket shopping an emotional struggle between the caregiver and child. Caregivers should read labels carefully before making a purchase.

Cultural Snapshot

Food preferences, likes, and dislikes are seen in many cultures. Take these variations into consideration when helping family caregivers make nutritious food choices for snacks and meals.

Preschoolers need guidance in choosing foods and are strongly influenced by the example of family members and peers. Food should never be used as a reward or bribe; otherwise, the child will continue to use food as a means to manipulate the environment and the behavior of others.

Preschoolers have definite food preferences. They generally do not like highly spiced foods, often will eat raw vegetables but not cooked ones, and prefer plain foods, rather than casseroles. New foods may be accepted but should be introduced one at a time to avoid overwhelming the child.

The preschooler shows growing independence and skill in eating. The 3-year-old child tries to mimic adult behavior at the table but often reverts to eating with the fingers, spilling liquids, and squirming. The 4-year-old is more skilled with the use of utensils, although an occasional misjudgment of abilities results in a mess. The 5-year-old uses utensils well, often can cut his or her own food, and can be taught to practice sophisticated table manners (Fig. 25-5). Rituals, such as using the same plate, cereal bowl, cup, or place mat, may become important to the child's mealtime happiness.

HEALTH PROMOTION AND MAINTENANCE

Routine checkups, family teaching, and accident and infection prevention are important aspects of health promotion and maintenance for the preschool child.

Routine Checkups

Preschoolers with up-to-date immunizations need boosters of diphtheria–tetanus–pertussis, polio vaccine,

---

Box 25-1 ▌ SUGGESTED SNACKS FOR THE PRESCHOOLER

Raw vegetables: carrots,* cucumbers, celery,* green beans, green pepper, mushrooms, turnips, broccoli, cauliflower, tomatoes
Fresh fruits: apples, oranges, pears, peaches, grapes,* cherries,* melons
Unsalted whole-grain crackers
Whole-grain bread: cut to finger-sized sticks; plain, toasted, or with peanut butter
Small sandwiches: cut into quarters
Natural cheese: cut into cubes
Cooked meat: cut into small chunks or sliced thinly
*Nuts**
*Sunflower seeds**
Cookies: made with lightly sweetened whole grains
*Plain popcorn**
Yogurt: plain or with fresh fruit added

*Children younger than 2 years of age may choke on nuts, seeds, popcorn, celery strings, or carrot sticks. Avoid these until preschool years and then always cut into small, bite-sized pieces.

■ **Figure 25-5** The 5-year-old can use a spoon well to feed herself.

and measles–mumps–rubella (MMR) vaccine and varicella vaccine between 4 and 6 years of age. These are required as preschool boosters for entrance into kindergarten.

An annual health examination is recommended to monitor the child's growth and development and to screen for potential health problems. Children who attend nursery school or a day care program are sometimes required to have an annual examination, but children who stay at home may not have this advantage. Recommended screening procedures include urinalysis, hematocrit, lead level, tuberculin skin testing, and Denver Developmental Screening Test. The practitioner should pay particular attention to the child's vision and hearing so that any problems can be treated before he or she enters school at age 5 or 6. A semiannual dental examination is also recommended.

It is wise for the caregiver to tell the preschool child in advance about the upcoming examination. The caregiver should use simple explanations and provide an opportunity for the child to ask questions and voice anxieties. A number of books available through public libraries are excellent for this purpose.

Family Teaching

Use routine checkups and any other opportunities to teach caregivers about common aspects of everyday life with a preschooler. Preschoolers are busy learning and showing initiative as they are involved in their day-to-day lives. Preschoolers are usually a pleasure to be around because they are so eager to learn anything new and are full of questions.

Bathing

Although preschoolers view themselves as "grown-up," they still need continual supervision while bathing. The caregiver should run the bath water. The hot water heater should be turned to no higher than 120°F (49°C), to avoid the danger of burns. Caregivers should teach

children to leave the faucets alone. Preschoolers can generally wash themselves with supervision. Ears, necks, and faces are spots that often need extra attention. Hands and fingernails often get soaked clean in the tub, but fingernails do need to be checked by the caregiver.

Preschoolers cannot wash their own hair, so this can be a time of tension between the child and caregiver. Shampooing in the tub with a nonirritating children's shampoo may work best. The child can lean the head back, look at the ceiling, and hold a washcloth on the forehead to keep water and soap from getting into the eyes. Shampoo protectors (clear plastic brims with no crowns) can be purchased if desired.

Bath time can be rather lengthy if the preschooler gets involved in playing with bath toys. This is something the caregiver can negotiate if limits need to be set. Some children this age are interested in taking a shower and may do so with adult supervision.

When washing their hands before meals or before or after going to the bathroom, preschoolers often wash only the fronts while ignoring the backs. If not supervised, the child may use only cold water and no soap. Again, the caregiver should turn the water on to a warm temperature to avoid burns.

Dressing

The preschooler may have definite ideas about what he or she wants to wear. Giving the child the opportunity to choose what to wear each day is an excellent way to begin fostering a sense of control and to help the child learn to make decisions. Preschoolers do not have very good taste in what matches, so some interesting outfits may result! Nevertheless, the child should be permitted to make these choices, and the caregivers (as well as older siblings and other adults) should accept the choices without negative comments. When it does matter—for the adults—how the child is dressed, the best plan is to give the child limited choices that will suit the occasion.

Dental Care

The caregiver needs to supervise the preschool child in tooth brushing. Although the preschooler can brush well, the caregiver should check the cleanliness of the child's teeth. The caregiver should be responsible for flossing because the preschooler does not have the necessary motor skills. To help prevent tooth decay, the preschooler should be encouraged to eat healthy snacks, such as fruits, raw vegetables, and natural cheeses, rather than candy, cakes, or sugar-filled gum. The preschool child should continue the use of fluoridated water or fluoride supplements.

Toileting

By the preschool years, almost all children have succeeded in toilet training, although an occasional accident may occur. When the child does have an accident, treating it in a matter-of-fact way and providing the child with clean, dry clothing is best. The preschooler needs continual reminders to wash the hands before and after toileting. Little girls should be taught to wipe from front to back. Preschoolers may still need to be checked for careful wiping, especially after a bowel movement.

Bed-wetting is not uncommon for young preschoolers and is not a concern unless it continues past the age of 5 to 7 (see Chapter 39 for further discussion).

Sleep

Preschoolers are often ready to give up their nap. This may depend partially on if they go to a preschool program that has a rest time. Often preschoolers will just curl up and fall asleep on a chair, a couch, or the floor. Bedtime can still be a challenge, but leading up to it with a period of quiet activities or stories encourages the child to wind down for the day.

Creativity can be useful.

One mother found a creative solution for her child's fear of going to sleep. The child was afraid of a monster in the closet or under the bed. The mother acknowledged the child's fears and purchased a spray can of room air freshener. At bedtime, she ceremoniously sprayed around the room, in the closet, and under the bed. She assured the child that it was a special spray to kill monsters, just like bug spray kills bugs. The reassured child slept without fear.

Dreams and nightmares are common during the preschool period. Caregivers need to explain that "it was only a dream" and offer love and understanding until the fear has subsided. Fear of the dark is another common problem during these years. Children may be afraid to go to sleep in a dark bedroom. These are very real fears to the child. A small night light may be reassuring to the child.

Accident Prevention

Adults caring for preschoolers need to be just as attentive as they are with toddlers because a child's curiosity at this stage still exceeds his or her judgment. Burns, poisoning, and falls are common accidents. Preschoolers are often victims of motor vehicle accidents either because they dart into the street or driveway or fail to wear proper restraints. All states have laws that define safety seat and restraint requirements for children. Adults must teach and reinforce these rules. One primary responsibility of adults is always to wear seat belts themselves and to make certain that the child always is in a safety seat or has a seat belt on when in a motor vehicle. Caregivers can calmly teach a child that the vehicle "won't go" unless the child is properly restrained.

By the age of 5, many preschoolers move from riding a tricycle to riding a bicycle. If the preschooler is not already

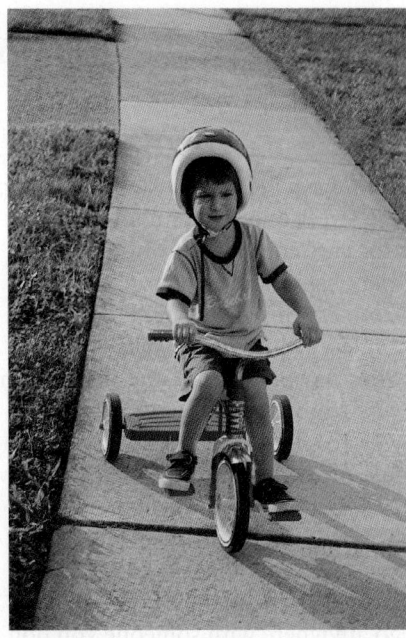

■ Figure 25-6 This preschooler has learned to always wear a proper safety helmet.

wearing a bicycle helmet, it is important to educate caregivers that safety helmets are a necessary safety precaution. Lightweight, child-sized safety helmets that fit properly can be purchased, and the child should be taught that the helmet must be worn when riding a bike (Fig. 25-6). Adults who wear helmets provide the best incentive to children. Safety rules for bicycle riding should be reinforced. The preschool child should be limited to protected areas for riding and should have adult supervision.

The preschool age is an excellent time to begin teaching safety rules. The rules for crossing the street and playing in an area near traffic are of vital importance. Adults who care for preschool children should be careful to serve as good role models. These safety rules should extend into all aspects of the child's life. See Family Teaching Tips: Safety Suggestions for Preschoolers.

Test Yourself

✔ What are some of the reasons preschool children need close supervision while bathing?

✔ What are the major causes of accidents in the preschool child?

✔ List measures preschoolers should be taught to prevent accidents.

Infection Prevention

Preschoolers who enjoy sound nutrition and adequate rest, exercise, and shelter usually are not seriously affected by simple childhood infections. Children who live in less than adequate economic circumstances, however,

Family Teaching Tips

SAFETY SUGGESTIONS FOR PRESCHOOLERS

- Look both ways before crossing the street.
- Cross the street only with an adult.
- Watch for cars coming out of driveways.
- Never play behind a car or truck.
- Watch for cars or trucks backing up.
- Wear a safety helmet when bike riding.
- Learn your name, address, and phone number.
- Stay away from strange dogs.
- Stay away from any dog while it's eating.
- Take only medicine that your caregiver gives you.
- Don't play with matches or lighters.
- Stay away from fires.
- Don't run near a swimming pool.
- Only swim when with an adult.
- Don't go anywhere with someone you don't know.
- Don't let anyone touch you in a way you don't like.

can be severely threatened by even a simple illness, such as diarrhea or chickenpox. Immunizations are available for many childhood communicable diseases, but some caregivers do not have their children immunized until it is required for entrance to school. As a result, some children suffer unnecessary illnesses.

Preschoolers are just learning to share, and that can mean sharing infections with the entire family—and playmates as well. Teaching them basic precautions can help prevent the spread of infections. See Family Teaching Tips: Preventing Infections.

Family Teaching Tips

PREVENTING INFECTIONS

- Cover your mouth when coughing or sneezing.
- Throw away tissues used for nose blowing.
- Wipe carefully after bowel movements (girls wipe front to back).
- Wash hands after going to the bathroom or blowing your nose.
- Wash hands before eating.
- Do not share food that you have partly eaten.
- If an eating utensil falls on the floor, wash it right away.
- If food falls on the floor, do not eat it.
- Do not drink from another person's cup.
- Do not share a toothbrush with someone else.

THE PRESCHOOLER IN THE HEALTH CARE FACILITY

The preschooler may view hospitalization as an exciting new adventure or as a frightening, dangerous experience, depending on the preparation by caregivers and health professionals. As mentioned, play is an effective way to let children act out their anxieties and to learn what to expect from the hospital situation. Preschoolers are frightened about intrusive procedures; therefore, it is preferable to take the temperature with an oral or tympanic thermometer, rather than with a rectal one.

The hospitalized preschooler may revert to bed-wetting but should not be scolded for it. Assure the family that this is normal. Explanations of where the bathrooms are and how to use the call light or bell to get help can help avoid problems with bed-wetting. If a child is afraid of the dark, a night light can be provided.

Hospital routines should follow home routines as closely as possible. Allow the child to participate in the care, even though this may take longer. Carefully explain all procedures to the child in words appropriate for the child's age, repeat the information as necessary.

If the child is ambulatory and not on infection-control precautions, the playroom can offer diversionary activities. If not, play materials can be provided for use in bed (Fig. 25-7).

Some nurses find this approach helpful.
Children are less anxious about procedures if they are allowed to handle equipment beforehand and perhaps "use" it on a doll or another toy.

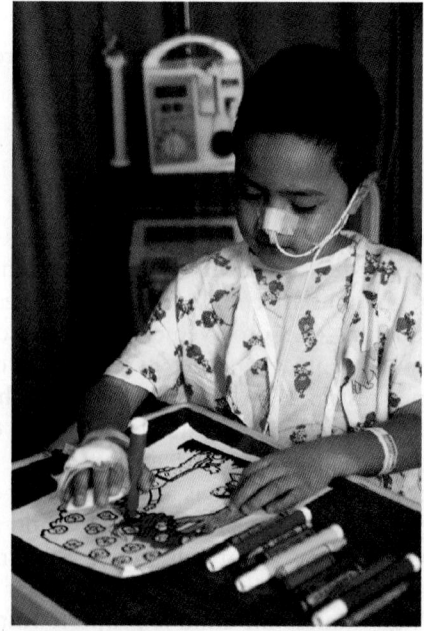

▮ Figure 25-7 This hospitalized child can enjoy age-appropriate activities, even when on bed rest.

Key Points

- According to Erikson, the major developmental task for the preschool-aged group is initiative versus guilt. Preschoolers try to find ways to do things to help, but they may feel guilty if scolded when they fail because of inexperience or lack of skill.
- During the preschool years, physical growth slows. The child gains about 3 to 5 lb each year (1.4–2.3 kg) and grows about 2.5 in (6.3 cm). Toward the end of the preschool stage, deciduous teeth begin to be replaced by permanent teeth. By the age of 6, children usually have achieved 20/20 vision. The greatest amount of skeletal growth in the preschooler occurs in the feet and legs.
- Language develops rapidly during the preschool period. Reading to the child, engaging the child in conversation, and offering encouragement contribute to language development. Language development may be delayed because of hearing impairment or physical problems, lack of stimulation, overprotection, or lack of parental support.
- Magical thinking and imagination contribute to fears and anxieties of the preschooler because these make it difficult for the child to separate fantasy from reality. Caregivers must acknowledge these concerns, be patient with explanations, and offer reassurance to the child.
- A preschooler's sexual curiosity and exploration of his or her genitalia is normal. A calm, understanding caregiver can help the child develop positive attitudes about herself or himself as a sexual being.
- Dramatic play allows for acting out troubling situations. Cooperative play is when children play in organized groups, and associative play occurs when children engage in similar activity but there is no organization or rules. When children play apart from others, it is solitary independent play. Watching TV is a form of onlooker play. In unoccupied behavior, the child is often daydreaming without specific purpose.
- The preschooler may show verbal aggression by name-calling and physical aggression by pushing, hitting, or kicking. Caregivers' need to help the child understand that aggressive behavior is not socially acceptable. Caregivers also serve as role models.
- The caregiver disciplines by setting limits and helping the child to develop inner control and take responsibility for his/her actions.
- The disadvantaged child who has not been able to develop a sense of trust needs understanding, acceptance, and guidance to develop appropriately. Programs such as Head Start give children opportunities to promote development.
- Even though the preschool child has a decreased and erratic appetite, adequate protein, nutritious snacks, and avoidance of foods that lack nutritional value are important.
- Preschoolers should have annual routine checkups to monitor growth, administer immunizations, and perform screening.
- Preschoolers need supervision while bathing and tooth brushing and need help with flossing. Fluoride supplements should be continued. Preschoolers may want to dress themselves. The preschooler needs continual reminders to wash the hands before and after toileting. Girls should be taught to wipe from front to back. Dreams, nightmares, and fear of the dark are common and caregivers need to be reminded to reassure and offer understanding to the child.
- Seat belt use, wearing bicycle safety helmets, and practicing street safety will help in prevention of accidents in the preschooler. Stranger, fire, and swimming safety should also be taught.
- The preschooler learns to share with family and playmates and in the process often shares infections. To prevent infection, the child is taught to cover his or her mouth when coughing or sneezing, proper disposal of tissues, correct wiping after bowel movements, good hand washing, and not to share cups, utensils, food, or toothbrushes.
- Keep in mind the preschooler's developmental tasks and needs. Play is an effective way to let children act out their anxieties and to learn what to expect from the hospital situation. Explain procedures in words appropriate for the child's age.

INTERNET RESOURCES

Head Start Programs

www.acf.hhs.gov/ohs
www.ecewebguide.com
www.earlychildhood.com

Workbook

■ NCLEX-STYLE REVIEW QUESTIONS

1. The nurse is assisting with a well-child visit for a 5½-year-old child. This child's records show that at the age of 3 years, this child weighed 32 lb, was 35.5 in tall, had 20 teeth, and slept 11 hours a day. If this child is following a normal pattern of growth and development, which of the following would the nurse expect to find in this visit?

   a. The child weighs 54 lb.
   b. The child measures 40 in tall.
   c. The child has two permanent teeth.
   d. The child sleeps 2 hours for a morning nap.

2. In working with a group of preschool children, which of the following activities would this age child *most* likely be doing?

   a. Pretending to be television characters.
   b. Playing a game with large balls and blocks.
   c. Participating in a group activity.
   d. Collecting stamps or coins.

3. The nurse is talking with a group of caregivers of preschool-aged children. Which of the following statements made by a caregiver would require further data collection?

   a. "My child calls her sister bad names when she doesn't get her way."
   b. "She told me her imaginary friend broke my favorite picture frame."
   c. "My son always wants to eat cookies for lunch and for snacks."
   d. "Even when his friends are over to play, he wants to play by himself."

4. A caregiver of a preschool-aged child says to the nurse, "My 4-year-old touches her genitals sometimes when she is resting." Which of the following statements would be appropriate for the nurse to respond?

   a. "Masturbation is embarrassing to the parents; scolding the child will stop the behavior."
   b. "When children are angry or upset, they often masturbate."
   c. "When this age child masturbates, it can be unhealthy and dangerous."
   d. "Masturbation is a normal behavior, so providing another activity for the child would be appropriate."

5. In working with the preschool-aged child and this child's family, teaching regarding prevention of infection is important. Which of the following are true regarding prevention of infection? Select all that apply.

   a. Girls should be taught to wipe from front to back after a bowel movement.
   b. Sharing foods or utensils with family members is acceptable.
   c. It is important to wash hands after coughing, sneezing, or blowing your nose.
   d. Each person should have her/his own toothbrush and use only that one.
   e. When washing hands, cold water works as well as warm water.

■ STUDY ACTIVITIES

1. List and compare the fine motor skills, gross motor skills, and language development in each of the following ages:

	3 Years	4 Years	5 Years
Fine motor skills			
Gross motor skills			
Language development			

2. Describe the guidelines you would give a family to help children develop good eating habits and encourage the trying of new foods. Write a 1-day menu, including snacks, for a preschooler.

3. You are working with the staff in a day care facility to help them develop activities for their preschool program. Using your knowledge of preschool growth and development, make a list of behaviors you would teach the staff to look for in the preschooler. What activities would you suggest to encourage normal preschool growth and development?

4. Do an Internet search on "child dental health."

   a. Make a list of three sites you find related to child dental health.
   b. What topics are discussed on these sites?
   c. What did you learn that you can share with peers, children, and family caregivers related to child dental health?

■ CRITICAL THINKING: WHAT WOULD YOU DO?

1. Clara has noticed her 5-year-old son Ted masturbating. She is upset and comes to you for help.

   a. What reactions and concerns might Clara express regarding masturbation in her preschool child?
   b. What will you tell Clara to help her understand preschoolers and masturbation?
   c. What actions would you suggest for Clara to do when she notices Ted is masturbating?

2. Jenny reports that her 3.5-year-old daughter, Krista, wakes up screaming in the middle of the night. This is causing the family to lose sleep.

   a. What concerns do you think Jenny might have regarding this situation?
   b. What characteristics of a preschooler might be causing Krista to wake up at night screaming?
   c. What would you suggest Jenny do and say to Krista when this happens?

3. A group of caregivers of 4-year-olds are discussing their children and the behaviors they are noticing.

One of the caregivers states, "My child is so frustrating." Several of the other caregivers nod their heads in agreement.

   a. What characteristics of preschoolers might lead to these caregivers' feelings of frustration?
   b. What explanations would you offer these caregivers as to the reasons they are seeing these behaviors in their children?
   c. How would you suggest these caregivers respond when they feel frustrated by these preschoolers?

26 Growth and Development of the School-Aged Child: 6 to 10 Years

KEY TERMS

classification
conservation
decentration
deliriants
epiphyses
hierarchical arrangement
inhalants
reversibility
scoliosis

LEARNING OBJECTIVES

On completion of this chapter, you should be able to:

1. State the major developmental task of the school-aged group according to Erikson.
2. Discuss the physical growth patterns during the school-aged years.
3. Describe dentition in school-aged children.
4. Discuss the psychosocial development of the school-aged child.
5. Explain the cognitive development seen in the school-aged child regarding (a) conservation, (b) decentration, (c) reversibility, and (d) classification.
6. Identify nutritional influences on the school-aged child, including (a) family attitudes, (b) mealtime atmosphere, (c) snacks, and (d) school's role.
7. List three factors that contribute to obesity in the school-aged child.
8. State two appropriate ways to help an obese child control weight.
9. Discuss recommended health promotion and maintenance for the school-aged child, including: (a) scoliosis screening, (b) vision and hearing screening, (c) dental hygiene, (d) exercise, and (e) sleep.
10. Discuss the need for sex education in the school-aged group and describe the role of the family, school, and others in this education.
11. Describe principles that a family caregiver can use to teach children about substance abuse.
12. Identify common inhalant products that children may use as deliriants.
13. Describe safety education appropriate for the school-aged group.
14. Discuss the effects of the progression in the 6- to 10-year-old child's concept of biology, including the concepts of (a) birth, (b) death, (c) human body, (d) health, and (e) illness.
15. Identify factors that may influence the school-aged child in the health care facility.

THE FIRST DAY of school marks a major milestone in a child's development, opening a new world of learning and growth. Between the ages of 6 and 10 years, dramatic changes occur in the child's thinking process, social skills, activities, attitudes, and use of language. The squirmy, boisterous 6-year-old child with a limited attention span bears little resemblance to the more reserved 10-year-old child who can become absorbed in a solitary craft activity for several hours.

Moving from the small circle of family into the school and community, children begin to see differences in their own lives and the lives of others. They constantly compare their families with other children's families and observe the way other children are disciplined, the foods they eat, the way they dress, and their homes. Every aspect of lifestyle is subject to comparison.

Most children reach school age with the necessary skills, abilities, and independence to function successfully in this new environment. They can feed and dress themselves, use the primary language of their culture to communicate their needs and feelings, and separate from their caregivers for extended periods. They show increasing interest in group activities and in making things. Children of this age work at many activities that involve motor, cognitive, and social skills. Success in these activities provides the child with self-confidence and a feeling of competence. Erikson's developmental task for this age group is industry versus inferiority. Children who are unsuccessful in completing activities during this stage, whether from physical, social, or cognitive disadvantages, develop a feeling of inferiority.

The health of the school-aged child is no longer the exclusive concern of the family but of the community as well. Before admittance, most schools require that children have a physical examination and that immunizations meet state requirements. Generally, this is a healthy period in the child's life, although minor respiratory disorders and other communicable diseases can spread quickly within a classroom. Few major diseases have their onset during this period. Accidents still pose a serious hazard; therefore, safety measures are an important part of learning.

PHYSICAL DEVELOPMENT

The physical development of the school-aged child includes changes in weight and height, as well as changes in dentition and the eruption of permanent teeth. The school-aged child's skeletal growth and changes are evident during this period.

Weight and Height

Between the ages of 6 and 10 years, growth is slow and steady. Average annual weight gain is about 5 to 6 lb (2–3 kg). By age 7, the child weighs about seven times as much as at birth. Annual height increase is about 2.5 in (6 cm). This period ends in the preadolescent growth spurt, in girls at about age 10 and in boys at about age 12.

Dentition

At about age 6, the child starts to lose the deciduous ("baby") teeth, usually beginning with the lower incisors. At about the same time, the first permanent teeth, the 6-year molars, appear directly behind the deciduous molars (Fig. 26-1). These 6-year molars are of the utmost importance: They are the key or pivot teeth that help to shape the jaw and affect the alignment of the permanent teeth. If these molars are allowed to decay so severely that they must be removed, the child will have dental problems later. (More information on care of the teeth is given later in this chapter.)

Skeletal Growth

The 6-year-old's silhouette is characterized by a flatter but still protruding abdomen and lordosis (sway-back). By the time the child has reached the age of 10 years, the spine is

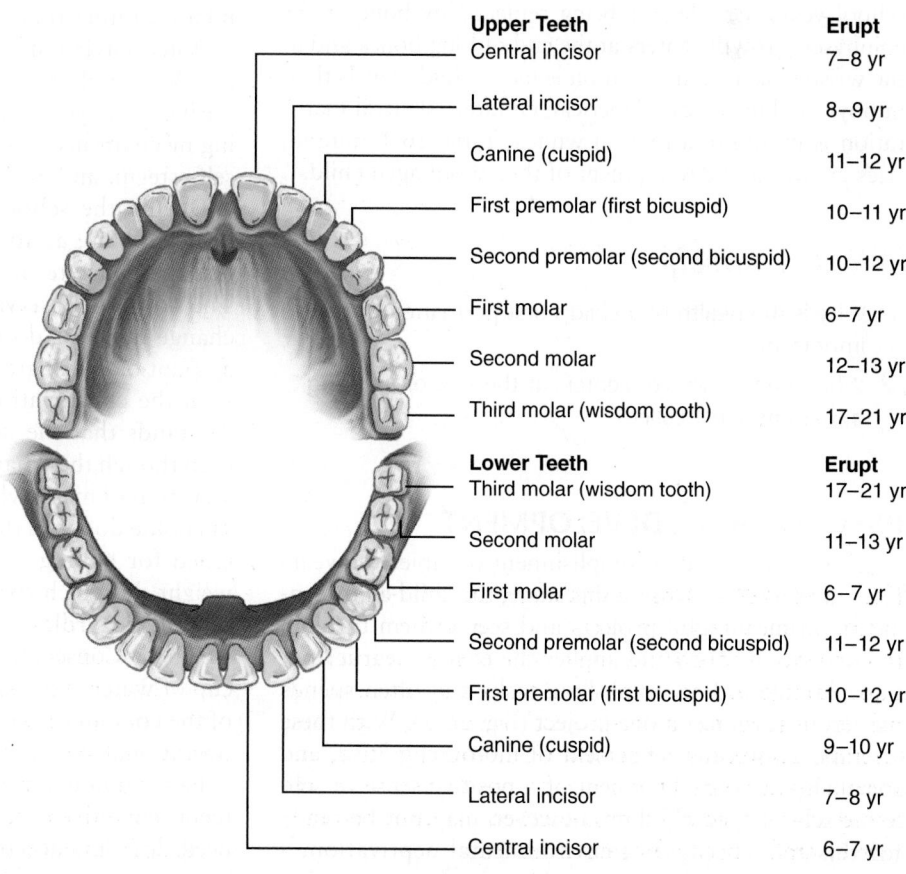

Upper Teeth	Erupt
Central incisor	7–8 yr
Lateral incisor	8–9 yr
Canine (cuspid)	11–12 yr
First premolar (first bicuspid)	10–11 yr
Second premolar (second bicuspid)	10–12 yr
First molar	6–7 yr
Second molar	12–13 yr
Third molar (wisdom tooth)	17–21 yr

Lower Teeth	Erupt
Third molar (wisdom tooth)	17–21 yr
Second molar	11–13 yr
First molar	6–7 yr
Second premolar (second bicuspid)	11–12 yr
First premolar (first bicuspid)	10–12 yr
Canine (cuspid)	9–10 yr
Lateral incisor	7–8 yr
Central incisor	6–7 yr

■ **Figure 26-1** The usual sequence of eruption of permanent teeth.

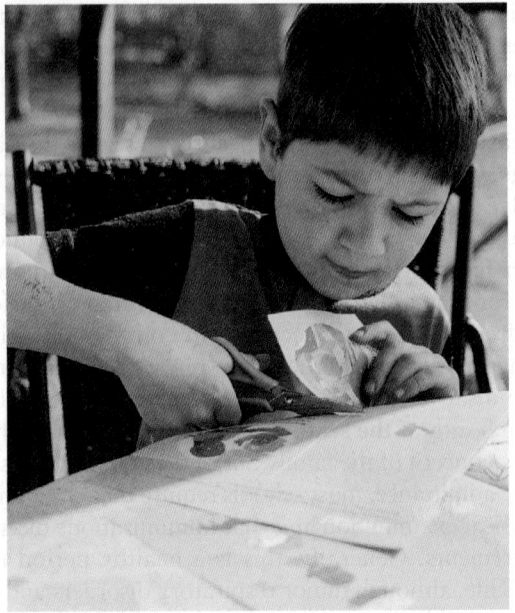

■ **Figure 26-3** This 6-year-old focuses on cutting out shapes with safety scissors to complete a craft project.

■ **Figure 26-2** (**Left**) Profile of a 6-year-old showing protuberant abdomen. (**Right**) Profile of a 10-year-old showing flat abdomen and four curves of adult-like spine.

straighter, the abdomen flatter, and the body generally more slender and long-legged (Fig. 26-2). Bone growth occurs mostly in the long bones and is gradual during the school years. Cartilage is being replaced by bone at the **epiphyses** (growth centers at the end of long bones and at the wrists). Skeletal maturation is more rapid in girls than in boys, and in African American children, skeletal maturation is more rapid than in whites. Table 26-1 summarizes growth and development of the school-aged child.

> *Test Yourself*
>
> ✔ Why is the health of a child's first permanent molars important?
> ✔ What are the growth centers at the end of the long bones and wrist called?

PSYCHOSOCIAL DEVELOPMENT

A sense of duty and accomplishment occupies the years from ages 6 to 10. During this stage, the child enjoys engaging in meaningful projects and seeing them through to completion. The child applies the energies earlier put into play toward accomplishing tasks and often spends numerous sessions on one project (Fig. 26-3). With these attempts comes the refinement of motor, cognitive, and social skills and development of a positive sense of self. Some school-aged children, however, may not be ready for this stage because of environmental deprivation, a

dysfunctional family, insecure attachment to parents, immaturity, or other reasons. Entering school at a disadvantage, these children may not be ready to be productive. Excessive or unrealistic goals set by a teacher or caregiver who is insensitive to this child's needs will defeat such a child and possibly lead to the child's feeling inferior, rather than self-confident.

When environmental support is adequate, the child should complete several personality development tasks during these years. These tasks include developing coping mechanisms, a sense of right and wrong, a feeling of self-esteem, and an ability to care for oneself.

During the school-aged years, the child's cognitive skills develop; at about the age of 7 years, the child enters the concrete operational stage identified by Piaget. The skills of **conservation** (the ability to recognize that a change in shape does not necessarily mean a change in amount or mass) are significant in this stage. This begins with the conservation of numbers, when the child understands that the number of cookies does not change even though they may be rearranged, along with the conservation of mass, when the child can see that an amount of cookie dough is the same whether in ball form or flattened for baking. This is followed by conservation of weight, in which the child recognizes that a pound is a pound, regardless of whether plastic or bricks are weighed. Conservation of volume (for instance, a half-cup of water is the same amount regardless of the shape of the container) does not come until late in the concrete operational stage, at about 11 or 12 years of age.

Each child is a product of personal heredity, environment, cognitive ability, and physical health. Every child needs love and acceptance, with understanding, support,

Table 26-1 ▊ DEVELOPMENTAL MILESTONES FOR THE SCHOOL-AGED CHILD

Age (yr)	Physical	Motor	Personal-Social	Language	Perceptual	Cognitive
6	Average height 45 in (116 cm) Average weight 46 lb (21 kg) Loses first tooth (upper incisors) Six-year molars erupt Food "jags" Appetite increased	Tie shoes Can use scissors (see Fig. 26-3) Runs, jumps, climbs, skips Can ride bicycle Can't sit for long periods Cuts, pastes, prints, draws with some detail	Increased need to socialize with same sex Egocentric—believes everyone thinks as they do Still in pre-operational stage until age 7	Uses every form of sentence structure Vocabulary of 2,500 words Sentence length about 5 words	Knows right from left May reverse letters Can discriminate vertical horizontal, and oblique Perceives pictures in parts or whole but not both	Recognizes simple words Conservation of number Defines objects by use Can group according to an attribute to form subclasses
7	Weight is seven times birth weight Gains 4.4–6.6 lb/yr (2–3 kg) Grows 2–2.5 in/yr (5–6 cm)	More cautious Swims Printing smaller than 6-year-old's Activity level lower than 6-year-old's	More cooperative Same-sex play group and friends Less egocentric	Can name day, month, season Produces all language sounds	b, p, d, q confusion resolved Can copy a diamond	Begins to use simple logic Can group in ascending order Grasps basic idea of addition and subtraction Conservation of substance Can tell time
8	Average height 49.5 in (127 cm) Average weight 55 lb (25 kg)	Movements more graceful Writes in cursive Can throw and hit a baseball Has symmetric balance and can hop	Adheres to simple rules Hero worship begins Same-sex peer group	Gives precise definitions Articulation near adult level	Can catch a ball Visual acuity 20/20 Perceives pictures in parts and whole	Increasing memory span Interest in causal relation Conservation of length Can put thoughts in a chronological sequence
9–10	Average height 51.5–53.5 in (132–137 cm) Average weight 59.5–77 lb (27–35 kg)	Good coordination Can achieve the strength and speed needed for most sports	Enjoys team competition Moves from group to best friend Hero worship intensifies	Can use language to convey thoughts and look at other's point of view	Eye–hand coordination almost perfect	Classifies objects Understands explanations Conservation of area and weight Describes characteristics of objects Can group in descending order

and concern when mistakes are made. Children thrive on praise and recognition and will work to earn them (see Family Teaching Tips: Guiding Your School-aged Child).

This is important.
The school-aged child needs consistent rules, positive attention, and clear expectations in order to develop self-confidence.

Development From Ages 6 to 7 Years

Children in the age group of 6 to 7 years are still characterized by magical thinking—believing in the tooth fairy, Santa Claus, the Easter Bunny, and others. Keen imaginations contribute to fears, especially at night, about remote, fanciful, or imaginary events. Trouble distinguishing fantasy from reality can contribute to lying to escape punishment or to boost self-confidence.

Family Teaching Tips

GUIDING YOUR SCHOOL-AGED CHILD

- Give your child consistent love and attention. Try to see the situation through your child's eyes. Do your best to avoid a hostile or angry reaction toward your child.
- Know where your child is at all times and who his or her friends are. Never leave your child home alone.
- Encourage your child to become involved in school and community activities. Become involved with your child's activities whenever possible. Encourage fair play and good sportsmanship.
- Show your children good examples by your behavior toward others.
- Never hit your children. Physical punishment shows them that it is all right to hit others and that they can solve problems in that way.
- Use positive nonphysical methods of discipline such as
  - "Time out"—1 minute per year is an appropriate amount of time.
  - "Grounding"—don't permit them to play with friends or take part in a special activity.
  - Take away a special privilege.
- Set these limits for brief periods only. Consistency is extremely important in setting these restrictions.
- Be consistent. Make a reasonable rule, let your child know the rule, and then stick with it. You can involve your children in helping to set rules.
- Treat your child with love and respect. Always try to find the "positives" and praise the child for those behaviors. Don't treat your child in a manner that you would not use with an adult friend.
- Let the child know what you expect of him or her. Children who have responsibilities (age-appropriate) learn self-discipline and self-control.
- When you have a problem with your child, try to sit down and solve it together. Help him or her figure out ways to solve problems nonviolently.

Children who have attended a day care center, preschool, kindergarten, or Head Start program usually make the transition into first grade with pleasure, excitement, and little anxiety. Those without that experience may find it helpful to visit the school to experience separation from home and caregivers and to try getting along with other children on a trial basis. Most 6-year-old children can sit still for short periods of time and understand about taking turns. Those who have not matured sufficiently for this experience will find school unpleasant and may not do well.

Group activities are important to most 6-year-old children, even if the groups include only two or three children. They delight in learning and show an intense interest in every experience. Judgment about acceptable and unacceptable behavior is not well developed and possibly results in name-calling and the use of vulgar words.

Between the ages of 6 and 8 years, children begin to enjoy participating in real-life activities, such as helping with gardening, housework, and other chores. They love making things, such as drawings, paintings, and craft projects (Fig. 26-4).

Development From Ages 7 to 10 Years

Between the seventh and eighth birthdays, children begin to shake off their acceptance of parental standards as the ultimate authority and become more impressed by the behavior of their peers. Interest in group play increases, and acceptance by the group is tremendously important.

These groups quickly become all-boy or all-girl groups and are often project oriented, such as Scout troops or athletic teams. Private clubs with homemade clubhouses, secret codes, and languages are popular. Individual friendships also form, and "best friends" are intensely loyal, if only for short periods. Table games, arts and crafts requiring skill and dexterity, computer games,

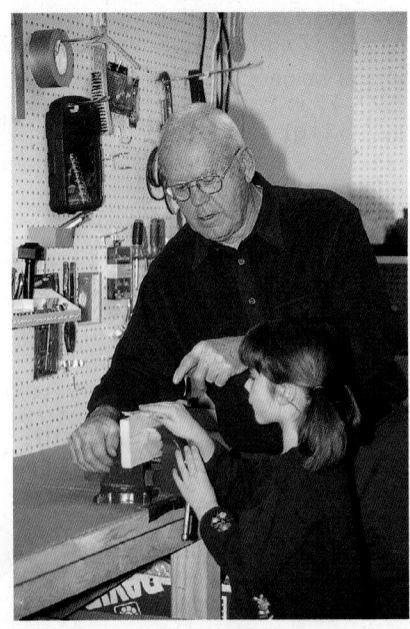

▪ **Figure 26-4** A 6-year-old works with her grandfather on a woodworking project.

■ **Figure 26-5** These 8-year-olds enjoy being part of a sports team.

school science projects, and science fairs are popular, as are more active pursuits. This period includes the beginning of many neighborhood team sports, including Little League, softball, football, and soccer (Fig. 26-5). Both boys and girls are actively involved in many of these sports.

Even though parents are no longer considered the ultimate authority, their standards have become part of the child's personality and conscience. Although the child may cheat, lie, or steal on occasion, he or she suffers considerable guilt if he or she learns that these are unacceptable behaviors.

Important changes occur in a child's thinking processes at about age 7 years, when there is movement from preoperational, egocentric thinking to concrete, operational, decentered thought. For the first time, children can see the world from someone else's point of view. **Decentration** means being able to see several aspects of a problem at the same time and to understand the relation of various parts to the whole situation. Cause-and-effect relations become clear; consequently, magical thinking begins to disappear.

During the seventh or eighth year, children have an increased understanding of the conservation of continuous quantity. Understanding conservation depends on **reversibility,** the ability to think in either direction. Seven-year-old children can add and subtract, count forward and backward, and see how it is possible to put some-

Cultural Snapshot

In some cultures, children are pressured to achieve high scores in school, as well as on college entrance exams, to bring value and pride to the family and culture. These children sometimes are pushed to study rather than to play and have normal relationships with their peers.

thing back the way it was. A 7- or 8-year-old can understand that illness is probably only temporary, whereas a 6-year-old may think it is permanent.

Another important change in thinking during this period is **classification,** the ability to group objects into a **hierarchical arrangement** (grouping by some common system). Children in this age group love to collect sports cards, insects, rocks, stamps, coins, or anything else that strikes their fancy. These collections may be only a short-term interest, but some can develop into lifetime hobbies.

This tip will be fun and useful.

The school-aged child loves to collect and count objects. Checking the child's pockets after school can be quite an adventure!

Test Yourself

✔ How is the developmental task of industry attained in the school-aged child?

✔ What sex are most of the school-aged child's friends and play groups?

NUTRITION

As coordination improves, the child becomes increasingly active and requires more food to supply necessary energy. The nutritional needs of the school-aged child should be met by choosing foods from all the food groups with the appropriate number of servings from each group in the child's daily diet (Table 26-2). (See also MyPyramid for Kids in Figure 22-3 in Chapter 22.) Increased appetite and a tendency to go on food "jags" (the desire for only one kind of food for a while) are typical of the 6-year-old child. This stage soon passes and is unimportant if the child generally gets the necessary nutrients. As the child's tastes develop, once-disliked foods may become favorites unless earlier battles have been waged over the food. Children are more likely to learn to eat most foods if everyone else accepts them in a matter-of-fact way.

Offering choices can make a difference.

Allowing the child to express food dislikes and permitting refusal of a disliked food item is usually the best way to handle the school-aged child.

Children learn by the examples that caregivers and others set for them. They will accept more readily the importance of manners, calm voices, appropriate table

Table 26-2 ∎ **DAILY NUTRITIONAL NEEDS OF THE 6- TO 10-YEAR-OLD**				
For a 1,400- to 2,200-calorie diet, the school-aged child needs the amounts below from each food group. School-aged children should be moderately active for 60 minutes every day, or most days.				
Grains	Vegetables	Fruits	Milk	Meat and Beans
5–7 oz	1.5–3 cups	1.5–2 cups	3 cups	4–6 oz

conversation, and courtesy if they see them carried out consistently at home. To keep mealtime a positive and pleasant time, mealtime should never be used for nagging, finding fault, correcting manners, or discussing a poor report card. Hygiene should be taught in a cheerful but firm manner, even if the child must leave the table more than once to wash his or her hands adequately.

Most children prefer simple, plain foods and are good judges of their own needs if they are not coaxed, nagged, bribed, rewarded, or influenced by television commercials. Disease or strong emotions may cause loss of appetite. Forcing the child to eat is not helpful and can have harmful effects.

Caregivers must carefully supervise children's snacking habits to be sure that snacks are nutritious and not too frequent. Children should avoid junk food; continual nibbling can cause lack of interest at mealtime. Caregivers should encourage children to eat a good breakfast to provide the energy and nutrients needed to perform well in school. Children need a clearly planned schedule that allows time for a good breakfast and tooth brushing before leaving for school.

Obesity can be a concern during this age. Some children may have a genetic tendency to obesity; environment and a sedentary lifestyle also play a part. In many families, caregivers urge children to "clean your plate." In addition, many families eat fast foods several times a week; fast foods tend to have high fat and calorie content and contribute to obesity. Other children, especially in the later elementary grades, can be unkind to overweight children by teasing them, not choosing them in games, or avoiding them as friends. The child who becomes sensitive to being overweight is often miserable.

Encouraging physical activity and limiting dietary fat intake to no more than 35% of total calories help control the child's weight. Popular fad diets must be avoided because they do not supply adequate nutrients for the growing child. Caregivers must avoid nagging and creating feelings of inferiority or guilt because the child may simply rebel. The child who is pressured to much too lose weight may sneak food, setting up patterns that will be harmful later in life. In addition, anorexia nervosa (see Chapter 42) has become a problem for some girls in the older school-aged group.

Health teaching at school should reinforce the importance of a proper diet. Family and cultural food patterns are strong, however, and tend to persist despite nutrition education. Some families are making a positive effort to reduce fat and cholesterol when preparing meals. Most schools have subsidized lunch programs for eligible children, and some have breakfast programs. These provide well-balanced meals, but often children eat only part of what they are offered. Some families post the school lunch menu on the refrigerator or kitchen bulletin board so that children can decide whether to eat the school's lunch or pack their own on any particular day. This way the child can avoid lunches he or she dislikes or simply refuses to eat. School-aged children are old enough to be at least partially responsible for preparing their own lunches.

Test Yourself

✔ List the factors that may contribute to obesity in the school-aged child.

✔ What can be suggested as ways to control a school-aged child's weight?

HEALTH PROMOTION AND MAINTENANCE

The school years are generally healthy years for most children. However, routine health care and health education, including health habits, safety, sex education, and substance abuse, are very important aspects of well-planned health promotion and maintenance programs for school-aged children.

Routine Checkups

The school-aged child should have a physical examination by a physician or other health care provider every year. Additional visits are commonly made throughout the year for minor illness. The school-aged child should visit the dentist at least twice a year for a cleaning and application of fluoride (Fig. 26-6).

Most states have immunization requirements that must be met when the child enters school. A booster of

■ **Figure 26-6** Visiting the dentist twice a year is important for school-aged children.

tetanus-diphtheria vaccine is recommended every 10 years throughout life. The Human papillomavirus (HPV) vaccine is now recommended for adolescent females, and the first dose may be given as early as 9 years of age (see Appendix J). In addition, physical and dental examinations may be required at specific intervals during the elementary school years. During a physical examination at about the age of 10 to 11 years, the child undergoes initial examination for signs of **scoliosis** (lateral curvature of the spine). The child is monitored on an ongoing basis and reexamined during adolescence (Fig. 26-7; refer to Chapter 40). Vision and hearing screening should be performed before entrance to school and on a periodic basis (annual or biannual) thereafter. The school nurse often conducts these examinations.

Elementary school children generally are healthy, with only minor illnesses that are usually respiratory or gastrointestinal in nature. The leading cause of death in this age group continues to be accidents.

Family Teaching

The school-aged child generally incorporates healthy habits into his or her daily routine but still needs reinforcement by caregivers. Education for the care of the teeth with particular attention to the 6-year molars is important. Proper dental hygiene includes a routine inspection and conscientious brushing after meals. A well-balanced diet with plenty of calcium and phosphorus and minimal sugar is important to healthy teeth. Foods containing sugar should be eaten only at mealtimes and should be followed immediately by proper brushing (Fig. 26-8).

Exercise and sufficient rest also are important during this period. Caregivers need to help school-aged children to balance their rest needs and their extracurricular activities. Extracurricular activities help the child remain fit, bond with peers, and establish positive, lifelong attitudes toward exercise. The school-aged child needs 10 to 12 hours of sleep per night. The 6-year-old needs 12 hours of sleep and should be provided with a quiet time after school to recharge after a busy day in the classroom. Highlight these important aspects of daily health care to both the caregivers and child.

■ **Figure 26-7** Scoliosis checkup.
(**A**) Viewing from the back, the examiner checks the symmetry of the girl's shoulders. She will also look for a prominent shoulder blade, an unequal distance between the girl's arms and waist, a higher or more prominent hip, and curvature of the spinal column.
(**B**) With the child bending over and touching her toes, the examiner checks for a curvature of the spinal column. She will also look for a rib hump.

A

B

▪ **Figure 26-8** The school-aged child needs encouragement to brush teeth after meals and at bedtime as part of a good dental hygiene program.

Health Education

Health teaching in the home and at school is essential. Caregivers have a responsibility to teach the child about basic hygiene, sexual functioning, substance abuse, and accident prevention. Schools must include these topics in the curriculum because many families are not informed well enough to cover them adequately. Some schools offer health classes taught by a health educator at each grade level. In other schools, health and sex education are integrated into the curriculum and taught by each classroom teacher. Nurses should become active in their community to ensure that these kinds of programs are available to children.

Sex Education

Children learn about femininity and masculinity from the time they are born. Behaviors, attitudes, and actions of the men and women in the child's life, especially their actions toward the child and toward each other, form impressions in the child that last a lifetime. The proper time and place for formal sex education have been very controversial. Part of the problem seems to be that many people automatically think that sex education means just adult sexuality and reproduction. However, sex education includes helping children develop positive attitudes toward their own bodies, their own sex, and their own sexual role to achieve optimum satisfaction in being a boy or a girl.

In some schools, sex education is limited to one class, usually in the fifth grade, in which children watch films about menstruation and their developing bodies; schools often offer separate classes for boys and girls. Some health educators strongly recommend that sex education

begin in kindergarten and develop gradually over the successive grades. Learning about reproduction of plants and animals, about birth and nurturing in other animals, and about the roles of the male and the female in family units can lead to the natural introduction of human reproduction, male and female roles, families, and nurturing. If all children grew up in secure, loving, ideal families, much of this could be learned at home. However, many children do not have this type of home, so they need healthy, positive information to help them develop healthy attitudes about their own sexuality. Feelings of self-worth woven into these lessons help children feel good about themselves and who they are.

Caregivers who feel uncomfortable discussing sex with their children may find it helpful to use books or pamphlets available for various age groups. Generally, a female caregiver finds it easier to discuss sex with a girl, and a male caregiver feels more comfortable with a boy. This can pose special problems for the single caregiver with a child of the opposite sex. Again, printed materials may be helpful. As a nurse, you may be called on to help a caregiver provide information, and it is important to be comfortable with your own sexuality to handle these discussions well.

At a young age, children are exposed to a large amount of sexually provocative information through the media. Children who do not get accurate information at home or at school will learn what they want to know from their peers; this information is often inaccurate, which makes sex education even more urgent. In addition, the U.S. Centers for Disease Control and Prevention currently recommends that elementary school children be taught about human immunodeficiency virus and acquired immunodeficiency syndrome and how it is spread. Many school districts are working hard to integrate this information into the health curriculum at all grade levels in a sensitive, age-appropriate manner.

Substance Abuse Education

In addition to nutrition, health practices, safety, and sex education, school-aged children also need substance abuse education. Programs that teach children to "just say no" are one way that children can learn that they are in control of the choices they make regarding substance abuse. Children as young as elementary school age may try cigarette smoking, chewing tobacco, alcohol, and other substances. Teaching children the unhealthy aspects of tobacco and alcohol use and drug abuse should begin in elementary school as a good foundation for more advanced information in adolescence.

Children may experiment with **inhalants** (substances whose volatile vapors can be abused) because they are readily available and may seem no more threatening than an innocent prank. Inhalants classified as **deliriants** contain chemicals that give off fumes that can produce symptoms of confusion, disorientation, excitement, and hallucinations. Many inhalants are commonly found in

A Personal Glimpse

When we had the program on drugs at school, I learned some things. Like when you take drugs, you can get sick or even die. In one part of the lesson, we watched a video where a kid took drugs and almost died and during the other part the school nurse showed us samples of drugs. Even though I learned about drugs from the program, I think that all children should be taught this subject by their parent or guardian.

Stephen, age 10

Learning Opportunity: What do you think is the most effective way to teach school-aged children about the dangers of substance abuse? List some ways you can help to reduce substance abuse among school-aged children.

right and wrong, set and enforce rules for acceptable behavior of family members, learn facts about drugs and alcohol, and actively listen to the children in the family (see Family Teaching Tips: Guidelines to Prevent Substance Abuse). An excellent reference for family caregivers is *Tips for Parents on Keeping Children Drug Free*, which is published by the U.S. Department of Education and is available for free (1-877-433-7827 or www.ed.gov/parents/academic/involve/drugfree/index.html).

Test Yourself

✔ How is a child screened for scoliosis? At what age is a child usually initially examined for signs of scoliosis?

✔ List substances that school-aged children might abuse.

the home (Box 26-1). The fumes are mind altering when inhaled. The child initially may experience a temporary high, giddiness, nausea, coughing, nosebleed, fatigue, lack of coordination, or loss of appetite. Overdose can cause loss of consciousness and possible death from suffocation by replacing oxygen in the lungs or depressing the central nervous system, thereby causing respiratory arrest. Permanent damage to the lungs, the nervous system, or the liver can result. Children who experiment with inhalants may proceed to abuse other drugs in an attempt to get similar effects. Addiction occurs in younger children more rapidly than in adults.

Family caregivers must work to develop a strong, loving relationship with the children in the family, teach the children the family's values and the difference between

Family Teaching Tips

GUIDELINES TO PREVENT SUBSTANCE ABUSE

- Openly communicate values by talking about the importance of honesty, responsibility, and self-reliance. Encourage decision making. Help children see how each decision builds on previous decisions.
- Provide a good role model for the child to copy. Children tend to copy parent's habits of smoking and drinking alcohol and attitudes about drug use, whether they are over-the-counter, prescription, or illicit drugs.
- Avoid conflicts between what you say and what you do. For example, don't ask the child to lie that you are not home when you are or encourage the child to lie about age when trying to get a lower admission price at amusement centers.
- Talk about values during family times. Give the child "what if" examples, and discuss the best responses when faced with a difficult situation. For example, "What would you do if you found money that someone dropped?"
- Set strong rules about using alcohol and other drugs. Make specific rules with specific punishments. Discuss these rules and the reasons for them.
- Be consistent in applying the rules that you set.
- Be reasonable; don't make wild threats. Respond calmly and carry out the expected punishment.
- Get the facts about alcohol and other drugs, and provide children with current, correct information. This helps you in discussions with children and also helps you to recognize symptoms if a child has been using them.

Box 26-1 ▌ COMMON PRODUCTS INHALED AS DELIRIANTS

Model glue
Rubber cement
Cleaning fluids
Kerosene vapors
Gasoline vapors
Butane lighter fluid
Paint sprays
Paint thinner
Varnish
Shellac
Hair spray
Nail polish remover
Liquid typing correction fluid
Propellant in whipped-cream spray cans
Aerosol paint cans
Upholstery-fabric-protection spray cans
Solvents

■ **Figure 26-9** Helmets are an important aspect of bike safety. Parents can be role models for their children by also wearing bike helmets.

Family Teaching Tips

SAFETY TOPICS FOR ELEMENTARY SCHOOL-AGED CHILDREN

- Traffic signals and safe pedestrian practices
- Safety belt use for car passengers
- Bicycle safety
  a. Wear a helmet.
  b. Use hand signals.
  c. Ride with traffic.
  d. Be sure others see you.
- Skateboard and skating safety
  a. Wear a helmet.
  b. Wear elbow and knee pads.
  c. Skate only in safe skating areas.
- Swimming safety
  a. Learn to swim.
  b. Never swim alone.
  c. Always know the water depth.
  d. Don't dive head first.
  e. No running or horseplay at a pool.
- Danger of projectile toys
- Danger of all-terrain vehicles
- Use of life jacket when boating
- Stranger safety
  a. Who is a stranger?
  b. Never accept a ride from someone you don't know.
  c. If offered a ride, check the vehicle license number and try to remember it.
  d. Never accept food or gifts from someone you don't know.
- Good touch and bad touch

Accident Prevention

As stated, accidents continue to be a leading cause of death during this period. Even though school-aged children do not require constant supervision, they must learn certain safety rules and practice them until they are routine (Fig. 26-9). They should understand the function of traffic lights. Family members should obey traffic lights as a matter of course because example is the best teacher for any child. Every child should know her or his full name, the caregivers' names, and his or her own home address and telephone number. Children should be taught the appropriate way to call for emergency help in their community (911 in a community that has such a system). Many communities have safe-home programs that designate homes where children can go if they have a problem on the way home from school. These homes are clearly marked in a way that children are taught to recognize. In many communities, local police officers or firefighters are interested in coming into the classroom to help teach safety. Children benefit from meeting police officers and understanding that the officer's duty is to help children, not to punish them. Safety rules should be stressed at home and at school. Family Teaching Tips: Safety Topics for Elementary School-Aged Children summarizes important safety considerations for school-aged children.

THE SCHOOL-AGED CHILD IN THE HEALTH CARE FACILITY

Increased understanding of their bodies, continuing curiosity about how things work, and development of concrete thinking all contribute to helping school-aged children understand and accept a health care experience better than younger children do. They can communicate better with health care providers, understand cause and effect, and tolerate longer separations from their family.

As a nurse caring for school-aged children, you should understand how concepts about birth, death, the body, health, and illness change between the ages of 6 and 10 years (Table 26-3). Explain all procedures to children and their families; showing the equipment and materials to be used (or pictures of them) and outlining realistic expectations of procedures and treatments are helpful. It is important to answer children's questions, including those about pain, truthfully. Children of this age have anxieties about looking different from other children. An opportunity to verbalize these anxieties will help a child deal with them. School-aged children need privacy more than younger children do

Table 26-3 ▮ CHILDREN'S CONCEPT OF BIOLOGY

Concept	6–8 Years	8–10 Years	Implications for Nursing
Birth	Gradually see babies as the result of three factors: social and sexual intercourse and biogenetic fusion Tend to see baby as emerging from female only; many still see baby as manufactured by outside force—created whole Boys less knowledgeable about baby formation than girls	Begin to put three components together; recognize that sperm and egg come together but may not be sure why Fewer discrepancies in knowledge based on sex differences	Cultural and educational factors play a part in development of where babies come from. Nurse should assess children's ideas about birth and if they can understand where babies come from and how before teaching. Explanations about roles of both parents can begin, but the idea of sperm and egg union may not be understood until 8 or 9 years of age.
Death	May be viewed as reversible Animism (attribution of life) may be seen in some children; death is viewed as result of outside force Experiences with death facilitate concept development	Considered irreversible Ideas about what happens after death unclear; related to concreteness of thinking and socio-religious upbringing	Change from vague view of death as reversible and caused by external forces to awareness of irreversibility and bodily causes Fears about death more common at 8; adults should be alert to this. Explanations about death, the fact that their thoughts will not cause a death, and they will not die (if illness is not fatal) are needed.
Human body	Know body holds everything inside Use outside world to explain Aware of major organs Interested in visible functions of body	Can understand physiology; use general principles to explain body functions; interested in invisible functions of body	Cultural factors may play a part in ability and willingness to discuss bodily functions. Educational programs can be very effective because of natural interest. Assess knowledge of body by using diagrams before teaching.
Health	See health as doing desired activities List concrete practices as components of health Many do not see sickness as related to health; may not consider cause and effect	See health as doing desired activities Understand cause and effect Believe it is possible to be part healthy and part not at the same time; can reverse from health to sickness and back to health	Need assistance in seeing cause and effect. Capitalize on positiveness of concept; health lets you do what you really want to do. Young children who are sick may feel they will never get well again.
Illness	Sick children may see illness as punishment; evidence suggests that healthy children do not see illness as punishment. Highly anxious children more likely to view illness as disruptive. Sickness is a diffuse state; rely on others to tell them when they are ill	Same as 6–8 years of age; can identify illness states, report bodily discomfort, recognize that illness is caused by specific factors	Social factors play a part in illness concept. Recognize that some see illness as punishment. Encourage self-care and self-help behavior, especially in older children.

and may not want to have physical contact with adults; this wish should be respected. Boys may be uncomfortable having a female nurse bathe them, and girls may feel uncomfortable with a male nurse. These attitudes should be recognized and handled in a way that ensures as much privacy as possible.

Family caregivers may feel guilty about the child's need for hospitalization and, as a result, may overindulge the child. The child may regress in response to this, but this regression should not be encouraged. Sometimes the family needs as much reassurance as the child does.

Discipline and rules have a place on a pediatric unit. Inform families and children about the rules as part of the admission routine. Opportunities for interaction with peers, learning situations, and doing crafts and projects can help make the child's experience more tolerable (Fig. 26-10).

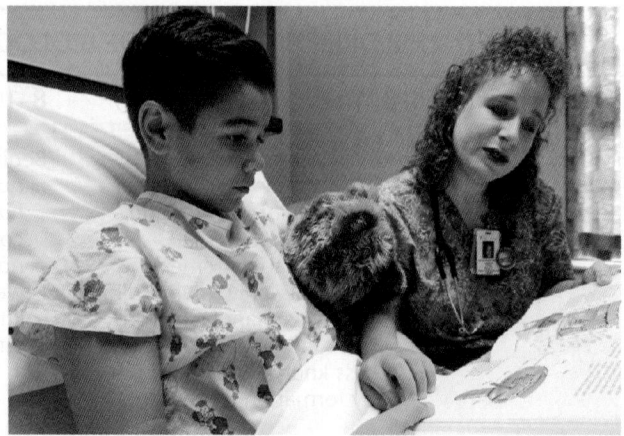

▪ Figure 26-10 School-aged children still like to listen to stories, in either the hospital or the home setting.

Key Points

➤ According to Erikson, the developmental task of school-aged children is industry versus inferiority. Success in activities using motor, cognitive, and social skills is necessary for the child to develop a sense of competency.

➤ Physical growth is slow and steady during the school-aged years. Average annual weight gain is about 5 to 6 lb (2–3 kg). The child begins to lose deciduous teeth and the first permanent teeth appear at about 6 years of age. Bone growth occurs mostly in the long bones and is gradual. By the time the child has reached the age of 10 years, the spine is straighter, the abdomen flatter, and the body generally more slender and long-legged.

➤ During this stage, the child is interested in engaging in meaningful projects and seeing them through to completion. Excessive or unrealistic goals defeat the child and possibly lead to feeling inferior, rather than self-confident. With positive support, the child develops a sense of right and wrong, a feeling of self-esteem, and an ability to care for one's self. Even though family is still a major influence, the school-aged child has a need to be accepted by groups of peers, often spends time in activities with children of the same sex, and enjoys team sports.

➤ The school-aged child develops the cognitive skills to understand *conservation* of numbers, mass, weight, and volume. The child can understand *decentration*, meaning they can see several aspects of a problem at the same time and understand the relation of various parts to the whole situation. Cause-and-effect relations become clear. They can think in either direction, so they learn to count forward and backward as well as add and subtract (the process of *reversibility*). Thinking also includes *classification*, the ability to group objects into a hierarchical arrangement (grouping by some common system).

➤ By allowing expression of food likes and dislikes and by setting good examples, caregivers can help the school-aged child develop good nutrition habits to be followed at home and school for meals as well as snacks.

➤ Obesity in the school-aged child can be related to genetic, environmental, or sedentary lifestyle factors. Appropriate physical activity, limiting fat intake, and positive caregiver support can be helpful in decreasing obesity.

➤ About the age of 10 to 11 years, the child is initially examined for signs of scoliosis (lateral curvature of the spine). Vision and hearing screening should be performed before entrance to school and on a periodic basis. Routine inspection, a well-balanced diet with adequate calcium and phosphorus, brushing after meals, and eating foods containing sugar only at mealtimes contribute to good dental health. Exercise and sufficient rest are important. The school-aged child needs 10 to 12 hours of sleep each night.

➤ Sex education regarding sexuality, reproduction, and positive attitudes regarding sexuality are important roles that families and schools often share.

➤ Substance abuse is an ever-increasing concern in school-aged children, especially the use of products that can be inhaled and used as deliriants. Family caregivers must make every effort to develop strong; loving relationships; teach family values; set and enforce rules for acceptable behavior; learn facts about drugs and alcohol; listen to what their children are saying; and teach the child about the unhealthy aspects of tobacco, alcohol, and other substances. As well, caregivers need to be alert to children's use of inhalants, deliriants, alcohol, or tobacco and to talk with the school-aged child about the abuse of substances.

➤ Children may use common inhalant products found in the home as deliriants (see Box 26-1).

➤ Safety issues for the school-aged child include teaching regarding traffic safety, especially in bicycle riding and skateboarding, seat belt use, and stranger safety.

➤ The changes in a school-aged child's understanding of birth, death, the human body, health, and illness influence the child's view of his or her own health care. Understanding these concepts is necessary to plan nursing care for the school-aged child. The child in the health care facility needs explanations and privacy.

INTERNET RESOURCES

Substance Abuse
www.toughlove.org

Family Support Groups
www.keepkidshealthy.com/schoolage

Workbook

∎ NCLEX-STYLE REVIEW QUESTIONS

1. The nurse is assisting with a well-child visit for a 7-year-old. This child's records show that at birth this child weighed 7 lbs 8 oz. At the age of 6 years, this child was 45 in tall. If this child is following a normal pattern of growth and development, which of the following would the nurse expect to find in this visit?

   a. The child weighs 54 lbs.
   b. The child measures 50 in in height.
   c. The child has four molars in the lower jaw.
   d. The child has an apical pulse of 60 beats a minute.

2. In working with a group of school-aged children, which of the following activities would this age child most likely be doing?

   a. Pretending to be television characters
   b. Playing a game with large balls
   c. Participating in a group activity
   d. Telling stories about themselves

3. During the school-aged years, according to Erikson, the child is in the stage of growth and development known as industry versus inferiority. If the caregivers of a group of children made the following statements, which statement reflects that the child is developing industry?

   a. "When my child falls down, he tries so hard to just get up and not cry."
   b. "My child was so excited when she finished her science project all by herself."
   c. "Every night my child follows the same routine at bedtime."
   d. "My child loves to make up stories about tall, big buildings."

4. In teaching caregivers of school-aged children, the nurse would reinforce that which of the following would be most important for this age group?

   a. Encouragement to brush teeth.
   b. Basic sex education.
   c. Screening for scoliosis.
   d. Wearing a bicycle helmet.

5. In working with the school-aged child and this child's family, teaching is an important role of the nurse. Which of the following are important to teach the school-aged child and family? Select all that apply.

   a. Food "jags" are common at this age.
   b. Eating foods that are disliked is important.
   c. Obesity can be a concern at this age.
   d. Scoliosis screening should be done.
   e. Foods containing sugar can be eaten as snacks.
   f. Sex education is best taught in the home.

∎ STUDY ACTIVITIES

1. List and compare the motor skills, social skills, and cognitive development in each of the following ages:

	6 Years	7 Years	8 Years	9–10 Years
Motor skills				
Social skills				
Cognitive development				

2. Make a safety poster or teaching aid to use in an elementary school classroom. Perhaps you can make this a class project and donate the posters to your pediatric unit or nearby school.

3. Survey your home and make a list of all the products available that a child could use as an inhalant for a deliriant effect.

4. Research the Internet for "tips on bicycle safety."

   a. Make a list of things you would suggest as a bike safety checklist.
   b. Describe how a bicycle helmet works.
   c. After reading this information, how would you answer the parent of a school-aged child who asks, "Does my child really need a bicycle helmet?"

∎ CRITICAL THINKING: WHAT WOULD YOU DO?

1. Delsey, the mother of 6-year-old Jasmine, is upset because Jasmine is a picky eater and often does not want to eat what Delsey has prepared.

   a. What eating patterns are seen in most school-aged children?
   b. What information would you share with Delsey about the normal nutrition requirements for Jasmine?
   c. What suggestions would you give Delsey regarding what she might offer Jasmine at meal and snack times?
   d. How could Delsey involve Jasmine in developing good nutritional patterns?

2. Steve, the primary family caregiver of 8-year-old Rebekah, feels that he should offer her sex education and asks for your advice.

   a. What topics need to be included in sex education for the school-aged child?
   b. How would you suggest Steve go about giving his daughter the sex education she needs?
   c. What resources would you offer to Steve to help him in teaching his daughter?

d. Why is it important for the family to be part of the sex education training of a child?

3. You have been asked to teach a school-aged program regarding substance abuse, including alcohol and tobacco use.

   a. What areas would you include in your teaching plan?

b. What would be the most effective teaching methods for you to use to present this material to school-aged children?

c. What questions and concerns would you anticipate from these children?

27 *Growth and Development of the Adolescent: 11 to 18 Years*

KEY TERMS

early adolescence
heterosexual
homosexual
malocclusion
menarche
nocturnal emissions
orthodontia
puberty

LEARNING OBJECTIVES

On completion of this chapter, you should be able to:

1. State the ages of the preadolescent and the adolescent.
2. Discuss the physical changes that occur in early or preadolescence.
3. Describe the psychosocial development of the adolescent.
4. List the secondary sexual characteristics that appear in adolescent boys and in adolescent girls.
5. Discuss (a) the major cognitive task of the adolescent according to Piaget and (b) the major developmental task according to Erikson.
6. Explain some problems that adolescents face when making career choices today.
7. Explain the role of intimacy in adolescence in preparation for long-term relationships.
8. Discuss the adolescent's need to conform to peers.
9. Discuss the influence of peer pressure on psychosocial development.
10. Discuss adolescent body image and associated problems.
11. Describe adolescent nutritional concerns, including (a) daily minimum needs and deficiencies, (b) habits and fads, (c) cultural influences, and (d) vegetarian diets.
12. Explain recommended health maintenance and promotion, as well as health concerns for the adolescent.
13. Discuss the aspects of sexual maturity that affect the need for health education in the adolescent.
14. Discuss the issues that the adolescent faces in making decisions related to sexual responsibility, substance use, mental health, and accident prevention.
15. State factors that may influence the adolescent's hospital experience.

"ADOLESCENCE" comes from the Latin word meaning "to come to maturity," a fitting description of this stage of life. The adolescent is maturing physically and emotionally, growing from childhood toward adulthood, and seeking to understand what it means to be grown up.

Early adolescence (preadolescence, pubescence) begins with a dramatic growth spurt that signals the advent of **puberty** (reproductive maturity). It is usually between ages 10 and 12 years. This early period ends and true adolescence begins with the onset of menstruation in the female and the production of sperm in the male. Adolescence usually spans ages 13 to 18 years.

Adolescents are fascinated and sometimes fearful and confused by the changes occurring in their bodies and their thinking processes. Body image is critical. Health problems that threaten body image, such as acne, obesity, dental or vision problems, and trauma, can seriously interfere with development.

Adolescents begin to look grown up, but they do not have the judgment or independence to participate in society as an adult. These young people are strongly

■ **Figure 27-1** The development of self-identity in adolescence involves developing interests and goals and becoming emotionally independent.

influenced by their peer group and often resent parental authority. Roller-coaster emotions characterize this age group, as does intense interest in romantic relationships.

The uncertainty and turmoil of adolescence often creates conflict between family caregivers and children. If these conflicts are resolved, normal development can

continue. Unresolved conflicts can foster delays in development and prevent the young person from maturing into a fully functioning adult.

Erikson describes the developmental task of adolescence as "identity versus role confusion." Adolescents confront marked physical and emotional changes and the knowledge that soon they will be responsible for their own lives. They must develop their own personal identity—a sense of being independent people with unique ideals and goals (Fig. 27-1). If parents, caregivers, and other adults refuse to grant that independence, adolescents may break rules just to prove that they can. Stress, anxiety, and mood swings are typical of this phase and add to the feelings of role confusion.

PREADOLESCENT DEVELOPMENT

Between 10 and 12 years of age, the rate of growth varies greatly in boys and girls. This variability in growth and maturation can be a concern to the child who develops rapidly or the one who develops more slowly than his or her peers. Children of this age do not want to be different from their friends. The developmental characteristics of the preadolescent child in late school-aged stage overlap with those of early adolescence; nevertheless, there are unique characteristics to set this stage apart (Table 27-1).

Physical Development

Preadolescence begins in the female between ages 9 and 11 years and is marked by a growth spurt that lasts for

Table 27-1 ■ GROWTH AND DEVELOPMENT OF THE PREADOLESCENT: 10 TO 13 YEARS

Physical	Motor	Personal–Social	Language	Perceptual	Cognitive
Average height 56.75–59 in (144–150 cm) Average weight 77–88 lb (35–40 kg) Pubescence may begin Girls may surpass boys in height Remaining permanent teeth erupt	Refines gross and fine motor skills May have difficulty with some fine motor coordination due to growth of large muscles before that of small muscle growth; hands and feet are first structures to increase in size; thus, actions may appear uncoordinated during early preadolescence Can do crafts Uses tools increasingly well	Attends school primarily for peer association Peer relationships of greatest importance Intolerant of violation of group norms Can follow rules of group and adapt to another point of view Can use stored knowledge to make independent judgments	Fluent in spoken language Vocabulary 50,000 words for reading; oral vocabulary of 7,200 words Uses slang words and terms, vulgarities, jeers, jokes, and sayings	Can catch or intercept ball thrown from a distance Possible growth spurts may cause myopia	Begins abstract thinking Conservation of volume Understands relations among time, speed, and distance Ability to sympathize, love, and reason are all evolving Right and wrong become logically clear

about 18 months. Girls grow about 3 in each year until **menarche** (the beginning of menstruation), after which growth slows considerably. Early in adolescence, girls begin to develop a figure, the pelvis broadens, and axillary and pubic hair begins to appear along with many changes in hormone levels. The variation between girls is great and often is a cause for much concern by the "early bloomer" or the "late bloomer." Young girls who begin to develop physically as early as 9 years of age are often embarrassed by these physical changes. In girls, the onset of menarche marks the end of the preadolescent period.

Boys enter preadolescence a little later, usually between 11 and 13 years of age, and grow generally at a slower, steadier rate than do girls. During this time, the scrotum and testes begin to enlarge, the skin of the scrotum begins to change in coloring and texture, and sparse hair begins to show at the base of the penis. Boys who start their growth spurt later often are concerned about being shorter than their peers. In boys, the appearance of **nocturnal emissions** ("wet dreams") is often used as the indication that the preadolescent period has ended.

Preparation for Adolescence

Preadolescents need information about their changing bodies and feelings. Sex education that includes information about the hormonal changes that are occurring or will be occurring is necessary to help them through this developmental stage.

Girls need information that will help them handle their early menstrual periods with minimal apprehension. Most girls have irregular periods for the first year or so; they need to know that this is not a cause for worry. They have many questions about protection during the menstrual period and the advisability of using sanitary pads or tampons. They may fear that "everybody will know" when they have their first period and must be allowed to express this fear and be reassured.

Boys also need information about their bodies. Erections and nocturnal emissions are topics they need to discuss, as well as the development of other male secondary sex characteristics.

Both boys and girls need information about changes in the opposite sex, including discussions that address their questions. This kind of information helps them increase their understanding of human sexuality. School programs may provide a good foundation for sex education, but each preadolescent needs an adult to turn to with particular questions. Even a well-planned program does not address all the needs of the preadolescent. The best school program begins early and builds from year to year as the child's needs progress (see Chapter 26).

Preadolescence is an appropriate time for discussions that will help the young teen resist pressures to become sexually active too early. Family caregivers may turn to a nurse acquaintance for guidance in preparing their child. Perhaps the most important aspect of discussions about sexuality is that honest, straightforward answers must be given in an atmosphere of caring concern. Children whose need for information is not met through family, school, or community programs will get the information—often inaccurate—from peers, movies, television, or other media.

ADOLESCENT DEVELOPMENT

Adolescence spans the ages of about 13 to 18 years. Some males do not complete adolescence until they are 20 years old. The rate of development during adolescence varies greatly from one teen to another. It is a time of many physical, emotional, and social changes. During this period, the adolescent struggles to master the developmental tasks that lead to successful completion of this stage of development (Table 27-2). Completion of the developmental tasks of earlier developmental stages is a prerequisite for the completion of these tasks.

Physical Development

Rapid growth occurs during adolescence. Girls begin growing more rapidly during the preadolescent period and achieve 98% of their adult height by the age of 16. Boys start their growth spurt, a period of rapid growth, around 13 years of age and may continue to grow until 20 years of age. The skeletal system's rapid growth, which outpaces muscular system growth, causes the long and lanky appearance of many teens and contributes to the clumsiness often seen during this age. The bone growth that began during intrauterine life continues through adolescence and is usually completed by the end of this period.

The adolescent's body begins to take on adultlike contours, the primary sex organs enlarge, secondary sexual characteristics appear, and hormonal activity increases. During the first menstrual cycles for girls, ovulation does not usually occur because increased estrogen levels are needed to produce an ovum mature enough to be released. However, at 13 to 15 years of age, the cycle becomes ovulatory, and pregnancy is possible. The girl's breasts take on an adult appearance by age 16, and pubic hair is curly and abundant.

By the age of 16 years, the male's penis, testes, and scrotum are adult in size and shape, and mature spermatozoa are produced. Male pubic hair also is adult in appearance and amount. After age 13, muscle strength and coordination develop rapidly. The larynx and vocal cords enlarge, and the voice deepens. The "change of voice" makes the teenage male's voice vary unexpectedly, which occasionally causes embarrassment for the teen.

Psychosocial Development

Adolescence is a time of transition from childhood to adulthood. Between the ages of 10 and 18 years, adolescents move from Freud's latency stage to the genital stage, from Erikson's industry versus inferiority to identity versus role confusion, and from Piaget's concrete operational

Table 27-2 ▮ DEVELOPMENTAL TASKS OF ADOLESCENCE

Basic Task	Associated Tasks
Appreciate own uniqueness*	Identify interests, skills, and talents Identify differences from peers Accept strengths and limitations Challenge own skill levels
Develop independent internal identity*	Value self as a person Separate physical self from psychological self Differentiate personal worth from cultural stereotypes Separate internal value from societal feedback
Determine own value system*	Identify options Establish priorities Commit self to decisions made Translate values into behaviors Resist peer and cultural pressures to conform to their value system Find comfortable balance between own and peer/cultural standards, behaviors, and needs
Develop self-evaluation skills*	Develop basis for self-evaluation and monitoring Evaluate quality of products Assess approach to tasks and responsibilities Develop sensitivity to intrapersonal relationships Evaluate dynamics of interpersonal relationships
Assume increasing responsibility for own behavior*	Quality of work, chores Emotional tone Money management Time management Decision making Personal habits Social behaviors
Find meaning in life	Accept and integrate meaning of death Develop philosophy of life Begin to identify life or career goals
Acquire skills essential for adult living	Acquire skills essential to independent living Develop social and emotional abilities and temperament Refine sociocultural amenities Identify and experiment with alternatives for facing life Acquire employment skills Seek growth-inducing activities
Seek affiliations outside of family	Seek companionship with compatible peers Affiliate with organizations that support uniqueness Actively seek models or mentors Identify potential emotional support systems Differentiate between acquaintances and friends Identify ways to express sexuality
Adapt to adult body functioning	Adapt to somatic (body) changes Refine balance and coordination Develop physical strength Consider sexuality and reproduction issues

*Tasks deemed crucial to continued maturation

thinking to formal operational thought. Adolescents develop a sense of moral judgment and a system of values and beliefs that will affect their entire lives. The foundation provided by family, religious groups, school, and community experiences is still a strong influence, but the peer group exerts tremendous power. Trends and fads among adolescents dictate clothing choices, hairstyles, music, and other recreational choices (Fig. 27-2). The adolescent whose family caregivers make it difficult to conform are adding another stress to an already emotion-laden period. Peer pressure to experiment with potentially dangerous practices, such as drugs, alcohol, and reckless driving, also can be strong; adolescents may need careful guidance and understanding support to help resist this peer influence.

■ **Figure 27-2** For many teens, hanging out with friends is an important way to share common interests and gain a sense of belonging.

■ **Figure 27-3** Intense interest in the opposite sex characterizes adolescence.

Personality Development

Erikson considered the central task of adolescence to be the establishment of identity. Adolescents spend a lot of time asking themselves, "Who am I as a person? What will I do with my life? Marry? Have children? Will I go to college? If so, where? If not, why not? What kind of career should I choose?"

Adolescents are confronted with a greater variety of choices than ever before. Sex role stereotypes have been shattered in most careers and professions. More women are becoming lawyers, physicians, plumbers, and carpenters; more men are entering nursing or choosing to become stay-at-home fathers while their wives earn the primary family income. Transportation has made greater geographic mobility possible, so many youngsters can spend summers or a full school year in a foreign country, plan to attend college thousands of miles from home, and begin a career in an even more remote location. Making decisions and choices is never simple. With such a tremendous variety of options, it is understandable that adolescents often are preoccupied with their own concerns.

When identity has been established, generally between the ages of 16 and 18 years, adolescents seek intimate relationships, usually with members of the opposite sex (Fig. 27-3). Intimacy, which is mutual sharing of one's deepest feelings with another person, is impossible unless both persons have established a sense of trust and a sense of identity. Intimate relationships are a preparation for long-term relationships, and people who fail to achieve intimacy may develop feelings of isolation and experience chronic difficulty in communicating with others.

Most intimate relationships during adolescence are **heterosexual,** or between members of the opposite sex. Sometimes, however, young people form intimate attachments with members of the same sex, or **homosexual** relationships. Because our culture is predominately heterosexual and is still struggling to understand homosexual relationships, these relationships can cause great anxiety for family caregivers and children. Although some parts of American society are beginning to accept homosexual relationships as no more than another lifestyle, prejudice still exists. So great a stigma has been attached to homosexuality that many adolescents fear they are homosexual if they are uncomfortable about heterosexual intimacy. However, this discomfort is normal as adolescents move from same-sex peer group activities to dating peers of the opposite sex.

Body Image

Body image is closely related to self-esteem. Seeing one's body as attractive and functional contributes to a positive sense of self-esteem. During adolescence, the desire not to be different can extend to feelings about one's body and can cause adolescents to feel that their bodies are inadequate, even though they are actually healthy and attractive.

American culture tends to equate a slender figure with feminine beauty and acceptability and a lean, tall, muscular figure with masculine virility and strength. Adolescents, particularly males, who feel that they are underdeveloped suffer great anxiety. Adolescent girls have even undergone plastic surgery to augment their breasts to relieve this anxiety. Girls in this age group often feel that they are too fat and try strange, nutritionally unsound diets to reduce their weight. Some literally starve themselves. Even after their bodies have become emaciated, they truly believe that they are still

Table 27-3 ▮ DAILY NUTRITIONAL NEEDS OF THE 11– TO 18–YEAR–OLD				
Males (M) need 2000–2800 calories/day; Females (F) need 1,800–2,000 calories/day. The moderately active adolescent needs the amounts below from each food group.				
Grains	Vegetables	Fruits	Milk	Meat and Beans
M: 6–10 oz F: 6 oz	M: 2.5–3.5 cups F: 2.5 cups	M: 2–2.5 cups F: 1.5–2 cups	M: 3 cups F: 3 cups	M: 5.5–7 oz F: 5–5.5 oz

fat and, therefore, unattractive. This condition is called *anorexia nervosa* and is discussed further in Chapter 42.

Adolescents need to establish a positive body image by the end of their developmental stage. Because bone growth is completed during adolescence, a person's height will remain basically the same throughout adult life, even though weight can fluctuate greatly. Tall girls who long to be petite and boys who would like to be 6 ft tall may need guidance and support to bring their expectations in line with reality and learn to have positive feelings about their bodies and accept them the way they are.

Test Yourself

✔ What are the secondary sex characteristics that develop in the (a) adolescent boy and the (b) adolescent girl?

✔ Why is body image so important for the adolescent?

NUTRITION

Adolescents need a balanced diet consisting of servings from each of the food groups (Table 27-3). (See also MyPyramid for Kids in Fig. 22-3 in Chapter 22.) Nutritional requirements greatly increase during periods of rapid growth. Adolescent boys need more calories than do girls throughout the growth period. Appetites increase, and most teens eat frequently. Families with teenage boys often jokingly say that they cannot keep the refrigerator filled. Nutritional needs are related to growth and sexual maturity, rather than age.

Even though adolescents understand something about nutrition, they may not relate this understanding to their dietary habits. Their accelerated growth rate and increased physical activities, for some, mean that they need more food to meet their energy requirements. Because adolescents are seeking to establish

their independence, their food choices are sometimes not wise and tend to be influenced by peer preference, rather than parental advice. Teens frequently skip meals, especially breakfast, snack on foods that provide empty calories, and eat a lot of fast foods. The era of fast food meals has given adolescents easy access to high-calorie, nutritionally unbalanced meals. Too many fast-food meals and nutritionally empty snacks can result in nutritional deficiencies (Fig. 27-4).

Nutrients that are often deficient in the teen's diet include calcium; iron; zinc; vitamins A, D, and B_6; and folic acid. Calcium needs increase during skeletal growth. Girls need additional iron because of losses during menstruation. Boys also need additional iron during this growth period (Table 27-4). When good nutritional habits have been established in early childhood, adolescent nutrition is likely to be better balanced than when nutritional teaching has been insufficient. Being part of a family that practices sound nutrition helps ensure that occasional lapses into sweets, fast foods, and other peer group food preferences will not create serious deficiencies.

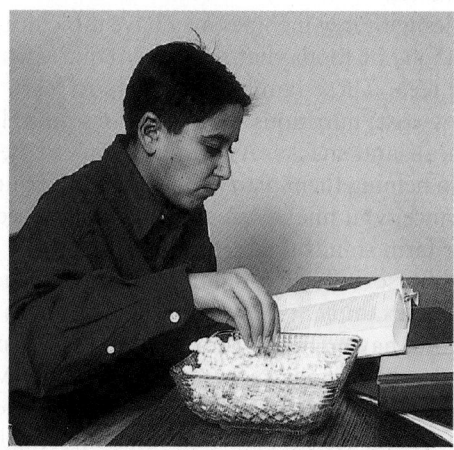

▮ Figure 27-4 Teens are always hungry, but often choose convenient junk foods, which lack nutritional value.

Table 27-4 ■ FOOD SOURCES OF NUTRIENTS COMMONLY DEFICIENT IN PREADOLESCENT AND ADOLESCENT DIETS

Common Nutrient Deficiencies	Food Sources
Vitamin A	Liver, whole milk, butter, cheese; sources of carotene such as yellow vegetables, green leafy vegetables, tomatoes, yellow fruits
Vitamin D	Fortified milk, egg yolk, butter
Vitamin B_6 (pyridoxine)	Chicken, fish, peanuts, bananas, pork, egg yolk, whole-grain cereals
Folate (folic acid)	Green leafy vegetables, enriched cereals, liver, dried peas and beans, whole grains
Calcium	Milk, hard cheese, yogurt, ice cream, small fish eaten with bones (e.g., sardines), dark-green vegetables, tofu, soybeans, calcium-enriched orange juice
Iron	Lean meats, liver, legumes, dried fruits, green leafy vegetables, whole-grain and fortified cereals
Zinc	Oysters, herring, meat, liver, fish, milk, whole grains, nuts, legumes

In their quest for identity and independence, some adolescents experiment with food fads and diets. Adolescent girls, worried about being fat, fall prey to a variety of fad diets. Athletes also may follow fad diets that may include supplements in the belief that these diets enhance bodybuilding. These diets often include increased amounts of protein and amino acids that cause diuresis and calcium loss. Carbohydrate loading, which some practice during the week before an athletic event, increases the muscle glycogen level to two to three times normal and may hinder heart function. A meal that is low in fat and high in complex carbohydrates eaten 3 to 4 hours before an event is much more appropriate for the teen athlete.

Adolescents often resist pressure from family members to eat balanced meals; all family caregivers can do is to provide nutritious meals and snacks and regular mealtimes. A good example may be the best teacher at this point. A refrigerator stocked with ready-to-eat nutritious snacks can be a good weapon against snacking on empty calories.

Families with low incomes may have difficulty providing the kinds of foods that meet the requirements for a growing teen. These families need help to learn how to make low-cost, nutritious food selections and plan adequate meals and snacks. As a nurse, you can be instrumental in helping them plan appropriate food purchases. For instance, you might recommend fruit and vegetable stores or farm stands that accept food stamps.

Culture also influences adolescent food choices and habits. For example, many Mexican Americans are accustomed to having their big meal at noon. When school lunches do not provide such a heavy meal, the Mexican American adolescent may supplement the lunch with sweets or fast foods. In the Asian community, milk is not a popular drink; this can result in a calcium deficiency. Many Asians are lactose intolerant; therefore, you can

recommend other products high in calcium, such as tofu (soybean curd), soybeans, and greens to increase calcium intake.

A person may follow a vegetarian diet for religious, ecologic, or philosophic reasons. If planned with care, vegetarian diets can provide needed nutrients. The most common types of vegetarian diets are the following:

- *Semivegetarian* includes dairy products, eggs, and fish; excludes red meat and possibly poultry.
- *Lacto-ovovegetarian* includes eggs and dairy products but excludes meat, poultry, and fish.
- *Lactovegetarian* includes dairy products and excludes meat, fish, poultry, and eggs.
- *Vegan* excludes all food of animal origin, including dairy products, eggs, fish, meat, and poultry.

Vegan diets may not provide adequate nutrients without careful planning. All vegetarians should include whole-grain products, legumes, nuts, seeds, and fortified soy substitutes if low-fat dairy products are unacceptable.

HEALTH PROMOTION AND MAINTENANCE

Adolescents have much the same need for regular health checkups, protection against infection, and prevention of accidents as do younger children. They also have special needs that can best be met by health professionals with

Cultural Snapshot

Be alert to cultural dietary influences on the adolescent; take these into consideration when helping the adolescent and the family devise an adequate food plan.

in-depth knowledge and understanding of adolescent concerns. The number of adolescent clinics and health centers has increased along with innovative health services, such as school-based clinics, crisis hotlines, homes for runaways, and rehabilitation centers for adolescents who have been involved with alcohol or other drugs or with prostitution. Staff members in these programs provide teens with services needed for healthy growth.

Routine Checkups

A routine physical examination is recommended at least twice during the teen years, although annual physical examinations are encouraged. At this time, a complete history of developmental milestones, school problems, behavioral problems, family relationships, and immunizations should be completed. Immunizations, which have not been administered at the recommended age, should be administered in order to catch-up the adolescent (see Appendix J). A urine pregnancy screening is advisable before the rubella vaccine is administered to a girl of childbearing age because administration of the vaccine during pregnancy can cause serious risks to the developing fetus. Tuberculin testing is included in at least one visit and, depending on the community, may be recommended at both visits if there is an interval of several years between visits.

Measure and record height, weight, and blood pressure. Vision and hearing screening are done if they have not been part of a regular school screening program. Adolescents to the age of 16 years need to be screened for scoliosis. Thyroid enlargement should be checked through age 14. Sexually active girls must have a pelvic examination, screening for sexually transmitted infections (STIs), and a Papanicolaou smear. Urinalysis is performed on all female adolescents, and a urine culture is performed if the girl has any symptoms of a urinary tract infection, such as urgency or burning and pain on urination. A routine physical is an excellent time for you to counsel the adolescent about sexual activity, STIs, and human immunodeficiency virus (HIV) infection.

Body piercing and tattoos are becoming more common in the adolescent population. Piercings are seen in ears, eyebrows, noses, lips, chins, breasts, navels—in almost every part of the body. Tattoos of all designs are seen in the adolescent. The adolescent with piercing and tattoos needs to be aware of the signs and symptoms of infection (redness, swelling, warmness, drainage, discomfort) and that these must be reported immediately if they occur. Sharing needles for piercing or tattooing needs to be discussed, and the adolescent needs to be taught that sharing needles carries the same risks as sharing needles with IV drug users.

Adolescents must be given privacy, individualized attention, confidentiality, and the right to participate in decisions about their health care. They may feel uncomfortable and out of place in a pediatrician's waiting room, where most of the patients are 3 ft tall, or in a waiting room filled with adults. Some clinics and providers specialize in adolescent

A Personal Glimpse

Every year around our birthdays, my little brother and I always go to our pediatrician's office. After being called by the nurse, we both go down to a tiny room with bright walls, baby pictures, and the kind of mobiles hung over a crib, the same kind of decorations that cover the entire office. I suppose the room itself is comforting, but then I have to strip down to my underwear right in front of my 6-year-old brother. To make matters worse, I have to put on a skimpy little gown that hardly covers my underwear and wait in a room with huge windows and blinds that don't close, overlooking the next building's parking lot. It's so embarrassing, having to climb up onto the examining table with a gown falling down underneath me. Why can't the gowns be longer? It isn't just 6-year-olds who have to wear them!

Jessica, age 12

Learning Opportunity: What do nurses and health care providers need to take into consideration regarding the privacy needs of adolescents? What specific things would you do in this situation to acknowledge and respect the needs of this adolescent girl?

health care, but many adolescents do not have these facilities available to them.

Continuity of care helps build the adolescent's confidence in the service and the caregivers. Professionals dealing with teens should recognize that the physical symptoms offered as the reason for seeking care are often not the most significant problem about which the adolescent is concerned. An attitude of nonjudgmental acceptance on the part of health care personnel can often encourage the adolescent to ask questions and share feelings and concerns about a troubling matter. Family members may accompany adolescents to the health care facility, but it is important to provide an opportunity to interview the adolescent alone (Fig. 27-5). Asking questions in a way that is concrete and specific will encourage the adolescent to give direct answers. The interviewer must be alert to verbal and nonverbal clues.

A little sensitivity is in order.
Adolescents who are given privacy and respect feel safer to share their feelings and concerns with adults.

Dental Checkups

Adolescents need continued regular dental checkups every 6 months. Dental **malocclusion** (improper alignment of the teeth) is a common condition that affects the way the teeth and jaws function. Correction of the

■ **Figure 27-5** Interviewing the adolescent in private and conveying a nonjudgmental attitude will encourage her to ask questions and express concerns about a troubling matter. Adolescents need to be included in plans and decisions regarding their health care.

malocclusion with dental braces improves chewing ability and appearance. The treatment of the malocclusion with dental braces is called **orthodontia**. Braces have become very common among adolescents because about half of them have malocclusions that can be corrected. Orthodontic treatment usually begins in early adolescence or late school age. The use of braces has become very widespread, and braces are readily accepted among teens, although many teens still feel awkward and self-conscious during their orthodontic treatment. Tongue piercing among adolescents has increased, and during dental checkups is a good time to discuss concerns of possible infections and teeth damage that can occur when an adolescent has a pierced tongue.

Family Teaching

The adolescent years are difficult for the maturing young person and often are just as difficult for the family caregiver. Caregivers must allow the independent teen to flourish while continuing to safeguard him or her from risky and immature behavior. Caregivers and adolescents struggle with issues related to sexuality, substance abuse, accidents, discipline, poor nutrition, and volatile emotions.

Learning about adolescent physical and psychosocial developments can help caregivers struggling to understand their teen. Caregivers will find information on sexuality

and substance abuse enlightening and useful. Attending workshops or consulting counselors, teachers, religious leaders, or health care workers may enhance the caregiver's communication skills. Good communication between adolescents and their caregivers is essential to fostering healthy relationships between them. Caregivers may need both guidance in preparing their teen for adulthood and emotional support to feel successful in this difficult period. Take every opportunity to provide the family caregiver with information and support.

Health Education and Counseling

Before adolescents can take an active role in their own health care, they need information and guidance on the need for health care and how to meet that need most effectively. Education and counseling about sexuality, STIs, contraception, and substance abuse are a vital part of adolescent health care. Some of this teaching should and sometimes does come from family caregivers.

> **You can make the difference.**
> Family caregivers' lack of information or discomfort in discussing certain topics with adolescents sometimes means that the job will have to be done by health professionals.

Sexuality

A good foundation in sex education can help the adolescent take pride in having reached sexual maturity; otherwise, puberty can be a frightening, shameful experience. Girls who have not been taught about menstruation until it occurs are understandably alarmed. Those who have been taught to regard it as "the curse," rather than an entrance into womanhood, will not have positive feelings about this part of their sexuality.

Boys who are unprepared for nocturnal emissions may feel guilty, believing that they have caused these "wet dreams" by sexual fantasies or masturbation. They need to understand that this is a normal occurrence and simply the body's method of getting rid of surplus semen.

Assuming that adolescents are adequately prepared for the events of puberty, sex education during adolescence can deal with the important issues of responsible sexuality, contraception, and STIs. More adolescents today are sexually active than ever, resulting in an alarmingly rapid increase in teenage pregnancies and STIs. The incidence of HIV infection is particularly increasing among adolescents.

Girls need to learn the importance of regular pelvic examinations and Pap smears and the technique for the monthly self-care procedure of breast self-examination (Family Teaching Tips: Breast Self-Examination). Boys need to learn that testicular cancer is one of the most common cancers in young men between the ages of 15 and 34 years and must be taught how and when to

Family Teaching Tips

BREAST SELF-EXAMINATION

INSTRUCTIONS

The best time to do the breast self-exam is about a week after your period ends. The breast is not as tender or swollen at this point in the menstrual cycle.

1. Lie down with a pillow under your right shoulder. Place your right arm behind your head (Fig. *A*).

A

2. Use the sensitive finger pads (where your fingerprints are, not the tips) of the middle three fingers on your left hand to feel for lumps in the right breast (Fig. *B*). Use overlapping dime-sized circular motions of the finger pads to feel the breast tissue. Powder, oil, or lotion can be applied to the breast to make it easier for the fingers to glide over the surface and feel changes.

B

3. Use three different levels of pressure to feel the breast tissue. First, light pressure to just move the skin without jostling the tissue beneath, then medium pressure pressing midway into the tissue, and finally firm pressure to probe more deeply down to the chest and ribs or to the point just short of discomfort. Use each pressure level to feel the breast tissue before moving on to the next spot.

4. Move your fingers around the breast in an up and down pattern (called the vertical pattern), starting at an imaginary line drawn straight down your side

from the underarm and moving across the breast to the middle of the chest bone (sternum or breastbone). Check the entire breast using each of the pressures described above. Completely feel all of the breast and chest area up under your armpit, up to the collarbone and all the way over to your shoulder to cover breast tissue that extends toward the shoulder (Fig. *C*).

C

5. Repeat the exam on your left breast using the finger pads of your right hand, with a pillow under your left shoulder.

6. While standing in front of a mirror, with your hands pressing firmly down on your hips (this position shows more clearly any breast changes), look at your breasts for any change in size, shape, contour, dimpling of the skin, changes in the nipple, redness, or spontaneous nipple discharge (Fig. D).

D

(continues on page 614)

BREAST SELF-EXAMINATION (Continued)

7. Examine each underarm while sitting or standing, with your arm only slightly raised (raising your arm straight tightens the tissue and makes it difficult to examine). The upright position makes it easier to check the upper and outer parts of the breasts (toward your armpits). You may want to do this part of the exam while showering. It's easy to slide soapy hands over your skin, and to feel anything unusual (Fig. E).

Breast self-examination from the American Cancer Society. Retrieved April 2008, from www.cancer.org.

perform testicular self-examination (Family Teaching Tips: Testicular Self-Examination).

Adolescents' growing awareness of their sexuality, sexually provocative material in the media, and lack of acceptable means to gratify sexual desires make masturbation a common practice during adolescence. Unlike young children's genital exploration, adolescent masturbation can produce orgasm in the female and ejaculation in the male. Generally, it is a private and solitary activity, but occasionally it occurs with other members of the peer group. Health professionals recognize masturbation as a positive way to release sexual tension and increase one's knowledge of body sensations. Reassure adolescents that masturbation is common in both males and females and is a normal outlet for sexual urges.

Sexual Responsibility

Not all adolescents are sexually active, but the number of those who are increases with each year of age. Although abstinence is the only completely successful protection, all adolescents need to have information concerning safe sex practices to be prepared for the occasion when they wish to be sexually intimate with someone. Adolescents do not have a good record of using contraceptives to prevent pregnancy. Many teens give excuses such as "sex shouldn't be planned," because if it is planned, it is wrong or they feel guilty. They need to feel that it "just happened" in the heat of the moment, not because they really wanted or planned it. Many adolescents are beginning to realize that much more than pregnancy may be at risk, but their attitude of "it won't happen to me," which is typical of their developmental age, continues to contribute to their increasing sexual activity.

Some adults continue to resist providing contraceptive information to adolescents in school, believing that such information encourages teens to become sexually active. However, as HIV infection becomes a greater threat to every sexually active person, this argument becomes harder to defend. Adolescents need contraceptive information to prevent pregnancy, but more importantly, they need straightforward information about using condoms to protect them against HIV and other infections. Both male and female adolescents need this information, and girls must be advised to carry their own condoms if they believe that there is any possibility of having sexual intercourse.

When condoms are used consistently and correctly, they are highly effective in preventing pregnancy and sexually transmitted infections. Condoms used with spermicidal foam have an even greater effective rate against pregnancy. The safest condom is one made of latex with a prelubricated tip or reservoir and pretreated with nonoxynol-9 spermicide. Family Teaching Tips: Safe Condom Use and Figure 4-6, both in Chapter 4, provide guidelines for use of male and female condoms, respectively.

TESTICULAR SELF-EXAMINATION

INSTRUCTIONS

Perform the examination once a month after a warm bath or shower. The scrotum is relaxed from the warmth. Select a day that is easy to remember, such as the first or last day of the month.

1. Stand in front of a mirror, if possible, and look for any swelling on the skin of the scrotum.
2. Examine each testicle, one at a time, using both hands.
3. Place the index and middle fingers under the testicle and the thumbs on top. Roll each testicle gently between the thumbs and fingers (Fig. A). One testicle is normally larger than the other.
4. The epididymis is the soft, tubelike structure located at the back of the testicle that collects and carries sperm (Fig. B). This must not be mistaken for an abnormal lump.
5. Most lumps are found on the sides of the testicle, although they may also appear on the front. Look and feel for any hard lumps or nodules (smooth, rounded masses) or any change in the size, shape, or consistency of the testes.
6. Report any lump to your health care provider at once. Testicular cancer is highly curable when treated promptly.

SIGNS OF TESTICULAR CANCER

- Small, painless lump in a testicle.
- Enlargement of a testicle. It is normal for one testicle to be slightly larger than the other.
- Significant loss in size of a testicle.
- A feeling of scrotal heaviness.
- A dull ache in the lower abdomen or groin.
- Testicular or scrotal pain or discomfort.
- Sudden accumulation of blood or fluid in the scrotum.
- Enlargement or tenderness of the breasts.

A

B

Epididymis

Testicle

Other STIs that sexually active adolescents need to know about are syphilis, gonorrhea, genital herpes, genital warts, and chlamydial and trichomonal infections. Prevention of STIs is the primary aim of education for adolescents. If prevention proves ineffective, however, the most important factor is referral for treatment. Many adolescents are reluctant to seek treatment, fearing that their family caregivers will discover their activity. Crisis hotlines are valuable resources to assure adolescents that treatment is vital for them and their partners and that confidentiality is ensured.

Health care personnel who work with adolescents seeking treatment for an STI must be nonjudgmental, supportive, and understanding. The adolescents need treatment and information about preventing spread of the STI to others, as well as how to prevent contracting another STI. See Chapter 41 for a thorough discussion of STIs and related nursing care.

Many adolescents are not sexually active, but most spend time dating or socializing with peers. In recent years, the use of Rohypnol, also known as the "date rape drug," has become a concern for the adolescent. Rohypnol is not sold legally in the United States, but it is brought in from countries where it is sold legally. The drug, especially in combination with alcohol, causes memory loss, blackouts, and an inability to resist sexual attacks. Often, the drug is secretly slipped into a person's drink. The drug has no taste or odor, but within a few minutes after ingesting the drug, the person feels dizzy, disoriented, and nauseated, and then rapidly passes out. After several hours, the person awakens and has no memories of what happened while under the influence of the drug. The adolescent needs to be encouraged to stay aware and alert to avoid becoming a victim of date rape. He or she should be taught to avoid using alcohol and never to leave any drink unattended.

Substance Abuse

As adolescents search for identity and independence, they are susceptible to many pressures from society and their peers. Adolescents may experiment with substances that may be habit forming or addictive and ultimately will harm them. This may be done "just for kicks," to "go along with the crowd" (peer group), or to rebel against the authority of family caregivers or other adults. Some substances abused by adolescents also are abused by many adults; so to some adolescents, using these substances may appear sophisticated.

Alcohol and certain other drugs provide an escape, however brief, from pressures the adolescent may feel. Alcohol is the mind-altering substance most commonly abused by adolescents. Other substances that adolescents may abuse are tobacco (including smokeless tobacco), marijuana, cocaine or "crack," heroin, "Ecstasy," other street drugs, and prescription drugs. (See Chapter 42 for further discussion of substance abuse.) Adolescents can often obtain tobacco products, despite federal legislation to enforce strict age limitations on their sale.

Programs developed to educate students about substance abuse meet with varying success. Health care personnel must stress to adolescents that use of alcohol or mind-altering chemicals is often accompanied by irresponsible sexual behavior that could further complicate their lives. Chapter 42 discusses these problems in more detail.

Test Yourself

✔ What nutrients are often missing in the adolescent diet?

✔ List the topics of health education that should be discussed with the adolescent.

Mental Health

The turmoil that adolescents experience while searching for self-esteem and self-confidence can cause stress that may lead to depression, suicide, and conduct disorders. Academic and social pressures add to that stress. The family also may be under stress due to unemployment or economic difficulties, separation, divorce, or death of a caregiver. Health care personnel must be sensitive to signs

that the adolescent is having problems. Adolescents need the opportunity to express their fears, concerns, and frustrations. The rapport between family caregivers and teens may not be such that the adolescent can express these feelings to the family. Many schools have mental health personnel on staff that can provide counseling when needed. Adolescents need counseling to work through troublesome situations and to avoid chronic mental health problems. Mental health assessment is an important part of the adolescent's total health assessment.

With the increased use of computers and the Internet, Internet safety is an important aspect of adolescent mental health. Parents need to be aware of their adolescent's computer activities and the sites they access, especially communication sites such as chat rooms. Discussions with adolescents regarding safety concerns on Internet sites help to increase their awareness and decrease potential dangers. See Family Teaching Tips: Internet Safety.

Accident Prevention

In every part of society, increasing numbers of adolescents are dying as a result of violence, which includes motor vehicle accidents, homicide, suicide, and other causes. Unintentional injuries and homicide rank as the leading causes of death for 15- to 19-year-old minority youth, regardless of gender (Joffe, 2006). Statistics

Family Teaching Tips

INTERNET SAFETY

Signs that might indicate online risks in a child or adolescent:
- Spends large amounts of time online, especially at night
- Has pornography on computer
- Receives phone calls from adults you don't know
- Makes calls, especially long distance, to numbers you don't recognize
- Receives mail, gifts, packages from someone you don't know
- Turns computer monitor off or changes screen when you enter room
- Becomes withdrawn from family

To minimize online concerns:
- Communicate and talk with child; openly discuss concerns and dangers.
- Spend time with child online.
- Use blocking software and devices.
- Use caller ID to determine who is calling your child.
- Maintain access to child's online account and monitor activity.

Adapted from FBI publication, *A parent's guide to Internet safety,* http://www.fbi.gov/publications/pguide/pguidee.htm

regarding adolescents are difficult to interpret, but death among adolescents is often related to risky behaviors. These behaviors include the unintentional (motor vehicles, fires) as well as the intentional (violence, suicide) injuries, alcohol and other drug use, sexual behaviors, tobacco use, and dietary behaviors. Alcohol and other drugs are often involved in fatal accidents. Death is not the only negative outcome of violence: Many adolescents are injured and hospitalized or treated in emergency departments, and many adolescents suffer psychological injury from being victims of violence.

Violence is also on the rise in schools—not just inner-city schools. Weapons are detected on students in schools all over the country. Guns and knives are the weapons most often found. The problem has become so serious that some schools have installed metal detectors to protect students.

Adolescents also are victims of violence in their own homes in greater numbers than any other age group of children. Date rape and other violence in a dating relationship are common.

Students have formed groups such as Students Against Drunk Driving to promote safety in driving (Web site: www.saddonline.com). Many schools provide support groups that help students to work through their grief after schoolmates have met with violent death.

Much work needs to be done to understand the reason for this increasing violence. One factor in adolescents is that they often act recklessly without benefit of mature judgment. Adolescents have relatively easy access to guns and often use them as a means to solve problems. Efforts to control and regulate gun sales are nationally discussed topics. Acts of terror and violence in the world increase the confusion and anxiety that adolescents have regarding conflicts and conflict resolution.

Nurses who have any contact with adolescents must make every effort to help them work through their problems in nonviolent ways. As a nurse, you can become involved at the school or community level by becoming an advocate for adolescents and an educator to promote safe driving, as well as wearing a helmet and safety practices when using a motorcycle, all-terrain vehicle, bicycle, skateboard, or in-line skates. You can also work with support groups that offer counseling to adolescents involved in date violence. As a community member and a health care worker, you can provide a positive role model for adolescents.

THE ADOLESCENT IN THE HEALTH CARE FACILITY

When adolescents are hospitalized, it is usually because of a major health problem such as an injury from violence or from a motor vehicle accident, substance abuse, attempted suicide, or a chronic health problem intensified by the physiologic changes of adolescence. Adolescents must cope with the stress of hospitalization, possible dramatic alterations in body image, partial or total inability to conform to peer group norms, and an interrupted search for identity.

Adolescents fear loss of control and loss of privacy. Provide opportunities for the adolescent to make choices, whenever possible. Providing screening and adequate covering during procedures helps to protect the adolescent's privacy.

Adolescents may react with anger and refuse to cooperate when their privacy or feelings of control are threatened. Be aware of this possible reaction and avoid labeling such an adolescent as a difficult patient.

The admission interview for an adolescent may be more successful if the family caregiver and the adolescent are interviewed separately. This provides the opportunity to gain information that the adolescent may not want to reveal in the presence of the family caregiver. It is important to thoroughly explore the adolescent's developmental level, listen carefully with empathy to his or her concerns, encourage maximum participation in self-care, and provide sufficient information to make this participation possible.

This is critical to remember. In working with adolescents, as with all patients, clear, honest explanations about treatments and procedures are essential.

During the admission interview, advise the adolescent of the unit's rules. Adolescents need to know what limits are set for their behavior while they are in the hospital. To share feelings and gain information, many find it helpful to discuss their health problem with a peer who has had the same or a related problem.

Adolescents need access to a telephone to contact peers and keep up social contacts. Recreation areas are important. In settings specifically designed for adolescents, recreation rooms can provide an area where teens can gather to do school work, play games and cards, and socialize. In many hospitals with adolescent units, video games as well as television are provided in each patient room. Access to a computer and electronic mail might also help the teen stay connected to peers. Supervision is important to decrease misuse of computer privileges. Teens are encouraged to wear their own clothes. They can be encouraged to shampoo and style their hair, and girls can wear their usual makeup.

The adolescent's health problem may require a lengthy hospitalization and intense rehabilitation efforts. Adequate preparation and guidance can help make that difficult experience easier and less damaging to normal growth and development.

Test Yourself

✔ What are the most frequent causes of accidents in adolescents?

✔ Give examples of how hospitalized adolescents can be given choices and control.

Key Points

➤ The preadolescent period is between ages 10 and 12 years, and adolescence spans ages 13 to 18 years.

➤ In preadolescence, the child's body begins to take on adultlike contours, the primary sex organs enlarge, secondary sexual characteristics appear, and hormonal activity increases. This early period ends with the onset of menstruation in the female and the production of sperm in the male. The rapid growth of the skeletal system outpaces the growth of the muscular system, contributing to the clumsiness sometimes noted in the adolescent.

➤ During adolescence, children go through many psychosocial changes on their way to adulthood. They are fascinated and sometimes fearful and confused by the changes occurring in their bodies and their thinking processes. The adolescent begins to look grown up, but lacks the judgment or independence to participate in society as an adult. They are strongly influenced by their peer group and often resent parental authority. Roller-coaster emotions characterize this age group, as does intense interest in romantic relationships.

➤ Secondary sexual characteristics seen in the adolescent boy include penis, testes, and scrotum reaching adult size and shape, as well as pubic hair, increased strength, and a deepening of the voice. Adolescent girls develop breasts and pubic hair and begin ovulation and menstruation.

➤ According to Piaget, the adolescent moves from concrete operational thinking to formal operational thought. Erikson's stage of development in the adolescent is referred to as identity versus role confusion. The adolescent's task is to establish his or her own identity and to find a place in society.

➤ Changing sex role stereotypes, geographic mobility, and abundant career opportunities and options add to the adolescent's difficulties in making a career choice.

➤ Intimacy or mutual sharing of deep feelings with another person occurs when people have developed trust and their own sense of identity. Intimate relationships in adolescents help in preparation for long-term relationships.

➤ In trying to develop their own sense of self and identity, adolescents begin the process of separating from family caregivers. The peers exert influence, and the adolescent feels a need to conform and to "fit" with peers. This peer pressure may be extremely influential in affecting the adolescent's attitudes and behaviors. A strong support system is important to help the adolescent through this stressful stage of development.

➤ Body image and self-esteem are closely related, and the adolescent struggles with wanting to be attractive and accepted. This drive can create anxiety in the adolescent, which can lead to unhealthy behavior, practices, and conditions.

➤ Appetites increase and most teens eat frequently. It is important for the adolescent to maintain a balanced diet with healthy food choices. Their food choices are sometimes not wise and tend to be influenced by peers. Adolescent diets are often deficient in calcium; iron; zinc; vitamins A, D, and B_6; and folic acid. Culture influences food choices and habits, as does the choice to follow a vegetarian diet.

➤ Routine physical examinations, including history of developmental milestones, school problems, behavioral problems, family relationships, and immunizations should be completed. Discussion of signs and symptoms of infection related to piercing and tattoos needs to be part of health promotion. Dental checkups every 6 months, correction of dental malocclusion with dental braces, and discussion of tongue piercing concerns is important. Female adolescents need regular pelvic examinations, Pap smears, and teaching regarding breast self-examination. Males must be taught how and when to perform testicular self-examination. Mental health assessment is an important part of the adolescent's total health assessment.

➤ Health education in the adolescent needs to include information regarding sexuality, sexual responsibility, sexually transmitted infections, and contraception, as well as teaching about substance abuse and mental health issues. Adolescents face peer pressure, personal values and beliefs, and societal influences in making decisions related to sexual responsibility, substance use, and other risk taking behaviors.

➤ In the health care facility, the adolescent fears loss of control and loss of privacy. Be sensitive to the hospitalized adolescent's needs, provide supportive care, and encourage as much participation by the adolescent as possible. Health problems that threaten the adolescent's body image may threaten the satisfactory completion of developmental tasks.

INTERNET RESOURCES

Testicular Exam/Cancer
www.cancerlinksusa.com

Breast Self-Exam
www.cancer.org

Drug-Resistance Activities
www.health.org/features/kidsarea

Workbook

■ NCLEX-STYLE REVIEW QUESTIONS

1. The nurse is assisting with a physical exam on a 12-year-old girl. Her record indicates that at age 9 she was 51 in tall and weighed 72 lbs. Which of the following would the nurse *most likely* find if the child were following a normal pattern of growth and development?

   a. The adolescent weighs 94 lbs.
   b. The adolescent measures 53 in in height.
   c. The adolescent has a small amount of pubic hair.
   d. The adolescent has well-developed breasts.

2. The nurse is working with a group of caregivers of adolescents who are discussing normal adolescent growth and development. Which of the following statements made by a caregiver would indicate a need for follow-up?

   a. "He wants to be a nurse after he finishes college."
   b. "She has her own money to spend now because she has a job."
   c. "My son has been spending at least half an hour to 1 hour in front of the mirror the last 3 months getting ready for school."
   d. "My daughter is so slim and trim, she has lost 10 lb in the last 6 weeks."

3. The nurse is teaching a group of adolescent girls about good nutrition habits and eating foods that will help to increase the deficient nutrients in the adolescent diet. Which of the following statements made by the girls in the group is correct?

   a. "Eating lots of broccoli will help increase the iron in my diet."
   b. "If I drink three glasses of milk each day, I will get plenty of vitamin C."
   c. "Even though I don't like eggs, if I eat four eggs a week I will get enough calcium."
   d. "I am sure I get enough vitamin A since I eat bread at every meal."

4. In working with adolescent children, the nurse would know that if the adolescents were following normal development patterns, this age child would *most* likely be involved in which of the following activities?

   a. Working to establish a career
   b. Playing a board game with siblings
   c. Participating in activities with peers
   d. Volunteering in community projects

5. The nurse is teaching a group of adolescent girls how to perform a breast self-exam. Which of the following actions should the nurse teach regarding the breast self-exam? Select all that apply.

   a. Perform the breast exam each month.
   b. Do the breast exam just before your period starts.
   c. Use the pads of the fingers to examine the breast.
   d. Use the same pattern to feel every part of the breast.
   e. Stand in front of a mirror to look for changes in breasts
   f. Examine the breasts while in the bathtub.

■ STUDY ACTIVITIES

1. List and compare the 15-year-old girl and the 15-year-old boy in regard to physical development, psychosocial development, personality development, and their feelings about body image.

Area of Development	15-Year-Old Female	15-Year-Old Male
Physical development		
Psychosocial development		
Personality development		
Body image		

2. Mattie is the mother of 13-year-old Chantal. Chantal has decided she will not eat meat or poultry because animals had to be killed to obtain it. Mattie is concerned about Chantal's nutrition. Develop a teaching plan, including a menu for a day for Mattie. Be sure your plan provides nutrients often deficient in adolescents and that it supports Chantal in her choice to not eat meat and poultry.

3. You are working with a group of adolescents in a school-based clinic and plan to have a discussion about substance abuse and sexually transmitted infections. Make a list of questions that you think the adolescents might want to ask but are uncomfortable asking. Discuss with your peers the answers you could give to each of these questions.

4. Go to the following Web site: www.kidshealth.org/teen Click on "Your Body" on the left side of the screen. Click on "Body Piercing." Read this section and answer the following.

   a. Why is it a concern to pierce the mouth or nose? Tongue? Lip?
   b. What specifically can make piercing more safe?
   c. List 10 risks related to body piercing.

▮ CRITICAL THINKING: WHAT WOULD YOU DO?

1. You have the opportunity to talk with a group of 16-year-old girls. The topics you have decided to focus on during this talk are breast self-examination and Pap smears.

   a. What are the reasons adolescent girls should do a breast self-exam and have routine Pap smears?

   b. What steps will you teach these girls to follow when doing a breast self-exam?

   c. What areas of concern would you anticipate these girls would have regarding breast self-exams and Pap smears?

   d. What would your responses to these concerns be?

2. Jamal is an adolescent athlete. He has told you he is planning to use a carbohydrate-loading diet before a big track meet.

   a. What reasons do you think Jamal will give you for wanting to follow this diet before his track meet?

   b. What concerns would you share with Jamal about his plan?

   c. What alternate suggestions and guidance could you offer to Jamal that would be more appropriate for him to follow?

3. Fifteen-year-old Caitlin is in a group discussing condom use. She scornfully tells you that girls don't need to know anything about condoms.

   a. How would you respond to Caitlin?

   b. What are your ideas regarding what you think should and should not be part of health education in high school settings?

   c. What are your rationales for your ideas for question b?

FOUNDATIONS OF PEDIATRIC NURSING

28 Assessment of the Child (Data Collection)

KEY TERMS

accommodation
chief complaint
nutrition history
personal history
pinna
point of maximum impulse (PMI)
school history
social history
symmetry

LEARNING OBJECTIVES

On completion of this chapter, you should be able to:

1. Describe the process for collecting subjective data from caregivers and children.
2. Discuss what should be included when obtaining a client history.
3. Define chief complaint.
4. Explain the purpose of doing a review of systems when gathering data.
5. State how the family caregiver may be involved in the collection of objective data regarding the child.
6. Discuss how the collection of objective data regarding general appearance, psychological status, and behavior provides indicators of health or illness in children.
7. Discuss the reasons that height, weight, and head circumference are measured on an ongoing basis.
8. Discuss the appropriate use of growth charts.
9. Explain the purpose and processes for obtaining vital signs, including (a) temperature, (b) pulse, (c) respirations, and (d) blood pressure.
10. List the types of patients on whom a rectal temperature should not be taken.
11. Identify the five types of respiratory retractions and the location of each.
12. State the purpose of pulse oximetry.
13. Describe components of a physical exam.
14. Identify the purpose of using the Glasgow coma scale for neurologic assessment.

WHETHER THE setting is a hospital or other health care facility, it is important to gather information regarding the child's history and current status. Although data collection is continuous throughout a child's care, most data are collected during the interview, the physical examination, and from the results of diagnostic tests and studies.

COLLECTING SUBJECTIVE DATA

Information spoken by the child or family is called *subjective data*. Interviewing the family caregiver and child allows you to collect information that can be used to develop a plan of care for the child. Communicating with the child and family caregiver requires knowledge of growth and development and an understanding of communication techniques (see Chapter 22).

Conducting the Client Interview

Most subjective data are collected through interviewing the family caregiver and the child. The interview helps you establish relationships with the child and family. Listening and using appropriate communication techniques help promote a good interview (see Chapter 22). Using focused questions and allowing time for answering help the child and family feel comfortable. A private, quiet setting decreases distractions during the interview.

Think about this.

The interview process is goal directed, unlike a social conversation. The focus is on the child and caregiver and their needs.

■ **Figure 28-1** The child sits on the caregiver's lap during the interview process.

Introduce yourself to the child and caregiver and state the purpose of the interview. A calm, reassuring manner helps to establish trust and comfort. Past experiences with health care may influence the interview. The caregiver and the interviewer should be comfortably seated, and the child should be included in the interview process (Fig. 28-1). The child may sit on the caregiver's lap or, if a crib is available, the child can be placed in the crib with the side rails up. This positioning will help to ensure the safety of the infant or child during the interview.

Interviewing Family Caregivers

The family caregiver provides most of the information needed in caring for the child, especially the infant or toddler. Rather than simply asking the caregiver to fill out a form, it may be helpful to ask the questions and write down the answers; this process gives the opportunity to observe the reactions of the child and the caregiver as they interact with each other and answer the questions. In addition, this approach eases the problem of the caregiver who cannot read or write. It is important to be nonjudgmental, being careful not to indicate disapproval by verbal or nonverbal responses. While gathering information about the child's physical condition, allow the caregiver to express concerns and anxieties. If

Here's a helpful hint.
Age-appropriate and safe toys and activities to keep young children occupied will allow the caregiver to focus on the questions asked.

Cultural Snapshot

Be aware of the primary language spoken an interpreter when needed help in gaining accurate information. It is important to note and respect various cultural patterns, such as avoiding eye contact.

a certain topic seems uncomfortable for the caregiver to discuss in front of the child, discuss that topic later when the child cannot hear what is being said.

Interviewing the Child

Include the preschool child and the older child in the interview. Use age-appropriate questions when talking with the child. Showing interest in the child and what she or he says helps both the child and caregiver to feel comfortable. Being honest when answering the child's questions helps to establish trust with the child. Using stories or books written at a child's level helps with understanding what the child is thinking or feeling. Listen attentively to the child's comments and make the child feel important in the interview.

Check out this tip.
Using a doll or stuffed animal that the child is familiar with can help involve the child in the interview process.

Interviewing the Adolescent

Adolescents can provide information about themselves. Interviewing them in private often encourages them to share information that they might not contribute in front of their caregivers. This is especially true when asking questions of a sensitive nature, such as information regarding the adolescent's drug use or sexual practices.

Test Yourself

✔ Define subjective data. How is subjective data collected?

✔ Why is it important to interview the family caregiver when caring for children?

✔ In what ways does interviewing the adolescent differ from interviewing the child?

Obtaining a Client History

When a child arrives in any health care setting, it is important to gather information regarding the child's current condition, as well as past medical history. This information is used to develop a plan of care for the child. In obtaining information from the child and caregiver, you are developing a relationship, as well as noting what the child and family know and understand about the child's health. Observations of the caregiver–child relationship can also provide important information.

Biographical Data

To begin obtaining a client history, collect and record identifying information about the child, including the child's name, address, and phone number, as well as information about the caregiver. This information is part of the legal record and should be treated as confidential. A questionnaire often is used to gather information, such as the child's nickname, feeding habits, food likes and dislikes, allergies, sleeping schedule, and toilet-training status (Fig. 28-2). Any

PEDIATRIC NURSING ASSESSMENT FORM

1. Name _____ Date/Time of Admission _____ Via _____
2. Birth Date _____ Information obtained from: _____ Relationship to child _____
3. Child's legal guardian: _____ Child's Nickname: _____

VITAL SIGNS	Temp	Apical Pulse	Radial Pulse	Respirations	BP	Height	Weight	Head Circum

CURRENT CHIEF COMPLAINT/DIAGNOSIS:
Symptoms and Duration

Child's/Caregivers' Understanding of Condition:

PREVIOUS ILLNESS/INJURIES/DIAGNOSIS:
Illness, Symptoms, and Duration

Injuries or Surgery:

Anesthesia Complications?

Allergies and Reactions:

Immunizations	Dates:	Exposure to Infectious Disease (chicken pox, measles, etc.)	Date
DTaP (DT)			
Polio			
Hepatitis B			
Hib (type)			
MMR (measles, mumps, rubella)			
TB skin test Result			

Medications:

Name:	Dose	Frequency	Time of Last Dose

Child's reaction to previous hospitalizations: _____

Special fears of child about hospitalization? _____

Family History: (Check all that apply—indicate relationship to child)

_____ Cancer _____	_____ Seizures _____	_____ TB _____
_____ Heart disease _____	_____ Asthma _____	_____ Anesthesia complications _____
_____ Allergy _____	_____ Smoking _____	_____ Other (specify) _____
_____ Diabetes _____	_____ Hypertension _____	_____

■ **Figure 28-2** A sample pediatric nursing assessment form. *(continued)*

Living Facilities (check)

_____ House   _____ Apartment   _____ Trailer   _____ Steps to travel? _____

Who does child live with? _____

Names, ages, of siblings in home _____

Names, ages of other children in home _____

Other persons in home _____

Special interests, toys, games, hobbies: _____

_____

Security object: _____ Was it brought to hospital? _____

Bowel/Bladder Habits:

Toilet Training (if applicable)

    Started   _____ Yes _____ No

    Completed   _____ Yes _____ No

Diapers:

    Day   _____ Yes _____ No

    Night   _____ Yes _____ No

Potty Chair: _____ Yes _____ No

Toilet: _____ Yes _____ No

Bedwetter: _____ Yes _____ No

Terms Used for:

    Bowel Movement _____ Urination _____

    Frequency of BM _____ Color _____ Consistency _____

    Does child have problems with diarrhea or constipation? _____

_____

    Does child have urinary frequency, burning, discomfort: _____ Yes _____ No

    If yes, please explain: _____

_____

_____

Patterns of:

Sleep/rest:

Bedtime _____ Wakeup _____

Nap _____ Yes _____ No — When? _____

Activity:

Does infant roll over? _____

Does child stand/walk? _____

Does child climb? _____

Does child dress self? _____

Does child go up and down stairs? _____

Does child talk in formed sentences? _____

Eating Habits:

    Does child: Feed self _____ Yes _____ No

    Does child need help to eat? _____

Food and beverage:

    Likes: _____

_____

    Dislikes: _____

    Usual appetite? _____

    Appetite now? _____

Last time child had food or beverage: _____

Items brought to hospital:

Glasses   _____ Yes _____ No

Contacts   _____ Yes _____ No

Hearing Aid _____ Yes _____ No

Dentures   _____ Yes _____ No

Braces   _____ Yes _____ No

Retainer   _____ Yes _____ No

Special bottle _____ Yes _____ No

Own pacifier _____ Yes _____ No

Does child smoke or drink alcoholic beverages? _____ Yes _____ No

    If yes, please give details _____

_____

Does child use street drugs? _____ Yes _____ No

    If yes, please give details _____

_____

Other behavior habits of the child (Please check)

    Thumbsucking _____ ; Nailbiting _____ ; Headbanging _____

    Rituals (Explain) _____

_____

    Disposition (Describe) _____

_____

Skin Assessment:

_____ Jaundice _____ Cyanosis _____ Pallor _____ Redness

_____ Cool _____ Warm _____ Clammy _____ Dry

_____ Normal appearance

Describe: (Location and character)

Rash _____

Abrasions _____

Lacerations _____

Contusions _____

Respiratory Assessment:

_____ Clear _____ Stridor _____ Rales (___moist, ___ dry) _____ Wheezing

_____ Rhonchi _____ Retractions (type) _____

_____ Coughing, Sneezing _____ Nasal Discharge (describe) _____

Child/Caregiver oriented to unit? _____ Yes _____ No; understanding verbalized by child _____, caregiver _____

Reviewed safety measures with child _____, caregiver _____; understanding verbalized by child _____, caregiver _____

Additional information nursing staff should know:

■ **Figure 28-2** Continued

special words the child uses or understands to indicate needs or desires, such as words used for urinating and bowel movements, are included on the questionnaire.

Chief Complaint

The reason for the child's visit to the health care setting is called the **chief complaint**. In a well-child setting, this reason might be a routine check or immunizations, whereas an illness or other condition might be the reason in another setting. The caregiver's primary concern is his or her reason for seeking health care for the child. To best care for the child, it is important to get the most complete explanation of what brought the child to the health care setting. Repeating the caregiver's statement regarding the child's chief complaint helps to ensure a correct understanding of what the caregiver has said.

History of Present Health Concern

To help discover the child's needs, elicit information about the current situation, including the child's symptoms, when they began, how long the symptoms have been present, a description of the symptoms, their intensity and frequency, and treatments to this time. Ask questions in a way that encourages the caregiver to be specific. This is also the time to ask the caregiver about any other concerns regarding the child.

Health History

Information regarding the mother's pregnancy and prenatal history are included in a health history for the child. Any occurrences during the delivery can contribute to the child's health concerns. The child's mother is usually the best source of this information. Other areas to ask questions about include common childhood, serious, or chronic illnesses; immunizations and health maintenance; feeding and nutrition; as well as hospitalizations and injuries.

Family Health History

Some diseases and conditions are seen in families and are important areas for prevention, as well as detection, for the child. The caregiver can usually provide information regarding family health history. Use this information to do preventative teaching with the child and family. Certain risk factors in families contribute to the development of health care concerns; monitoring or changing risk factors early in a child's life can decrease the child's risk of getting these diseases or conditions.

> ## Test Yourself
> ✔ Why is it important to collect biographical data when developing a plan of care for a child?
> ✔ Explain what is meant by the "chief complaint."
> ✔ What are the reasons it is important to ask about a child's present, past, and family health history?

Review of Systems for Current Health Problem

While collecting subjective data, ask the caregiver or child questions about each body system. Gathering this information helps to focus the physical exam and to get an overall picture of the child's current status. Review the body system involved in the chief complaint in detail. As other body systems are discussed, reassure the caregiver that the chief complaint has not been forgotten or ignored. Table 28-1 lists areas to include in a review of the body systems.

Pay attention to the details.

Using a head-to-toe approach is an organized way to gather subjective data.

Table 28-1 ▌ REVIEW OF SYSTEMS

	Areas to Be Reviewed
General	Weight gain or loss, fatigue, colds, illnesses, behavior changes, edema
Skin	Itching, dryness, rash, color change
Head and neck	Headache, dizziness, injury, stiff neck, swollen neck glands
Eyes	Drainage, trouble focusing or seeing, rubbing, redness
Ears	Pulling, pain, drainage, difficulty hearing
Nose, mouth, throat	Nosebleeds, drainage, trouble breathing, toothache, sore throat, trouble swallowing
Chest and lungs—respiratory	Coughing, wheezing, shortness of breath, sputum, breast development, pain
Heart—cardiovascular	Cyanosis, fatigue, anemia, heart murmurs
Abdomen—gastrointestinal	Nausea, vomiting, pain
Genitalia and rectum	Pain or burning when voiding, blood in urine or stool, constipation, diarrhea
Back and extremities Musculoskeletal	Extremities—pain, difficult movement, swollen joints, broken bones, muscle sprains
Neurologic	Seizures, loss of consciousness

Allergies, Medications, and Substance Abuse

Discuss allergic reactions to any foods, medications, or any other known allergies to prevent the child being given any medications or substances that might cause an allergic reaction. Record medications the child is taking or has taken, whether prescribed by a care provider or over the counter. This information will help avoid the possibility of overmedicating or causing drug interactions. It is important, especially in the adolescent, to assess the use of substances, such as tobacco, alcohol, or illegal drugs (substance abuse is discussed in Chapters 27 and 42).

This could save a life.
Always discuss a child's allergies with the caregiver. Document this information in the child's record.

Lifestyle

School history includes information regarding the child's current grade level and academic performance, as well as behavior at school. The child's interactions with teachers and peers often give insight into areas of concern that might affect the child's health.

Social history offers information about the child's environment, including the home setting, parents' occupations, siblings, family pets, religious affiliations, and economic factors. The persons who live in the home and those who care for the child are important data, especially in cases of separation or divorce.

Personal history relates to data collected about such things as the child's hygiene, sleeping, and elimination patterns. Activities, exercise, special interests, and the child's favorite toys or objects are included. Questions about relationships and how the child emotionally handles certain situations can help in understanding the child. Discuss any behaviors such as thumb sucking, nail biting, or temper tantrums.

Nutrition history of the child includes information regarding eating habits and preferences, as well as nutrition concerns that might indicate illness.

Developmental Level

To gather information about the child's developmental level, ask questions directly related to growth and development milestones. These milestones are discussed in detail in the growth and development chapters (Chapters 23–27) of this text. Knowing normal development patterns will help you determine if there are concerns that should be further assessed regarding the child's development.

COLLECTING OBJECTIVE DATA

Information you observe directly is called *objective data*. Objective data to collect include baseline measurements of the child's height, weight, temperature, pulse, respiration, and blood pressure. Data are also collected by examination of the body systems. Often the exam for a child does not proceed in a head-to-toe manner as in adults but rather in an order that takes the child's age and developmental needs into consideration. Aspects of the exam that might be more traumatic or uncomfortable for the child are done last.

This advice could save the day.
Examining the nose and mouth may be uncomfortable and traumatic for the child; save these for last.

The procedure of the physical exam may be familiar from previous health care visits. If comfortable with helping, the caregiver may help with the data collection. For example, the caregiver might help take a young child's temperature and obtain a urine specimen. Arrangements should be made so that the caregiver also may be present, if possible, for tests or examinations that need to be performed. Included in this initial exam is an inspection of the child's body. Record all observations and carefully describe in detail any finding that is not within normal limits.

Conduct or assist in conducting a complete physical exam with special attention to any symptoms that the caregiver has identified. As the practical/vocational nurse, your primary role in the complete assessment may be to support the child. All the information gathered is used to plan the child's care.

Test Yourself

✔ What approach is used to do a review of systems in a child? Why is this approach used?

✔ What is included when collecting information about the child's lifestyle?

✔ Define objective data. How is objective data collected?

Noting General Status

Use knowledge of normal growth and development to note if the child appears to fit the characteristics of the stated age. Interactions the child has with caregivers and siblings provide information about these relationships. Note the child's overall general appearance, facial expressions, speech, and behavior as you begin collecting information about the child.

General Appearance

Observing physical appearance and condition can give clues to the child's overall health. The infant or child's face and body should be symmetrical (i.e., well balanced). Observations provide information related to

Table 28-2 ▮ COMPARISON OF OBSERVATIONS OF AN INFANT'S PHYSICAL AND EMOTIONAL BEHAVIOR

Observation	Healthy Activity	Behavior Indicating Illness*
Activity	Constantly active; some infants are more intense and curious than others.	Lies quietly; little or no interest in surroundings; may stay in the same position
State of muscular tension	Muscular state is tense; grasp is tight; head is raised when prone; kicks are vigorous. When supine, there is a space between the mattress and the infant's back.	Lies relaxed with arms and legs straight and lax; makes no attempt to turn or raise head if placed in prone position; does not move about in crib
Constancy of reaction	Shows a constancy in reaction; does not regress in development; peppy and vigorous; interested in food; responds to caregiver's presence or voice.	Not as peppy as usual; responds to discomfort and pain in apathetic manner; turns away from food that had once interested; turns head and cries instead of usual response
Behavior indicating pain	Appreciates being picked up. Activity is not restlessness. Shows activity in every part of body.	Cries or protests when handled; seems to want to be left alone. May cry when picked up, but settles down after being held for a time, indicating something hurts when moved Turns head fretfully from side to side; pulls ear or rubs head; turns and rolls constantly; seemingly to try to get away from pain
Cry	Strong, vigorous cry	Weak, feeble cry or whimper High-pitched cry; shrill cry may indicate increased intracranial pressure
Skin color	Healthy tint to skin; nail beds, oral mucosa, conjunctiva, and tongue are reddish-pink	Light-skinned babies may show unusual pallor or blueness around the eyes and nose. All babies may have dark or cyanotic nail beds; pale oral mucosa, conjunctiva, and tongue.
Appetite or feeding pattern	Exhibits an eagerness and impatience to satisfy hunger	May show indifference toward formula; sucks half-heartedly; vomits feeding; habitually regurgitates. May exhibit discomfort after feeding
Bizarre behavior		Any behavior that differs from expected for level of development; unusually good, or passive when in strange surroundings; responds with rejection to every overture, friendly or otherwise; extremely clinging, never satisfied with amount of attention received

*Any *one* manifestation in itself may not be significant. The important thing is whether this behavior is consistent with this particular child or is a change from previous behavior. The significance depends greatly on the constancy of the behavior.

nutritional status, hygiene, mental alertness, and body posture and movements. Examine the skin for color, lesions, bruises, scars, and birthmarks. Observe hair texture, thickness, and distribution.

Psychological Status and Behavior

Carefully observing the child's behavior and recording those observations provide vital clues to a child's condition. When recording observed behavior, include factors that influence the behavior and how often the behavior is repeated. Note physical behavior as well as emotional and intellectual responses. Behavior may depend on the child's age and developmental level, the abnormal environment of the health care facility, and whether the child has been hospitalized previously, or otherwise separated from family caregivers. Note if the behavior is consistent or unpredictable and any apparent reasons for changed behavior.

Observation of the infant's behavior is critical because infants cannot articulate information regarding their health status. Table 28-2 compares characteristic behaviors of the healthy infant with behaviors that may indicate signs of illness. Be cautious when using the type of information shown in such a table because occasional evidence of one or more of the behaviors may not be significant.

Any instance of behavior indicating illness needs to be documented and further evaluated in light of the behavior frequency, as well as the child's usual behavior. If the caregiver indicates in the interview or on further questioning that this behavior is not out of the ordinary for the child, it may not be indicative of a problem.

Measuring Height and Weight

The child's height and weight are helpful indicators of growth and development. Height and weight should be measured and recorded each time the child has a routine physical examination, as well as at other health care visits. These measurements must be charted and compared with norms for the child's age (see Appendix G). Plotting the child's growth on a growth chart gives a good indication of the child's health status. This process gives a picture of how the child is progressing and often indicates wellness. Although the charts are indicators, the size of other family members, the child's illnesses, general nutritional status, and developmental milestones also must be considered.

In a hospital setting, weigh the infant or child at the same time each day on the same scales in the same amount of clothing. The young child is weighed nude. The infant is weighed lying on an infant scale; the toddler who is able to sit can be weighed while sitting (Fig. 28-3A and B). Keep a hand within 1 in of the child at all times to be ready to protect the child from injury. Cover the scale with a fresh paper towel or clean sheet of paper, as a means of infection control (Nursing Procedure 28-1). A child who can stand alone steadily is weighed without shoes on platform-type scales. Bed scales may be used if the child cannot get out of bed. Record weights in grams and kilograms or pounds and ounces.

The child who can stand usually is measured for height at the same time. The standing scales have a useful, adjustable measuring device (Fig. 28-3C). To measure the height of a child who is not able to stand alone steadily, usually younger than the age of about 2, place the child flat, with the knees held flat, on an examining table. Measure the child's height by straightening the child's body and measuring from the top of the head to the bottom of the foot. Sometimes examining tables have a measuring device mounted along the side of the table or have a measuring board attached (Fig. 28-4). If using a measuring board, place the child's head at the top of the board and the heels against the footboard. If not

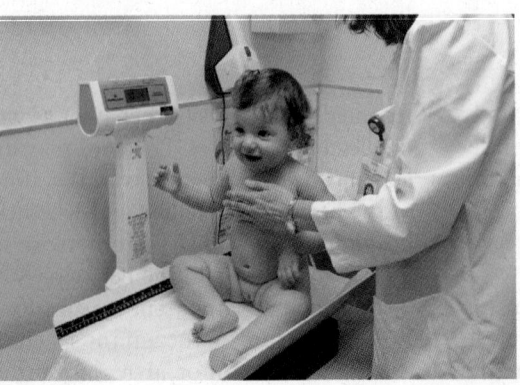

■ Figure 28-3 The nurse keeps a hand close while weighing (A) the infant or (B) the toddler. (C) The nurse measures the older child for weight and height on a standing scale.

Nursing Procedure 28-1
WEIGHING THE INFANT OR CHILD

EQUIPMENT

Scale appropriate for child's age and ability to sit or stand
Disposable paper covering for scale
Paper and pen to record weight
Cleaning solution and equipment, according to facility policy

PROCEDURE

1. Explain procedure to child and family caregiver.
2. Wash hands.
3. Place paper on scale.
4. Balance scale to a reading of "0."

5. Weigh the hospitalized child at the same time, using same scale, same amount of clothing each time child is weighed.
6. Weigh infant with no clothing, older child in underwear or lightweight gown; child should not wear shoes.
7. **Always** hold one hand within 1 in of the child for safety.
8. Pick up the child or have older child step off scale.
9. Remove and discard paper scale cover.
10. Read the weight on the scale.
11. Record the weight on paper to be transferred to permanent document.
12. Clean the scale according to the facility's policy.
13. Report weight as appropriate.

using a measuring device, make marks on the paper table covering and then measure between the marks. Record height in centimeters or inches according to the practice of the health care facility; it is important to know which measuring system is used.

Measuring Head Circumference

The head circumference is measured routinely in children up to the age of 2 or 3 years or in any child with a neurologic concern. Place a paper or plastic tape measure around the largest part of the head, just above the eyebrows, and around the most prominent part of the back of the head (Fig. 28-5). Record and plot this measurement on a growth chart to monitor the growth

of the child's head. During childhood, the chest exceeds the head circumference by 2 to 3 in.

Taking Vital Signs

Vital signs, including temperature, pulse, respirations, and blood pressure, are taken at each visit and compared with the normal values for children of the same age, as well as to that child's previous recordings. In a hospital setting, closely monitor and record the vital signs, report any changes. Keeping in mind the child's developmental needs will increase your ability to take accurate vital sign measurements. It is usually less traumatic for the infant to count the respirations before disturbing the child and to then take the pulse and the temperature.

■ **Figure 28-4** The measuring board is the most accurate method for obtaining the length of the infant or toddler.

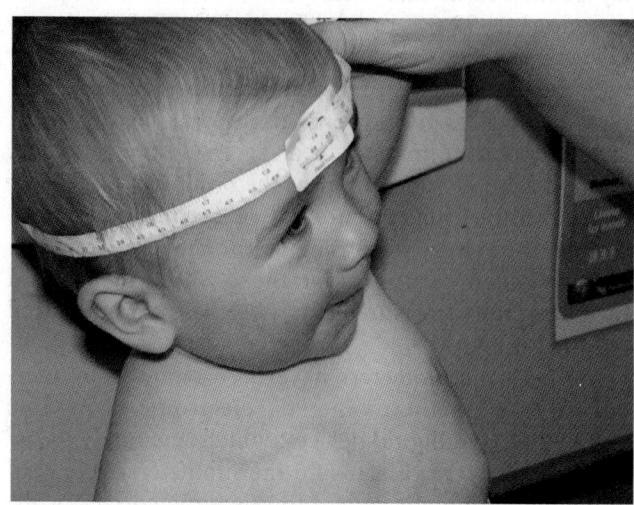

■ **Figure 28-5** Measuring the head circumference.

A Personal Glimpse

I am 11 years old, and I have already been in the hospital for four surgeries. I think I could be a nurse. One time a student nurse and her teacher came to do my vital signs. The teacher left, and the student named Joan told me I was her first patient ever. She tried three of those electronic thermometers to take my temperature, but she said they were all broken. Then she tried to take my blood pressure with the blood pressure machine and she said it was broken. Then she used another blood pressure cuff, and this time she put it on backwards. I knew it was wrong, but I just let her pump it up and up until it exploded off my arm. I laughed, but she almost cried. I showed her how to do it right, and she seemed pretty glad that she finally got it to work. I was kind of happy when she left because I didn't know if I could teach her everything. A little while later, she came back with her teacher and the teacher said, "Joan is going to give you your shot." "Uh Oh!" I thought, "here comes trouble." I just held my breath and hoped she won't do that wrong too. It wasn't too bad. Later, before she went home she brought me a pear. I am pretty sure she was relieved the day was over and I was too.

Abigail, age 11

Learning Opportunity: What could this student nurse have done to be better prepared to take care of this patient? What feelings do you think this child might have had when the nurse came in with the medication?

Temperature

The method of measuring a child's temperature is commonly set by the policy of the health care setting. The temperature can be measured by the oral, tympanic, temporal, rectal, or axillary method. Temperatures are recorded in Celsius or Fahrenheit, according to the policy of the health care facility. A normal oral temperature range is 97.6°F to 99.3°F (36.4°C–37.4°C). A rectal temperature is usually 0.5° to 1.0° higher than the oral measurement. An axillary temperature usually measures 0.5° to 1.0° lower than the oral measurement. The temperature measurement taken by the tympanic method is in the same range as the oral method. Report any deviation from the normal range of temperature. Temperatures vary according to the method by which they are taken, so it is important to record the method of temperature measurement, as well as the measured temperature.

Mercury thermometers have been replaced by mercury-free glass thermometers, electronic, tympanic membrane, and digital devices, which accurately measure temperatures. Electronic thermometers have oral and rectal probes. Be careful to select the correct probe when using the thermometer.

Oral Temperatures

Oral temperatures usually are taken only on children older than 4 to 6 years of age who are conscious and cooperative. Place oral thermometers under the tongue, toward the side of the child's mouth. Do not leave the child unattended while any temperature is being taken.

Tympanic Temperatures

Tympanic thermometers are now used in many health care settings (Fig. 28-6A). The tympanic thermometer records the temperature rapidly (registering in about 2 seconds), is noninvasive, and causes little disturbance to the child. A tympanic measurement often can be obtained without awakening a sleeping infant or child. Use tympanic thermometers according to the manufacturer's directions and the facility's policy. Use a disposable speculum for each child.

Temporal Temperatures

Temporal temperatures are a newer method of measuring temperature in the child. An infrared sensor probe is scanned across the skin on the forehead. The sensor measures heat from blood flow in the temporal artery. Use of this noninvasive procedure is becoming more common, especially as a screening tool and in detecting rapid temperature changes, but it is still not widely accepted as a reliable measurement of temperature in all ages and situations.

Rectal Temperatures

Rectal temperatures may be taken in children but usually only if another method cannot be used. They are not desirable in the newborn because of the danger of irritation to the rectal mucosa or in children who have had rectal surgery or who have diarrhea. When taking a rectal temperature, lubricate the end of the thermometer with a water-soluble lubricant. Place the child in a prone position, gently separate the buttocks with one hand, and gently insert the thermometer about ¼ to ½ in into the rectum. If you feel any resistance, remove the thermometer immediately, take the temperature by some other method, and notify the physician about the resistance. Keep one hand on the child's buttocks and the other on the thermometer during the entire time the rectal thermometer is in place. Remove an electronic thermometer as soon as it signals a recorded temperature.

Axillary Temperatures

Axillary temperatures are taken on newborns and on infants and children with diarrhea or when a rectal

> **Be alert for patient safety.**
> Some caregivers might still have a mercury thermometer at home. Advise them to replace it with a nonmercury thermometer, which can easily be purchased at many pharmacies or super stores.

A   **B**

▮ **Figure 28-6 (A)** Many facilities use a tympanic thermometer sensor to take the child's temperature. **(B)** Taking an axillary temperature on a newborn. (Photo B © B. Proud.)

temperature is contraindicated. When taking an axillary temperature on an infant or child, be certain to place the thermometer tip well into the armpit and bring the child's arm down close to the body (Fig. 28-6B). Check to see that there is skin-to-skin contact with no clothing in the way. Leave the thermometer in place until the electronic thermometer signals.

Pulse

Counting an apical rate is the preferred method to determine the pulse in an infant or young child. Try to accomplish this while the child is quiet.

Count the apical pulse before the child is disturbed for other procedures. A caregiver can hold the child on his or her lap for security for the full minute that the pulse is counted. Place the stethoscope between the child's left nipple and sternum. A radial pulse may be taken on an older child. This pulse may be counted for 30 seconds and multiplied by two. If a pulse is unusual in quality, rate, or rhythm, count it for a full minute. Report any rate that deviates from the normal rate. Pulse rates vary with age: from 100 to 180 beats per minute for a neonate (birth to 28 days old) to 50 to 95 beats per minute for the 14- to 18-year-old adolescent (Table 28-3).

> **Some nurses find this tip helpful.**
> When checking an apical pulse, approach the child in a soothing, calm, quiet manner.

Cardiac monitors are used to detect changes in cardiac function. Many of these monitors have a visual display of the cardiac actions. Electrodes must be placed properly to obtain accurate readings of the cardiac system. Cleanse the skin with alcohol to remove oil, dirt, lotions, and powder. Alarms are set to maximum and minimum settings above and below the child's resting heart rate. Check the electrode sites every 2 hours to detect any skin redness or irritation and to determine that the electrodes are secure. The child's cardiac status must be checked immediately when the alarm sounds. Sometimes the monitor used will monitor both cardiac and respiratory function. Apnea monitors, which monitor respiratory function, are discussed later in this chapter.

Respirations

Respirations of an infant or young child also must be counted during a quiet time. Observe the child while he or she is lying or sitting quietly. Infants are abdominal breathers; therefore, observe the movement of the infant's abdomen to count respirations.

Table 28-3 ▮ NORMAL PULSE RANGES IN CHILDREN

Age	Normal Range	Average
0–24 hr	70–170 bpm	120 bpm
1–7 d	100–180 bpm	140 bpm
1 mo	110–188 bpm	160 bpm
1 mo–1 yr	80–180 bpm	120–130 bpm
2 yr	80–140 bpm	110 bpm
4 yr	80–120 bpm	100 bpm
6 yr	70–115 bpm	100 bpm
10 yr	70–110 bpm	90 bpm
12–14 yr	60–110 bpm	85–90 bpm
14–18 yr	50–95 bpm	70–75 bpm

bpm = beats per minute

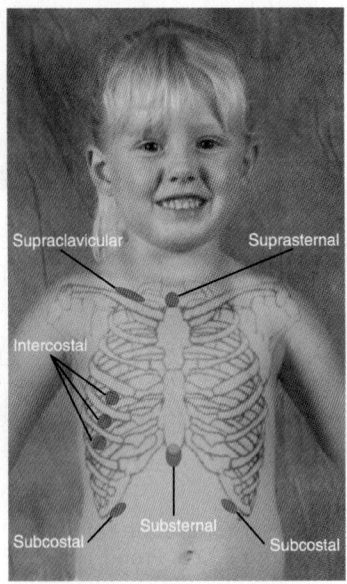

■ **Figure 28-7** Sites of respiratory retraction.

Observe the older child's chest, much as you would an adult's. The infant's respirations must be counted for a full minute because of normal irregularity. Observe the chest of the infant or young child for retractions that indicate respiratory distress. Note retractions as substernal (below the sternum), subcostal (below the ribs), intercostal (between the ribs), suprasternal (above the sternum), or supraclavicular (above the clavicle) (Fig. 28-7).

Pulse Oximetry

Pulse oximetry measures the oxygen saturation of arterial hemoglobin. The probe of the oximetry unit can be placed on the finger, toe, or clipped on the ear lobe. In an infant, the foot or toe is often used (Fig. 28-8). Take the pulse oximetry and record it with other vital signs. In certain situations, the probe is left in place to continually monitor the oxygen saturation. Check the site every 2 hours to ensure that the probe is secure and tissue perfusion is adequate. Change the site at least every 4 hours to prevent skin irritation. Alarms can be set to sound when oxygen saturation registers lower than a predetermined limit. At the beginning of each shift and after transport of the patient, check that alarms are accurately set and have not been inadvertently changed. This is true for all types of monitors.

Apnea Monitor

An apnea monitor detects the infant's respiratory movement. Place the electrodes or belt on the infant's chest where the greatest amount of respiratory movement is detected; the electrodes are attached to the monitor by a cable (Fig. 28-9). Set the limits on the alarm to sound when the infant does not breathe for a predetermined number of seconds.

These monitors can be used in a hospital setting and often are used in the home for an infant who is at risk for apnea or who has a tracheostomy. Family caregivers learn to stimulate the infant when the monitor sounds and to perform cardiopulmonary resuscitation if the infant does not begin breathing.

> **Warning, be alert for patient safety.**
> Respond immediately when the alarm on the apnea monitor sounds. The child must be observed to determine what caused the alarm to sound.

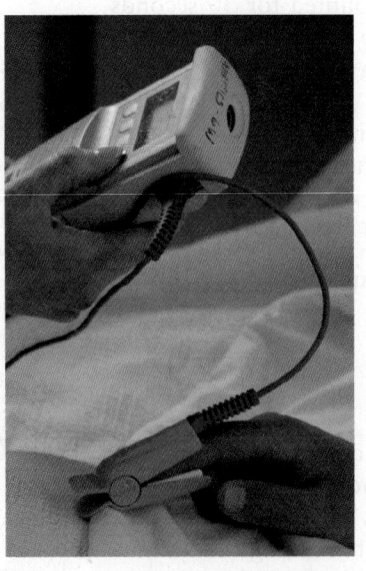

■ **Figure 28-8** The pulse oximetry sensor measuring the oxygen saturation in the **(A)** infant and **(B)** older child.

A   **B**

Midaxillary line

Electrode

Electrode placement

Figure 28-9 Placement of electrodes for apnea monitoring. Electrodes are placed 2 fingerbreadths below the nipple.

Table 28-4 ▮ NORMAL BLOOD PRESSURE RANGES (mm hg)		
Age	Systolic	Diastolic
Newborn—12 hr (<1,000 g)	39–59	16–36
Newborn—12 hr (3,000 g)	50–70	24–45
Newborn—96 hr (3,000 g)	60–90	20–60
Infant	74–100	50–70
Toddler	80–112	50–80
Preschooler	82–110	50–78
School-age	84–120	54–80
Adolescent	94–140	62–88

Blood Pressure

For children 3 years of age and older, blood pressure monitoring is part of routine and ongoing data collection. Take a baseline blood pressure for a child of any age who presents to a health care facility. Explain the procedure to the child in terms the young child can understand. First taking a blood pressure on a stuffed animal or doll will further show the child the procedure is not to be feared.

Obtaining a blood pressure measurement in an infant or small child is difficult, but equipment of the proper size helps ease the problem. The most common sites used to obtain a blood pressure reading in children are the upper arm, lower arm or forearm, thigh, and calf or ankle (Fig. 28-10). When the upper arm is used, the cuff should be wide enough to cover about two thirds of the upper arm and long enough to encircle the extremity without overlapping. If other sites are used, the size of the cuff is determined by the size of the extremity; a smaller cuff is used on the forearm, whereas a larger cuff is used on the thigh or calf.

Try this approach.
Referring to the blood pressure cuff as "giving your arm a hug" will help explain taking the blood pressure.

Take the blood pressure by the auscultation, palpation, or Doppler or electronic method (Nursing Procedure 28-2). The Doppler method is used with increasing frequency to monitor pediatric blood pressure, but the cuff still must be the correct size. Electronic blood pressure recording devices are used frequently in health care settings and provide accurate measurement. Normal blood pressure values gradually increase from infancy through adolescence (Table 28-4).

A   B   C   D

Brachial artery

Radial artery

Popliteal artery

Dorsalis pedis artery

Posterior tibial artery

Figure 28-10 Various positions of cuff placement and auscultation area for obtaining blood pressure: **(A)** upper arm, **(B)** lower arm, **(C)** thigh, **(D)** calf/ankle.

Nursing Procedure 28-2
METHODS FOR MEASURING PEDIATRIC BLOOD PRESSURE

EQUIPMENT

Stethoscope, pediatric preferred
Blood pressure cuff, appropriate size for child
   Wide enough to cover 2/3 of child's upper arm
   Long enough to encircle child's arm
Doppler or electronic monitor
Paper and pen to record blood pressure

PROCEDURE

1. Explain procedure to child and family caregiver.
2. Wash hands.
3. Allow child to handle equipment when appropriate.
4. Use terminology appropriate to child's age.
5. Encourage preschool or school-aged child to use equipment to "take" blood pressure on a doll or stuffed animal.
6. Record blood pressure on paper to be transferred to permanent document.
7. Report blood pressure as appropriate.

AUSCULTATION

1. Place the correct size of cuff on the infant's or child's bare arm.

2. Locate the artery by palpating the antecubital fossa.
3. Inflate the cuff until radial pulse disappears or about 30 mm Hg above expected systolic reading.
4. Place stethoscope lightly over the artery and slowly release air until pulse is heard.
5. Record readings as in adults.

PALPATION

1. Follow steps 1 and 2 above.
2. Keep the palpating finger over the artery and inflate the cuff as above.
3. The point at which the pulse is felt is recorded as the systolic pressure.

DOPPLER OR ELECTRONIC MONITOR

1. Obtain the monitor, dual air hose, and proper cuff size.
2. If monitor is not on a mobile stand, be certain that it is placed on a firm surface.
3. Plug in monitor (unless battery-operated) and attach dual hose if necessary.
4. Attach appropriate-size blood pressure cuff and wrap around child's limb.
5. Turn on power switch. Record the reading.

Test Yourself

✔ How is comparing behaviors seen in a healthy child to behaviors that might indicate illness helpful in caring for the child?

✔ Why should height and weight be routinely measured and monitored in children?

✔ What is the purpose in doing pulse oximetry when obtaining vital signs?

✔ Describe the methods used to obtain a blood pressure in a child.

Conducting or Assisting with a Physical Examination

Data are also collected by examining the body systems of the child. You may be responsible for performing the physical exam or assisting the health care provider in doing the physical exam.

Head and Neck

The head's general shape and movement should be observed. The features of the face and the head should have **symmetry** or balance. Observe the child's ability to control the head and the range of motion. To see full range of motion, ask the older child to move her or his head in all directions. Gently move the infant's head to observe for any stiffness in the neck. Feel the infant's skull to determine if the fontanels are open or closed and to check for any swelling or depression.

Eyes

Observe the eyes for symmetry and location in relationship to the nose. Note any redness, evidence of rubbing, or drainage. Observe pupils for equality, roundness, and reaction to light. When a light is quickly shined toward the eye, the pupil constricts. As the light is moved away, the pupil should expand. **Accommodation** occurs when the pupils constrict in order to bring an object into focus. When a bright object is held at a distance and then quickly moved toward the face, the pupil will constrict, and thus accommodate. Normal pupil reactions are recorded as PERRLA (pupils equal, round, react to light, and accommodation). Neurologic considerations are discussed later in this chapter. Routine vision screening occurs in school or clinic settings. Screening helps identify vision concerns in children; with early detection, appropriate visual aids can be provided.

Ears

Note the alignment of the ears by drawing an imaginary line from the inner to the outer canthus of the eye and continuing past the ear; the top of the ear, known as the **pinna**, should be even with or above this line (see Fig. 13-6 in Chapter 13). Ears that are set low often indicate mental retardation (see Chapter 35). Note the child's ability to hear during normal conversation. A child who speaks loudly, responds inappropriately, or does not speak clearly may have hearing difficulties that should be explored. Note any drainage or swelling.

Nose, Mouth, and Throat

The nose is in the middle of the face. If an imaginary line were drawn down the middle, both sides of the nose should be symmetrical. Flaring of the nostrils might indicate respiratory distress and should be reported immediately. Observe for swelling, drainage, or bleeding. To observe the mouth and throat, have the older child hold her or his mouth wide open and move the tongue from side to side. With the infant or toddler, use a tongue blade to see the mouth and throat. Gently place the tongue blade on the side of the tongue to hold it down (Fig. 28-11). A light will help visualize the mouth and throat. Observe the mucous membranes for color, moisture, and any patchy areas that might indicate infection. Observe the number and condition of the child's teeth.

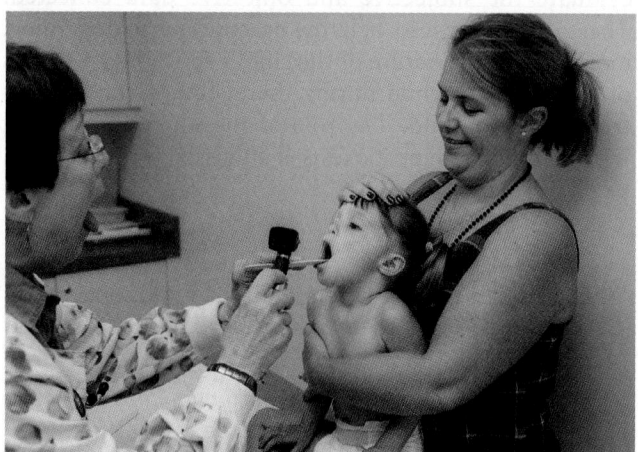

■ **Figure 28-11** The young child may need to be gently restrained to safely observe the mouth and throat.

The lips should be moist and pink. Note any difficulty in swallowing.

Chest and Lungs

Chest measurements are done on infants and children to determine normal growth rate. Take the measurement at the nipple level with a tape measure. Observe the chest for size, shape, movement of the chest with breathing, and any retractions (see respirations in this chapter). In the older school-aged child or adolescent, note evidence of breast development. Evaluate respiratory rate, rhythm, and depth. Report any noisy or grunting respirations. Using a stethoscope, listen to breath sounds in each lobe of the lung, anterior and posterior, while the child inhales and exhales. Describe, document, and report absent or diminished breath sounds, as well as unusual sounds, such as crackling or wheezing. If the child is coughing or bringing up sputum, record the frequency, color, and consistency of sputum.

Heart

In some infants and children, a pulsation can be seen in the chest that indicates the heart beat. This point is called the **point of maximum impulse (PMI)**. This point is where the heart beat can be heard the best with a stethoscope. Listen for the rhythm of the heart sounds and count the rate for 1 full minute. Abnormal or unusual heart sounds or irregular rhythms might indicate the child has a heart murmur, heart condition, or other abnormality that should be reported. The heart is responsible for circulating blood to the body. Assess the pulses in various parts of the body to determine the effectiveness of the heart function (Fig. 28-12). Other indicators of good cardiac function are included in this textbook's discussions of specific disorders.

Abdomen

The abdomen may protrude slightly in infants and small children. To describe the abdomen, divide the area into four sections and label sections with the terms left upper quadrant (LUQ), left lower quadrant (LLQ), right upper quadrant (RUQ), and right lower quadrant (RLQ). Using a stethoscope, listen for bowel sounds or evidence of peristalsis in each section of the abdomen and record what is heard. Observe the umbilicus for cleanliness and any abnormalities. Infants and young children sometimes have protrusions in the umbilicus or inguinal canal that are called hernias (see Chapter 21). Report a tense or firm abdomen or unusual tenderness.

Genitalia and Rectum

When inspecting the genitalia and rectum, it is important to respect the child's privacy and take into account the child's age and the stage of growth and development.

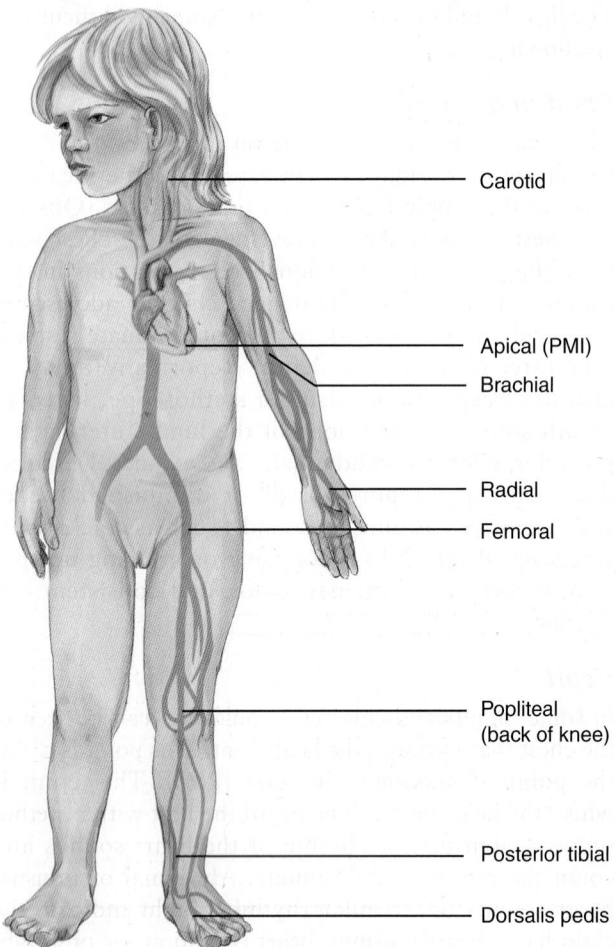

Carotid

Apical (PMI)

Brachial

Radial

Femoral

Popliteal
(back of knee)

Posterior tibial

Dorsalis pedis

▮ **Figure 28-12** Sites in the child where pulses can be felt.

While wearing gloves, inspect the genitalia and rectum. Observe the area for any sores or lesions, swelling, or discharge. In male children, the testes descend at varying times during childhood; if the testes cannot be palpated, report this information. Be aware that unusual findings, such as bruises in soft tissue, bruises with a clear outline of an object, or unexplained injuries, might indicate child abuse and should be further investigated (see Chapter 33).

Sensitivity is essential.
Keeping the child covered as much as possible when examining the genitalia and rectum is important in respecting the child's privacy.

Back and Extremities

Observe the back for symmetry and for the curvature of the spine. In infants, the spine is rounded and flexible. As the child grows and develops motor skills, the spine further develops. Screening is done in school-aged children to detect abnormal curvatures of the spine, such as scoliosis

(see Chapter 40). Note gait and posture when the child enters or is walking in the room. The extremities should be warm, have good color, and be symmetrical. When observing the child's movements during the exam, note range of motion, movement of the joints, and muscle strength. In infants, examine the hips and report any dislocation or asymmetry of gluteal skin folds. These could indicate a congenital hip dislocation (see Chapter 21).

Neurologic

Assessing the neurologic status of the infant and child is the most complex aspect of the physical exam. All the body systems function in relationship to the nervous system. The practitioner in the health care setting assesses the neurologic status of the child by doing a complete neurologic exam. This exam includes detailed examination of the reflex responses, as well as the functioning of each of the cranial nerves. The practitioner will perform a neurologic exam on children after a head injury or seizure or on children who have metabolic conditions, such as diabetes mellitus, drug ingestion, severe hemorrhage, or dehydration, which might affect neurologic status. A neurologic assessment determines the level of the child's neurologic functioning.

As the nurse, you may be responsible for using neurologic assessment tools, such as the Glasgow coma scale, to monitor a child's neurologic status after the initial neurologic exam. The use of a standard scale for monitoring permits the comparison of results from one time to another and from one examiner to another. Use this tool to monitor various aspects of the child's neurologic functioning (Fig. 28-13). If a child is hospitalized with a neurologic concern, closely monitor the neurologic status, and use a neurologic assessment tool every 1 or 2 hours to observe for significant changes.

Assisting With Common Diagnostic Tests

Diagnostic tests and studies often are done to further evaluate the subjective and objective data collected. These diagnostic tests help the practitioner to determine, more clearly, the nature of the child's concern. The needs of the infant or child during these studies vary greatly from child to child. The role of the nurse in assisting with common diagnostic tests is discussed in Chapter 30.

Test Yourself

✔ Explain the term symmetry and the importance of observing for symmetry when doing a physical exam on a child.

✔ What does the term *point of maximum impulse (PMI)* mean and how does it relate to the physical exam in children?

✔ What is included when doing a neurologic exam on a child?

GLASGOW COMA SCALES			MODIFIED COMA SCALE FOR INFANTS		
ACTIVITY	BEST RESPONSE		ACTIVITY	BEST RESPONSE	
Eye Opening	Spontaneous	4	Eye Opening	Spontaneous	4
	To speech	3		To speech	3
	To pain	2		To pain	2
	None	1		None	1
Verbal	Oriented	5	Verbal	Coos, babbles	5
	Confused	4		Irritable	4
	Inappropriate words	3		Cries to pain	3
	Nonspecific sounds	2		Moans to pain	2
	None	1		None	1
Motor	Follows commands	6	Motor	Normal spontaneous movements	6
	Localizes pain	5		Withdraws to touch	5
	Withdraws to pain	4		Withdraws to pain	4
	Abnormal flexion	3		Abnormal flexion	3
	Extend	2		Abnormal extension	2
	None	1		None	1

PUPIL SIZE:

6 mm ●   5 mm ●   4 mm ●

3 mm ●   2 mm ●   1 mm ●

REACTION: **N**–normal, **S**–sluggish, **F**–fixed

		PUPIL SIZE		PUPIL REACTION		EXTREMITY MOVEMENT/ RESPONSE				GLASGOW COMA SCALE			VITAL SIGNS		
DATE	TIME	R	L	R	L	RA	LA	RL	LL	VERBAL RESP.	MOTOR RESP.	EYE OPENING	BP	PULSE	RESP.

GUIDE TO NEUROLOGIC EVALUATION

Pupils

Pupils should be examined in dim light
1. Compare each pupil with the size chart and record pupil size.
2. Use a bright flashlight to check the reaction of each pupil. Hold the flashlight to the outer aspect of the eye. While watching the pupil, turn the flashlight on and bring it directly over the pupil. Record the reaction. Repeat for the other eye. Report if either pupil is fixed or dilated.

Extremities

1. Observe the child for quality and strength of muscle tone in each upper extremity. Have child squeeze nurse's hand. Have child raise arms. Ask child to turn palms up, then palms down. Infant is observed for movement and position of arms when stroked or lightly pinched.
2. The child should be able to move each leg on command, and push against nurse's hands with each foot. Infant is observed for movement of legs and feet when stroked or lightly pinched.
3. Score the extremities using the motor scale appropriate for age (below).

Glasgow Coma Scale

Assess each response according to age

Eye opening
4 Opens eyes spontaneously when approached
3 Opens eyes to spoken or shouted speech

2 Opens eyes only to painful stimuli (nail bed pressure)
1 Does not open eyes in response to pain

Verbal
5 Oriented to time, place, person; infant responds by cooing and babbling, recognizes parent
4 Talks, not oriented to time, place, person; infant irritable, doesn't recognize parent
3 Words senseless, unintelligible; infant cries in response to pain
2 Responds with moaning and groaning, no intelligible words; infant moans to pain
1 No response

Motor
6 Responds to commands; infant smiles, responds
5 Tries to remove painful stimuli with hands; infant withdraws from touch
4 Attempts to withdraw from painful stimuli; infant withdraws from pain source
3 Flexes arms at elbows and wrists in response to pain (decorticate rigidity)
2 Extends arms at elbows in response to pain (cerebrate rigidity)
1 No motor response to pain

Check infant's fontanelle for bulging and record results

■ **Figure 28-13** Neurologic flow sheet and neurologic evaluation guide.

Key Points

> Interviewing the caregiver and the child is important to collect subjective data regarding the child that can be used to develop a plan of care.

> Biographical data, chief complaint, history of the present health concern, and child and family health history are included in obtaining a client history. A review of each body system and related information gives an overall picture of the current status. Information related to allergies, medications being taken, or concerns of substance abuse are gathered. School, social, personal, and nutritional history as well as assessing the developmental level of the child adds additional information for the care provider.

> The chief complaint is the reason the child was brought to the health care setting and should be fully explored with the child and caregiver.

> When doing a review of systems, ask questions about each of the body systems, using a head-to-toe approach to gather data to get an overall picture of the child's current status.

> The caregiver may be involved in collecting objective data by being a support to the child as well as assisting with tasks such as obtaining a temperature or urine specimen.

> Observing and recording the child's general appearance, behavior, and emotional and intellectual responses provides indications of overall health status. Possible indications of illness in children include the child being quieter or less active than usual, crying or acting uncomfortable, refusing to eat, exhibiting behaviors that are different from expected for the child's level of development, and having changes in skin coloration.

> Height, weight, and head circumference are assessed on an ongoing basis because they are good indicators of the child's growth and development, as well as the child's health status.

> Growth charts are used to establish a standard to compare an individual child's growth progress.

> Vital signs are taken and compared with normal values for children the same age, as well as to that child's previous recordings. Temperatures are taken by oral, tympanic, temporal, rectal, or axillary methods. An apical pulse is taken on infants and small children. Cardiac monitors may be used in some situations. Respirations are counted for a full minute when the child is lying or sitting quietly. Apnea monitors are used when indicated. Blood pressure measurement can be obtained by auscultation, palpation, and Doppler or electronic methods.

> A rectal temperature should not be taken on newborns, on children who have had rectal surgery or who have diarrhea, or if any resistance is noted when inserting the thermometer.

> Respiratory retractions are substernal (below the sternum), subcostal (below the ribs), intercostal (between the ribs), suprasternal (above the sternum), or supraclavicular (above the clavicle).

> Pulse oximetry measures the oxygen saturation of arterial hemoglobin.

> To collect objective data, a physical exam is done on a child, using knowledge of normal growth and development as a basis for the exam. Unlike the head-to-toe exam in the adult, the exam in the child proceeds from the less traumatic areas to be examined to the areas that are more traumatic or uncomfortable to the child. Range of motion is observed in the head and neck, and facial features are noted for balance or symmetry. The chest is measured and respiratory characteristics noted. Heart sounds are listened to at the point of maximum impulse (PMI), and pulses throughout the body are assessed. The abdomen is assessed for abnormalities. Bowel sounds in the four quadrants are noted. The genitalia and rectum are inspected as well as the back and extremities.

> The Glasgow coma scale is used as a tool for neurologic assessment and to consistently monitor the child's neurologic functioning.

INTERNET RESOURCES

Pediatric Nursing
www.pediatricnursing.com

National Institute of Child Health and Human Development
www.nichd.nih.gov

Workbook

■ NCLEX-STYLE REVIEW QUESTIONS

1. The nurse is doing an admission interview with a toddler and the child's caregiver. Which of the following statements that the nurse makes to the caregiver indicates the nurse has an understanding of this child's growth and development needs?

   a. "You can sit in one chair and your child can sit in the other chair."

   b. "It would be best if you let the child play in the playroom while we are talking."

   c. "If you would like to hold your child on your lap, that would be fine."

   d. "I can find someone to take your child for a walk for a while."

2. When interviewing an adolescent, which of the following is the *most* important for the nurse to keep in mind?

   a. The adolescent will be able to give accurate details regarding her or his history.

   b. The adolescent may feel more comfortable discussing some issues in private.

   c. The adolescent may have a better understanding if books and pamphlets are provided.

   d. The adolescent will be more cooperative if age-appropriate questions are asked.

3. In taking vital signs on a 6-month-old infant, the nurse obtains the following vital sign measurements. Which set of vital signs would the nurse be *most* concerned about?

   a. Pulse 94 beats per minute (bpm), temperature 36.9°C, blood pressure 80/50 mm Hg

   b. Pulse 118 bpm, temperature 37.6°C, blood pressure 88/60 mm Hg

   c. Pulse 134 bpm, temperature 38.0°C, blood pressure 92/62 mm Hg

   d. Pulse 152 bpm, temperature 38.5°C, blood pressure 96/56 mm Hg

4. When doing a physical exam on an infant, an understanding of this child's developmental needs are recognized when the exam is done by examining the

   a. heart before the abdomen.

   b. chest before the nose.

   c. legs before the feet.

   d. neurologic status before the back.

5. The nurse is measuring an 18-month-old child's height and weight. Which of the following actions should the nurse implement? Select all that apply.

   a. Plot the measurements on a growth chart.

   b. Wear a gown and mask during the procedure.

   c. Keep a hand within 1 in of the child.

   d. Encourage the parent to gently hold the child's legs.

   e. Have the child wear the same amount of clothing each time the procedure is done.

   f. Cover the scale with a clean sheet of paper before placing the child on the scale.

6. The nurse is performing an assessment on a child who has a respiratory condition. Identify the area where the nurse will observe this child for substernal respiratory retractions by marking an X on the spot where substernal retractions are noted.

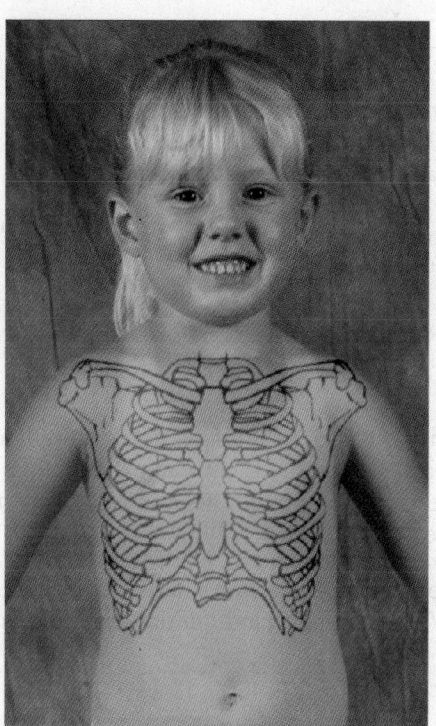

■ STUDY ACTIVITIES

1. Explain the step-by-step procedure you would follow to take vital signs on a 3-month-old infant. List the order in which you would take the vital signs and explain why you would do them in that order.

2. For each of the following body parts or systems, write a question that would be appropriate to ask a

patient or caregiver when doing a review of systems as part of an interview.

Body Part or System	Question to Ask
General	
Skin	
Head and neck	
Eyes	
Ears	
Nose, mouth, throat	
Chest and lungs—respiratory	
Heart—cardiovascular	
Abdomen—gastrointestinal	
Genitalia and rectum	
Back and extremities—musculoskeletal	
Neurologic	

3. List five methods of taking a temperature and describe each method. Give an example of a reason that each method might be used to take a child's temperature.

4. Go to the following Web site: www.luhs.org/depts/emsc/Teaching.pdf. Find "Initial Pediatric Assessment Teaching Tool." Scroll down to section III "General Approach to the Stable Pediatric Patient."
   a. List five suggestions for the nurse to use in approaching the pediatric patient. Scroll down to section V "Initial Inspection."
   b. List five observations that the nurse would make when first approaching the child.

▮ CRITICAL THINKING: WHAT WOULD YOU DO?

1. You are conducting an interview with the caregiver of a preschool-aged child.
   a. What would you discuss with the caregiver?
   b. What would you say and do with the caregiver to get the important information you need to care for the child?
   c. What would you say to the preschool-aged child during the interview with the caregiver?

2. As the nurse in a pediatric outpatient setting, you are responsible for obtaining the child's height and weight at each visit.
   a. What would you explain to the caregiver when you are asked why the height and weight of a child are measured at each health care visit?
   b. What information would you record and document on the child's growth record?
   c. What is the purpose and significance of plotting height and weight on a pediatric growth chart?

3. You are assisting in doing a physical exam on a toddler.
   a. What is the process of doing a physical exam on a child?
   b. How does the exam on a child differ from that of an adult?
   c. What are the most important considerations to keep in mind when doing a physical exam on a child?

29 Care of the Hospitalized Child

KEY TERMS

anuria
child-life program
patient-controlled analgesia
play therapy
rooming-in
therapeutic play

LEARNING OBJECTIVES

On completion of this chapter, you should be able to:

1. List nine possible influences on the family's response to a child's illness.
2. Explain the family caregivers' role in educating the young child about hospitals.
3. Describe ways in which pediatric units differ from adult care settings.
4. Explain safety concerns in the pediatric hospital setting and why special precautions are needed in times of stress, such as hospitalization.
5. Identify four ways that pathogens are transmitted and give an example of each.
6. Differentiate standard precautions and transmission-based precautions and state the role that hand washing plays in infection control.
7. Describe how to help ease the feelings of isolation a child may have when segregated because of transmission-based precautions.
8. Identify and differentiate the three stages of a child's response to separation from family caregivers.
9. Explain why and how caregivers participate in the care of the hospitalized child.
10. Explain how a planned admission with a preadmission visit differs from an emergency admission.
11. State the role of the caregiver in the child's admission process.
12. Outline topics that should be covered in family teaching before the child is discharged from the hospital.
13. Describe how health professionals can help the adjustment of the child scheduled for surgery through preoperative teaching.
14. Discuss variations in preoperative preparation for children, including skin, gastrointestinal, urinary, and medication preparation.
15. Discuss postoperative care of the child.
16. Describe pain management in children and identify behavioral characteristics that may indicate an infant or a young child is in pain.
17. Discuss the role of play for the hospitalized child including (a) play room or area, (b) play therapy, (c) therapeutic play, and (d) play materials.

HOSPITALIZATION MAY cause anxiety and stress at any age. Fear of the unknown is always threatening. The child who faces hospitalization is no exception. Children are often too young to understand what is happening or are afraid to ask questions. Short hospital stays occur more frequently than extended hospitalization, but even during a short stay, the child is often apprehensive. In addition, the child may pick up on the fears of family caregivers, and these negative emotions may hinder the child's progress.

The child's family suffers stress for a number of reasons. The cause of the illness, its treatment, guilt about the illness, past experiences of illness and hospitalization, disruption in family

This is important to keep in mind.
Children are tuned in to the feelings and emotions of their caregivers. By supporting the caregiver, you are also supporting the child.

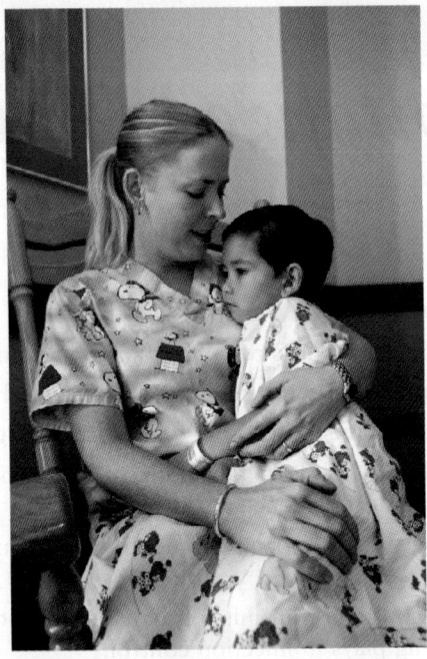

Figure 29-1 Holding and rocking the younger child helps alleviate the anxiety of hospitalization, especially when caregivers are not able to be with the child.

Figure 29-2 A nurse helps children learn what to expect from hospitalization during a prehospital program and tour of the facility.

life, the threat to the child's long-term health, cultural or religious influences, coping methods within the family, and financial impact of the hospitalization all may affect how the family responds to the child's illness. Although some of these are concerns of the family and not specifically the child, they nevertheless influence how the child feels.

The child's developmental level also plays an important role in determining how he or she handles the stress of illness and hospitalization. When you understand the child's developmental needs, you may significantly improve the child's hospital stay and overall recovery (Fig. 29-1).

Many hospitals have a **child-life program** to make hospitalization less threatening for children and their parents. These programs are usually under the direction of a child-life specialist whose background is in psychology and early childhood development. This person works with nurses, physicians, and other health team members to help them meet the developmental, emotional, and intellectual needs of hospitalized children. The child-life specialist also works with students interested in child health care to help further their education. Sometimes, however, the best way to ease the stress of hospitalization is to ensure that the child has been well prepared for the hospital experience.

THE PEDIATRIC HOSPITAL SETTING
Early Childhood Education About Hospitals

Hospitals are part of the child's community, just as police and fire departments are. When the child is capable of understanding the basic functions of community re-

sources and the people who staff them, it is time for an explanation. Some hospitals have regular open house programs for healthy children. Children may attend with parents or caregivers or in an organized community or school group. A room is set aside where children can handle equipment, try out call bells, try on masks and gowns, have their blood pressure taken to feel the squeeze of the blood pressure cuff, and see a hospital pediatric bed and compare it with their bed at home. Hospital staff members explain simple procedures and answer children's questions. A tour of the pediatric department, including the playroom, may be offered (Fig. 29-2). Some hospitals have puppet shows or show slides or videos about admission and care. Child-life specialists, nurses, and volunteers help with these orientation programs.

Families are encouraged to help children at an early age develop a positive attitude about hospitals. The family should avoid negative attitudes about hospitals. Young children need to know that the hospital is more than a place where "mommies go to get babies"; it is also important to avoid fostering the view of the hospital as a place where people go to die. This is a particular concern if the child knows someone who died in the hospital. A careful explanation of the person's illness and simple, honest answers to questions about the death are necessary.

The Pediatric Unit Atmosphere

An effort by pediatric units and hospitals to create friendly, warm surroundings for children has produced many attractive, colorful pediatric settings. Walls are colorful, often decorated with murals, wall-

Good News.
In pediatric units, furniture is attractive, appropriate in size, and designed with safety in mind. A variety of colors helps decrease the child's anxiety.

paper, photos, and paintings specifically designed for children. Curtains and drapes in appealing colors and designs are often coordinated with wall coverings.

The staff members of the pediatric unit often wear colored tops, colorful sweatshirts, or printed scrub suits. Children often are encouraged to wear their own clothing during the day. Colorful printed pajamas are provided for children who need to wear hospital clothing.

Treatments are performed in a treatment room, not in the child's room. Using a separate room to perform procedures promotes the concept that the child's bed is a "safe" place. All treatments, with no exceptions, should be performed in the treatment room to reassure the child.

A playroom or play area is a vital part of all pediatric units (see later discussion of The Hospital Play Program). The playroom should be a place that is safe from any kind of procedures.

Most pediatric settings encourage parents or family caregivers to visit as frequently as possible. This approach helps minimize the separation anxiety of the young child in particular. Care-

Here's a helpful tip.
Caregivers can be supportive and helpful in the pediatric unit. They provide comfort and reassurance to the child.

givers are involved in much of the young child's care.

Many pediatric units use primary nursing assignments so that the same nurse is with a child as much as possible. This approach provides the opportunity to establish a trusting relationship with the child.

Planning meals that include the child's favorite foods, within the limitations of any special dietary restrictions, may perk up a poor appetite. In addition, when space permits, several children may eat together at a small table. Younger children can be seated in high chairs or other suitable seats and should always be supervised by an adult. Meals should be served out of bed, if possible, and in a pleasant atmosphere. Some pediatric units use the playroom to serve meals to ambulatory children.

Test Yourself

✔ What are some of the reasons the child and family of a hospitalized child might suffer from stress?

✔ What are some advantages of children having an opportunity to tour or visit a hospital setting before they are hospitalized?

✔ Describe some differences that might be seen between a pediatric unit and an adult hospital unit.

 A Personal Glimpse

Hi, my name is Jenni. I am 15 years old and would like to tell you about my experience in the hospital.

I am an asthmatic. I have been since my early childhood because of allergies to many things. Whenever I get a cold, it sometimes aggravates my asthma. I recently had an episode where I needed to be hospitalized because of an asthma attack.

I don't like hospitals. I could not wait until I was released. The IV hurt and needed to be put back in. The nurse had dry, scaly hands. It looked like she worked on a farm and then came to work at the hospital. The food was not too great either, not like Pizza Hut or McDonald's.

The person who made the whole ordeal tolerable was the respiratory therapist. I needed regular nebulizer treatments, and it was a dream when he came into the room. Yes, he was good looking, but what made the difference was his personality and sense of humor. It makes a big difference when it seems as if the staff person wants to be there and really cares, rather than being cared for by someone who is there just because it's a job and can't wait until the shift ends.

Jenni, age 15 years

Learning Opportunity: What do you think are three important behaviors by the nurse or health care professional that indicate to a patient that he or she is cared about as a person?

Pediatric Intensive Care Units

A child's admission to a pediatric intensive care unit may be overwhelming for both the child and the family, especially if the admission is unexpected. Highly technical equipment, bright lights, and the crisis atmosphere may be frightening. Visiting may be restricted. The many stressors present increase the effects on the child and the family. Pediatric intensive care unit nurses should take great care to prepare the family for how the child will look when they first visit. The family should be given a schedule of visiting hours so that they may plan permitted visits. Visiting hours should be flexible enough to accommodate the child's best interests. The family can bring in a special doll or child's toy to provide comfort and security. The child's developmental level must be assessed so that the nursing staff can provide appropriate explanations and reassurances before and during procedures. Positive reinforcements, such as stickers and small badges, may provide symbols of courage. Interpret technical information for family members. Promote the relationship between the family caregiver and the child as much as possible. Encourage the caregiver to touch and talk to the child. If possible, the caregiver may hold and rock the child; if not, he or she can comfort the child by caressing and stroking.

Safety

Safety is an essential aspect of pediatric nursing care. Accidents occur more often when people are in stressful situations; infants, children, and their caregivers experience additional stress when a child is hospitalized. They are removed from a familiar home environment, faced with anxieties and fear, and must adjust to an unfamiliar schedule. Consciously assessing every situation for accident potential, you must have safety in mind at all times as a pediatric nurse.

The pediatric environment should meet all the safety standards appropriate for other areas of the facility, including good lighting, dry floors with no obstacles that may cause falls, electrical equipment checked for hazards, safe bath and shower facilities, and beds in low position for ambulatory patients.

Additional safety considerations depend on the child's age and developmental level. Toddlers are explorers whose developmental task is to develop autonomy. Toddlers love to put small objects into equally small openings, whether the opening is in their bodies, the oxygen tent, or elsewhere in the pediatric unit. Careful observation to eliminate dangers may prevent the toddler from having access to small objects. Toddlers are also often climbers and must be protected from climbing and falling. Toddlers and preschoolers must be watched to protect them from danger. Hospital staff must encourage family members to keep the crib sides up when not directly caring for the infant in the crib. One unguarded moment may mean that the infant falls out of a crib. Box 29-1 presents a summary of pediatric safety precautions.

Infection Control

Infection control is important in the pediatric hospital setting. The ill child may be especially vulnerable to pathogenic (disease-carrying) microorganisms. Precautions must be taken to protect the children, families, and personnel. Microorganisms are spread by contact (direct, indirect, or droplet), vehicle (food, water, blood, or contaminated products), airborne (dust particles in the air), or vector (mosquitoes, vermin) means of transmission. Each type of microorganism is transmitted in a specific way, so precautions are tailored to prevent the spread of specific microorganisms.

The U.S. Centers for Disease Control and Prevention and the Hospital Infection Control Practices Advisory Committee publish guidelines for isolation practices in hospitals. The guidelines include two levels of precautions: standard precautions and transmission-based precautions (see Appendix A). Health care facilities follow these guidelines.

Standard Precautions

Standard precautions blend the primary characteristics of universal precautions and body substance isolation. Standard precautions apply to blood; all body

---

Box 29-1 ▪ SAFETY PRECAUTIONS FOR PEDIATRIC UNITS

- Cover electrical outlets.
- Keep floor dry and free of clutter.
- Use tape or Velcro closures when possible.
- Always close safety pins when not in use.
- Inspect toys (child's or hospital's) for loose or small parts, sharp edges, dangerous cords, or other hazards.
- Do not permit friction toys where oxygen is in use.
- Do not leave child unattended in high chair.
- Keep crib sides up all the way except when caring for child.
- If the crib side is down, keep hand firmly on infant at all times.
- Use crib with top if child stands or climbs.
- Always check temperature of bath water to prevent burns.
- Never leave infant or child unattended in bath water.
- Keep beds of ambulatory children locked in low position.
- Turn off motor of electric bed if young children might have access to controls.
- Always use safety belts or straps for children in infant seats, feeding chairs, strollers, wheelchairs, or stretchers.
- Use restraints only when necessary.
- When restraints are used, remove and check for skin integrity, circulation, and correct application at least every hour or 2.
- Never tie a restraint to the crib side; tie to bed frame only.
- Keep medications securely locked in designated area; children should never be permitted in this area.
- Set limits and enforce them consistently; do not let children get out of control.
- Place needles and syringes in sharps containers; make sure children have no access to these containers.
- Always pick up any equipment after a procedure.
- Never leave scissors or other sharp instruments within child's reach.
- Do not allow sleepy family caregivers to hold a sleeping child as they may fall asleep and drop the child.

---

fluids, secretions, and excretions, except sweat; nonintact skin; and mucous membranes. Standard precautions are intended to reduce the risk of transmission of microorganisms from recognized or unrecognized sources of infection in hospitals. Health care providers follow standard precautions in the care of all patients.

Transmission-Based Precautions

For patients documented or suspected of having highly transmissible pathogens, health care providers must follow transmission-based precautions. These precautions are in addition to the standard precautions.

> **This is critical to remember.**
>
> Hand washing is the cornerstone of all infection control. Wash your hands conscientiously between seeing each patient, even when gloves are worn for a procedure.

Transmission-based precautions include three types: airborne precautions, droplet precautions, and contact precautions. Certain diseases may require more than one type of precaution. See Nursing Care Plan 29-1: The Child Placed on Transmission-Based Precautions.

The child who is segregated because of transmission-based precautions is subject to social isolation. Make every effort to help reduce the child's feelings of loneliness and depression. The child must not think that being in a room alone is a punishment. Arrange to spend extra time in the room when performing treatments and procedures. While in the room, you might read a story, play a game, or just talk with the child, rather than going quickly in and out of the room.

Encourage family caregivers to spend time with the child. Help them with gowning and other necessary precaution procedures so that they become more comfortable in the situation. Caregivers may need reminders about precaution measures, including hand washing, gowning, and masking as necessary. Encourage the family to bring the child's favorite dolls, stuffed animals, or toys. Most of these items can be sterilized after use. For the older child, electronic toys may help provide stimulation to ease the loneliness. Positioning the child's bed near a window may help reduce feelings of isolation. Encourage the child to make phone calls to friends or family members to keep up social contacts. For the school-aged child, family caregivers might contact the child's teacher so that classmates can send cards and other school items to keep the child involved.

If masks or gloves are part of the necessary precautions, the child may experience even greater feelings of isolation. Before putting on the mask, allow the child to see your face; that process will help the child easily identify you. Gloves prevent the child from experiencing skin-to-skin contact; talk to the child to draw out any of the child's feelings about this. Explaining at the child's level of understanding why gloves are necessary may help the child accept them. If the child is upset by the fact that caregivers must wear gowns, a careful explanation should help the child accept this. No matter what

precautions are necessary, always be alert to the child's loneliness and sadness and be prepared to meet these needs.

Importance of Caregiver Participation

Research has shown that separating young children from their family caregivers, especially during times of stress, may have damaging effects. Young children have no concept of time, so separation from their primary caregivers is especially difficult for them to understand.

Children often go through three characteristic stages of response to the separation: protest, despair, and denial. During the first stage (*protest*), the young child cries, often refuses to be comforted by others, and constantly seeks the primary caregiver at every sight and sound. When the caregiver does not appear, the child enters the second stage (*despair*) and becomes apathetic and listless. Health care personnel often interpret this as a sign that the child is accepting the situation, but this is not the case; the child has given up. In the third stage (*denial*), the child begins taking interest in the surroundings and appears to accept the situation. However, when the caregivers do visit, the child often turns away from them, showing distrust and rejection. It may take a long time before the child accepts them again, and even then, remnants of the damage linger. The child may always have a memory of being "abandoned" at the hospital. Regardless of how mistaken they may be, childhood impressions have a deep effect.

Most pediatric settings provide **rooming-in** facilities, where the caregiver can stay in the room with the child (Fig 29-3). Rooming-in helps minimize the hospitalized child's separation anxiety and depression. Although separation from primary caregivers is thought to cause the greatest upset in children younger than 5 years of age, children of all ages should be considered when setting up a rooming-in system.

One advantage of rooming-in is the measure of security the child feels as a result of the caregiver's care and attention. The primary caregiver may participate in bathing, dressing, and feeding; preparing the child for

■ **Figure 29-3** Rooming-in helps alleviate separation anxiety for both the child and the caregiver.

Nursing Care Plan 29-1

THE CHILD PLACED ON TRANSMISSION-BASED PRECAUTIONS

TS is a 5-year-old girl who has a highly infectious illness resulting from an airborne microorganism. The child is placed on Airborne Transmission-Based Precautions.

NURSING DIAGNOSIS
Risk for Loneliness related to transmission-based precautions

GOAL: The child will have adequate social contact.

EXPECTED OUTCOMES
• The child interacts with nursing staff and family.
• The child visits with friends and family via telephone.

Nursing Interventions	Rationale
Identify ways in which the child can communicate with staff, family, and friends. Facilitate the use of telephone for the child to talk with friends. Suggest family caregivers ask the child's preschool friends to send notes and drawings.	Frequent contact with family and staff helps to decrease the child's feeling of isolation. Use of the telephone helps child feel connected with her friends. Notes, photos, and drawings are concrete signs to the child that her friends are thinking of her. It helps her stay in touch with her preschool.

NURSING DIAGNOSIS
Deficient Diversional Activity related to monotony of restrictions

GOAL: The child will be engaged in age-appropriate activities.

EXPECTED OUTCOMES
• The child participates in age-appropriate activities.
• The child approaches planned activities with enthusiasm.

Nursing Interventions	Rationale
Gather a collection of age-appropriate books, puzzles, and games. Consult with play therapist if available. Encourage family caregivers to engage the child in activities she enjoys. Audiotapes can be made for (or by) playmates. Plan nursing care to include time for reading or playing a game with the child. Encourage physical exercise within the restrictions of the child's condition.	A variety of appropriate activities provide diversion and entertainment without boredom. Family caregivers can use visiting time to help alleviate the monotony of isolation. Audiotapes make friends seem closer. Activities with a variety of persons (besides family caregivers) are welcome to the child. Physical activity helps to improve circulation and feelings of well-being.

NURSING DIAGNOSIS
Powerlessness related to separation resulting from required precautions

GOAL: The child will have control over some aspects of the situation.

EXPECTED OUTCOMES
• The child will make choices about some of her daily routine.
• The child's family caregivers and the staff keep their promises about planned activities.

Nursing Interventions	Rationale
Include the child in planning for daily activities such as bath routine, food choices, timing of meals and snacks, and other flexible activities. Maintain the schedule after making the plan. Plan a special activity with the child each day and keep your promise.	The child will feel some control over her life if she is included in ways where she can have a choice. Keeping the schedule reinforces for the child that she really does have some control. When the child can depend on the word of those in control, she is reassured about her own value.

bed; and providing recreational activities. If treatments are to be continued at home, rooming-in creates an excellent opportunity for the caregiver to observe and practice before leaving the hospital.

Rules should be clearly understood before admission, and facilities for caregivers should be clearly explained. The hospital may provide a foldout bed or reclining chair in the child's room. Provision for meals should be explained to the caregiver.

Avoid creating a situation in which you appear to be expecting the primary caregivers to perform as health care technicians. The primary caregiver's basic role is to provide security and stability for the child.

Nursing judgment is in order.

Rooming-in should not be used to relieve staff shortage. The role of the caregiver is to help the child feel safe and secure.

Many pediatric units also allow siblings to visit the ill child. This policy benefits both the ill child and the sibling. The sibling at home may be imagining a much more serious illness than is actually the case. Visiting policies usually require that a family adult accompany and be responsible for the sibling and that the visiting period is not too long. Visiting siblings must not have a cold or other contagious illness and must have up-to-date immunizations.

While encouraging caregiver participation, the nursing staff also should be aware of the caregiver's needs. The caregiver needs to be encouraged to take a break, leave for a meal, or to occasionally go home, if possible, for a shower and rest. The caregiver may give a personal possession to the child to help reassure him or her that

This advice could be a lifesaver.

Some hospitals provide pagers for family caregivers so that they can leave the immediate area of the child's room or waiting area but can be quickly paged to return, if needed. Having caregivers' mobile phone numbers easily accessible is also helpful in contacting them.

the caregiver will return. Having a way to contact the family quickly gives the family freedom and reassurance. This is particularly useful during periods when the caregivers must wait for procedures, surgery, or other activities.

Test Yourself

✔ Why is infection control especially important in the pediatric setting?

✔ Explain the difference between standard precautions and transmission-based precautions.

✔ Why is caregiver participation important in the pediatric hospital setting?

ADMISSION AND DISCHARGE PLANNING

Although admission may be a frightening experience, the child feels in much better control of the situation if the person taking the child to the hospital has explained where they are going and why, and has answered questions truthfully. When the caregiver and the child arrive on the nursing unit, they should be greeted in a warm, friendly manner and taken to the child's room, or to a room set aside specifically for the admission procedure. The caregiver and the child need to be oriented to the child's room, the nursing unit, and regulations (Box 29-2).

Planned Admissions

Preadmission preparation may make the experience less threatening and the adjustment to admission as smooth as possible. Children who are candidates for hospital admission may attend open house programs or other special programs that are more detailed and specifically related to their upcoming experience. It is important for family caregivers and siblings to attend the preadmission tour with the future patient to reduce anxiety in all family members.

Box 29-2 ▌ GUIDELINES TO ORIENT CHILD TO PEDIATRIC UNIT

1. Introduce the primary nurse.
2. Orient to the child's room:
   a. Demonstrate bed, bed controls, side rails.
   b. Demonstrate call light.
   c. Demonstrate television; include cost, if any.
   d. Show bathroom facilities.
   e. Explain telephone and rules that apply.
3. Introduce to roommate(s); include families.
4. Give directions to or show "special" rooms:
   a. Playroom—rules that apply, hours available, toys or equipment that may be taken to child's room.
   b. Treatment room—explain purpose.
   c. Unit kitchen—rules that apply.
   d. Other special rooms.
5. Explain pediatric rules; give written rules if available:
   a. Visiting hours, who may visit.
   b. Mealtimes, rules about bringing in food.
   c. Bedtimes, naptimes, or quiet time.
   d. Rooming-in arrangements.
6. Explain daily routines:
   a. Vital signs routine.
   b. Bath routine.
   c. Other routines.
7. Provide guidelines for involvement of family caregiver.

■ **Figure 29-4** The child who is going to have surgery may act out the procedure on a doll, thereby reducing some of her fear. (© B. Proud.)

During the preadmission visit, children may be given surgical masks, caps, shoe covers, and the opportunity to "operate" on a doll or other stuffed toy specifically designed for teaching purposes (Fig. 29-4). Many hospitals have developed special coloring books to help prepare children for tonsillectomy or other specific surgical procedures. These books are given to children during the preadmission visit, or they are sent to children at home before admission. During the visit, children and their families often are hesitant to ask questions or express feelings; the staff must be sensitive to this problem and discuss common questions and feelings. Children are told that some things will hurt but that doctors and nurses will do everything they can to make the hurt go away. Honesty must be a keynote to any program of this kind. The preadmission orientation staff also must be sensitive to cultural and language differences and make adjustments whenever appropriate.

Emergency Admissions

Emergencies leave little time for explanation. The emergency itself is frightening to the child and the family, and the need for treatment is urgent. Even though a caregiver tries to act calm and composed, the child often may sense the anxiety. If the hospital is still a great unknown, it will only add to the child's fear and panic. If the child has even a basic understanding about hospitals and what happens there, the emergency may seem a little less frightening.

In an emergency, physical needs assume priority over emotional needs. When possible, the presence of a family caregiver who can conceal his or her own fear often is comforting to the child; however, the child may be angry that the caregiver does not prevent invasive procedures from being performed. Sometimes, however, it is impossible for the caregiver to stay with the child. The family caregiver may provide a staff member with information about the child while the child receives treatment. This helps the family member to feel involved in the child's care.

Emergency department nurses must be sensitive to the needs of the child and the family. Recognizing the child's cognitive level and how it affects the child's reactions is important. In addition, the staff must explain procedures and conduct themselves in a caring, calm manner to reassure both the child and the family.

The Admission Interview

An admission interview is conducted as soon as possible after the child has been admitted. See Chapter 28 for specific information related to the client interview and history. During the interview, an identification bracelet is placed on the child's wrist. If the child has allergies, an allergy bracelet must be placed on the wrist as well. The child must be prepared for even this simple procedure with an explanation of why it is necessary.

When receiving the child on the pediatric unit, it is important to be friendly and casual, remembering that even a well-informed child may be shy and suspicious of excessive friendliness.

Through careful questioning, the interviewer tries to determine what the family's previous experience has been with hospitals and health care providers. It is also important to ascertain how much the caregiver and the child understand about the child's condition and their expectations of this hospitalization, what support systems are available when the child returns home, and any disturbing or threatening concerns on the part of the caregiver or the child. These findings, in addition to the client history and physical exam (see Chapter 28), form the basis for the patient's total plan of care while hospitalized.

> **Pay attention to this.**
> The child who reacts with fear to your well-meaning advances and who clings to the caregiver is telling you to go more slowly with the acquaintance process. Children who know that the caregiver may stay with them are more quickly put at ease.

The Admission Physical Examination

After the child has been oriented to the new surroundings by perhaps clinging to the family caregiver's hand or carrying a favorite toy or blanket, the caregiver may undress the child for the physical examination. This procedure may be familiar from previous health care visits. If comfortable with helping, the caregiver may stay with the child during the physical exam. See Chapter 28 for specific information related to the physical exam.

Discharge Planning

Planning for the child's discharge and care at home begins early in the hospital experience. Nurses and other health team members must assess the levels of understanding of the child and family and their abilities to learn about the child's condition and the care necessary after the child goes home. Giving medications, using special equipment, and enforcing necessary restrictions must be discussed with the person who will be the primary caregiver and with one other person, if possible. Specific, written instructions should be provided for reference at home; the anxiety and strangeness of hospitalization often limit the amount of information retained from teaching sessions. Be certain the caregiver can understand the written materials too. If the treatment necessary at home appears too complex for the caregiver to manage, it may be helpful to arrange for a visiting nurse to assist for a period after the child is sent home.

Shortly before the child is discharged from the hospital, a conference may be arranged to review information and procedures with the family caregivers. This conference may or may not include the child, depending on his or her age and cognitive level. Health care providers must deal with questions and concerns honestly and offer a resource such as a telephone number the caregiver can call for questions that arise after discharge.

The return home may be a difficult period of adjustment for the entire family. The preschool child may be aloof at first, followed by a period of clinging, demanding behavior. Other behaviors, such as regression, temper tantrums, excessive attachment to a toy or blanket, night waking, and nightmares, may demonstrate fear of another separation. The older child may demonstrate anger or jealousy of siblings. The family may be advised to encourage positive behavior and avoid making the child the center of attention because of the illness. Discipline should be firm, loving, and consistent. The child may express feelings verbally or in play activities. Reassure the family that this is not unusual.

THE CHILD UNDERGOING SURGERY

Surgery frightens most adults, even though they understand why it is necessary and how it helps correct their health problems. Young children do not have this understanding and may become frightened of even a minor surgical procedure. If properly prepared, older children and adolescents are capable of understanding the need for surgery and what it will accomplish.

Many minor surgical procedures are performed in outpatient surgery facilities that permit the patient to return home the day of the operation. These facilities reduce or eliminate the separation of parents and children, one of the most stressful factors in surgery for infants and young children. Whether admitted for less than 1 day or for several weeks, the child who has surgery needs compassionate and thorough preoperative and postoperative care.

Preoperative Care

Specific physical and psychological preparation of the child and the family varies according to the type of surgery planned. General aspects of care include patient teaching, skin preparation, preparation of the gastrointestinal and urinary systems, and preoperative medication.

Patient Teaching

The child admitted for planned surgery probably has had some preadmission preparation by the health care provider and family caregivers. Many families, however, have an unclear understanding of the surgery and what it involves, or they may be too anxious to be helpful. The health professionals involved in the child's care must determine how much the child knows and is capable of learning, help correct any misunderstandings, explain the preparation for surgery and what the surgery will "fix," as well as how the child will feel after surgery. This preparation must be based on the child's age, developmental level, previous experiences, and caregiver support. All explanations should be clear and honest and expressed in terms the child and the family caregivers can understand. Encourage questions to ensure that the child and the family caregivers correctly understand all the information. When the child is too young to benefit from preoperative teaching, direct explanations to family caregivers to help relieve their anxiety and to prepare them to participate in the child's care after surgery.

Balance is the order of the day.

If possible, conduct preoperative teaching in short sessions, rather than trying to discuss everything at once.

Children need to be prepared for standard preoperative tests and procedures, such as radiographs and blood and urine tests. Explain the reason for withholding food and fluids before surgery, so children do not feel they are being neglected or punished when others receive meal trays.

Children sometimes interpret surgery as punishment and should be reassured that they did not cause the condition. They also fear mutilation or death and must be able to explore those feelings, while recognizing them as acceptable fears. Children deserve careful explanation that the physician is going to repair only the affected body part.

Cultural Snapshot

Surgery and surgical procedures are feared in some cultures. Anxiety over anesthesia and being "put to sleep" causes such concern in some cultures that surgery is refused. Careful explanations of procedures and the benefits to the patient are important. Using an interpreter when language barriers exist is helpful.

■ **Figure 29-5** Before surgery, these children work with a child-life specialist using a model of the body organs.

Therapeutic play, discussed later in this chapter, is useful in preparing the child for surgery. Using drawings to identify the area of the body to be operated on helps the child have a better understanding of what is going to happen. Role playing, adjusted to the child's age and understanding, is helpful. This approach may include a trip on a stretcher and pretending to go to surgery. If the child requests, you or the play leader can pretend to be the patient.

The older child or adolescent may have a greater interest in the surgery itself, what is wrong and why, how the repair is done, and the expected postoperative results. Models of a child's internal organs or individual organs, such as a heart, are useful for demonstration, or the patient may be involved in making the drawing (Fig. 29-5).

Emphasize to the child that he or she will not feel anything during surgery because of the special sleep that anesthesia causes. Describing the postanesthesia care unit (PACU or wake-up room) and any tubes, bandages, or appliances that will be in place after surgery lets the child know what to expect. If possible, the child should see and handle the anesthesia mask (if this is the method to be used) and equipment that will be part of the postoperative experience. A preoperative tour of the intensive care unit (ICU) or postanesthesia care unit is also helpful.

A child needs to understand that several people will be involved in preoperative, surgical, and postoperative care. If possible, staff members from the anesthesia department and the operating room, recovery room, or the ICU should visit the child before surgery. Explaining what the people will be wearing (caps, masks, and gloves) and what equipment will be used (including bright lights) helps make the operating room experience less frightening.

Most patients experience postoperative pain, and children should be prepared for this experience. They also need to know when they may expect to be allowed to have fluids and food after surgery.

■ **Figure 29-6** The preoperative teaching this adolescent received helps him splint his abdomen after surgery.

Children should learn to practice coughing and deep-breathing exercises. Deep-breathing practice may be done with games that encourage blowing. Teaching children to splint the operative site with a pillow helps reassure them that the sutures will not break and allow the wound to open (Fig. 29-6).

Tell children where their family will be during and after surgery, and make every effort to minimize separation. Encourage family caregivers to be present when the child leaves for the operating room.

Skin Preparation

Depending on the type of surgery, skin preparation may include a tub bath or shower and certainly includes special cleaning and inspection of the operative site. Any necessary shaving usually is performed in the operating room. If fingers or toes are involved, the nails are carefully trimmed. The operative site may be cleansed with a special antiseptic solution as an extra precaution against infection, depending on the physician's orders and the procedures of the hospital.

Gastrointestinal and Urinary System Preparation

The surgeon may order a cleansing enema the night before surgery (see Chapter 30). An enema is an intrusive procedure and must be explained to the child before it is given. If old enough, the child should understand the reason for the enema.

Children usually receive nothing by mouth (NPO) for a period of 4 to 12 hours before surgery because any food or fluids in the stomach may cause vomiting and aspiration, particularly during general anesthesia.

The NPO period varies according to the child's age; infants become dehydrated more rapidly than older children and thus require a shorter NPO period before surgery. Pediatric NPO orders should be accompanied by an intravenous (IV) fluid initiation order. Loose teeth are also a potential hazard and should be counted and recorded according to hospital policy.

In some instances, urinary catheterization may be performed before surgery, but usually it is done while the child is in the operating room. The catheter is often removed immediately after surgery but can be left in place for several hours or days. Children who are not catheterized before surgery should be encouraged to void before the administration of preoperative medication.

Preoperative Medication

Depending on the physician's order, preoperative medications usually are given in two stages: a sedative is administered about 1.5 to 2 hours before surgery, and an analgesic-atropine mixture may be administered immediately before the patient leaves for the operating room. When the sedative has been given, dimming the lights and minimizing noise help the child relax and rest. Family caregivers and the child should be aware that atropine could cause a blotchy rash and a flushed face.

Bring preoperative medication to the child's room when it is time for administration. Tell the child that it is time for medication and that another nurse has come along to help the child hold still. Administer medication carefully and quickly because delays only increase the child's anxiety.

If hospital regulations permit, family caregivers should accompany the child to the operating room and wait until the child is anesthetized. If this is impossible, the nurse who has been caring for the child can go along to the operating room and introduce the child to personnel there.

Postoperative Care

During the immediate postoperative period, the child receives care in the postanesthesia care unit or the surgical ICU. Meanwhile, the room in the pediatric unit should be prepared with appropriate equipment for the child's return. Depending on the type of surgery performed, it may be necessary to have suctioning, resuscitation, or other equipment at the bedside.

When the child returns to the room, nursing care focuses on careful observation for any signs or symptoms of complications: shock, hemorrhage, or respiratory distress. Monitor and record vital signs according to postoperative orders. Keep the child warm with blankets, as needed. Take note of any dressings, IV apparatus, urinary catheters, and any other appliances. An IV flow sheet is used to document the type of fluid, the amount of fluid to be absorbed, the rate of flow, any additive medications, the site, and the site's appearance and condition. The IV flow sheet may be separate or incorporated into a general flow sheet for the pediatric patient.

The first voiding is an important milestone in the child's postoperative progress because it indicates the adequacy of blood flow and urinary output. An inadequate amount of urine voided might indicate possible urinary retention. Also note any irritation or burning, and notify the physician if **anuria** (absence of urine) persists longer than 6 hours.

Postoperative orders may provide for ice chips or clear liquids to prevent dehydration; these may be administered with a spoon or in a small medicine cup. Frequent repositioning is necessary to prevent skin breakdown, orthostatic pneumonia, and decreased circulation. Coughing, deep breathing, and position changes are performed at least every 2 hours (Fig. 29-7).

Pain Management

Pain is a concern of postoperative patients in any age group. Most adult patients can verbally express the pain they feel, so they request relief. However, infants and young children cannot adequately express themselves and need help to tell where or how great the pain is. Longstanding beliefs that children do not have the same amount of pain that adults have or that they tolerate pain

▮ **Figure 29-7** The nurse encourages this child to deep breathe after surgery by using a pinwheel.

better than adults, have contributed to undermedicating infants and children in pain. Research has shown that infants and children do experience pain.

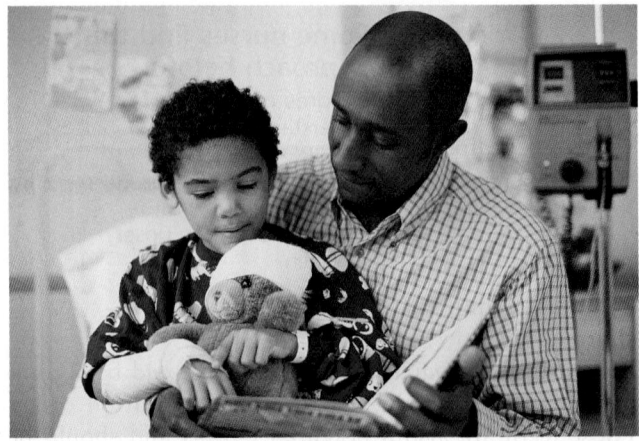
Figure 29-9 Distraction supplements pain control while a child is using patient-controlled analgesia.

Nursing judgment is in order.

Some children may try to hide pain because they fear an injection or because they are afraid that admitting to pain will increase the time they have to stay in the hospital.

Be alert to indications of pain, especially in young patients. Careful assessment is necessary—for example, noting changes in behavior such as rigidity, thrashing, facial expressions, loud crying or screaming, flexion of knees (indicating abdominal pain), restlessness, and irritability. Physiologic changes, such as increased pulse rate and blood pressure, sweating palms, dilated pupils, flushed or moist skin, and loss of appetite, also may indicate pain.

Various tools have been devised to help children express the amount of pain they feel. The tools also allow you to measure the effectiveness of pain management efforts. These tools include the faces scale, the numeric scale, and the color scale. The faces and numeric scales are useful primarily with children 7 years of age and older (Fig. 29-8). To use the color scale, the young child is given crayons ranging from yellow to red or black. Yellow represents no pain, and the darkest color (or red) represents the most pain. The child selects the color that represents the amount of pain felt.

Pain medication may be administered orally, by routine intramuscular or IV routes, or by **patient-controlled analgesia,** a programmed IV infusion of narcotic analgesia that the child may control within set limits. A low-level dose of analgesia may be administered, with the child able to administer a bolus as needed. Patient-controlled analgesia may be used for children 7 years of age or older who have no cognitive impairment and undergo a careful evaluation. Intramuscular injections are avoided if possible

because they can be traumatic and painful for the child. Monitor vital signs and document the child's level of consciousness frequently, following the standards of the facility.

Comfort measures should be used along with the administration of analgesics. No child should suffer pain unnecessarily. Appropriate nonpharmacologic comfort measures may include position changes, massage, distraction, play, soothing touch, talk, coddling, and affection. Activities provided for distraction must be appropriate for the child's age, level of development, and interests (Fig. 29-9).

Surgical Dressings

Postoperative care includes close observation of any dressings for signs of drainage or hemorrhage and reinforcing or changing dressings as ordered. Wet dressings can increase the possibility of contamination; clean, dry dressings increase the child's comfort. If there is no physician's order to change the dressing, reinforce the moist original dressing by covering it with a dry dressing and taping the second dressing in place. If bloody drainage is present, draw around the outline of the drainage with a marker and record the time and date. In this way, the amount of additional drainage can be assessed when the dressings are inspected later.

Supplies needed for changing dressings vary according to the wound site and the physician's orders that specify the sterile or antiseptic technique to be used. Detailed procedures for these techniques and the supplies to be used can be found in the facility's procedures manual.

As with all procedures, explain to the child what will be done and why, before beginning the dressing change. Some dressing changes are painful; if so, tell the child that it will hurt and offer praise for behavior that shows courage and cooperation.

Patient Teaching

Postoperative patient teaching is as important as preoperative teaching. It is important to repeat some explanations and instructions given before surgery because the child's earlier anxiety may have prevented thorough

A   No pain   Worst pain

      0   1   2   3   4   5   6   7   8   9   10

B

      0   1   2   3   4   5
   NO HURT   HURTS   HURTS   HURTS   HURTS   HURTS
             LITTLE   LITTLE   EVEN   WHOLE   WORST
             BIT   MORE   MORE   LOT

Alternate
coding 0   2   4   6   8   10

Figure 29-8 Pain scales: **(A)** Numeric scale. **(B)** Faces rating scale. (From Hockenberry, M. J., Wilson, D., & Winkelstein, M. L. [2005]. *Wong's essentials of pediatric nursing* [7th ed., p.1259]. St. Louis, MO: Mosby. © Mosby. Used with permission.)

understanding. Now that tubes, restraints, and dressings are part of the child's reality, they need to be discussed again: Why they are important and how they affect the child's activities.

Family caregivers want to know how they can help care for the child and what limitations are placed on the child's activity. If caregivers know what to expect and how to aid in their child's recovery, they will be cooperative during the postoperative period.

As the child recuperates, encourage the caregivers and child to share their feelings about the surgery, any changes in body image, and their expectations for recovery and rehabilitation.

When the sutures are removed, reassure the child that the opening has healed and the child's insides will not "fall out," which is a common fear.

Before the child is discharged from the hospital, teaching focuses on home care, use of any special equipment or appliances, medications, diet, restrictions on activities, and therapeutic exercise (Fig. 29-10). Caregivers should demonstrate the procedures or repeat information to confirm that learning has occurred. Use the nursing process to assess the needs of the child and the family to plan appropriate postoperative care and teaching.

Test Yourself

✔ Why is preoperative teaching important for the child and family caregivers?

✔ What preparation procedures might the child have before surgery?

✔ What factors are important in pain management for the child after surgery?

✔ What might be included in postoperative teaching for the child and family?

THE HOSPITAL PLAY PROGRAM

Play is the business of children and a principal way in which they learn, grow, develop, and act out feelings and problems. Playing is a normal activity; the more it can be part of hospital care, the more normal and more comfortable this environment becomes.

Play helps children come to terms with the hurts, anxieties, and separation that accompany hospitalization. In the hospital playroom, children may express frustrations, hostilities, and aggressions through play without the fear of being scolded by the nursing staff. Children who keep these negative emotions bottled up suffer much greater damage than do those who are allowed to express them where they may be handled constructively. Children must feel secure enough in the situation to express negative emotions without fear of disapproval.

Children, however, must not be allowed to harm themselves or others. Although it is important to express acceptable or unacceptable feelings, unlimited permissiveness is as harmful as excessive strictness. Children rely on adults to guide them and set limits for behavior because this means the adults care about them. When behavior correction is necessary, it is important to make it clear that the child's action, not the child, is being disapproved.

The Hospital Play Environment

An organized and well-planned play area is important in the overall care of the hospitalized child. The play area should be large enough to accommodate cribs, wheelchairs, IV poles, and children in casts. It should provide a variety of play materials suitable for the ages and needs of all children (Fig. 29-11). Play is usually unstructured; the child chooses the toy and the kind of play needed or desired. However, all children should participate, and the play leaders should ignore no one.

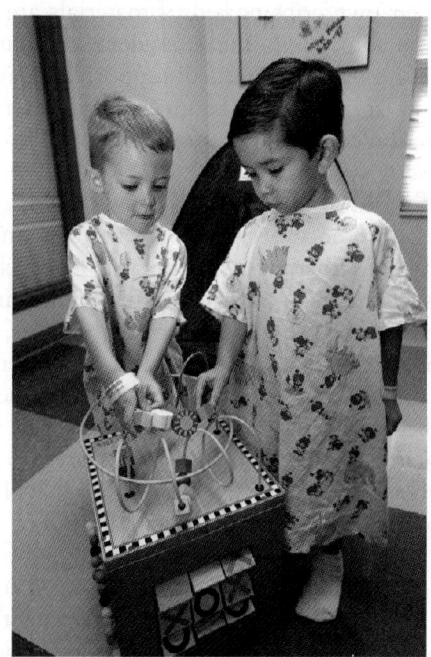

■ Figure 29-11 Children occupied in a hospital playroom. It is important to provide age-appropriate activities for children.

■ Figure 29-10 The nurse uses charts with pictures to perform patient teaching before the child goes home.

■ **Figure 29-12** This adolescent enjoys playing on the computer in the adolescent room on the pediatric unit.

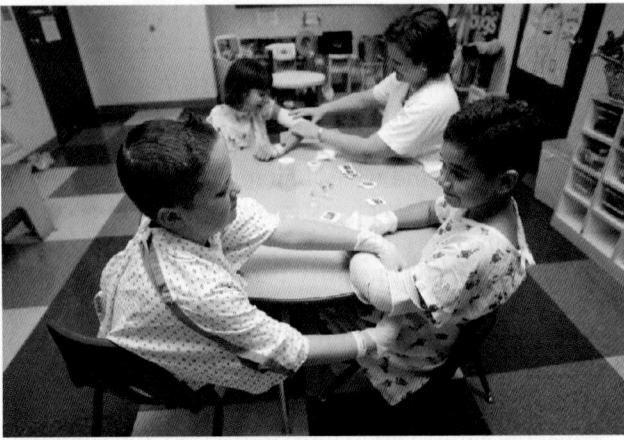

■ **Figure 29-13** This group of children is involved in therapeutic play with the supervision of the child-life specialist.

If possible, adolescents should have a separate recreation room or area away from young children. Ideally, this is an area where adolescents may gather to talk, play pool or table tennis, watch television and movies, use a computer, drink soft drinks (if permitted), and eat snacks (Fig. 29-12). Tables and chairs should be provided to encourage interaction among the adolescents. Rules may be clearly spelled out and posted. If adolescents must share the same recreation area with younger children, the area should be referred to as the "activity center," rather than the "playroom."

Although a well-equipped playroom is of major importance in any pediatric department, some children cannot be brought to the playroom, or some play programs may be cut because of cost-containment efforts. In these situations, be creative in providing play opportunities for children. Children may act out their fantasies and emotions in their own cribs or beds if materials are brought to them and someone (a nurse, student, or volunteer) is available to give them needed support and attention. Children in isolation may be given play material, provided infection control precautions are strictly followed.

Therapeutic Play

There is a difference between play therapy and therapeutic play. **Play therapy** is a technique of psychoanalysis that psychiatrists or psychiatric nurse clinicians use to uncover a disturbed child's underlying thoughts, feelings, and motivations to help understand them better. The therapist might have the child act out experiences using dolls as the participants in the experience.

Therapeutic play is a play technique used to help the child have a better understanding of what will be happening to him or her in a specific situation. For instance, the child who will be having an IV started before surgery might be given the materials and encouraged to "start" an IV on a stuffed animal or doll. By observing the child, you can often note concerns, fears, and anxieties the child might express. Therapeutic play is a play technique

that play therapists, nurses, child-life specialists, or trained volunteers may use to help the child express feelings, fears, and concerns (Fig. 29-13).

The play leader should be alert to the needs of the child who is afraid to act independently as a result of strict home discipline. Even normally sociable children may carry their fears of the hospital environment into the playroom. It could be some time before timid, fearful, or nonassertive children feel free enough to take advantage of the play opportunities. Too much enthusiasm on the part of the play leader in trying to get the child to participate may defeat the purpose and make the child withdraw. The leader must decide carefully whether to initiate an activity for a child or let the child advance at a self-set pace.

Often other children provide the best incentive by doing something interesting, so that the timid child forgets his or her apprehensions and tries it, or another child says, "Come and help me with this," and soon the other child becomes involved. A fearful child trusts a peer before trusting an adult, who represents authority. Nevertheless, the adult should not ignore the child's presence. The leader shows the child around the playroom, indicating that the children are free to play with whatever they wish and that the leader is there to answer questions and to help when a child wishes help.

When initiating group play, the leader may invite but not insist that the timid child participate. The leader must give the child time to adjust and gain confidence.

Play Material

Play material should be chosen with safety in mind; there should be no sharp edges and no small parts that can be swallowed or aspirated. Toys and equipment should be inspected regularly for broken parts or sharp edges.

One important playroom function is that it gives the child opportunities to dramatize hospital experiences. Providing hospital equipment, miniature or real, as play material gives the child an opportunity to act out feelings about the hospital environment and treatments.

Stethoscopes, simulated thermometers, stretchers, wheelchairs, examining tables, instruments, bandages, and other medical and hospital equipment are useful for this purpose.

Dolls or puppets dressed to represent the people with whom the child comes in contact daily—a boy, girl, infant, adult family members, nurses, physicians, therapists, and other personnel—should be available. Hospital scrub suits, scrub caps, isolation-type gowns, masks, or other types of uniforms may be provided for children to use in acting out their hospital experiences. These simulated hospitals also serve an educational purpose: They may help a child who is to have surgery, tests, or special treatments to understand the procedures and why they are done.

Hand puppets can be useful to orient or reassure a hospitalized child. The doctor or nurse puppet on the play leader's hand answers questions (and discusses feelings) that the puppet on the child's hand has asked. A child often finds it easier to express feelings, fears,

Be alert for patient safety.
Constant supervision of children while they are playing is necessary for safety.

and questions through a puppet than to verbalize them directly. The child can make believe that the puppet is really expressing things that he or she hesitates to ask.

Other useful play materials include clay, paints, markers, crayons, stamps, stickers, sand art, cut-out books, construction paper, puzzles, building sets, and board games. Tricycles, small sliding boards, and seesaws may be fun for children who can be more physically active. Books for all age groups are also important.

Sometimes only a little imagination is needed to initiate an interesting playtime. Table 29-1 suggests activities for various age levels, most of which may be played in the child's room. These are especially useful for the child who cannot go to the playroom.

Test Yourself

✔ Why is play an important part of the hospitalization of children?

✔ Explain the difference between play therapy and therapeutic play.

✔ What is the most important factor to keep in mind when choosing play materials as well as other activities on the pediatric unit?

Table 29-1 ▌ GAMES AND ACTIVITIES USING MATERIALS AVAILABLE ON A NURSING UNIT

Age	Activity
Infant	Make a mobile from roller gauze and tongue blades to hang over a crib.
	Ask the pharmacy or central supply for different size boxes to use for put-in, take-out toys. (Do not use round vials from pharmacy; if accidentally aspirated, these can completely occlude the airway.)
	Blow up a glove as a balloon; draw a smiling face on it with a marker. Hang it out of infant's reach.
	Play "patty cake," "So Big," "Peek-a-boo."
Toddler	Ask central supply for boxes to use as blocks for stacking.
	Tie roller gauze to a glove box for a pull toy.
	Sing or recite familiar nursery rhymes such as "Peter, Peter, Pumpkin Eater."
Preschool	Play "Simon Says" or "Mother, May I?"
	Draw a picture of a dog; ask child to close eyes; add an additional feature to the dog; ask child to guess the added part, repeat until a full picture is drawn.
	Make a puppet from a lunch bag or draw a face on your hand with a marker.
	Cut out a picture from a newspaper or a magazine (or draw a picture); cut it into large puzzle pieces.
	Pour breakfast cereal into a basin; furnish boxes to pour and spoons to dig.
	Furnish chart paper and a magic marker for coloring.
	Make modeling clay from 1 cup salt, 1/2 cup flour, 1/2 cup water from diet kitchen.
	Play "Ring-Around-the-Rosey" or "London Bridge."
School-age	Play "I Spy" or charades.
	Make a deck of cards to play "Go Fish" or "Old Maid"; invent cards such as Nicholas Nurse, Doctor Dolittle, Irene Intern, Polly Patient.
	Play "Hangman."
	Furnish scale or table paper and a magic marker for a hug drawing or sign.
	Hide an object in the child's room and have the child look for it (have the child name places for you to look if the child cannot be out of bed).
Adolescent	Color squares on a chart form to make a checker board.
	Have adolescent make a deck of cards to use for "Hearts" or "Rummy."
	Compete to see how many words the adolescent can make from the letters in his or her name.
	Compete to guess whether the next person to enter the room will be a man or woman, next car to go by window will be red or black, and so forth.
	Compete to see who can name the characters in current television shows or movies.

Key Points

- The cause of the illness, its treatment, guilt about the illness, past experiences of illness and hospitalization, disruption in family life, the threat to the child's long-term health, cultural or religious influences, coping methods within the family, and financial impact of the hospitalization all may affect how the family responds to the child's illness.

- The family caregivers' role in educating the child about hospitals includes helping the child develop a positive attitude about hospitals, hospitalization, and illness and giving children simple, honest answers to their questions.

- Pediatric units are developed to create a comfortable and safe atmosphere for children and are decorated with a variety of colors. Treatments are done in treatment rooms rather than the child's room. Playrooms encourage activities for promoting normal age-related development.

- Safety is an essential aspect of pediatric care. The stress that infants, children, and their caregivers experience when a child is hospitalized may increase the frequency of accidents. Understanding the growth and development levels of each age group helps you to be alert to possible dangers for each child.

- Microorganisms are spread by contact (direct, indirect, or droplet), vehicle (food, water, blood, or contaminated products), airborne (dust particles in the air), or vector (mosquitoes, vermin) means.

- Standard precautions reduce the risk of transmission of microorganisms from recognized or unrecognized sources of infection. Transmission-based precautions are used for patients documented or suspected of having highly transmissible pathogens that require additional precautions. Hand washing is the cornerstone of all infection control. Wash hands conscientiously between seeing each patient, even when gloves are worn for a procedure.

- For a child placed on transmission-based precautions, spending extra time in the room when performing treatments and procedures, reading a story, playing a game, or talking with the child can help ease feelings of isolation.

- The three stages of response to separation seen in the child include *protest* (the child cries, refuses to be comforted, and constantly seeks the primary caregiver), *despair* (the child becomes apathetic and listless when the caregiver does not appear), and *denial* (the child appears to accept the situation, but ignores the primary caregiver when he or she returns).

- Family caregiver participation is important to relieve the child's separation anxiety. Rooming-in is encouraged to make the child feel more secure and to provide opportunities to teach family caregivers about how to care for the child after discharge. Encourage caregivers to take breaks from the child when needed.

- In a planned admission, preadmission education helps prepare the child for hospitalization. There is time to explain procedures to the child and let the child play with equipment to become familiar with it. In an emergency admission, there may be little time for explanations because physical needs are the priority.

- The family caregiver is a vital participant in the care of an ill child. The caregiver participates in the admission interview and should be included in the planning of nursing care.

- Discharge planning includes teaching the child and the family about the care needed after discharge from the hospital. Written instructions should be provided. Teaching also includes information about how the child may respond after discharge. The family should encourage positive behavior, avoid making the child the center of attention, and provide loving but firm discipline.

- In preoperative teaching, health professionals determine how much the child knows and is capable of learning, help correct any misunderstandings, explain the preparation for surgery, and explain how the child will feel after surgery. Teaching must be based on the child's age, developmental level, previous experiences, and caregiver support.

- Preoperative preparation for the child may include skin preparation, such as a tub bath or shower, shaving the surgical site, administering enemas, keeping the child NPO, urinary catheterization, and administering preoperative medications.

- Postoperative care of the child following surgery includes careful observation and assessing for complications, close monitoring of vital signs, dressings, intake and output, following postoperative orders, and providing patient and family teaching.

- Assessment and treatment of pain is important in caring for children. Use of assessment tools helps children express the amount of pain they are having. Behaviors such as rigidity, thrashing, facial expressions, loud crying or screaming, flexion of knees (indicating abdominal pain), restlessness, and irritability may indicate the child is in pain. Physiologic changes, such as increased pulse rate and blood pressure, sweating palms, dilated pupils, flushed or moist skin, and loss of appetite, also may indicate pain.

➤ Play is the principal way in which children learn, grow, develop, and act out feelings and problems. In hospital play programs, children may express frustrations, hostilities, and aggressions through play without the fear of being scolded. A well-planned hospital play area with safe play materials and activities for children of all ages is important. Play therapy is a technique used to uncover a disturbed child's underlying thoughts, feelings, and motivations to help understand them better. Therapeutic play is a play technique used to help the child have a better understanding of what will be happening to him or her in a specific situation.

INTERNET RESOURCES

Virtual Pediatric Hospital
www.virtualpediatrichospital.org

Hospitalization
http://kidshealth.org

Discovery Health
http://health.discovery.com

Workbook

■ NCLEX-STYLE REVIEW QUESTIONS

1. When caring for a child in a pediatric setting, which of the following actions by the nurse indicates an understanding of standard precautions?

   a. Carrying used syringes immediately to the sharps container in the medication room

   b. Wearing one pair of gloves while doing all care for a patient

   c. Leaving an isolation gown hanging inside the patient's room to reuse for the next treatment or procedure

   d. Cleaning reusable equipment before using it for another patient

2. When discussing postoperative pain management with a caregiver of a school-aged child, which of the following statements by the caregiver indicates a need for further teaching?

   a. "My child can push the patient-controlled analgesia pump button without any help."

   b. "After the last surgery, they gave my child pain medicine shots in the leg."

   c. "Talking or singing seems to decrease the amount of pain medication my child needs."

   d. "I am relieved to know my child will have less pain than adults do."

3. A 5-year-old child placed on transmission-based precautions has a nursing diagnosis of "Risk for loneliness" as part of the child's care plan. Which of the following would best help the child cope with the loneliness?

   a. Talking to the child about how he or she feels being alone

   b. Answering the call light over the intercom immediately

   c. Encouraging the child to talk to friends on the telephone

   d. Providing age-appropriate activities that can be played alone

4. The hospitalized child away from her or his home and normal environment goes through stages of separation. Which of the following behaviors by the child might indicate the child is in the "denial" stage of separation?

   a. Crying loudly even when being held by the nurse

   b. Searching for the caregiver to arrive

   c. Ignoring caregivers when they visit

   d. Quietly lying in the crib when no one is in the room

5. After the discharge of a preschool-aged child from the hospital, which of the following behaviors by the child might indicate he or she is afraid of another separation?

   a. The child plays with siblings for long periods of time.

   b. The child carries a favorite blanket around the house.

   c. The child requests to go visit the nurses at the hospital.

   d. The child wakes up very early in the morning.

6. The nurse is following standard precautions when caring for a child on the pediatric unit when the nurse does which of the following? Select all that apply.

   a. Washes hands when gloves are removed.

   b. Wears gloves when touching contaminated articles.

   c. Cleans reusable equipment with hot water before using on another patient.

   d. Removes needle from syringe immediately after medication administration.

   e. Wears protective eye covering when secretions are likely to splash.

   f. Removes disposable gown promptly if soiling has occurred.

■ STUDY ACTIVITIES

1. Design an ideal teen activity room. List all furniture and equipment you would have, and state the use(s) for each.

2. Discuss how rooming-in can be helpful in discharge planning.

3. Plan an orientation visit for a group of preschoolers from a nursery school. Check and use what is available in the pediatric unit where you have your clinical experience.

4. Do an Internet search on "preparing children for surgery." After exploring some of the sites you find, answer the following.

   a. What are some of the sites you found?

   b. What books did you find that you think might help a caregiver prepare a child who will be having a planned surgery?

   c. What other information on these sites do you think would be helpful in preparing a child for hospitalization?

■ CRITICAL THINKING: WHAT WOULD YOU DO?

1. Your neighbor's daughter, 3-year-old Angela, is going to be admitted to the pediatric unit for tests and possible surgery.

   a. What will you say to Angela to help prepare her for the tests that will be done?

b. What activities will you suggest Angela's mother might do to prepare her daughter for this event?

c. What will you tell Angela when she asks you what surgery is?

2. Edgar, the 4-year-old son of migrant workers, is hurt in a farming accident. You are working in the emergency department when he is brought in for treatment. His grandmother, who speaks little English, is with him.

a. What will you include in Edgar's plan of care that will help both the child and his grandmother?

b. What can you do to further communication between you, Edgar, and his grandmother?

3. On a playground, you hear a child's caregiver say, "If you don't stop that, you're going to hurt yourself and end up in the hospital!"

a. What are your feelings about this statement?

b. What would you say if you had the opportunity to respond to this caregiver after this statement was made?

c. What statement do you think would have been more appropriate for the caregiver to say in this situation?

30 *Procedures and Treatments*

KEY TERMS

bolus feeding
clove hitch restraint
colostomy
elbow restraint
enteral tube feeding
gastrostomy tube
gavage feeding
ileostomy
jacket restraint
mummy restraint
papoose board
tracheostomy
urostomy

LEARNING OBJECTIVES

On completion of this chapter, you should be able to:

1. Describe nursing responsibilities when preparing the child for a procedure or treatment.
2. Describe nursing responsibilities after the child undergoes a procedure or treatment.
3. Explain different types of restraints, their uses, and safety measures to consider in children.
4. Describe appropriate positioning of the child for holding, transporting, and sleeping.
5. List methods of reducing an elevated body temperature in children.
6. Explain the reason for monitoring accurate intake and output measurements when caring for children.
7. Discuss the reasons and procedure for inserting a feeding tube and administering a gavage feeding.
8. Explain the use of gastrostomy feeding in children and how it is different from gavage feeding.
9. Describe oxygen administration methods and safety considerations for children.
10. Describe nasal or oral suctioning to improve the child's respiratory function.
11. Explain basic components of tracheostomy care for the child.
12. Discuss the use of hot or cold therapy in children in relationship to circulation.
13. Describe nursing care for three types of ostomies that are created in children with problems related to elimination.
14. Explain how and why nose and throat specimens may be collected from the child.
15. Describe four methods of urine specimen collection.
16. Explain the method of stool collection for the child.
17. Discuss the role of the nurse in assisting with procedures related to blood collection, lumbar puncture, and diagnostic tests and studies in children.

NURSE'S ROLE IN PREPARATION AND FOLLOW-UP

As a pediatric nurse, your role in performing or assisting with procedures and treatments includes following guidelines set by the healthcare institution. These guidelines include the preparation before the procedure, as well as the follow-up needed when the procedure is completed. You are also responsible for following facility policies and ensuring patient safety before, during, and after all procedures and treatments.

Preparation for Procedures

An important role in preparation for pediatric procedures is supporting the child and family. It is also important to follow the facility's policies to ensure that legal requirements and safety precautions are met.

■ **Figure 30-1** The nurse explains the procedure to the older child in a calm, reassuring manner and allows him to ask questions. This open communication helps minimize the child's stress related to the procedure.

Psychological or Emotional Support

Many procedures in highly technological health care facilities may be frightening and painful to children. You can be an important source of comfort to children who must undergo these procedures, even though it is difficult to assist with or perform procedures that cause discomfort or pain. Explain the procedure and its purpose to the caregiver to help decrease anxiety.

Explain the procedure to the child in a manner appropriate for the child's age and level of development. If the child is old enough to understand, explain the purpose of the procedure and the expected benefit. Encourage the child to ask questions and give complete answers (Fig. 30-1). Toddlers require some explanation of procedures and what to expect, but their understanding will be limited. Even when toddlers grasp the words, they are not likely to fully understand the meaning. The reality is the pain that occurs. For infants, help to soothe and comfort before and after the procedure.

Sometimes children's interest can be diverted so that they may forget their fear. They must be allowed to cry if necessary, and they should always be listened to and have their questions answered. It takes maturity and experience to know exactly which questions are stalling techniques and which call for firmness and action. Children need someone to take charge in a kind, firm manner that tells them the decision is not in their

Here's an important tip.

When the caregiver's anxiety and concerns decrease, the child in turn often will have less anxiety.

hands. They are too young to take this responsibility for themselves.

Legal and Safety Factors

When preparing to perform or assist with any procedures or treatments, there are certain steps to follow no matter what the health care setting is. Most procedures require a written order before they are done. Clarify orders when needed. Always identify the child before any treatment or procedure; check the child's identification band and verify that information by having the child or caregiver state the child's name. Follow institution policies and, if consent is needed, see that the form is completed, signed, and witnessed. As stated earlier, discuss the procedure with the child and family caregiver and answer any questions. Washing hands before and after any procedure helps prevent or control the spread of microorganisms. Gather the needed supplies and equipment and review the steps for beginning the procedure. Safety for the child (see Chapter 29) is a priority. Standard precautions are followed for all procedures (see Appendix A).

Follow-up for Procedures

When the procedure is completed, leave the child in a safe position with side rails raised and bed lowered. For the older child, place the call light within reach. Comforting and reassuring the child is important, particularly if the procedure has been uncomfortable or traumatic. The caregiver might also have concerns or questions to discuss.

Remove equipment and supplies and dispose of them properly. Handle contaminated linens according to facility policy. If a specimen is to be taken to another department, label the specimen with the patient's name, identifying information, and the type of specimen in the container. Follow the appropriate facility policies. Often paperwork must go with the specimen, and certain precautions are taken to prevent any exposure from the specimen. Documentation includes the procedure, the child's response, and the description and characteristics of any specimen obtained. If specimens are sent to another department in the facility, also record this information.

Nurses have conflicting thoughts about the merit of giving the child some reward after a treatment. Careful thought is necessary. If a child receives a reward, it is not for being brave or good; it is simply a part of the entire treatment. The unpleasant part is mitigated by the pleasant. An older person's

Good news.

Children given a treat or a small toy after an uncomfortable procedure tend to remember the experience as not totally bad.

reward is contemplating the improved health that the procedure may provide, but the child does not have sufficient reasoning ability to understand future benefits.

Test Yourself

✔ What are two important nursing responsibilities when performing or assisting with procedures and treatments?

✔ Explain why written orders are required before doing a procedure.

✔ How should you identify the child before performing or assisting with a procedure?

✔ What are the important factors to remember for a child after a procedure?

PERFORMING PROCEDURES RELATED TO POSITION

Safety is the most important nursing responsibility when performing procedures related to positioning a child. The child's safety and comfort must be a priority when using restraints or transporting children. Safety is also an important factor when holding, transporting, or positioning children for sleep.

Using Restraints

Restraints are often needed to protect a child from injury during a procedure or an examination or to ensure the infant's or child's safety and comfort. Restraints should never be used as a form of punishment. It is important to follow the health care facility's procedure and policy regarding restraints. In addition, The Joint Commission's guidelines and standards for the use of restraints must be followed. Many settings require a written order and have a set procedure of releasing the restraint at least every 2 hours and documenting this and any findings. When possible, restraining by hand is the best method. However, mechanical restraints must be used to secure a child during intravenous infusions; to protect a surgical site from injury, such as cleft lip and cleft palate; or when restraint by hand is impractical.

Be alert to family concerns when the child is in restraints. Explanations about the need for restraints help the family understand and be cooperative. The caregiver may wish to restrain the child by hand to prevent the

Be alert for patient safety.
Safety is *always* a priority when performing any procedure on children. The importance of observing a child closely cannot be overemphasized.

use of restraints, and this action is often possible. Each situation must be judged individually.

Various types of restraints may be used for children (Fig. 30-2). Whatever the type of restraint, close observation is a necessary part of nursing care.

Mummy Restraints and Papoose Boards

Mummy restraints are snug wraps used to restrain an infant or small child during a procedure. This device is effective when performing a scalp venipuncture, inserting a nasogastric tube, or performing other procedures that involve only the head or neck. **Papoose boards** are used with toddlers or preschoolers for similar purposes.

Clove Hitch Restraints

Clove hitch restraints are used to secure an arm or leg, most often when a child is receiving an intravenous infusion. The restraint is made of soft cloth formed in a figure-of-eight. Padding under the restraint is desirable if the child puts any pull on it. Loosen the restraint and check the site at least every 1 to 2 hours. Commercial restraints also are available for this purpose. Secure this restraint to the lower part of the crib or bed, not to the side rail, to avoid possibly causing injury when the side rail is raised or lowered.

Elbow Restraints

Elbow restraints are wrapped around the child's arm and tied securely to prevent the child from bending the elbow. They are often made of muslin or other materials in two layers. Pockets wide enough to hold tongue depressors are placed vertically in the width of the fabric. The top flap folds over to close the pockets. Care must be taken to ensure that the elbow restraints fit the child properly. They should not be too high under the axillae. They may be pinned to the child's shirt to keep them from slipping. Commercially made elbow restraints may also be used.

Jacket Restraints

Jacket restraints are used to secure the child from climbing out of bed or a chair or to keep the child in a horizontal position. The restraint must be the correct size for the child. Monitor the child in a jacket restraint closely to prevent him or her from slipping and choking on the neck of the jacket. Ties must be secured to the bed frame, not the side rails, so that the jacket is not pulled when the side rails are moved up and down.

Crib Top Restraints

A crib top bubble restraint is a clear plastic covering attached to the top of the crib. This type of restraint is used for older infants and toddlers who are able to stand and climb to prevent them from climbing over the side of the bed and falling.

▮ Figure 30-2 **(A)** Mummy restraint. **(B)** Papoose board. **(C)** Clove hitch restraint. **(D)** Elbow restraint. **(E)** Commercial elbow restraint. **(F)** Jacket restraint. **(G)** Crib top restraint.

Test Yourself

✔ What are the different types of restraints used in children?

✔ When are each of the different types of restraints used?

Holding

When a child is held, he or she needs to be safe and feel secure. The three most common methods of holding a child are the horizontal position, upright position, or the football hold (Fig. 30-3). When holding an infant, always support the infant's head and back.

■ Figure 30-3 Positions to hold an infant or child: (A) horizontal position, (B) upright position, and (C) football hold.

During and after feedings, hold the infant in a sitting position on the lap for burping. Lean the infant forward against one hand and use the thumb and finger to support the infant's head; this leaves the other hand free to gently pat the infant's back (Fig. 30-4).

Transporting

When moving infants and small children in a health care setting, the safety of the child is the biggest concern. It is best to carry the infant or place him or her in a crib or bassinet. The toddler may be transported in a crib with high side rails or a high-topped crib. Strollers or wheelchairs are used when the child is able to sit. Many pediatric settings use wagons to transport children.

Older children are placed on stretchers or may be moved in their beds; often a hospitalized child who is in traction, which cannot be removed, can go to the playroom or other areas in the hospital in this manner.

Seat belts or safety straps should always be used when transporting the child.

Have some fun with this.
When transporting a child, a wagon ride is functional, as well as enjoyable for the child.

Positioning for Sleep

Position infants on their backs or supported on their sides for sleeping. These positions seem to have decreased the incidence of crib death or sudden infant death syndrome (see Chapter 20) in infants. Teach and reinforce this information to family caregivers.

PERFORMING PROCEDURES RELATED TO ELEVATED BODY TEMPERATURE

Significant alterations in body temperature can have severe consequences for children. "Normal" body temperature varies from 97.6°F (36.4°C) orally to 100.3°F (37.9°C) rectally. The body temperature generally should be maintained below 101°F (38.3°C) orally or 102°F (38.9°C) rectally, although the health care facility or practitioner may set lower limits. Methods used to reduce fever include maintaining hydration by encouraging fluids and administering acetaminophen. Because of

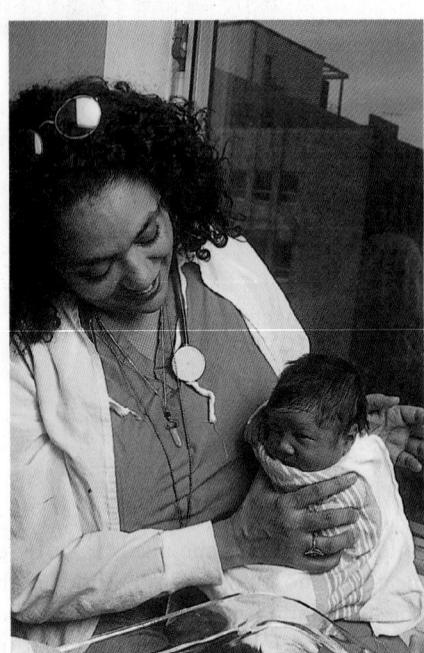

■ Figure 30-4 The nurse holds the infant in a sitting position to burp the baby.

Family Teaching Tips

REDUCING FEVER

- Do not overdress or heavily cover child. Diaper, light sheet, or light pajamas are sufficient.
- Encourage child to drink fluids.
- Keep room environment cool.
- Use acetaminophen or other antipyretics according to the care provider's directions. Do not give aspirin.
- Wait for 30 minutes and take temperature again.
- Call care provider at once if child's temperature is 105°F (40.6°C) or higher.
- Call care provider if child has history of febrile seizures.

their ineffectiveness in reducing fever and the discomfort they cause, tepid sponge baths are no longer recommended for reducing fever. Because many children have a fever but do not need hospitalization, family caregivers need instructions on fever reduction (see Family Teaching Tips: Reducing Fever).

Control of Environmental Factors

Removing excess coverings from the child with fever permits additional cooling through evaporation. Changing to lightweight clothes, removing clothes, lowering the room temperature, or applying cool compresses to the forehead may help to lower the temperature. If a child begins to shiver, whatever method is being used to lower the temperature should be stopped. Shivering indicates the child is chilling, which will cause the body temperature to increase.

Cooling Devices

A cooling device, such as a hypothermia pad or blanket, can lower or maintain the child's body temperature. The blanket is always covered before being placed next to the child's skin so moisture can be absorbed from the skin. Closely monitor the child's temperature by checking it frequently with a regular thermometer. Document the child's baseline temperature and additional temperature measurements, as well as information regarding the child's response to the treatment.

PERFORMING PROCEDURES RELATED TO FEEDING AND NUTRITION

Monitoring the intake of fluids and nutrients is important in both maintaining and promoting appropriate growth in children. As the nurse, you are responsible for accurately documenting both a child's intake and output. If a child is unable to consume adequate amounts of

fluid or foods, gavage or gastrostomy feedings are given to meet the child's nutrient needs and promote normal growth.

Intake and Output Measurements

Accurately measuring and recording intake and output are especially important in working with the ill or hospitalized child to monitor and maintain the child's fluid balance. In a well-child setting, the caregiver can provide information about the child's usual patterns of intake and output. With the ill or hospitalized child, more exact measurements of fluid intake and output are required. In many settings, these measurements are recorded as often as every hour, and a running total is kept to closely monitor the child.

Oral fluids, feeding tube intake, intravenous fluids, and foods that become liquid at room temperature (e.g., frozen foods such as popsicles) are all measured and recorded as intake. Urine, vomitus, diarrhea, gastric suctioning, and any other liquid drainage are measured and considered output. Also, describe and record the color and characteristics of the output.

To measure the output of an infant wearing a diaper, weigh the wet diaper and subtract the weight of a dry diaper; the difference is the amount to record.

Gavage Feeding

Sometimes infants or children who have had surgery or have a chronic or serious condition are unable to take adequate food and fluid by mouth. These children must receive nourishment by means of tube or gavage feedings. **Gavage feeding,** also called **enteral tube feeding,** provides nourishment directly through a tube passed into the stomach through the nose or mouth (Nursing Procedure 30-1). This procedure is particularly appropriate in infants, but also may be used in the older child. These feedings may be given intermittently as a **bolus feeding,** or may be given continuously at a slower rate over a longer period of time. If feedings will be given continuously, a *gastrostomy tube* is often placed (see later discussion). If gavage or enteral feedings are not well tolerated, report it and await alternate orders from the provider.

Warning.
Verifying positioning of the feeding tube by inserting air (using an Asepto syringe) and listening with a stethoscope for sounds in the stomach is considered an *unreliable* method of checking for tube placement and is no longer recommended.

Gastrostomy Feeding

Whereas a gavage feeding tube is inserted into the stomach through the nose or mouth, a **gastrostomy tube** is surgically inserted through the abdominal wall into the

Nursing Procedure 30-1
GAVAGE FEEDING

EQUIPMENT

Feeding tube
Nonsterile gloves
Sterile water or water-soluble lubricating jelly
Tape or marking pen
Catheter-tip syringe (bulb or Asepto syringe)
pH tape
Feeding solution

PROCEDURE

Inserting a Gavage Feeding Tube

1. Explain procedure to child and family caregiver.
2. Wash hands.
3. Position the infant in a supine position with a towel or pillow under the shoulders to elevate the head. Position the child in a sitting position, if possible.
4. Determine the length of tubing to use by measuring from the tip of the child's nose to the earlobe, and from the earlobe down to the tip of the sternum (Fig. A).

A

5. Mark this length on the tube with tape or a marking pen.
6. Put on nonsterile gloves.
7. Lubricate the end of the tube to be inserted with sterile water or water-soluble lubricating jelly (never an oily substance because of the danger of oil aspiration into the lungs).

8. Insert tube nasally (nasogastric) or orally (orogastric).
9. Confirm placement by radiologic confirmation, the most accurate method of verifying tube placement and position. Because of the risks of repeated radiation exposure, this procedure cannot be used before each feeding (see procedure for checking placement before feeding below).
10. Secure tubing to the child's nose using adhesive tape (Fig. B).

B

11. Further secure tubing for the child's comfort by gently placing tubing behind the ear and securing to the child's cheek (Fig. C).

C

Nursing Procedure 30-1

GAVAGE FEEDING *(continued)*

Administering Gavage Feeding

1. Verify order for gavage feeding and gather supplies.
2. Wash hands.
3. Warm feeding to room temperature.
4. Explain procedure to child and family caregiver.
5. Elevate the child's head and shoulders.
6. Place a rolled-up diaper or towel behind the neck.
7. Turn the child's head and align the body to the right.
8. Put on nonsterile gloves.
9. Insert the feeding syringe (bulb or Asepto syringe) into feeding tube.
10. Verify position of tube to ensure that the tube is in the stomach by aspirating stomach contents.
11. Check the pH of the fluids aspirated. The pH of gastric contents is acidic, rather than alkaline, which would be noted if the fluid were respiratory in nature.
12. Measure and replace stomach contents that have been aspirated. In a very small infant, subtract this amount from the amount ordered for that particular feeding.
13. Slowly administer feeding over 15 to 30 minutes, letting it flow by gravity.
14. Observe for signs of distress, such as gasping, coughing, or cyanosis, which might indicate tube is incorrectly placed in the airway. Stop the feeding and withdraw the tube if any of these signs are noted.
15. Flush the tube with water after the feeding to maintain the patency of the tube.
16. Burp the infant.
17. Position the infant or child on the right side for at least 1 hour to prevent regurgitation and aspiration.
18. Discard any leftover feeding at the completion of the procedure.
19. Document:
    a. Date and time of feeding
    b. Type and size of tubing used
    c. Verify the method of placement and tube patency
    d. Type and amount of contents aspirated, pH of residual
    e. Type and amount of feeding given
    f. Child's response to and tolerance of procedure
    g. Positioning of child following feeding

stomach (Fig. 30-5A). The tube is inserted with the child under general anesthesia. Gastrostomy tubes are used in children who must receive tube feedings over a long period of time. They are also used in children who have obstructions or surgical repairs in the mouth, pharynx, esophagus, or cardiac sphincter of the stomach, or who are respirator dependent.

The surgeon inserts a catheter, usually a Foley or mushroom, that is left unclamped and connected to gravity drainage for 24 hours. Meticulous care of the wound site is necessary to prevent infection and irritation. Until healing is complete, the area must be covered with a sterile dressing. Ointment, Stomahesive, or other skin preparations may be ordered for application to the site. The child may need to be restrained to prevent pulling on the catheter, which may cause leakage of caustic gastric juices.

For long-term gastrostomy feedings, a gastrostomy button may be inserted (Fig. 30-5B). Some advantages of buttons are that they are more desirable cosmetically, are simple to care for, and cause less skin irritation.

▮ **Figure 30-5 (A)** A gastrostomy tube or **(B)** gastrostomy button is placed when long-term feedings will be needed.

A

B

Procedures for positioning and feeding the child with a gastrostomy tube are similar to those for gavage feedings. Aspirate, measure, and replace the residual stomach contents at the beginning of the procedure. Elevate the child's head and shoulders during the feeding. Following the feeding, flush the tube with water to clear the tubing and prevent the feeding solution from occluding the tube. After each feeding, place the child on the right side or in Fowler's position.

In some cases, a continuous feeding is administered at a slow rate over a period of time. These feedings are administered using a feeding pump set at a specific rate. Many times, continuous feedings are given through the night to allow the child to be disconnected from the feeding during the day. This allows the child to be less restricted in daytime activities.

Take note.

Both gavage and gastrostomy tubes can also be used to administer liquid or dissolved forms of oral medications (see Chapter 31). Following medication administration, always flush the tube adequately with water to prevent the tube from being occluded.

When regular oral feedings are resumed, the tube is surgically removed, and the opening usually closes spontaneously.

Test Yourself

✔ When might a cooling device be used?

✔ Why is it important to monitor and document a child's intake?

✔ When are gavage or gastrostomy feedings used?

✔ What is the difference between a gavage tube and a gastrostomy tube?

PERFORMING PROCEDURES RELATED TO RESPIRATION

Oxygen administration, nasal and oral suctionings, and caring for the child with a tracheostomy are procedures you might be called on to perform for the child with a respiratory condition. Monitoring and maintaining adequate oxygenation are nursing responsibilities.

Oxygen Administration

Oxygen is administered to treat symptoms of respiratory distress or when the oxygen saturation level in the blood is below normal (see Chapter 28 for measurement of oxygen saturation). Depending on the child's age and oxygen needs, many different methods are used to deliver oxygen (Table 30-1). Infants, as well as older children, might have oxygen administered by nasal cannula or prongs, mask, or via an oxygen hood. Oxygen tents may also be used. The oxygen concentration is more difficult to maintain in the tent because it is opened many times throughout the day. The tent may be frightening to children, so they must be reassured frequently (Fig. 30-6).

Whatever equipment is used to administer oxygen, explain the procedure and equipment to the child and the caregiver. Letting the child hold and feel the equipment and flow of oxygen through the device helps decrease the child's fear and anxiety about the procedure. The device warms and humidifies oxygen to prevent the recipient's nasal passages from becoming dry. Closely monitor children receiving oxygen therapy;

Don't forget.

An advantage of using an oxygen tent for the toddler and school-age child is that no device has to be put over the child's nose or face.

Table 30-1 ▌ **METHODS OF OXYGEN ADMINISTRATION**

Method	Age or Reason to Use	Nursing Concerns When Using
Nasal prongs/cannula	Many sizes available Nasal prongs fit into child's nose Toddlers may pull out of nose, other method better	Not humidified; causes dryness Keep nasal prongs clean and clear of secretions Monitor nostrils for irritation
Mask	Various sizes available Covers mouth and nose, not eyes Humidified, decreases dryness	Not used in comatose children
Hood	Fits over head and neck of child Clear so child can be seen	May be frightening for child
Oxygen tent/croupette	Equipment does not come in contact with face Allows for movement inside tent	Difficult to see child in tent Difficult for child to see out Child feels isolated Change clothing and linen often Keep siderails up
Tracheostomy	Used in emergencies or when long-term oxygen is needed	Must be kept clean with airway patent Suction when needed

■ **Figure 30-6** The child in the oxygen tent needs frequent reassurance. Side rails are always raised when the child is unattended.

■ **Figure 30-7** A bulb syringe is used to remove secretions from the nose and mouth.

when oxygen is to be discontinued, it is done so gradually. Check equipment frequently to ensure proper functioning, cleanliness, and correct oxygen content. Exposure to high concentrations of oxygen can be dangerous to small infants and children with respiratory diseases.

Many times children are cared for in a home setting while receiving oxygen. Teach the family caregiver regarding oxygen administration, equipment, and safety measures (see Family Teaching Tips: Oxygen Safety).

Nasal/Oral Suctioning

Excess secretions in the nose or mouth can obstruct the infant's or child's airway and decrease respiratory function. Coughing often clears the airway, but when the infant or child is unable to remove secretions, they are removed by suctioning. Use a bulb syringe to remove secretions from the nose and mouth (Fig. 30-7). Sterile normal saline drops may be used to loosen dried nasal secretions. Nasotracheal suctioning with a sterile suction

catheter may be needed if secretions cannot be removed by other methods.

Tracheostomy Care

A **tracheostomy** is a surgical procedure in which an opening is made into the trachea so that a child with a respiratory obstruction can breathe. A tracheostomy is performed in emergency situations or in conditions in which infants or children have a blocked airway. Mechanical ventilation and oxygen can be supplied using a ventilator, when needed.

Children with a tracheostomy are cared for initially in a hospital setting; children with a long-term condition often are cared for at home or in long-term care facilities. The tracheostomy tube is suctioned to remove mucus and secretions and to keep the airway patent. The plastic or metal tracheostomy tube must be cleaned often to decrease the possibility of infection. Care of the skin around the site will prevent breakdown. A tracheostomy collar or mist tent provides moisture and humidity. The tracheostomy prevents the child from being able to cry or speak, so monitor closely and find alternative methods of communicating with the child.

PERFORMING PROCEDURES RELATED TO CIRCULATION

Heat or cold therapy may be used to treat problems associated with circulation. After a provider has written an order for heat or cold therapy, you may be responsible for applying the treatment, closely monitoring the effects of the treatment, and documenting those observations.

Heat Therapy

The local application of heat increases circulation by vasodilatation and promotes muscle relaxation, thereby relieving pain and congestion. It also speeds the formation and drainage of superficial abscesses.

Artificial heat should never be applied to the child's skin without a specific order. Tissue damage can occur, particularly in fair-skinned people or in those who have

Family Teaching Tips

OXYGEN SAFETY

- Keep equipment clean. Dirty equipment can be a source of bacteria.
- Use signs noting that oxygen is in use.
- Give good mouth care. Use swabs and mouthwash.
- Offer fluids frequently.
- Keep nose clean.
- Don't use electric or battery-powered toys.
- Don't allow smoking, matches, or lighters nearby.
- Don't keep flammable solutions in room.
- Don't use wool or synthetic blankets.

experienced sensory loss or impaired circulation. Children require close monitoring, and none should receive heat treatments longer than 20 minutes at a time, unless specifically ordered by the provider.

Moist heat produces faster results than does dry heat and is usually applied in the form of a warm compress or soak.

Dry heat may be applied by means of an electric heating pad, a K-pad (a unit that circulates warm water through plastic-enclosed tubing), or a hot water bottle. Many children have been burned because of the improper use of hot water bottles; therefore, these devices are not recommended. Electric heating pads and K-pads should be covered with a pillowcase, towel, or stockinette. Document the application type, start time, therapy duration, and the skin's condition before and after the application.

Be alert for patient safety.

If towels are used to provide moist heat, they should not be warmed in the microwave because the microwave may unevenly heat the towels, which in turn may burn the child.

Cold Therapy

As with heat, a provider must order the use of cold applications. In addition to reducing body temperature (see the section on Cooling Devices), the local application of cold also may help prevent swelling, control hemorrhage, and provide an anesthetic effect. Intervals of about 20 minutes are recommended for both dry cold (ice bag and commercial instant-cold preparation) and moist cold (compress, soak, and bath) treatments. Lightly cover dry cold applications to protect the child's skin from direct contact. Because cold decreases circulation, prolonged chilling may result in frostbite and gangrene.

Inspect the child's skin before and after the cold application to detect skin redness or irritation. Document the application type, start time, therapy duration, and the skin's condition before and after the application.

Detailed instructions for the therapeutic application of cold and heat may be obtained in the procedures manual of each facility and from manufacturers of commercial devices.

Test Yourself

✔ What are some methods used to administer oxygen to children?

✔ What is a tracheostomy, and when would one be used?

✔ For what reasons might heat therapy be used?

✔ For what reasons might cold therapy be used?

PERFORMING PROCEDURES RELATED TO ELIMINATION

As the nurse in the pediatric setting, you may be responsible for performing procedures related to elimination. You might administer an enema to a child as a treatment or as a preoperative procedure. When a child has a colostomy, ileostomy, or urostomy, you may care for the ostomy site and document the output from the ostomy.

Enema Administration

An enema may be used in an infant or child as treatment for some disorders or before a diagnostic or surgical procedure. Administering the enema can be uncomfortable and threatening, so it is important to discuss the procedure with the child before giving the enema. The type and amount of fluid, as well as the distance the tube is inserted, vary according to age. Lubricate the tube with a water-soluble jelly before insertion. Because the infant or younger child cannot retain the solution, hold the buttocks for a short time to prevent the fluid from being expelled. With an explanation before the procedure, the older child can usually hold the solution. A diaper or bedpan is used, and the child's back and head are supported by a pillow. Make sure a bedpan or bathroom is available before starting the enema.

Ostomy Care

Infants and children may have an ostomy created for various disorders and conditions that prevent the child from having normal bowel or bladder elimination. A **colostomy** is made by bringing a part of the colon through the abdominal wall to create an outlet for fecal material elimination. Colostomies can be temporary or permanent. A new colostomy may be left to open air or a bag, pouch, or appliance used to collect the stool. An **ileostomy** is a similar opening in the small intestine. The drainage from the ileostomy contains digestive enzymes, so the stoma must be fitted with a collection device to prevent skin irritation and breakdown. It is important to teach the child or caregiver how to care for the stoma and skin with any ostomy. Preventing skin breakdown is a priority. A **urostomy** may be created to help in the elimination of urine.

Check ostomy bags for leakage, empty them frequently, and change the bags when needed. A variety of collection bags and devices are available to be used with ostomies. Review and follow institution procedures regarding the products used and the procedure for changing the bags or appliances. The output from any ostomy must be recorded accurately.

PERFORMING PROCEDURES FOR SPECIMEN COLLECTION

Collecting or assisting in the collection of specimens is often a nursing responsibility. Standard precautions (see Appendix A) are followed in collecting and transporting specimens, no matter what the source of the specimen.

Nose and Throat Specimens

Specimens from the nose and throat are used to help diagnose infection. To diagnose respiratory syncytial virus (Chapter 36), a nasal washing may be done. A small amount of saline is instilled into the nose; then the fluid is aspirated and placed into a sterile specimen container.

To collect a nasal or throat specimen, swab the nose or the back of the throat and tonsils with a special collection swab. The swab is placed directly into a culture tube and taken to the lab for analysis. If epiglottitis (Chapter 36) is suspected, a throat culture should not be done because of possible trauma and airway occlusion.

Urine Specimens

Urine is collected for a variety of reasons, including urinalysis, urine cultures, specific gravity, and dip sticking urine for glucose, protein, and pH. Several methods can be used to obtain specimens. To monitor the intake and output, all urine is collected and measured, whether voided into a diaper, urinal, bedpan, or toilet collection device (see Intake and Output Measurement). If urine specimens are needed for diagnostic purposes, other methods of collection may be used. Cotton balls can be placed in the diaper of an infant; the urine squeezed from the cotton ball can be collected and used for many urine tests. Because toddlers and young children cannot usually void on command, offer them fluids 15 to 20 minutes before the urine specimen is needed. Offering privacy to the older child and adolescent is important when obtaining a urine specimen.

This advice could save the day!

When requesting a specimen, use the word the child knows to identify urination, such as "pee-pee" or "potty," so the child will understand.

In preparation for collecting a urine specimen, position the infant or child so that the genitalia are exposed and the area can be cleansed. On the male patient, wipe the tip of the penis with a soapy cotton ball, followed by a rinse with a cotton ball saturated with sterile water or wiped with a commercial cleaning pad. In the female patient, clean the labia majora front to back using

■ **Figure 30-8** The nurse cleans the perineal area of the female from front to back.

one cotton pad for each wipe. Then expose and clean the labia minora in the same fashion (Fig. 30-8). Rinse the area with a cotton ball saturated with sterile water. Allow the male or female genitalia to air-dry before collection methods are followed (see later discussion).

After the collection, the specimen may be sent to the laboratory in the plastic collection container or in a specimen container preferred by the laboratory. Appropriate documentation includes the time of specimen collection, the amount and color of the urine, the test to be performed, and the condition of the perineal area.

Collection Bag

To collect a urine specimen from infants and toddlers who are not potty trained, use a pediatric urine collection bag (Fig. 30-9A). For the collection bag to stay in place, the skin must be clean, dry, and free of lotions, oils, and powder. The device is a small plastic bag with a self-adhesive material to apply it to the child's skin. Remove the paper backing from the urine collection container, and apply the adhesive surface over the penis in

A

B

■ **Figure 30-9 (A)** The skin must be clean and dry in order for the urine collection bag to adhere to the child's skin. **(B)** The urine collection bag should be removed as soon as the child voids.

the male and the vulva in the female. Replace the child's diaper. Usually within a short period of time, the child will void and the specimen can be obtained. Remove the collection device as soon as the child voids (Fig. 30-9B).

Clean Catch

If a urine specimen is needed for a culture, the older child may be able to cooperate in the collection of a midstream specimen. Instruct the child as to the procedure so she or he understands what to do. The genital area is cleaned (as described earlier), the child urinates a small amount, stops the flow, then continues to void into a specimen container.

Catheterization

Occasionally, children must be catheterized to obtain a specimen, particularly if a sterile specimen is required. If the catheter is only needed to get a specimen, often a small sterile feeding tube is used. If an indwelling or Foley catheter is needed after catheterization, the catheter is left in place, the balloon inflated, and a collection bag attached.

24-Hour Urine Collection

Timed urine collections are sometimes done for a period of as long as 24 hours. The caregiver can often assist and should be instructed in the procedure. The urine is kept on ice in a special bag or container during the collection time period. At the end of the timed collection, the entire specimen is sent to the lab.

Stool Specimens

Stool specimens are tested for various reasons, including the presence of occult blood, ova and parasites, bacteria, glucose, or excess fat. Put on gloves and use a tongue blade to collect these specimens from a diaper or bedpan. Place the specimens in clean specimen containers. Stool specimens must not be contaminated with urine, and they must be labeled and delivered to the laboratory promptly. Document the time of specimen collection; stool color, amount, consistency, and odor; the test to be performed; and the skin condition.

ASSISTING WITH PROCEDURES RELATED TO COLLECTION OF BLOOD AND SPINAL FLUID

As a pediatric nurse, one of your roles is to assist with procedures performed on children. You might assist with the collection of blood samples or in holding and supporting a child during a lumbar puncture.

Blood Collection

Blood tests are part of almost every hospitalization experience and many times must be done in other settings to help with diagnosis. Although laboratory personnel or a physician usually obtains the specimens, you must be familiar with the general procedure to explain it to the child. You may be asked to help hold or restrain the child during the procedure. Blood specimens are obtained either by pricking the heel, great toe, earlobe, or finger or by venipuncture. In infants, the jugular or scalp veins are most commonly used; sometimes the femoral vein is used (Fig. 30-10). In older children, the veins in the arm are used.

A Personal Glimpse

I have been sick so many times that I don't know which one to write about. When I had hepatitis, I was very sick for a very long time. I missed a lot of school. I had to get blood tests, urine tests, and medications all the time, and I slept a lot because I felt tired all the time. Every time I had to get a blood test, I would cry because I didn't want to go. After a very long time, I got well enough to go back to school, but I couldn't play any gym games or activities because I couldn't get hit in my belly.

Justin, age 9 years

Learning Opportunity: What approach would be appropriate for the nurse to take with this patient if he were to become ill again and need medical care? What would you say to him before any treatment or procedure was done?

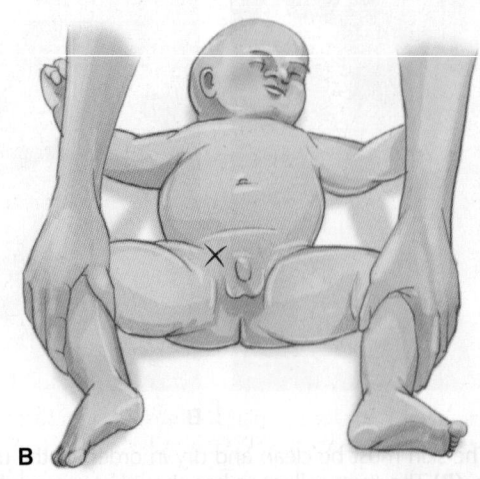

■ **Figure 30-10** **(A)** Position of infant for jugular venipuncture. **(B)** Position of infant for femoral venipuncture.

A   B

Lumbar Puncture

When analysis of cerebrospinal fluid is necessary, a lumbar puncture is performed. Children undergoing this procedure may be too young to understand its explanation. Tell the child, however, that it is important to hold still and the child will have help to do this. During the procedure, restrain the child in the position shown in Figure 30-11 until the procedure is completed. Grasp the child's hands with the hand that has passed under the child's lower extremities and hold the child snugly against your chest. This position enlarges the intervertebral spaces for easier access with the aspiration needle. The lumbar puncture is performed with strict asepsis. A sterile dressing is applied when the procedure is complete. The child must remain quiet for 1 hour after the procedure. Monitor vital signs, level of consciousness, and motor activity frequently for several hours after the procedure.

ASSISTING WITH PROCEDURES RELATED TO DIAGNOSTIC TESTS AND STUDIES

A variety of health care personnel in the radiology, nuclear imaging, and other departments of the health care setting perform many diagnostic tests and procedures. These diagnostic studies include x-rays, arteriograms, computed tomography scans, intravenous pyelograms, bone or brain scans, electrocardiograms, electroencephalograms, magnetic resonance imaging scans, and cardiac catheterizations.

A

B

C

D

▌ **Figure 30-11** Positions of infant or child for lumbar puncture: **(A)** Infant side-lying. **(B)** Infant sitting. **(C)** Child side-lying. **(D)** Child sitting.

As the nurse, your role for these tests often is to teach and prepare the child and the caregiver for the procedures. After orders have been written, request and schedule the tests or studies to be done. See that the required paperwork is completed and consents are signed. If the child must receive nothing by mouth (NPO) before the study, ensure that the NPO status is maintained. Clarify and document any allergies on the consent and requisition forms. During the procedure, you might be called on to support and comfort or restrain the child. After the procedure, perform and document the care needed.

Test Yourself

✔ How do a colostomy, an ileostomy, and a urostomy differ?

✔ How are nose and throat specimens obtained?

✔ Describe various methods for obtaining urine specimens in children.

✔ What are the reasons a stool specimen might be obtained?

Key Points

➤ When preparing for a procedure, nursing responsibilities include supporting and teaching the child and family to decrease their anxiety. Follow guidelines and policies of the health care setting, such as checking the child's identification band and ensuring signed consent is obtained.

➤ After any procedure or treatment, nursing responsibilities include ensuring the child is in a safe position, comforting and reassuring the child, answering questions, and following documentation and procedure policies of the health care setting.

➤ Types of restraints used for children include mummy restraints, papoose boards, clove hitch restraints, elbow restraints, and jacket restraints. Children in restraints require regular, careful observation to prevent injury. Family caregivers need explanations about the need for restraints.

➤ The three most common methods of holding a child are the horizontal position, upright position, or the football hold. Always support the infant's head and back. When transporting a child, the child should be held or placed in a crib, bassinet, bed, wagon, wheelchair, or stroller; use seat belts or safety straps. Position infants on their backs or supported on their sides for sleeping.

➤ Methods of reducing an elevated body temperature include not overdressing or heavily covering the child, encouraging the child to drink fluids, keeping the room environment cool, and using acetaminophen or other antipyretics, according to the provider's instructions. A cooling device may also be used. With any method, closely monitor the child's temperature.

➤ Accurately measuring and recording intake and output are especially important in working with the ill or hospitalized child to monitor and maintain the child's fluid balance.

➤ A nasogastric (through the nose) or orogastric (through the mouth) tube is used to administer gavage feedings directly into the stomach for a child who is unable to get adequate food and fluid by mouth. Refer to Nursing Procedure 30-1.

➤ If tube feedings are needed for a long period of time, a gastrostomy tube may be surgically inserted into the stomach through the abdominal wall. After the incision is made, a catheter is inserted and used as the feeding tube.

➤ The infant often receives oxygen while in an isolette or incubator. Other methods of oxygen administration include nasal cannula or prongs, mask, oxygen hood, or oxygen tent. High concentrations of oxygen can be dangerous to children, so close monitoring is needed. Oxygen safety measures are taught to caregivers and followed by care providers.

➤ Oral and nasal secretions can obstruct the airway and are removed by coughing or suctioning.

➤ In emergency situations, a tracheostomy is surgically performed to create an opening in the trachea to allow breathing. The tracheostomy must be monitored closely, suctioned, and kept clean to decrease possibilities of infection. The tracheostomy prevents the child from being able to cry or speak. Close observation and finding ways to communicate with the child are important.

➤ Local application of heat increases circulation by vasodilatation and promotes muscle relaxation, thereby relieving pain and congestion. It also speeds the formation and drainage of superficial abscesses. The local application of cold may help prevent swelling, control hemorrhage, and provide an anesthetic effect.

➤ A colostomy is created as an outlet for fecal material elimination. An ileostomy is a similar opening in the small intestine, and the drainage contains digestive enzymes. A urostomy may be created to help in the elimination of urine.

➤ Nasal washings and specimens taken from the nose or throat may be used to diagnose infection.

➤ To collect a urine specimen from an infant, place cotton balls in the diaper and squeeze urine from the cotton ball. Other urine collection methods include using a pediatric urine collection bag, or collecting a midstream specimen (clean catch), catheterization, and 24-hour collection.

➤ Wear gloves and use a tongue blade to collect a stool specimen from the diaper or bedpan.

➤ For blood collection or lumbar puncture, explain the procedure to the child and family and help hold the child still. For diagnostic tests and studies, assist by supporting and teaching the child and caregiver, preparing the child for the procedure, completing required paperwork, getting consents signed, maintaining NPO status, clarifying allergies, and documenting what has been done.

INTERNET RESOURCES

www.kidswithtubes.org
www.tracheostomy.com
www.aboutkidsgi.org

Workbook

▪ NCLEX-STYLE REVIEW QUESTIONS

1. When the nurse is performing or assisting the care provider with a procedure, which of the following actions by the nurse would be the highest priority?

   a. Explain the procedure to the child.
   b. Gather the needed supplies.
   c. Identify the child before beginning the procedure.
   d. Document the procedure immediately after completion.

2. The nurse is inserting a nasogastric tube on a toddler. Which of the following restraints would be the most appropriate for the nurse to use with this child during this procedure?

   a. Mummy restraint
   b. Clove hitch restraint
   c. Elbow restraint
   d. Jacket restraint

3. After giving instructions to the child's caregiver regarding methods used to reduce an elevated temperature, the caregiver makes the following statements. Which statement would require follow-up by the nurse?

   a. "The last time my child had immunizations, I gave her Tylenol."
   b. "When my older child had a fever, I always gave him a cold bath."
   c. "I have had trouble getting my child to drink juice."
   d. "My child does not like lots of blankets over her."

4. When caring for a 3½-year-old child who is receiving oxygen in an oxygen tent, which of the following toys or activities would be best to offer this child?

   a. A radio playing soothing music
   b. Age-appropriate books
   c. A favorite blanket belonging to the child
   d. Board games the child can play alone

5. The practical nurse is participating in the development of a plan of care for a child who has a new ileostomy. Of the following nursing diagnoses, which would be the highest priority for this child?

   a. Risk for altered development
   b. Ineffective family coping
   c. Bowel incontinence
   d. Risk for impaired skin integrity

6. The nurse needs to calculate the intake and output during the 7:00 A.M. to 7:00 P.M. shift. The child is receiving supplemental gavage feedings in addition to oral intake. The child had a bowl of cereal with 2 oz of milk and a 3-oz glass of orange juice for breakfast. At 10:00 A.M., the child voided 75 mL of urine. The child refused lunch and was given a gavage feeding of 120 mL of supplemental feeding. Early in the afternoon, the child had an emesis of 50 mL. Throughout the afternoon, the child sucked on 4 oz of ice chips. At 3:00 P.M., the child had 25 mL of apple juice and several crackers. At 4:00 P.M., the child voided 45 mL of urine and had a small formed stool. The child again refused to eat any supper and was given a 120-mL gavage feeding. Calculate the child's 12-hour intake and output.

▪ STUDY ACTIVITIES

1. Using the table below, list the types of restraints, describe each restraint, and explain the purpose of using this type of restraint in the pediatric patient.

Type of Restraint	Description	Purpose

2. Develop a teaching plan to be used in teaching a group of caregivers about caring for a child who has a fever. Include in your plan when and how to take a temperature, what to do to reduce the fever, and when it would be important for the caregiver to call the health care provider.

3. Make a list of games and activities that a child who is in an oxygen tent could play or do.

4. Do an Internet search using the key term "fever management." Find sites that would be helpful for the pediatric nurse. Answer the questions below and discuss what you found with your peers.

   a. At what body temperature is it considered that a child has an elevated temperature?
   b. What are some ways to treat a fever without using medications?

▪ CRITICAL THINKING: WHAT WOULD YOU DO?

1. Three-year-old Denise has an elevated temperature of 104.4°F (40.2°C).

   a. What specific steps would you follow in caring for this child?

b. What explanations would you give this child and caregiver about what you are doing?

c. What would be your highest priority for this child?

d. What complication would you be most concerned about for this child?

2. The caregiver of a 2-year-old child seems upset when you enter the patient's room. The child has a feeding tube in place, as well as an intravenous line. The caregiver says, "My child does not like to have her hands tied down. Why don't you just untie her?"

a. What explanation would you give to the caregiver?

b. What could you do to help reassure this caregiver?

c. What could you do to support this child?

3. You are the nurse on the pediatric unit teaching a group of your peers about caring for children in oxygen tents.

a. What will you teach regarding the reasons the child might be in an oxygen tent versus receiving oxygen by a different method?

b. What factors must be considered when providing activities for a child who must be in an oxygen tent?

c. Why must these factors be considered?

31 Medication Administration and Intravenous Therapy

KEY TERMS

acid-base balance
acidosis
alkalosis
azotemia
body surface area (BSA) method
body weight method
electrolytes
extracellular fluid
extravasation
homeostasis
induration
infiltration
intermittent infusion device
interstitial fluid
intracellular fluid
intravascular fluid
total parenteral nutrition (TPN)
West nomogram

LEARNING OBJECTIVES

On completion of this chapter, you should be able to:

1. Discuss the six "rights" of medication administration.
2. Describe developmental behaviors and nursing actions to consider when giving medications to children.
3. Explain the body weight method of calculating pediatric drug dosages.
4. Calculate low and high safe dosages of medications for children using body weight.
5. Explain the body surface area method of calculating pediatric drug dosages.
6. Discuss various routes of medication administration used in children.
7. Identify the muscle preferred for intramuscular injections in the infant and explain the process of administering the intramuscular injection in that muscle.
8. Discuss the importance of maintaining a fluid and electrolyte balance in children.
9. Differentiate between intracellular fluid and extracellular fluid.
10. Identify the reasons children might receive intravenous therapy.
11. Discuss what needs to be observed for and monitored in the child receiving intravenous therapy.
12. State the reason infusion controls, such as a control chamber or buretrol, are used in pediatric intravenous infusions.

As a PEDIATRIC nurse, your role in medication administration and caring for the child undergoing intravenous (IV) therapy includes following guidelines set by the healthcare institution as well as the guidelines related to your scope of practice. Medication administration includes following safe and accurate procedure. Your knowledge and understanding of the principles of IV therapy when caring for the child undergoing IV therapy are important.

MEDICATION ADMINISTRATION

Caring for children who are ill challenges every nurse to function at the highest level of professional competence. Giving medications is one of the most important nursing responsibilities. Medication administration calls for accuracy, precision, and considerable psychological skill.

Rights and Guidelines

Basic to administering medications to a person of any age are the following six "rights" of medication administration:

- *The right medication.* Check the drug label to confirm that it is the correct drug. Do not use a drug that is not clearly labeled. Check the expiration date of the drug.
- *The right patient.* Check the identification bracelet each time that a medication is given to confirm identification of the patient. In settings where such bracelets are not worn, always verify the child's name with the caregiver.
- *The right dose.* Always double-check the dose by calculating the dosage according to the child's weight. Question the order if it is unclear. Have another qualified person double-check any time that a

divided dosage is to be given or for insulin, digoxin, and other agents governed by the facility's policy. Use drug references or check with a physician or pharmacist for the appropriateness of the dose. Orders must be questioned before the drug is given.

- *The right route.* Give the drug only by the route ordered. Question the order if it is unclear or confusing. If a child is vomiting or a drug needs to be given by an alternate route, always get an order from the provider before administration.
- *The right time.* Administering a drug at the correct time helps to maintain the desired blood level of the drug. When giving an as needed medication, always check the last time it was given, and clarify how much has been given during the past 24 hours.
- *The right documentation.* Recording the administration of the medication, especially as needed medications, is critical to avoiding potential errors in medication administration.

Administering medications to children is much more complex than these guidelines indicate. Accurate administration of medications to children is especially critical because of the variable responses to drugs that children have as a result of immature body systems. It is important to understand the factors that influence or alter how the child absorbs, metabolizes, and excretes the medication and any allergies the child has. As the nurse, you may be responsible for the administration of medications. You may also be responsible for teaching the patient and family caregivers about the effects and possible side effects of medications given.

Ten rules to guide medication administration are presented in Box 31-1. Evaluate each child from a developmental point of view to administer medications successfully. Understanding, planning, and implementing nursing care that considers the child's developmental level and coping mechanisms helps to minimize trauma to the child receiving medication (Table 31-1).

Medication errors can occur because nurses are human and not perfect. To admit an error is often difficult, especially if there has been carelessness concerning the rules. A person may be strongly tempted to adopt a "wait and see" attitude, which is the gravest error of all. It is important to accept responsibility for your actions. Serious consequences for the child may be avoided if a mistake is disclosed promptly.

A word of caution is in order.
As a nurse, you are legally liable for errors of medication.

Box 31-1 ▮ RULES OF MEDICATION ADMINISTRATION IN CHILDREN

- Never give a child a choice of whether or not to receive medicine. The medication is ordered and is necessary for recovery; therefore, there is no choice to be made.
- Do give choices that allow the child some control over the situation, such as the kind of juice or the number of bandages.
- Never lie. Do not tell a child that an injection will not hurt.
- Keep explanations simple and brief. Use words that the child will understand.
- Assure the child that it is all right to be afraid and that it is okay to cry.
- Do not talk in front of the child as though he or she were not there. Include the child in the conversation when talking to family caregivers.
- Be positive in approaching the child. Be firm and assertive when explaining to the child what will happen.
- Keep the time between explanation and execution to a minimum. The younger the child, the shorter the time should be.
- Preparations, such as setting up an injection, solutions, or instrument trays, should be done out of the child's sight.
- Obtain cooperation from family caregivers. They may be able to calm a frightened child, persuade the child to take the medication, and achieve cooperation for care.

Test Yourself

✔ What are the six "rights" of medication administration?

✔ Why are the six "rights" especially important when administering medication to children?

✔ Why is it necessary for the nurse to always calculate and have another nurse double-check medication dosages for children?

Pediatric Dosage Calculation

Commercial unit-dose packaging sometimes does not include dosages for children, so you must calculate the correct dosage. Two methods of computing dosages are used to determine accurate pediatric medication dosages. As the nurse, you must use these methods to verify that the dosages ordered are appropriate and accurate. The first method uses the child's weight in kilograms to determine dosage. The second method uses the child's body surface area.

Table 31-1 ■ DEVELOPMENTAL CONSIDERATIONS IN MEDICATION ADMINISTRATION

Age	Behaviors	Nursing Actions
Birth–3 mo	Reaches randomly toward mouth and has a strong reflex to grasp objects	The infant's hands must be held to prevent spilling of medications.
	Poor head control	The infant's head must be supported while medications are given.
	Tongue movement may force medication out of mouth	A syringe or dropper should be placed along the side of the mouth.
	Sucks as a reflex with stimulation	Use this natural sucking desire by placing oral medications into a nipple and administering in that manner.
	Stops sucking when full	Administer medications before feeding when infant is hungry. Be aware that some medications' absorption is affected by food.
	Responds to tactile stimulations	The likelihood that the medication is taken will increase if the infant is held in a feeding position.
3–12 mo	Begins to develop fine muscle control and advances from sitting to crawling	Medication must be kept out of reach to avoid accidental ingestion.
	Tongue may protrude when swallowing	Administer medication with a syringe.
	Responds to tactile stimuli	Physical comfort (holding) given after a medication is helpful.
12–30 mo	Advances from independent walking to running without falling	Allow the toddler to choose position for taking medication.
	Advances from messy self-feeding to proficient feeding with minimal spilling	Allow the toddler to take medicine from a cup or spoon.
	Has voluntary tongue control; begins to drink from a cup	Disguise medication in a small amount of corn syrup to decrease incidence of spitting out medication.
	Develops second molars	Chewable tablets may be an alternative.
	Exhibits independence and self-assertiveness	Allow as much freedom as possible. Use games to gain confidence. Use a consistent, firm approach. Give immediate praise for cooperation.
	Responds to sense of time and simple direction	Give direction to "Drink this now" and "Open your mouth."
	Responds to and participates in routines of daily living	Involve the family caregivers and include the toddler in medicine routines.
	Expresses feelings easily	Allow for expression through play.
30 mo–6 yr	Knows full name	Ask the child his or her name before giving medicine.
	Is easily influenced by others when responding to new foods or tastes	Approach the child in a calm, positive manner when giving medications.
	Has a good sense of time and a tolerance of frustration	Use correct immediate rewards for the young child and delayed gratification for the older child.
	Enjoys making decisions	Give choices when possible.
	Has many fantasies; has fear of mutilation	Give simple explanations. Stress that the medication is not being given because the child is bad.
	Is more coordinated	Child can hold cup and may be able to master pill-taking.
	Begins to lose teeth	Chewable tablets may be inappropriate because of loose teeth.
6–12 yr	Strives for independence	Give acceptable choices. Respect the need for regression during hospitalization.
	Has concern for bodily mutilation	Give reassurance that medication, especially injectables, will not cause harm. Reinforce that medications should be taken only when given by nurse or family caregiver.
	Can tell time	Include the child in daily schedule of medication. Make the child a poster of medications and time due so he or she can be involved in care.
	Is concerned with body image and privacy	Provide private area for administration of medication, especially injections.
	Peer support and interaction are important	Allow child to share experiences with others.
12 + yr	Strives for independence	Write a contract with the adolescent, spelling out expectations for self-medication.
	Can understand abstract theories	Explain why medications are given and how they work.

Table 31-1 ■ DEVELOPMENTAL CONSIDERATIONS IN MEDICATION ADMINISTRATION *(continued)*

Age	Behaviors	Nursing Actions
12 + yr	Decisions are influenced by peers	Encourage teens to talk with their peers in a support group. Work with teens to plan medication schedule around their activities. Differentiate pill-taking from drug-taking.
	Questions authority figures	Be honest and provide medication information in writing.
	Is concerned with sex and sexuality	Explain relationships among illness, medications, and sexuality. For example, emphasize, "This medication will not react with your birth-control pills."

Body Weight Method

The **body weight method** uses the child's weight as a basis for computing the medication dosage. You must first convert the child's weight to kilograms if it is recorded in pounds. Often drug companies provide a dosage range of milligrams of a medication to number of kilograms the child weighs. To calculate a safe dose range for a child, use the child's weight in kilograms and the dosage range provided by the drug manufacturer.

Converting Pounds to Kilograms

To use the body weight method of dosage calculation, you must first convert a child's weight into kilograms if the weight has been recorded in pounds. To do this, set up a proportion using the number of pounds in a kilogram in one fraction and the known weight in pounds and the unknown weight in kilograms in the other fraction. For a child weighing 42 lb, set up the conversion as follows:

$$2.2 \text{ lb}/1 \text{ kg} = 42 \text{ lb}/X \text{ kg}$$

Then cross-multiply the fractions:

$$2.2 \text{ lb} \times X \text{ kg} = 1 \text{ kg} \times 42 \text{ lb}$$

Solve the problem for X. Divide each side by 2.2, and cancel the units that are in both the numerator and the denominator.

$$(2.2 \text{ lb} \times X \text{ kg})/2.2 \text{ lb} = (1 \text{ kg} \times 42 \text{ lb})/2.2 \text{ lb}$$
$$X = 42/2.2$$
$$X = 19 \text{ kg}$$

The child who weighs 42 lb weighs 19 kg.

Calculating Dosage Using Body Weight Method

After converting the child's weight into kilograms, calculate a safe dose range for that child. For example, if a dosage range of 10 to 30 mg/kg of body weight is a safe dosage range and a child weighs 20 kg, calculate the low safe dose using the following:

$$10 \text{ mg}/1 \text{ kg} = X \text{ mg}/20 \text{ kg}$$

Cross-multiply the fractions:

$$10 \text{ mg} \times 20 \text{ kg} = 1 \text{ kg} \times X \text{ mg}$$

Solve for X by dividing each side of the equation by 1 (canceling the units that are in both the numerator and the denominator):

$$(10 \text{ mg} \times 20 \text{ kg})/1 \text{ kg} = (1 \text{ kg} \times X \text{ mg})/1 \text{ kg}$$
$$200 \times 1 = 1X$$
$$200 = X$$

The low safe dose range of this medication for the child who weighs 20 kg is 200 mg.

To calculate the high safe dose for this child, use the following:

$$30 \text{ mg}/1 \text{ kg} = X \text{ mg}/20 \text{ kg}$$

Cross-multiply the fractions:

$$30 \text{ mg} \times 20 \text{ kg} = 1 \text{ kg} \times X \text{ mg}$$

Solve for X by dividing each side of the equation by 1 (canceling the units that are in both the numerator and the denominator):

$$30 \text{ mg} \times 20 \text{ kg} = 1 \text{ kg} \times X \text{ mg}/1 \text{ kg}$$
$$600 \times 1 = 1X$$
$$600 = X$$

The high safe dose range of this medication for the child who weighs 20 kg is 600 mg.

The safe dose range for this medication for the child who weighs 20 kg is 200 mg to 600 mg.

Body Surface Area Method

The second formula used to calculate dosages is the **body surface area (BSA) method.** The **West nomogram,** commonly used to calculate BSA, is a graph with several scales arranged so that when two values are known, the third can be plotted by drawing a line with a straight edge (Fig. 31-1). Mark the child's weight on the right scale, and mark the height on the left scale. Use a straight edge to draw a line between the two marks. The point where the lines cross the column labeled SA (surface area)

HEIGHT		SURFACE AREA	WEIGHT	
feet	centimeters	in square meters	pounds	kilograms

■ **Figure 31-1** West nomogram for estimating body surface area of infants and young children. To determine the body surface area, draw a straight line between the point representing the child's height on the left scale to the child's weight on the right scale. The point at which this line intersects the middle scale is the child's body surface area in square meters.

is the BSA, expressed in square meters (m^2). The average adult BSA is 1.7 m^2; thus, the formula to calculate the appropriate dosage for a child is:

$$\text{Estimated child's dose} = \text{child's BSA } (m^2)/1.7 \ m^2 \text{ (adult BSA)} \times \text{usual adult dose}$$

For example, a child is 37 in (95 cm) tall and weighs 34 lb (15.5 kg). The usual adult dose of the medication is 500 mg. Place and hold one end of a straight edge on the first column at 37 in and move it so that it lines up with 34 lb in the far right column. On the SA column, the straight edge falls across 0.64 (m^2). You are ready to do the calculation.

$$\begin{aligned}\text{Estimated child's dose} &= 0.64 \ m^2/1.7 \ m^2 \times 500 \text{ mg} \\ &= 0.38 \times 500 \text{ mg} \\ &= 190 \text{ mg}\end{aligned}$$

Dividing the child's BSA by the average adult BSA tells you that this child's BSA is 0.38 times that of the average adult. Multiplying 0.38 times 500 mg (the usual adult dose) gives you the child's dose. The child's dose is 190 mg.

After computing any dosage, always have the computation checked by another staff person qualified to give medication or by someone in the department who is delegated for this purpose. Errors are easy to make and easy to overlook. A second person should do the computation separately; then both results should be compared.

Oral Administration

Oral medications come in liquids, powders, capsules, and tablets. The age of the child and the type of medication helps to determine the form in which it is given. For example, small babies who are hungry may suck almost anything liquid, including liquid medicines, through a nipple unless the medicine is bitter. Medications that are available in syrup or fruit-flavored suspensions are easily administered this way. Many devices are used to give liquid oral medications to children (Fig. 31-2). One method of administering oral medications is to drop them slowly into the child's mouth with a plastic medicine dropper or oral syringe. When using a syringe, place it on the side of the tongue and slowly drip the medication into the child's mouth (Fig. 31-3). To avoid aspiration, keep the infant or child in an upright position while giving oral medications. Medication cups and spoons can be used to administer liquid medications to the older child.

Liquid medications may be in the form of elixirs, syrups, or suspensions. Elixirs contain alcohol and may cause choking unless they are diluted. Syrups and suspensions are thick and may need dilution to ensure that the child gets the full dose. Always check with the pharmacist before diluting any medication. To ensure the liquid medication is evenly distributed, some medications, especially suspensions, must be shaken well before the dose is given.

■ **Figure 31-2** Examples of devices used to administer oral medications to children.

■ **Figure 31-3** A syringe may be used to administer an oral medication by placing the syringe at the side of the tongue.

When a child is old enough to swallow a capsule or tablet, make sure that the pill is actually swallowed. When asked to open their mouths, children usually cooperate so well and open so wide that their tonsils can be inspected. While the mouth is open, look under the tongue to be sure the medication is not hidden.

It usually is best to give medicine in solution form to a small child. Some tablets can be crushed and some capsules can be opened and dissolved in a small amount of water or liquid. Consult the pharmacist before crushing a tablet or opening a capsule to be sure it is safe to administer the medication this way. Enteric-coated and time-release forms of medications can deliver an incorrect and even dangerous dosage of medication if crushed or opened and thus, should never be crushed or opened to administer. Do not use orange juice for a solvent unless specifically ordered to do so; the child may always associate the taste of orange juice with the unpleasant medicine. If the medicine is bitter, corn syrup may disguise the taste. The child may develop a dislike for corn syrup, but that is not as problematic as a lifelong dislike of orange juice.

As a general rule, medications should not be given in food because if the child does not consume the entire amount of food, the dosage of medication will not be accurate. In addition, if given with food, the child may eventually associate the bad taste of the medication with food and may refuse to eat that food. If a medication is ever given with food, it should be only a small amount of a nonessential food (such as applesauce) and the entire amount needs to be eaten.

Do not restrain the child and force medication down the child's throat. The danger of aspiration is real. Of even

Check out this tip.
When available, chewable tablets work well for the preschool child.

greater importance are the antagonism and helplessness that build up in the child subjected to such a procedure. A child's sense of dignity must be respected as much as that of an adult. Refer to Table 31-1 to review the developmental characteristics to consider at each age. For guidelines to teach caregivers administering oral medications at home, see the Family Teaching Tips: Giving Oral Medications.

Ophthalmic, Otic, Nasal, and Rectal Administration

Medications are also commonly administered through the ophthalmic (eye), otic (ear), nasal (nose), or rectal (rectum) routes. With few variations, the principles of administering medications by these routes are much the same as those for adults. Eye, ear, and nose drops should be warmed to room temperature before being administered. The infant or young child may need to be restrained for safe administration. This restraint may be accomplished with a mummy restraint or the assistance of a second person. It is important to realize that these are invasive procedures and that the young child may be resistant. Approaching the child with patience, explanations, and praise for cooperation helps gain the child's cooperation. Documentation must be completed after the administration of any medication.

Ophthalmic

To administer eye drops or ointment, place the child in a supine position. To instill drops, pull the lower lid down to form a pocket, and drop the solution into the pocket. Have the child hold the eye shut briefly, if possible, to help distribute the medication to the conjunctiva. Apply gentle pressure to the inner canthus to decrease systemic absorption. Ointment is applied from the inner to the outer canthus, with care not to touch the eye with the tip of the dropper or tube (Fig. 31-4).

■ **Figure 31-4** Administering eye ointment. Gently pull the lower lid down to form a pocket, and apply the ointment from the inner to the outer canthus with care not to touch the eye with the tip of the dropper or tube.

Family Teaching Tips

GIVING ORAL MEDICATIONS

Before giving the medication know
- The name of the medication
- What the drug is and what it is used for
- How the medication will help your child
- How often and for how long your child will need to take it
- If it should be taken with meals or on an empty stomach
- What the correct dose is and how it is given
- How soon the medication will start working
- What the possible side effects are and when the care provider should be called
- What to do if a dose is missed, spit up, or vomited
- If there are any concerns about your child taking this medication and other medications

When giving the medication
- Read the entire label and instructions each time it is given
- Check the medicine's expiration date
- Give the right dose at the right time interval
- Use a dosing instrument that will administer an exact dose such as the following:
  - Plastic medication cup
  - Hypodermic syringe without the needle
  - Oral syringe or dropper
  - Cylindrical dosing spoon
- Measure the medication carefully and read at eye level
- **ALWAYS** remove the cap on the syringe before giving the medication

- Throw the cap away or place it out of the reach of children
- Squirt it in the back of the child's mouth or along the side of the cheek (a little at a time)
- Blowing gently on your child's face after giving the medication will cause him to swallow, if he is reluctant
- Make the medication more palatable by mixing it with a small amount of liquid or soft food (such as applesauce or yogurt); use only a small amount of food and make sure your child eats the entire portion. (*Always* check with your child's pharmacist before doing so, however, because the effectiveness of some drugs may be compromised.)
- *Never* tell your child the medication is candy to get the child to take it

After the medication is given
- **If the child is wheezing, has trouble breathing, or has severe pain after taking a medication, seek emergency help by calling 911 or going to the emergency department <u>immediately</u>**
- Watch closely for side effects or allergic reactions
- **ALWAYS** use child-resistant caps and store all medications in a safe place
- Refrigerate the medication if required to do so
- Don't give medication prescribed for one child to another child
- Keep a chart and mark it each time your child takes the medication

Otic

To administer ear drops, place the infant or young child in a side-lying position with the affected ear up. In an infant or toddler, pull the pinna (the outer part of the ear) down and back to straighten the ear canal. In a child older than 3 years of age, pull the pinna up and back, as with adults, to straighten the canal (Fig. 31-5). After instilling the drops, gently massage the area in front of the ear. Keep the child in a position with the affected ear up for 5 to 10 minutes. A cotton ball may be loosely inserted into the ear to prevent leakage of medication.

Nasal

Before nose drops are instilled, the nostrils should be wiped free of mucus. For instillation, hold an infant with his or her head hyperextended over your arm. For a toddler or older child, place the head over a pillow while the child is lying flat. The infant or child should maintain the position for at least 1 minute to ensure distribution of the medication.

Rectal

To administer rectal medications, place the child in a side-lying position and wear gloves or a finger cot. Lubricate the suppository and then insert it into the rectum, followed by a finger, up to the first knuckle joint. The little finger should be used for insertion in infants. After the insertion of the suppository, hold the buttocks tightly together for 1 or 2 minutes until the child's urge to expel the suppository passes.

Intramuscular Administration

Children have the same fear of needles as adults. Inexperienced nurses are reluctant to hurt children and often cause the pain they are trying to prevent by inserting the needle slowly. When giving intramuscular (IM) or other injections, a swift, sure thrust with insertion is the best way to minimize pain, but it is important to stay calm and sure and be prepared for the child's squirming. Have a second nurse help hold the child if he or she is younger than school age or if this is his or her first injection.

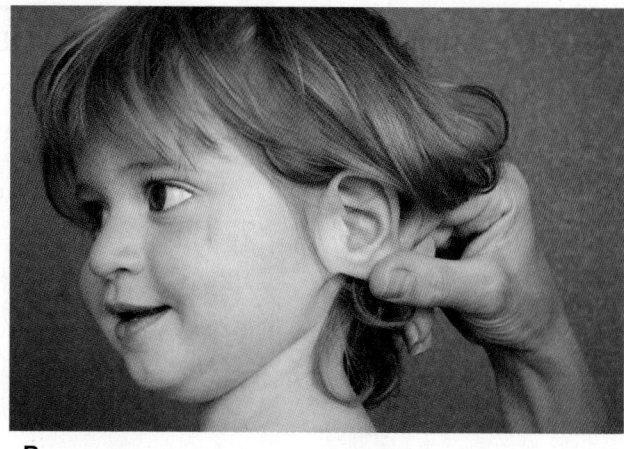

A   B

■ **Figure 31-5** Positioning for administering ear drops. **(A)** In the child older than 3 years, pull the pinna up and back. **(B)** In the child younger than 3 years, the pinna is pulled down and back.

Have an adhesive bandage ready to cover the injection site. This technique prevents young children from worrying that they might "leak out" of the hole, and the bandage serves as a badge of courage or bravery for the older child.

Table 31-2 describes IM injection sites, how to locate them, the suggested needle size, and the amount of medication to inject.

Something to always remember.

Whenever possible, give injections and do treatments in the treatment room. Keep the bed and playroom as "safe" places for the child.

Subcutaneous and Intradermal Administration

Subcutaneous injections are often used to administer insulin, allergy shots, and some immunizations. The medication is injected into the fatty tissue between the skin and the muscle. Sites most frequently used are the upper arm, abdomen, and the anterior thigh. The needles used for subcutaneous injections are small in gauge (26–30 gauge) and short in length (3/8–5/8 in). The angle of administration is either 45 or 90 degrees, depending on the size of the needle and the size of the child.

Intradermal injections are most often used for tuberculosis screening and allergy testing. The forearm is the site most often used. The needle is inserted just under the skin and a small amount of solution administered. A short and small gauged needle is used.

Intravenous Administration

Medications are often administered intravenously to pediatric patients by registered nurses. Some drugs must be administered intravenously to be effective; in some patients, the quick response gained from IV administration is important. Delivering medications intravenously is actually less traumatic than administering multiple IM injections. Extra caution is necessary to observe for irritation of small pediatric veins from irritating medications. Double-checking the medication label before hanging the IV fluid bottle is important to ensure that the medication is correct for the correct patient, that it is being administered at the correct time, and that it is not outdated. IV devices and sites are covered in the discussion of IV therapy that follows.

A Personal Glimpse

When I was 5 years old, I went to the doctor's office. I had to get shots my Mom said were for school. I don't know what they were for. I felt scared before I went. My Mom told me ideas to think about when I got the shots so I wouldn't think about it hurting. She told me to think about my puppy dog and flowers and sailing ships. The nurse told me it would hurt a little. It hurt when the nurse stuck a needle in my leg. It didn't hurt as much as I thought it would. The nurse was nice and told me I was a brave girl. I am glad I thought about my dog Cheeto. I was happy to go to kindergarten.

Adriel, age 6

Learning Opportunity: Why is it important to prepare children for medication administration? What would you include when teaching a child before giving IM injections?

Test Yourself

✔ What are some methods of administering oral medications to children?

✔ What is the procedure for administering eye drops to children?

✔ What are the important factors to remember when administering ear drops to children of different ages?

✔ What sites are used in children to administer IM injections?

Table 31-2 ▪ INTRAMUSCULAR INJECTION SITES

Muscle Site	Needle Size	Maximum Amount	Procedures
Vastus lateralis	Infant: 25 gauge, ⅝ in or 23 gauge, 1 in	1 mL	This main thigh muscle is used almost exclusively in infants for intramuscular injections but is used frequently in children for all ages. Locate the trochanter (hip joint) and knee as landmarks. Divide the area between landmarks into thirds. Inject into the middle third section, using the lateral aspect. Inject at a 90-degree angle.
	Older: 22 gauge, 1–1.5 in	2 mL	
Ventrogluteal	Assess child's muscle mass. 22–25 gauge, ⅝–1 in		With thumb facing the front of child, place forefinger on the anterior superior iliac spine with middle finger on the iliac crest and the palm centered over the greater trochanter. Inject at a 90-degree angle below the iliac crest within the triangle defined. No important nerves are in this area.
	Infant:	½–¾ mL	
	Toddler:	1 mL	
	School-age and older:	1½–2 mL	
Deltoid	Not recommended for infants		Expose entire arm. Locate the acromion process at the top of the arm. Give the injection in the densest part of the muscle below the acromion process and above the armpit. Not recommended for repeated injections. Can be used for one-time immunizations. Angle needle slightly toward the shoulder.
	Older: 22–25 gauge, 0.5–1in	Small muscle limits amount to ½–1 mL	

Labels on Vastus lateralis illustration: Greater trochanter; Site of injection (vastus lateralis); Knee joint

Labels on Ventrogluteal illustration: Iliac crest; Anterior superior iliac spine; Site of injection; Palm over greater trochanter

Labels on Deltoid illustration: Acromion process; Deltoid muscle; Site of injection

Table 31-2 ▌ INTRAMUSCULAR INJECTION SITES

Muscle Site	Needle Size	Maximum Amount	Procedures
Dorsogluteal Posterior superior iliac spine Greater trochanter of femur Gluteus maximus muscle A B	This site is not recommended in children who have not been walking for at least 1–2 yr. Not recommended for infant or toddler. School-age and older: 20–25 gauge, 0.5–1.5 in	1½–2 mL	Because of the location of the sciatic nerve, use of this site is discouraged in younger children. Place child on abdomen with toes pointing in; this relaxes the gluteus. Locate the posterior superior iliac crest and the greater trochanter of the femur. Draw an imaginary line between the two. Give the injection above and to the outside of this line. The needle should be inserted at a 90-degree angle. The accompanying figure shows **(A)** how to locate the dorsogluteal intramuscular injection site and **(B)** a child in position for a dorsogluteal injection. The site is marked by an X.

INTRAVENOUS THERAPY

IV therapy is commonly administered in the pediatric patient for the following reasons:

- To administer fluids to maintain fluid and electrolyte balance
- To administer medications, especially antibiotics, pain medication, and chemotherapy or anticancer drugs
- To administer blood or blood products
- To administer nutrients

Candidates for IV therapy include children who have poor gastrointestinal absorption caused by diarrhea, vomiting, and dehydration; those who need a high serum concentration of a drug; those who have resistant infections that require IV medications; those with emergency problems; and those who need continuous pain relief.

Planning nursing care for the child receiving IV therapy requires knowledge of the physiology of fluids and electrolytes. It also requires understanding of the child's developmental level and the emotional aspects of IV therapy for children.

Fundamentals of Fluid and Electrolyte Balance

Maintenance of fluid balance in the body tissues is essential to health. Uncorrected, severe imbalance causes death,

as in patients with serious dehydration resulting from severe diarrhea, vomiting, or loss of fluids in extensive burns. The fundamental concepts of fluid and electrolyte balance in body tissue are reviewed briefly to illustrate the importance of adequate fluid therapy for the sick child.

Water

A continuous supply of water is necessary for life. At birth, water accounts for about 77% of body weight. Between ages 1 and 2 years, this proportion decreases to the adult level of about 60%.

In health, the body's water requirement is met through the normal intake of fluids and foods. Intake is regulated by the person's thirst and hunger. Normal body losses of fluid occur through the lungs (breathing) and the skin (sweating) and in the urine and feces. In the normal state of health, intake and output amounts balance each other, and the body is said to be in a state of **homeostasis** (a uniform state). Homeostasis signifies, biologically, the dynamic equilibrium of the healthy organism. This balance is achieved by appropriate shifts in fluid and electrolytes across the cellular membrane and by elimination of the end products of metabolism and excess electrolytes.

Body water, which contains electrolytes, is situated within the cells, in the spaces between the cells, and in the plasma and blood. Imbalance (failure to maintain homeostasis) may be the result of some pathologic process in the body. Some of the disorders associated with imbalance are pyloric stenosis, high fever, persistent or severe diarrhea and vomiting, and extensive burns. Retention of fluid may occur through impaired kidney action or altered metabolism.

Intracellular Fluid

Intracellular fluid is contained within the body cells. Nearly half the volume of body water in the infant is intracellular. Intracellular fluid accounts for about 40% of body weight in both infants and adults. Each cell must be supplied with oxygen and nutrients to keep the body healthy. In addition, the body's water and sodium levels must be kept constant within narrow parameters.

A semipermeable membrane that retains protein and other large constituents within the cell surrounds cells. Water, certain salts and minerals, nutrients, and oxygen enter the cell through this membrane. Waste products and useful substances produced within the cell are excreted or secreted into the surrounding spaces.

Extracellular Fluid

Extracellular fluid is situated outside the cells. It may be **interstitial fluid** (situated within the spaces or gaps of body tissue) or **intravascular fluid** (situated within the blood vessels or blood plasma). Blood plasma contains protein within the walls of the blood vessels and water and mineral salts that flow freely from the vascular system into the surrounding tissues.

Interstitial fluid (also called intercellular or tissue fluid) has a composition similar to plasma, except that it contains almost no protein. In the infant, about 25% to 35% of body weight is attributable to interstitial fluid. In the adult, interstitial fluid accounts for only about 15% of body weight (Fig. 31-6). This reservoir of fluid outside the body cells decreases or increases easily in response to disease. An increase in interstitial fluid results in edema. Dehydration depletes this fluid before the intracellular and plasma supplies are affected.

Infants and children can become dehydrated in a short amount of time. In part, this dehydration occurs because of a greater fluid exchange caused by the rapid metabolic activity associated with infants' growth. It also occurs because of the increased BSA relative to the body fluid volume; the ratio is two or three times that in adults. Because of this, larger quantities of fluid are lost through the skin in the infant.

Because of these factors, the infant who is taking in no fluid loses an amount of body fluid equal to the extracellular volume in about 5 days, or twice as rapidly as does an adult. The

Remember this.
Infants and children become dehydrated much more quickly than do adults.

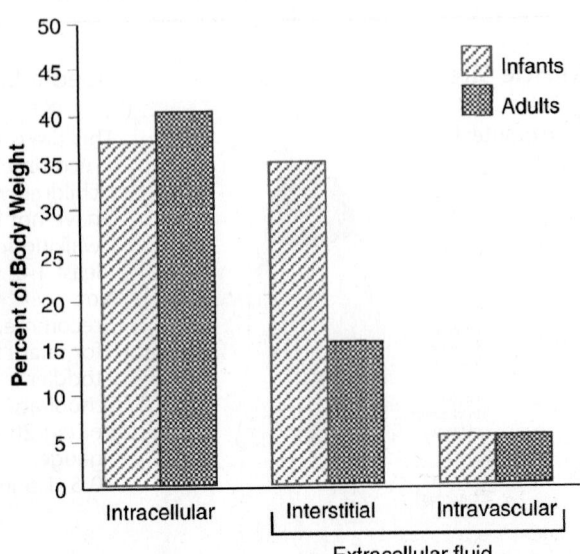

Fluid Distribution in Body

■ Figure 31-6 Distribution of fluid in body compartments. Comparison between the infant and adult fluid distribution in body compartments shows that the adult total is about 60% of body weight, whereas the infant total is more than 70% of body weight.

infant's relatively larger volume of extracellular fluid may be designed to compensate partially for this greater loss.

Test Yourself

✔ What are different reasons children might receive IV therapy?

✔ What are some disorders that might cause an imbalance of water in children?

✔ What is the difference between intracellular and extracellular fluid?

Electrolytes

Electrolytes are chemical compounds (minerals) that break down into ions when placed in water. An ion is an atom with a positive or a negative electrical charge. Important electrolytes in body fluids are sodium (Na^+), potassium (K^+), magnesium (Mg^{++}), calcium (Ca^{++}), chloride (Cl^-), phosphate (PO_4^-), and bicarbonate (HCO_3^-). Electrolytes have the important function of maintaining acid-base balance. Each water compartment of the body has its own normal electrolyte composition.

Acid-Base Balance

Acid-base balance is a state of equilibrium between the acidity and the alkalinity of body fluids. The acidity of a solution is determined by the concentration of hydrogen (H^+) ions. Acidity is expressed by the symbol pH. Neutral fluids have a pH of 7.0, acid fluids lower than 7.0, and alkaline fluids higher than 7.0. Normally, body fluids are slightly alkaline. Internal body fluids have a pH of 7.35 to 7.45. Body excretions, however, are products of metabolism and become acid; the normal pH of urine, for example, is 5.5 to 6.5.

Defects in the acid-base balance result either in **acidosis** (excessive acidity of body fluids) or **alkalosis** (excessive alkalinity of body fluids). Acidosis may occur in conditions such as diabetes, kidney failure, and diarrhea. Hyperventilation is a frequent cause of alkalosis.

Regulation of Fluids and Electrolytes

In normal health, the fluid and electrolyte balance is maintained through the intake of a well-balanced diet. The kidneys play an important part in regulating concentrations of electrolytes in the various fluid compartments. In illness, the balance may be disturbed because of excessive losses of certain electrolytes. Replacement of these minerals is necessary to restore health and maintain life. When the infant or child can take sufficient fluids orally, that is the preferred route; often though it is necessary to administer IV fluids.

IV Therapy Administration

IV fluids are administered to provide water, electrolytes, and nutrients that the child needs. As stated earlier, blood products, medications, and parenteral nutrition (see discussion that follows) are also administered intravenously. The type and purpose of IV therapy influence the equipment and site used.

Peripheral Intravenous Access

IV infusions may be administered through a peripheral vein. Over-the-needle catheters or winged-infusion needles, sometimes called "butterflies" or scalp vein needles are used. Site selection in the pediatric patient varies with the child's age. The best choice of sites is the one that least restricts the child's movements. Sites used include the hand, wrist, forearm, foot, and ankle. The

antecubital fossa, which restricts movement, is sometimes used only if other sites are not available. The scalp vein may be used if no other site can be accessed. This site has an abundant supply of superficial veins in infants and toddlers. When a scalp vein is used, the child's hair is shaved over a small area; family caregivers can be reassured that the child's hair will grow back quickly.

Older children may be permitted some choice of site, if possible. The child should be involved in all aspects of the procedure within age-appropriate capabilities. The preschool child often can cooperate if given adequate explanation. Play therapy in preparation for IV therapy may be helpful. Honesty is essential with children of any age. The older school-aged child and adolescent may have many questions that should be answered at his or her level of understanding. Family caregivers also need explanations and should be included in the preparation for the procedure. By their presence and reassurance, family caregivers may provide the emotional support the child needs and may help the child remain calm throughout the procedure.

In preparation for starting a peripheral IV line, all the equipment that may be needed should be collected. This equipment includes the IV tubing; any necessary extension tubing; the container of solution; the equipment to stabilize the site; a tourniquet; cleansing supplies used by the institution, such as povidone-iodine or alcohol swabs; sterile gauze; adhesive tape; cling roll gauze; an IV pole; an infusion pump or controller; and a plastic cannula or winged small-vein needle, usually between 21-gauge and 25-gauge (depending on the child's size).

To protect the IV site, an inverted medicine cup or a paper cup with the bottom cut out is often taped over the site. The needle is stabilized with U-shaped taping, and a loop of the tubing is taped so that if the child pulls on the tubing, the loop will absorb the pull and the site will remain intact (Fig. 31-7A and B). The older infant's hands may need to be restrained. If a site in the hand, foot, or arm is used, the limb should be stabilized on an arm board before insertion is attempted (Fig. 31-7C and D). These sites restrict the child's movement much more than the scalp site.

A   **B**   **C**   **D**

■ **Figure 31-7** Protection of the IV site: **(A)** Paper cup taped over IV site. **(B)** Scalp vein IV site with U-shaped tubing taped so that if the child pulls on the tubing, the loop will absorb the pull and the site will remain intact. **(C)** Armboard restraint used when IV site is in the hand. **(D)** IV House over the site on an infant's foot.

■ **Figure 31-8** The heparin lock allows for more freedom of movement between uses.

If the child does not require continuous IV fluid infusion but may still require IV fluids or medications intermittently, an **intermittent infusion device,** sometimes referred to as a heparin lock, may be used. This method frees the child from IV tubing between medication administrations. The veins on the back of the hand are often used for heparin lock insertion (Fig. 31-8). Medication is administered through the lock; when the administration is completed, the needle and tubing are removed and the heparin lock is flushed. A self-healing rubber stopper closes the heparin lock so that it does not leak between administrations. This method also may be used for a child who must have frequent blood samples drawn. The heparin lock is flushed every 4 to 8 hours with saline or heparin, according to the facility's procedure.

Only nurses skilled in the procedure should start an IV infusion in children. An unskilled nurse should not attempt the procedure unless under the direct supervision of a person skilled in pediatric IV administration. It is sometimes difficult to gain access to children's small veins, and they may easily be "blown." Venipuncture requires practice and expertise. If you are the staff nurse, you may serve as the child's advocate when the physician or IV nurse comes to start an infusion. If you have cared for the child, you may have the child's confidence and know the child's preferences.

Central Intravenous Access

Some solutions are administered through a central IV access line. Central venous infusions are administered through a large vein such as the jugular or subclavian vein. The line is inserted by surgical technique and is sutured into place. These catheters may exit through a tunnel in the subcutaneous tissue on the chest. Some brand names of central venous lines are Hickman, Broviac, or Groshong catheters. Caring for a child with a central venous line calls for skilled nursing care because of the danger of complications, such as contamination, thrombosis, dislodgement of the catheter, and **extravasation** (fluid

escaping into surrounding tissue). The infant or child must be closely monitored for hyperglycemia, dehydration, or **azotemia** (nitrogen-containing compounds in the blood).

Another type of central venous access is a vascular access port. Examples are brands such as Port-A-Cath and Infus-A-Port, small plastic devices that are implanted under the skin and are used for medication administration or for long-term fluid administration. Special needles are used to access these ports. The advantages of vascular access ports are that blood samples can be removed through the port, they are not visible, and they do not need a dressing over them.

When assisting with the insertion of a central IV line, gather the equipment required for the procedure. Your role will be to support the child during the procedure and be available to assist in the procedure. Dressing changes are routinely performed on the external site of a central venous device. The institution's policies must always be clarified and followed; practical nurses often assist with this dressing change. This is a sterile procedure, so sterile gloves and forceps are used. After the dressing change, the procedure is documented, as is skin condition, including any redness, swelling, drainage, or irritation.

Infusion Control

A variety of IV infusion pumps are suitable for pediatric use. The rate of infusion for infants and children must be carefully monitored. To avoid overloading the circulation and inducing cardiac failure, the IV drip rate must be slow for the small child. In addition to infusion pumps, various adapting devices are available that decrease the size of the drop to a "mini" or "micro" drop of 1/50 mL or 1/60 mL, thus delivering 50 or 60 minidrops or microdrops per milliliter, rather than the 15 drops per milliliter of a regular set. Many IV sets also contain a control chamber (or buretrol) that holds 100 to 150 mL of fluid; this chamber is designed to deliver controlled volumes of fluid to avoid the accidental entrance of too great a fluid volume into the child's system (Fig. 31-9). A syringe pump that can be programmed to deliver a small amount of fluid over a period of time may be used for IV medication administration.

Regardless of the control systems and safeguards, the child and the IV infusion require monitoring as frequently as every hour. Check the IV site to see that it is intact and observe for redness, pain, **induration** (hardness), flow rate, moisture at the site, and swelling. Documentation is sometimes done on an IV flow sheet that lists the flow rate, the amount in the bottle, the amount in the burette, the amount infused, and the condition of the site. It is important to accurately document IV fluid intake on any child undergoing IV therapy.

Parenteral Nutrition Administration

Total parenteral nutrition (TPN) is the administration of dextrose, lipids, amino acids, electrolytes, vitamins, minerals, and trace elements into the circulatory system to

■ **Figure 31-9** An infant with an infusion pump and an infusion chamber. The infusion chamber has a "mini" dropper to reduce the size of the drops.

meet the nutritional needs of a child whose needs cannot be met through the gastrointestinal tract.

Peripheral vein parenteral nutrition may occasionally be used on a short-term basis. Extra care must be taken to avoid **infiltration,** fluid leaking into the surrounding tissues, because tissue injury and sloughing may be severe.

For long-term administration of TPN, a central venous access device may be inserted (see discussion of central venous access earlier in the text). Children can be discharged from the hospital on TPN therapy after family caregivers have been instructed in the care of the device, thus reducing hospital time and expense.

Test Yourself

✔ What is the difference between peripheral and central IV access?

✔ What sites might be used for peripheral IV therapy in children?

✔ Why is it important to use an infusion control device for IV therapy in children?

Key Points

➤ The six "rights" of medication administration include the right medication, patient, dose, route, time, and documentation.

➤ Administering medications to children is complex because of their immature body systems and varying sizes. Age-related behaviors and developmental considerations should be kept in mind, and age-appropriate nursing actions should be used when administering medications to children.

➤ To use the body weight method of pediatric dosage calculation, always calculate the child's weight in kilograms if the medication is ordered as a dose per kilogram. Then calculate the safe low and high doses by using the child's body weight. Always have another person check computations of drug dosage before administering medications to children.

➤ The BSA method can also be used to calculate pediatric dosages. A West nomogram is used to determine the child's BSA based on his or her height and weight. Then use the BSA and usual adult dosage of the medication to calculate the child's dose.

➤ Routes of pediatric medication administration are oral, ophthalmic, otic, nasal, rectal, IM, subcutaneous, intradermal, and IV. Oral is the most common route.

➤ The muscle preferred for IM injections in the infant is the vastus lateralis. To use the vastus lateralis muscle for an IM injection, locate the trochanter (hip joint) and knee as landmarks. Divide the area between landmarks into thirds. Using the middle section of the three sections, follow correct procedure for drawing up the medication and inject the needle into the lateral aspect of the leg at a 90-degree angle.

➤ Maintaining fluid balance in the body tissues is essential to health. Severe imbalance can occur rapidly in children because they dehydrate much faster than do adults. Serious dehydration can result from diarrhea, vomiting, or loss of fluids in extensive burns. Electrolytes help maintain the acid-base balance in the body, so the electrolyte balance in the body is also essential.

➤ Intracellular fluid is contained within the body cells and makes up 40% of body weight in children and adults. Extracellular fluid is situated outside the cells and is either interstitial fluid (situated within the spaces or gaps of body tissue) or intravascular fluid (situated within the blood vessels or blood plasma).

➤ IV therapy might be administered to children to provide water, electrolytes, blood products, medications, or nutrients (TPN) the child needs.

➤ IV fluid administration requires careful observation of the child's appearance, vital signs, intake and output, and the fluid's flow rate.

➤ IV flow rate is regulated by the use of a control chamber or buretrol in order to closely monitor the rate of infusion. IV infusion sites must be monitored to avoid infiltration and tissue damage.

INTERNET RESOURCES

Dosage Calculation
http://home.roadrunner.com/~nurdosagecal

Medication Administration
www.fda.gov/FDAC/features/196_kid.html
http://nrc.uchsc.edu/SPINOFF/MED/MED.htm

Workbook

▪ NCLEX-STYLE REVIEW QUESTIONS

1. The pediatric nurse is administering oral liquid medications to a 4-year-old child. Which of the following statements by the nurse indicates an understanding of the child's developmental level?

   a. "Your Mom will help me hold your hands."
   b. "Would you like orange or apple juice to drink after you take your medicine?"
   c. "You can make a poster of the schedule for all your medications."
   d. "This booklet tells all about how this medicine works."

2. The nurse is calculating a medication dosage for an infant who weighs 16 lb. How many kilograms does the child weigh?

   a. 0.72 kg
   b. 1.7 kg
   c. 7.3 kg
   d. 9.0 kg

3. The dosage range of Demerol for a school-aged child is 1.1 mg/kg to 1.8 mg/kg. Of the following, which dosage would be appropriate to give a school-age child who weighs 76 lb?

   a. 24.4 mg
   b. 30.0 mg
   c. 60 mg
   d. 110 mg

4. When administering an IM injection to a 4-month-old infant, the best injection site to use would be the

   a. vastus lateralis.
   b. ventrogluteal.
   c. deltoid.
   d. dorsogluteal.

5. Infusion pumps and volume control devices are used when children are given IV fluids. The most important reason these devices are used is to

   a. regulate the rate of the infusion.
   b. decrease the size of the drops delivered.
   c. reduce the chance of infiltration.
   d. administer medications.

6. The nurse is administering an IM injection using the vastus lateralis muscle. Mark an X on the

location of the vastus lateralis muscle in this child's right leg.

▪ STUDY ACTIVITIES

1. Caitlin weighs 28.5 lb (13 kg) and measures 35.5 in (90 cm). Find her BSA using the West nomogram. Calculate the dose of a medication for her if the adult dosage is 750 mg.

2. Describe how you would approach each of the following children when giving oral medications and IM medications.

	Oral Medications	Intramuscular Medications
6-month-old Kristi		
18-month-old Jared		
3-year-old Sarah		
4.5-year-old Miguel		
8-year-old Danika		
16-year-old Jon		

3. Identify each of the IM injection sites, state how to locate each of the sites, and name the landmarks used.

4. Go to the following Web site: www.findarticles.com. In the space next to "Find," type in "Recommendations for preventing medication errors in children" and press "Enter." Click on the link for the article by this name, and read the article.

   a. What is the recommendation for liquid medications?

   b. What does the author say should always be written before a decimal for doses that are less than 1?

■ CRITICAL THINKING: WHAT WOULD YOU DO?

1. You have been asked to lead a discussion with a group of your peers about medicating children.

   a. What is the importance of following the six "rights" of medication administration?

   b. What do you think are the most important responsibilities of the nurse when medicating children?

   c. How does medicating children differ from medicating adults?

   d. What steps would you take if you discovered that you had made a medication error?

   e. What are your legal responsibilities related to medication errors?

SPECIAL CONCERNS OF PEDIATRIC NURSING

UNIT

SPECIAL CONCERNS OF PEDIATRIC NURSING

32 The Child With a Chronic Health Problem

KEY TERMS

chronic illness
denial
gradual acceptance
overprotection
rejection
respite care
stigma

LEARNING OBJECTIVES

On completion of this chapter, you should be able to:

1. Identify 10 conditions that cause chronic illness in children.
2. Explain 10 concerns common to many families of a child with a chronic illness.
3. Discuss the effects chronic illness may have on the child's parents.
4. Discuss the effects chronic illness may have on the child's growth and development.
5. Describe the effects the child's chronic illness may have on well siblings in the family, including siblings' positive and negative responses.
6. Identify ways the nurse may encourage growth and development, self-care, and socialization in the child with a chronic illness.
7. Describe how the nurse can help the family adjust to the child's chronic condition.
8. Discuss general guidelines for preparing the family for home care of the child with a chronic condition.

A CHRONIC illness is a condition of long duration or one that progresses slowly, shows little change, and often interferes with daily functioning. Chronic illness during childhood may affect a child's physical, psychosocial, and cognitive development. The illness also affects the entire family. As a nurse, you may be involved in caring for these children and their families at the stage of diagnosis and as they continue to experience ongoing and long-term needs over many years. Therefore, you can play a vital role in helping the family adjust to the condition.

CAUSES OF CHRONIC ILLNESS IN CHILDREN

Chronic illness is a leading health problem in the United States. The numbers of chronically ill children are growing as more infants and children survive prematurity, difficult births, congenital anomalies, accidents, and illnesses that once were fatal. Most children experience only brief, acute episodes of illness; however, a significant number are affected by chronic health problems.

Diseases that cause chronic illness in children include congenital heart disease, cystic fibrosis, juvenile arthritis, asthma, hemophilia, muscular dystrophy, leukemia,

other malignancies, spina bifida, and immunodeficiency syndromes. These specific chronic health problems of children are discussed in chapters throughout this text. Each requires individualized management based on the disease process and the abilities of the patient and family to understand and comply with the treatment regimen.

EFFECTS OF CHRONIC ILLNESS ON THE FAMILY

The diagnosis of a chronic health problem causes a crisis in the family, whether it happens during the first few hours or days of the child's life or much later. Although the specific disorders that cause chronic illness are varied, all chronic health problems create some common challenges for patients and families. Some of these concerns include:

- Financial concerns such as payment for treatment, living expenses at a distant health care facility, or caregiver's job loss because of time not at work
- Administration of treatments and medications at home
- Disruption of family life such as vacations, family goals, and careers
- Educational opportunities for the child

699

- Social isolation because of the child's condition
- Family adjustments because of the disease's changing course
- Reaction of well siblings
- Stress among caregivers
- Guilt about and acceptance of the chronic condition
- Care of the child when family caregivers can no longer provide care

The effects of these challenges on the family depend, in part, on family members' coping abilities. How families cope with chronic illness varies greatly from one family to another. Families who have a strong support system usually are better able to meet these challenges.

Parents and Chronic Illness

When family caregivers learn of the child's diagnosis, their first reactions may be shock, disbelief, and denial. These reactions may last for a varied amount of time, from days to months. The initial response may be one of mourning for the "perfect" child they lost, combined with guilt, blame, and rationalization. The caregivers may seek advice from other professionals and actually may go "shopping" for another health care provider, hoping to find the diagnosis is incorrect or not as serious as they have been told. They may refuse to accept the diagnosis or talk about it, or they may delay seeking or agreeing to treatment. Gradually, however, they adjust to the diagnosis. They may enter a period of chronic sorrow when they adapt to the child's state of chronic illness but do not necessarily accept it. They often waver between the stages, and they experience emotional highs and lows as they care for the child and meet the challenges of daily life.

Several typical caregiver responses have been identified: overprotection, rejection, denial, and gradual acceptance. Caregivers responding with **overprotection** try to protect the child at all costs: They hover, which prevents the child from learning new skills; they fail to use discipline; and they use any means to prevent the child from experiencing any frustration. Caregivers in **rejection** distance themselves emotionally from the child. Although they provide physical care, they tend to scold and correct the child continuously. Caregivers in **denial** behave as though the condition does not exist, and they encourage the child to overcompensate for any disabilities. Caregivers who respond with **gradual acceptance** take a common-sense approach to the child's condition; they help the child to set realistic goals for self-care and independence and encourage the child to achieve social and physical skills within his or her capability (Fig. 32-1).

Economic pressures can become overwhelming to the families of chronically ill children. If the family does not have adequate health insurance, the costs of treatment may be enormous. Away-from-home living costs may become a problem if the child must go to a distant hospital for further diagnosis or treatment. To keep health insurance benefits, a family caregiver may feel tied to a job, which creates additional stress. The time required to

■ **Figure 32-1** This father and brother encourage a child with a disability to participate in outdoor activities.

take the child to medical appointments can be excessive and may threaten job security because of the time lost from the job.

Families must make many adjustments to care for the chronically ill child. The family caregivers may have to learn to perform treatments and give medications. Family life is often disrupted. Vacations may be nonexistent, and the family may be limited in how they can spend their leisure time. Families may have difficulty finding babysitters and have little opportunity for a break from the routine. Some families become isolated from customary social activities because of the responsibilities of caring for their child. **Respite care** (care of the ill child so that the caregivers can have a period of rest and refreshment) is often desperately needed but is not readily available in many communities. Families in which both parents work may have to forgo a second income so that one adult can stay home with the child.

As the child grows, concerns about education may become foremost among the caregivers' worries. These concerns include the availability of appropriate education, early learning opportunities, physical accessibility of the facilities, acceptance of the child by school personnel and classmates, inclusive versus segregated classes, availability and quality of homebound teaching, and general flexibility of the school's teachers and administrators. Few schools are prepared to accommodate treatments at school that would otherwise require the child to leave during the school day. Family caregivers often must become the child's advocate to preserve as much normalcy as possible in the child's educational experience.

As the child's condition changes, the family must make additional changes. All of these stressors may strain a marriage, and couples may have little time left for each other when caring for a chronically ill child. Sometimes partners in relationships blame each other for the child's problems, which further strains the relationship. Single-parent families have significant needs to which health care personnel must be especially sensitive.

The Child and Chronic Illness

The child with a chronic illness may face many problems that interfere with normal growth and development. These problems vary with the diagnosis and condition. For example, some conditions require the child to be immobilized; if this occurs for a school-aged child during the stage of industry and inferiority, the child cannot complete tasks of industry, such as helping with household chores or working on special projects with siblings or peers. The child's attitude toward the condition is a critical element in its long-term management and the family's adjustment.

The child's response to the chronic condition is influenced by the response of family caregivers. Whether

A Personal Glimpse

I am 16 years old, and I was diagnosed with cystic fibrosis at birth. Every morning, I wake up and have many things that I have to accomplish; taking a breathing treatment, having percussion done, and taking many pills. I guess it isn't so bad if you are used to doing it every day, but it is a bit annoying having the same routine all the time. I have been doing all of this for 16 years. I sometimes feel that I am very different from other people. My friends don't feel it is weird having me as a friend, but they know that I have this disease and they are afraid of what can happen to me. My friends don't treat me any different. I think that is the most important thing. It is good that I have friends who can care so much that they don't let it bother them.

I don't like it when I have to cough all the time; everyone stares at me. When I am in school, at lunch I have to take pills before I eat. Everyone is always asking me why I am taking the pills. Even when I go to a friend's house, I have to take my medication and get my percussions done. My friends usually help out with the percussions.

A lot of times, I feel very lonely because I am the only one in my family that has this disease. No one knows what I am feeling, and that sometimes makes me very lonely and afraid. I have a twin brother who really cares for me a lot. When anyone asks about my illness, he is usually the person to explain it to them. He has always been there for me when I needed him. When I have to go in the hospital, he gets my work for me. We are very close. I am glad to have a brother like him.

I am very lucky to have a family that cares for me and loves me like they do. They are always helping me when I need percussions done and they are very supportive. I don't know what I would do without their help. They all took care of me when I couldn't. They still do now. I owe them a lot of credit. I love them very much and always will.

Gretchen, age 16

Learning Opportunity: Do you think this adolescent has accepted her disease? What are the things she shared that you think show that she has or has not accepted her condition? What are your thoughts about her family and friends?

caregivers respond with overprotection, rejection, denial, or gradual acceptance, as discussed earlier, may greatly affect the child's attitude and motivation to participate in self-care activities.

As with any illness, children may perceive a chronic illness as punishment for a bad thought or action, depending on the child's developmental stage at the time of diagnosis. This perception is also influenced by the attitudes of parents and peers. Rejection by caregivers, for example, may further convince the child that the illness is a punishment. The child's perception is also shaped by whether the dysfunctional body part is visible. Problems such as asthma, allergies, and epilepsy are difficult for young children to understand because "what's wrong" is inside, not outside.

The child's family, peers, and school personnel comprise the support system that can affect the child's adaptation. Sometimes the efforts necessary to meet the child's physical needs are so great that finding time and energy to meet the child's emotional needs can be difficult for members of the support team. The older child with a chronic illness also has developing sexual needs that should not be ignored but must be acknowledged and respected.

Disease progression can add additional stresses over time. For instance, Hodgkin's disease can be successfully treated for a time with chemotherapy and radiation therapy, but this adds the side effects of treatment (steroid-induced acne, edema, and alopecia) to the disease manifestations of night sweats, chronic fatigue, pruritus, and gastrointestinal bleeding. The child with Duchenne muscular dystrophy gradually weakens so that in adolescence he or she is wheelchair-bound, when peers are actively involved in sports and exploring sexual relationships. These stresses can add up to more than one young person can cope with for long.

Discrimination continues to be present in the life of the chronically ill child and the family. Discrimination can occur in relationships among children, and social exclusion of the chronically ill child is common. Physical barriers may present problems that families must struggle to help their child overcome. Sometimes hurtful discrimination is as simple as being stared at in public places.

Siblings and Chronic Illness

Some degree of sibling rivalry can be found in most families with healthy children, so it is not surprising that a child with a chronic health problem can seriously disrupt the lives of brothers and sisters. Much of the family caregivers' time, attention, and money are directed toward management of the ill child's problem. This can cause anger, resentment, and jealousy in the well siblings. The caregivers' failure to set limits for the ill child's behavior while maintaining discipline for the healthy siblings can cause further resentment. Some family caregivers unknowingly create feelings of guilt in the healthy children by overemphasizing the ill child's needs.

Family Teaching Tips

HELPING SIBLINGS COPE WITH A CHRONIC ILLNESS

- Find time for special activities with the healthy children.
- Explain the ill child's condition as simply as possible.
- Involve the healthy siblings in the care of the ill child according to his or her developmental ability.
- Set behavioral limits for all children in the family.

Siblings may feel that having a brother or sister with a chronic illness is a **stigma**, a mark of embarrassment or shame, especially if the ill child has a physical disfigurement or apparent cognitive deficit. Siblings may choose not to tell others about the ill child or may be selective in whom they tell, choosing to tell only persons they can trust. An older sibling is more likely to tell others than a younger one, perhaps because the older child tends to understand more about the illness and its effect.

Both positive and negative influences can be found in the behaviors of well siblings. Some siblings react with anger, hostility, jealousy, increased competition for attention, social withdrawal, and poor school performance. On the other hand, many siblings demonstrate positive behaviors such as caring and concern for the ill sibling, cooperating with family caregivers in helping care for the ill child, protecting the ill child from negative reaction of others, and including the ill child in activities with peers.

How well siblings react to a chronically ill sibling may ultimately depend on how the family copes with stress and how its members feel about one another. This delicate balance is challenging and takes great effort and caring for a family to sustain, but the results are well worth it. See Family Teaching Tips: Helping Siblings Cope With a Chronic Illness for additional information.

Test Yourself

✔ What effect does chronic illness have on the parents of the chronically ill child?

✔ What problems might the child with a chronic illness face?

✔ What effect does chronic illness have on the siblings of the chronically ill child?

THE ROLE OF THE NURSE

As the nurse, you play an important role in providing care for the child with a chronic illness and in helping the child and family learn to cope. Be aware of individual needs and abilities to cope with the illness. Encourage the child and family to share their feelings and reactions to the situation. Support by listening and providing appropriate interventions.

Nursing Process for the Family and the Child With a Chronic Illness

Assessment

The assessment of the family and the child with a disability or chronic illness is an ongoing process by the health care team. The information and data collected are reviewed and updated with each visit the child makes to the health care facility. Include the child in the admission and ongoing interview processes if he or she is old enough and able to participate. Unless the child is newly diagnosed, the family caregivers may have a good understanding of the condition. Observe for evidence of the family's knowledge and understanding so that plans can be made to supplement it as needed.

> **Something to think about!**
> The child may have had many visits and treatments in the past that have left negative memories, so approach the child in a low-key, kind, gentle manner to gain cooperation.

During any interview with the child or family caregivers, determine how the family is coping with the child's condition and observe for the family's strengths, weaknesses, and acceptance of the diagnosis. Identify the needs that change with the child's condition and include them in planning care. Also, consider needs that change with the child's growth and development.

Adjust the physical exam to correspond with the child's illness and current condition. Throughout the physical exam, make every effort to gain the child's cooperation and explain what is being done in terms that the child can understand. Praise the child for cooperation throughout the process to gain the child's (and the family caregivers') goodwill.

Selected Nursing Diagnoses

- Delayed Growth and Development related to impaired ability to achieve developmental tasks or family caregivers' reactions to the child's condition
- Self-Care Deficit related to limitations of illness or disability
- Anxiety related to procedures, tests, or hospitalization
- Risk for Social Isolation of the child or family related to the child's condition
- Grieving of family caregiver related to possible losses secondary to condition
- Interrupted Family Processes related to adjustment requirements for the child with chronic illness or disability

■ Health-Seeking Behaviors by caregivers related to home care of the child

Outcome Identification and Planning

Major goals for the chronically ill child are to accomplish growth and development milestones, perform self-care tasks, decrease anxiety, and experience more social interaction. Goals for the caregiver or family are to increase their social interaction; decrease their feelings of grief, anger, and guilt; increase their adjustment to living with a chronically ill child; and teach them about caring for the chronically ill or disabled child.

Implementation

Encouraging Optimal Growth and Development

The family caregivers may become overprotective and prevent the ill child from exhibiting growth and development appropriate for his or her age and disability. Help the caregivers recognize the child's potential and set realistic growth and development goals. Consistent care by the same staff helps to provide a sense of routine in which the child can be encouraged to have some control and perform age-appropriate tasks within the limitations of the disability. Set age-appropriate limits and enforce appropriate discipline. Accomplish this gradually by displaying a kind and caring attitude. Give the child choices within the limits of treatments and other aspects of required care. Encourage the child to wear regular clothes, rather than stay in pajamas, to reduce feelings of being an invalid. Encourage the child to learn about the condition. Introducing the child to other children with the same or a similar condition can help dispel feelings that he or she is the only person with such a condition.

An older child or adolescent benefits from social interaction with peers with and without disabilities (Fig. 32-2). Encourage family caregivers to help the adolescent join in age-appropriate activities. The adolescent also may need

■ **Figure 32-2** The adolescent with disabilities benefits from social interaction

some help dressing or using makeup to improve his or her appearance and minimize any physical disability.

Promoting Self-care

To encourage the child to assist in self-care, devise aids to ease tasks. When appropriate, integrate play and toys into the care to help encourage cooperation. Do not expect the child to perform tasks beyond his or her capabilities. Make certain that the child is well rested before he or she attempts any energy-taxing tasks. Remember these tasks are often hard work for the child. Praise and reward the child genuinely and generously for tasks attempted, even if they are not totally completed.

> **Try this!**
> Use a chart or other visual aid with listed tasks as a tool to help the child reach a desired goal. Stickers can record the child's progress. School-aged children often respond well to contracts. For instance, a special privilege or other incentive is awarded when a set number of stickers are earned.

Reducing Anxiety About Procedures and Treatments

Periodically the child may need to undergo procedures, tests, and treatments. The child may also be hospitalized frequently. Many of the procedures may be painful or at least uncomfortable. Explain the tests, treatments, and procedures to the child ahead of time and encourage the child to ask questions. Acknowledge to the child that a particular procedure is painful and help him or her to plan ways to cope with the pain. Advise family caregivers that they should also help the child to prepare for hospitalization ahead of time, whenever possible.

Preventing Social Isolation

The chronically ill child may feel isolated from peers. When the child is hospitalized, consider arranging for contact with peers by phone, in writing, or through visits. Many pediatric units have special programs that help children deal with chronic conditions and hospitalizations. Encourage regular school attendance as soon as the child is physically able. If the child is a member of an inclusive classroom, suggest that the caregiver make arrangements with the school for rest periods, as needed. Ask the child about interests; these may give some clues about suitable after-school activities that will increase the child's interactions with peers. Make suggestions and confer with family caregivers to ensure that proposed plans are carried out.

> **Listen carefully!**
> The child's discussions about social activities can help you gain insight into his or her feelings about socialization.

Family caregivers may also be at risk for social isolation. Having a child who requires constant or frequent attention often can be exhausting. The care requirements and exhaustion may leave little time for the caregivers to socialize. The family with no close extended family and few close friends may find getting away for rest and relaxation, even for an evening, almost impossible. Help the family caregivers find resources for respite care. Any caregiver, no matter how devoted, needs to have a break from everyday cares and concerns. Refer the family to social services where they can get help. Sometimes a caregiver may feel that another person cannot care for the child adequately. Encourage this caregiver to express fears and anxieties about leaving the child. This helps the caregiver to work through some of these anxieties and feel more confident about getting away for a period of rest.

Aiding Caregivers' Acceptance of the Condition

When anyone suffers a serious loss, a grief reaction occurs. This is true of family caregivers when they first learn that their child has a chronic or disabling illness. Encourage family caregivers to express these feelings and help them to understand that this reaction is common and acceptable.

Denial is usually the first reaction that family caregivers have to the diagnosis. This is a time when they say, "How could this be?" or "Why my child?" Let them express their emotions, and respond in a nonjudgmental way. Staying with them and offering quiet, accepting support may be helpful. Statements such as "It will seem better in time" are inappropriate. Acknowledge the caregivers' feelings as acceptable and reasonable.

During the next stage, called guilt, listen to the caregivers express their feelings of guilt and remorse. Again, acknowledging their feelings is useful. Accept expressions of anger by family caregivers without viewing them as a personal attack. Using active listening techniques that reflect the caregivers' feelings, such as "You sound very angry," are a helpful method of handling these emotions.

Grief reactions also may occur when the family caregivers are informed that their child is deteriorating or has had a setback. Although caregivers usually cycle through these reactions much more quickly by this time, the same methods are useful.

Helping the Family Adjust to the Child's Condition

The family's adjustment to the condition is assessed during initial and ongoing interviews. Adjustment may depend on how recently the child has been diagnosed or on the current status of the child's condition. After determining the family's needs, provide an opportunity for the family members to express their feelings and anxieties. Help them explore any feelings of guilt or blame about the child's condition. Encourage them to express doubts they may have about their ability to cope with the child's future. Help the caregivers look realistically at their resources, and give them suggestions about ways to cope. Serve as a role model when caring for the child, expressing a positive attitude toward the child and the illness or disability.

Question the family to determine the resources and support systems available to them. Remind them that these support systems may include immediate family members, extended family, friends, community services, and health care providers.

Encourage the caregivers to discuss the needs of the well siblings and their adjustment to the ill child's condition. Help the family meet the needs of the well siblings, and help the siblings feel comfortable with the ill child's problems and needs. Assist the family in setting reasonable expectations for all their children.

Planning for Home Care

Home care planning begins when the child is admitted to the health care facility and continues until discharge. Focus plans for care at home on the continuing care, medications, and treatments the child will need. During a health care visit or hospitalization, include family caregivers when caring for the child so that they become comfortable with the care. Demonstrate the use of special equipment and treatments and give the family caregivers a chance to perform the treatments under guidance and supervision. A discussion of the home's facilities may be appropriate to help the family accommodate any special needs the child may have. Give the caregivers a list of community services and organizations that they can turn to for help and support, including appropriate disease- or disability-specific organizations.

Teach the caregivers about growth and development guidelines so that they have a realistic concept of what to expect as the child develops. Throughout the child's hospital stay, encourage caregivers to express their concerns to help solve whatever problems the family anticipates having while caring for the child at home. Give the family the name and telephone number of a contact person they can call for support.

> **You can make a difference!**
> Families face many hurdles while caring for a chronically ill child, but they are more likely to feel that they can competently face the future with the reassurance that help is just a telephone call away.

Caring for a chronically ill child can be an overwhelming task that requires cooperation by all involved with the child and the family. Family caregivers deserve all the help they can get (see Nursing Care Plan 32-1).

Nursing Care Plan 32-1

THE CHRONICALLY ILL CHILD AND FAMILY

CASE SCENARIO
Billy is a 10-year-old who has Duchenne muscular dystrophy. His condition has worsened, and he has recently begun to use a walker. He has gradually begun to need more assistance in his activities of daily living. He has a sister who is 8 years old and a 5-year-old brother. Both parents live at home.

NURSING DIAGNOSIS
Delayed Growth and Development related to impaired ability to achieve developmental tasks or family caregivers' reactions to the child's condition

GOAL: The child will achieve the highest levels of growth and development within constraints of illness, and the family caregivers will acknowledge appropriate growth and development expectations.

EXPECTED OUTCOMES
- The child attains growth and development milestones within his capabilities.
- The family encourages the child to reach his potential.
- The family sets realistic developmental goals for the child.

Nursing Interventions	*Rationale*
Encourage the child to participate in growth and development activities to the best of his abilities.	Milestones of growth and development are attained when activities are offered to help the child develop those skills.
Discuss with the child's family the effects of overprotectiveness on his development.	Many families react to a child's long-term illness by shielding the child from challenges that the child could cope with if allowed to do so.
Help the child's family recognize his potential and help them to set realistic goals; encourage them to set age-appropriate limits for activities with appropriate discipline for violations.	Family caregivers may not know what to expect in terms of their child's development and may tend to overprotect the child, which prevents him from reaching his potential; it is important to allow him to reach for his potential without overprotection.

NURSING DIAGNOSIS
Self-Care Deficit related to limitations of illness or disability

GOAL: The child will become involved in self-care activities.

EXPECTED OUTCOMES
- The child participates in self-care as appropriate for his age and capabilities.
- The child demonstrates evidence of using creative problem-solving techniques.
- The child demonstrates a positive outlook about his achievements.

Nursing Interventions	*Rationale*
Generously praise any self-care the child performs; carefully avoid expecting him to do tasks beyond his capabilities.	Positive reinforcement gives the child self-confidence and pride in his accomplishments.
When the child finds a task difficult to accomplish, assist him by devising aids to help him with the task, rather than doing it for him.	Difficult accomplishments reinforce the importance of self-care and independence; demonstrating creative problem-solving techniques provides skills that the child can use in the future.
Encourage the child to carry out self-care appropriate for his age and stage of mobility; allow him to make as many choices as possible.	The child will have a better feeling of control and self-worth; he will be encouraged to try new things and not let his illness unnecessarily stop him.

(continues on page 706)

Nursing Care Plan 32-1 (continued)

THE CHRONICALLY ILL CHILD AND FAMILY

NURSING DIAGNOSIS
Risk for Social Isolation of the child or family related to the child's condition

GOAL: The child and the family will actively socialize with others.

EXPECTED OUTCOMES
- The child participates in activities with his peers.
- The child's family finds adequate respite care for Billy.
- The child's family gets away for a break with minimal anxieties.

Nursing Interventions	*Rationale*
Encourage the family to establish and maintain the child's contacts with his peers. Advise the family that it may take advance planning and creative solutions for him to participate in activities such as team sports.	The child needs to feel that he is part of the world in which his schoolmates and friends are involved; he needs activities to look forward to.
Help family caregivers find resources for respite care by making referrals to social services or other resources as necessary.	Family caregivers who periodically get away from the responsibilities of caring for the child will be re-energized and return with a refreshed spirit.
Encourage the family caregivers to express anxieties about leaving the child with someone else.	Talking with the family about such fears helps them to work through anxieties, dismiss unrealistic fears, and make specific plans for legitimate ones. This helps the family to have a more restful time when away.

NURSING DIAGNOSIS
Interrupted Family Processes related to adjustment requirements for the child with chronic illness or disability

GOAL: The family caregivers will deal with their feelings of anger, grief, guilt, and loss.

EXPECTED OUTCOMES
- The family members express fears and anxieties about the child's weakening condition.
- The family verbalizes a positive attitude to the child about his adaptations to his growing weakness.
- The child's family expresses feelings of guilt about his illness and deals with them positively.

Nursing Interventions	*Rationale*
Provide opportunities for family members to express feelings, including fears about his or her weakening condition.	The family may need encouragement to talk about some of their fears and anxieties.
Maintain a positive but realistic attitude about the child's growing disabilities both when providing care and when discussing the impact of the child's illness on the family.	The nurse serves as a role model for the family; modeling a positive attitude will help family caregivers take the same approach.
Explore with the child's family their feelings of guilt.	The family needs to resolve their feelings of guilt.
Provide the family with resources and support systems. Encourage them to talk with their younger children about their feelings concerning the child's illness.	The family needs to use community resources and support systems to help them with the long-term needs of the entire family.

NURSING DIAGNOSIS
Health-Seeking Behaviors by caregivers related to home care of the child

GOAL: The family caregivers will actively participate in the child's home care.

Nursing Care Plan 32-1 (continued)

THE CHRONICALLY ILL CHILD AND FAMILY

EXPECTED OUTCOMES
- The family members ask appropriate questions about the child's care.
- The family members demonstrate the ability to perform the child's care and treatment.
- The family members make contact with support groups and community services.

Nursing Interventions	*Rationale*
Explain and demonstrate any equipment used in the child's care; demonstrate treatments or therapy that the family will need to do at home; provide opportunities for practice under the guidance of a nurse or therapist.	Watching someone who knows how to perform a technique well and performing that technique yourself are very different matters. Practice and opportunities for questions are essential.
Provide the family with a list of community services and organizations where they can turn for help and support; include the name and telephone number of a contact person at the health care facility whom the family can call with questions or concerns.	Knowing whom to contact and how to reach that person gives the family reassurance that help is close by and increases their self-confidence about being able to handle their child's care.

Evaluation: Goals and Expected Outcomes

Goals: The child will achieve highest level of growth and development within constraints of illness, and the family caregivers will acknowledge appropriate growth and development expectations.

Expected Outcomes:

- The child attains growth and development milestones within her or his capabilities.
- The family caregivers acknowledge the child's capabilities, encourage the child, and set realistic goals for the child.

Goal: The child will become involved in self-care activities.

Expected Outcome: The child participates in self-care as appropriate for age and capabilities.

Goal: The child's anxiety will be decreased.

Expected Outcome: The child's anxiety is minimized as evidenced by cooperation with care and treatments.

Goal: The child and the family will actively socialize with others.

Expected Outcomes:

- The child and family use opportunities to socialize with others.
- The family seeks and finds adequate respite care for the child.

Goal: The family will deal with their feelings of anger, grief, guilt, and loss.

Expected Outcomes: The family caregivers

- express their feelings of guilt, fears, and anxieties.

- receive support while working toward accepting the child's condition.

Goal: The family caregivers will adjust to the requirements of caring for the child with chronic illness or disability.

Expected Outcomes: The family caregivers

- express ways they can cope with their child's condition.
- list the resources and support systems available to them.

Goal: The family caregivers will actively participate in the child's home care.

Expected Outcomes: The family caregivers

- ask pertinent questions.
- contact support groups and community agencies for help.
- demonstrate their ability to perform care and treatments.

Test Yourself

✔ How might a chronic illness affect a child's growth and development?

✔ What can you do to help decrease the social isolation of the chronically ill child?

✔ Why is it important for you to try to determine how the family and child are coping with a chronic illness?

Key Points

➤ Diseases that cause chronic illness in children include congenital heart disease, cystic fibrosis, juvenile arthritis, asthma, hemophilia, muscular dystrophy, leukemia, other malignancies, spina bifida, and immunodeficiency syndromes.

➤ Concerns common to many families of a child with a chronic illness include financial, administration of treatments and medications at home, disruption of family life, educational opportunities for the child, social isolation, family adjustments, reaction of siblings, stress among caregivers, guilt about and acceptance of the chronic condition, and care of the child when family caregivers can no longer provide care.

➤ Economic pressures, such as adequate health insurance; away-from-home living costs; the stress of having to keep a job, especially when the child needs the caregiver's time and attention; and the threat to job security because of time away from the job, can become overwhelming to the families of chronically ill children.

➤ Respite care is important so that family caregivers can have time away from the ill child and a break in the routine. Time away will help keep the caregivers from becoming isolated and enable them to participate in normal social activities.

➤ Caregivers of children with a chronic illness may respond by overprotecting the child, which may prevent the child from learning new skills. Sometimes caregivers distance themselves emotionally (rejection) or are in denial and behave as though the condition does not exist. Caregivers with acceptance are able to help the child set realistic goals.

➤ A chronic illness may interfere with normal growth and development depending on the diagnosis; age

of the child when diagnosed; and the overall condition, severity, and long-term disability the illness may cause.

➤ Well siblings may respond negatively to the child's illness by showing anger, hostility, jealousy, increased competition for attention, social withdrawal, and poor school performance. Positive responses many siblings demonstrate include caring and concern for the ill sibling, helping care for the ill child, protecting the ill child from negative reaction of others, and including the ill child in activities with peers.

➤ To help promote normal growth and development, encourage the child to participate in age-appropriate activities and to do tasks within the limitations of the child's disability. Encourage self-care by the child by devising aids to ease tasks; integrating play and toys into the care; praising the child for tasks attempted; being sure the child is well rested before attempting tasks; and by using charts, visual aids, and stickers as ways to reward the child.

➤ Help the family adjust to the child's condition by encouraging the family caregivers to express their feelings of anger, guilt, fear, and remorse by responding in a nonjudgmental way. Encourage the family to express doubts they may have about their ability to cope with the child's future and to look realistically at their resources. Offer suggestions about ways to cope, be a role model when caring for the child, and have a positive attitude.

➤ Preparing the family for home care of the child may include having the family caregivers observe the nurse when caring for the child so that they become comfortable performing continuing care, using equipment, giving medications, and doing treatments when the child goes home.

INTERNET RESOURCES

Make a Wish Foundation
www.wish.org

The Fathers Network
www.fathersnetwork.org

CoachArt
www.coachart.org

The Dream Factory of Kansas City
www.kcdream.org

Workbook

▮ NCLEX-STYLE REVIEW QUESTIONS

1. In planning nursing care for a child with a chronic illness, which of the following goals would *most likely* be part of this child's plan of care?

   a. The child will achieve the highest levels of growth and development.

   b. The child will participate in age-appropriate activities.

   c. The child will eat at least 75% of each meal.

   d. The child will share feelings about changes in body image.

2. The nurse is working with the family caregivers of a child who has a chronic illness. Which of the following statements made by the child's caregivers is an example of the common response called overprotection?

   a. "My child was born with this and it will always be part of our lives."

   b. "She should be punished when she breaks things because she knows better."

   c. "I know I should let her try new activities, but she just gets frustrated."

   d. "My child just isn't what I expected when I decided to become a parent."

3. The nurse is working with the caregivers of a child who has a chronic illness. Which of the following statements made by the child's caregivers is an example of the common response called acceptance?

   a. "My child was born with this and it will always be part of our lives."

   b. "She should be punished when she breaks things because she knows better."

   c. "I know I should let her try new activities, but she just gets frustrated."

   d. "My child just isn't what I expected when I decided to become a parent."

4. In working with families of children who have chronic illnesses, an important nursing intervention would be for the nurse to encourage family members to do which of the following?

   a. Refrain from talking about the condition.

   b. Openly express their feelings.

   c. Prevent the child from overhearing conversations.

   d. Tell stories about themselves.

5. In working with siblings of children who have chronic illnesses, it is important for the nurse to recognize that which of the following may be true about the siblings in many cases?

   a. Siblings may feel embarrassed about their brother's or sister's condition.

   b. Siblings are the primary caregiver for the sick child.

   c. Siblings excel in school in an effort to decrease the family stress.

   d. Siblings get jobs at a young age to help support the family.

6. When working with the family caregivers of a child with a chronic health concern, the nurse may note the family experiences a grief reaction before coming to an acceptance of the child's condition. Which of the following behaviors by the nurse would be helpful in working with these family caregivers? Select all that apply.

   a. Encouraging the family to express their feelings.

   b. Responding in a nonjudgmental way.

   c. Stating, "It won't be so hard as time goes on."

   d. Reminding the family that anger is inappropriate.

   e. Staying quietly with the family.

▮ STUDY ACTIVITIES

1. Lena and Josh are the young parents of Nina, a 12-month-old girl with meningomyelocele (spina bifida). Nina must be catheterized at least four times a day and also has mobility problems. Describe some of the economic and other stresses that this young couple faces.

2. Using your local telephone book, make a list of agencies to which you could refer families for assistance and support in the care of a chronically ill child.

3. Eight-year-old Jason, a patient in your pediatric unit, is undergoing chemotherapy. He seems very lonely and sad, although his family visits him regularly. You decide he may need contact with children his own age. Describe plans that you will make to provide contact with peers.

4. Go to the following Internet site: www.lehman.cuny.edu/faculty/jfleitas/bandaides/. See "Bandaides and Blackboards." Click on "Kids." Click on the star next to the section "To tell or not to tell," and read this section.

   a. List five reasons kids choose *not* to tell others that they have a chronic health condition.

   b. List five reasons kids choose to tell others that they have a chronic health condition.

▮ CRITICAL THINKING: WHAT WOULD YOU DO?

1. You are caring for 5-year-old Abby, who has cystic fibrosis. Her mother, Mattie, has been overprotective and has always done everything for her.

a. What will you do to involve Abby in caring for herself?

b. What will you say or do to help and encourage Mattie to encourage Abby to do more of her own care?

c. What are the reasons you think Mattie is overprotective of her child?

2. Nine-year-old Tyson is angry. He tells you that he hates his 6-year-old brother, Josh, who has Down syndrome.

a. What would you say to Tyson to begin a discussion with him about his feelings?

b. What are some of the factors you think might be causing Tyson to be angry?

c. What would you say or suggest if you had the opportunity to talk to Tyson and Josh's family caregiver?

3. Cassie is a 16-year-old girl with cerebral palsy. She wants to go to the school prom, but her family caregivers are very resistant to the idea. Cassie pleads with you to talk to them.

a. How will you approach this problem?

b. What are your responses to Cassie and to her caregivers?

33 Abuse in the Family

KEY TERMS

child abuse
child neglect
codependent parent
dysfunctional family
incest
sexual abuse
sexual assault

LEARNING OBJECTIVES

On completion of this chapter, you should be able to:

1. Discuss factors that may lead to child abuse.
2. Identify the circumstances under which physical punishment can be classified as abusive.
3. Describe the differences between bruises that occur accidentally to a child and those that result from physical abuse.
4. Explain the injuries that occur with shaken baby syndrome.
5. Describe Munchausen syndrome by proxy.
6. Discuss how a child may be emotionally abused.
7. Explain child neglect.
8. Discuss sexual abuse and the effects on the child.
9. Describe the nursing responsibilities for the child who has been abused.
10. Discuss how domestic violence in the family may affect a child.
11. Describe the unpredictable behavior of a parent with substance addiction and its effect on the child.
12. Identify behaviors that suggest there is an addiction problem in the child's family.

EVERY FAMILY faces many types of stress at one time or another. Events that create stress for a family include illness, job loss, economic crisis or poverty, relocation, birth, death, and trauma. How the family handles these stresses affects greatly the emotional, social, and physical health of each member of the family. A **dysfunctional family** is one that cannot resolve these stresses and work through them in a positive, socially acceptable manner. Families often face multiple pressures at the same time; this dynamic creates additional stress and adds to the risk of dysfunctional coping. The atmosphere in a dysfunctional family creates additional stress for all family members. Because of the lack of support within the dysfunctional family for individual members, these members respond negatively to real or perceived problems. This family climate may set the stage for abuse and other unhealthy coping behaviors.

Abuse in the family can take various forms. Parents or caregivers may abuse the child, spouses or other family members, or substances. Child abuse can have a significant negative impact on the child's growth and development and physical and emotional health. Likewise, the family problems of domestic violence or parental sub-stance abuse negatively affect the child. In some cases, domestic violence or parental substance abuse may lead to child abuse, but this is not always the case. As the nurse, you must be alert to signs of abuse in the family and be aware of the potential effects on the child.

CHILD ABUSE

Although child abuse has occurred throughout history, the evolution of cultural practices in the United States during the last few decades of the 20th century emphasized the rights of children. Thus, any sort of mistreatment and abuse of children is regarded as unacceptable. The term **child abuse** has come to mean any intentional act of physical, emotional, or sexual abuse, including acts of negligence, committed by a person responsible for the care of the child.

Each year, increasing numbers of child abuse cases are brought to the attention of authorities. Estimates of the number of children treated in emergency departments after an episode of abuse range from 500,000 to 1 million annually. However, the actual number of abused children may be much higher because many more cases may go undetected.

Child abuse is not limited to one age group and can be detected at any age. The courts have even viewed fetal exposure to drugs and alcohol as child abuse. The age group of children from birth to 3 years has the highest number of victims of child abuse, with girls being abused more frequently than boys (Reece, 2006).

Abusive parents can be found at all socioeconomic levels, but families with greater financial means may be able to evade detection more easily. Low-income families show greater evidence of violence, neglect, and sexual abuse according to some studies. Commonly, abusive parents have inadequate parenting skills; if they have unrealistic expectations of the child, they may not respond appropriately to the child's behavior.

State laws require health care personnel to report suspected child abuse. This requirement overrides the concern for confidentiality. Laws have been enacted that protect the nurse who reports suspected child abuse from reprisal by a caregiver (e.g., being sued for slander), even if it is found that the child's situation is not a result of abuse. If you do not report suspected child abuse, the penalty can be loss of your nursing license.

If abuse is suspected, the health care facility can hold the child for a certain period of time, and then a court holds a hearing to determine if the charges are true and to decide where the child should be placed.

> **This is critical to remember.**
> A health care facility can usually hold a child for 72 hours after suspected abuse has been reported so that a caseworker can investigate the charge.

Types of Child Abuse

Physical Abuse

Physical abuse may occur when the caregiver is unfamiliar with normal child behavior. Inexperienced caregivers may not know what normal behavior is for a child and become frustrated when the child does not respond in the way they expect. If inexperience is coupled with dysfunctional coping, the caregiver may physically abuse the child. Some young women become pregnant to have a child to love, and they expect that love to be returned in full measure. When the child resists the caregiver's control or seems to do the opposite of what is expected, the caregiver may take it as a personal affront and become angry, possibly responding with physical punishment. Some cultures support physical punishment for children, citing the principle "spare the rod, spoil the child." Despite evidence that physical punishment often results in negative behavior and that other forms of punishment are more effective, corporal punishment continues to be approved occasionally, even in some schools. However, physical punishment that leaves marks, causes injury, or threatens the child's physical or emotional well-being is considered abusive.

When a child's physical injury requires medical attention, family caregivers may attribute the injury to some action of the child's that is not in keeping with the child's age or level of development. For example, the caregiver may attribute an injury to the child's playing in a competitive sport that the child is too young to play. The caregiver may also attribute the injury to an action of a sibling. When the child's symptoms do not match the injury the caregiver describes, be alert for possible abuse. However, do not accuse the caregiver before a complete investigation takes place.

> **Pay attention to what you see.**
> An important role of the health care team is to identify abusive or potentially abusive situations as early as possible.

Young, active children often have a number of bruises that occur from their usual activities. Most of these bruises occur over bony areas such as the knees, elbows, shins, and forehead. Bruises that occur in areas of soft tissue, such as the abdomen, buttocks, genitalia, thighs, and mouth, may be suspect (Fig. 33-1). Bruises in the inner aspect of the upper arms may indicate that the child raised the arms to protect the face and head from blows.

Bruises may be distinctive in outline, clearly indicating the instrument that was used. Cigarettes, hangers, belt buckles, electrical cords, handprints, teeth (from biting), and sticks leave identifiable marks (Fig. 33-2). The injuries may be in varying stages of healing, indicating that not all the injuries occurred during one episode.

Signs or possible evidence of child abuse can be further evaluated by the use of technology. On a radiograph, bone fractures in various stages of healing may be noted. Spiral fractures of the long bones of a young child are not common, and their presence might indicate possible abuse. Children who have been harshly shaken may not show a clear picture of abuse, but computed tomography may demonstrate cerebral edema or cerebral hemorrhage.

Burns are another common type of injury seen in the abused child (Fig. 33-3). Although burns may be accidental in young children, certain types of burns are highly suspicious. Cigarette burns, for example, are common abuse injuries. Burns from immersion of a hand in hot liquid, a hot register (as evidenced by the grid pattern), a steam iron, or a curling iron are other common abuse injuries. Caregivers have been known to immerse the buttocks of a child in hot water if they thought the child was uncooperative in toilet training. Caregivers are often unaware of how quickly a child can be seriously burned. A burn that is neglected or not immediately reported must be considered suspicious until all the facts can be gathered and examined.

Common nonaccidental injury sites

A

B

▮ **Figure 33-1** **(A)** Injury sites that are suspicious for physical abuse. **(B)** Example of suspicious bruises.

Shaken Baby Syndrome

Shaken baby syndrome occurs when a small child is shaken by the arms or shoulders in a repetitive, violent manner. Shaking causes a whiplash-type injury to the child's neck. In addition, the child may have edema to the brain stem and retinal or brain hemorrhages. Loss of vision, mental retardation, or even death may occur in these children. Clinical manifestations may include lethargy, irritability, vomiting, and seizures, but often the signs of this form of child abuse are not easily observed and may be missed during physical examination. Internal symptoms are detected by the use of computed tomography and magnetic resonance imaging.

Munchausen Syndrome by Proxy

In Munchausen syndrome by proxy, one person either fabricates or induces illness in another to get attention. When a caregiver has this syndrome, he or she frequently brings the child to a health care facility and reports symptoms of illness when the child is actually well. The child's mother is most often the person who has the syndrome. Often the mother injures the child to get the attention of medical personnel. She may slowly poison the child with prescription drugs, alcohol, or other drugs, or she may suffocate the child to cause apnea. Many times, the symptoms, such as seizures or abdominal pain, are not easy to find on physical exam but are reported as history. The mother appears very attentive to the child and is often familiar with medical terminology. This situation is frustrating for health care personnel because it is difficult to catch the suspect in the act of endangering the child. Close observation of the caregiver's interactions with the child is necessary. For instance, if episodes of apnea occur only in the presence of the caregiver, be alert for this syndrome. The caregiver who suffers from this syndrome must receive psychiatric help.

Emotional Abuse

Injury from emotional abuse can be just as serious and lasting as that from physical abuse, but it is much more difficult to identify. Several types of emotional abuse can occur, including:

- Verbal abuse such as humiliation, scapegoating, unrealistic expectations with belittling, and erratic discipline
- Emotional unavailability when caregivers are absorbed in their own problems
- Insufficient or poor nurturing, or threatening to leave the child or otherwise end the relationship
- Role reversal in which the child must take on the role of parenting the parent and is blamed for the parent's problems

Children may show evidence of emotional abuse by appearing worried or fearful or having vague complaints of illness or nightmares. Caregivers may display signs of inappropriate expectations of the child when in the health care facility by sometimes mocking or belittling the child for age-appropriate behavior. In young children, failure to thrive may be a sign of emotional abuse. In the older child, poor school performance and attendance, poor self-esteem, and poor peer relationships may be clues.

Neglect

Child neglect is failure to provide adequate hygiene, health care, education, nutrition, love, nurturing, and

■ **Figure 33-2** Physical injuries may have distinctive outlines that indicate the instrument of abuse. **(A)** Cigarette burn on child's foot. **(B)** Imprint from a radiator cover. **(C)** Rope burn from being tied to crib rail. **(D)** Imprint from a looped electrical cord.

supervision needed for growth and development. If a child is not given adequate care for a serious medical condition, the caregivers are considered neglectful. For example, if a child is seriously burned, even accidentally, and the caregivers do not take the child for evaluation and treatment until several days later, they may be judged to be neglectful. Often, the child with failure to thrive as a result of being underfed, deprived of love, or constantly criticized can be classified as neglected; however, be careful not to make an unsubstantiated accusation of neglect.

Sexual Abuse

The Federal Child Abuse Prevention and Treatment Act defines **sexual abuse** as "the employment, use, persua-sion, inducement, enticement, or coercion of any child to engage in, or assist any other person to engage in, any sexually explicit conduct or simulation of such conduct for the purpose of producing a visual depiction of such conduct; or the rape, and in cases of caretaker or inter-familial relationships, statutory rape, molestation, pros-titution, or other form of sexual exploitation of children, or incest with children" (*Child Abuse Prevention and Treatment Act as Amended by the Keeping Children and Families Safe Act of 2003*).

Sexual abuse of children has existed in all ages and cultures, but it has seldom been admitted when perpe-trated by parents or other relatives in the home. **Incest** (sexually arousing physical contact between family mem-bers not married to each other) occurs in an estimated

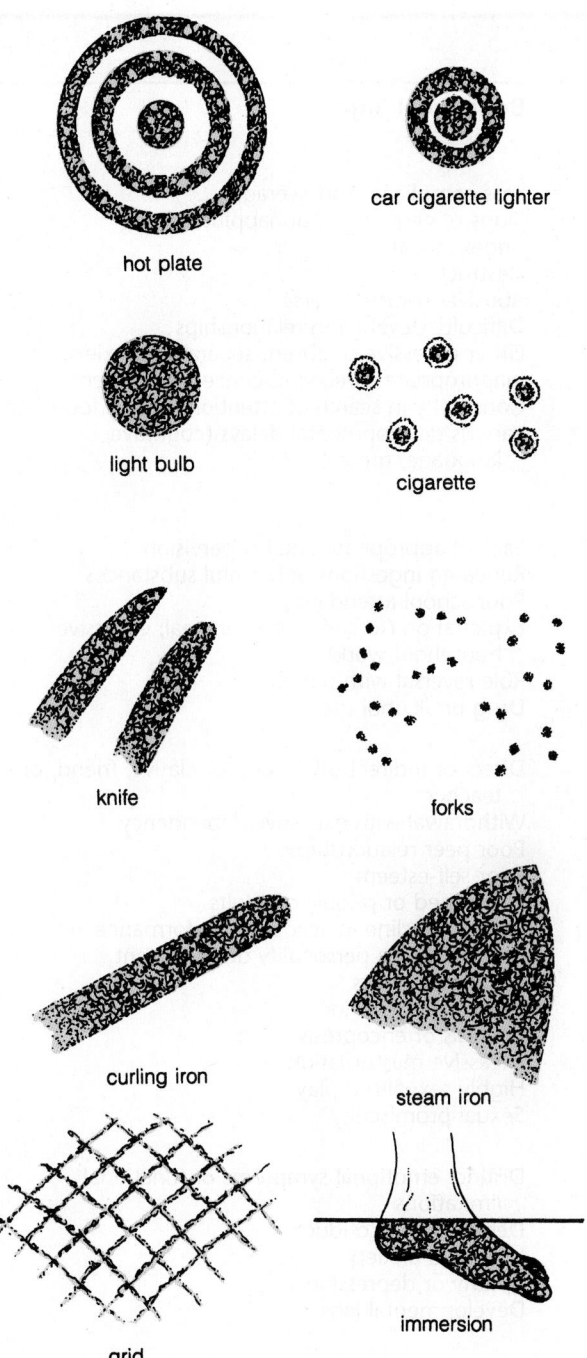

■ **Figure 33-3** Burn patterns from objects used for inflicting burns in child abuse.

contact, exhibitionism, and voyeurism. From a legal viewpoint, sexual contact between a child and another person in a caregiving position, such as a parent, babysitter, or teacher, is classified as sexual abuse. A sexual contact made by someone who is not functioning in a caregiver role is classified as **sexual assault.** When a person has power or control over a child, that person, even if a child, can be a sexual abuser.

When a child is sexually assaulted by a stranger, the caregivers usually become aware of the incident, promptly report it, and take the child for a physical examination. However, in the case of incest, the child rarely tells another person what is happening; the family member committing the acts often intimidates the child with threats, appeals to the child's desire to be loved and to please, and convinces the child of the importance of keeping the act secret. The child may exhibit physical complaints such as various aches and pains, gastrointestinal upsets, changes in bowel and bladder habits (including enuresis), nightmares, and acts of aggression or hostility. Some of these complaints or behaviors may be the presenting problem when a health care provider sees the child.

Regardless of the relationship of the perpetrator to the child, the outcome of the abuse is devastating. Sexual abuse by a person the child trusts seems to be the most damaging type.

Effects on the Child and Family

Child abuse has long-term as well as immediate effects. The abused child may be hyperactive; may exhibit angry, antisocial behavior; or may be especially withdrawn. When child abuse is suspected or confirmed, the child may be removed from the home or separated from the family for protection. Abusive parents often were abused themselves as children; thus, the problem of child abuse continues in a cyclical fashion from generation to generation.

240,000 to 1 million American families annually, and that number is growing each year. As with other types of child abuse, sexual abuse knows no socioeconomic, racial, religious, or ethnic boundaries. However, substance abuse, job loss, and poverty are contributing factors. Like other forms of child abuse, sexual abuse is being recognized and reported more often.

Several terms are commonly used when sexual abuse is discussed. *Sexual contact* includes fondling of breasts or genitalia, intercourse (vaginal or anal), oral–genital

Test Yourself
✔ What are the different types of child abuse often seen?
✔ What differentiates punishment for inappropriate behavior from child abuse?
✔ Who is the person who usually has the disease in Munchausen syndrome by proxy?

Table 33-1 ■ SIGNS OF ABUSE IN CHILDREN

Physical Signs	Behavioral Signs
Physical Abuse	
Bruises and welts: may be on multiple body surfaces or soft tissue; may form regular pattern (e.g., belt buckle)	Less compliant than average
	Signs of negativism, unhappiness
Burns: cigar or cigarette, immersion (stocking/glovelike on extremities or doughnut-shaped on buttocks or genitals), or patterned as an electrical appliance (e.g., iron)	Anger, isolation
	Destructive
	Abusive toward others
	Difficulty developing relationships
Fractures: single or multiple; may be in various stages of healing	Either excessive or absent separation anxiety
	Inappropriate caregiving concern for parent
Lacerations or abrasions: rope burns; tears in and around mouth, eyes, ears, genitalia	Constantly in search of attention, favors, food, etc.
	Various developmental delays (cognitive, language, motor)
Abdominal injuries: ruptured or injured internal organs	
Central nervous system injuries: subdural hematoma, retinal or subarachnoid hemorrhage	
Physical Neglect	
Malnutrition	Lack of appropriate adult supervision
Repeated episodes of pica	Repeated ingestions of harmful substances
Constant fatigue of listlessness	Poor school attendance
Poor hygiene	Exploitation (forced to beg or steal; excessive household work)
Inadequate clothing for circumstances	Role reversal with parent
Inadequate medical or dental care	Drug or alcohol use
Sexual Abuse	
Difficulty walking or sitting	Direct or indirect disclosure to relative, friend, or teacher
Thickening or hyperpigmentation of labial skin	Withdrawal with excessive dependency
Vaginal opening measures >4 mm horizontally in preadolescence	Poor peer relationships
	Poor self-esteem
Torn, stained, or bloody underclothing	Frightened or phobic of adults
Bruises or bleeding of genitalia or perianal area	Sudden decline in academic performance
Lax rectal tone	Pseudomature personality development
Vaginal discharge	Suicide attempts
Recurrent urinary tract infections	Regressive behavior
Nonspecific vaginitis	Enuresis or encopresis
Venereal disease	Excessive masturbation
Sperm or acid phosphatase on body or clothes	Highly sexualized play
Pregnancy	Sexual promiscuity
Emotional Abuse	
Delays in physical development	Distinct emotional symptoms or functional limitations
Failure to thrive	Deteriorating conduct
	Increased anxiety
	Apathy or depression
	Developmental lags

Nursing Process for the Child Who Is Abused

Assessment

When assessing a child who may have been abused or neglected, it is important to observe and document thoroughly and completely. The child should have a complete physical exam; carefully describe and accurately document all bruises, blemishes, lacerations, areas of redness and irritation, and marks of any kind on the child's body. It may be necessary to request that photographs be taken.

Observe the interaction between the child and the caregiver, and carefully document your observations using nonjudgmental terms. The child's body language may be revealing, so be alert for significant information. For example, if the child shrinks away from contact by the caregiver or health care practitioner or, on the other hand, is especially clinging to the caregiver, watch for other signs of inappropriate behavior. These assessments vary with the child's age (Table 33-1).

Perhaps the most difficult part may be to maintain a nonjudgmental attitude throughout the interview and examination. Be calm and reassuring with the child; let the child lead the way when possible.

Selected Nursing Diagnoses

■ Anxiety, Fear by child related to history of abuse, and fear of abuse from others

- Impaired Parenting related to situational stressors or poor coping skills
- Disabled Family Coping related to unrealistic expectations of the child by the parent
- Ineffective Coping by the nonabusive parent related to fear of violence from abusive partner or feelings of powerlessness

Outcome Identification and Planning

Major goals for the abused child include caring for any injuries the child has sustained as well as relieving anxiety and fear. An important family goal is to improve parenting and coping skills of the caregiver or family.

Implementation

Relieving the Child's Anxiety and Fear

Observe the child for behavior that indicates anxiety or fear such as withdrawal, ducking or shying away from the nurse or caregivers, and avoiding eye contact. One nurse should be assigned to care for the child so that the child can relate to one person consistently. Provide physical contact, such as hugging, rocking, and caressing, only if the child accepts it. Identify nursing actions that seem to comfort the child and use them consistently. Use a calm, reassuring, and kind manner, and provide a safe atmosphere in which the child has an opportunity to express feelings and fears. Use play to help the child express some of these emotions. Be careful not to do anything that might alarm or upset the child. Psychological support is provided through social services or an abuse team.

Observing Interaction Between the Caregiver and Child

While caring for the abused child when the caregiver is present, take the opportunity to observe how the caregiver relates to the child and how the child reacts to the caregiver. Give the caregiver the same courtesy extended to all caregivers. Offer a compliment when the caregiver does something well in caring for the child. Give the caregiver an opportunity to discuss in private any concerns; during this time, you may be able to gain his or her confidence.

Promoting Parenting Skills and Coping

Abuse often occurs when a caregiver is unfamiliar with normal growth and development and the behaviors common to a particular stage of development. Help the caregiver develop realistic expectations of the child. To help accomplish this goal, design a teaching plan and include the caregiver in caring for the child. Teach the caregiver the child's expected responses and help him or her learn about normal development. Praise the caregiver for displaying positive behaviors. Point out specific behaviors of the child and explain them to the caregiver. Explore the reasons for the caregiver's absence when he or she does not visit regularly. Discuss specific behaviors of the child that are upsetting to the caregiver and explain that these are common for the child's age.

The caregiver may be facing temporary or permanent placement of the child in another home. Help the caregiver and the child accept this change. Emotions that a caregiver has had for a long period cannot be easily eliminated. The assistance of social services and a child life specialist is beneficial in these situations. Act as a member of the team to aid in the transition. The foster parents may need support from the nursing staff to help ease the child's transition to the new home. Abused children must be followed up carefully after discharge from the health care facility to ensure that their well-being is protected.

Supporting the Nonabusive Caregiver

In some cases, one caregiver in the family may be an abuser and the other is not. The nonabusive caregiver is a victim, as is the child. Give the nonabusive caregiver an opportunity to express fears and anxieties. He or she may feel powerless in the situation. Support the passive caregiver in deciding whether to continue or leave the relationship with the abuser. Try to preserve the caregiver's self-esteem because this is not an easy decision to make. Remember that building trust is essential when discussing the problems and issues of the situation.

Evaluation: Goals and Expected Outcomes

Goal: The child will exhibit decreased signs of anxiety and fear.
Expected Outcomes: The child

- demonstrates relaxed play, facial expressions, and posture.
- displays no withdrawal or guarding during contacts with the nursing staff.

Goal: The caregiver will exhibit positive interaction with the child.
Expected Outcomes: The caregiver

- talks with the child and is sensitive to his or her needs.
- refrains from making unreasonable demands on the child.

Goal: The caregiver will be involved in the child's care and will verbalize examples of normal growth and development and ways to handle the child's misbehavior.
Expected Outcomes: The caregiver

- states age-appropriate behavior for the child.
- discusses ways to handle the child's irritating behavior.
- is involved in counseling or other discharge plans.

Goal: The nonabusive caregiver will begin to cope with fears and feelings of powerlessness.
Expected Outcomes: The nonabusive caregiver

- expresses fears and concerns.
- makes plans to resolve problems.

DOMESTIC VIOLENCE IN THE FAMILY

Millions of children are exposed to domestic violence each year (American Bar Association). Sometimes referred to as family violence, domestic violence is a serious concern seen in families of all races, socioeconomic groups, and educational backgrounds. In cases of domestic violence, a person uses power and control over a person who is a partner or family member. Physical violence, threats, emotional abuse, harassment, and stalking are forms of violence often seen. Children who are exposed to or witness domestic violence are greatly impacted.

Effects on the Child and Family

The impact of domestic violence on the family is great. Even if all family members are not victims of the violence, each family member is affected. The child may witness domestic violence, overhear it from another room, or see physical evidence, such as bruises or broken bones on the victimized parent. The child may even be injured during an episode of violence. In most cases, the victim of domestic violence is the mother, but not always. The older child, especially adolescent males, may feel a need to intervene to protect the mother. The person who is violent toward a spouse will often abuse his or her children as well.

Clinical Manifestations in the Child

Children affected by domestic violence may show signs and symptoms that result from the violent situation. These symptoms may be referred to as symptoms of post-traumatic stress disorder and may include inability to sleep, bedwetting, temper tantrums, withdrawal, and feelings of guilt for not being able to protect the victim. The school-aged child may have academic problems, frequent absences, behavior issues, or self-isolation. The older child will often use drugs or alcohol; get into legal trouble, many times by committing a crime against another person; or attempt or commit suicide. Children who witness domestic violence in their homes may become victims or perpetrators as they grow into adulthood.

As a nurse, you must be aware of the signs and symptoms that families affected by domestic violence might exhibit. Shame and embarrassment may prevent children from talking about the violent behavior they have witnessed. Sometimes the abuser has threatened further violence if anyone in the family tells others about the situation. Asking direct and specific questions when domestic violence is suspected will encourage the child or family member to be honest about the situation.

Members of the family may have to seek emergency help from relatives, friends, or community shelters in order to be safe. Shelters for battered women and their children are available in many communities. The National Domestic Violence Hotline (1-800-799-SAFE [7233]) is available for families and victims. The child needs support to deal with the fear and disruption these events cause. In cases where the child becomes a victim of the domestic violence, the child may even be removed from the home, causing even further trauma.

PARENTAL SUBSTANCE ABUSE

The problem of substance abuse has grown to alarming proportions since the early 1980s. More than 10% of children come from a home affected by the alcoholism of one or both parents. Alcoholism exacts a terrible toll on the functioning of the family. Children of alcoholics have an increased risk of becoming alcoholics themselves. When other substances are included, the number of affected homes increases substantially. Adverse childhood experiences, such as physical, emotional, or sexual abuse, have a strong influence on alcohol and drug abuse as adults.

Effects on the Child and Family

Substance abuse is a family problem. If one member of the family abuses alcohol and/or drugs, every member of that family is affected. Children who have at least one parent who is a substance abuser are at risk for a variety of problems that researchers relate to substance abuse in the family. Developmental delays occur in young children of substance abusers. Infants of cocaine abusers avoid the caregiver's gaze, which contributes further to bonding delays.

The parent who is addicted may be so involved in procuring the drug that he or she forgets any parenting responsibilities. Caught in the ups and downs of addiction, the parent is not dependable and cannot provide any stability for the child. The parent may waver between overindulgence—smothering the child with attention, leniency, and gifts—and the opposite behavior of irritability, unreasonable accusations, threats, and anger. This unpredictable behavior has a severe negative impact on relationships in the family.

Children of substance-abusing parents often become loners and avoid relationships with others for fear that the substance-abusing parent might do or say something to embarrass them in front of their peers.

As the parent's substance abuse worsens, the family's dysfunction and social isolation increase. The **codependent parent** supports, directly or indirectly, the addictive behavior of the other parent. This behavior usually involves making excuses for the addict's actions and expecting others (i.e., the children) to overlook the parent's moodiness, erratic behavior, and consumption of alcohol or drugs. Codependency adds to the dilemma of children living with an addicted parent.

Clinical Manifestations in the Child

Children react to parental substance addiction in a variety of ways. Children rarely talk about the parent's problem even to the other parent. These children often experience guilt, anxiety, confusion, anger, depression, and addictive behavior. An older child, often a girl, may take on the responsibility of running the household, taking care of the younger children, making meals, and per-

A Personal Glimpse

When I was little, we had such happy times. We used to go places together and even when we stayed home, we laughed and had fun. My brother was born when I was 3 and then my little sister was born when I was 8. Sometimes after she was born, I could hear my parents arguing and shouting downstairs when they thought I was asleep. I couldn't usually hear the words they were saying but it scared me to hear them. The next day they would act like nothing had happened and things were fine. I thought the way they argued was just what parents did. I worked hard in school, got good grades, and never got into trouble. I helped take care of my little brother and sister. I kept my room clean and helped with cooking and laundry. I noticed my mom always had a glass in her hand; I thought it was soda when I was little. As I got older, I realized that my mom was drinking. Sometimes when my parents were arguing it was so loud, I tried to cover my ears and my brother's and sister's ears so they wouldn't hear. Words like alcoholic, drunk, drinking, were always part of the screaming. If I ever asked my dad about my mom, he would always excuse her behavior or apologize to me and tell me he would talk to her and things would be better.

By the time I was in eighth grade, I was used to walking home from school because my mother forgot to pick me up. When I would get home, she would be passed out on the couch. I made excuses to my friends why they couldn't come to my house. I was so afraid my mom would show up at a school meeting drunk that I didn't even tell her about the meetings. She would get mad and blame me for things I didn't do and then turn around and promise me she would take me places or do things with me. I would get excited and think finally things with my mom would be better. Over and over, she would forget her promise and I would feel hurt again.

By the time I was in high school, I just couldn't wait to get away from home. I was so embarrassed, I never told anyone my mom drank or what really happened at my house. I worked so hard to keep our secret. My brother was always in trouble, and one day the school counselor called me in to her office. She asked me how things were at my house and finally I couldn't keep the pain inside anymore. I am thankful she listened. We started to go to counseling, and my dad started going to Al-Anon. I wish I could say my mom stopped drinking. My parents got a divorce and we live with my dad. I hope someday my mom will get help.

Caitlyn, age 17

Learning Opportunity: What are some of the things this father did that added to the addictive behavior of this mother? What are some ways that children deal with a parent's substance abuse?

Another child in the family may try to deflect the embarrassment and anger of the other siblings by trying to make everyone feel good. As these children become adolescents or young adults, they may have problems, such as substance abuse or eating disorders. The child in the family who "acts out" and engages in delinquent behavior is most likely to come to the attention of social services and be identified as a child who needs help.

Behaviors that may alert nurses and other health care personnel to an addiction problem in the family include:

- The loner child who avoids interaction with classmates
- The child who is failing in school or has numerous episodes of unexcused absences or truancy
- The child with frequent minor physical complaints, such as headaches or stomachaches
- The child who steals or commits acts of violence
- The aggressive child
- The child who abuses drugs or alcohol

Nurses and others who work with children must be alert to these signals for help. Children can benefit from programs that support them and help them understand what is happening in the home. Such a program may include group therapy sessions at school in which the child learns that others have the same problems; this reduces his or her feelings of isolation. Other programs may include the whole family, perhaps as part of the program for the addicted parent who is trying to break the addiction. Professional help is necessary to prevent the child from developing more serious problems. The earlier the child can be identified and treatment begun, the better the prognosis. Family Teaching Tips: Resources for Information and Help with Drugs and Alcohol Problems in Chapter 42 provides a list of resources for information and help with drug and alcohol problems.

Don't be afraid to speak up.

There is help for the child in a home where substance abuse is an issue. You can provide referrals and support that benefit the child and family.

Test Yourself

- ✔ What are some examples of the forms of domestic violence often seen?
- ✔ The signs and symptoms seen in children as a result of a violent situation may be referred to as symptoms of what?
- ✔ What term is used to describe the parent who supports, directly or indirectly, the addictive behavior of the other parent?

forming the tasks that the parent normally should do. These children may become overachievers in school but remain isolated emotionally from their peers and teachers. This child does not usually bring negative attention to the family, and substance abuse in the family is not often suspected based on the behavior of this child.

Key Points

➤ Family stressors and how the family handles these stresses may lead to child abuse. Poor parenting skills may lead to child abuse if the parent has unrealistic expectations of the child or dysfunctional coping skills.

➤ Physical punishment can be classified as abusive if it leaves marks, causes injury, or threatens the child's physical or emotional well-being.

➤ Bruises that occur accidentally to a child appear over bony areas such as the knees, elbows, shin, and forehead. Those that have been inflicted in an abusive manner are found in soft tissue such as the abdomen, buttocks, genitalia, thighs, and mouth.

➤ Shaken baby syndrome causes a whiplash-type injury in the neck. In addition, the child may have edema to the brain stem, brain hemorrhages, loss of vision, mental retardation, or even death. The child might have clinical manifestations of lethargy, irritability, vomiting, and seizures or have no easily noted symptoms.

➤ Munchausen syndrome by proxy occurs when one person, commonly the mother, either fabricates or induces illness in another (usually the child) to get attention.

➤ A child may be emotionally abused verbally or by emotional unavailability of the caregiver, poor nurturing, threats involving leaving the child, or role reversal, in which the child must take on the role of parenting or is blamed for the parent's problems.

➤ Child neglect is failure to provide adequate hygiene, health care, nutrition, love, nurturing, and supervision.

➤ Sexual abuse can be incest, sexual contact, or sexual assault and occurs in all socioeconomic, racial,

religious, and ethnic groups. Substance abuse, job loss, and poverty are often contributing factors.

➤ Nursing care goals for the child who has been abused focus on caring for any injuries the child has sustained as well as relieving anxiety and fear. Nursing care that promotes parenting skills and coping benefits the child as well.

➤ In cases of domestic violence, the child may have witnessed, heard, or seen evidence of the violence. The child may be injured or have symptoms such as inability to sleep, bedwetting, temper tantrums, withdrawal, and feelings of guilt. He or she may have academic problems, frequent absences, behavior issues, or isolate from others. The older child may use drugs or alcohol, commit crimes, or attempt or commit suicide. These children may become victims or perpetrators of domestic violence as adults.

➤ The parent with substance addiction is not dependable and cannot provide stability for the child. The parent may waver between overindulgence and the opposite—unreasonable and unpredictable behavior toward the child.

➤ Behaviors seen in children who have an addicted parent include avoidance of interaction with classmates, failing in school, unexcused absences or truancy, frequent minor physical complaints, stealing or committing acts of violence, aggressive behavior, and abuse of drugs or alcohol. Sometimes children behave in a positive manner to prevent attention being drawn to the family. These children may take on the responsibilities the adult would normally take on, may become overachievers in school, or they may attempt to deflect the behaviors of their siblings by trying to make everyone feel good.

INTERNET RESOURCES

Child Welfare Information Gateway
www.childwelfare.gov

Prevent Child Abuse America
www.preventchildabuse.org

Tennyson Center for Children at Colorado Christian Home
www.childabuse.org

Workbook

■ NCLEX-STYLE REVIEW QUESTIONS

1. The nurse is assisting with a physical exam on a child who has been admitted with a diagnosis of possible child abuse. Which of the following findings in the child might alert the nurse to the possibility that the child has been abused?

   a. A fractured bone.
   b. Bruises on the knees and elbows.
   c. Hyperactive and angry behavior.
   d. A burn that has not been treated.

2. The nurse is interviewing the caregiver of a 5-year-old child who has been admitted with bruises on the abdomen and thighs as well as additional bruises in various stages of healing. Which of the following statements made by the caregiver might alert the health care team to the possibility of child abuse?

   a. "His brother just plays too rough with him."
   b. "My child goes to the day care after school."
   c. "He just learned to ride his bicycle."
   d. "When he is in trouble, I make him go to his room."

3. In caring for a child who has been admitted after being sexually abused, which of the following interventions would be included in the child's plan of care?

   a. Observe for signs of anxiety.
   b. Weigh on the same scale each day.
   c. Encourage frequent family visits.
   d. Test the urine for glucose upon admission.

■ STUDY ACTIVITIES

1. You are on duty in the emergency department when an infant is admitted with injuries that cause you to suspect abuse. The mother says her boyfriend was babysitting for her. State how you feel about this. Describe the observations that you will make when assessing the infant. What are your plans to approach the mother? Write out an effective communication you might have with the mother.

2. Children react differently to living with a family caregiver who is addicted. Make a list of the behaviors you might see that would cause you to be alert to a child with such a family problem. Research your community for resources available to children from families where addiction is a problem. Share the information you find with your classmates.

3. Research the Internet to find at least three reliable websites that give information regarding substance abuse in parents and how a child is affected by a parent's use of substances.

■ CRITICAL THINKING: WHAT WOULD YOU DO?

1. Your neighbor, 17-year-old Holly, has an active 18-month-old toddler named Jason. You overhear Holly screaming at him and saying, "I'm going to beat you if you don't listen to me!"

   a. Describe your feelings about the comment the mother made.
   b. What might be some factors that contributed to this situation?
   c. What would you say and do regarding this situation?

2. At a well-child visit, a mother confides in you that her husband's drinking is a concern to her. She tells you she has tried to get him to stop drinking because she thinks his drinking is affecting the children.

   a. Explain how the codependent parent supports, either directly or indirectly, the addictive behavior of the other parent.
   b. What are some behaviors that might be seen in the children in this family?
   c. What would you say to this mother?

34 *The Dying Child*

KEY TERMS

anticipatory grief
hospice
thanatologist
unfinished business

LEARNING OBJECTIVES

On completion of this chapter, you should be able to:

1. Discuss reasons why nurses may have difficulty working effectively with dying children.
2. Identify how a nurse can personally prepare to care for a dying child.
3. Explain factors that affect the child's understanding of death.
4. Describe how a child's understanding of death changes at each developmental level.
5. Describe the role of anticipatory grief in the grieving process.
6. Describe the reactions of family caregivers when a child has a terminal illness.
7. Describe why a family may suffer excessive grief and guilt when a child dies suddenly.
8. Describe possible reactions in a child when a sibling dies.
9. Identify settings for caring for the dying child and the advantages and disadvantages of each.
10. Discuss the role of the nurse in caring for the dying child and the child's family.

DEATH IS A tragic reality for thousands of children each year. Accidents are the leading cause of death in children between the ages of 1 and 14 years; cancer is the number one fatal disease in this age group (National Childhood Cancer Foundation, 2007). Nearly all these children leave behind at least one grieving family caregiver and perhaps brothers, sisters, and grandparents. As a nurse caring for children and families, you must be prepared for encounters with the dying and the bereaved.

Death of a child is the most difficult death to accept. We may more easily accept that elderly patients have lived a full life and that life must end, but the life of a child still holds the hopes, dreams, and promises of the future. When a child's life ends early, whether abruptly, such as the result of an accident, or after a prolonged illness, we ask ourselves, "Why? What's the justice of this?"

Caring for a family facing the death of their child calls on all your personal and professional skills as a nurse. It means offering sensitive, gentle, and physical care and comfort measures for the child and continuing emotional support for the child, the family caregivers, and the siblings. This kind of caring demands an understanding of your own feelings about death and dying, knowledge of the grieving process that patients and their families experience during a terminal illness or when facing an unexpected death, and a willingness to become involved.

Like chronic illness, terminal illness creates a family crisis that can either destroy or strengthen the family as a unit and as individuals. Nurses and other health professionals who can offer knowledgeable, sensitive care to these families help to make the remainder of the child's life more meaningful and the family's mourning experience more healing. Helping a family struggle through this crisis and emerge stronger and closer can yield deep satisfaction.

You can make a difference.
Caring for a dying child and his or her family is stressful but can also be extremely rewarding.

THE NURSE'S REACTION TO DEATH AND DYING

Health care workers often are uncomfortable with dying patients, so they avoid them and are afraid that the patients will ask questions they cannot or should not answer. These caregivers signal by their behavior that the patient should

A Personal Glimpse

I am a student nurse. I am dying. I write this to you who are and will become nurses in the hope that by my sharing my feelings with you, you may someday be better able to help those who share my experience. . . . You slip in and out of my room, give me medications and check my blood pressure. Is it because I am a student nurse, myself, or just a human being, that I sense your fright? And your fears enhance mine. Why are you afraid? I am the one who is dying!

I know you feel insecure, don't know what to say, don't know what to do. But please believe me, if you care, you can't go wrong. Just admit that you care. . . . Don't run away—wait—all I want to know is that there will be someone to hold my hand when I need it. . . . If only we could be honest, both admit our fears, touch one another. If you really care, would you lose so much of your valuable professionalism if you even cried with me? Just person to person? Then it might not be so hard to die in a hospital—with friends close by.

(American Journal of Nursing, 1970)

Learning Opportunity: Describe your feelings about the student nurse's story. How might this person's experience influence your approach to caring for the dying patient?

avoid the fact of his or her impending death and should keep up a show of bravery. In effect, they are asking the patient to meet their needs, instead of trying to meet the patient's needs.

Death reminds us of our own mortality, a thought with which many of us are uncomfortable. The thought that someone even younger than we are is about to die makes us feel more vulnerable.

Something to think about.

Every nurse needs to examine his or her own feelings about death and the reasons for these feelings.

How have you reacted to the death of a friend or a family member? When growing up, was talking and thinking about death avoided because of your family's attitudes? Admitting that death is a part of life and that patients should be helped to live each day to the fullest until death are steps toward understanding and being able to communicate with those who are dying. Attending a workshop, conference, or seminar in which you can explore your own feelings about life and death is useful in preparing you to provide nursing care for the dying child and family (Box 34-1).

Learning to care for the dying patient requires talking with other professionals, sharing concerns, and comforting each other in stressful times. It calls for reading stud-

Box 34-1 ▮ QUESTIONS TO COVER IN A SELF-EXAMINATION ABOUT DEATH

The following questions can be used in a group with a hospice or other facilitator. They can be used to help heighten your awareness of yourself: who are you; how you have gotten to where you are today; what you are doing with your life and why; how you would change the way you live; your feelings about death in general, in relation to your friends and family, and in regard to your own death.

Some Considerations in the Resolution of Death and Dying

- What was your first conscious memory of death? What were your feelings and reactions?
- What is your most recent memory of death? How was it the same or different from your first memory?
- What experience of death had the most effect on you? Why?

Get Comfortable and Imagine Now

- You have just been told you have 6 months to live. What is your first reaction to that news?
- *3 months later*—What relationships might require you to tie up loose ends? What unfinished business do you have to deal with? You and your significant other are trying to cope with the news, what changes occur in your relationship?
- *1 month remains*—What do you need to have happen in the remaining time? What hopes, dreams, and plans can or need to be fulfilled?
- *1 week remains*—You are very weak and barely have enough energy to talk. You don't even want to look at yourself. Nausea and vomiting are constant companions. Write a letter to the one person you feel would be the most affected by your dying.
- *24 hours remain*—You are dying. Breathing is difficult, you feel very hot inside, and overwhelming fatigue is ever-present. How would you like to spend this last day?

Courtesy of Ruth Anne Sieber, from Hospice: The Bridge, Lewistown, PA.

ies about death to discover how dying patients feel about their care, their illness, their families, and how they want to spend the rest of their lives. It also requires being a sensitive, empathic, nonjudgmental listener to patients and families who need to express their feelings, even if they may not be able to express them to each other. Caring for the dying is usually a team effort that may involve a nurse, a physician, a chaplain, a social worker, a psychiatrist, a hospice nurse, or a **thanatologist** (a person, sometimes a nurse, trained especially to work with the dying and their families), but the nurse is often the person who coordinates the care.

THE CHILD'S UNDERSTANDING OF DEATH

Stage of development, cognitive ability, and experiences all influence children's understanding of death. The child's first experience with death may be the death of a pet or a family member. How the family deals with the experience has a great impact on the child's understanding of death, but children usually do not have a realistic comprehension of the finality of death until they near preadolescence. Although the dying child may be unable to understand death, the emotions of family caregivers and others alert the child that something is threatening his or her secure world. Dealing with the child's anxieties with openness and honesty restores the child's trust and comfort.

Developmental Stage

Infants and Toddlers

Infants and toddlers have little if any understanding of death. The toddler may fear separation from beloved caregivers but have no recognition of the fact that death is nearing and irreversible. A toddler may say, "Gramma's gone bye-bye to be with God" or "Grampy went to heaven" and a few moments later ask to go visit the deceased person. This is an opportunity to explain to the child that Gramma or Grampy is in a special place and cannot be visited, but the family has many memories of him or her that they will always treasure. The child should not be scolded for not understanding. Questions are best answered simply and honestly.

If the infant's or toddler's own death is approaching, family caregivers can be encouraged to stay with the child to provide comfort, love, and security. Maintaining routines as much as possible helps to give the toddler a greater sense of security.

Preschool Children

The egocentric thinking of preschool children contributes to the belief that they may have caused a person or pet to die by thinking angry thoughts. Magical thinking also plays an important part in the preschooler's beliefs about death. It is not unusual for a preschool child to insist on burying a dead pet or bird, then in a few hours or a day or two dig up the corpse to see if it is still there. This may be especially true if the child has been told that it will "go to heaven." Many preschoolers think of death as a kind of sleep; they do not understand that the dead person will not wake up. They may fear going to sleep after the death of a close family member because they fear that they may not wake up. Family caregivers must watch for this kind of reaction and encourage children to talk about their fears while reassuring them that they need not fear dying while sleeping. The child's feelings must be acknowledged as real, and the child must

be helped to resolve them. The feelings must never be ridiculed.

A preschool child may view personal illness as punishment for thoughts or actions. Because preschoolers do not have an accurate concept of death, they fear separation from family caregivers. Caregivers can provide security and comfort by staying with the child as much as possible.

> ## Test Yourself
>
> ✔ Why is it important for the nurse to examine his or her own feelings about death?
>
> ✔ What does the toddler fear in relationship to death and dying?
>
> ✔ How does magical thinking in preschool children relate to their understanding of death?

School-aged Children

The child who is 6 or 7 years old is still in the magical thinking stage and continues to think of death in the same way as the preschool child does. At about 8 or 9 years of age, children gain the concept that death is universal and irreversible. Around this age, death is personified—that is, it is given characteristics of a person and may be called the devil, God, a monster, or the bogeyman. Children of this age often believe they can protect themselves from death by running past a cemetery while holding their breath, keeping doors locked, staying out of dark rooms, staying away from funeral homes and dead people, or avoiding stepping on cracks in the sidewalk.

When faced with the prospect of their own death, school-aged children are usually sad that they will be leaving their family and the people they love (Fig. 34-1).

■ **Figure 34-1** School-aged children are often sad when faced with their own death and leaving their family.

Family Teaching Tips

TALKING TO CHILDREN ABOUT DEATH

- Encourage children to talk about the topic of death
- Talk about the subject when the child wants to talk
- Share information at the child's level of understanding
- Listen to what the child is saying and to what they are asking
- Accept the child's feelings
- Be open and honest, and give simple, brief answers, especially when talking with the younger child
- Answer the question each time the child asks, sometimes children need to ask the same question more than once
- Say "I don't know" to questions you don't have answers for
- Use the words "death," "died," and "dying"
- Talk about death when less emotion is involved, such as dead flowers, trees, insects, and birds
- Explain death in terms of the absence of things that occur in everyday life, such as when people die they don't breathe, eat, talk, think, or feel

They may be apprehensive about how they will manage when they no longer have their parents around to help them. They often view death as another new experience, like going to school, leaving for camp, or flying in an airplane for the first time. They may fear the loss of control that death represents to them and express this fear through vocal aggression. Family caregivers and nurses must recognize this as an expression of their fear and avoid scolding or disciplining them for this behavior. This is a time when the people close to the child can help him or her voice anxieties about the future and provide an outlet for these aggressive feelings. The presence of family members and maintenance of relatively normal routines help to give the child a sense of security. Family Teaching Tips: Talking to Children About Death provides help for caregivers in talking with their children about death.

Adolescents

Adolescents have an adult understanding of death but feel that they are immortal—that is, death will happen to others but not to them. This belief contributes to adolescents' sometimes dangerous, life-threatening behavior. This denial also may contribute to an adolescent's delay in reporting symptoms or seeking help.

Diagnosis of a life-threatening or terminal illness creates a crisis for the adolescent. To cope with the illness, the adolescent must draw on cognitive functioning, past experiences, family support, and problem-solving ability. The adolescent with a terminal illness may express help-lessness, anger, fear of pain, hopelessness, and depression. Adolescents often try to live the fullest lives they can in the time they have.

Adolescents may be upset by the results of treatments that make them feel weak and alter their appearance such as alopecia, edema resulting from steroid therapy, and pallor. They may need assistance in presenting themselves as attractively as possible to their peers. Adolescents need opportunities to acknowledge their impending death and can be encouraged to express fears and anxieties and ask questions about death. Participating in their usual activities helps adolescents feel in control.

> **This is important to remember.**
> A child's understanding of death and dying is affected by the child's stage of growth and development, so it is important for you to be aware of what the child may understand and think.

Test Yourself

- ✔ At what age does the child understand the concept that death is universal and irreversible?
- ✔ What belief do adolescents have regarding dying that allows them to sometimes participate in dangerous, life-threatening behaviors?

Experience With Death and Loss

Every death that touches the life of a child makes an impression that affects the way the child thinks about every other death, including his or her own. Attitudes of family members are powerful influences. Family caregivers must be able to discuss death with children when a grandparent or other family member dies, even though the discussion may be painful. Otherwise, the child thinks that death is a forbidden topic; avoiding the subject leaves room for fantasy and distortion in the child's imagination.

Many books are available to help a child deal with loss and death. *A Balloon Story*, a simply produced 13-page coloring storybook by hospice nurse Ruth Anne Sieber, is an introduction to loss, appropriate for the young child. This story of two children who go to a fair with their mothers is illustrated with large line drawings to color. The children each select and purchase a helium balloon of which they are quite proud. Unfortunately, Nathan's balloon slips from his hand and floats away forever. Nathan displays typical grief reactions of protest, anger, and finally acceptance (Fig. 34-2). Reading the story to a child provides the adult with the perfect opening to discuss loss. A small booklet for caregivers accompanies *A Balloon Story* and contains excellent guidelines for discussing death and loss with a

Figure 34-2 Nathan cried and kept jumping and reaching after everyone else had given up. (Courtesy of Ruth Anne Sieber.)

Figure 34-3 Drawings done by fourth-grade students after a presentation about death that included a reading of *Water Bugs and Dragonflies*. **(A)** In the s[t]ages of life, we change. At the center of the drawing is a pond with three lily pads. The stems at the end represent plants that waterbugs crawl up on before turning into dragonflies. **(B)** Nobody lives forever. (Courtesy of Ruth Anne Sieber.)

child. *A Balloon Story* can be obtained from Hospice: The Bridge, Lewistown Hospital, Lewistown, Pennsylvania 17044.

Another small booklet that is excellent to use with any age group is *Water Bugs and Dragonflies*. This story approaches life and death as stages of existence by illustrating that after a water bug turns into a dragonfly, he can no longer go back and tell the other curious water bugs what life is like in this beautiful new world to which he has gone. This story can serve as the foundation for further discussion about death (Fig. 34-3).

Available books on death vary in their approaches. A number of books focus on the death of an animal or pet. Many stories deal with death as a result of old age. Several books have an accident as the cause of death. Most of the books are fiction, but several nonfiction books are available for older children (Table 34-1). There is no discussion of one's own death in these books, which is consistent with the Western philosophy of handling death as something that happens to others but not to oneself.

Awareness of Impending Death

Children know when they are dying. They sense and fear what is going to happen, even if they cannot identify it by name. Their play activities, artwork, dreams, and symbolic language demonstrate this knowledge.

Family caregivers who insist that a child not learn the truth about his or her illness place health care professionals at a disadvantage because they are not free to help the child deal with fears and concerns. If caregivers permit openness and honesty in communication with a dying child, the health care staff can meet the child's needs more effectively, dispel misunderstandings, and see that the child and the family are able to resolve any problems or **unfinished business**. Completing unfinished business may mean spending more time with the child, helping siblings to understand the child's illness and impending death, and giving family members a chance to share their love with the child. Allowing openness does not mean that nurses and other personnel offer information not requested by the child but simply means that the child be given the information desired gently and directly in words the child can understand. The truth can be kind as well as cruel.

Table 34-1 ▮ BOOKS ABOUT DEATH FOR CHILDREN

Author	Book	Publisher	Who Dies	Age Appropriate
Blume, Judy	*Tiger Eyes*	Scarsdale, NY: Bradbury Press	Father	11–15
Bunting, E.	*The Happy Funeral*	New York: Harper and Row	Grandfather	3–7
Carrick, C.	*The Accident*	New York: Houghton Mifflin, Clarion Books	Dog	6–11
Claudy, A.F.	*Dusty Was My Friend*	Human Sciences Press	Friend	6–11
Edleman, Hope	*Motherless Daughters*	Dell Publishing Company	Mother	14 and up
Graeber, C.	*Mustard*	New York: MacMillian Publishing Co.	Cat	6–10
Hemery, Kathleen	*The Brightest Star*	Omaha, NE: Centering Corporation	Mother	4–8
Henkes, Kevin	*Sun & Spoon*	New York: Greenwillow Books	Grandmother	9–13
Hermes, P.	*You Shouldn't Have to Say Goodbye*	New York: Harcourt Brace Jovanovich	Mother	9–13
Hesse, K.	*Poppy's Chair*	New York: MacMillian Publishing Co.	Grandfather	6–11
Hickman, M. W.	*Last Week My Brother Anthony Died*	Abington Press	Brother	3–7
Holmes, Margaret and Mudlaff, Sasha	*Molly's Mom Died*	Omaha, NE: Centering Corporation	Mother	5–9
Lorenzen, K.	*Lanky Longlegs*	New York: Atheneum. A Margaret K. McElderry Book	Brother	9–13
Lowden, Stephanie Golightly	*Emily's Sadhappy Season*	Omaha, NE: Centering Corporation	Father	4–8
Schotter, R.	*A Matter of Time*	New York: Collins Press	Mother	14 and up
Scrivani, Mark	*I Heard Your Mommy Died*	Omaha, NE: Centering Corporation	Mother	3–7
Scrivani, Mark	*I Heard Your Daddy Died*	Omaha, NE: Centering Corporation	Father	3–7
Scrivani, Mark	*When Death Walks In: For Teens Facing Grief*	Omaha, NE: Centering Corporation		13 and up
Shook-Hazen, B.	*Why Did Grandpa Die*	Racine, WI: Western Publishing Co.	Grandfather	3–7
Smith, D. B.	*A Taste of Blackberries*	Boston: Thomas Crowell Company	Friend	6–11
Thomas, J. R.	*Saying Goodbye to Grandma*	New York: Clarion Books	Grandmother	6–11
Tiffault, Benette	*A Quilt for Elizabeth*	Omaha, NE: Centering Corporation	Father	4–8
Vigna, Judith	*Saying Goodbye to Daddy*	Morton Grove, IL: Albert Whitman & Co.	Father	6–9

Cultural Snapshot

Death and dying are not discussed openly in many cultures. In some cultures, the fact that a person is dying is discussed only in very private settings and often not with the dying individual. In front of the dying child for instance, the atmosphere might be jovial, with eating, joking, playing games, and singing.

Adolescents usually are sensitive to what is happening to them and may need you to be an advocate for them if they have wishes they want to fulfill before dying. An adolescent who senses your willingness and ability may discuss feelings that he or she is uncomfortable discussing with family members. You can talk with the adoles-

Acceptance is not as hard as you think.

When working with the child who is dying, as well as the child's family, honest, specific answers leave less room for misinterpretation and distortion.

cent and work with the family to help them understand the adolescent's desires and needs. You can call on hospice workers, social or psychiatric services, or a member of the clergy to help the family express and resolve their concerns and recognize the adolescent's needs.

THE FAMILY'S REACTION TO DYING AND DEATH

The death of a child sends feelings of shock, disbelief, and guilt through every family member. Family members typically go through the stages of the grieving process: denial and isolation, anger, bargaining, depression and acute grief, and, finally, acceptance. Not every child or family will complete the process because each family, as well as each death, is personal and unique.

When death is expected, as in a terminal illness, the family begins to mourn in anticipation of the death, a phenomenon called **anticipatory grief**. For some people, this shortens the period of acute grief and loss after the child's death. Anticipatory grief begins when a potentially fatal disease (such as acquired immunodeficiency syndrome, cystic fibrosis, or cancer) is diagnosed and continues until remission or death. When the disease rapidly advances, anticipatory grief may be short-lived as the child's death nears. In cases of accidental or sudden death, the family has no time to anticipate or begin grieving the loss of the child. Their grief may last longer and be more difficult to resolve.

Grief for the death of a child is not limited in time but may continue for years. Sometimes professional counseling is necessary to help family members work through grief. The support of others who have experienced the same sort of loss can be helpful. Two national organizations founded to offer support are the Candlelighters Childhood Cancer Foundation and The Compassionate Friends (see Internet Resources at the end of the chapter). These organizations have many local chapters.

Family Caregivers' Reactions

Family caregivers may grieve for the death of a child that follows a terminal illness or that is sudden and unexpected.

Terminal Illness

The family caregivers of children in the final stages of a terminal illness may have had to cope with many hospital admissions between periods at home. During this time, the family may face decisions about the child's physical care, as well as learning to live with a dying child. As the child's condition deteriorates, you can encourage the family to talk to their child about dying. This is a task they may find very difficult. Support from a religious counselor, hospice nurse, or social service or psychiatric worker can help them through this difficult task. Family caregivers can be encouraged to provide as much normalcy as possible in the child's schedule. School attendance and special trips can be encouraged within the child's capabilities and desires.

During this time, family caregivers may go through a grieving process of anger, depression, ambivalence, and bargaining over and over again. The caregivers may direct anger at the hospital staff, themselves (because of guilt), each other, or the child. Reassure the caregivers that this is a normal reaction, but avoid taking sides.

If the child improves enough to go home again, parents may find themselves overprotecting the child. As in chronic illness, this overprotective attitude reinforces the child's sick behavior and dependency and is usually accompanied by a lack of discipline. Failure to set limits accentuates the child's feelings of being different and creates problems with siblings. The child learns to manipulate family members, only to find that this kind of behavior does not bring positive results when attempted with peers or health care personnel.

When the child has to return to the hospital because of increasing symptoms, family caregivers may once again experience all stages of the grieving process. The family members dread the child's approaching death and fear that the child will be in great pain or may die when they are not present. You can help relieve these fears by keeping the family informed about the child's condition, making the child as comfortable as possible, and reassuring the family members that they will be summoned if death appears to be near.

When death comes, it is perfectly appropriate to share the family's grief, crying with them then giving them privacy to express their sorrow. You can stay with the family for a while, remaining quietly supportive with an attitude of a comforting listener. An appropriate comment may be, "I am so sorry" or "This is a very sad time." Keep the focus on the family's grief and what you can do to support them.

The family may want to hold the child to say a final goodbye, and you can encourage and assist them in this. Intravenous lines and other equipment can be removed to make holding the child easier. The family may be left alone during this time if they desire. Be sensitive to the family's needs and desires to provide them with comfort.

> **A little sensitivity is in order.**
> When a child dies, it is not an appropriate time for you to share personal experiences of loss.

Test Yourself

✔ What does the term *anticipatory grief* mean?

✔ How is anticipatory grief helpful to the family who has lost a child by death?

✔ Why is it important for family caregivers to refrain from being overprotective with the dying child?

Sudden or Unexpected Death

When a child dies suddenly and unexpectedly, the family is not able to prepare for the death as they could with a terminal illness. They do not have the opportunity to complete unfinished business or go through anticipatory grief. Such a family may have excessive guilt and remorse for something they felt they left unsaid or undone. Even if a child has had a traumatic death with disfigurement, the family must be given the opportunity to be with, see, and hold the child to help with closure of the child's life. You can prepare the family for seeing the child, explaining why parts of the body may be covered. Viewing the child, even if the body is severely mutilated, helps the family to have a realistic view of the child and aids in the grief process.

The family may face a number of decisions that must be made rather quickly, especially when the child's death is unexpected. Families of terminally ill children usually have made some plans for the child's death and may know exactly what they want done. However, when the child dies unexpectedly, decisions may be necessary concerning organ donation, funeral arrangements, and an autopsy. If the death has been the result of violence or is unexplained, law requires an autopsy, but there may be other reasons that an autopsy is desired. An autopsy might be helpful in finding causes and treatments for other children diagnosed with the same disease, especially if it is a diagnosis about which little research is available. Organ donation can be discussed with the family by the hospital's organ donor coordinator or other designated person. The family needs to be well informed and must be supported throughout these difficult decisions.

The Child's Reaction

The child who has a terminal illness also experiences anticipatory grief. Even young children are aware of the seriousness of their illness because of the actions and emotions of the people around them. The child realizes that he is going to die and that there is no cure for him. Sadness and depression are common. The child may have fears about dying as well as concerns for the family members who will be left behind. It is important for the

 ## A Personal Glimpse

As I sit here each morning after losing my little girl, I know I'll make it through another day. I know this because I told her every day how happy I was that she was my child. As she was developing into a young woman, I never forgot to say how gorgeous she looked. I also know in my heart I can sleep each night hereafter, because from the day I gave birth to her I told her to always come back to me. Don't get me wrong! I always worried endlessly, but I felt it was important for her not to know these fears. As parents, we hope our kids will always do the right thing. I wanted my children, and still do Michael, to know that whatever they did or do I would stand behind them, beside them, and always in my heart near them. I spent every waking day with Nicole and Michael as they were growing. I enjoyed all their developmental years. I reveled in their games, ideas, and thoughts. I know now that I was growing vicariously through them. Not a day went by that I didn't want them with me. Maybe because of this I was not as good a wife as I should have been, but I can sleep at night knowing that I was and am a great mother to my children.

You are all saying how strong I am. This is not strength. This is the power of knowing I tried through it all to be supportive and share with them what little knowledge I had. I understood that these little bodies were given to me to mold and build into productive, loving, caring human beings and with that I held the future so that my grandchildren would be better people. Nicole would have definitely gone on to bigger and better things. I know her part in society would have made a difference. Her impact on the future would have changed things for the better. Cry? I really can't cry, for I know my Nikki will never leave me. I'll always see her smile. I'll always remember her voice. I'll always remember all the little things she needed to cultivate to become the adult that she would have become.

Sunday night the skies were in such turmoil. I found deep solace in that for I knew that they were letting her in. She was probably fighting with others and found her way to the front of the line. I know in my heart that once she got there she began checking the situation carefully and assessing what needed to be done and the tasks that she wanted to take on to make a difference up there. How do I know this? The skies were rumbling, the lightning was crashing, and then a heavy downpour began. I knew the angels were crying—so happy and confused as to why someone with so much to give on Earth would be up in Heaven so early. This went on for a good 10 minutes. It was pouring like crazy and then in my Nikki's infinite wisdom she spoke to them, explained the stupidity of that night, and everyone settled down. I also found great comfort, for at this time the sun, which hadn't appeared all day, broke through the clouds and shined on me. I was sitting where she knows I always sit when I need quiet time and through an opening in these clouds she spoke directly to me and said "Ma, I'm here. It's okay. I tried to get home. I would have told you some of the things of how my night was. But, Ma, I screwed up and I'll be waiting here for all of you!" This, my friend, is what has given me comfort. To love has many different meanings, but I am by far a better person for having her in memories with me always. Thanks Nikki. I will always love you.

Marie (after losing her 16-yr-old daughter, Nicole, in a car accident)

Learning Opportunity: What are some of the experiences this mother shared that gave her strength in dealing with her daughter's death? What are your feelings about the death of a child or teenager?

child to have the opportunity to talk about fears, anger, and concerns, as well as to be able to express feelings about the joys and happiness in his or her life. When the child is ready to talk about these things, encourage him or her to do so. The child needs support, honesty, and answers to questions regarding her illness, treatment, and prognosis. Children should be encouraged to express their feelings through crying, playing, acting out, or drawing. The child may fear that pain is a part of death and should be reassured that medications can be used to control pain and keep the child comfortable. Religious and spiritual beliefs can help the child deal with feelings regarding separation from family. Reassure the child that he will not be alone at the time of death.

The dying child may have a decreased level of consciousness, although hearing remains intact. Family members at the bedside and health care personnel may need to be reminded to avoid saying anything that would not be said if the child were fully conscious. Gentle touching and caressing may provide comfort to the child.

Excellent nursing care is required. Medications for pain are given intravenously because they are poorly absorbed from muscle due to poor circulation. Keep mucous membranes clean, and apply petroleum jelly (Vaseline) to the lips to prevent drying and cracking. Moisten the conjunctiva of the eyes with normal saline eye drops, such as Artificial Tears, if drying occurs. Keep the skin clean and dry, and turn and position the child regularly to provide comfort and to prevent skin breakdown. While caring for the child, talk to the child and explain everything that is being done.

As death approaches, the internal body temperature increases; thus, dying patients seem to be unaware of cold even though their skin feels cool. Explain this to family members so they do not think the child needs additional covering. Just before death, the child who has remained conscious may become restless, followed by a time of peace and calm. Be aware of these reactions and know that death is near; keep family members informed as well.

Test Yourself

✔ What feelings might the family of a child who dies suddenly and unexpectedly have?

✔ For what reason should caregivers and families never say anything in the presence of a comatose child that they would not say if the child were alert?

Siblings' Reactions

The siblings of a child who is dying of a terminal illness have an opportunity to themselves go through a period of anticipatory grieving. If a sibling dies suddenly, the sibling begins the process of grief at the time of the death. Siblings may feel confused, lonely, and frightened about the sudden loss of their brother or sister. The unexpected change in the atmosphere of the household can be upsetting.

Just as in the case of chronic illness, siblings resent the attention given to the ill child and are angry about the disruption in the family. Reaction varies according to the sibling's developmental age and parental attitudes and actions. Younger children find it almost impossible to understand what is happening; it is difficult even for older children to grasp. Reaction to the illness and its accompanying stresses can cause classroom problems for school-aged siblings; these may be incorrectly labeled as learning disabilities or behavioral disorders unless school personnel are aware of the family situation.

When the child dies, young siblings who are still prone to magical thinking may feel guilty, particularly if a strong degree of rivalry existed before the illness. These children need continued reassurance that they did not cause or help to cause their sibling's death.

The decision of whether or not a sibling should attend funeral services for the child may be difficult. Although there has been little research, the current thinking among many health professionals supports the presence of the sibling. The sibling may be encouraged to leave a token of love and good-bye with the child—a drawing, note, toy, or another special memento. Siblings can visit the dead child in privacy with few other mourners present. Dealing with the realities of the brother's or sister's death openly is likely to be more beneficial than avoiding the issue and allowing the sibling to use his or her imagination about death (Box 34-2).

SETTINGS FOR CARE OF THE DYING CHILD

Where the child dies can greatly influence the family's response to and acceptance of a child's death. In a hospital, the child may receive the most professional care and the most technologically advanced treatment. However, having a child in the hospital can contribute to family separation, a feeling of loss of control, and a sense of isolation. An increasing number of families are choosing to keep the child at home to die.

Hospice Care

In medieval times, a **hospice** was a refuge for various travelers—not only those traveling through the countryside, but also the terminally ill who were leaving this life for another. Hospices often were operated by religious orders and became havens for the dying. The current hospice movement in health care began in England,

Box 34-2 ▌ GUIDELINES FOR HELPING CHILDREN COPE WITH DEATH

DO

- Know your own beliefs.
- Begin where the child is.
- Be there.
- Confront reality.
- Encourage expression of feelings.
- Be truthful.
- Include the child in family rituals.
- Encourage remembrance.
- Admit when you don't know the answer.
- Use touch to communicate.
- Start death education early, simply, using naturally occurring events.
- Recognize symptoms of grief and deal with the grief.
- Accept differing reactions to death.

DON'T

- Praise stoicism (detached, unemotional behavior).
- Use euphemisms (mild expressions substituted for ones that might be offensive).
- Be nonchalant.
- Glamorize death.
- Tell fairy tales or half-truths.
- Close the door to questions.
- Be judgmental of feelings and behaviors.
- Protect the child from exposure to experiences with death.
- Encourage forgetting the deceased.
- Encourage the child to be like the deceased.

---

when Dr. Cicely Saunders founded St. Christopher's Hospice in London in 1967. This institution has become the model for others in the United States and Canada, with an emphasis on sensitive, humane care for the dying. Hospice principles of care include relief of pain, attention to the needs of the total person, and absence of heroic life-saving measures.

The first hospice in the United States was the New Haven Hospice in Connecticut. Many communities now have hospice programs that may or may not be affiliated with a hospital. Some programs offer a hospice setting to which patients go in terminal stages of illness; others provide support and guidance for the patient and family while the patient remains in the hospital or is cared for at home. Most of these hospice programs are established primarily for adults, but some programs also accept children as patients.

Children's Hospice International, founded in 1983, is an organization dedicated to hospice support of children. Through an individualized plan of care, Children's Hospice addresses the physical, developmental, psychological, social, and spiritual needs of children and families in a comprehensive and consistent way. It serves as a resource and advocacy center, providing education for parents and professionals. The organization conducts seminars and conferences, publishes training manuals, and supports a clearinghouse of information available through a national hotline (1-800-24-CHILD). Its Web site (www.chionline.org) provides information for adults, as well as games, books, and an excellent list of Web sites for children.

Home Care

Caring for the dying patient, young or old, at home has become increasingly common in recent years. More families are choosing to keep their child at home during the terminal stage of illness. Factors that contribute to the decision to care for a child at home include:

- Concerns about costs for hospitalization and nonmedical expenses such as the family's travel, housing, and food
- Stress from repeated family separations
- Loss of control over the care of the child and family life

Families feel that the more loving, caring environment of the home draws the family closer and helps to reduce the guilt that often is a part of bereavement. All family members can be involved to some extent in the child's care and in this way gain a feeling of usefulness. Family caregivers feel that they remain in control.

There are disadvantages of home care, however. Costs that would have been covered by health insurance if the child were hospitalized may not be covered if the child is cared for at home. Caring for a dying child can be extremely difficult emotionally and physically. Not every family has someone who can carry out the procedures that may need to be performed regularly. In some instances, home nursing assistance is available, but this varies from community to community. Usually the home care nurse visits several days a week and may be on call the rest of the time. In some communities, hospice nurses may provide the teaching and support that families need.

■ **Figure 34-4** The nurse helps support the dying child in the hospital setting.

Deciding whether or not to care for a dying child at home is an extremely difficult decision for a family. Family members need support and guidance from health care personnel when they are trying to make the decision, after the decision is made, and even after the child dies.

Hospital Care

Dying in a hospital has both limitations and advantages. The child and the family may find support from others in the same situation. Family members may not have the physical or emotional strength to cope with total care of the child at home, but they can participate in care supported by the hospital staff (Fig. 34-4). Hospital care is much more expensive, but this may not be important to some families, especially those with health insurance. The hospital is still the culturally accepted place to die, and this is important to some people. Patients and families who choose hospital care need to know that they have rights and can exert some control over what happens to them.

Test Yourself

✔ What are the principles of hospice care for the dying child?

✔ What factors contribute to the decision to care for a dying child at home?

✔ What might be helpful for the family of a dying child, if the child is hospitalized?

THE ROLE OF THE NURSE

As the nurse, you play an important role in providing both physical care for the child who is dying and emotional care for both the child and family. Provide information as clearly and simply as possible. Open, honest communication is important. Encourage the child and family to share their feelings and reactions to the situation and to ask questions. Support by listening and providing appropriate interventions.

Nursing Process for The Dying Child

Assessment

The assessment of the terminally ill child and family is an ongoing process developed over a period of time by the health care team. The health care team's assessment covers the child's developmental level, the influence of cultural and spiritual concerns, the family's support system, present indications of grieving (e.g., anticipatory grief), interactions among family members, and unfinished business. To understand the child's view of death, consider the child's previous experiences, developmental level, and cognitive ability.

Selected Nursing Diagnoses

Nursing diagnoses for the dying child include those appropriate for the child's illness, as well as the following, which are specific to the dying process:

- Acute Pain related to illness and weakened condition
- Risk for Social Isolation related to terminal illness
- Anxiety related to condition and prognosis
- Compromised Family Coping related to approaching death
- Powerlessness of family caregivers related to inability to control child's condition

Outcome Identification and Planning

Goals and plans of care depend on the stage of the illness, the child's and the family's acceptance of the illness, and their attitudes and beliefs about death and dying. Major goals for the child include minimizing pain, diminishing feelings of abandonment by peers and friends, and relieving anxiety about the future. Goals for the family include helping cope with the impending death and identifying feelings of powerlessness.

Implementation

Relieving Pain and Discomfort

The child may be in pain for many reasons such as chemotherapy; nausea, vomiting, and gastrointestinal cramping; pressure caused by positioning; or constipation. Until the child is comfortable and relatively pain free, all other nursing interventions are fruitless: Pain becomes the child's primary focus until relief is provided. Nursing measures to relieve pain may include positioning, using pillows as needed; changing linens; providing conscientious skin and mouth care; protecting skin surfaces from rubbing together; offering back rubs and massages; and administering antiemetics, analgesics, and stool softeners as appropriate.

Providing Appropriate Social Interactions

Encourage the child's siblings and friends to maintain contact. Provide opportunities for peers to visit, write, or telephone, as the child is able. Read to the child and engage in other activities that he or she finds interesting and physically tolerable. When possible, encourage the child to make decisions to foster a feeling of control. Explain all procedures and how they will affect the child. Provide the child with privacy, but do not neglect him or her. Provide ample periods of rest. Continue to talk to and tell the child what you are doing, even though the child may seem unresponsive.

Easing the Child's Anxiety

Ask family caregivers about the child's understanding of death and previous experiences with death. Observe how the child exhibits fear, and ask family caregivers for any additional information. Encourage the child to use a doll, a pillow, or another special "warm fuzzy" for comfort. Use words such as "dead" or "dying," if appropriate, in conversation because this may give the child an opening to talk about death. Nighttime is especially frightening for children because they often think they will die at night. Provide company and comfort, and be alert for periods of wakefulness when the child may need someone to talk with. Be honest and straightforward, and avoid injecting your beliefs into the conversation. If appropriate, read a book about death to the child to initiate conversation (although ideally this would have been done much earlier in the child's care).

Helping the Family Cope

Family caregivers may need encouragement to discuss their feelings about the child. Acknowledge emotions and fears and reassure caregivers that their reactions are normal. The support of a member of the clergy may be helpful during this time. Help family members contact their own spiritual counselor, or offer to contact the hospital chaplain if the family desires. Encourage family caregivers to eat and rest properly so they will not become ill or exhausted, themselves. Explain the child's condition to the family and answer any questions. Reassure the family that everything is being done to keep the child as comfortable and pain free as possible. Interpret signs of approaching death for the family.

If appropriate, ask the family about the siblings: what they know, how much they understand, and if the family has discussed the approaching death. Offer to help the caregivers talk with siblings.

Helping the Family Feel Involved in the Child's Care

Respond to the family's need to feel some control over the situation by suggesting specific measures they can perform to provide comfort for the child such as positioning, moistening lips, and reading or telling a favorite story. Encourage the caregivers to talk to the child even if the child does not respond. Discourage whispered conversations in the room. Encourage and help the family to carry out cultural customs if they wish. Help the family complete any unfinished business on the agenda; this may include the need for the child to go home to die. Help family contact support persons such as hospice workers or social services. (See Nursing Care Plan 34-1.)

Evaluation: Goals and Expected Outcomes

Goal: The child will have minimal pain.
Expected Outcomes: The child

- rests quietly.
- reports no pain when asked.

Goal: The child will have social interaction with others.
Expected Outcome:

- Within physical capabilities, the child engages in activities with peers, family, and others.

Goal: The child will express feelings of anxiety and use available supports to cope with anxiety.
Expected Outcomes:

- The child keeps a "warm fuzzy" close by for comfort and talks about death to the nurse or family.
- When awake at night, the child is comforted by the presence of someone to talk with.

Goal: The family members will develop ways to cope with the child's approaching death.
Expected Outcomes:

- The family members express their feelings; identify signs that indicate approaching death; and use available support systems and people.
- The siblings visit and talk about their feelings regarding the approaching death of their sister or brother.

Goal: The family members will be involved in the child's care to decrease feelings of powerlessness.
Expected Outcomes: The family members

- provide comfort measures for the child and talk to the child.
- complete unfinished business with the child.

Nursing Care Plan 34-1

THE DYING CHILD AND FAMILY

CASE SCENARIO
JR is a 7-year-old who has a terminal illness. She is not expected to live more than a few more weeks. She has a brother who is 10 and a sister who is 4. A family member is with her continuously.

NURSING DIAGNOSIS
Acute Pain related to illness and weakened condition

GOAL: The child will have minimal pain.

EXPECTED OUTCOMES
• The child has uninterrupted periods of quiet rest.
• Using a pain scale, the child indicates that she experiences relief from pain.

Nursing Interventions	*Rationale*
Pain relief must be the primary focus of all nursing care until the child is comfortable.	Pain is the child's primary focus; until pain is relieved, all other nursing interventions are fruitless.
Administer pain relief medication, but also include such nursing measures as positioning, providing back rubs and massages, changing linens, providing conscientious skin and mouth care, and protecting skin surfaces from rubbing together to increase child's comfort.	Each child's pain experience is unique, and it may vary from one time to another. Some measures may relieve pain in one situation but not another. Discover the measures that work most frequently for this child.

NURSING DIAGNOSIS
Risk for Social Isolation related to terminal illness

GOAL: The child will have social interaction with others.

EXPECTED OUTCOMES
• The child engages in social interaction with her classmates and other peers.
• The family caregivers and others play games with or read to child within her physical limitations.
• The caregivers talk with child when giving care regardless of her apparent level of consciousness.

Nursing Interventions	*Rationale*
Encourage child's siblings and peers (including school friends) to maintain contact; provide opportunities for such contact by arranging for convenient visiting hours, providing paper and pens for writing, and making a telephone available.	The child needs to feel that she is not cut off from everyone and everything. This helps relieve boredom and also diverts the child's attention from her condition.
Spend time with and talk to the child, even when you are not sure she is responsive.	Hearing is often the last sense to shut down; the child will feel reassured by your voice and presence.

NURSING DIAGNOSIS
Anxiety related to condition and prognosis

GOAL: The child will express feelings of anxiety and use available supports to cope with anxiety.

EXPECTED OUTCOMES
• The child talks to her family or the nurse about death.
• The child has a "warm fuzzy" close by.
• The child freely expresses her fears about dying, especially fears about nighttime.

Nursing Care Plan 34-1 (continued)

THE DYING CHILD AND FAMILY

Nursing Interventions	Rationale
Discuss with the family the child's understanding of death, and note how she exhibits fear. Use straightforward terminology when discussing death.	The child may or may not have discussed death with the family, and it is important for the nurse to respond to the child appropriately. The nurse is able at the same time to get a sense of how family members view the child's death and what sort of help they may need to discuss the topic with their child and each other.
Encourage the child to keep a favorite object or "warm fuzzy" for comfort and reassurance. Provide company and comfort particularly at night. Keep a night light on to ease anxieties.	Many children think they will die at night; periods of wakefulness are common. If the child is left alone, fears may compound. A night light provides some sense of security.

NURSING DIAGNOSIS
Compromised Family Coping related to approaching death

GOAL: The family members will develop ways to cope with the child's approaching death.

EXPECTED OUTCOMES
- The family caregivers express their feelings and anxieties.
- The family caregivers contact a spiritual advisor for support.
- The family caregivers identify signs in the child that indicate approaching death.

Nursing Interventions	Rationale
Encourage family caregivers to discuss their feelings about the child and to acknowledge their fears and emotions; reassure them that their reactions are normal.	It may be very difficult for family members to talk about their child's death; they may feel they need to "keep up a brave front" for the child and siblings. However, it is important for them to acknowledge the death and begin to express some of their emotions.
Help the family contact their spiritual advisor or a hospital chaplain, if they desire.	The support of a spiritual counselor, particularly one known to the family, may be helpful.
Help the family recognize and acknowledge signs of the child's impending death. Help them talk with her siblings.	Acknowledging the impending signs of death helps the family caregivers to be realistic about the approaching death. They also may need support and guidance to know how to talk with the other children.
Make sure family caregivers are resting and eating adequately.	The family caregivers must avoid exhaustion; lack of sleep and inadequate nutrition will only make it harder for them to cope.

NURSING DIAGNOSIS
Powerlessness of family caregivers related to inability to control child's condition

GOAL: The family members will be involved in child's care to decrease feelings of powerlessness.

EXPECTED OUTCOMES
- The family caregivers provide comfort measures for the child.
- The family caregivers talk with child and complete unfinished business with her.

(continues on page 736)

Nursing Care Plan 34-1 (continued)

THE DYING CHILD AND FAMILY

Nursing Interventions	*Rationale*
Suggest specific care measures that family members might perform to comfort the child; encourage the family to carry out cultural practices if they desire.	Caregivers need to feel they are doing something to help their child; performing meaningful cultural customs helps the family express feelings and provides a feeling of continuity.
Explain "unfinished business" to the family and encourage them to complete any unfinished business on their agenda.	Discussion of unfinished business provides another opportunity for family members to engage in meaningful activity with their child before the child's death.
Encourage family members to talk to the child even when she seems unresponsive.	The child may be able to hear voices even when unable to respond; family caregivers will feel better when they can still communicate love and support.

Key Points

➤ Anticipatory grief shortens the period of acute grief and loss after the child's death.

➤ Nurses and other health care workers often are uncomfortable with dying patients because they are afraid that the patients will ask questions they cannot or should not answer. In addition, death reminds us of our own mortality, a thought with which many of us are uncomfortable. It is important to examine your own feelings about death and the reasons for these feelings.

➤ You can personally prepare to care for dying children by exploring your own feelings about life and death. Attending a workshop, conference, or seminar in which one's own feelings about death are explored can be helpful. Talking with other professionals, sharing concerns, comforting each other in stressful times, and reading studies about death to discover how dying patients feel about their situation also can be helpful in preparing to work with dying patients.

➤ Factors that affect the child's understanding of death include his/her stage of development, cognitive ability, experiences, and how the family deals with death. Most children do not understand the finality of death until they near preadolescence.

➤ Infants and toddlers have little understanding of death; the toddler may fear separation but has no recognition of the fact that death is nearing and irreversible. The preschool child may believe that death happens because of angry thoughts. Magical thinking about death and thinking of death as a kind of sleep are seen in preschool-aged children until about 8 or 9 years of age. After age 9, children gain the

concept that death is universal and irreversible. Adolescents have an adult understanding of death, but feel that they are immortal—that is, death will happen to others but not to them.

➤ When a child has a terminal illness, family caregivers go through anticipatory grieving. Families have the opportunity to complete unfinished business by spending time with the dying child, helping siblings to understand the child's illness and impending death, and giving family members a chance to share their love with the child.

➤ When a child dies suddenly, a family may suffer excessive grief and guilt for something they felt they left unsaid or undone.

➤ When a sibling dies, possible reactions seen in children depend on the stage of development of that sibling. Young siblings find death impossible to understand. School-aged siblings may have classroom problems, behavioral disorders, and feelings of guilt about the death of their sibling. Dealing with the realities of the brother's or sister's death openly is likely to be more beneficial than avoiding the issue.

➤ Settings for caring for the dying child include the home, hospice, and hospital settings. The home provides a loving, caring environment and may decrease costs and family separations. Home settings may prevent some expenses from being covered and may be difficult emotionally and physically for the family. Hospice principles of care include relief of pain, attention to the needs of the total person, and absence of heroic life-saving measures. In the hospital setting, the child and the family may find support from others in the same situation, support from the hospital staff, and technologically advanced treatment. Hospital care is much more expensive, but this may not be important to some families. The hospital is still the culturally accepted place to die, but having a child in the hospital can contribute to family separation, a feeling of loss of control, and a sense of isolation.

➤ Nursing care for the dying child focuses on minimizing pain, diminishing feelings of abandonment by the child's peers and friends, and relieving anxiety about the future. Care also aims to help the family find ways to cope with the impending death and to identify feelings of powerlessness.

INTERNET RESOURCES

Candlelighters Childhood Cancer Foundation
www.candlelighters.org

Children's Hospice International
www.chionline.org

The Compassionate Friends
www.compassionatefriends.org

Hospice
www.hospicenet.org

Workbook

▉ NCLEX-STYLE REVIEW QUESTIONS

1. While the nurse is working with the family of a child who is terminally ill, the child's siblings make the following statements to the nurse. Which statement is an example of the stage of grief referred to as bargaining?

   a. "I just want him to come to my birthday party next month."

   b. "It makes me mad that they said my brother is going to die."

   c. "I think he will get well now that he has a new medicine."

   d. "When he dies, at least he won't have any more pain."

2. When working with the family of a child who is terminally ill, the child's siblings make the following statements to the nurse. Which statement is an example of the stage of grief referred to as denial?

   a. "I just want him to come to my birthday party next month."

   b. "It makes me mad that they said my brother is going to die."

   c. "I think he will get well now that he has a new medicine."

   d. "When he dies, at least he won't have any more pain."

3. The nurse is working with a group of 4- and 5-year-old children who are talking about death and dying. One child in the group recently experienced the death of the family pet. Which of the following statements would the nurse expect a 5-year-old child to say about the death of the pet?

   a. "I think he was sad to leave us."

   b. "He's only a little dead."

   c. "A monster came and took him during the night."

   d. "I will be real good so I won't die."

4. The nurse is discussing the subject of death and dying with a group of adolescents. Which of the following statements made by an adolescent would be expected considering her or his stage of growth and development?

   a. "I always hold my breath and run past the cemetery to protect myself."

   b. "It would be sad to die because my girlfriend would really miss me."

   c. "Others die in car wrecks, but even if I had a wreck, I wouldn't be killed."

   d. "It makes me nervous to go to sleep. I am afraid I won't wake up."

5. The nurse is with a family whose terminally ill child has just died. Which of the following statements made by the nurse would be the *most* therapeutic statement?

   a. "It will not hurt as much as time passes."

   b. "My sister died when I was a teenager. I know how you feel."

   c. "I will leave the call light here. Call me if you need me."

   d. "This is a really sad and difficult time."

6. The family of a child with a terminal illness might go through a process known as anticipatory grief. Which of the following might occur for the family during this process? Select all that apply.

   a. Having an opportunity to complete unfinished business

   b. Preparing for the eventual death of the child

   c. Having no feelings of guilt or remorse

   d. Beginning the process of preparing for the funeral

   e. Helping the child's siblings deal with the coming death

▉ STUDY ACTIVITIES

1. List and compare thoughts and ideas a child of each of the following ages would most likely have regarding death and dying:

Toddler	Preschool	School-aged	Adolescent

2. Research your community to find the procedure for organ donation. Make arrangements for a speaker from the organization to discuss organ donation with your class. If such a person is not available, research organ donation on the Internet and share your findings with your class.

3. Survey your community to see if there is a hospice available. Describe how it functions. Find out if it accepts children as patients and if there are any restrictions concerning children. Discuss your findings with your peers.

4. Do an Internet search on "sibling loss." Find a site dealing with ways to help children deal with the loss of a sibling.

■ CRITICAL THINKING: WHAT WOULD YOU DO?

1. The Andrews family has an 8-year-old daughter with a terminal illness.

   a. What factors do you think the family needs to consider when deciding if they will care for the child at home?

   b. What feelings do you think the family might be dealing with?

2. The Andrews decide they cannot care for the child at home.

   a. What are your feelings about this decision?

   b. What would you say to this family to support them in their decision?

UNIT X

THE CHILD WITH A HEALTH DISORDER

35

The Child With a Sensory/ Neurological Disorder

KEY TERMS

amblyopia
astigmatism
ataxia
aura
binocular vision
cataract
clonus
conjunctivitis
diplopia
dysarthria
esotropia
exotropia
febrile seizures
goniotomy
hordeolum
hyperopia
lacrimation
myopia
myringotomy
nuchal rigidity
opisthotonos
orthoptics
partial seizures
photophobia
purpuric rash
refraction
strabismus

LEARNING OBJECTIVES

On completion of this chapter, you should be able to:

1. Discuss ways the infant and child's eyes, ears, and nervous system differ from the adult's.
2. Compare different types of vision impairment.
3. Describe eye conditions and treatment for these conditions.
4. Differentiate types of hearing impairment and explain the difference between a child who is hard of hearing and one who is deaf.
5. Explain otitis media including the behavior of the child with acute otitis media.
6. Discuss the symptoms, diagnosis, and treatment of Reye syndrome.
7. Discuss nursing care for a child with acute or nonrecurrent seizures.
8. Discuss seizure disorders and the nursing care specific to a child at high risk for seizures.
9. Describe (a) simple partial motor seizures, (b) simple partial sensory seizures, and (c) complex partial (psychomotor) seizures.
10. Describe (a) tonic-clonic seizures, (b) absence seizures, (c) atonic or akinetic seizures, (d) myoclonic seizures, and (e) infantile spasms.
11. Explain status epilepticus and the treatment for this disorder.
12. Discuss *Haemophilus influenzae* meningitis including the potential complications.
13. Describe cerebral palsy and its causes.
14. Differentiate between types of cerebral palsy.
15. Identify the health care professionals involved in the care of the child with cerebral palsy.
16. List the possible causes of mental retardation.
17. Discuss the nursing care of the child with cognitive impairment.
18. Describe head injuries seen in children.
19. Discuss drowning in children and the immediate care of a drowning victim.

NEUROLOGIC disorders can be caused by many different factors. Nerve cells do not regenerate, and complications from these disorders can be serious and permanent. If neurologic damage has occurred, your role as the nurse is often one of support and guidance to the child and family dealing with the neurologic disorder.

Children learn about the world they live in through their senses. Any disorder related to the eyes and ears can have significant impact on the normal growth and development of the child.

GROWTH AND DEVELOPMENT OF THE EYES, EARS, AND NERVOUS SYSTEM
The Nervous System

The nervous system is the communication network of the body. The central nervous system is made up of the brain and spinal cord. The peripheral nervous system is made up of the nerves throughout the body. A fluid known as cerebrospinal fluid flows through the chambers of the brain and through the spinal cord, serving as a cushion and protective mechanism for nerve cells.

Maybe this will jog your memory on an exam.
Cerebrospinal fluid continually forms, circulates, and is reabsorbed. Many neurologic disorders relate to this aspect of the functioning of the nervous system.

Nerves go from the brain and spinal cord to all parts of the body. These nerves quickly transmit information from the central nervous system. Stimuli of all types cause signals called nerve impulses to occur. These nerve impulses activate, coordinate, integrate, and control all of the body functions.

A part of the peripheral nervous system, the autonomic nervous system, regulates the involuntary functions of the body, such as the heart rate. At birth, the nervous system is immature. As the child grows, the quality of the nerve impulses sent through the nervous system develops and matures. As these nerve impulses become more mature, the child's gross and fine motor skills increase in complexity. The child becomes more coordinated and able to develop motor skills.

Sensory Organs

The eyes and ears are specialized organs of the nervous system. These organs transmit impulses to the central nervous system.

Eyes

The eye is a sensory organ that detects light, the stimuli, from the environment. Parts of the eye respond to the light and produce and transmit a nerve impulse to the brain. That information and image is interpreted in the brain, and thus the person "sees" the object.

Newborns do not focus clearly, but will stare at a human face directly in front of them. By 2 months of age, the infant can focus and follow an object with the eyes (Fig. 35-1). By 7 months of age, depth perception has matured enough so that the infant can transfer objects back and forth between his or her hands. Visual acuity of children gradually increases from birth, when the visual acuity is usually between 20/100 and 20/400 until about 7 years of age, when most children have 20/20 vision (Traboulsi, 2006).

Ears

Ears function as the sensory organ of hearing, as well as the organ responsible in part for equilibrium and balance. Sounds waves, vibrations, and fluid movements create nerve impulses that the brain ultimately distinguishes as sounds.

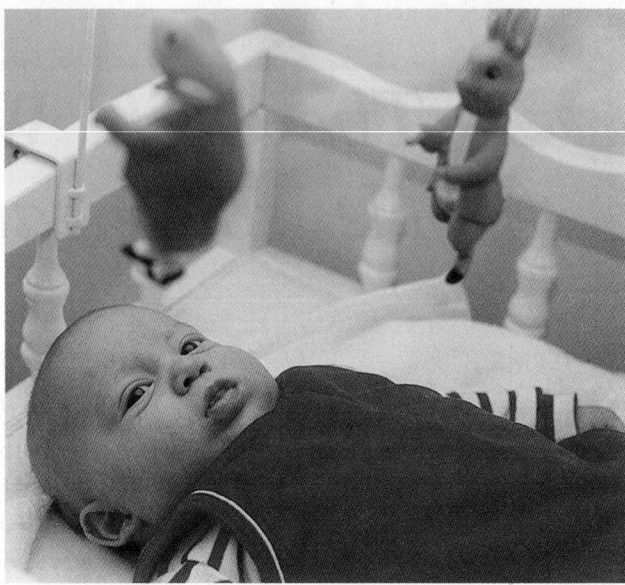

■ **Figure 35-1** A 2-month-old focusing on a simple mobile.

The ear is made up of the external, middle, and inner ear. The eardrum or tympanic membrane is in the external ear. In the middle ear, the eustachian tube connects the throat with the middle ear. In infants and young children, this tube is straighter, shorter, and wider than in the older child and adult (Fig. 35-2). Hearing in children is acute, and the infant will respond to sounds within the first month of life.

VISION IMPAIRMENT

Good vision is essential to a child's normal development. How well a child sees affects his or her learning process, social development, coordination, and safety. One in 1,000 children of school age has serious vision impairment. The sooner these impairments are corrected, the better a child's chances are for normal or near-normal development.

Children with vision impairments are classified as sighted with eye problems, partially sighted, or legally blind.

Types of Vision Impairment
Refractive Errors

Among sighted children with eye problems, errors of **refraction** (the way light rays bend as they pass through the lens to the retina) are the most common. About 10% of school-aged children have **myopia** (nearsightedness), which means that the child can see objects clearly at close range but not at a distance. When proper lenses are fitted, vision is corrected to normal. If uncorrected, this defect may cause a child to be labeled inattentive or mentally disabled. Myopia tends to be seen in families; it often progresses into adolescence and then levels off.

Hyperopia (farsightedness) is a refractive condition in which the person can see objects better at a distance than

A Eustachian tube (adult)

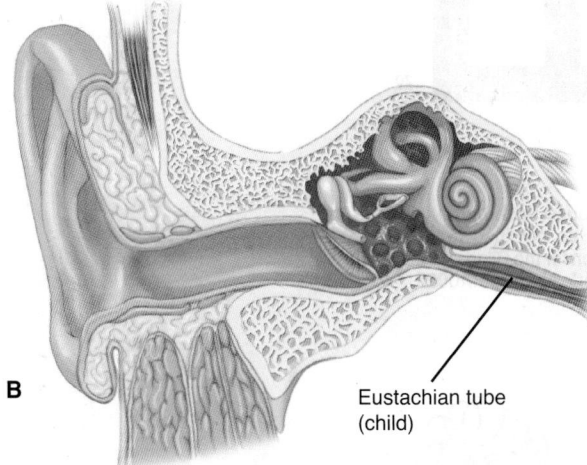

B Eustachian tube (child)

■ **Figure 35-2** Comparison of the eustachian tube **(A)** in the adult and **(B)** in the infant or young child. Note the child's shorter, wider, and more horizontal eustachian tube.

close up. It is common in young children and often persists into the first grade or even later. The ocular specialist examining the child must decide whether or not corrective lenses are needed on an individual basis. Usually correction is not needed in a preschooler. Teachers and parents should be aware that considerable eye fatigue might result from efforts at accommodation for close work.

Astigmatism, which may occur with or without myopia or hyperopia, is caused by unequal curvatures in the cornea that bend the light rays in different directions; this produces a blurred image. Slight astigmatism often does not require correction, moderate degrees usually require glasses for reading and watching television and movies, and severe astigmatism requires glasses at all times.

Partial Sight

Children with partial sight have a visual acuity between 20/20 and 20/200 in the better eye after all necessary medical or surgical correction. These children also have a high incidence of refractive errors, particularly

myopia. Eye injuries also cause loss of vision, as do conditions such as cataracts, which can be improved by treatment but result in diminished sight.

Blindness

Blindness is legally defined as a corrected vision of 20/200 or less, or peripheral vision of less than 20 degrees in the better eye. Many causes of blindness, such as retrolental fibroplasia (caused by excessive oxygen concentrations in newborns) and trachoma, a viral infection, have been reduced or eliminated. Maternal infections are still a common cause of blindness.

Between the ages of 5 and 7 years, children begin to form and retain visual images; they have memory with pictures. Children who become blind before 5 years of age are missing this crucial element in their development.

Good news.
The incidence of maternal rubella causing blindness in infants has decreased since the immunization for measles, mumps, and rubella has been given.

Blindness can seriously hamper the child's ability to form human attachments; learn coordination, balance, and locomotion; distinguish fantasy from reality; and interpret the surrounding world. How well the blind child learns to cope depends on the family's ability to communicate, teach, and foster a sense of independence in the child.

Clinical Manifestations and Diagnosis

Squinting and frowning while trying to read a blackboard or other material at a distance, tearing, red-rimmed eyes, holding work too close to the eyes while reading or writing, and rubbing the eyes are all signs of possible vision impairment. Although blindness is likely to be detected in early infancy, partial sightedness or correctable vision problems may go unrecognized until a child enters school, unless vision screening is part of routine health maintenance (Fig. 35-3).

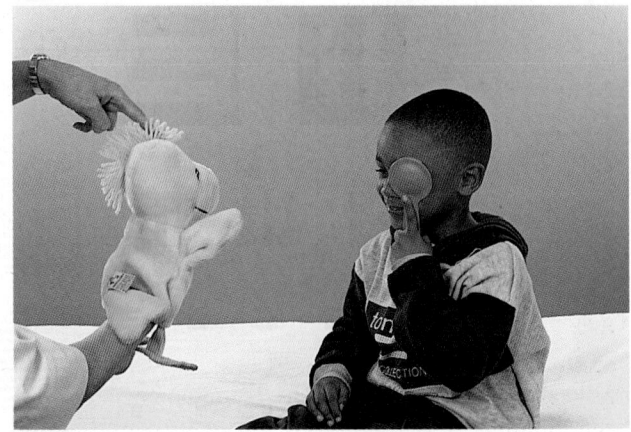

■ **Figure 35-3** Vision screening on a preschool child as part of a routine exam.

A simple test kit for young children is available for home use by family caregivers or visiting nurses (Fig. 35-4). This kit is an adaptation of the Snellen E chart used for testing children who have not learned to read. To use the E chart, the child covers one eye and then points the fingers in the same direction as the "fingers" on each E, beginning with the largest. Some examiners refer to these as "legs on a table."

The Snellen chart is a familiar test in which the letters on each line are smaller than those on the line above. If the child can read the 20-foot line standing 20 feet away from the chart, visual acuity is stated as 20/20. If the child can read only the line marked 100, acuity is stated as 20/100. The chart should be placed at eye level with good lighting and in a room free from distractions. One eye is tested at a time, with the other eye covered.

Lighthouse flash-card vision test. This test may be obtained from the New York Association for the Blind, 111 East 59th Street, New York, New York 10022.

■ **Figure 35-4** Home testing kit. This allows the young child to take the test in surroundings that are more familiar. The test may be obtained at www.preventblindness. org/children or by calling 1-800-331-2020.

Picture charts for identification also are used but are not considered as accurate. An intelligent child can memorize the pictures and guess from the general shape without being able to see distinctly.

Treatment and Education

Significant medical and surgical advances have occurred in the treatment of cataracts, strabismus, and amblyopia. The earlier the child is treated, the better the child's chances of adequate vision for normal development and function. Errors of refraction are usually correctable. Corrective lenses for minor vision impairments should be prescribed early and checked regularly to be sure they still provide adequate correction.

Children who are partially sighted or totally blind benefit from association with normally sighted children. In most communities, education for these special children is provided within the regular school or in special classes that offer the child more specialized equipment and instruction.

Specialized equipment includes printed material with large print, pencils with large leads for darker lines, tape recordings, magnifying glasses, and keyboards. For children with a serious impairment that sharply curtails participation in regular activities, talking books, raised maps, and Braille equipment are needed as well. These devices prevent isolation of the visually impaired child and minimize any differences from the other children.

Nursing Care

Children with a visual impairment have the same needs as other children and these should not be overlooked. The child who is blind needs emotional comfort and sensory stimulation, most of which must be communicated by touch, sound, and smell. Explain sounds and other sensations that are new to the child, and let him or her touch the equipment that will be used in procedures. A tactile tour of the room helps orient the child to the location of furniture and other facilities.

Identify yourself when you enter the room and tell the child when you leave. Explanations of what is going to happen reduce the child's fear, anxiety, and the possibility of being startled by an unexpected touch. The child with a visual impairment should be involved with as many peers and their activities as possible. The child also should be encouraged to be as

independent as possible. One step is to provide the child with finger foods and encourage self-feeding after orienting the child to the plate. A small bowl, instead of a plate, is useful so that food can be scooped against the side to get it on the spoon. Eating can be a time-consuming and messy affair, but having the opportunity to learn to feed themselves is essential to the growth of independence in all children.

EYE CONDITIONS

Vision screening is part of routine health maintenance. Cataracts, congenital infantile glaucoma, and strabismus are disease conditions that may need to be dealt with during childhood. Eye injuries can occur when children are exploring their environment or playing. In addition, eye infections may occur because exploring hands can easily carry infectious organisms to the eyes.

Cataracts

A **cataract** is a development of opacity in the crystalline lens that prevents light rays from entering the eye. Congenital cataracts may be hereditary, or they may be complications of maternal rubella infection during the first trimester of pregnancy. Cataracts also may develop later in infancy or childhood from eye injury or from metabolic disturbances, such as galactosemia and diabetes.

Surgical extraction of the cataracts can be performed at an early age. With early removal, the prognosis for good vision is improved. The child is fitted with a contact lens. If only one eye is affected, the "good" eye is patched to prevent amblyopia (see discussion in the Strabismus section). As the child gets older, numerous lens changes are needed to modify the strength of the lens.

Glaucoma

There are three types of glaucoma in children. The congenital infantile type occurs in children younger than 3 years of age; the juvenile type shows clinical manifestations after 3 years; and the secondary type results from injury or disease. Increased intraocular pressure caused by overproduction of aqueous fluid causes the eyeball to enlarge and the cornea to become large, thin, and sometimes cloudy. Untreated, the disease slowly progresses to blindness. Pain may be present.

Goniotomy (surgical opening into Schlemm's canal) provides drainage of the aqueous humor and is often effective in relieving intraocular pressure. Goniotomy may need to be performed multiple times to control intraocular pressure. Surgery is performed as early as possible to prevent permanent damage.

Strabismus

Strabismus is the failure of the two eyes to direct their gaze at the same object simultaneously. This condition is commonly called "squint" or "crossed eyes" (Fig. 35-5).

Normally, **binocular** (normal) **vision** is maintained through the muscular coordination of eye movements,

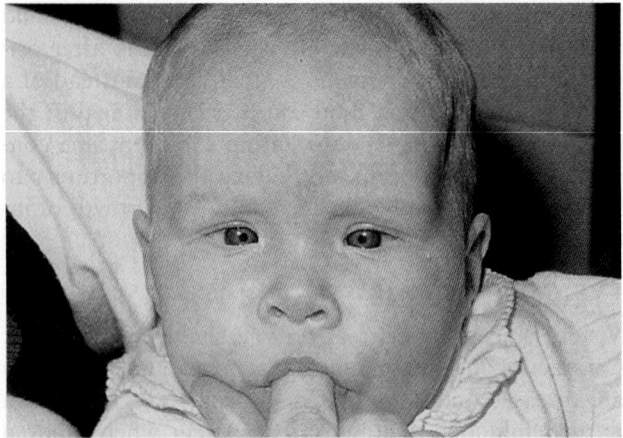

■ **Figure 35-5** Strabismus in an infant.

so that a single vision results. In strabismus, the visual axes are not parallel, and **diplopia** (double vision) results. In an effort to avoid seeing two images, the child's central nervous system suppresses vision in the deviant eye, causing **amblyopia** (dimness of vision from disuse of the eye), which is sometimes called "lazy eye."

A wide variation in the manifestation of strabismus exists; there are lateral, vertical, and mixed lateral and vertical types. There may be monocular strabismus, in which one eye deviates while the other eye is used, or alternating strabismus, in which deviation alternates from one eye to the other. The term **esotropia** is used when the eye deviates toward the other eye; **exotropia** denotes a turning away from the other eye (Fig. 35-6).

Treatment depends on the type of strabismus present. In monocular strabismus, occlusion of the better eye by patching to force the use of the deviating eye should be initiated at an early age. Patching is continued for weeks or months. The younger the child is, the more rapid the improvement. The patching may be for set periods of time or be continuous, depending on the child's age. For example, an older child usually needs continuous periods of patching, whereas

> **Some nurses find this approach helpful.**
> For the child who must have one eye patched, encourage the child to use the unpatched eye. Promote activities such as doing puzzles, drawing, and sewing.

a younger one may respond quickly to short periods of patching.

Glasses can correct a refractive error if amblyopia is not present. **Orthoptics** (therapeutic ocular muscle exercises) to improve the quality of vision may be prescribed to supplement the use of glasses or surgery.

Early detection and treatment of strabismus are essential for a successful outcome. Surgery on the eye muscle to correct the defect is necessary for children who do not respond to glasses and exercises. Many children need surgery after amblyopia has been corrected. The surgical correction is believed to be necessary before the child reaches age 6 years or the visual damage may be permanent. However, some authorities believe that correction can be successful up to age 10 years.

Eye Injury and Foreign Objects in the Eye

Eye injuries are fairly common, particularly in older children. Ecchymosis of the eye (black eye) is of no great importance unless the eyeball is involved. A penetrating wound of the eyeball is potentially serious—BB shots in particular are dangerous—and requires the ophthalmologist's attention. With any history of an injury, a thorough examination of the entire eye is necessary.

Sympathetic ophthalmia, an inflammatory reaction of the uninjured eye, may follow perforation wounds of the globe, even if the perforations are small. Sympathetic ophthalmia often includes **photophobia** (intolerance to light), **lacrimation** (secretion of tears), pain, and some dimness of vision. The retina may become detached, and atrophy of the eyeball may occur. Prompt and skillful treatment at the time of the injury is essential to avoiding involvement of the other eye.

Small foreign objects, such as specks of dust that have lodged inside the eyelid, may be removed by rolling the lid back and exposing the object. If the object cannot be easily removed with a small piece of moistened cotton or soft clean cloth or flushed out with saline solution, the child should be seen by a care provider.

> **A word of caution is in order.**
> Cotton-tipped applicators should not be used to remove small objects that have lodged inside the eyelid because of the danger of sudden movement and possible perforation of the eye.

A   B

■ **Figure 35-6** Types of strabismus. **(A)** Esotropia. **(B)** Exotropia.

Eye Infections

Hordeolum, known commonly as a stye, is a purulent infection of the follicle of an eyelash, generally caused by Staphylococcus aureus. Localized swelling, tenderness, pain, and a reddened lid edge are present. The maximal tenderness is over the infected site. The lesion progresses to suppuration, with eventual discharge of the purulent material. Warm saline compresses applied for about 15 minutes three or four times daily give some relief and hasten resolution, but recurrence is common. The stye should never be squeezed. Antibiotic ointment may help prevent accompanying conjunctivitis and recurrence.

Conjunctivitis is an acute inflammation of the conjunctiva. In children, a virus, bacteria, allergy, or foreign body may be the cause. Most commonly, conjunctivitis is caused by bacteria. The purulent drainage, a common characteristic, can be cultured to determine the causative organism. Because of the danger of spreading infection, bacterial conjunctivitis is treated with ophthalmic antibacterial agents.

Here's a pharmacology fact.

Erythromycin, bacitracin, sulfacetamide, and polymyxin are often used to treat bacterial eye infections.

Because ointments blur vision, eye drops are used during the day and ointments are used at night. Before medication is applied, warm moist compresses can be used to remove the crusts that form on the eyes. The child who has bacterial conjunctivitis should be kept separate from other children until the condition has been treated. The use of separate washcloths, towels, and disposable tissues is important in preventing the spread of infection among family members.

Nursing Care for the Child Undergoing Eye Surgery

When a child undergoes eye surgery, sensory deprivation is possible. Anyone experiencing sensory deprivation finds it difficult to stay in touch with reality.

A child who wakens from surgery to total darkness may go into a state of panic. Observation of the child returning from surgery may reveal panic and anxiety evidenced by trembling and nervousness. The child needs a family caregiver or loved one to stay during the time when vision is restricted.

Think about this.

A child whose eyes are covered is particularly vulnerable to sensory deprivation. Nurses who have not experienced this deprivation do not always appreciate the implications of not being able to see. To better understand, cover one eye for a period of time and note the effects of this experience!

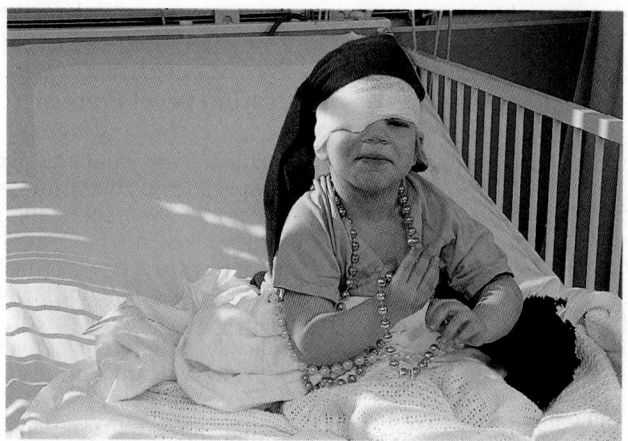

■ Figure 35-7 Pretending to be a pirate enables this toddler to find enjoyment in wearing an eye patch.

The child needs to be as well prepared for the event as possible. However, the small child has no experience to help in understanding what actually is going to happen. The darkness, pain, and total strangeness of the situation can be overwhelming. Using play can be helpful. For example, one preoperative preparation might be to play a game with a blindfold to help the child become accustomed to having his or her eyes covered (Fig. 35-7).

Restraints should not be used indiscriminately. However, most small children need some reminder to keep their hands away from the affected eye, unless someone is beside them to prevent them from rubbing it or from removing eye dressings. Elbow restraints are useful, although they do not prevent rubbing the eye with the arm. Flannel strips applied to the wrists in clove-hitch fashion can be tied to the bedsides in such a manner as to allow freedom of arm movement but to prevent the child from causing damage to the operative site.

Speak to the child to alert him or her as you approach. The child needs tactile stimulation; therefore, after speaking, you may stroke or pat the child. If permitted, hold the child for additional reassurance.

HEARING IMPAIRMENT

Hearing loss is one of the most common disabilities in the United States. About 2 or 3 of every 1,000 children are born with hearing impairments (O'Reiley, 2006). Depending on the degree of hearing loss and the age at detection, a child's development can be moderately to severely impaired. Development of speech, human relationships, and understanding of the environment all depend on the ability to hear. Infants at high risk for hearing loss should be screened when they are between 3 and 6 months of age.

Hearing loss ranges from mild (hard of hearing) to profound (deaf) (Table 35-1). A child who is hard of hearing has a loss of hearing acuity but can learn speech and language by imitating sounds. A deaf child has no hearing ability.

Table 35-1 ▌ LEVELS OF HEARING IMPAIRMENT

Decibel Level	Hearing Level Present
Slight (<30 dB)	Unable to hear whispered word or faint speech No speech impairment present May not be aware of hearing difficulty Achieves well in school and home by compensating by leaning forward, speaking loudly
Mild (30–50 dB)	Beginning speech impairment may be present Difficulty hearing if not facing speaker; some difficulty with normal conversation
Moderate (55–70 dB)	Speech impairment present; may require speech therapy Difficulty with normal conversation
Severe (70–90 dB)	Difficulty with any but nearby loud voice Hears vowels easier than consonants Requires speech therapy for clear speech May still hear loud sounds, such as jets or a train
Profound (>90 dB)	Hears almost no sound

From Pillitteri, A. (2007). *Maternal and child health nursing* (5th ed.). Philadelphia: Lippincott Williams & Wilkins.

Types of Hearing Impairment

There are four types of hearing loss: conductive, sensorineural, mixed, and central.

Conductive Hearing Loss

In conductive hearing loss, middle ear structures fail to carry sound waves to the inner ear. This type of impairment most often results from chronic serous otitis media or other infection and can make hearing levels fluctuate. Chronic middle ear infection can destroy part of the eardrum or the ossicles, which leads to conductive deafness. This type of deafness is seldom complete and responds well to treatment.

Sensorineural (Perceptive) Hearing Loss

Sensorineural (perceptive) hearing loss may result from damage to the nerve endings in the cochlea or to the nerve pathways leading to the brain. It is generally severe and unresponsive to medical treatment. Diseases such as meningitis and encephalitis, hereditary or congenital factors, and toxic reactions to certain drugs (such as streptomycin) may cause sensorineural hearing loss. Maternal rubella is also believed to be one of the common causes.

Mixed Hearing Loss

Mixed hearing loss combines both conductive and sensorineural hearing impairments. In these instances, the conduction level determines how well the child can hear.

Central Auditory Dysfunction

Although the child with central auditory dysfunction may have normal hearing, damage to or faulty development of the proper brain centers makes this child unable to use the auditory information received.

Clinical Manifestations

Mild to moderate hearing loss often remains undetected until the child moves outside the family circle into nursery school or kindergarten. The hearing loss may have been gradual, and the child may have become such a skilled lip reader that neither the child nor the family is aware of the partial deafness.

Certain reactions and mannerisms characterize a child with hearing loss. Observe the child for an apparent inability to locate a sound and a turning of the head to one side when listening. The child who fails to comprehend when spoken to, who gives inappropriate answers to questions, who consistently turns up the volume on the television or radio, or who cannot whisper or talk softly may have hearing loss.

Don't be too quick to judge.
Caregivers and teachers should be aware of the possibility of hearing loss in children who appear to be inattentive and noisy and who create disturbances in the classroom.

Diagnosis

Children who are profoundly deaf are more likely to be diagnosed before 1 year of age than are children with mild to moderate hearing losses. The child who is suspected of having a hearing loss should be referred for a complete audiologic assessment, including pure-tone audiometric, speech reception, and speech discrimination tests. Children with sensorineural impairment generally have a greater loss of hearing acuity, which may vary from slight to complete, in the high-pitched tones. Children with a conductive loss are more likely to have equal losses over a wide range of frequencies.

A child's hearing should be tested at all frequencies by a pure-tone audiometer in a soundproof room. Speech reception and speech discrimination tests measure the amount of hearing impairment for both speech and communication. Accurate measurements usually can be made in children as young as 3 years of age if the test is introduced as a game.

Infants and very young children must be tested in different ways. An infant with normal hearing should be able to locate a sound at 28 weeks, imitate sounds at 36 weeks, and associate sounds with people or objects at 1 year of age. A commonly used screening test for very young children uses noisemakers of varying intensity and pitch. The examiner stands beside or behind the child who has been given a toy. As the examiner produces sounds with a rattle, buzzer, bell, or other noisemaker, a hearing child is distracted and turns to the source of the new sound, whereas a deaf child does not react in a particular way.

Deafness, mental retardation, and autism are sometimes incorrectly diagnosed because the symptoms can be similar. Deaf children may fail to respond to sound or develop speech because they cannot hear. Children with mental retardation or autism may show the same lack of response and development, even though they do not have a hearing loss.

Treatment and Education

When the type and degree of hearing loss have been established, the child, or even the infant, may be fitted with a hearing aid. Hearing aids are helpful only in conductive deafness, not in sensorineural or central auditory dysfunction. These devices only amplify sound; they do not localize or clarify it. Many models are available, including those that are worn in the ear or behind the ear, incorporated in glasses, or worn on the body with a wire connection to the ear. FM receiver units also are available that can broadcast the speaker's voice from a greater distance and cut out the background noise. When the FM transmitter is turned off, this type of unit functions as an ordinary hearing aid.

Deaf children can best be taught to communicate by a combination of lip reading, sign language, and oral speech (Fig. 35-8). The family members are the child's first teachers; they must be aware of all phases of development—physical, emotional, social, intellectual, and language—and seek to aid this development.

A deaf child depends on sight to interpret the environment and to communicate. Thus, it is important to be sure that the child's vision is normal and, if it is not, to correct that problem. The child with a hearing loss is twice as likely to also have some vision impairment. Training in the use of all the other senses—sight, smell, taste, and touch—makes the deaf child better able to use any available hearing. Some researchers believe that most deaf children do have some hearing ability.

■ **Figure 35-8** A young deaf girl learns to use the computer with the help of a speech therapist.

Preschool classes for deaf children exist in many large communities. These classes attempt to create an environment in which a deaf child can have the same experiences and activities that hearing preschoolers have. Children are generally enrolled at age 2.5 years.

The John Tracy Clinic in Los Angeles, founded in 1943, is dedicated to young children (birth through age 5 years) born with severe hearing loss or those who have lost hearing through illness before acquiring speech and language. The clinic's purpose is "to find, encourage, guide, and train the parents of deaf and hard-of-hearing children, first in order to reach and help the children, and second to help the parents themselves." With early diagnosis and intervention, hearing-impaired children can develop language and communication skills in the critical preschool period that enable many of them to speech-read (lip-read) and to speak. All services to parents and children are free. Full audiologic testing, parent–child education, demonstration nursery school, parent education classes, and parent groups are offered. Many medical residents, nurses, and allied health care professionals observe the model programs at the clinic to see the benefits of early diagnosis.

The clinic also provides a correspondence course for parents. Three courses are available for deaf infants, deaf preschoolers, and deaf-blind children. These courses, which are provided in both English and Spanish and include written materials and videotapes, guide parents in encouraging their child to develop auditory awareness, speech-reading skills, and expressive language. Information about the clinic can be obtained by calling toll-free (800) 522–4582 or on the Internet at www.johntracyclinic.org.

Federal law requires free and appropriate education for all disabled children. Children with a hearing loss who cannot successfully function in regular classrooms are provided with supplementary services (speech therapist, speech interpreter, and signer) in special classrooms or in a residential school.

Nursing Care

When the deaf child is in a health care facility, the child's primary caregiver should be present during the stay. Caregiver presence is encouraged to help the child communicate needs and feelings, not as a convenience to the nursing staff.

The deaf child's anxiety about unfamiliar situations and procedures can be greater than that of the child with normal hearing. When speaking to the deaf child, stand or sit face to face on the child's level. Be certain that a deaf child can see you before you touch him or her. Demonstrate each procedure before it is performed, showing the child the equipment or pictures of the equipment to be used. Follow demonstrations with explanations to be sure the child understands. Keep a night light in the child's room because sight is a critical sense to the deaf child.

A little sensitivity is in order.
To understand the deaf child's helpless feeling, imagine being in a soundless, dark room. Be sure the child's room is well lighted.

Hearing aids are expensive, so learning how to take care of and maintain them is important. Put the aid in a safe place when the child is not wearing it. Check linens before putting them into the laundry so as not to discard a hearing aid along with the dirty linens.

Use family members as important resources to learn about the child's habits and communication patterns. In many communities, signing classes are available for those working with hearing-impaired children and adults.

Test Yourself
✔ What are five types of vision impairment?
✔ What term is commonly used to describe strabismus?
✔ What are four types of hearing loss?
✔ What are four examples of nursing interventions used when working with deaf children?

OTITIS MEDIA

Otitis media is one of the most common infectious diseases of childhood. Two of every three children have at least one episode of otitis media by the time they are 1 year of age (Schwarzwald & Kline, 2006). Because the eustachian tube in an infant is shorter, wider, and straighter than in the older child or adult (Fig. 35-2), nasopharyngeal secretions are able to enter the middle ear more easily. *Haemophilus influenzae* is an important causative agent of otitis media in infants and children.

Clinical Manifestations

A restless infant who repeatedly shakes the head and rubs or pulls at one ear should be checked for an ear infection. These behaviors often indicate that the infant is having pain in the ears. Older children can express and describe the pain they are experiencing. In addition to pain, symptoms may include fever, irritability, and hearing impairment. Vomiting or diarrhea may occur.

Diagnosis

The infant's ear is examined with an otoscope by pulling the ear down and back to straighten the ear canal. In the older child, the ear is pulled up and back. The exam reveals a bright-red, bulging eardrum in otitis media. Spontaneous rupture of the eardrum may occur, in which case there will be purulent drainage, and the pain caused by the pressure build-up in the ear will be relieved. If present, purulent drainage is cultured to determine the causative organism and appropriate antibiotic.

Treatment and Nursing Care

Antibiotics are used during the period of infection and for several days after to prevent mastoiditis or chronic infection. A 10-day course of amoxicillin is a common treatment. Most children respond well to antibiotics.

Some children have repeated episodes of otitis media. Children with chronic otitis media may be put on a prophylactic course of an oral penicillin or sulfonamide drug. **Myringotomy** (incision of the eardrum) may be performed to establish drainage and to insert tiny tubes into the tympanic membrane, to facilitate drainage. In most cases, the tubes eventually fall out spontaneously. Attention to chronic otitis media is essential because permanent hearing loss can result from frequent occurrences.

Mastoiditis, infection of the mastoid sinus, is a possible complication of untreated acute otitis media. Mastoiditis was much more common before the advent of antibiotics. Currently it is seen only in children who have an untreated ruptured eardrum or inadequate treatment (through noncompliance of caregivers or improper care) of an acute episode.

Most infants and children with otitis media are cared for at home; therefore, your primary nursing responsibility is to teach the family caregivers about prevention and the care of the child (see Family Teaching Tips: Otitis Media).

INSERTION OF FOREIGN BODIES INTO THE EAR OR NOSE

Children, especially toddlers and preschool-aged children, may insert small objects into their ears or noses.

OTITIS MEDIA

The eustachian tube is a connection between the nasal passages and the middle ear. The eustachian tube is wider, shorter, and straighter in the infant, allowing organisms from respiratory infections to travel into the middle ear to cause infection (otitis media).

PREVENTION

- Hold infant in an upright position or with head slightly elevated while feeding, to prevent formula from draining into the middle ear through the wide eustachian tube.
- Never prop a bottle.
- Do not give infant a bottle in bed. This allows fluid to pool in the middle ear, encouraging organisms to grow.
- Protect child from exposure to others with upper respiratory infections.
- Protect child from passive smoke; don't permit smoking in child's presence.
- Remove sources of allergies from the home.
- Observe for clues to ear infection: shaking head, rubbing or pulling at ears, and fever combined with restlessness or screaming and crying.
- Be alert to signs of hearing difficulty in toddlers and preschoolers. This may be the first sign of an ear infection.
- Teach toddler or preschooler gentle nose blowing.

CARE OF CHILD WITH OTITIS MEDIA

- Have child with upper respiratory infection who shows symptoms of ear discomfort checked by a health care professional.
- Complete the entire amount of antibiotic prescribed, even though the child seems better.
- Use heat (such as a heating pad on low setting) to provide comfort, but an adult must stay with the child.
- Soothe, rock, and comfort child to help relieve discomfort. The child is more comfortable sleeping on side of infected ear.
- Give pain medications (such as acetaminophen) as directed. Never give aspirin.
- Provide liquid or soft foods; chewing causes pain.
- Know that hearing loss may last up to 6 months after infection.
- Schedule follow-up with hearing test as advised

Irrigation of the ear may remove small objects, except paper, which becomes impacted as it absorbs moisture. The physician generally uses small forceps to remove objects not dislodged by irrigation.

This is important and can be dangerous!

Children often put small objects, such as peas or beans, crumpled paper, beads, and small toys, into their ears or noses.

The child may have placed a foreign body in the nose just inside the nares, but manipulation may push it in further. If the object remains in the nose for any length of time, infection may occur. When the object is discovered, a care provider should inspect with a speculum and remove the object.

REYE SYNDROME

Reye syndrome (rhymes with "eye") is characterized by acute encephalopathy and fatty degeneration of the liver and other abdominal organs. It occurs in children of all ages but is seen more frequently in young school-aged children than in any other age group. Reye syndrome usually occurs after a viral illness, particularly after an upper respiratory infection or varicella (chickenpox). Administration of aspirin during the viral illness has been implicated as a contributing factor. As a result, the American Academy of Pediatrics recommends that aspirin or aspirin compounds not be given to children with viral infections.

Clinical Manifestations

The symptoms appear within 3 to 5 days after the initial illness. The child is recuperating unremarkably when symptoms of severe vomiting, irritability, lethargy, and confusion occur. Immediate intervention is needed to prevent cerebral edema with increased intracranial pressure (IICP) and the possibility of respiratory arrest (Table 35-2).

Diagnosis

The history of a viral illness is an immediate clue. Liver function tests, including aspartate aminotransferase (AST; serum glutamic oxaloacetic transaminase [SGOT]), alanine aminotransferase (ALT; serum glutamic pyruvic transaminase (SGPT]), lactic dehydrogenase (LDH), and serum ammonia levels are elevated because of poor liver function. The child is hypoglycemic and has delayed prothrombin time.

Treatment

The child with Reye syndrome often is cared for in the intensive care unit because the disease may progress rapidly. Medical management focuses on supportive measures—improving respiratory function, reducing cerebral edema, and controlling hypoglycemia. Osmotic diuretics

Table 35-2 ▪ STAGING OF REYE SYNDROME

Stage	Symptoms Seen in Stage
Stage I	Lethargic, follows verbal commands, normal posture, purposeful response to pain
Stage II	Combative or stuporous, inappropriate verbalizing, normal posture
Stage III	Comatose, decorticate posture, and response to pain
Stage IV	Comatose, decerebrate posture, and response to pain
Stage V	Comatose, flaccid, no pupillary response, no response to pain

Adapted from the National Institutes of Health Staging System, Louis, P. T. (2006). Reye syndrome. In J. McMillan, R. Feigin, C. DeAngelis, & M. Jones. *Oski's pediatrics: Principles and practice* (4th ed.). Philadelphia: Lippincott Williams & Wilkins.

(e.g., mannitol) may be administered to reduce cerebral edema. The specific treatment is determined by the staging of the symptoms (Table 35-2).

Nursing Care

Carefully observe the child for overall physical status and any change in neurologic status. This observation is essential in evaluating the progression of the illness. Accurate intake and output determinations are necessary to determine when fluids need to be adjusted to control cerebral edema and prevent dehydration. Monitor the blood glucose level and bleeding time. Low blood glucose levels can lead to seizures quickly in young children, and a prolonged bleeding time can indicate coagulation problems, as a result of liver dysfunction.

This hospitalization period is a traumatic time for family members, so give them opportunities to deal with their feelings. In addition, keep the family well informed about the child's care. Having a child in intensive care is a frightening experience for the family, so make every effort to reassure them with sincerity and honesty.

Since the American Academy of Pediatrics made its recommendation to avoid giving aspirin to children, especially during viral illnesses, the number of cases of Reye syndrome has steadily decreased. The prognosis for children with Reye syndrome is greatly improved with early diagnosis and vigorous treatment. Teach family caregivers to avoid the use of aspirin in children.

Don't!
Don't give children aspirin, especially if they have a viral illness.

Test Yourself

✔ What is the physiologic reason otitis media occurs more often in young children than in older children and adults?

✔ What has greatly decreased the incidence of Reye syndrome?

ACUTE OR NONRECURRENT SEIZURES

A seizure (convulsion) may be a symptom of a wide variety of disorders. In children between the age of 6 months and 3 years, **febrile seizures** (seizures resulting from fever) are the most common. Febrile seizures usually occur in the form of a generalized seizure early in the course of a fever. Although commonly associated with high fever (102°F–106°F [38.9°C–41.1°C]), some children appear to have a low seizure threshold and convulse when a fever of 100°F to 102°F (37.8°C–38.9°C) is present. These seizures are often one of the initial symptoms of an acute infection somewhere in the body.

Less common causes of convulsions are intracranial infections, such as meningitis, and toxic reactions to certain drugs or minerals such as lead, metabolic disorders, and various brain disorders.

Clinical Manifestations and Diagnosis

A seizure may occur suddenly without warning; however, restlessness and irritability may precede an episode. The body stiffens, and the child loses consciousness. In a few seconds, clonic movements occur. These movements are quick, jerking movements of the arms, legs, and facial muscles. Breathing is irregular, and the child cannot swallow saliva. These symptoms prompt immediate treatment; further evaluation is made after the urgency of the seizure has passed.

Treatment

Emergency care to protect the child during the seizure is the primary concern. If the seizure activity continues, diazepam (Valium) may be administered IV to control the seizure. Acetaminophen is administered to reduce the temperature.

Nursing Process for the Child at Risk For Seizures

Assessment

During the family caregiver interview, ask about any history of seizure activity. Have the caregivers describe any previous episodes, including the child's temperature, how the child behaved immediately before the seizure, movements during the seizure, and any other information they believe to be relevant. Ask about the presence of any fever during the present illness and any indications of seizure activity before this admission. Promptly institute seizure precautions. A child whose fever or other symptoms indicate that a seizure may be anticipated should be placed under constant observation.

During the physical exam, obtain a baseline temperature. Using a neurologic tool, observe the child's neurologic status, and make other observations appropriate for the present illness.

Selected Nursing Diagnoses

- Risk for Aspiration during seizure related to decreased level of consciousness
- Risk for Injury related to uncontrolled muscular activity during seizure
- Compromised Family Coping related to the child's seizure activity
- Deficient Knowledge of caregivers related to seizure prevention and precautions during seizures

Outcome Identification and Planning

The immediate goals for the child during a seizure are preventing aspiration and preventing injury. Goals for the family include promoting coping and increasing knowledge about seizures. With safety in mind, develop the nursing plan of care according to these goals.

Implementation

Preventing Aspiration

When convulsions begin, position the child to one side to prevent aspiration of saliva or vomitus. Remove blankets, pillows, or other items that may block the child's airway. Have oxygen and suction equipment readily available for emergency use.

> **Do you know the why of it?**
>
> If a child has a seizure, do not put anything in the child's mouth; doing so could cause injury to the child or to you.

Promoting Safety

Keep the child who has a history of seizures under close observation. Pad the crib sides, and keep sharp or hard items out of the crib. Do not, however, completely hide the view of the surroundings outside the crib because this could make the child feel isolated. During the seizure, stay with the child to protect, but not restrain, him or her. Loosen any tight clothing. If the child is not in bed when the seizure starts, move him or her to a flat surface.

Document the seizure completely after the episode. Document the type of movements (rigidity, jerking, and twitching), the body parts involved, the duration of the seizure, pulse and respirations, the child's color, and any deviant eye movements or other notable signs.

Promoting Family Coping

A convulsion or seizure is very frightening to family caregivers. With a calm, confident attitude reassure caregivers that the child is in good hands. Explain that febrile seizures are not uncommon in small children. Reassure caregivers that the provider will evaluate the child to determine if the seizure has any cause other than nervous system irritation resulting from the high fever.

Providing Family Teaching

Teach family caregivers seizure precautions so they can handle a seizure that occurs at home. Also, instruct them on what observations to make during a seizure so they can report these to the physician to help in evaluating the child. Explain methods to control fever, cautioning caregivers to avoid using aspirin for fever reduction. Refer to Family Teaching Tips: Reducing Fever, in Chapter 30, when teaching caregivers how to reduce fevers at home.

Evaluation: Goals and Expected Outcomes

Goal: The child's airway will remain patent throughout the seizure.
Expected Outcome: The child's airway is patent with no aspiration of saliva or vomitus.
Goal: The child will remain free from injury during the seizure.
Expected Outcome: The child is free from bruises, abrasions, concussions, or fractures after the seizure.
Goal: The family caregivers' anxiety will be reduced.
Expected Outcome: The family caregivers verbalize their concerns and relate an understanding of febrile seizures.
Goal: The family caregivers will verbalize an understanding of seizure precautions.
Expected Outcome: The family caregivers state methods to reduce fevers and handle seizures at home.

SEIZURE DISORDERS

Seizure disorders, also referred to as convulsive disorders, are common in children and may result from a variety of causes. Unlike the acute febrile seizure that occurs with fevers and acute infections, epilepsy is a recurrent and chronic seizure disorder. Epilepsy can be classified as primary (idiopathic), with no known cause, or secondary, resulting from infection, head trauma, hemorrhage, tumor, or other organic or degenerative factors. Primary epilepsy is the most common; its onset generally occurs between ages 4 and 8 years.

Clinical Manifestations

Seizures are the characteristic clinical manifestation of both types of epilepsy and may be either partial (focal) or generalized. **Partial seizures** are limited to a particular area of the brain; generalized seizures involve both hemispheres of the brain.

Partial Seizures

Manifestations of partial seizures vary depending on the area of the brain from which they arise. Loss of consciousness or awareness may not occur. Partial seizures are classified as simple partial motor, simple partial sensory, or complex partial (psychomotor).

Simple Partial Seizures

Simple partial motor seizures cause a localized motor activity such as shaking of an arm, leg, or other part of the body. These may be limited to one side of the body or may spread to other parts.

Simple partial sensory seizures may include sensory symptoms called an **aura** (a sensation that signals an impending attack) involving sight, sound, taste, smell, touch, or emotions (a feeling of fear, for example). The child may also have numbness, tingling, paresthesia, or pain.

Complex Partial Seizures

Complex partial seizures, also called psychomotor seizures, also begin in a small area of the brain and change or alter consciousness. They cause memory loss and staring. Nonpurposeful movements, such as hand rubbing, lip smacking, arm dropping, and swallowing, may occur. After the seizure, the child may sleep or may be confused for a few minutes. The child is often unaware of the seizure. These can be the most difficult seizures to control.

Generalized Seizures

Types of generalized seizures include tonic-clonic (formerly called grand mal), absence (formerly called petit mal), atonic or akinetic (formerly called "drop attacks"), myoclonic, and infantile spasms.

Tonic-Clonic Seizures

Tonic-clonic seizures consist of four stages: the prodromal period, which can last for days or hours; the aura, which is a warning immediately before the seizure; the tonic-clonic movements; and the postictal stage. Not all these stages occur with every seizure; the seizure may just begin with a sudden loss of consciousness. During the prodromal period, the child might be drowsy, dizzy, or have a lack of coordination. If the seizure is preceded by an aura, it is identified as a generalized seizure secondary to a partial seizure. The aura may reflect in which part of the brain the seizure originates. Young children may have difficulty describing an aura but may cry out in response to it. In the tonic phase, the child's muscles contract, the child may fall, and the child's extremities may stiffen. The contraction of respiratory muscles during the tonic phase may cause the child to become cyanotic and appear briefly to have respiratory arrest. The eyes roll upward, and the child might utter a guttural cry. The initial rigidity of the tonic phase changes rapidly to generalized jerking muscle movements in the clonic phase. The child may bite the tongue or lose control of bladder and bowel functions. The jerking movements gradually diminish and then disappear, and the child relaxes. The seizure can be brief, lasting less than 1 minute, or protracted, lasting 30 minutes or longer. The period after the tonic-clonic phase is called the postictal period. The child may sleep soundly for several hours during this stage or return rapidly to an alert state. Many children have a period of confusion, and others experience a prolonged period of stupor.

Absence Seizures

Absence seizures rarely last longer than 20 seconds. The child loses awareness and stares straight ahead, but does not fall. The child may have blinking or twitching of the mouth or an extremity along with the staring. Immediately after the seizure, the child is alert and continues conversation but does not know what was said or done during the episode. Absence seizures can recur frequently, sometimes as often as 50 to 100 a day. If seizures are not fully controlled, the caregiver needs to be especially aware of dangerous situations that might occur in the child's day, such as crossing a street on the way to school. These seizures often decrease significantly or stop entirely at adolescence.

Atonic or Akinetic Seizures

Atonic or akinetic seizures cause a sudden momentary loss of consciousness, muscle tone, and postural control and can cause the child to fall. They can result in serious facial, head, or shoulder injuries. They may recur frequently, particularly in the morning. After the seizure, the child can stand and walk as normal.

Myoclonic Seizures

Myoclonic seizures are characterized by a sudden jerking of a muscle or group of muscles, often in the arms or legs, without loss of consciousness. Myoclonus occurs during the early stages of falling asleep in people who do not have epilepsy.

Infantile Spasms

Infantile spasms occur between 3 and 12 months of age, and they almost always indicate a cerebral defect and have a poor prognosis despite treatment. These seizures occur twice as often in boys as in girls and are preceded or followed by a cry. Muscle contractions are sudden, brief, symmetrical, and accompanied by rolling eyes. Loss of consciousness does not always occur.

Status Epilepticus

Status epilepticus is the term used to describe a seizure that lasts longer than 30 minutes or a series of seizures, in which the child does not return to his or her previous normal level of consciousness. Immediate treatment decreases the likelihood of permanent brain injury, respiratory failure, or even death.

> **Take note!**
> Status epilepticus is an emergency situation and requires immediate treatment. The drugs diazepam, given rectally or intravenously (IV), and lorazepam are used to treat the condition.

Diagnosis

The types of seizures can be differentiated through the use of electroencephalography, video and ambulatory electroencephalography, skull radiography, computed tomography, magnetic resonance imaging, brain scan, and physical and neurologic assessments. The child's seizure history is an important part of determining the diagnosis.

Treatment

The main goal of treatment, complete control of seizures, can be achieved for most people through the use of anticonvulsant drug therapy. A number of anticonvulsant drugs are available (Table 35-3). The drug is chosen based on its effectiveness in controlling seizures and side effects and on its degree of toxicity. Chewable or tablet forms of the medications are often used because suspensions separate and sometimes are not shaken well, causing the possibility of inaccurate dosage. The oldest and most popular drug is phenytoin (Dilantin).

> **Here's a pharmacology fact.**
> Be aware that the drug phenytoin (Dilantin) can cause hypertrophy of the gums (gingival hyperplasia) after prolonged use. Encourage good oral hygiene and frequent dental checkups.

A few children may be candidates for surgical intervention when the focal point of the seizures is in an area of the brain that is accessible surgically and not critical to functioning. If the cause of the seizures is a tumor or other lesion, surgical removal is sometimes possible.

Ketogenic diets (high in fat and low in carbohydrates and protein) cause the child to have high levels of ketones, which help to reduce seizure activity. These diets are prescribed, but long-term maintenance is difficult because the diets are difficult to follow and may be unappealing to the child.

Nursing Care

In the hospital or home setting, keeping the child safe during a seizure is the highest priority. Teach the caregiver of a child who has a seizure disorder how to prevent injury if the child has a seizure (see Family Teaching Tips: Precautions Before and During Seizures). In the hospital setting, the side rails are padded, objects that could cause harm are kept away from the bed, oxygen and suction are kept at the bedside, the side rails are in the raised position, and the bed lowered when the child is sleeping or resting.

If the child begins to have a seizure, place the child on her or his side with the head turned toward one side. Stay calm, remove any objects from around the child, protect the child's head, and loosen tight clothing. During the seizure, note the following:

- Time the seizure started
- What the child was doing when the seizure began
- Any factor present just before the seizure (bright light, noise)
- Part of the body where seizure activity began
- Movement and parts of the body involved
- Any cyanosis
- Eye position and movement
- Incontinence of urine or stool
- Time seizure ended
- Child's activity after the seizure

When the seizure ends, monitor the child, paying close attention to his or her level of consciousness, motor functions, and behavior. Document the information noted during the seizure activity. If the child is able to describe the aura, this information is important to document.

> **Be sure to ask.**
> The child may be able to describe the aura or sensation that occurred just before a seizure.

Education and counseling are important parts of nursing care. The child and family caregivers need complete and accurate information about the disorder and the results that can be realistically expected from treatment. Epilepsy does not lead inevitably to mental retardation, but continued and uncontrolled seizures do increase its possibility. Thus, early diagnosis and control of seizures are very important.

Table 35-3 ■ ANTIEPILEPTIC-ANTICONVULSIVE THERAPEUTIC AGENTS

Drug	Indication	Side Effects	Nursing Implications
carbamazepine (Tegretol)	Generalized tonic-clonic, simple partial, complex partial	Drowsiness, dry mouth, vomiting, double vision, leukopenia, gastrointestinal upset, thrombocytopenia	There may be dizziness and drowsiness with initial doses. This should subside within 3–14 days.
clonazepam (Klonopin)	Absence seizures, generalized tonic-clonic, myoclonic, simple partial, complex partial	Double vision, drowsiness, increased salivation, changes in behavior, bone marrow depression	Obtain periodic liver function tests and complete blood count. Monitor for drowsiness, lethargy.
ethosuximide (Zarontin)	Absence seizures, myoclonic	Dry mouth, anorexia, dizziness, headache, nausea, vomiting, gastrointestinal upset, lethargy, bone marrow depression	Use with caution in hepatic or renal disease.
phenobarbital (Luminol)	Generalized tonic-clonic, myoclonic, simple partial, complex partial	Drowsiness, alteration in sleep patterns, irritability, respiratory and cardiac depression, restlessness, headache	Alcohol can enhance the effects of phenobarbital. Monitor blood levels of drug. Liver function studies are necessary with prolonged use.
phenytoin (Dilantin)	Generalized tonic-clonic, simple partial, complex partial	Double vision, blurred vision, slurred speech, nystagmus, ataxia, gingival hyperplasia, hirsutism, cardiac arrhythmias, bone marrow depression	Alcohol, antacids, and folic acid decrease the effect of phenytoin. Instruct the child or caregiver to notify the dentist that he or she is taking phenytoin to monitor hyperplasia of the gums. Inform the child or caregiver that the drug may color the urine pink to red-brown.
primidone (Mysoline)	Generalized tonic-clonic, simple partial, complex partial	Behavior changes, drowsiness, hyperactivity, ataxia, bone marrow depression	Adverse effects are the same as for phenobarbital. Sedation and dizziness may be severe during initial therapy; dosage may need to be adjusted by the physician.
valproic acid (Depakene)	Absence, generalized tonic-clonic, myoclonic, simple partial, complex partial	Nausea, vomiting, or increased appetite, tremors, elevated liver enzymes, constipation, headaches, depression, lymphocytosis, leukopenia, increased prothrombin time	Physical dependency may result when used for prolonged period. Tablets and capsules should be taken whole. Elixir should be taken alone, not mixed with carbonated beverages. Increased toxicity may occur with administration of salicylates (aspirin).

General Nursing Considerations With Anticonvulsant Therapy
General nursing considerations with anticonvulsant therapy that apply to all or most of drugs given to children include:
1. Warn the patient and family that patients should avoid activities that require alertness and complex psychomotor coordination (e.g., climbing).
2. Medication can be given with meals to minimize gastric irritation.
3. The anticonvulsant medications should not be discontinued abruptly, as this can precipitate status epilepticus.
4. Anticonvulsant medications generally have a cumulative effect, both therapeutically and adversely.
5. Alcohol ingestion increases the effects of anticonvulsant drugs, exaggerating central nervous system depression.
6. Many of the drugs can cause bone marrow depression (leukopenia, thrombocytopenia, neutropenia, megaloblastic anemia). Regular complete blood cell counts, including white blood cells, red blood cells, and platelets, are necessary to evaluate bone marrow production.
7. The child should receive periodic blood tests to monitor therapeutic levels as opposed to toxic levels.

Although the outlook for a normal, well-adjusted life is favorable, inform the child and family about restrictions they may encounter. Children with epilepsy should be encouraged to participate in physical activities but should not participate in sports in which a fall could cause serious injury. In many states, a person with uncontrolled epilepsy is legally forbidden to drive a motor vehicle; this could limit choice of vocation and lifestyle. Despite attempts to educate the general public about epilepsy, many people remain prejudiced

Family Teaching Tips

PRECAUTIONS BEFORE AND DURING SEIZURES

BEFORE

- Have the child swim with a companion.
- Have the child use protective helmet and padding for bicycle riding and skateboarding.
- Supervise when using power equipment.
- Carry or wear medical identification bracelet.
- Discuss the child's condition with teachers and school nurse.
- Know factors that trigger seizure activity.

DURING

- Stay calm.
- Move furniture or objects that could cause injury.
- Turn the child on side with head turned to one side.
- Remove glasses.
- Protect the child's head.
- Do not restrain the child.
- Do not try to put anything between the child's teeth.
- Keep people from crowding around the child.
- After seizure, notify care provider for follow-up.
- If seizures continue without stopping, call for emergency help.

about this disorder, and this can limit the epileptic person's social and vocational acceptance.

HAEMOPHILUS INFLUENZAE MENINGITIS

Purulent meningitis in infancy and childhood is caused by a variety of agents, including meningococci, the tubercle bacillus, and the *Haemophilus influenzae* type B bacillus. Of these, the most common form is *H. influenzae* meningitis. Transmission of the infection varies. For example, meningococcal and *H. influenzae* meningitis are spread by means of droplet infection from an infected person; all other forms are contracted by invasion of the meninges via the bloodstream from an infection elsewhere.

Peak occurrence of *H. influenzae* meningitis is between the ages of 6 and 12 months. It is rare during the first 2 months of life and is seldom seen after the 4th year. Purulent meningitis is an infectious disease. In addition to standard precautions, droplet transmission precautions should be observed for 24 hours after the start of effective antimicrobial therapy or until pathogens can no longer be cultured from nasopharyngeal secretions. Current immunizations include the HIB vaccine, given at 2 months and

repeated at 4, 6, and 12 months, which offers protection against the bacterium (see Appendix J).

Clinical Manifestations

The onset may be either gradual or abrupt after an upper respiratory infection. Children with meningitis may have a characteristic high-pitched cry, fever, and irritability. Other symptoms include headache, **nuchal rigidity** (stiff neck) that may progress to **opisthotonos** (arching of the back), and delirium. Projectile vomiting may be present. Generalized convulsions are common in children. Coma may occur early, particularly in the older child. Meningococcal meningitis, which tends to occur as epidemics in older children, produces a **purpuric rash** (caused by bleeding under the skin), in addition to the other symptoms.

Diagnosis

Early diagnosis and treatment are essential for uncomplicated recovery. A lumbar puncture (spinal tap) is performed promptly whenever symptoms raise a suspicion of meningitis. For accurate results, the procedure is done before antibiotics are administered. Assist by holding the child in the proper position (see Fig. 30-11 in Chapter 30). The spinal fluid is under increased pressure, and laboratory examination of the fluid reveals increased protein and decreased glucose content. Early in the disease, the spinal fluid may be clear, but it rapidly becomes purulent. The causative organism usually can be determined from stained smears of the spinal fluid, enabling specific medication to be started early without waiting for growths of organisms on culture media.

Treatment

The child is initially isolated and treatment is started using IV administration of antibiotics. Third-generation cephalosporins, such as ceftriaxone (Rocephin), are commonly used, often in combination with other antibiotics. Antibiotics chosen for treatment depend on sensitivity studies. Later in the disease, medications may be given orally. Treatment depends on the progress of the condition and continues as long as there is fever or signs of subdural effusion or otitis media. The administration of IV steroids early in the course has decreased the incidence of deafness as a complication. If seizures occur, anticonvulsants are often given.

Subdural effusion may complicate the condition in children during the course of the disease. Fluid accumulates in the subdural space between the dura and the brain. Needle aspiration through the open suture lines in the infant or burr holes in the skull of the older child are used to remove the fluid. Repeated aspirations may be required.

Complications of *H. influenzae* meningitis with long-term implications are hydrocephalus, nerve deafness, mental retardation, and paralysis. The risk of complications is lessened when appropriate medication is started early in the disease.

Test Yourself

✔ What are seven types of seizures seen in children?
✔ What 10 factors should the nurse document after a seizure?
✔ How can *H. influenzae* meningitis be prevented?

Nursing Process for the Child With Meningitis

Assessment

The child with meningitis is extremely sick, and the anxiety level of the family caregivers is understandably high. Be patient and sensitive to their feelings when doing an interview. Obtain a complete history with particular emphasis on the present illness, including any recent upper respiratory infection or middle ear infection. Information on other children in the family and their ages is also important.

The physical exam of the child includes obtaining temperature, pulse, and respirations; use a neurologic evaluation tool to monitor neurologic status, including the child's level of consciousness (see the section on neurologic evaluation, Chapter 28). Examine the infant for a bulging fontanelle and measure the head circumference for a baseline. Perform this exam after the lumbar puncture is completed and IV fluids and antibiotics are initiated because those procedures take precedence over everything else.

Selected Nursing Diagnoses

- Decreased Intracranial Adaptive Capacity related to infection and seizure activity
- Risk for Aspiration related to decreased level of consciousness
- Risk for Injury related to seizure activity
- Risk for Deficient Fluid Volume related to vomiting, fever, and fluid restrictions
- Excess Fluid Volume related to syndrome of inappropriate antidiuretic hormone
- Deficient Knowledge of family caregivers related to airborne transmission exposure to others
- Compromised Family Coping related to the child's condition and prognosis

Outcome Identification and Planning

The goals for the child with meningitis include monitoring for complications related to neurologic compromise, preventing aspiration, keeping the child safe from injury during a seizure, and monitoring fluid balance. The goals for the family include teaching ways of preventing the transmission of infection and promoting family coping. The nursing care plan includes interventions, such as eliminating the infection by administering antibiotics and observing for signs of increased intracranial pressure.

Implementation

Monitoring for Complications

Because of the child's neurologic status, closely monitor the child for signs of increased intracranial pressure (IICP), including increased head size; headache; bulging fontanelle; decreased pulse; vomiting; seizures; high-pitched cry; increased blood pressure; change in eyes; level of consciousness, or in pupil response; and irritability or other behavioral changes. Vital signs also require close monitoring. An increase in blood pressure, decrease in pulse, change in neurologic signs, or signs of respiratory distress must be reported at once. Measure the infant's head circumference at least every 4 hours to detect complications of subdural effusion or obstructive hydrocephalus. Keep the child's room quiet and darkened to decrease stimulation that may cause seizures. While in the room, speak softly, avoid sudden movements, move quietly, and raise and lower side rails carefully. The head of the bed can be elevated.

Preventing Aspiration

Position the child in a side-lying position with the neck supported for comfort and the head elevated. Remove pillows, blankets, and soft toys that might obstruct the airway. Watch for and remove excessive mucus, as much as possible. Use suction sparingly.

Promoting Safety

Keep the child under close observation. Implement seizure precautions and observe the child for seizure activity. At least every 2 hours, monitor vital signs, neurologic signs, and observe for change in level of consciousness. Pad the crib sides, and keep sharp or hard items out of the crib.

Loosen any tight clothing (see Nursing Process for the Child at Risk for Seizures in this Chapter).

> **Don't forget.**
> During a seizure stay with the child, protect the child from injury, but *DO NOT* restrain him or her.

Monitoring Fluid Balance

Fluid balance is an important aspect of this child's care. Strict intake and output measurements are critical. Methods of reducing fever may be used as needed. Administer IV fluids while observing and monitoring the IV infusion site and following safety precautions to maintain the site.

The infectious process may increase secretion of the antidiuretic hormone produced by the posterior pituitary gland. As a result, the child may not excrete urine adequately, and body fluid volume excess will occur, further emphasizing the need for strict measurement of intake and output. Also, monitor daily weight and electrolyte levels. Signs that must be reported immediately are decreased urinary output, hyponatremia, increased weight, nausea, and irritability. The child is placed on fluid restrictions if these signs occur.

Providing Family Teaching Regarding Spread of Infection

H. influenzae is a highly contagious organism that may spread to other people by means of droplet transmission. Droplet transmission precautions must be maintained for the first 24 hours after the antibiotic is administered. Staff members and family caregivers must follow proper precautions, including standard precautions. Meticulous hand washing is also a key precaution. Other children in the family may need to be examined to determine if they should receive prophylactic antibiotics.

Promoting Family Coping

Teach the caregivers isolation procedures and good hand-washing technique and encourage them to stay with their child, if possible. Support family caregivers through every step of the process. Their anxiety about procedures, the child's seizures and condition, and the possible complications are all serious concerns. Family caregivers must be included and made to feel useful. If they are not too apprehensive, help them find small things they can do for their child. Keep them advised about the child's progress at all times.

Evaluation: Goals and Expected Outcomes

Goal: The child will have a normal neurologic status.
Expected Outcomes: The child's

- vital signs are within normal limits.
- neurologic status is stable.

Goal: The child's airway will remain patent and clear.
Expected Outcomes: The child's

- position is side-lying with neck supported and head elevated.
- airway remains patent with no aspiration of saliva or vomitus.

Goal: The child will remain free from injury.
Expected Outcome: The child is free from bruises, abrasions, concussions, or fractures during seizure activity.
Goal: The child will maintain normal fluid balance.
Expected Outcomes: The child's

- intake and output are within normal limits.
- temperature is 98.6°F to 100°F (37°C–37.8°C).
- assessment shows no signs of dehydration.

Goal: The child will maintain normal weight and have adequate urinary output.
Expected Outcomes: The child's

- weight and electrolyte levels are within normal limits.
- hourly urine output is 2 to 3 mL/kg.

Goal: The family caregivers will follow measures to prevent the transmission of *H. influenzae* bacteria to others.

Expected Outcomes: The family caregivers

- identify measures for preventing the spread of bacteria.
- discuss the need for isolation of the ill child.

Goal: The family caregivers' anxiety will decrease.
Expected Outcomes: The family caregivers

- verbalize understanding of the disease process.
- relate the child's progress throughout the crisis.

CEREBRAL PALSY

Cerebral palsy (CP) is a group of disorders arising from a malfunction of motor centers and neural pathways in the brain. It is one of the most complex of the common permanent disabling conditions and often can be accompanied by seizures, mental retardation, sensory defects, and behavior disorders. Research in this area is directed at adapting biomedical technology to help people with cerebral palsy cope with the activities of daily living and achieve maximum function and independence.

Causes

Although the cause of CP cannot be identified in many cases, several causes are possible. It may be caused by damage to the parts of the brain that control movement; this damage generally occurs during the fetal or perinatal period, particularly in premature infants.

Common *prenatal* causes are

- Any process that interferes with the oxygen supply to the brain such as separation of the placenta, compression of the cord, or bleeding
- Maternal infection (e.g., cytomegalovirus, toxoplasmosis, rubella)
- Nutritional deficiencies that may affect brain growth
- Kernicterus (brain damage caused by jaundice) resulting from Rh incompatibility
- Teratogenic factors, such as drugs and radiation

Common *perinatal* causes are

- Anoxia immediately before, during, and after birth
- Intracranial bleeding
- Asphyxia or interference with respiratory function
- Maternal analgesia (e.g., morphine) that depresses the sensitive neonate's respiratory center
- Birth trauma
- Prematurity because immature blood vessels predispose the neonate to cerebral hemorrhage

About 10% to 20% of cases occur after birth. Common *postnatal* causes are

- Head trauma (e.g., due to a fall, motor vehicle accident)
- Infection (e.g., encephalitis, meningitis)
- Neoplasms
- Cerebrovascular accident

Prevention

Because brain damage in CP is irreversible, prevention is the most important aspect of care. Prevention of CP focuses on

- Prenatal care to improve nutrition, prevent infection, and decrease the incidence of prematurity
- Perinatal monitoring with appropriate interventions to decrease birth trauma
- Postnatal prevention of infection through breast-feeding, improved nutrition, and immunizations
- Protection from trauma of motor vehicle accidents, child abuse, and other childhood accidents

Clinical Manifestations and Types

Difficulty in controlling voluntary muscle movements is one manifestation of the central nervous system damage. Seizures, mental retardation, hearing and vision impairments, and behavior disorders often accompany the major problem. Delayed gross motor development, abnormal motor performance (e.g., poor sucking and feeding behaviors), abnormal postures, and persistence of primitive reflexes are other signs of CP. Diagnosis of CP seldom occurs before 2 months of age and may be delayed until the 2nd or 3rd year, when the toddler attempts to walk and caregivers notice an obvious lag in motor development. Diagnosis is based on observations of delayed growth and development through a process that rules out other diagnoses.

Several major types of CP occur; each has distinctive clinical manifestations.

Spastic Type

Spastic CP is the most common type and is characterized by

- A hyperactive stretch reflex in associated muscle groups
- Increased activity of the deep tendon reflexes
- **Clonus** (rapid involuntary muscle contraction and relaxation)
- Contractures affecting the extensor muscles, especially the heel cord
- Scissoring caused by severe hip adduction. When scissoring is present, the child's legs are crossed and the toes are pointed down (Fig. 35-9). When standing, the child is on her or his toes. It is difficult for this child to walk on the heels or to run.

Athetoid Type

Athetoid CP is marked by involuntary, uncoordinated motion with varying degrees of muscle tension. Children with this disorder are constantly in motion, and the whole body is in a state of slow, writhing muscle contractions whenever voluntary movement is attempted. Facial grimacing, poor swallowing, and tongue move-

■ Figure 35-9 The physical therapist works with a child who has cerebral palsy. Note the scissoring of the legs.

ments causing drooling and **dysarthria** (poor speech articulation) also are present. These children are likely to have average or above average intelligence, despite their abnormal appearance. Hearing loss is most common in this group.

Ataxic Type

Ataxia is essentially a lack of coordination caused by disturbances in the kinesthetic and balance senses. The least common type of CP, ataxic CP may not be diagnosed until the child starts to walk: The gait is awkward and wide-based.

Rigidity Type

Rigidity CP is uncommon and is characterized by rigid postures and lack of active movement.

Mixed Type

Children with signs of more than one type of CP, termed mixed type, are usually severely disabled. The disorder may have been caused by postnatal injury.

Diagnosis

Children with CP may not be diagnosed with certainty until they have difficulties when attempting to walk. They may show signs of mental retardation, attention deficit disorder, or recurrent convulsions. Computed tomography, magnetic resonance imaging, and ultrasonography for infants before closure of skull sutures may be used to help determine the cause of CP.

Treatment and Special Aids

Treatment of CP focuses on helping the child to make the best use of residual abilities and achieve maximum satisfaction and enrichment in life. A team of health care professionals—physician, surgeon, physical therapist, occupational therapist, speech therapist, and perhaps a social worker—works with the family to set realistic goals. Dental care is important because enamel hypoplasia is common, and children whose seizure disorders are controlled with phenytoin (Dilantin) are likely to develop gingival hypertrophy. Medications, such as baclofen, diazepam, and dantrolene, may be used to help decrease spasticity.

Physical Therapy

Body control needed for purposeful physical activity is learned automatically by a normal child but must be consciously learned by a child who has problems with physical mobility. Physical therapists attempt to teach activities of daily living that the child has been unable to accomplish. Methods must be suited to the needs of each child, as well as to the general needs arising from the condition. These methods are based on principles of conditioning, relaxation, use of residual patterns, stimulation of contraction and relaxation of antagonistic muscles, and others. Various techniques are used. Because there are many variations in the disabilities caused by CP, each child must be considered individually and treated appropriately.

Orthopedic Management

Braces are used as supportive and control measures to facilitate muscle training, to reinforce weak or paralyzed muscles, or to counteract the pull of antagonistic muscles. Various types are available; each is designed for a specific purpose (Fig. 35-10). Orthopedic surgery sometimes is used to improve function and to correct deformities, such as the release of contractures and the lengthening of tight heel cords.

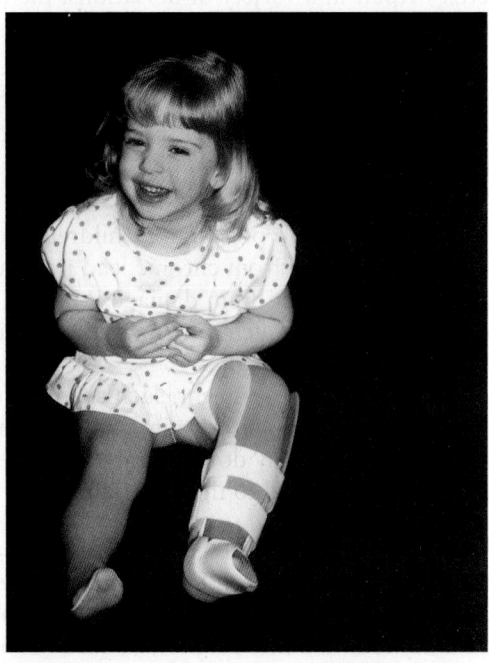

■ **Figure 35-10** Ankle-foot braces are being used for this child with cerebral palsy to give support for walking.

Technological Aids for Daily Living

Biomedical engineering, particularly in the field of electronics, has perfected a number of devices to help make the disabled person more functional and less dependent on others. The devices range from simple items, such as wheelchairs and specially constructed toilet seats, to completely electronic cottages furnished with a computer (even including a voice synthesizer), a tape recorder, a calculator, and other equipment that facilitates independence and useful study or work. Many of these devices can be controlled by a mouth stick, which is an extremely useful feature for people with poor hand coordination.

A child who has difficulty maintaining balance while sitting may need a high-backed chair with sidepieces and a foot platform. Feeding may be a challenge, so caregivers may need help finding a method that works for feeding their child. Sometimes controlling and stabilizing the jaw by hand will help with feeding. Feeding aids include spoons with enlarged handles for easy grasping or with bent handles that allow the spoon to be brought easily to the mouth. Plates with high rims and suction devices to prevent slipping enable a child to eat with little assistance. Covered cups set in holders with a hole in the lid to admit a straw help a child who does not have hand control (Fig. 35-11). The severely disabled child may need a nasogastric or gastrostomy tube.

Manual skill can be aided by games that must be manipulated, such as pegboards and cards.

Computer programs have been designed to enable these children to communicate and improve their learning skills. Special keyboards, joysticks, and electronic devices help the child to have fun and gain a sense of achievement while learning. Computers also have expanded the opportunities for future employment for these children.

Good news.
Keyboarding is an ego-boosting alternative for a child whose disability is too severe to permit legible writing.

Nursing Care

The child with CP may be seen in the health care setting at any age level. Interview and observe the child and the family to determine the child's needs, the level of development, and the stage of family acceptance and to set realistic long-range goals. The child with a new diagnosis and the family may have more potential nursing diagnoses than the child and family who have been successfully dealing with CP for a long time.

To ease the change of environment when the child is hospitalized, communicate with the family to learn as much as possible about the child's activities at home. Encourage the child to maintain current self-care activities and set goals for attaining new ones. Positioning to prevent contractures, providing modified feeding utensils,

■ Figure 35-11 Feeding aids and devices: **(A)** cups, **(B)** utensils, and **(C)** dishes.

and suggesting appropriate educational play activities are all important aspects of the child's care. If the child has been admitted for surgery, the child and family need appropriate preoperative and postoperative teaching, emotional support, and assistance in setting realistic expectations. The family may need help to explore educational opportunities for the child.

Like any chronic condition, CP can become a devastating drain on the family's emotional and financial resources. The child's future depends on many variables: family attitudes; economic and therapeutic resources; the child's intelligence; and the availability of competent, understanding health care professionals. Some children, when given the emotional and physical support they need, can achieve a satisfactory degree of independence. Some have been able to attend college and find fulfilling work. Vocational training is also available to an increasing number of these young people. Some people with CP will always need a significant amount of nursing care with the possibility of institutionalized care when their families can no longer care for them.

The outlook for these children and their families is improving, but a great deal of work remains to be done. Working as a community member, the health care professional can play a vital role in promoting educational opportunities, rehabilitation, and acceptance for disabled children.

MENTAL RETARDATION

Mental retardation is defined in the *Diagnostic and Statistical Manual of Mental Disorders* (DSM-IV-TR) (American Psychiatric Association, 2000) using two criteria: significantly subaverage general intellectual functioning—an intelligence quotient (IQ) of 70 or lower—and concurrent deficits in adaptive functioning. Adaptive functioning refers to how well people can meet the standards of independence (activities of daily living) and social responsibility expected for their age and cultural group. Mental retardation often occurs in combination with other physical disorders.

Causes

Many factors can cause mental retardation. Prenatal causes include

- Inborn errors of metabolism such as phenylketonuria, galactosemia, or congenital hypothyroidism. Damage often can be prevented by early detection and treatment.
- Prenatal infection, such as toxoplasmosis or cytomegalovirus. Microcephaly, hydrocephalus, cerebral palsy, and other brain damage can result from intrauterine infections.
- Teratogenic agents, such as drugs, radiation, and alcohol, can have devastating effects on the central nervous system of a developing fetus.
- Genetic factors—inborn variations of chromosomal patterns—result in a variety of deviations, the most common of which is Down syndrome.

Perinatal causes of mental retardation include birth trauma, anoxia from various causes, prematurity, and difficult birth. In some instances, prenatal factors may have influenced the perinatal complications.

Postnatal causes include

- Poisoning, such as lead poisoning. Children who develop encephalopathy from chronic lead poisoning usually have significant brain damage.
- Infections and trauma such as meningitis, convulsive disorders, and hydrocephalus.
- Impoverished early environment, such as inadequate nutrition and a lack of sensory stimulation. Emotional rejection in early life may do irreparable damage to a child's ability to respond to the environment.

Clinical Manifestations and Diagnosis

About 3% of all children born in the United States have some level of cognitive impairment. About 20% of these are so severely retarded that diagnosis is made at birth or during the first year. Most of the other children are diagnosed when they begin school.

The most common classification of mental retardation is based on IQ. Although controversy exists about the validity of tests that measure intelligence, this system is still the most useful for grouping these children.

The child with an IQ of 70 to 50 is considered to have mild mental retardation. This child is a slow learner but can acquire basic skills. The child can learn to read, write, and do arithmetic to a fourth- or fifth-grade level but is slower than average in learning to walk, talk, and feed himself or herself. Retardation may not be obvious to casual acquaintances. With support and guidance, this child usually can develop social and vocational skills adequate for self-maintenance. About 80% of children with mental retardation are classified in this category.

The child with an IQ of 55 to 35 has moderate mental retardation. This child has little, if any, ability to attain independence and academic skills and is referred to as trainable. Motor development and speech are noticeably delayed, but training in self-help activities is possible. This child may be able to learn repetitive skills in sheltered workshops. Some children may learn to travel alone, but few become capable of assuming complete self-maintenance. About 10% of cases of mental retardation fall in the moderate category.

The child who tests in the IQ range of 40 to 20 has severe mental retardation. This child's development is markedly delayed during the first year of life. The child cannot learn academic skills, but may be able to learn some self-care activities if sensorimotor stimulation is begun early. Eventually this child will probably learn to walk and develop some speech; however, a sheltered environment and careful supervision always will be required.

The child with an IQ lower than 20 has profound mental retardation. This child has minimal capacity for functioning and needs continuing care. Eventually the child may learn to walk and develop a primitive speech but will never be able to perform self-care activities. Only about 1% of children with mental retardation are in this category.

Treatment and Education

Knowledge about teaching children with cognitive impairment has increased dramatically, and new teaching methods have been yielding encouraging results. People with mild and moderate retardation are taught to perform tasks that enable them to achieve some degree of independence. More and better services are available for all cognitively impaired children and adults.

The child with cognitive impairment may not be identified until well into the preschool stage, because slow development often can be excused in one way or another. The family may be the best judge of the child's development, and health care personnel must listen carefully to any concerns or questions that caregivers express.

When family members are faced with the fact that their child is retarded, they need to go through a grieving process, as do family members of any other child with a serious disorder. They need to mourn the loss of the normal child that was expected and resolve to give this child the best opportunities to develop his or her potential.

Early diagnosis and intervention are important. Tests done during infancy are difficult to administer and the results are inaccurate, but they may provide the family with some idea about the child's potential. The family must be aware that these are only predictions based on unreliable test data.

The child is usually kept at home in the family environment. The current philosophy of care for such a child is to approach teaching in an aggressive manner by encouraging learning in a supportive home environment where the child can relate closely to a few people whose role is to stimulate and encourage maximum development. The individual attention, security, and sense of belonging to a family are important factors in every child's growth and development.

Nursing Process for the Child With Cognitive Impairment

Assessment

The child who has a cognitive impairment is seen in the health care setting for diagnosis, treatment, and follow-up, as well as the usual health maintenance visits. During these visits, communicating with the child may be a challenge. A thorough interview with the child's caregiver can be helpful in learning about the child and family. Listen carefully to the caregiver, paying particular attention to any comments or concerns he or she has.

The interview and physical exam may be lengthy and detailed, depending partially on the circumstances of the child's primary need for health care. Aside from the data collection needed as dictated by the current health care needs, also collect information about the child's habits, routines, and personal terminology (such as nicknames and toileting terms). Be careful to communicate at the child's level of understanding, and do not talk down to the child during the interview. Treat the child with respect. This approach helps gain cooperation from both the family and the child. Arrange the initial interview and physical exam so that they can be conducted in an unhurried atmosphere that avoids placing undue stress on the child or the family.

Selected Nursing Diagnoses

- Delayed Growth and Development related to physical and mental disability
- Bathing/Hygiene, Dressing/Grooming, Feeding, and Toileting Self-Care Deficit related to cognitive or neuromuscular impairment (or both)
- Impaired Verbal Communication related to impaired receptive or expressive skills
- Risk for Injury related to physical or neurologic impairment (or both)

- Compromised Family Coping related to emotional stress or grief
- Risk for Social Isolation (family or child) related to fear of and embarrassment about the child's behavior or appearance

Outcome Identification and Planning

The major goals for the cognitively impaired child depend entirely on the child's abilities as determined during data collection and the interview. Common goals include promoting growth and development to reach the highest level of functioning (within the child's ability), promoting self-care (within the child's ability), fostering communication with caregivers and nurses, and preventing injury. Goals for the family include promoting family coping and preventing social isolation.

Implementation

Promoting Growth and Development

The child with cognitive impairment often has physical disabilities that affect growth and development. All but the most profoundly impaired children go through the sequence of normal development with delays at each stage; their abilities level off as the children reach the limits of their capabilities. A cognitively impaired child proceeds according to mental age, rather than chronological age. Thus, an impaired 6-year-old child may be functioning on a mental level of 2 years, and the expected behavior must be essentially that of a 2-year-old child. Teach the family caregivers about the important landmarks of normal growth and development to help them understand the progressive nature of maturation and to improve planning for the child.

Environmental stimulation is essential for development in all children, but the cognitively impaired child needs much more environmental enrichment than does the average child. Suggested activities for providing this enrichment are summarized in Table 35-4.

Whether at home or in a health care facility, the child with cognitive impairment needs to know which behaviors are acceptable and which are unacceptable. Discipline is as important to this child as to any other. The limited ability of these children to adapt to varying circumstances makes consistent discipline essential, with instructions given in simple, direct, concise language. Using a positive approach with many examples and demonstrations achieves better results than a constant stream of "don't touch" or "stop that."

Obedience is an important part of discipline, especially for the child with faulty reasoning ability, but the objectives of discipline should be much broader than simply obedience. The child needs to know what to expect and finds security and support in routines and consistency. Use kindness, love, understanding, and physical comforting as a major part of discipline.

If discipline is needed, be certain it follows the misdeed immediately so that the cause-and-effect relationship is clear. Taking the child away from the group for a short time may help restore self-control. If the child is using misbehavior to get attention, praise and approval for good behavior may eliminate the need for wrongdoing.

Promoting Self-Care

Teaching the child with mental retardation can be time-consuming, frustrating, challenging, and rewarding. When the child is first seen in a health care setting, a teaching program that reflects his or her developmental level must be designed. Be certain that all personnel who care for the child and any involved family members are aware of the program. Break each element of care to be taught into small segments and repeat those steps over and over.

> **Most nurses find this approach helpful.** Patience is one of the most important aspects of teaching a cognitively impaired child.

Use praise generously, and give small material rewards as useful tools to aid in teaching. Challenge the child, but make the immediate small goals realistic and attainable. Brushing teeth, brushing or combing the hair, bathing, washing the hands and face, feeding oneself, dressing independently, and basic safety are all self-care areas in which the child needs instruction and positive reinforcement.

Teaching the cognitively impaired child requires the same principles used in teaching any child: Work at a level appropriate to the stage of the child's maturation, not the chronological age. If the child has physical disabilities in addition to mental retardation, the rate of physical development is also affected. One factor that makes the child with cognitive impairment different from the average child is the lack of ability to reason abstractly. This prevents transfer of learning or application of abstract principles to varied situations. Learning takes place by habit formation and emphasizing the "three Rs": routine, repetition, and relaxation. Most cognitively impaired children increase in mental age, although slowly and to a limited level. Therefore, each child needs to be watched for evidence of readiness for a new skill.

Fostering Communication Skills

The child with cognitive impairment often has major problems with language skills. The child may have problems forming various speech sounds because of an enlarged tongue or other physical deviations, including hearing impairment. These problems can frustrate attempts at communication. In addition, the child may not be able to process the spoken word, which compounds communication problems. A speech therapist can evaluate the child and develop a program to help caregivers work

Table 35-4 ▮ EXAMPLES OF DEVELOPMENTAL STIMULATION AND SENSORIMOTOR TEACHING FOR INFANTS AND YOUNG CHILDREN WITH MENTAL RETARDATION

Developmental Sequence	Possible Activities to Encourage Development
Sitting	
1. Sit with support in caregiver's lap	Hold child in sitting position on lap, supporting under armpits. Do several times a day, gradually lessening the support.
2. Sit independently when propped	Place child in sitting position against firm surface with pillow behind the back and on either side. Leave the child alone several times a day.
3. Sit with increasingly less support	Allow child to sit on equipment that provides increasingly less support such as baby swing, feeder, walker, high chair.
4. Sit in chair without assistance	Place child in a chair with arms. Provide balance support at first, and then gradually withdraw. Leave for 10 minutes at a time.
5. Sit without support	Place child on floor. Gradually withdraw assistance.
Self-Feeding	
1. Sucking	Encourage child to suck by putting food on pacifier, putting a drop on tongue, and so forth.
2. Drink from a cup	Put small amount of fluid in a baby cup. Raise cup to mouth by placing hands under child.
3. Grasp piece of food and place in mouth	Place bit of favorite food in child's hand. Guide hand and food to mouth. Gradually reduce support.
4. Transfer food from spoon to mouth	Move spoon to child's mouth with hand supporting baby's mouth. Gradually reduce support.
5. Scoop up food and transfer to mouth	Have child hold spoon by handle, scoop up food, and transfer to mouth. Do not allow child to use fingers. Progress from bowl to flat plate.
Stimulation of Touch	
1. Body sensation	Hold, cuddle, rock child.
2. Explore environment through touch	Brush skin with objects of various textures (feathers, silk, sandpaper). Place objects of different textures near child. Move hand to object.
3. Explore environment through mouth	Give child objects that can be chewed. Guide hand to mouth at first.
4. Explore tactile sensations	Expose child to hard, soft, warm, and cold objects.
5. Explore with water	Place hands or feet in water.

with the child to improve both the child's understanding of what is said and the child's ability to use language.

Preventing Injury

The child with cognitive impairment has faulty reasoning ability and a short attention span. As a result, the caregivers must be responsible for protecting the child. The health care facility and the home must be made safe. Teach elementary safety rules and reinforce them continuously.

Promoting Family Coping

Before effective treatment can begin, the family must accept the reality of the child's problem and must want to cope with the difficult task of helping the child develop to his or her full potential. Diagnosis made at birth or during the first year affords the greatest hope of early acceptance and beginning education and training.

The family's first reaction to learning that the child may have cognitive impairment is grief because this is not the perfect child of their dreams. A parent may feel shame, assuming that he or she cannot produce a perfect child. Some rejection of the child is almost inevitable, at least in the initial stages, but this must be worked through for the family to cope. Some parents compensate

for their early hostile feelings by overprotection or over concern, making the child unnecessarily helpless and perhaps taking out their anger and frustration on the normal siblings. The family begins to function effectively only when the caregivers accept the child as another family member to be helped, loved, and disciplined.

Preventing Social Isolation

Family members need to know that their feelings are normal. Talking with other families of impaired children can offer some of the best support and guidance, as caregivers seek information to help them deal with the problem. One group that includes both families and health care professionals is the National Association of Retarded Citizens, a volunteer organization with chapters in many communities (Web site www.thearc.org). The National Down Syndrome Society is another excellent resource for the family of a child with Down syndrome (Web site www.ndss.org). Participating in the Special Olympics is a good way for children to begin to gain self-confidence.

Evaluation: Goals and Expected Outcomes

Goal: The child will attain the milestones of his or her stage of growth and development according to mental

A Personal Glimpse

The mother of a developmentally delayed child knows her child has a problem before any doctor notices. Visually my son looked perfect. There were no outward signs of retardation. He was a beautiful baby but he was often ill—severe croup, pneumonia, bronchitis, grand mal seizures due to fever, hospital stays, EEGs, spinal taps, tests and more tests—but he always bounced back, much better than his parents recovered.

Slowly, I started to notice that he was not the same as other kids his age. His vocabulary was Mom and DaDa where other 3-year-olds were starting to put words together into little sentences. Everyone said he didn't talk because I spoiled him and got him everything he needed before he asked for it. I would try to believe people, including doctors, who would say, "Don't worry; you are just being an overprotective mother. Your son will be fine." You try to hide from the truth, but slowly you realize you have to get others to see what you see. You have to get help for your child—someone has to listen to you.

Finally I forced my pediatrician to try some physical dexterity tests. My son failed these tests. I heard the doctor say the words that broke my heart: "I am sorry. I thought you were just another hysterical mother—but there is something wrong with your child. We must schedule him for more testing." Then I cried.

Patricia

Learning Opportunity: What are some feelings parents of children diagnosed with mental retardation might have? What are some ways that the nurse can support the mother and the child in the above situation?

age; family caregivers verbalize an understanding of the child's level of development.

Expected Outcomes:

- The child attains the highest level of functioning for his or her mental age.
- Family caregivers identify the child's developmental level and set realistic goals.

Goal: The child will develop skills to meet self-care needs within her or his ability.

Expected Outcome: The child practices basic hygiene habits, as well as dressing/grooming, feeding, and toileting skills within his or her abilities with support and supervision.

Goal: The child's communication skills will improve.

Expected Outcome: The child can communicate basic needs to staff and family.

Goal: The child will be free from injury by caregivers and will learn basic safety rules.

Expected Outcome: The child remains free from injury and cooperates with basic safety rules within his or her abilities.

Goal: The family will effectively cope with the child's diagnosis.

Expected Outcomes: The family

- verbalizes feelings and mourns the loss of the "perfect child."
- provides appropriate care to help the child reach optimum functioning.

Goal: The family will interact with social groups and support networks.

Expected Outcomes: The family

- freely voices feelings and concerns about the child and makes contact with support systems.
- establishes relationships with families of other cognitively impaired children.

Test Yourself

✔ What is the difference between the five types of cerebral palsy?

✔ What is the most common way to classify mental retardation?

✔ What is usually seen in the growth and development of a child with cognitive impairment?

HEAD INJURIES

Head injuries are a significant cause of serious injury or death in children of all ages. The primary cause of a head injury varies with the child's age. Toddlers and young children may receive a head injury from a fall or child abuse; school-aged children and adolescents usually experience such an injury as a result of a bicycling, inline skating, or motor vehicle accident.

Children, especially young children, seem to receive many head injuries. Fortunately, most of them are not serious, but they are often frightening to the caregiver. If a scalp laceration is involved, the caregiver may be quite alarmed by the amount of bleeding because of the large blood supply to the head and scalp. The caregiver can apply an ice pack and pressure until the bleeding is controlled. Applying ice cubes in a zip-closure sandwich bag wrapped in a washcloth works well at home. An open wound should be cleaned with soap and water and a sterile dressing applied. For an injury without a break in the skin, the caregiver can apply ice for an hour or so to decrease the amount of swelling.

The caregiver should observe the child for at least 6 hours for vomiting or a change in the child's level of consciousness. If the child falls asleep, he or she should be awakened every 1 to 2 hours to determine that the level of consciousness has not changed. No analgesics or sedatives should be administered during this period of observation. The child's pupils are checked for reaction to light every 4 hours for

48 hours. The caregiver should notify the health care provider immediately if the child vomits more than three times, has pupillary changes, has double or blurred vision, has a change in level of consciousness, acts strange or confused, has trouble walking, or has a headache that becomes more severe or wakes him or her from sleep; these instructions should be provided in written form to the caregiver.

Family caregivers are wise to take the child to a health care facility to have the injury evaluated if they have any doubt about its seriousness. Complications of head injuries with or without skull fractures can include cerebral hemorrhage, cerebral edema, and increased intracranial pressure. These conditions require highly skilled intensive care, and victims are usually cared for in a pediatric neurologic or intensive care unit.

Shaken baby syndrome, a form of child abuse that can cause head injury without external signs of head trauma, is discussed in Chapter 33.

DROWNING

Drowning is the second leading cause of accidental death in children. Toddlers and older adolescents have the highest actual rate of death from drowning. Drowning in children often occurs when the child has been left unattended in a body of water. Infants more commonly drown in a bathtub; toddlers and preschoolers drown in pools or small bodies of water. A pail of

---

Table 35-5 ▌ SUMMARY OF BASIC LIFE SUPPORT MANEUVERS IN INFANTS AND CHILDREN

Maneuver	Infant (<1 yr)	Child (1–8 yrs)
Activate		
Emergency Response Number (lone rescuer)	Activate after performing 5 cycles of CPR	Activate after performing 5 cycles of CPR
	For sudden, witnessed collapse, activate after verifying that victim is unresponsive	For sudden, witnessed collapse, activate after verifying that victim is unresponsive
Airway		
	Head tilt–chin lift (unless trauma present)	Head tilt–chin lift (unless trauma present)
	Jaw thrust (if suspected trauma)	Jaw thrust (if suspected trauma)
Breaths		
Initial	2 effective breaths at 1 sec/breath	2 effective breaths at 1 sec/breath
Rescue breathing without chest compressions	12–20 breaths/min (approximately 1 breath every 3 to 5 seconds)	12–20 breaths/min (approximately 1 breath every 3–5 seconds)
Rescue breaths for CPR with advanced airway	8–10 breaths/min (approximately 1 breath every 6–8 seconds)	8–10 breaths/min (approximately 1 breath every 6–8 seconds)
Foreign-body airway obstruction	Back slaps and chest thrusts	Abdominal thrusts
Circulation		
Pulse check (≤10 sec)	Brachial/femoral	Carotid/femoral
Compression landmarks	Just below nipple line	Center of chest, between nipples
Compression method (Push hard and fast; allow complete recoil)	1 rescuer: 2 fingers 2 rescuers: 2 thumb-encircling hands	2 Hands: Heel of 1 hand with second on top or 1 Hand: Heel of 1 hand only
Compression depth	Approximately 1/3 to 1/2 the depth of the chest	Approximately 1/3 to 1/2 the depth of the chest
Compression Rate	Approximately 100/min	Approximately 100/min
Compression-ventilation ratio	30:2 (single rescuer) 15:2 (two rescuers)	30:2 (single rescuer) 15:2 (two rescuers)
Defibrillation		
AED	No recommendations for infants <1 year of age	Use AED as soon as available for sudden collapse and in-hospital Use after 5 cycles of CPR if out-of-hospital Use child pads/child system for child 1 to 8 years, if available; if child pads/system not available, use adult AED and pads

Source: American Heart Association. (2005). American Heart Association Guidelines for Cardiopulmonary Resuscitation and Emergency Cardiovascular Care. International Consensus on Science. *Circulation, 112,* IV-1–IV-211.

A. Opening the airway with the head tilt- chin lift maneuver. One hand is used to tilt the head, extensing the neck. The index finger of the rescuer's other hand lifts the mandible outward by lifting of the chin. Head tilit should not be preformed if cervical spine injury is suspected.

B. Opening the airway with the jaw-thrust maneuver. The airway is open by lifting the angle of the mandible. The rescuer uses two fingers of each hand to lift the jaw while other fingers guide the jaw upward.

C. Rescue breathing in an infant. The rescuer's mouth covers the infant's nose and mouth, creating a seal. One hand performs head tilt while the other hand lifts the infant's jaw. Avoid head tilt if the infant has sustained head or neck trauma.

D. The rescue breathing in a child. The rescuer's mouth covers the mouth of the child creating a mouth-to-mouth seal. One hand maintains the head tilt; the thumb and forefinger of the same hand are used to pinch the childs nose.

E. Locating and palpating the carotid artery pulse in a child.

F. Palpating the brachial artery pulse.

G. Cardiac compressions. Top: infant supine on palm of rescuer's hand. Bottom: Performing CPR while carrying the infant or small child. Note that the head is kept level with torso. (compare with H)

H. Locating the proper finger position for chest compression in infant. Note that the rescuer's other hand is used to maintain head position to facilitate ventilation.

I. Locating Hand position for chest compression in child.

J. Lift fingers to avoid pressing on child's ribs. Note that the hand not performing chest compressions is used to maintain head position and ventilation.

■ Figure 35-12 Cardiopulmonary resuscitation. (Adapted from American Heart Association [2001]. *Basic life support for healthcare providers*. Dallas, TX: Author.)

water may become something for the toddler to investigate, which could lead to accidental death. Many drowning deaths in this age group occur in home pools; including spas, hot tubs, and whirlpools. Drowning in older children often occurs because the child is playing or acting in an unsafe manner.

A responsible adult must continuously supervise all infants and young children when they are near any source of water. Older children and adolescents should not play alone around any body of water. Swimming in undesig-nated swimming areas, such as creeks, quarries, and rivers, is especially hazardous for older children and adolescents.

When a drowning victim of any age is discovered, cardiopulmonary resuscitation (CPR) should be started immediately and continued until the victim can be transported to a medical facility for additional care. Intensive care is carried out according to the patient's needs. All adults who care for children in any capacity must learn CPR and be ready to perform it immediately (Table 35-5 and Fig. 35-12).

Key Points

- At birth, the nervous system is immature. As the child grows, the quality of the nerve impulses sent through the nervous system develops and matures, allowing for the development of gross and fine motor skills.

- Visual acuity of children gradually increases from birth until about 7 years of age, when most children have 20/20 vision. Hearing in children is acute, and the infant will respond to sounds within the first month of life.

- Vision impairment includes myopia (nearsightedness), hyperopia (farsightedness), astigmatism, partial sight, or blindness. Adequate vision and normal development are more likely with early treatment. Specialized equipment helps prevent isolation.

- Cataracts, glaucoma, and strabismus may be detected and treated, sometimes surgically, during childhood. Eye injuries and infections are common. Bacterial conjunctivitis is treated with ophthalmic antibacterial agents such as erythromycin, bacitracin, sulfacetamide, and polymyxin.

- Types of hearing loss and the treatment depend on the part of the ear or brain that is affected. A child who is hard of hearing has a loss of hearing but is able to learn speech and language. A child who is deaf has no hearing ability.

- The child with acute otitis media is usually restless, shakes the head, and rubs or pulls at the ear. The child may also have fever, irritability, and hearing impairment. Antibiotics or a Myringotomy, incision of the eardrum with tiny tubes placed in the tympanic membrane, are used to treat otitis media.

- Reye syndrome usually occurs after a viral infection. The child has severe vomiting, irritability, lethargy, and confusion. The disease can progress rapidly. The symptoms are classified by stages and supportive measures are used to treat the disease.

- Nursing care for the child at high risk for seizures includes monitoring for complications, such as signs of increased intracranial pressure (IICP), as well as preventing aspiration, keeping the child safe, monitoring intake and output, and supporting the child's family.

- A simple partial motor seizure causes a localized motor activity such as shaking of an arm, leg, or other body part. Simple partial sensory seizures may include sensory symptoms, called an aura, which signals an impending attack. Complex partial (psychomotor) seizures begin in a small area of the brain and can cause memory loss and staring.

- Tonic-clonic seizures consist of four stages. In the prodromal period, the child may be drowsy or dizzy. An aura is a warning and occurs immediately before the seizure. During the tonic phase, the muscles contract and the extremities stiffen. The initial rigidity of the tonic phase changes to generalized jerking muscle movements in the clonic phase. The jerking movements gradually diminish then disappear. Sleep usually occurs during the postictal stage.

- In absence seizures, there is lose of awareness and eye blinking or twitching, but the child does not fall. After the seizure, the child is alert and continues conversation. Atonic or akinetic seizures cause a sudden momentary loss of consciousness, muscle tone, and postural control, and the child may fall. In myoclonic seizures, there is a sudden jerking of a muscle or group of muscles, often in the arms or legs. Infantile spasms usually indicate a cerebral defect and consist of muscle contractions and rolling of the eyes.

- Status epilepticus describes a seizure that lasts longer than 30 minutes or a series of seizures, in which the child does not return to a normal level of consciousness. Drug therapy is used to stop and control the seizure activity.

- *Haemophilus influenzae* meningitis is spread by droplet infection. Symptoms include high-pitched cry, fever, irritability, headache, nuchal rigidity (stiff neck) that may progress to opisthotonos (arching of the back), and delirium. Projectile vomiting may be present. Generalized convulsions are common. The four complications of *Haemophilus influenzae* meningitis are hydrocephalus, nerve deafness, mental retardation, and paralysis.

➤ Cerebral palsy is a group of disorders arising from a malfunction of motor centers and neural pathways in the brain, often accompanied by seizures, mental retardation, sensory defects, and behavior disorders.

➤ Prenatal causes of cerebral palsy include oxygen deprivation, maternal infection, nutritional deficiencies, Rh incompatibility, and teratogenic agents, such as drugs and radiation. Perinatal causes include anoxia, intracranial bleeding, asphyxia, maternal analgesia, trauma, and prematurity. Postnatal head trauma, infection, neoplasms, or cerebrovascular accident can also cause CP.

➤ Spastic type CP is characterized by a hyperactive stretch reflex in associated muscle groups; increased activity of the deep tendon reflexes; clonus; contractures of the extensor muscles, especially the heel cord, and scissoring caused by hip adduction. Athetoid type CP is marked by involuntary, uncoordinated motion with muscle tension; the child is in constant motion. Ataxic CP is a lack of coordination caused by disturbances in the kinesthetic and balance senses. Rigidity CP is characterized by rigid postures and lack of active movement.

➤ Health care professionals involved in the care of the child with cerebral palsy include a physical therapist, as well as individuals who specialize in orthopedic and technological aids to help in activities of daily living.

➤ Prenatal causes of mental retardation include inborn errors of metabolism; prenatal infection; teratogenic agents, such as drugs, radiation, and alcohol; and genetic factors. Birth trauma, anoxia, prematurity, and difficult birth are perinatal causes. Postnatal causes include poisoning, such as lead poisoning, infections, trauma, inadequate nutrition, and a lack of sensory stimulation.

➤ Promoting self-care, fostering communication with caregivers and nurses, promoting growth and development to reach the highest level of functioning (within the child's ability), and preventing injury are the goals when working with cognitively impaired children.

➤ Head injuries are a significant cause of serious injury or death in children of all ages. Toddlers and young children may receive a head injury from a fall or child abuse; school-aged children and adolescents usually experience such an injury as a result of a bicycling, inline skating, or motor vehicle accident. The child is monitored closely following a head injury and any change in the child is reported immediately.

➤ Drowning is the second leading cause of accidental death in children. Toddlers and older adolescents have the highest actual rate of death from drowning. Drowning in children often occurs when the child has been left unattended in a body of water. Cardiopulmonary resuscitation (CPR) should be started immediately when a drowning victim is discovered.

INTERNET RESOURCES

Epilepsy
www.efa.org

Febrile Seizures
www.ninds.nih.gov/disorders/febrile_seizures/detail_febrile_seizures.htm

Hearing Loss
www.johntracyclinic.org

Mental Retardation
www.aamr.org

Otitis Media
www.nidcd.nih.gov/health/hearing/otitismedia.asp

Reye Syndrome
www.reyessyndrome.org

Workbook

■ NCLEX-STYLE REVIEW QUESTIONS

1. If a child has a febrile seizure, what is the *highest* priority for the nurse?
   a. Document the child's behavior during the seizure.
   b. Teach the caregivers about fever reduction methods.
   c. Protect the child during the seizure activity.
   d. Reassure the caregivers that seizures are common.

2. After discussing ways to lower a fever with the caregiver of an infant, the caregiver makes the following statements. Which statement requires further teaching?
   a. "I won't give my child baby aspirin when she has a fever."
   b. "I know I need to dress my baby lightly if she has a fever."
   c. "When my baby has a fever, I will sponge her in cool water for 20 minutes."
   d. "I need to recheck my baby's temperature until it is below 101."

3. The nurse admits a child with a diagnosis of meningitis. The child is being monitored for signs of increased intracranial pressure (IICP). Of the following signs and symptoms, which would *most* likely be seen in the child with IICP?
   a. High-pitched cry, headache
   b. Itching, swelling around eyes
   c. Weight gain or loss
   d. Decreased head size, sunken fontanel

4. The nurse has admitted a 6-year-old child who has received a diagnosis of a seizure disorder and has frequent tonic-clonic seizures. Which of the following are characteristics of tonic-clonic seizures? Select all that apply.
   a. The seizure activity might be preceded by a sight, sound, taste, or smell.
   b. The seizure activity is usually limited to one side of the body.
   c. The seizure activity involves a phase in which the muscles are rigid.
   d. The seizure activity causes memory loss and staring.
   e. The seizure activity involves a phase in which there are jerking muscle movements.
   f. The seizure activity often is followed by a loss of control of bowel and bladder.

5. The nurse has admitted a 9-year-old child who is blind. Of the following nursing actions, which

would be important for the nurse to implement? Select all that apply.
   a. Identify self when entering the room.
   b. Quietly walk out of the room when he or she leaves.
   c. Involve the child in activities with younger children.
   d. Encourage the child to be as independent as possible.
   e. Provide the child with only finger foods.
   f. Encourage self-feeding after orienting the child to the plate.

■ STUDY ACTIVITIES

1. Research your community for financial resources, supplies and equipment, and support groups available to children and families with the following disorders. Complete the following table and share the information with your peers.

Condition	Financial Resources	Supplies and Equipment	Support Groups
Vision impairment			
Hearing impairment			
Cerebral palsy			
Mental retardation			

2. Create a poster or teaching aid to be used in teaching family caregivers of children who have seizure disorders. Include safety precautions, what to do when a child has a seizure and after the seizure, and medication considerations.

3. Go to the following Web site: www.preventblindness.org.
   a. Click on the section titled, "Your Child's Sight."
   b. Click on "Home eye tests for children"
   c. Click on "Distance Vision Test for Younger Children"
   d. Print a copy of the Distance Vision Chart.
   e. Following the instructions given, administer the distance vision test to a preschooler.
   f. What did you discover about this child's vision?

■ CRITICAL THINKING: WHAT WOULD YOU DO?

1. Four-year-old Todd is blind. You are the nurse helping with his care. He is going to have surgery and will be hospitalized for 3 to 4 days.
   a. What will you do to orient him to the pediatric unit?

b. What things will you teach him and do to prepare him for his hospital stay?

c. What age-appropriate activities will you offer to him before and after surgery?

2. You are caring for 10-year-old Missy, who has a mild hearing impairment. She and her father have returned to the pediatric clinic for a follow-up visit.

a. What information do you need to ask Missy's father that will help you in communicating with Missy?

b. What will you do to adapt your nursing care to improve your communication with her?

3. You and your friend are working with a group of children with physical limitations. One of the children has cerebral palsy. Your friend asks you if cerebral palsy is inherited and if it can be prevented.

a. What explanation will you give your friend regarding the causes of cerebral palsy?

b. How will you answer the question regarding whether or not CP can be prevented?

c. What will you tell your friend about the types of cerebral palsy that children might have?

4. Dosage calculation: An infant with a diagnosis of otitis media is being treated with amoxicillin. The child weighs 13.2 lb. The usual dosage of this medication is 40 mg/kg per day in divided doses, every 8 hours. Answer the following:

a. How many kilograms does the child weigh?

b. How much amoxicillin will be given in a 24-hour time period?

c. How many milligrams per dose will be given?

d. How many doses will the child receive in a day?

5. Dosage calculation: A school-aged child with a diagnosis of a seizure disorder is being treated with Dilantin. The child weighs 58 lbs. The child is being given a dose of 6 mg/kg a day in three divided doses. Answer the following:

a. How many kilograms does the child's weigh?

b. How many milligrams of Dilantin will the child receive in a 24-hour period of time?

c. How many milligrams of Dilantin will the child receive in each dose?

d. If the dose is increased by 20 mg a dose, how many milligrams will then be in each dose?

e. How many milligrams will the child receive in a 24-hour period, after the dose has been increased?

36 The Child With a Respiratory Disorder

KEY TERMS

achylia
adenoids
circumoral
coryza
croup
dysphagia
emetic
hypochylia
metered-dose inhaler
nebulizer
stridor
teratogenicity
tonsils
wheezing

LEARNING OBJECTIVES

On completion of this chapter, you should be able to:

1. Discuss ways the infant and child's respiratory system differs from the adult's system.
2. Name the most common complication of acute nasopharyngitis.
3. Discuss nursing care of the child with allergic rhinitis.
4. Discuss nursing care of the child with tonsillitis and adenoiditis.
5. Explain the most common complication of a tonsillectomy and list the signs requiring observation.
6. Compare the croup syndrome disorders including: (a) spasmodic laryngitis, (b) acute laryngotracheobronchitis, and (c) epiglottitis.
7. Discuss the symptoms, diagnosis, and treatment of acute bronchiolitis/respiratory syncytial virus (RSV) infection.
8. Describe asthma including (a) factors that can trigger an asthma attack, (b) the physiologic response that occurs in the respiratory tract during an asthma attack, (c) treatment, and (d) nursing care.
9. Explain the diagnosis of pneumonia including the treatment and nursing care.
10. Identify the basic defect and organs affected by cystic fibrosis, along with diagnostic procedures.
11. Name the most common type of complication in cystic fibrosis and describe the dietary and pulmonary treatments of the disorder.
12. Discuss how tuberculosis is detected and treated.

RESPIRATORY disorders in infants and children are common. They range from mild to serious, even life threatening. They can be acute or chronic in nature. Sometimes these problems require hospitalization, which interrupts development of the child–family relationship and the child's patterns of sleeping, eating, and stimulation. Although the illness might be acute, if recovery is rapid and the hospitalization brief, the child probably will experience few, if any, long-term effects. However, if the condition is chronic or so serious that it requires long-term care, both child and family may suffer serious consequences.

GROWTH AND DEVELOPMENT OF THE RESPIRATORY SYSTEM

The respiratory system is made up of the nose, pharynx, larynx, trachea, epiglottis, bronchi, bronchioles, and the lungs. These structures are involved in the exchange of oxygen and carbon dioxide and the distribution of the oxygen to the body cells. Tiny, thin-walled sacs called alveoli are responsible for distributing air into the bloodstream. It is also through the alveoli that carbon dioxide is removed from the bloodstream and exhaled through the respiratory system. The structures and organs found in the respiratory system cleanse, warm, and humidify the air that enters the body.

This is critical to remember.

The diameter of the infant and child's trachea is about the size of the child's little finger. This small diameter makes it extremely important to be aware that something can easily lodge in this small passageway and obstruct the child's airway.

Respiratory problems occur more often and with greater severity in infants and children than in adults because of their immature body defenses and small, undeveloped anatomical structures. The respiratory tract grows and changes until the child is about 12 years of age. During the first 5 years, the child's airway increases in length but not in diameter.

Infants and young children have larger tongues in proportion to their mouths, shorter necks, narrower airways, and the structures are closer together. This leads to the possibility of respiratory obstruction, especially if there is edema, swelling, or increased mucus in the airways. The ability to breathe through the mouth when the nose is blocked is not automatic but develops as the child's neurologic development increases.

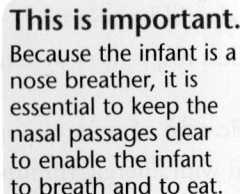

This is important.
Because the infant is a nose breather, it is essential to keep the nasal passages clear to enable the infant to breath and to eat.

The tonsillar tissue is enlarged in the early school-age child, but the pharynx, which contains the tonsils, is still small, so the possibility of obstruction of the upper airway is more likely. In children older than 2 years of age, the right bronchus is shorter, wider, and more vertical than the left.

Infants use the diaphragm and abdominal muscles to breathe. Beginning at about age 2 to 3 years, the child starts using the thoracic muscles to breath. The change from using abdominal to using thoracic muscles for respiration is completed by the age of 7 years. Because accessory muscles are used for breathing, weakness of these muscles can cause respiratory failure (Fig. 36-1).

Think about this.
If the child inhales a foreign body, it is more likely to be drawn into the right bronchus rather than the left.

ACUTE NASOPHARYNGITIS (COMMON COLD)

The common cold is one of the most common infectious conditions of childhood. The young infant is as susceptible as the older child but generally is not exposed as frequently.

The illness is of viral origin such as rhinoviruses, Coxsackie virus, respiratory syncytial virus (RSV), influenza virus, parainfluenza virus, or adenovirus. Bacterial invasion of the tissues might cause complications such as ear, mastoid, and lung infections. The child appears to be more susceptible to complications than is an adult. The infant should be protected from people who have colds because complications in the infant can be serious.

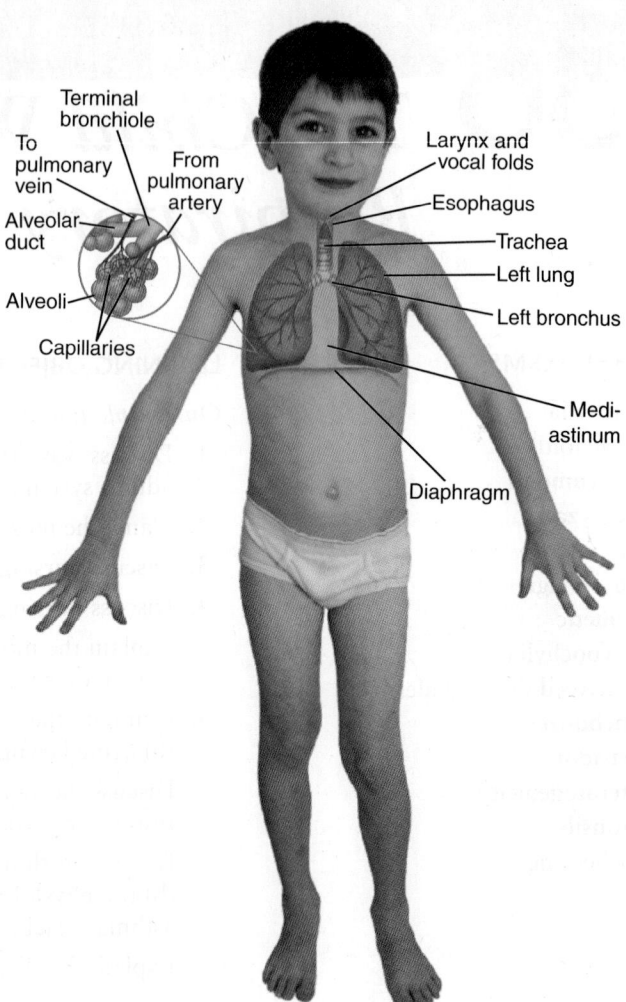

■ **Figure 36-1** Anatomy of the child's respiratory tract.

Clinical Manifestations

The child older than age 3 months usually develops fever early in the course of the infection, often as high as 102°F to 104°F (38.9°C–40°C). Younger infants usually are afebrile. The child sneezes and becomes irritable and restless. The congested nasal passages can interfere with nursing, increasing the infant's irritability. Because the older child can mouth breathe, nasal congestion is not as great a concern as in the infant. The child might have vomiting or diarrhea, which might be caused by mucous drainage into the digestive system.

Diagnosis

This nasopharyngeal condition might appear as the first symptom of many childhood contagious diseases, such as measles, and must be observed carefully. The common cold also needs to be differentiated from allergic rhinitis.

Treatment and Nursing Care

The child with an uncomplicated cold may not need any treatment in addition to rest, increased fluids and adequate nutrition, normal saline nose drops, suction with a bulb syringe, and a humidified environment. In the older child, acetaminophen or children's ibuprofen can be administered as an analgesic and antipyretic. It is best if aspirin is avoided. If the nares or upper lip become irritated, cold cream or petrolatum (Vaseline) can be used. The child needs to be comforted by holding, rocking, and soothing. If the symptoms persist for several days, the child must be seen by a physician to rule out complications, such as otitis media.

ALLERGIC RHINITIS (HAY FEVER)

Allergic rhinitis in children is most often caused by sensitization to animal dander, house dust, pollens, and molds. Pollen allergy seldom appears before 4 or 5 years of age.

Clinical Manifestations

A watery nasal discharge, postnasal drip, sneezing, and allergic conjunctivitis are the usual symptoms of allergic rhinitis. Continued sniffing, itching of the nose and palate, and the "allergic salute," in which the child pushes his or her nose upward and backward to relieve itching and open the air passages in the nose, are common complaints. Because of congestion in the nose, there is backpressure to the blood circulation around the eyes, and dark circles are visible under the eyes (Fig. 36-2). Headaches are common in older children.

Treatment and Nursing Care

When possible, offending allergens are avoided or removed from the environment. Antihistamine–decongestant

■ **Figure 36-2** Back pressure to blood circulation around the eyes leads to dark areas under the eyes in the child with allergic rhinitis. The child pushes the nose upward in the "allergic salute" to relieve itching and open the airway.

preparations, such as Dimetapp and Actifed, can be helpful for some patients. Hyposensitization can be implemented, particularly if antihistamines are not helpful or are needed chronically. Be sure to teach parents the importance of avoiding allergens and administering antihistamines to decrease symptoms.

TONSILLITIS AND ADENOIDITIS

Tonsillitis is a common illness in childhood resulting from pharyngitis. A brief description of the location and functions of the tonsils and adenoids serves as an introduction to the discussion of their infection and medical and surgical treatments.

A ring of lymphoid tissue encircles the pharynx, forming a protective barrier against upper respiratory infection. This ring consists of groups of lymphoid tonsils, including the faucial, the commonly known **tonsils;** pharyngeal, known as the **adenoids;** and lingual tonsils. Lymphoid tissue normally enlarges progressively in childhood between the ages of 2 and 10 years and shrinks during preadolescence. If the tissue itself becomes a site of acute or chronic infection, it may become hypertrophied and can interfere with breathing, cause partial deafness, or become a source of infection in itself.

Clinical Manifestations and Diagnosis

The child with tonsillitis may have a fever of 101°F (38.4°C) or more; a sore throat, often with **dysphagia** (difficulty swallowing); hypertrophied tonsils; and erythema of the soft palate. Exudate may be visible on the tonsils. The symptoms vary somewhat with the causative organism. Throat cultures are performed to diagnose tonsillitis and the causative organism. Frequently the cause of tonsillitis is viral, although beta-hemolytic streptococcal infection also may be the cause.

Treatment and Nursing Care

Medical treatment of tonsillitis consists of analgesics for pain, antipyretics for fever, and an antibiotic in the case of streptococcal infection.

Teach parents that a soft or liquid diet is easier for the child to swallow, and to encourage the child to maintain good fluid intake. A cool-mist vaporizer may be used to ease respirations.

> **Here's a pharmacology fact.**
>
> A standard 10-day course of antibiotics is often recommended for the treatment of tonsillitis. Stress the importance of completing the full prescription of antibiotic to ensure that the streptococcal infection is eliminated.

Tonsillectomies and adenoidectomies are controversial. One can be performed independent of the other, but they are often done together. No conclusive evidence has been found that a tonsillectomy in itself improves a child's health by reducing the number of respiratory infections, increasing the appetite, or improving general well-being. Currently, tonsillectomies generally are not performed unless other measures are ineffective or the tonsils are so hypertrophied that breathing and eating are difficult. Tonsillectomies are not performed while the tonsils are infected. The adenoids are more susceptible to chronic infection. An indication for adenoidectomy is hypertrophy of the tissue to the extent of impairing hearing or interfering with breathing. Performing only an adenoidectomy if the tonsil tissue appears to be healthy is an increasingly common practice. Tonsillectomy is postponed until after the age of 4 or 5 years, except in the rare instance when it appears it is urgently needed. Often when a child has reached the acceptable age, the apparent need for the tonsillectomy has disappeared.

Nursing Process for the Child Having a Tonsillectomy

Assessment

Much of the preoperative preparation, such as complete blood count, bleeding and clotting time, and urinalysis, is done on a preadmission outpatient basis. In many facilities, the child is admitted on the day of surgery or the procedure is done in a day surgery setting. Psychological preparation is often accomplished through preadmission orientation. Acting out the forthcoming experience, particularly in a group, with the use of puppets, dolls, and play-doctor or play-nurse material helps the child develop security. The amount and the timing of preparation before admission depend on the child's age. The child may become frightened about losing a body part. Telling the child that the troublesome tonsils are going to be "fixed" is a much better choice than saying that they are going to be "taken out." Include the child and the caregiver in the admission interview. Ask about any bleeding tendencies because postoperative bleeding is a concern. Carefully explain all procedures to the child and be sensitive to the child's apprehension. Take and record vital signs to establish a baseline for postoperative monitoring. The temperature is an important part of the data collection to determine that the child has no upper respiratory infection. Observe the child for loose teeth that could cause a problem during administration of anesthesia, document findings.

Selected Nursing Diagnoses

- Risk for Aspiration postoperatively related to impaired swallowing and bleeding at the operative site
- Acute Pain related to surgical procedure
- Deficient Fluid Volume related to inadequate oral intake secondary to painful swallowing
- Deficient Knowledge related to caregivers understanding of postdischarge home care and signs and symptoms of complications

Outcome Identification and Planning

The major postoperative goals for the child include preventing aspiration; relieving pain, especially while swallowing; and improving fluid intake. The major goal for the family is to increase knowledge and understanding of postdischarge care and possible complications. Design the plan of care with these goals in mind.

Implementation

Preventing Aspiration Postoperatively

Immediately after a tonsillectomy, place the child in a partially prone position with head turned to one side until the child is completely awake. This position can be accomplished by turning the child partially over and by flexing the knee where the child is not resting to help maintain the position. Keeping the head slightly lower than the chest helps facilitate drainage of secretions. Avoid placing pillows under the chest and abdomen, which may hamper respiration. Encourage the child to expectorate all secretions, and place an ample supply of tissues and a waste container near him or her. Discourage the child from coughing. Check vital signs every 10 to 15 minutes until the child is fully awake and then check every 30 minutes to 1 hour. Note the child's preoperative baseline vital signs to interpret the vital signs correctly. Hemorrhage is the most common complication of a tonsillectomy. Bleeding is most often a concern within the first 24 hours after surgery and the fifth to seventh postoperative day. During the 24 hours after surgery, observe, document, and report any unusual restlessness or anxiety, frequent swallowing, or rapid pulse that may indicate bleeding. Vomiting dark, old blood may be expected, but bright, red-flecked emesis or oozing indicates fresh bleeding. Observe the pharynx with a flashlight each time vital signs are checked. Bleeding can occur when the clots dissolve between the fifth and seventh postoperative days if new tissue is not yet present. Because the child is cared for at home by this time, give the family caregivers information concerning signs and symptoms for which to watch.

Providing Comfort and Relieving Pain

Apply an ice collar postoperatively; however, remove the collar if the child is uncomfortable with it. Administer pain medication as ordered. Liquid acetaminophen with codeine is often prescribed. Rectal or intravenous analgesics may be used. Encourage the caregiver to remain at the bedside to provide soothing reassurance. Crying irritates the raw throat and increases the child's discomfort; thus, it should be avoided if possible. Teach the caregiver what may be expected in drainage and signs that should be reported immediately to the nursing staff.

Encouraging Fluid Intake

When the child is fully awake from surgery, give small amounts of clear fluids or ice chips. Synthetic juices, carbonated beverages that are "flat," and frozen juice popsicles are good choices.

Avoid irritating liquids, such as orange juice and lemonade. Milk and ice cream products tend to cling to the surgical site and make swallowing more difficult; thus, they are poor choices, despite the old tradition of offering ice cream after a tonsillectomy. Continue administration of intravenous fluid and record intake and output until adequate oral intake is established.

Here's a helpful hint.
After a tonsillectomy, offer the child liquids that are not red in color to eliminate confusion with bloody discharge.

Providing Family Teaching

The child typically is discharged on the day of or the day after surgery if no complications are present. Instruct the caregiver to keep the child relatively quiet for a few days after discharge. Recommend giving soft foods and non-irritating liquids for the first few days. Teach family members that if at any time after the surgery they note any signs of hemorrhage (bright red bleeding, frequent swallowing, restlessness), they should notify the care provider. Provide written instructions and telephone numbers before discharge. Advise the caregivers that a mild earache may be expected about the third day.

Evaluation: Goals and Expected Outcomes

Goal: The child's airway will remain patent after surgery.
Expected Outcomes: The child

- shows signs of an open and clear airway.
- expectorates saliva and drainage with no aspiration.

Goal: The child will show signs of being comfortable.
Expected Outcomes: The child

- rests quietly and does not cry.
- exhibits pulse rate that is regular and normal for their age.
- states that pain is lessened.

Goal: The child's fluid intake will be adequate for their age.
Expected Outcomes: The child's

- skin turgor is good.
- mucous membranes are moist.
- hourly urinary output is at least 20 to 30 mL.
- parenteral fluids are maintained until oral fluid intake is adequate.

Goal: Family caregivers will verbalize an understanding of postdischarge care.
Expected Outcomes: Family caregivers

- give appropriate responses when questioned about care at home.
- verbalize signs and symptoms of complications and ask appropriate questions for clarification.

CROUP SYNDROMES

Croup is not a disease, but a group of disorders typically involving a barking cough, hoarseness, and inspiratory **stridor** (shrill, harsh respiratory sound). The disorders are named for the respiratory structures involved. Acute laryngotracheobronchitis, for instance, affects the larynx, trachea, and major bronchi.

SPASMODIC LARYNGITIS

Spasmodic laryngitis occurs in children between ages 1 and 3 years. The cause is undetermined; it may be of infectious or allergic origin, but certain children seem to develop severe laryngospasm with little, if any, apparent cause.

Clinical Manifestations and Diagnosis

The attack may be preceded by **coryza** (runny nose) and hoarseness or by no apparent signs of respiratory irregularity during the evening. The child awakens after a few hours of sleep with a bark-like cough, increasing respiratory difficulty, and stridor. The child becomes anxious, restless, and markedly hoarse. A low-grade fever and mild upper respiratory infection may be present.

This condition is not serious but is frightening both to the child and to the family. The episode subsides after a few hours; little evidence remains the next day when an anxious caregiver takes the child to the physician. Attacks frequently occur 2 or 3 nights in succession.

Treatment and Nursing Care

Humidified air is helpful in reducing laryngospasm. Humidifiers may be used in the child's bedroom to provide high humidity. Cool humidifiers are recommended, but vaporizers also may be used. If a vaporizer is used, caution must be taken to place it out of the child's reach to protect the child from being burned. Cool-mist humidifiers provide safe humidity. Humidifiers and vaporizers must be cleaned regularly to prevent the growth of undesirable organisms. Sometimes the spasm is relieved by exposure to cold air—when, for instance, the child is taken out into the night to go to the emergency department or to see the care provider. The physician may prescribe an **emetic** (an agent that causes vomiting) in a dosage less than that needed to produce vomiting; this usually gives relief by helping to reduce spasms of the larynx.

Good news.
Although frightening to the child and family, spasmodic laryngitis is not serious and can often be lessened quickly by taking the child into the bathroom, shutting the door, and turning on the hot water tap. This fills the room with steam or humidified air and relieves the child's symptoms.

It is important to explain which symptoms can be treated at home (hoarseness, croupy cough, and inspiratory

stridor) and which symptoms might indicate a more serious condition in which the child needs to be seen by
the care provider (continuous stridor, use of accessory
muscles, labored breathing, lower-rib retractions, restlessness, pallor, and rapid respirations). The family
must be aware that recurrence of these conditions may
occur.

ACUTE LARYNGOTRACHEOBRONCHITIS

Laryngeal infections are common in small children, and
they often involve tracheobronchial areas as well. Acute
laryngotracheobronchitis (bacterial tracheitis or laryngotracheobronchitis) may progress rapidly and become a
serious problem within a matter of hours. The toddler is
the most frequently affected age group. This condition is
usually of viral origin, but bacterial invasion, usually
staphylococcal, follows the original infection. It generally occurs after an upper respiratory infection with
fairly mild rhinitis and pharyngitis.

Clinical Manifestations and Diagnosis

The child develops hoarseness and a barking cough with
a fever that may reach 104°F to 105°F (40°C–40.6°C).
As the disease progresses, marked laryngeal edema occurs, and the child's breathing becomes difficult, the
pulse is rapid, and cyanosis may appear. Heart failure
and acute respiratory embarrassment can result.

Treatment and Nursing Care

The major goal of treatment for acute laryngotracheobronchitis is to maintain an airway and adequate air exchange. Antimicrobial therapy is ordered. The child is
placed in a supersaturated atmosphere, such as a
croupette or some other kind of mist tent, that also can
include the administration of oxygen. To achieve bronchodilation, racemic or nebulized epinephrine may be
administered, usually by a respiratory therapist. Nebulization is usually administered every 3 or 4 hours. Nebulization often produces rapid relief because it causes
vasoconstriction. However, the child requires careful observation for the reappearance of symptoms.

If necessary, intubation with a nasotracheal tube may
be performed for a child with severe distress unrelieved
by other measures. Tracheostomies, once performed frequently, are rarely performed today; intubation is preferred. Antibiotics are administered parenterally initially
and continued after the temperature has normalized.

Close and careful observation of the child is important. Observation includes checking the pulse, respirations, and color; listening for hoarseness and stridor; and
noting any restlessness that may indicate an impending
respiratory crisis. Pulse oximetry is used to determine the
degree of hypoxia.

EPIGLOTTITIS

Epiglottitis is acute inflammation of the epiglottis (the
cartilaginous flap that protects the opening of the

■ **Figure 36-3** The "tripod" position of the child with
epiglottitis.

larynx). Commonly caused by Haemophilus influenzae
type B, epiglottitis most often affects children ages 2 to
7 years. The epiglottis becomes inflamed and swollen
with edema. The edema decreases the ability of the
epiglottis to move freely, which results in blockage of the
airway and creates an emergency.

Clinical Manifestations and Diagnosis

The child may have been well or may have had a mild
upper respiratory infection before the development of a
sore throat, dysphagia (difficulty swallowing), and a
high fever of 102.2°F to 104°F (39°C–40°C). The dysphagia may cause drooling. A tongue blade should never
be used to initiate a gag reflex because complete obstruction may occur. The child is very anxious and
prefers to breathe by sitting up and leaning forward with
the mouth open and the tongue out. This is called the
"tripod" position (Fig. 36-3). Immediate emergency attention is necessary.

Treatment and Nursing Care

The child may need endotracheal intubation or a tracheostomy if the epiglottis is so swollen that intubation
cannot be performed. Moist air is necessary to help reduce the inflammation of the epiglottis. Pulse oximetry is
required to monitor oxygen requirements. Antibiotics
are administered intravenously. After 24 to 48 hours of
antibiotic therapy, the child may be extubated. Antibiotic therapy usually is continued for 10 days. This condition is not common, and it is extremely frightening for
the child and the family.

ACUTE BRONCHIOLITIS/RESPIRATORY SYNCYTIAL VIRUS INFECTION

Acute bronchiolitis (acute interstitial pneumonia) is most common during the first 6 months of life and is rarely seen after the age of 2 years. Most cases occur in infants who have been in contact with older children or adults with upper respiratory viral infections. It usually occurs in the winter and early spring.

Acute bronchiolitis is caused by a viral infection. The causative agent in more than 50% of cases has been shown to be RSV. Other viruses associated with the disease are parainfluenza virus, adenoviruses, and other viruses not always identified.

The bronchi and bronchioles become plugged with thick, viscid mucus, causing air to be trapped in the lungs. The child can breathe air in but has difficulty expelling it. This hinders the exchange of gases and cyanosis appears.

Clinical Manifestations

The onset of dyspnea is abrupt, sometimes preceded by a cough or nasal discharge. Manifestations include a dry and persistent cough, extremely shallow respirations, air hunger, and often marked cyanosis. Suprasternal and subcostal retractions are present. The chest becomes barrel-shaped from the trapped air. Respirations are 60 to 80 breaths per minute.

Fever is not extreme, seldom higher than 101°F to 102°F (38.3°C–38.9°C). Dehydration may become a serious factor if competent care is not given. The infant appears apprehensive, irritable, and restless.

Diagnosis

Diagnosis is made from clinical findings and can be confirmed by laboratory testing (enzyme-linked immunosorbent assay [ELISA]) of the mucus obtained by direct nasal aspiration or nasopharyngeal washing.

Treatment and Nursing Care

The child is usually hospitalized and treated with high humidity by mist tent (see Chapter 30, Fig. 30-6), rest, and increased fluids. Oxygen may be administered in addition to the mist tent. Monitoring of oxygenation may be done by means of capillary blood gases or pulse oximetry. Antibiotics are not prescribed because the causative organism is a virus. Intravenous fluids often are administered to ensure an adequate intake and to permit the infant to rest. The hospitalized child is placed on contact transmission precautions to prevent the spread of infection.

Ribavirin (Virazole) is an antiviral drug that may be used to treat certain children with RSV. It is administered as an inhalant by hood, mask, or tent. The American Academy of Pediatrics states that the use of ribavirin must be limited to children at high risk for severe or complicated RSV such as children with chronic lung disease, premature infants, transplant recipients, and children receiving chemotherapy. Ribavirin is classified as a category X drug, signifying a high risk for **teratogenicity** (causing damage to a fetus). Health care personnel and others may inhale the mist that escapes into the room, so care must be taken when the drug is administered.

Warning.
Women who might be pregnant should stay out of the room where ribavirin is being administered.

For children who are at high risk for getting RSV and having serious complications, there are some new drugs available that may be given to prevent RSV. These drugs are administered only in specific cases and are given intravenously or intramuscularly.

Test Yourself

✔ What is the most common complication after a tonsillectomy? What two time periods is bleeding a concern after a tonsillectomy? Explain the reasons these time periods are a concern for bleeding.

✔ What is a fast and effective way to reduce laryngospasm for the child with croup?

✔ What is a complication often seen in the infant with a respiratory infection?

✔ What is the causative agent in many cases of bronchiolitis?

ASTHMA

Asthma is a spasm of the bronchial tubes caused by hypersensitivity of the airways in the bronchial system and inflammation that leads to mucosal edema and mucous hypersecretion. Asthma is also sometimes referred to as reactive airway disease. This reversible obstructive airway disease affects millions of people in the United States, including 5% to 10% of all children in the United States.

Asthma attacks are often triggered by a hypersensitive response to allergens. In young children, asthma may be a response to certain foods. Asthma is often triggered by exercise, exposure to cold weather, irritants such as wood-burning stoves, cigarette smoke, dust, and pet dander and foods such as chocolate, milk, eggs, nuts, and grains. Infections, such as bronchitis and upper respiratory infection, can provoke asthma attacks. In children with asthmatic tendencies, emotional stress or anxiety can trigger an attack. Some children with asthma may have no evidence of an immunologic cause for the symptoms.

Asthma can be either intermittent, with extended periods when the child has no symptoms and does not need

Normal airway

Airway with inflammation

Airway with inflammation,
bronchospasm,
and mucus production

■ **Figure 36-4** Note airway edema, mucus production, and bronchospasm occurring with asthma.

medication, or chronic, with the need for frequent or continuous therapy. Chronic asthma affects the child's school performance and general activities and may contribute to poor self-confidence and dependency. Asthma accounts for one third of the missed school days in the United States (Eggleston, 2006).

Spasms of the smooth muscles cause the lumina of the bronchi and bronchioles to narrow. Edema of the mucous membranes lining these bronchial branches and increased production of thick mucus within them combine with the spasm to cause respiratory obstruction (Fig. 36-4).

Clinical Manifestations

The onset of an attack can be very abrupt or can progress over several days, as evidenced by a dry hacking cough, **wheezing** (the sound of expired air being pushed through obstructed bronchioles), and difficulty breathing. Asthma attacks often occur at night and awaken the child from sleep. The child must sit up and is totally preoccupied with efforts to breathe. Attacks might last for only a short time, or might continue for several days. Thick, tenacious mucus might be coughed up or vomited after a coughing episode. In some asthmatic patients, coughing is the major symptom, and wheezing occurs rarely if at all. Many children no longer have symptoms after puberty, but this is not predictable. Other allergies may develop in adulthood.

Diagnosis

The history and physical examination are of primary importance in diagnosing asthma. When observing the child's breathing, dyspnea and labored breathing may be noted, especially on expiration. When listening to the child's lung sounds (auscultation), the examiner hears wheezing, which is often generalized over all lung fields. Mucus production may be profuse. Pulmonary function tests are valuable diagnostic tools and indicate the amount of obstruction in the bronchial airways, especially in the smallest airways of the lungs. A definitive

diagnosis of asthma is made when the obstruction in the airways is reversed with bronchodilators.

Treatment

Children and their families must be taught to recognize the symptoms that lead to an acute attack so they can be treated as early as possible. These symptoms include respiratory retractions and wheezing and an increased amount of coughing at night, in the early morning, or with activity. Use of a peak flow meter is an objective way to measure airway obstruction, and children as young as 4 or 5 years of age can be taught to use one (see Family Teaching Tips: How to Use a Peak Flow Meter and Fig. 36-5). A peak flow diary should be maintained and also can include symptoms, exacerbations, actions taken, and outcomes. Families must make every effort to eliminate any possible allergens from the home.

Did you know?

Prevention is the most important aspect in the treatment of asthma.

■ **Figure 36-5** The child with asthma uses a peak flow meter and keeps track of readings on a daily basis.

Family Teaching Tips

HOW TO USE A PEAK FLOW METER

INTRODUCTION

Your child cannot feel early changes in the airway. By the time the child feels tightness in the chest or starts to wheeze, he or she is already far into an asthma episode. The most reliable early sign of an asthma episode is a drop in the child's peak expiratory flow rate, or the ability to breathe out quickly, which can be measured by a peak flow meter. Almost every asthmatic child over the age of 4 years can and should learn to use a peak flow meter (Figs. A and B.)

A

B

STEPS TO ACCURATE MEASUREMENTS

1. Remove gum or food from the mouth.
2. Move the pointer on the meter to zero.
3. Stand up and hold the meter horizontally with fingers away from the vent holes and marker.
4. With mouth wide open, slowly breathe in as much air as possible.
5. Put the mouthpiece on the tongue and place lips around it.
6. Blow out as hard and fast as you can. Give a short, sharp blast, not a slow blow. The meter measures the fastest puff, not the longest.
7. Repeat steps 1–6 three times. Wait at least 10 seconds between puffs. Move the pointer to zero after each puff.
8. Record the best reading.

GUIDELINES FOR TREATMENT

Each child has a unique pattern of asthma episodes. Most episodes begin gradually, and a drop in peak flow can alert you to start medications before the actual symptoms appear. This early treatment can prevent a flare-up from getting out of hand. One way to look at peak flow scores is to match the scores with three colors:

Green	Yellow	Red
80%–100% personal best	50%–80% personal best	Below 50% personal best
No symptoms	Mild to moderate symptoms	Serious distress
Full breathing reserve	Diminished reserve	Pulmonary function is significantly impaired
Mild trigger may not cause symptoms	A minor trigger produces noticeable symptoms	Any trigger may lead to severe distress
Continue current management	Augment present treatment regimen	Contact care provider

Remember, treatment should be adjusted to fit the individual's needs. Your care provider will develop a home management plan with you. When in doubt, consult your care provider.

The goals of asthma treatment include preventing symptoms, maintaining near-normal lung function and activity levels, preventing recurring exacerbations and hospitalizations, and providing the best medication treatment with the fewest adverse effects. Depending on the frequency and severity of symptoms and exacerbations, a stepwise approach to the treatment of asthma is used to manage the disease. The steps are used to determine combinations of medications to be used (Table 36-1).

Table 36-1 ▮ STEPWISE APPROACH TO TREATING ASTHMA

Steps	Symptoms
Step One Mild intermittent	Symptoms occur <2 times a week No symptoms between exacerbations Exacerbations brief Nighttime symptoms <2 times a month
Step Two Mild persistent	Symptoms occur >2 times a week but <1 time a day Exacerbations may affect activity Nighttime symptoms >2 times a month
Step Three Moderate persistent	Daily symptoms Daily use of inhaled short-acting beta-2 agonist Exacerbations affect activity Exacerbations >2 times a week, may last days Nighttime symptoms >1 time a week
Step Four Severe persistent	Continual symptoms Limited physical activity Frequent exacerbations Frequent nighttime symptoms

Medications used to treat asthma are divided into two categories: quick-relief medications for immediate treatment of symptoms and exacerbations and long-term control medications to achieve and maintain control of the symptoms. The classifications of drugs used to treat asthma include bronchodilators (sympathomimetics and xanthine derivatives) and other antiasthmatic drugs (corticosteroids, leukotriene inhibitors, and mast cell stabilizers). Table 36-2 lists some of the medications used to treat asthma. Many of these drugs can be given either by a **nebulizer** (tube attached to a wall unit or cylinder that delivers moist air via a face mask) or a **metered-dose inhaler** ([MDI]; a hand-held plastic device that delivers a premeasured dose). The MDI may have a spacer unit attached that makes it easier for the young child to use (Fig. 36-6).

Bronchodilators

Bronchodilators are used for quick relief of acute exacerbations of asthma symptoms. They are short acting and available in pill, liquid, or inhalant form. These drugs are administered every 6 to 8 hours or every 4 to 6 hours by inhalation if breathing difficulty continues. In severe attacks, epinephrine by subcutaneous injection often affords quick relief of symptoms. Some bronchodilators, such as salmeterol (Serevent), are used in long-term control.

Theophylline preparations have long been used in the treatment of asthma. The drug is available in short-acting and long-acting forms. The short-acting forms are given about every 6 hours. Because they enter the bloodstream quickly, they are most effective when used only as needed for intermittent episodes of asthma. Long-acting preparations of theophylline are given every 8 to 12 hours. Some of these preparations come in sustained-release forms. These are helpful in patients who continually need medication because these drugs sustain more consistent theophylline levels in the blood than do short-acting forms. Patients hospitalized for status asthmaticus may receive theophylline intravenously.

Corticosteroids

Corticosteroids are anti-inflammatory drugs used to control severe or chronic cases of asthma. Steroids may be given in inhaled form to decrease the systemic effects that accompany oral steroid administration.

Leukotriene Inhibitors

Leukotriene inhibitors are given by mouth along with other asthma medications for long-term control and prevention of mild, persistent asthma. Leukotrienes are bronchoconstrictive substances that are released in the body during the inflammatory process. These drugs inhibit leukotriene production, which helps with bronchodilation and decreases airway edema.

Mast Cell Stabilizers

Mast cell stabilizers help to stabilize the cell membrane by preventing mast cells from releasing the chemical mediators that cause bronchospasm and mucous membrane inflammation. They are used to help decrease wheezing and exercise-induced asthma attacks. These are nonsteroidal anti-inflammatory drugs and have relatively few side effects. A bronchodilator often is given to open up the airways just before the mast cell stabilizer is used. Children dislike the taste of the medication, but receiving sips of water after the administration minimizes the distaste.

Chest Physiotherapy

Because asthma has multiple causes, treatment and continued management of the disease require more than medication. Chest physiotherapy includes breathing exercises, physical training, and inhalation therapy. Studies have shown that breathing exercises to improve respiratory function and to control asthma

Check out this tip.

For the asthmatic child, if exercises can be taught as part of play activities, children are more likely to find them fun and to practice them more often.

Table 36-2 ▪ MEDICATIONS USED IN THE TREATMENT OF ASTHMA

Generic Name	Trade Name	Dose Form	Uses	Adverse Reactions/Side Effects
Bronchodilators				
Sympathomimetics (Beta-2-receptor Agonists)				
albuterol sulfate	Proventil, Ventolin	MDI PO Nebulizer	Quick relief	Restlessness, anxiety, fear, palpitations, insomnia, tremors
metaproterenol hydrochloride	Alupent, Metaprel	MDI PO Nebulizer	Quick relief Short-term control	Tremors, anxiety, insomnia, dizziness, tachycardia
terbutaline sulfate	Brethine	MDI PO	MDI—Quick relief PO—Long-term control	Tremors, anxiety, insomnia, dizziness, tachycardia
salmeterol	Serevent	MDI	Long-term control	Headache, tremors, tachycardia
Xanthine Derivative				
Theophylline	Slo-Phyllin, Elixophyllin Theo-Dur	PO Timed-release	Long-term control	Nausea, vomiting, headache, nervousness, irritability, insomnia
Antiasthma Drugs				
Corticosteroids				
beclomethasone	Beclovent	MDI	Long-term control	Throat irritation, cough, nausea, dizziness
triamcinolone	Azamacort	MDI	Long-term control	Throat irritation, cough, nausea, dizziness
Leukotriene Inhibitors				
Montelukast	Singulair	PO	Long-term control	Headache, nausea, abdominal pain, diarrhea
Mast Cell Stabilizers				
Cromolyn	Intal	Intranasal nebulizer	Long-term control	Nasal irritation, unpleasant taste, headache, nausea, dry throat

MDI = metered-dose inhaler

attacks can be an important adjunct to using medications for treatment. These exercises teach children how to help control their own symptoms and thereby build self-confidence, which is sometimes lacking in asthmatic children.

Nursing Process for the Child With Asthma
Assessment

Obtain information from the caregiver about the asthma history, the medications the child takes, and the medications

A

B

▪ Figure 36-6 **(A)** Girl using a nebulizer with a mask. **(B)** Boy using a metered-dose inhaler with spacer.

taken within the last 24 hours. Ask whether the child has vomited because vomiting would prevent absorption of oral medications. Ask about any history of respiratory infections; possible allergens in the household such as pets; type of furniture and toys; if there is a damp basement (which could contain mold spores); and a history of breathing problems after exercise.

In the physical exam, include vital signs, observation for diaphoresis and cyanosis, position, type of breathing, alertness, chest movement, intercostal retractions, and breath sounds. Note any wheezing.

If the child is old enough and alert enough to cooperate, involve him or her in gathering the history, and encourage the child to add information. Ask questions that can be answered "yes" or "no" to minimize tiring the distressed child.

Selected Nursing Diagnoses

- Ineffective Airway Clearance related to bronchospasm and increased pulmonary secretions
- Risk for Deficient Fluid Volume related to water loss from tachypnea and diaphoresis and reduced oral intake
- Fatigue related to dyspnea
- Anxiety related to sudden attacks of breathlessness
- Deficient Knowledge of the caregiver related to disease process, treatment, home care, and control of disease

Outcome Identification and Planning

The initial major goals for the child include maintaining a clear airway and an adequate fluid intake and relieving fatigue and anxiety. The family's goals include learning how to manage the child's life with asthma. Base the nursing plan of care on these goals.

Implementation

Monitoring Respiratory Function

Continuously monitor the child while he or she is in acute distress from an asthma attack using pulse oximetry and an electronic monitor. If this equipment is unavailable, take the child's respirations every 15 minutes during an acute attack and every 1 or 2 hours after the crisis is over. Listening to lung sounds should be done to further monitor the respiratory function. Observe for nasal flaring and chest retractions; observe the skin for color and diaphoresis.

Elevate the child's head. An older child may be more comfortable resting forward on a pillow placed on an over-bed table. Monitor the child for response to medications and their side effects such as restlessness, gastrointestinal upset, and seizures. Use humidified oxygen and suction as needed during periods of acute distress.

Monitoring and Improving Fluid Intake

During an acute attack, the child may lose a great quantity of fluid through the respiratory tract and may have a poor oral intake because of coughing and vomiting. Theophylline administration also has a diuretic effect, which compounds the problem. Monitor intake and output. Encourage oral fluids that the child likes. Intravenous (IV) fluids are administered as ordered. IV fluid intake is monitored, and all precautions for parenteral administration are followed. Note the skin turgor and observe the mucous membranes at least every 8 hours. Weigh the child daily to help determine fluid losses.

Promoting Energy Conservation

The child might become extremely tired from the exertion of trying to breathe. Activities and patient care should be spaced to provide maximum periods of uninterrupted rest. Provide quiet activities when the child needs diversion. Keep visitors to a minimum, and maintain a quiet environment.

Reducing Child and Parent Anxiety

The sudden onset of an asthma attack can be frightening to the child and the family caregivers. Respond quickly when the child has an attack. Reassure the child and the family during an episode of dyspnea.

 A Personal Glimpse

The first time I put Bobbie in the hospital it was very scary. I knew the nurses, but I was still afraid for him. I felt like someone was punishing me. I couldn't leave him for a minute. I was afraid he wouldn't be alive when I came back. I was also afraid he would be frightened. He was so small, he needed me to protect him, but I couldn't help him. We were in the hospital every couple of weeks. He would get better then have another attack. It got to the point where I would call the doctor and say that Bobbie was having another attack and they would just send us to admitting. After a few times, I got used to caring for him in the hospital. The nurses taught me how to keep his tent humidified and I could just take care of it myself. Finally I was able to go back to work during the day and care for him on my breaks and time off. It was very difficult each and every time, but we adjusted to hospital life. Although I was afraid for him, I knew he was a fighter and I had to be too. I feel this experience made him a stronger person. He is now 8 years old and has had no severe attacks since he was about 2 years old. He has had a few mild attacks, but it doesn't affect him or myself.

Tracee

Learning Opportunity: Give specific examples of what the nurse could do to support this mother and to help decrease the fear she had when her child was hospitalized.

Teach the child and the caregiver the symptoms of an impending attack and the immediate response needed to decrease the threat of an attack. This knowledge will help them to cope with impending attacks

Nursing judgment is in order.
The asthmatic child's fear of attacks can be increased by the caregiver's behavior.

and plan how to handle the attacks. When they are prepared with information, the child and family may be less fearful. Give the child examples of sports figures, entertainers, actors and actresses, and political leaders who have or have had asthma, for example, Olympic track and field athlete Jackie Joyner Kersee and President John F. Kennedy. Others include Jerome Bettis, professional football player; Amy Van Dyken, American swimming champion; Nancy Hogshead, Olympic gold medalist in swimming; Dennis Rodman, NBA basketball player; and Diane Keaton, actress.

Providing Family Teaching

Child and family caregiver teaching is of primary importance in the care of asthmatic children. Family caregivers might overprotect the child because of the fear that an attack will occur when the child is with a babysitter, at school, or anywhere away from the caregiver. Asthma attacks can be prevented or decreased by prompt and adequate intervention. Teach the caregiver and child, within the scope of the child's ability to understand, about the disease process, recognition of symptoms of an impending attack, environmental control, infection avoidance, exercise, drug therapy, and chest physiotherapy.

Teach the caregiver and the child how to use metered-dose inhaler medications and have them demonstrate correct usage (see Family Teaching Tips: How to Use a Metered-Dose Inhaler). Give instructions on home use of a peak flow meter. Urge them to maintain a diary to record the peak flow as well as asthma symptoms, onset of attacks, action taken, and results. Include instructions about administering premedication before the child is exposed to situations in which an attack may occur.

Inform caregivers of allergens that may be in the child's environment and encourage them to eliminate or control the allergens as needed. Stress the importance of quick response when the child has a respiratory infection. Give instructions for exercise and chest physiotherapy.

Stress to the caregivers the importance of informing the child's classroom teacher, physical education teacher, school nurse, babysitter, and others who are responsible for the child about the child's condition. With a physician's order, including directions for use, the child should

---

Family Teaching Tips

HOW TO USE A METERED-DOSE INHALER

- When ready to use, shake the inhaler well with the cap still on. The child should stand, if possible.
- Remove the cap.
- Hold the inhaler with the mouthpiece down, facing the child.
- Be sure the child's mouth is empty.
- Hold the mouthpiece about 1 to 1.5 in from the lips.*
- Breathe out normally. Open mouth wide and begin to breathe in.
- Press top of medication canister firmly while inhaling deeply. Hold breath as long as possible (at least 10 seconds—teach child to count slowly to 10).
- Breathe out *slowly* through nose or pursed lips.
- Relax 2 to 5 minutes repeat as directed by physician.

*The mouthpiece can also be put between the lips, with the lips forming an airtight seal, or a spacer can be attached to the inhaler and the mouthpiece held between the lips.

---

be permitted to bring medications to school and keep them so they can be used when needed.

Provide information on support groups available in the area. The American Lung Association has many materials available to families and can provide information about support groups, camps, and workshops (Web site: www. lungusa.org). The Asthma and Allergy Foundation of America (Web site: www.aafa.org) and the National Heart, Lung, and Blood Institute (Web site: www.nhlbi.nih.gov) are also resources.

Evaluation: Goals and Expected Outcomes

Goal: The child's airway will remain open.
Expected Outcomes: The child's

- breath sounds are clear with no wheezing, retractions, or nasal flaring.
- skin color is good.

Goal: The child's fluid intake will be adequate.
Expected Outcomes: The child's

- hourly urine output is 30 to 40 mL.
- mucous membranes are moist.
- skin turgor is good.
- weight remains stable.

Goal: The child will have increased energy levels.
Expected Outcomes: The child

- participates in age-appropriate activities.
- rests between activities.

Goal: The child's and caregivers' anxiety and fear related to impending attacks will be minimized.

Expected Outcomes: The child and the caregiver

- list symptoms of an impending attack.
- describe appropriate responses.
- display confidence in their ability to handle an attack.

Goal: The child and the caregiver will gain knowledge of how to live with asthma.

Expected Outcomes: The child and the caregiver

- verbalize an understanding of the disease process, treatment, and control.
- interact with health care personnel and ask and answer relevant questions.
- obtain information and makes contact with support groups.

Test Yourself

✔ What is the most important aspect in the treatment of asthma?

✔ What are the two categories of medications used in the treatment of asthma?

✔ What are the routes of administration for many of the medications used to treat asthma?

✔ Why is chest physiotherapy used in the treatment of asthma?

BACTERIAL PNEUMONIA

Pneumococcal pneumonia is the most common form of bacterial pneumonia in infants and children. Its incidence has decreased during the last several years. This disease occurs mainly during the late winter and early spring, principally in children younger than 4 years of age.

In the infant, pneumococcal pneumonia is generally of the bronchial type. In older children, pneumococcal pneumonia is generally of the lobar type. It is usually secondary to an upper respiratory viral infection. The most common finding in infants is a patchy infiltration of one or several lobes of the lung. Pleural effusion is often present. In the older child, the pneumonia may localize in a single lobe. Immunization with the pneumococcal vaccine (PCV) is currently recommended, beginning at 2 months of age.

H. influenzae pneumonia also occurs in infants and young children. Its clinical manifestations are similar to those of pneumococcal pneumonia, but its onset is more insidious, its clinical course is longer and less acute, and it is usually seen in the lobe of the lung. Complications in the infant are common—usually bacteremia, pericarditis, and empyema (pus in the lungs). The treatment is the same. Immunization with *H. influenzae* type B

conjugate vaccine (HIB) is currently recommended, beginning at 2 months of age.

Clinical Manifestations

The onset of the pneumonic process is usually abrupt, following a mild upper respiratory illness. Temperature increases rapidly to 103°F to 105°F (39.4°C–40.6°C). Respiratory distress is marked with obvious air hunger, flaring of the nostrils, **circumoral** (around the mouth) cyanosis, and chest retractions. Tachycardia and tachypnea are present, with a pulse rate frequently as high as 140 to 180 beats per minute and respirations as high as 80 breaths per minute.

Generalized convulsions may occur during the period of high fever. Cough may not be noticeable at the onset but may appear later. Abdominal distention caused by swallowed air or paralytic ileus commonly occurs.

Diagnosis

Diagnosis is based on clinical symptoms, chest radiograph, and culture of the organism from secretions. The white blood cell count may be elevated. The antistreptolysin titer (ASO titer) is usually elevated in children with staphylococcal pneumonia.

Treatment

The use of anti-infectives early in the disease gives a prompt and favorable response. Penicillin or ampicillin has proved to be the most effective treatment and is generally used unless the child has a penicillin allergy. Cephalosporin anti-infectives are also used. Oxygen started early in the disease process is important. In some instances, a croupette or mist tent is used. Some consider the use of mist tents without constant observation unsafe. Children have become cyanotic in mist tents, with subsequent arrest, because of the difficulty of seeing the child; therefore, a mask or hood is thought to be the better choice. Intravenous fluids are often necessary to supply the needed amount of fluids. Prognosis for recovery is excellent.

NURSING PROCESS FOR THE CHILD WITH PNEUMONIA

Assessment

Conduct a thorough interview with the caregiver. In addition to standard information, include specific data such as when the symptoms were first noticed, the course of the fever thus far, a description of respiratory difficulties, and the character of any cough. Collect data regarding how well the child has been taking nourishment and fluids. Ask about nausea, vomiting, urinary and bowel output, and history of exposure to other family members with respiratory infections.

Conduct a physical exam, including measurement of temperature, apical pulse, respirations (rate, respiratory effort, retractions [costal, intercostal, sternal, suprasternal, substernal], and flaring of nares) (see Chapter 28). Also note breath and lung sounds (crackles, wheezing), cough (dry, productive, hacking), irritability, restlessness, confusion, skin color (pallor, cyanosis), circumoral (around the mouth) cyanosis, cyanotic nail beds, skin turgor, anterior fontanelle (depressed or bulging), nasal passage congestion (color, consistency), mucous membranes (mouth dry, lips dry or cracked), and eyes (bright, glassy, sunken, moist, crusted). If the child is old enough to communicate verbally, ask questions to determine how the child feels.

Selected Nursing Diagnoses

- Ineffective Airway Clearance related to obstruction associated with edema, mucous secretions, nasal and chest congestion
- Impaired Gas Exchange related to inflammatory process
- Risk for Deficient Fluid Volume related to respiratory fluid loss, fever, and difficulty swallowing
- Hyperthermia related to infection process
- Risk for Further Infection related to location and anatomical structure of the eustachian tubes
- Activity Intolerance related to inadequate gas exchange
- Anxiety related to dyspnea, invasive procedures, and separation from caregiver
- Compromised Family Coping related to child's respiratory symptoms and child's illness
- Deficient Knowledge of the caregiver related to child's condition and home care

Outcome Identification and Planning

The major goals for the child with pneumonia are maintaining respiratory function, preventing fluid deficit, maintaining body temperature, preventing otitis media, conserving energy, and relieving anxiety. Goals for the family include relieving anxiety and improving caregiver knowledge.

The need for immediate intubation is always a possibility; thus, vigilance is essential. The child's energy must be conserved to reduce oxygen requirements. The child may need to be placed on infection control precautions, according to the policy of the health care facility, to prevent nosocomial spread of infection. Many children with a respiratory condition need to be placed in a croupette or mist tent, making additional nursing interventions necessary. If IV fluids are ordered, interventions that promote tissue and skin integrity are needed. To ensure that the child does not interfere with the IV infusion site, it may be necessary to prepare restraints. Intravenous administration and the use of restraints are discussed in Chapter 30 (see Nursing Care Plan 36-1: The Child With Pneumonia).

Implementation

Maintaining Airway Clearance

A humidified atmosphere is provided with an ice-cooled mist tent or cool vaporizer. The moisturized air helps thin the mucus in the respiratory tract to ease respirations. Suction or clear secretions as needed to keep the airway open. Position the child to provide maximum ventilation, and change positions at least every 2 hours. Use pillows and padding to maintain the child's position. Observe frequently for slumping, which causes crowding of the diaphragm. Avoid use of constricting clothes and bedding. Stuffed toys are not recommended in mist tents because they become saturated and provide an environment in which organisms flourish.

Monitoring Respiratory Function

Be continuously alert for warning signs of airway obstruction. Monitor the child at least every hour; uncover the child's chest and observe the child's breathing efforts. Observe for tachypnea (rapid respirations), and note the amount of chest movement, shallow breathing, and retractions. Listen with a stethoscope for breath sounds, particularly noting the amount of stridor, which indicates difficult breathing. Oxygen saturation levels are monitored using oximetry. Increasing hoarseness should be reported. In addition, observe for pallor, listlessness, circumoral cyanosis, cyanotic nail beds, and restlessness; these are indications of impaired oxygenation and should be reported at once. Cool, high humidity provides relief. Oxygen may be administered by hood, mist tent, or nasal cannula if the practitioner orders.

Promoting Adequate Fluid Intake

It is important to clear the nasal passages immediately before feeding. For the infant, use a bulb syringe. Administer normal saline nose drops to thin secretions about 10 to 15 minutes before feedings and at bedtime. Feed the child slowly, allowing frequent stops with suctioning during feeding, as needed. Avoid overtiring the infant or child during feeding.

Adequate hydration helps reduce thick mucus. Maintaining adequate fluid intake may be a problem for children of any age because the child may be too ill to want to eat. Offer warm, clear fluids to encourage oral intake. Between meals, offer juices and water appropriate for the infant or child's age. For infants, use a relatively small-holed nipple so he or she does not choke, but does not work too hard. Maintain accurate intake and output measurements. Observe carefully for aspiration, especially in severe respiratory distress. The child may need to be kept NPO to prevent this threat. Parenteral fluids may be administered to replace those lost through respiratory loss, fever, and anorexia. Follow all safety measures for administration of parenteral fluids. Observe patency, placement, site integrity, and flow rate, at least hourly. Fluid needs are determined by the amount

Nursing Care Plan 36-1

THE CHILD WITH PNEUMONIA

CASE SCENARIO:
CW, a 6-month-old child with pneumonia, has been brought to the hospital from the doctor's office by his mother. He has a copious amount of thick nasal discharge and has rapid, shallow respirations with substernal and intercostal retractions. His temperature is 101.5°F (39.1°C). His young mother appears very anxious.

NURSING DIAGNOSIS
Ineffective Airway Clearance related to infectious process

GOAL: The child's respiratory function will improve and airway will be patent.

EXPECTED OUTCOMES:
* The child no longer uses respiratory accessory muscles to aid in breathing.
* The child's breath sounds are clear and respirations are regular.
* Mucous secretions become thin and scant; nasal passages are clear.

Nursing Interventions	*Rationale*
Provide moist atmosphere by placing him in ice-cooled mist tent.	Moisture helps liquefy and thin secretions for easier respirations.
Keep nasal passages clear, using bulb syringe.	Open passages increase air flow.
Monitor respiratory function by observing for retractions, respiratory rate, and listening to breath sounds at least every 4 hours. Monitor more frequently if tachypnea or deep retractions are noted.	Changes in the child's breathing may be early indicators of respiratory distress.
Monitor child's bedding and clothing every 4 hours.	Clothing and bedding can become very wet from mist. Dry clothing and bedding help to prevent chilling.

NURSING DIAGNOSIS
Imbalanced Nutrition: Less Than Body Requirements related to inability to suck, drink, or swallow because of congested nasal passages or fatigue from difficulty breathing

GOAL: The child will have adequate food and fluid intake to maintain normal growth and development.

EXPECTED OUTCOMES:
* The child has an adequate caloric intake as evidenced by appropriate weight gain of 1 oz or more a day.
* The child is able to suck, drink, and swallow easily without tiring.
* Skin turgor returns to normal.

Nursing Interventions	*Rationale*
Clear nasal passages immediately before feeding. Teach family caregiver to use bulb syringe.	Infants are obligatory nasal breathers. Clearing eases child's breathing to permit adequate feeding. Family caregiver can use this technique at home, as needed.
Administer normal saline nose drops before feedings and at bedtime.	Normal saline nose drops help thin mucous secretions.
Weigh infant daily in morning before first feeding.	Child will maintain appropriate weight gain.

NURSING DIAGNOSIS
Risk for Further Infection (otitis media) related to current respiratory infection and the size and location of child's eustachian tube

GOAL: The child will remain free from further infection and complications of otitis media.

EXPECTED OUTCOMES:
* The child shows no signs of ear pain, such as irritability, shaking head, pulling on ears.

Nursing Care Plan 36-1 (continued)

THE CHILD WITH PNEUMONIA

Nursing Interventions	*Rationale*
Change child's position, turning from side to side every hour.	Turning child prevents mucus from pooling in the eustachian tubes.
Feed child in upright position.	Upright position improves drainage and helps open nasal passages.
Observe for irritability, shaking of head, or pulling at ears.	Early recognition of signs of otitis media promotes early diagnosis and treatment.

NURSING DIAGNOSIS
Compromised Family Coping related to child's illness

GOAL: The caregiver's anxiety will be reduced.

EXPECTED OUTCOMES:
* The family caregivers verbalize understanding of the child's condition and treatments.
* The family caregivers reflect confidence in the staff evidenced by cooperation and appropriate questions.

Nursing Interventions	*Rationale*
Actively listen to caregivers' concern.	Family members gain confidence when they feel their concerns are being heard.
Provide reassurance and explain what you are doing and why you are doing it when working with the child.	Understanding the disease and treatment methods helps family to feel that the child's illness is under control.
Involve caregivers in caring for child. Teach techniques of care that can be used at home.	Family caregivers feel valued and benefit from nursing care tips that they can use at home.

needed to maintain body weight with sufficient amounts added to replace the additional losses. Monitor daily weights and accurately record intake and output. Monitor serum electrolyte levels to ensure they are within normal limits. At least once per shift, observe and record skin turgor and the condition of mucous membranes. Observe the child for dehydration; skin turgor, anterior fontanelle (in infants), and urine output are good indicators of dehydration. For the infant, maintain diaper counts and weigh diapers to determine the amount of urine output (1 mL urine weighs 1 g).

Maintaining Body Temperature

Monitor the child's temperature frequently, at least every 2 hours if it is higher than 101.3°F (38.6°C). If the child has a fever, remove excess clothing and covering. Antipyretic medications may be ordered.

Promoting Energy Conservation

During an acute stage, allow the child to rest as much as possible. Plan work so that rest and sleep are interrupted no more than necessary.

Preventing Additional Infections

Turn the child from side to side every hour so that mucus is less likely to drain into the eustachian tubes, thereby reducing the risk for development of otitis media. An infant seat may help facilitate breathing and prevent the complication of otitis media in the younger child. Observe the child for irritability, shaking of the head, pulling at the ears, or complaints of ear pain. Do not give the infant a bottle while he or she is lying in bed. The best position for feeding is upright to avoid excessive drainage into the eustachian tubes.

Reducing the Child's Anxiety

When frightened or upset and crying, the child with a respiratory condition may hyperventilate, which causes additional respiratory distress. For this reason, maintain a calm, soothing manner while caring for the child. When possible, the child should be cared for by a constant caregiver with whom a trusting relationship has been achieved. Offering support to the child during invasive procedures, such as when an IV is being started, will help decrease the child's anxiety. The family can provide the child with a favorite blanket or toy. The family caregiver is encouraged to stay with the child if possible to provide reassurance and avoid separation anxiety in the child. Plan care to minimize interrupting the child's much-needed rest. Give the child age-appropriate explanations of treatment and procedures.

As the child's condition improves, provide age-appropriate diversional activities to help relieve anxiety and boredom. Make extra efforts to relieve the child's feelings of loneliness, especially when infection control precautions are being used.

Promoting Family Coping

Watching a child with severe respiratory symptoms is frightening for the parent or family caregiver. Family caregivers need teaching and reassurance. The parent or caregiver may feel helpless, and these feelings of anxiety and helplessness may be exhibited in a variety of ways. To alleviate these feelings, encourage the caregiver to discuss them. Using easily understood terminology, explain equipment, procedures, treatments, the illness, and the prognosis to the caregiver. Include the caregiver in the child's care as much as possible and encourage him or her to soothe and comfort the child. Actively listen to caregivers and use communication skills to respond to their worries.

Providing Family Teaching

Provide the caregiver with thorough explanations of the condition's signs and symptoms. Teach the use of cool humidifiers or vaporizers, including cleaning methods and safety measures to avoid burns when using a steam vaporizer. Explain the effects, administration, dosage, and side effects of medications. To be certain the information was understood, have the parent relate specific facts to you. Write the information down in a simple way so that it can be clearly understood, and determine that the parent can read and understand the written material. When appropriate, observe the caregiver demonstrating care of equipment and any treatments to be done at home. See Family Teaching Tips: Respiratory Infections.

Evaluation: Goals and Expected Outcomes

Goal: The child's airway will remain clear and patent.
Expected Outcomes: The child's

- airway is clear with no evidence of retractions, stridor, hoarseness, or cyanosis.
- mucous secretions are thin and scant.

Goal: The child's respiratory function will be within normal limits for age.
Expected Outcomes:

- The child's respiratory rate is 20 to 35 breaths per minute, normal range for child's age, regular, with breath sounds clear.

Family Teaching Tips

RESPIRATORY INFECTIONS

- Clear nasal passages with a bulb syringe for the infant.
- Feed the child slowly, allow the infant to breast-feed without tiring.
- Frequently burp the infant to expel swallowed air.
- Offer child extra fluids.
- Leave the child in mist tent except for feeding and bathing (unless otherwise indicated).
- Soothe and comfort child in mist or croup tent.
- Follow respiratory infection control precautions and good hand-washing techniques.
- Discourage persons with infections from visiting child.
- Use a humidifier at home after discharge.
- Clean humidifier properly and frequently.

- The infant no longer uses respiratory accessory muscles to aid in breathing.
- The child's oxygen saturation levels are within established limits.

Goal: The child's fluid intake will be adequate for age and weight.
Expected Outcomes: The child

- exhibits good skin turgor and moist, pink mucous membranes.
- has urine output of 1 to 3 mL/kg/hr.

Goal: The child will maintain a temperature within normal limits.
Expected Outcome:

- The child's temperature is 98.6°F to 100°F (37°C–37.8°C).

Goal: The child's energy will be conserved.
Expected Outcome:

- The child has extended periods of uninterrupted rest and tolerates increased activity.

Goal: The child will be free from complications of otitis media.
Expected Outcomes: The child

- shows no signs of ear pain such as irritability, shaking of the head, pulling on the ears.
- does not complain of ear pain.

Goal: The child will experience a reduction in anxiety.
Expected Outcomes: The child

- rests quietly with no evidence of hyperventilation.
- cooperates with care, cuddles a favorite toy for reassurance, smiles, and plays contentedly.

Goal: The family caregiver's anxiety will be reduced.
Expected Outcomes: The family caregivers

- cooperate with and participate in the child's care.
- appear more relaxed, verbalize his or her feelings, and soothe the child.

Goal: The family caregivers will verbalize an understanding of the child's condition and how to provide home care for the child.

Expected Outcomes: The family caregivers

- accurately describe facts about the child's condition.
- ask appropriate questions.
- relate signs and symptoms to observe in the child.
- name the effects, side effects, dosage, and administration of medications.

CYSTIC FIBROSIS

When first described, cystic fibrosis (CF) was called "fibrocystic disease of the pancreas." Additional research has revealed that this disorder represents a major dysfunction of all exocrine glands. The major organs affected are the lungs, pancreas, and liver. Because about half of all children with CF have pulmonary complications, this disorder is discussed here with other respiratory conditions.

CF is hereditary and transmitted as an autosomal recessive trait. Both parents must be carriers of the gene for CF to appear. With each pregnancy, the chance is one in four that the child will have the disease. In the United States, the incidence is about 1 in 3,300 in white children and 1 in 16,300 in African American children.

The normal gene produces a protein, cystic fibrosis transmembrane conductance regulator, which serves as a channel through which chloride enters and leaves cells. The mutated gene blocks chloride movement, which brings on the apparent signs of CF. The blocking of chloride transport results in a change in sodium transport; this in turn results in abnormal secretions of the exocrine (mucous-producing) glands that produce thick, tenacious mucus rather than the thin, free-flowing secretion normally produced. This abnormal mucus leads to obstruction of the secretory ducts of the pancreas, liver, and reproductive organs. Thick mucus obstructs the respiratory passages, causing trapped air and over inflation of the lungs. In addition, the sweat and salivary glands excrete excessive electrolytes, specifically sodium and chloride.

Clinical Manifestations

Meconium ileus is the presenting symptom of CF in 5% to 10% of the newborns who later develop additional manifestations. Depletion or absence of pancreatic enzymes before birth results in impaired digestive activity, and the meconium becomes viscid (thick) and mucilaginous (sticky). The inspissated (thickened) meconium fills the small intestine, causing complete obstruction. Clinical manifestations are bile-stained emesis, a distended abdomen, and an absence of stool. Intestinal perforation with symptoms of shock may occur. These newborns taste salty when kissed because of the high sodium chloride concentration in their sweat.

Initial symptoms of CF may occur at varying ages during infancy, childhood, or adolescence. A hard, nonproductive chronic cough may be the first sign. Later, frequent bronchial infections occur. Development of a barrel chest and clubbing of fingers (Fig. 36-7) indicate chronic lack of oxygen. The abdomen becomes distended, and body muscles become flabby.

> **Nutrition News**
> Despite an excellent appetite in the child with CF, malnutrition is apparent and becomes increasingly severe.

Pancreatic Involvement

Thick, tenacious mucus obstructs the pancreatic ducts, causing **hypochylia** (diminished flow of pancreatic enzymes) or **achylia** (absence of pancreatic enzymes). This achylia or hypochylia leads to intestinal malabsorption and severe malnutrition. The deficient pancreatic enzymes are lipase, trypsin, and amylase. Malabsorption of fats causes frequent steatorrhea. Anemia or rectal prolapse is common if the pancreatic condition remains untreated. The incidence of diabetes is greater in these children than in the general population, possibly because of changes in the pancreas. The incidence of diabetes in patients with CF is expected to increase because of their increasing life expectancy.

Pulmonary Involvement

The degree of lung involvement determines the prognosis for survival. The severity of pulmonary involvement differs in individual children, with a few showing only minor involvement. Now more than half of children with CF are expected to live beyond the age of 18 years, with increasing numbers living into adulthood.

Respiratory complications pose the greatest threat to children with CF. Abnormal amounts of thick, viscid mucus clog the bronchioles and provide an ideal medium

▮ **Figure 36-7** Clubbing of fingers indicates chronic lack of oxygen. **(A)** Normal angle; **(B)** early clubbing—flattened angle; **(C)** advanced clubbing—the nail is rounded over the end of the finger.

 A Normal

 B Early clubbing

 C Advanced clubbing

for bacterial growth. *Staphylococcus aureus* coagulase can be cultured from the nasopharynx and sputum of most patients. *Pseudomonas aeruginosa* and *H. influenzae* also are found frequently. However, the basic infection appears most often to be caused by *S. aureus*.

Numerous complications arise from severe respiratory infections. Atelectasis and small lung abscesses are common early complications. Bronchiectasis and emphysema may develop with pulmonary fibrosis and pneumonitis; this eventually leads to severe ventilatory insufficiency. In advanced disease, pneumothorax, right ventricular hypertrophy, and cor pulmonale are common complications. Cor pulmonale is a common cause of death.

Other Organ Involvement

The tears, saliva, and sweat of children with CF contain abnormally high concentrations of electrolytes, and most such children have enlarged submaxillary salivary glands. In hot weather, the loss of sodium chloride and fluid through sweating produces frequent heat prostration. Additional fluid and salt should be given in the diet as a preventive measure. In addition, males with CF who reach adulthood will most likely be sterile because of the blockage or absence of the vas deferens or other ducts. Females often have thick cervical secretions that prohibit the passage of sperm.

Diagnosis

Diagnosis is based on family history, elevated sodium chloride levels in the sweat, analysis of duodenal secretions (via a nasogastric tube) for trypsin content, a history of failure to thrive, chronic or recurrent respiratory infections, and radiologic findings of hyperinflation and bronchial wall thickening. In the event of a positive sodium chloride sweat test, at least one other criterion must be met to make a conclusive diagnosis.

The principal diagnostic test to confirm CF is a sweat chloride test using the pilocarpine iontophoresis method. This method induces sweating by using a small electric current that carries topically applied pilocarpine into a localized area of the skin. Elevations of 60 mEq/L or more are diagnostic, with values of 50 to 60 mEq/L highly suspect. Although the test itself is fairly simple, conducting the test on an infant is difficult, and false-positive results do occur.

Treatment

In the newborn, meconium ileus is treated with hyperosmolar enemas administered gently. If this does not resolve the blockage of thick, gummy meconium, surgery is necessary. During surgery, a mucolytic, such as Mucomyst, may be used to liquefy the meconium. If this procedure is successful, resection may not be necessary.

In the older child, treatment is aimed at correcting pancreatic deficiency, improving pulmonary function, and preventing respiratory infections. If bowel obstruc-

tion does occur (meconium ileus equivalent), the preferred management includes hyperosmolar enemas and an increase in fluids, dietary fiber, oral mucolytics, lactulose, and mineral oil.

The overall treatment goals are to improve the child's quality of life and to provide for long-term survival. A health care team is needed, including a primary care provider, a nurse, a respiratory therapist, a dietitian, and a social worker, to work together with the child and family. Treatment centers with a staff of specialists are becoming more common, particularly in larger medical centers.

> **Good news!!**
> With improved treatment, it is not unusual for a child with CF to grow into adulthood.

Dietary Treatment

Commercially prepared pancreatic enzymes given during meals or with snacks aid digestion and absorption of fat and protein. Because pancreatic enzymes are inactivated in the acidic environment of the stomach, microencapsulated capsules are used to deliver the enzymes to the duodenum, where they are activated. These enzymes come in capsules that can be swallowed or opened and sprinkled on the child's food. A powdered preparation is used for infants.

The child's diet should be high in carbohydrates and protein, with no restriction of fats. The child may need 1.5 to 2 times the normal caloric intake to promote growth. These children have large appetites unless they are acutely ill. However, even with their large appetites they can receive little nourishment without a pancreatic supplement. With proper diet and enzyme supplements, these children show evidence of improved nutrition, and their stools become relatively normal. Enteric-coated pancreatic enzymes essentially eliminate the need for dietary restriction of fat.

Because of the increased loss of sodium chloride, these children are allowed to use as much salt as they wish, even though onlookers may think it is too much. During hot weather, additional salt may be provided with pretzels, salted bread sticks, and saltine crackers.

Supplements of fat-soluble vitamins A, D, and E are necessary because of the poor digestion of fats. Vitamin K may be supplemented if the child has coagulation problems or is scheduled for surgery. Water-miscible preparations can be given to provide the needed supplement.

Pulmonary Treatment

The treatment goal is to prevent and treat respiratory infections. Respiratory drainage is provided by thinning the secretions and by mechanical means, such as postural drainage and clapping to loosen and drain secretions from the lungs. Antibacterial drugs for the treatment of infection are necessary as indicated. Some physicians prescribe a prophylactic antibiotic regimen when the child receives the diagnosis of CF. Antibiotics may be administered orally or parenterally, even in the home. With home parenteral administration of antibiotic therapy, a central venous access device is used. Immunization against childhood communicable diseases is extremely important for these chronically ill children. All immunization measures may be used and should be maintained at appropriate intervals.

Physical activity is essential because it improves mucous secretion and helps the child feel good. The child can be encouraged to participate in any aerobic activity he or she enjoys. Activity along with physical therapy should be limited only by the child's endurance.

Inhalation therapy can be preventive or therapeutic. A bronchodilator drug, such as theophylline or a beta-adrenergic agonist (metaproterenol, terbutaline, or albuterol), may be administered either orally or through nebulization. Recombinant human DNA (DNase, Pulmozyme) breaks down DNA molecules in sputum, breaking up the thick mucus in the airways. A mucolytic, such as Mucomyst, may be prescribed during acute infection. Hand-held nebulizers are easy to use and convenient for the ambulatory child.

Humidifiers provide a humidified atmosphere. In summer, a room air conditioner can help provide comfort and controlled humidity.

Chest physical therapy, a combination of postural drainage and chest percussion, is performed routinely at least every morning and evening, even if little drainage is apparent (Fig. 36-8). Performed correctly, chest percussion (clapping and vibrating of the affected areas) helps to loosen and move secretions out of the lungs. The physical therapist usually performs this procedure in the hospital and teaches it to the family. Chest physical therapy, although time consuming, is part of the ongoing, long-term treatment and should be continued at home.

Home Care

The home care for a child with CF places a tremendous burden on the family. This is not a one-time hospital treatment and there is no prospect of cure to brighten the horizon. Each day, much time is spent performing treatments. Family caregivers must learn to perform chest physical therapy, how to operate respiratory equipment, and administer IV antibiotics, when necessary. The child's diet must be planned with additional enzymes regulated according to need. Great care is needed to prevent exposure to infections.

Family caregivers must guard against overprotection and against undue limitation of their child's physical activity. Somehow, caregivers must preserve a good family relationship, also giving time and attention to other members of the family.

Physical activity is an important adjunct to the child's well-being and is necessary to get rid of secretions. Capacity for exercise is soon learned, and the child can be trusted to become self-limiting as necessary, especially if given an opportunity to learn the nature of the disease. The child may find postural drainage fun when a caregiver raises the child's feet in the air and walks the child around "wheelbarrow" fashion.

A little fun can be good. The older child with CF can learn to hang from a monkey bar by the knees, having fun and at the same time increasing postural drainage.

Providing as much normalcy as possible is always desirable. Hot-weather activity should be watched a little more closely, with additional attention to increased salt and fluid intake during exercise.

Caring for a child with CF places great stress on a family's financial resources. The expense of daily medications, frequent clinic or office visits, and sometimes lengthy hospitalizations can be devastating to an ordinary family budget, even with medical insurance coverage. The Cystic Fibrosis Foundation (www. cff.org), with chapters throughout the United States, is helpful in providing education and services. Some assistance may be available through local agencies or community groups.

Nursing Process for the Child With Cystic Fibrosis
Assessment

The collection of data on the child with CF varies, depending on the child's age and the circumstances of the admission. Conduct a complete parent interview that includes the standard information, as well as data concerning respiratory infections, the child's appetite and eating habits, stools, noticeable salty perspiration, history of bowel obstruction as an infant, and family history for CF, if known. Also determine the caregiver's knowledge of the condition.

When collecting data about vital signs, include observation of respirations, such as cough, breath sounds, and barrel chest; respiratory effort, such as retractions and nasal flaring; clubbing of the fingers; and signs of pancreatic involvement, such as failure to thrive and steatorrhea. Examine the skin around the rectum for irritation and breakdown from frequent foul stools. Involve the child in the interview process by asking age-appropriate questions, and determine the child's perception of the disease and this current illness.

Selected Nursing Diagnoses
- Ineffective Airway Clearance related to thick, tenacious mucus production
- Ineffective Breathing Pattern related to tracheobronchial obstruction

POSITION #1, for infants
UPPER LOBES, Apical segments

POSITION #1
UPPER LOBES, Apical segments

POSITION #2
UPPER LOBES, Posterior segments

POSITION #4
LINGULA

POSITION #3
UPPER LOBES, Anterior segments

POSITION #5
MIDDLE LOBE

POSITION #6
LOWER LOBES, Anterior basal segments

▪ **Figure 36-8** Positions for postural drainage.

POSITION #7
LOWER LOBES, Posterior basal segments

POSITION #8 & 9
LOWER LOBES, Lateral basal segments

POSITION #10
LOWER LOBES, Superior segments

■ **Figure 36-8** Continued

- Risk for Infection related to bacterial growth medium provided by pulmonary mucus and impaired body defenses
- Imbalanced Nutrition: Less Than Body Requirements related to impaired absorption of nutrients
- Anxiety related to hospitalization
- Compromised Family Coping related to child's chronic illness and its demands on caregivers
- Deficient Knowledge of the caregiver related to illness, treatment, and home care

Outcome Identification and Planning

As already stated, much depends on the reason for the specific admission and other factors discussed in Nursing Diagnoses. The child's age and ability for self-expression affect any goal setting the child can do. The major goals for the child include relieving immediate respiratory distress, maintaining adequate oxygenation, remaining free from infection, improving nutritional status, and relieving anxiety. The caregivers' primary goal may include relieving problems related to this admission. However, other goals may include concerns about stress on the family related to the illness, as well as a need for additional information about the disease, treatment, and prevention of complications.

Implementation

Improving Airway Clearance

Mucus obstructs the airways and diminishes gas exchange. Monitor the child for signs of respiratory distress, while observing for dyspnea, tachypnea, labored respirations with or without activity, retractions, nasal flaring, and color of nail beds. Perform aerosol treatments. Teach the child to cough effectively. Examine and document the mucus produced, noting the color, consistency, and odor. Send cultures to the laboratory, as appropriate. Increase fluid intake to help thin mucous secretions. Encourage the child to drink extra fluids and ask the child (or the caregiver if the child is too young) what favorite drinks might be appealing. Intravenous fluids may be necessary. Provide humidified air, either in the form of a cool mist humidifier or mist tent, as prescribed.

Improving Breathing

Maintain the child in a semi-Fowler's position, with the upper half of the body elevated about 30 degrees, or high Fowler's position, with the upper half of the body elevated about 90 degrees, to promote maximal lung expansion. Pulse oximetry may be used. Maintain oxygen saturation higher than 90%. Administer oxygen as ordered if the oxygen saturation falls below this level for an extended period. Administer mouth care every 2 to 4 hours, especially when oxygen is administered. Perform chest physical therapy every 2 to 4 hours, as ordered. If respiratory therapy technicians or physical therapists do these treatments, observe the child after the treatment to determine effectiveness and if more frequent treatments may be needed. Supervise the child who can self-administer nebulizer treatments to ensure correct use.

Conserve the child's energy. Plan nursing and therapeutic activities so that maximal rest time is provided for the child. Note dyspnea and respiratory distress in relation to any activities. Plan quiet diversional activities as the child's physical condition warrants. Help the child and family to understand that activity is excellent for the child not in an acute situation. Teach them that exercise helps loosen the thick mucus and also improves the child's self-image.

Preventing Infection

The child with CF has low resistance, especially to respiratory infections. For this reason, take care to protect the child from any exposure to infectious organisms. Good hand-washing techniques should be practiced by all; teach the child and family the importance of this first line of defense. Practice and teach other good hygiene habits. Carefully follow medical asepsis when caring for the child and the equipment. Monitor vital signs every 4 hours for any indication of an infectious process. Restrict people with an infection, such as staff, family members, other patients, and visitors, from contact with the child. Advise the family to keep the child's immunizations up to date. Administer antibiotics as prescribed, and teach the child or caregiver home administration, as needed. Also, teach the family the signs and symptoms of an impending infection so they can begin prophylactic measures at once.

Maintaining Adequate Nutrition

Adequate nutrition helps the child resist infections. Greatly increase the child's caloric intake to compensate for impaired absorption of nutrients and to provide adequate growth and development. In addition to increased caloric intake at meals, provide the child with high-calorie, high-protein snacks, such as peanut butter and cheese. Low-fat products can be selected, if desired. Administer pancreatic enzymes with all meals and snacks. In addition, multiple vitamins and iron may be prescribed. Reinforce the need for these supplements to both the child and the family. The child also may require additional salt in the diet. Encourage the child to eat salty snacks. If the child has bouts of diarrhea or constipation, the dosage of enzymes may need to be adjusted. Report any change in bowel movements. Weigh and measure the child. Plot growth on a chart so that progress can easily be visualized.

Reducing the Child's Anxiety

Provide age-appropriate activities to help alleviate anxiety and the boredom that can result from hospitalization. Choose activities such as reading or arts and crafts according to age. Schoolwork may help ease some anxiety. Some older children may enjoy a video game, if available, but watch the child for overexcitement. Encourage the family caregiver to stay with the child to help diminish some of the child's anxiety. Allow the child to have familiar toys or mementos from home. Stay with the child during acute episodes of coughing and dyspnea to reduce anxiety. Give the child age-appropriate information about CF. Quiz the child in a relaxed, friendly manner to help determine what the child knows and what teaching may be needed. Learning about CF can be turned into a game for some children, making it much more enjoyable.

Providing Family Support

The family with a child who has CF is faced with a long-term illness and may have already seen deterioration in the child's health. Give the family and the child opportunities to voice fears and anxieties. Respond with active-listening techniques to help authenticate their feelings. Provide emotional support throughout the entire hospital stay. Demonstrate an interest and willingness to talk to the family; do not make family members feel as though they are intruding on time needed to do other things. As the nurse, you are the person who can best provide overall support.

Providing Family Teaching

Evaluate the family's knowledge about CF to determine their teaching needs. The family may need to have all the information repeated or may need clarification in just a few areas. Provide information for resources such as the Cystic Fibrosis Foundation, the American Lung Association (www.lungusa.org), and other local organizations. The family may have questions about genetic counseling and may need referrals for counseling.

Evaluation: Goals and Expected Outcomes

Goal: The child's airway will be clear.
Expected Outcomes: The child

- effectively clears mucus from the airway and the airway remains patent.
- cooperates with chest physical therapy.

Goal: The child will exhibit adequate respiratory function.
Expected Outcomes: The child

- rests quietly with no dyspnea; the respiratory rate is even and appropriate for age.
- maintains oxygen saturation above 90%.

Goal: The child will remain free of signs and symptoms of infection.
Expected Outcomes:

- The child's vital signs are within normal limits for age.
- The child and family follow infection-control practices.

Goal: The child's nutritional intake will be adequate to compensate for decreased absorption of nutrients and to provide for adequate growth and development.

Expected Outcomes: The child

- demonstrates weight gain appropriate for age.
- exhibits normal growth as indicated by growth chart.

Goal: The child's anxiety will subside.

Expected Outcome:

- The child engages in age-appropriate activities and appears relaxed.

Goal: The family caregivers will verbalize feelings related to the child's chronic illness.

Expected Outcome:

- The family caregivers verbalize fears, anxieties, and other feelings related to the child's illness.

Goal: The family caregivers will verbalize an understanding of the child's illness and treatment.

Expected Outcomes: The family caregivers

- explain CF and describe treatments and possible complications.
- become involved in available support groups.

Test Yourself

✔ What two immunizations have decreased the incidence of bacterial pneumonia in children?

✔ What major organs are affected by CF?

✔ What is the dietary treatment for CF?

✔ For what type of infection is the child with CF most susceptible?

PULMONARY TUBERCULOSIS

Tuberculosis is present in all parts of the world and is the most important chronic infectious disease in terms of illness, death, and cost (Starke, 2006). The incidence of tuberculosis in the United States had declined steadily until about 1985. In the years since, there has been an increase in the number of cases reported in the United States. Several factors contribute to this increase; one factor is the number of people who have human immunodeficiency virus and have become infected with tuberculosis.

Cultural Snapshot

In some cultures, it is common for many people to live together in one home or in a close living arrangement. Respiratory illness is easily spread from person to person when people live in close contact with each other.

Tuberculosis is caused by *Mycobacterium tuberculosis*, a bacillus spread by droplets of infected mucus that become airborne when the infected person sneezes, coughs, or laughs. The bacilli, when airborne, are inhaled into the respiratory tract of the unsuspecting person and become implanted in lung tissue. This process is the beginning of the formation of a primary lesion.

Clinical Manifestations

Primary tuberculosis is the original infection that goes through various stages and ends with calcification. Primary lesions in children are generally unrecognized. The most common site of a primary lesion is the alveoli of the respiratory tract. Most cases arrest with the calcification of the primary infection. However, in children with poor nutrition or health, the primary infection may invade other tissues of the body, including the bones, joints, kidneys, lymph nodes, and meninges. This is called miliary tuberculosis. In the small number of children with miliary tuberculosis, general symptoms of chronic infection, such as fatigue, loss of weight, and low-grade fever, may occur accompanied by night sweats.

Secondary tuberculosis is a reactivation of a healed primary lesion. It often occurs in adults and contributes to the exposure of children to the organism. Although secondary lesions are more common in adults, they may occur in adolescents. Symptoms resemble those in an adult, including cough with expectoration, fever, weight loss, malaise, and night sweats.

Diagnosis

The tuberculin skin test is the primary means by which tuberculosis is detected. A skin test can be performed using a multipuncture device that deposits purified protein derivative intradermally (tine test) or by intradermal injection of 0.1 mL of purified protein derivative. Both tests are administered on the inner aspect of the forearm. The site is marked and read at 48 and 72 hours. Redness, swelling, induration, and itching of the site indicate a positive reaction. Persons with a positive reaction are further examined by radiographic evaluation. Sputum tests of young children are rarely helpful because children do not produce a good specimen. Screening by means of skin testing is recommended for all children at 12 months, before entering school, and in adolescence. Screening is recommended annually for children in high-risk situations or communities including children in whose family there is an active case; Native Americans; and children who recently immigrated from Central or South America, the Caribbean, Africa, Asia, or the Middle East. Other high-risk children are those infected with human immunodeficiency virus, those who are homeless or live in overcrowded conditions, and those immunosuppressed for any reason.

Treatment

Drug therapy for tuberculosis includes administration of isoniazid (INH), often in combination with rifampin. Although INH has been known to cause peripheral neuritis in children with poor nutrition, few problems occur in children whose diets are well balanced. Rifampin is tolerated well by children but causes body fluids such as urine, sweat, tears, and feces to turn orange-red. A possible disadvantage for adolescents is that it may permanently stain contact lenses. Rifamate is a combination of rifampin and INH. Other drugs that may be used are ethambutol, streptomycin, and pyrazinamide.

Drug therapy is continued for 9 to 18 months. After drug therapy has begun, the child or adolescent may return to school and normal activities unless clinical symptoms are evident. An annual chest radiograph is necessary from that time on.

Prevention

Prevention requires improvements in social conditions such as overcrowding, poverty, and poor health care. Also needed are health education; medical, laboratory, and radiographic facilities for examination; and control of contacts and persons suspected of infection.

A vaccine called bacilli Calmette-Guérin (BCG) is used in countries with a high incidence of tuberculosis. It is given to tuberculin-negative persons and is said to be effective for 12 years or longer. Mass vaccination is not considered necessary in parts of the world where the incidence of tuberculosis is low. After administration of BCG vaccine, the skin test will be positive, so screening is no longer an effective tool. The use of BCG vaccine remains controversial because of the effect it has on screening for the disease, as well as the questionable effectiveness of the vaccine.

Key Points

➤ An infant or child's respiratory system, because of its small size and underdeveloped anatomic structures, is more prone to respiratory problems. Smaller structures lead to a greater chance of obstruction and respiratory distress. As the child grows, the use of the thoracic muscles takes the place of the use of the diaphragm and abdominal muscles for breathing.

➤ The most common complication of acute nasopharyngitis (common cold) is otitis media.

➤ Avoiding or removing allergens is the best way to prevent allergic rhinitis. Antihistamines and hyposensitization may be helpful for some patients.

➤ The child with tonsillitis may have a fever, sore throat, difficulty swallowing, hypertrophied tonsils, and erythema of the soft palate. Exudate may be visible on the tonsils. Treatment of tonsillitis consists of analgesics, antipyretics, and antibiotics. Surgical removal of the tonsils and adenoids may be indicated.

➤ The most common complication of a tonsillectomy is hemorrhage or bleeding. The child must be observed, especially in the first 24 hours, after surgery and in the fifth to seventh postoperative days for unusual restlessness, anxiety, frequent swallowing, or rapid pulse. Vomiting bright, red-flecked emesis or bright red oozing or bleeding may indicate hemorrhage. If noted, these should be reported immediately.

➤ Spasmodic laryngitis may be of infectious or allergic origin. An attack is often preceded by a runny nose and hoarseness. The child awakens after a few hours of sleep with a bark-like cough; respiratory difficulty; stridor; and may be anxious, restless, and hoarse. Humidified air is used to decrease the laryngospasm. A low dose of an emetic may be used to reduce spasms of the larynx. Acute laryngotracheobronchitis is often caused by the staphylococcal bacterium. The child may become hoarse and have a barking cough and elevated temperature. Breathing difficulty, a rapid pulse, and cyanosis may occur. Antibiotics are given and the child is placed in a croupette or mist tent with oxygen. Epiglottitis is an acute inflammation of the epiglottis and is not commonly seen.

➤ Bronchiolitis/RSV is caused by a viral infection. Dyspnea occurs as well as a dry and persistent cough, extremely shallow respirations, air hunger, and cyanosis. Suprasternal and subcostal retractions are present with respirations as high as 60 to 80 breaths per minute. Diagnosis is made from clinical findings confirmed by laboratory testing (enzyme-linked immunosorbent assay [ELISA]). The child is hospitalized, placed on contact transmission precautions, and treated with high humidity by mist tent, rest, and increased fluids. Ribavirin (Virazole), an antiviral drug, may be used.

➤ An asthma attack can be triggered by a hypersensitive response to allergens; foods such as chocolate, milk, eggs, nuts, and grains; exercise; or exposure to cold or irritants such as wood-burning stoves, cigarette smoke, dust, and pet dander. Infections, stress, or anxiety can also trigger an asthma attack.

➤ During an asthma attack, the combination of smooth muscle spasms, which cause the lumina of the bronchi and bronchioles to narrow; edema; and increased mucus production causes respiratory obstruction.

➤ The goals of asthma treatment include preventing symptoms, maintaining near-normal lung function and activity levels, preventing recurring exacerbations and hospitalizations, and providing the best medication treatment with the fewest adverse effects. Nursing care is focused on maintaining a clear airway, maintaining an adequate fluid intake, and relieving fatigue and anxiety.

➤ Bacterial pneumonia is usually caused by pneumococcal or *H. influenzae* bacterium. The onset is usually abrupt, following a mild upper respiratory illness. Symptoms may include a high temperature, respiratory distress with air hunger, flaring of the nostrils, circumoral cyanosis, and chest retractions. Tachycardia and tachypnea are present, with a pulse rate as high as 140 to 180 beats per minute and respirations as high as 80 breaths per minute. Anti-infectives, such as penicillin or ampicillin, have proved to be the most effective in the treatment of pneumonia. If the child has a penicillin allergy, cephalosporin anti-infectives are also used. Nursing care is focused on maintaining respiratory function, preventing fluid deficit, maintaining body temperature, preventing otitis media, conserving energy, and relieving anxiety.

➤ CF causes the exocrine (mucous-producing) glands to produce thick, tenacious mucus, rather than thin, free-flowing secretions. These secretions obstruct the secretory ducts of the pancreas, liver, and reproductive organs.

➤ The sweat chloride test, which shows elevated sodium chloride levels in the sweat, is the principal diagnostic test used to confirm CF. Family history, analysis of duodenal secretions for trypsin content, history of failure to thrive, chronic or recurrent respiratory infections, and radiologic findings also help diagnose the disorder.

➤ The most common and serious complications of CF arise from respiratory infections, which may lead to severe respiratory concerns.

➤ Pancreatic enzymes given with meals and snacks are used in the dietary treatment of children with CF. The child's diet is high in protein and carbohydrates, and salt in large amounts is allowed. The use of chest physiotherapy, antibiotics, and inhalation therapy help in the prevention and treatment of respiratory infections.

➤ Tuberculosis can be detected by doing a tuberculin skin test using purified protein derivative. When a person has a positive reaction to the skin test, additional evaluation using radiography is done to confirm the disease. INH and Rifampin are used to treat tuberculosis and are given for 9 to 18 months.

INTERNET RESOURCES

Cystic Fibrosis Foundation
www.cff.org

National Heart, Lung, and Blood Institute
www.nhlbi.nih.gov

Asthma and Allergy
www.aafa.org

American Lung Association
www.lungusa.org

American Academy of Allergy Asthma and Immunology
www.aaaai.org

RSV
www.marchofdimes.com/pnhec/298_9546.asp

Workbook

■ NCLEX-STYLE REVIEW QUESTIONS

1. The nurse is doing teaching with the caregivers of a child who has had a tonsillectomy the previous day and is being discharged. The nurse would reinforce that which of the following should be reported *immediately* to the child's physician?

   a. The child complains of a sore throat on the third postoperative day.

   b. The child refuses to leave the ice collar on for more than 10 minutes.

   c. The child vomits dark, old blood within 4 hours after being discharged.

   d. The child has frequent swallowing around the sixth day after surgery.

2. A toddler with a diagnosis of a respiratory disorder has a fever and decreased urinary output. When planning care for this child, which of the following goals would be *most* appropriate for this toddler?

   a. The child's anxiety will be reduced.

   b. The child's fluid intake will be increased.

   c. The child's caregivers will talk about their concerns.

   d. The child's caloric intake will be adequate for age.

3. The nurse is teaching a group of caregivers of children who have asthma. The caregivers make the following statements. Which of these statements indicates a need for additional teaching?

   a. "We need to identify the things that trigger our child's attacks."

   b. "I always have him use his bronchodilator before he uses his steroid inhaler."

   c. "We will be sure our child does not exercise to prevent attacks."

   d. "She drinks lots of water, which I know helps to thin her secretions."

4. A child with cystic fibrosis will have which of the following interventions included in the child's plan of care?

   a. Maintain a flat lying position when in bed.

   b. Provide low protein snacks between meals.

   c. Perform postural drainage in the morning and evening.

   d. Teach infection control procedures when hospitalized.

5. After discussing the disease with the caregiver of a child with cystic fibrosis, the caregiver makes the following statements. Which of these statements indicates a need for additional teaching?

   a. "It is good to know that my other children won't have the disease."

   b. "I will be sure to give my child the medication every time she eats."

   c. "It is important to let my child play with the other kids when she is at school."

   d. "When she exercises, I will feed her a salty snack."

6. The nurse is completing the intake and output record for a toddler who has a respiratory infection. The dry weight of the child's diaper is 38 g. The child has had the following intake and output during the shift:

   Intake: 3 oz of apple juice
   ½ serving of pancakes
   5 oz of milk
   4 saltine crackers
   ¼ cup of chicken soup
   2 oz of gelatin
   130 cc of IV fluid
   Output: Diaper with urine weighing 87 f
   Diaper with stool only weighing 124 f
   Diaper with urine weighing 138 f
   Diaper with urine weighing 146 f
   Diaper with urine weighing 95 f

   a. How many milliliters should the nurse document as the child's total intake?

   b. How many milliliters should the nurse document as the child's urinary output?

■ STUDY ACTIVITIES

1. Draw a diagram to explain the heredity pattern of cystic fibrosis.

2. Research your community to find sources of help for families with children who have cystic fibrosis. What support groups and organizations are available that you might recommend to families of children with cystic fibrosis? Discuss with your peers what you found and make a list of resources to share.

3. Go to the following Web site: www.lungusa.org. Find the section on Asthma and on the drop down menu, click on "Asthma & Children." Click on "Early Warning Signals: Asthma Always Gives a Sign."

   a. List six areas covered on this site that you could share with a family of a child with asthma.

   b. What five suggestions are given in the area covering "What to Listen For?"

   c. Read the section on "How to Listen."

   d. Describe how you listen to the breath sounds in a child with asthma.

   e. What are five emergency signs that require immediate treatment?

❚ CRITICAL THINKING: WHAT WOULD YOU DO?

1. Sandy calls the 24-hour pediatric health line at 10:30 p.m. about her 2.5-year-old child Jared. Jared had gone to bed at his usual bedtime of 8:00 p.m. after an uneventful evening. He had awakened with a bark-like cough, respiratory difficulty, and a high-pitched harsh sound on inspiration.

   a. What questions would you ask this mother to further clarify Jared's situation?

   b. What would you suggest Sandy should do to decrease Jared's symptoms?

   c. What would you tell Sandy to watch for that might indicate Jared needs emergency attention?

2. Rachel, a 6-year-old girl, is brought to the clinic with a dry hacking cough, wheezing, and difficulty breathing. Rachel is coughing up thick mucus. Her parents are with her and are extremely anxious about Rachel's condition. The pediatrician examines Rachel, and a diagnosis of an acute asthma attack is made.

   a. What other findings might have been noted during a physical exam of Rachel?

   b. What will most likely be done to treat Rachel's current condition?

   c. What medications might have been given?

   d. What would you teach Rachel's parents about prevention of additional attacks?

3. Dosage calculation: A toddler with a diagnosis of cystic fibrosis is being treated with the bronchodilator Theophylline. The child weighs 32 lb. The usual dosage of this medication is 4 mg/kg/dose every 6 hours. Answer the following:

   a. How many kilograms does the child's weigh?

   b. How many milligrams per dose will be given?

   c. How many doses will the child receive in a day?

   d. How much Theophylline will be given in a 24-hour period?

37

The Child With a Cardiovascular/ Hematologic Disorder

KEY TERMS

adenopathy
alopecia
arthralgia
bradycardia
carditis
chorea
congestive heart failure
digitalization
granulocytes
hemarthrosis
hirsutism
intrathecal administration
leukemia
lymphoblast
lymphocytes
monocytes
petechiae
polyarthritis
purpura

LEARNING OBJECTIVES

On completion of this chapter, you should be able to:

1. Describe the cardiovascular and hematologic systems and how they function.
2. Discuss ways the child's cardiovascular and hematologic system differs from the adult's system.
3. Discuss congestive heart failure, including care of the child with CHF.
4. Name the bacterium usually responsible for the infection that leads to the development of rheumatic fever.
5. List the major manifestations of rheumatic fever and describe the nursing care.
6. Explain Kawasaki disease and state the most serious concern for the child with Kawasaki disease.
7. Discuss iron deficiency anemia and identify the common causes.
8. Explain how (a) sickle cell trait and (b) sickle cell anemia are inherited.
9. Describe the shape of the red blood cell and the effect it has on the circulation in sickle cell anemia.
10. Discuss the nursing care for the child with sickle cell anemia.
11. Discuss the common complications and prognosis for the child with thalassemia.
12. Name the most common types of hemophilia and state how they are inherited.
13. Discuss the treatment and nursing care for the child with hemophilia.
14. Describe the symptoms noted in the child with idiopathic thrombocytopenic purpura.
15. Explain the diagnosis of leukemia including the symptoms, treatment, and nursing care.

CARDIOVASCULAR system disorders and hematologic disorders, which are disorders having to do with the blood and blood-forming tissues, are usually serious and may be chronic or long-term conditions. Many of these conditions are hereditary and often present at birth. The congenital heart disorders are discussed in Chapter 21. The seriousness of disorders related to the cardiovascular system creates fear and concern in the child and family. An understanding of the cardiovascular system and how it functions can be helpful in decreasing the anxiety these families have.

GROWTH AND DEVELOPMENT OF THE CARDIOVASCULAR AND HEMATOLOGIC SYSTEMS

All systems of the body depend on the cardiovascular system. It works to carry the needed chemicals to and from the cells in the body so they can function properly. The major organ of the cardiovascular system is the heart, which is the pump that keeps the blood, containing oxygen and nutrients, circulating through the body. The hematologic system includes the blood and blood-forming tissues. The cardiovascular and hematologic systems work together to remove the waste products from the cells so they can be excreted from the body. The vessels, which carry the blood to and from the heart and through the body, include the arteries, veins, and capillaries. Arteries carry blood away from the heart to the body, and veins collect the blood and return it to the heart. Capillaries are the exchange vessels for the materials that flow through the body. Blood is a fluid composed of many elements, including plasma, red blood cells (RBCs), white blood cells (WBCs), and platelets. Each of these elements has a different function. These blood cells are formed in the bone marrow. The diseases and disorders of the circulatory system and the blood-forming tissues occur when the heart itself or the blood or blood-forming tissues are genetically altered, infection or damage has occurred, the organs or tissues are not shaped or functioning normally, or when the elements in the blood are increased or decreased in amount.

DIFFERENCES BETWEEN THE CHILD'S AND ADULT'S CARDIOVASCULAR AND HEMATOLOGIC SYSTEMS

Normal fetal circulation and the changes that occur in the cardiovascular system when the infant is born are covered in Chapter 21. Congenital heart disorders often occur in infants because the heart is not formed properly or the structures do not close at birth. At birth, both the right and left ventricles are about the same size, but by a few months of age, the left ventricle is about two times the size of the right. The infant's heart rate is higher than the older child's or adult's so that the infant's cardiac output can provide adequate oxygen to the body. If the infant has a fever, respiratory distress, or any increased need for oxygen, the pulse rate goes up to increase the cardiac output. Although the size is smaller by the time the child is 5 years old, the heart has matured, developed, and functions just as the adult's heart (Fig. 37-1). The blood volume in the body is proportionate to the body weight. The younger the child, the higher the blood volume is per kilogram of body weight.

CONGESTIVE HEART FAILURE

Congestive heart failure (CHF) occurs when blood and fluids accumulate in the organs and body tissues. This accumulation happens because the heart is not able to pump and circulate enough blood to supply the oxygen and nutrient needs of the body cells. Manifestations of CHF may appear in children with conditions such as congenital heart disorders (see Chapter 21 for additional discussion), rheumatic fever, or Kawasaki disease. The condition places an increased workload on the ventricles of the heart.

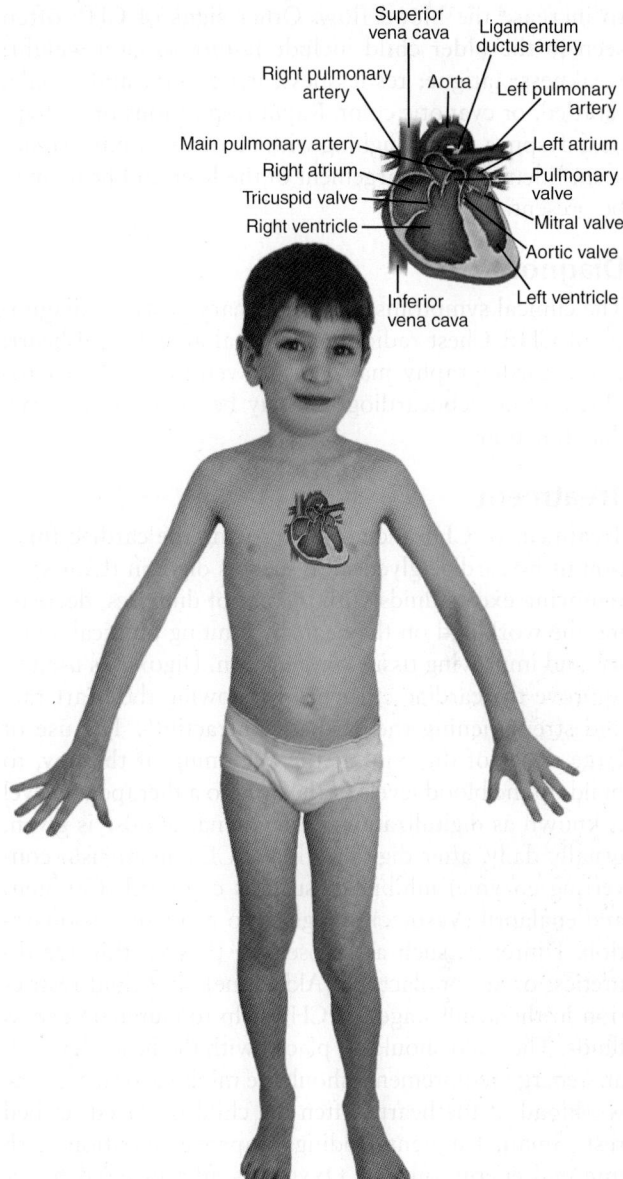

■ **Figure 37-1** Anatomy of the normal heart.

Clinical Manifestations

The indications of CHF vary in children of different ages. Signs in the infant may be hard to detect because they are subtle. These include easy fatigability, which is manifested by feeding problems. The infant tires easily; breathes hard; and may have rapid respirations with an expiratory grunt, flaring of the nares, and sternal retractions. The infant may refuse the bottle after just 1 or 2 oz, but soon becomes hungry again. During feeding, the infant may even become diaphoretic from the effort of feeding. Lying flat causes stress for the infant, who may appear more comfortable if held upright over an adult's shoulder. Periorbital edema may be present. A rapid weight gain may also indicate CHF.

In infants and older children, one of the first signs of CHF is tachycardia. The heart beats faster in an attempt to increase the blood flow. Other signs of CHF often seen in the older child include failure to gain weight; weakness; fatigue; restlessness; irritability; and a pale, mottled, or cyanotic color. Rapid respirations or tachypnea, dyspnea, and coughing with bloody sputum also are seen. Edema and enlargement of the liver and heart may be present.

Diagnosis

The clinical symptoms are the primary basis for diagnosis of CHF. Chest radiographs reveal an enlarged heart; electrocardiography may indicate ventricular hypertrophy, and an echocardiogram may be done to note cardiac function.

Treatment

Treatment of CHF includes improving the cardiac function using cardiac glycosides, such as digoxin (Lanoxin), removing excess fluids with the use of diuretics, decreasing the workload on the heart by limiting physical activity, and improving tissue oxygenation. Digoxin is used to improve the cardiac efficiency by slowing the heart rate and strengthening the cardiac contractility. The use of large doses of digoxin, at the beginning of therapy, to build up the blood levels of the drug to a therapeutic level is known as **digitalization.** A maintenance dose is given, usually daily, after digitalization. ACE (angiotensin-converting enzyme) inhibitors, such as captopril (Capoten) and enalapril (Vasotec), are given to increase vasodilatation. Diuretics, such as furosemide (Lasix), thiazide diuretics, or spironolactone (Aldactone), and fluid restriction in the acute stages of CHF help to eliminate excess fluids. The child should be placed with the head elevated, and energy requirements should be minimized to ease the workload of the heart. Often the child is placed on bed rest. Small, frequent feedings improve nutrition with minimal energy output. Oxygen is administered to increase oxygenation of tissues.

Nursing Process for the Child With Congestive Heart Failure

Assessment

An interview with the family caregiver of a child with CHF must include the gathering of information about the current illness and any previous episodes. Ask about any problems the child may have during feeding, episodes of rapid or difficult respirations, episodes of turning blue, and difficulty with lying flat. Determine if the child has been gaining weight. Avoid causing any feelings of guilt in the caregiver.

The physical examination of the child includes a complete measurement of vital signs. Note the quality and rhythm of the apical pulse. Observe respiratory status, including any use of accessory muscles, retractions, breath sounds, rate, and type of cry. Examine the skin and extremities for color, skin temperature, and evidence

of edema. Observe the child closely for signs of easy fatigability or an increase in symptoms on exertion.

Selected Nursing Diagnoses

- Decreased Cardiac Output related to structural defects or decreased cardiac functioning
- Ineffective Breathing Pattern related to pulmonary congestion and anxiety
- Risk for Imbalanced Nutrition: Less Than Body Requirements related to fatigue and dyspnea
- Activity Intolerance related to insufficient oxygenation
- Deficient Knowledge of caregivers related to the child's illness

Outcome Identification and Planning

The major goals include improving cardiac output and oxygenation, relieving inadequate respirations, maintaining adequate nutritional intake, and conserving energy. The family's goals include increasing understanding of the condition and its prognosis.

Implementation

Monitoring Vital Signs

Monitor vital signs regularly to detect symptoms of decreased cardiac output. Monitor pulse rates closely. Digoxin is frequently ordered for the child. Always check the dosage of digoxin with another nurse before administering it. Observe closely for any signs of digoxin toxicity, such as anorexia, nausea and vomiting, irregular pulse, or decreased pulse rate (**bradycardia**).

Regularly observe the child for evidence of periorbital or peripheral edema. Weigh the undressed child early in the morning before the first feeding of the day, using the same scale every time. Maintain careful intake and output measurements. If diuretics are administered, monitor serum electrolyte levels, especially potassium levels.

> **Here's a pharmacology fact.**
>
> If digoxin is ordered, count the apical pulse for a full minute before administering digoxin. Withhold digoxin and notify the physician if the apical rate is lower than the established norms for the child's age and baseline information (90–110 beats per minute for infants, 70–85 beats per minute for older children).

Improving Respiratory Function

Elevate the head of the crib mattress so that it is at a 30-degree to 45-degree angle. Do not allow the child to shift down in the crib and become "scrunched up," which causes decreased expansion room for the chest. Avoid constricting clothing. Administer oxygen as ordered. Monitor respirations at least every 4 hours, paying close attention to breath sounds, dyspnea, tachypnea, and retractions. Observe the child for cyanosis, especially noting the color of the nail beds and around the mouth, lips, hands, and feet. Monitor oxygen saturation levels with pulse oximetry. Respiratory infections can be a concern for the child with CHF. The child has a decreased resistance to these infections, and exposure to people who have respiratory infections should be avoided. Monitor closely for any signs of infection and report any findings.

Maintaining Adequate Nutrition

Give frequent feedings in small amounts to avoid overtiring the child. For the infant, use a soft nipple with a large opening to ease the child's workload. If adequate nutrition cannot be taken during feedings, gavage feedings may be necessary.

Promoting Energy Conservation

Nursing care is planned so that the child has long periods of uninterrupted rest. While carrying out nursing procedures, talk to the child softly and soothingly and handle him or her gently with care. Respond to the child's cries quickly to avoid tiring the child.

Providing Family Teaching

The family of this child has reason to be apprehensive and anxious. It is important that you are understanding, empathic, and nonjudgmental when communicating with them. Give them information about CHF in a way that they can understand. Repeat information about signs and symptoms and offer explanations as many times as necessary. Include teaching about medication, feeding and care techniques, growth and development expectations, and future plans for correction of the defect, if known. Involve the family in the child's care as much as possible within the limitations of the child's condition.

Evaluation: Goals and Expected Outcomes

Goal: The child's cardiac output will improve and be adequate to meet the child's needs.
Expected Outcomes: The child

- has a heart rate within the normal limits for his or her age.
- is free from arrhythmia or evidence of edema.
- maintains adequate peripheral perfusion.

Goal: The child's respiratory function will improve.
Expected Outcomes: The child's

- respirations are regular with no retractions.
- breath sounds are clear.
- oxygen saturation is within the acceptable range for the child's status.

Goal: The child's caloric intake will be adequate to maintain nutritional needs for growth.
Expected Outcomes: The child

- consumes most of the feeding each time and feeds with minimal tiring.
- has appropriate weight gain for age.

Goal: The child will have increased levels of energy.
Expected Outcomes: The child

- rests quietly during uninterrupted periods of rest.
- does not become overly tired when awake.

Goal: The family caregivers are prepared for the child's home care.
Expected Outcomes: The family

- verbalizes anxieties.
- asks appropriate questions.
- participates in the child's care.
- discusses the child's condition.

RHEUMATIC FEVER

Rheumatic fever is a chronic disease of childhood, affecting the connective tissue of the heart, joints, lungs, and brain. An autoimmune reaction to group A beta-hemolytic streptococcal infections, rheumatic fever occurs throughout the world, particularly in the temperate zones. It has become less common in developed countries, but there have been recent indications of increased occurrences in some areas of the United States.

Rheumatic fever is precipitated by a streptococcal infection, such as strep throat, tonsillitis, scarlet fever, or pharyngitis, which may be undiagnosed or untreated. The resultant rheumatic fever manifestation may be the first indication of trouble. However, an elevation of antistreptococcal antibodies that indicates recent streptococcal infection can be demonstrated in about 95% of the rheumatic fever patients tested within the first 2 months of onset. An antistreptolysin-O titer, or ASO titer, measures these antibodies.

Clinical Manifestations

A latent period of 1 to 5 weeks follows the initial infection. The onset is often slow and subtle. The child may be listless, anorectic, and pale. He or she may lose weight and complain of vague muscle, joint, or abdominal pains. Often there is a low-grade late afternoon fever. None of these is diagnostic by itself, but if such signs persist, the child should have a medical examination.

Major manifestations of rheumatic fever include carditis, polyarthritis, and chorea. The onset may be acute, rather than insidious, with severe carditis or arthritis as the presenting symptom. Chorea (disorder characterized by emotional instability, purposeless movements, and muscular weakness) generally has an insidious onset.

Carditis

Carditis refers to inflammation of the heart. It is the major cause of permanent heart damage and disability among children with rheumatic fever. Carditis may occur alone or as a complication of either arthritis or chorea. Presenting symptoms may be vague enough to be missed. The child may have a poor appetite, pallor, a low-grade fever, listlessness, or moderate anemia. Careful observation may reveal slight dyspnea on exertion. Physical examination shows a soft systolic murmur over the apex of the heart. Unfortunately, such a child may have been in poor physical health for some time before the murmur is discovered.

Acute carditis may be the presenting symptom, particularly in young children. An abrupt onset of high fever (perhaps as high as 104°F [40°C]), tachycardia, pallor, poor pulse quality, and a rapid decrease in hemoglobin are characteristic. Weakness, prostration, cyanosis, and intense precordial pain are common. Cardiac dilation usually occurs. The pericardium, myocardium, or endocardium may be affected.

Polyarthritis

Polyarthritis, or migratory arthritis, moves from one major joint to another (ankles, knees, hips, wrists, elbows, shoulders). The joint becomes painful to either touch or movement (**arthralgia**) and appears hot and swollen. Body temperature is moderately elevated; the erythrocyte sedimentation rate (ESR) is increased. Although extremely painful, this type of arthritis does not lead to the disabling deformities that occur in rheumatoid arthritis.

Chorea

Chorea is a disorder characterized by emotional instability, purposeless movements, and muscular weakness. The onset of chorea is gradual, with increasing incoordination, facial grimaces, and repetitive involuntary movements. Movements may be mild and remain so, or they may become increasingly severe. Active arthritis is rarely present when chorea is the major manifestation. Carditis occurs, although less commonly than when polyarthritis is the major condition. Attacks tend to be recurrent and prolonged, but are rare after puberty. It is seldom possible to demonstrate an increase in the antistreptococcal antibody level because of the generally prolonged latency period.

Diagnosis

Rheumatic fever is difficult to diagnose and sometimes impossible to differentiate from other diseases. The possible serious effects of the disease demand early and conscientious medical treatment. However, avoid causing apprehension and disruption of the child's life because the condition could prove to be something less serious. Do not attempt a diagnosis yourself, but understand the criteria on which a presumptive diagnosis is based.

The modified Jones criteria (Fig. 37-2) are generally accepted as a useful rule for guidance when deciding whether or not to treat the patient for rheumatic fever. The criteria are divided into major and minor categories. The presence of two major or one major and two minor criteria indicates a high probability of rheumatic fever if supported by evidence of a preceding streptococcal infection. This system is not infallible; however, because

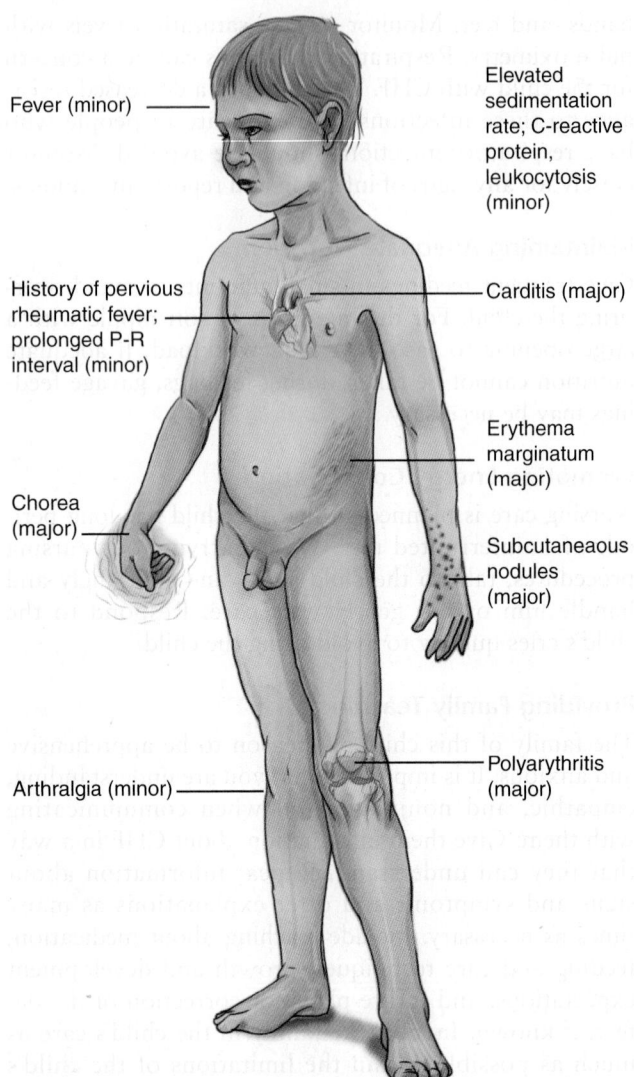

Fever (minor)

Elevated sedimentation rate; C-reactive protein, leukocytosis (minor)

History of pervious rheumatic fever; prolonged P-R interval (minor)

Carditis (major)

Erythema marginatum (major)

Chorea (major)

Subcutaneaous nodules (major)

Polyarythritis (major)

Arthralgia (minor)

■ **Figure 37-2** Major and minor manifestations of rheumatic fever.

no one criterion is specific to the disease, additional manifestations can help confirm the diagnosis.

Treatment

The chief concern in caring for a child with rheumatic fever is the prevention of residual heart disease. Bed rest is ordered, and the length of bed rest is determined by the degree of carditis present. This may be from 2 weeks to several weeks, depending on how long heart failure is present.

Residual heart disease is treated in accordance with its severity and its type with digitalis, restricted activities, diuretics, and a low-sodium diet, as indicated.

> **This could make a difference.**
>
> As long as the rheumatic process is active, progressive heart damage is possible, so bed rest is essential for the child with rheumatic fever to reduce the heart's workload.

Laboratory tests, although nonspecific, provide an evaluation of the disease activity to guide treatment. Two commonly used indicators are the ESR and the presence of C-reactive protein. The ESR is elevated in the presence of an inflammatory process and is nearly always increased in the polyarthritis or carditis manifestation of rheumatic fever. It remains elevated until clinical manifestations have ceased and any subclinical activity has subsided. It seldom increases in uncomplicated chorea. Therefore, ESR elevation in a choreic patient may indicate cardiac involvement.

C-reactive protein in the body indicates an inflammatory process is occurring. It appears in the serum of acutely ill people, including people ill with rheumatic fever. As the patient improves, C-reactive protein decreases or disappears.

Leukocytosis is also an indication of an inflammatory process. Until the leukocyte count returns to a normal level, the disease probably is still active.

Medications used in the treatment of rheumatic fever include penicillin, salicylates, and corticosteroids. Penicillin is administered to eliminate the hemolytic streptococci. If the child is allergic to penicillin, erythromycin is used. Penicillin administration continues after the acute phase of the illness to prevent the recurrence of rheumatic fever.

Here's a pharmacology fact.

Ensure that the child takes the complete prescription of penicillin (usually 10 days' supply). Even though the symptoms disappear and the child feels well, the infection can return if the entire course of antibiotics is not taken.

Salicylates are given in the form of acetylsalicylic acid (aspirin) to children, with the daily dosage calculated according to the child's weight. Aspirin relieves pain and reduces the inflammation of polyarthritis. It is also used for its antipyretic effect. The continued administration of a relatively large dosage may cause toxic effects; individual tolerance differs greatly.

For mild or severe carditis, corticosteroids appear to be the drug of choice because of their prompt and dramatic action.

Administration of salicylates or corticosteroids is not expected to alter the course of the disease, but the control of the toxic manifestations enhances the child's comfort and sense of well-being and helps reduce the burden on the heart. This is of particular importance in acute carditis with CHF. Diuretics may be administered when needed in severe carditis.

Corticosteroids and salicylates are of little value in the treatment of uncomplicated chorea. The child may be sedated with phenobarbital, chlorpromazine (Thorazine), haloperidol (Haldol), or diazepam (Valium). Bed rest is necessary, with protection such as padding of the sides of the bed if the movements are severe.

Prevention

Because the peak of onset of rheumatic fever occurs in school-aged children, health services for this age group take on added importance. The overall approach is to promote continuous health supervision for all children, including the school-aged child. The use of well-child conferences or clinics needs to increase to provide continuity of care for children. If you have contact in any way with school-aged children, you must be aware of the importance of teaching the public about the need to have upper respiratory infections evaluated for group A beta-hemolytic streptococcus and the need for treatment with penicillin.

Test Yourself

✔ What are the common symptoms and treatments for CHF?

✔ What type of infection would likely be found in the history of a child who has rheumatic fever?

✔ Explain the terms carditis, polyarthritis, and chorea.

✔ What are two important aspects in the prevention of rheumatic fever?

Nursing Process for the Child With Rheumatic Fever

Assessment

Conduct a thorough exam of the child. Begin with a careful review of all systems, and note the child's physical condition. Observe for any signs that may be classified as major or minor manifestations. In the physical exam, observe for elevated temperature and pulse and carefully examine for erythema marginatum, subcutaneous nodules, swollen or painful joints, or signs of chorea. A throat culture determines whether there is an active infection. Obtain a complete up-to-date history from the child and the caregiver. Ask about a recent sore throat or upper respiratory infection. Find out when the symptoms began, the extent of the illness, and what if any treatment was obtained. Include the school-aged child in the nursing interview to help contribute to the history.

Selected Nursing Diagnoses

- Acute Pain related to joint pain when extremities are touched or moved
- Deficient Diversional Activity related to prescribed bed rest
- Activity Intolerance related to carditis or arthralgia
- Risk for Injury related to chorea
- Risk for Noncompliance with prophylactic drug therapy related to financial or emotional burden of lifelong therapy
- Deficient Knowledge of caregiver related to the condition, need for long-term therapy, and risk factors

Outcome Identification and Planning

The goals are determined in cooperation with the child and the caregiver. Goals for the child include reducing pain, providing diversional activities and sensory stimulation, conserving energy, and preventing injury. Goals for the caregiver include complying with drug therapy and increasing knowledge about the long-term care of the child. Throughout planning and implementation, bear in mind the child's developmental stage.

Implementation

Providing Comfort Measures and Reducing Pain

Position the child to relieve joint pain. Large joints, including the knees, ankles, wrists, and elbows are usually involved. Carefully handle the joints when moving the child to help minimize pain. Warm baths and gentle range-of-motion exercises help to alleviate some of joint discomfort. Use pain indicator scales with children so they are able to express the level of their pain (see Fig. 29-8, Chapter 29).

Watch out.
Even the weight of blankets may cause pain for the child with rheumatic fever. Be alert to this possibility and improvise covering as needed.

Salicylates are administered in the form of aspirin to reduce fever and relieve joint inflammation and pain. Although salicylates as a general rule are not given to children, they continue to be the treatment of choice for rheumatic fever. Because of the risks of long-term administration of salicylates, note any signs of toxicity and record and report them promptly. Administer aspirin after meals or with a glass of milk to lessen gastrointestinal irritation. Enteric-coated aspirin is also available for patients who are sensitive to the effects of aspirin. Large doses may alter the prothrombin time and thus interfere with the clotting mechanism. Salicylate therapy is usually continued until all laboratory findings are normal.

Here's a pharmacology fact.
Tinnitus, nausea, vomiting, and headache are all important signs of toxicity when administering aspirin. Observe closely and report any of these symptoms.

The child whose pain is not controlled with salicylates may be administered corticosteroids. Side effects, such as **hirsutism** (abnormal hair growth) and "moon face," may be upsetting to the child and family. Toxic reactions, such as euphoria, insomnia, gastric irritation, and growth suppression, must be watched for and reported. Because premature withdrawal of a steroid drug is likely to cause a relapse, it is important to discontinue use of the drug gradually by decreasing dosages.

Providing Diversional Activities and Sensory Stimulation

Children vary greatly in how ill they feel during the acute phase of rheumatic fever. For those who do not feel very ill, bed rest can cause distress or resentment. Be creative in finding diversional activities that allow bed rest, but prevent restlessness and boredom. This may be a good time to choose a book that involves the child's imagination and that has enough excitement to create ongoing interest. Do not use the television as an all-day baby-sitter. Quiet games can provide some entertainment. Use of a computer can be beneficial, because both entertaining and educational games are available, and most children enjoy working with a computer. Simple needlework and model building are other useful diversional activities. Make efforts during the school year (or encourage the caregiver) to provide the child with a tutor and work from school; this helps relieve boredom and also maintains contact with peers. Plan all activities with the child's developmental stage in mind. The pain of arthralgia may be so great that the child will not want to be involved in any kind of activity. Administer analgesics as ordered to help decrease the inflammation of the joints and decrease the pain, so the child will want to participate in age-appropriate activities.

Promoting Energy Conservation

Provide rest periods between activities to help pace the child's energies and provide for maximum comfort. During times of increased cardiac involvement or exacerbations of joint pain, the child may want to rest and perhaps have someone read a story. Peers may be encouraged to visit, but these visits must be monitored so that the child is not overly tired. The child's classmates could be encouraged to write to the child to provide contact with everyday school activities and keep the child in touch. If the child has chorea, inform visitors that the child cannot control these movements, which may be as upsetting to others as they are to the child.

Preventing Injury

The child with chorea may be frustrated with his or her inability to control the movements. Provide an opportunity for the child to express feelings. Protect the child from injury by keeping the side rails up and padding them. Do not leave a child with chorea unattended in a wheelchair. Use all appropriate safety measures.

Promoting Compliance With Drug Therapy

A child does not become immune from future attacks of rheumatic fever after the first illness. Rheumatic fever can recur whenever the child has a group A beta-hemolytic streptococcal infection if the child is not properly treated. For this reason, the child who has had rheumatic fever must be maintained on prophylactic doses of penicillin for 5 years or longer. Whenever the child is to have oral surgery, including dental work, extra prophylactic precautions should be taken, even in adulthood. Because of this long-term therapy, noncompliance for both financial and emotional reasons can become a problem. Oral penicillin is usually prescribed, but if compliance is poor, monthly injections of Bicillin can be substituted. Encourage the family to contact the local chapter of the American Heart Association (Web site: www.american-heart.org) for help finding economical sources of penicillin. Become informed about other resources that may be available in your community. Emphasize to the child and the family the need to prevent recurrence of the disease because of the danger of heart damage. Follow-up care must be ongoing, even into adulthood.

Providing Family Teaching

Inform the family and child about the importance of having all upper respiratory infections checked by a health care provider to prevent another episode of a streptococcal infection. Be certain that they understand the child can have recurrences and that a future recurrence could have much more serious effects. If the child has had carditis and heart damage has occurred, instruct the caregiver that the child must receive regular follow-up evaluations of the damage. The child may need to be maintained on cardiac medications. Instruct the family about these medications. Mitral valve dysfunction is a common aftereffect of severe carditis. A girl who has had mitral valve damage from cardiac involvement may have problems in adulthood during pregnancy. Inform the caregiver that heart failure for such a girl is a possibility during pregnancy and that she should be monitored closely to determine heart problems in the event that a mitral valve replacement is needed.

Teaching time is an excellent opportunity to stress the importance of preventing rheumatic fever. Other children in the family may benefit if caregivers are given this information.

Evaluation: Goals and Expected Outcomes

Goal: The child's joint pain will be minimal.
Expected Outcome:

- The child verbalizes or indicates, by using a pain scale to express degree of pain, that the pain level is decreased.

Goal: The child will become engaged in activities while on bed rest.
Expected Outcomes: The child

- displays interest in participating in activities.
- is actively involved in age-appropriate activities.

Goal: The child will learn when and how to conserve energy.
Expected Outcomes: The child

- rests quietly during rest periods.
- identifies when he or she needs rest.
- engages in quiet diversional activities.

Goal: The child will remain free of injury from chorea movements and a safe environment is maintained.
Expected Outcomes: The child

- has no evidence of injury.
- follows safety measures.

Goal: The family caregivers will comply with follow-up drug therapy, and the child will take prophylactic medications.
Expected Outcomes: The child and family caregivers

- verbalize an understanding of the importance of prophylactic medication.
- identify means for obtaining medications.

Goal: The family caregivers will verbalize an understanding of the child's condition, need for long-term therapy, and risk factors.
Expected Outcomes: The caregivers

- discuss the child's condition and need for follow-up care for the child.
- indicate how they will obtain follow-up care.

KAWASAKI DISEASE

Kawasaki disease (mucocutaneous lymph node syndrome) is an acute, febrile disease that is most often seen in boys younger than 5 years of age. The etiology is unknown, but the disease appears to be caused by an infectious agent. After an infection, an alteration in the immune system occurs. Most cases occur in the late winter or early spring. The major concern for the child is development of cardiac involvement.

Clinical Manifestations

An elevated temperature (102°F–104°F [38.8°C–40°C]) is noted from the first day of the illness and may continue 1 to 3 weeks. Irritability; lethargy; inflammation in the conjunctiva in both eyes; strawberry colored tongue; dry, red, cracked lips; edema in the hands and feet; and red, swollen joints are seen. The skin on the fingers and toes peels in layers, and a rash covers the trunk and extremities. Cervical lymph nodes may be enlarged. Inflammation of the arteries, veins, and capillaries occurs, and this inflammation can lead to serious cardiac concerns, including aneurysms and thrombus. The child may report abdominal pain. The disease occurs in three stages:

- Acute—high fever that does not respond to antibiotics or antipyretics; child is irritable.
- Subacute—fever resolves, irritability continues; greatest risk for aneurysms.
- Convalescent—symptoms are gone; phase continues until lab values are normal and child's energy, appetite, and temperament have returned.

Diagnosis

For Kawasaki disease to be diagnosed, the child must have an elevated temperature and four of the following symptoms: cervical lymphadenopathy; conjunctivitis; dry, swollen, cracked lips; strawberry tongue; aneurysm; abdominal pain; peeling of hands and feet; trunk rash; or red, swollen joints. The WBC and ESR are elevated. During the subacute stage, the platelet count increases, this may lead to blood clotting and cardiac problems. Echocardiograms may show cardiac involvement.

Treatment and Nursing Care

A high dose of intravenous immunoglobulin therapy is given to relieve the symptoms and prevent coronary artery abnormalities. Aspirin is used to control inflammation and fever and is continued for as long as 1 year in lower doses as an antiplatelet.

Nursing care for the child with Kawasaki disease focuses on management of the symptoms. It is important that you relieve pain, discomfort, and itching. Closely monitor temperature, cardiac status, intake and output, and daily weight. Offer extra fluids and soft foods, and provide mouth and lip care to help decrease the soreness. Encourage use of passive range-of-motion exercises that increase joint movement. Dealing with the irritability may be difficult for you as well as the child's family. Promote rest and a quiet environment to help decrease irritability. It is essential that you encourage the parents to have times away from the child to help them cope with the stress of the illness. Include in discharge teaching information regarding the disease and symptoms, which may persist for a period of time. Also, discuss follow-up treatments, visits, medication routines, and side effects. Most children recover without long-term effects, but the cardiac involvement may not be seen for a period of time after the child's recovery.

Do you know the why of it?

Immunizations, especially live vaccines, such as measles, mumps, and rubella (MMR), should not be given for 3 to 6 months to a child who has been treated with immunoglobulin. The immunoglobulin prevents the body from building antibodies, so the vaccine will likely be ineffective in preventing the disease it is being given to prevent.

IRON DEFICIENCY ANEMIA

Iron deficiency anemia is a common nutritional deficiency in children. It is a hypochromic, microcytic anemia—in other words, the blood cells are deficient in production of hemoglobin and are smaller than normal—and is common between the ages of 9 and 24 months. The full-term newborn has a high hemoglobin level (needed during fetal life to provide adequate oxygenation) that decreases during the first 2 or 3 months of life. Considerable iron is reclaimed and stored, however, usually in sufficient quantity to last for 4 to 9 months of life.

A child needs to absorb 0.8 to 1.5 mg of iron per day. Because only 10% of dietary iron is absorbed, a diet containing 8 to 10 mg of iron is needed for good health. During the first years of life, obtaining this quantity of iron from food is often difficult for a child. If the diet is inadequate, anemia quickly results. (In addition, adolescent girls may have iron deficiency anemia because of improper dieting to lose weight.)

Babies with an inordinate fondness for milk can take in an astonishing amount and, with their appetites satisfied, show little interest in solid foods. These babies are prime candidates for iron deficiency anemia. They may have a history of consuming 2 or 3 quarts of milk daily while not accepting any other foods or, at best, only foods with a high carbohydrate content. Many caregivers incorrectly believe that milk is a perfect food and that they should let the baby have all the milk desired. These children are commonly known as milk babies. They have pale, almost translucent (porcelainlike) skin and are chubby and susceptible to infections.

Many children with iron deficiency anemia, however, are undernourished because of the family's economic problems. Along with the economic factor, a caregiver's knowledge deficit about nutrition is often present. The Women, Infants, and Children (WIC) program, discussed in Chapter 23, does much to alleviate this problem.

Clinical Manifestations

The signs of iron deficiency anemia include below-average body weight, pale mucous membranes, anorexia, growth retardation, and listlessness, in addition to the characteristics of milk babies described earlier.

Diagnosis

In blood tests that measure hemoglobin, a level <11 g/dL or a hematocrit <33% is highly suspect. Stool is tested for occult blood to rule out low gastrointestinal bleeding as a cause for the depleted hemoglobin and hematocrit.

Treatment and Nursing Care

Treatment consists of improved nutrition, with ferrous sulfate administered between meals with juice (preferably orange juice, because vitamin C aids in iron absorption). For best results, iron should not be given with meals. Tell the caregivers that ferrous sulfate can cause constipation or turn the child's stools black.

A few children have a hemoglobin level so low or anorexia so acute that they need additional therapy. An iron–dextran mixture (Imferon) for intramuscular use is administered. Because of its irritating nature, this medication should be administered in the vastus lateralis by the Z-track method to

Here's a tip to share with family caregivers.

To prevent staining, brush the child's teeth after administering iron preparations, such as ferrous sulfate.

Family Teaching Tips

IRON DEFICIENCY ANEMIA

- One of the most important things you can do for your child and family is to learn about the foods that will help them stay healthy.
- Milk is good for your child, but no more than a quart a day (four 8-oz bottles for the infant).
- Liquid iron preparations should be taken through a straw to prevent staining of teeth.

FOODS HIGH IN IRON

- Baby cereals fortified with iron.
- For older children, fortified instant oatmeal and cream of wheat are good sources of iron.
- Some infant formulas are iron fortified.
- Egg yolks are rich in iron. Avoid egg whites for young children because of allergies.
- Green, leafy vegetables are good sources of iron.
- Dried beans, dried peas, canned refried beans, and peanut butter provide good iron sources for toddlers and older children.
- Fruits that are iron-rich include peaches, prune juice, and raisins (do not give to a child younger than 3 years of age because of danger of choking).
- Read labels to check for iron content of processed foods.
- Organ meat, poultry, and fish are good iron sources.
- Orange juice helps the body absorb iron.

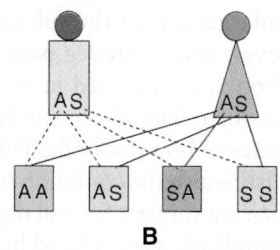

■ **Figure 37-3** Inheritance patterns. **(A)** Heterozygous type. One parent carries a hemoglobin S gene, and one does not. Two children will be free of the gene (AA), and two will be carriers (AS). **(B)** Homozygous type. Each parent is carrying one hemoglobin A gene and one hemoglobin S gene. One child is free of the gene (AA), two are carriers (AS), and one has sickle cell disease (SS).

avoid leakage into the subcutaneous tissues. For children who are seriously ill, refer to Nursing Process for the Child With Nutritional Problems in Chapter 38.

For most children with iron deficiency anemia, teaching for home care is needed. When teaching caregivers, remember that attitudes and food choices are often influenced by cultural differences. See Family Teaching Tips: Iron Deficiency Anemia.

SICKLE CELL DISEASE

Sickle cell disease is a hereditary trait occurring most commonly in African Americans. It is characterized by the production of abnormal hemoglobin that causes the red blood cells to assume a sickle shape. It appears as an asymptomatic trait when the sickling trait is inherited from one parent alone (heterozygous state). There is a 50% probability that each child born to one parent carrying the sickle cell trait will inherit the trait from that parent. When the trait is inherited from both parents (homozygous state), the child has sickle cell disease and anemia develops (Fig. 37-3). A rapid breakdown of red blood cells carrying hemoglobin S, the abnormal hemoglobin, causes a severe hemolytic anemia. Persons who inherit the gene for the sickle cell trait from only one

parent have no symptoms, normal hemoglobin levels, and normal red blood cell counts.

The sickling trait occurs in about 10% of African Americans; there is a much higher incidence in parts of Africa. In African Americans, the disease itself, sickle cell anemia, has an incidence of 0.3% to 1.3%. The tendency to sickle can be demonstrated by a laboratory test.

Clinical Manifestations

Clinical symptoms of the disease usually do not appear before the latter half of the first year of life because sufficient fetal hemoglobin is still present to prevent sickling. Sickle cell disease causes a chronic anemia, with a hemoglobin level of 6 to 9 g/dL (the normal level in an infant is 11–15 g/dL). The chronic anemia causes the child to be tired and have a poor appetite and pale mucous membranes.

Sickle cell crisis is the most severe manifestation of the condition. Normal red blood cells, which carry oxygen to the tissues, are disc shaped and normally move through the blood vessels while bending and flexing to flow through smoothly. The smooth, uniform shape of the red blood cells and the low viscosity (thickness) of the blood is such that these cells split relatively easily at Y-intersections and go single file through the capillaries with little or no clustering. The affected red blood cells (hemoglobin S) do much the same thing until an episode causes sickling. An episode (sickle cell crises) can be precipitated by low oxygen levels, which can be caused by a respiratory infection or extremely strenuous exercise, dehydration, acidosis, or stress. When sickling occurs, the affected red blood cells become crescent-shaped and, therefore, do not slip through as easily as do the disc-shaped cells. The viscosity of the blood increases (becomes thicker), causing slowdown and sludging of the red blood cells. The impaired circulation results in tissue damage and infarction.

A sickle cell crisis may be the first clinical manifestation of the disease and may recur frequently during early childhood. This disturbance presents a variety of symptoms. The most common symptom is severe, acute abdominal pain (caused by sludging, which leads to enlargement of the spleen) together with muscle spasm; fever; and severe leg pain that may be muscular, osseous (bony), or localized in the joints, which become hot and swollen. The abdomen becomes boardlike with an absence of bowel sounds. This makes it extremely difficult to distinguish the condition from an abdominal condition requiring surgery. Several days after a crisis, the child will be jaundiced, as evidenced by yellow sclera, as a result of the hemolysis. The crisis may have a fatal outcome caused by cerebral, cardiac, or hemolytic complications.

Diagnosis

Screening for the presence of hemoglobin S may be done with a test called Sickledex, a fingerstick screening test that gives results in 3 minutes. Definite diagnosis is made through hemoglobin electrophoresis ("fingerprinting"). If the Sickledex screening results are positive, diagnosis can be done to determine if the child is carrying the trait or has sickle cell disease.

Treatment

Prevention of crises is the goal between episodes. Adequate hydration is vital; fluid intake of 1,500 to 2,000 mL daily is desirable for a child weighing 20 kg and should be increased to 3,000 mL during the crisis. The child should avoid extremely strenuous activities that may cause oxygen depletion. These children should also avoid visiting areas of high altitude. Small blood transfusions help bring the hemoglobin to a near-normal level, temporarily. Iron preparations have no effect in sickle cell disease.

Treatment for a crisis is supportive for each presenting symptom, and bed rest is indicated. Oxygen may be administered. Analgesics are given for pain. Dehydration and acidosis are vigorously treated. Prognosis is guarded, depending on the severity of the disease.

Nursing Process for the Child With Sickle Cell Crisis

Assessment

The parents who have a child with sickle cell disease may experience a great deal of guilt for having passed the disease to their child. Take care not to increase this guilt, but help them cope with it. During the interview with the family caregivers, ask about activities or events that led to this crisis, obtain a history of the child's health and any previous episodes, and evaluate the caregivers' knowledge about the condition.

Data collection techniques vary somewhat, depending on the child's age. Record vital signs, particularly noting fever, abdominal pain, presence of bowel sounds, pain or swelling and warmth in the joints, and muscle spasms. Observe the young child for dactylitis (hand–foot syndrome), which results from soft-tissue swelling caused by interference with circulation. This swelling further impairs circulation.

Selected Nursing Diagnoses

- Acute Pain related to disease condition affecting abdominal organs or joints and muscles
- Deficient Fluid Volume related to low fluid intake, impaired renal function, or both
- Activity Intolerance related to oxygen depletion and pain
- Impaired Physical Mobility related to muscle and joint involvement
- Risk for Impaired Skin Integrity related to altered circulation
- Compromised Family Coping related to child's condition
- Deficient Knowledge of caregivers related to understanding of disorder and appropriate care measures

Outcome Identification and Planning

Maintaining comfort and relieving pain, increasing fluid intake, and conserving energy are major goals for the child with sickle cell disease. Other goals include improving physical mobility, maintaining skin integrity, and reducing the caregivers' anxiety. Another important goal is decreasing the number of future episodes by increasing the caregiver's knowledge about the causes of crisis episodes. Plan individualized nursing care according to these goals.

Implementation

Relieving Pain

The child in sickle cell crisis often has severe abdominal pain because of enlargement of the spleen (splenomegaly). Joint and muscle pain are also common because of poor perfusion of the tissues. Monitor the child's pain level, use nursing measures to relieve pain, and provide prompt administration of analgesics. The family caregivers can be involved, if they wish, in helping administer comfort measures to the child. Sometimes diverting activities can help alleviate perceived pain.

> **This is critical to remember.**
> Be assured that children with sickle cell anemia are in pain and need analgesics promptly.

Maintaining Fluid Intake

The child is prone to dehydration because of the kidneys' inability to concentrate urine. Observe for signs of dehydration, such as dry mucous membranes, weight loss, or, in the case of infants, sunken fontanelles. Strict intake and output measurements and daily weights are necessary. In sickle cell crisis, urine specific gravity is not a good indicator of dehydration. Teach the family caregivers that fluid intake is important, and intake should be maintained at 1,500 to 2,000 mL when the child is not in crisis. Offer the child appealing fluids, such as juices, popsicles, non-caffeinated soda, and favorite flavored gelatins. Teach family caregivers that increasing fluid intake as the child ages will help to avoid a crisis during the child's activities such as hiking, swimming, and sports. The child also needs increased fluids during episodes of infections.

Promoting Energy Conservation

The child may become dyspneic doing any kind of activity. Plan nursing care so that the child is disturbed as little as possible and can rest. Bed rest is necessary to decrease the demands of oxygen supply. Oxygen may be administered by mask or nasal cannula to improve tissue perfusion.

Improving Physical Mobility

Sickling that affects the muscles and joints causes a great deal of pain for the child. The child needs careful handling and should be moved slowly and gently. Joints can be supported with pillows. Warm soaks and massages may help relieve some of the discomfort. Administer analgesics before exercise and as needed. Passive exercises help prevent contractures and wasting of muscles.

Promoting Skin Integrity

Increased fluid intake and improved nutrition are important. Observe the child's skin regularly each shift, and provide good skin care consisting of lotion, massage, and skin-toughening agents, especially over bony prominences. Additional padding in the form of foam protectors and egg-crate pads or mattresses may be helpful when there is irritation from bedding.

Promoting Family Coping

Guilt plays an important part in the anxiety that the family caregivers experience. Explain procedures, planned treatments, and care to help the caregivers feel that they are being included in the care. Caregivers need to feel that they have some control over the disease.

Providing Family Teaching

Teach measures that may help alleviate pain or encourage fluid intake. Also, emphasize the importance of protecting the child from situations that may cause overexhaustion or that may otherwise deplete the child's oxygen supplies or lead to dehydration. This knowledge may give the family caregivers a feeling of control. In addition, caregivers may need more information concerning the disorder. If the child's diagnosis is not new, the caregivers should already have had information presented to them. In this instance, determine their knowledge level and supplement and reinforce that information.

Evaluation: Goals and Expected Outcomes

Goal: The child's pain will be reduced or eliminated.
Expected Outcome:

- The child rests quietly and, if possible, reports his or her comfort.

Goal: The child's fluid intake will improve.
Expected Outcome:

- The child has an intake of at least 3,000 mL/day.

Goal: The child's energy will be conserved.
Expected Outcomes: The child's

- activities are restricted to conserve energy.
- oxygen saturation is >90%.

Goal: The child's muscles and joints will remain flexible.
Expected Outcome:

- The child cooperates with daily passive exercises.

Goal: The child's skin integrity will be maintained.
Expected Outcome:

- The child's skin shows no signs of redness, irritation, or breakdown.

Goal: The family caregivers' anxiety will be reduced.
Expected Outcomes: The family caregivers

- exhibit self-confidence.
- cooperate with nursing personnel.

Goal: The family caregivers will express understanding of the disease process.
Expected Outcomes: The family caregivers

- verbalize an understanding of the disease process.
- state ways to prevent a crisis from occurring.

Cultural Snapshot

In working with children and families of children who have disorders that are passed through genetics, it is important that genetic counseling be done in a sensitive, nonthreatening manner. Some cultures believe that the mother or the parents caused a hereditary disease because of certain behaviors or actions. The parents often feel guilty, so a sensitive, objective approach is essential.

Test Yourself

✔ What are some reasons iron deficiency anemias might be seen in infants?
✔ Explain the shape of the red blood cell and how it affects the child with sickle cell anemia.
✔ What is the most common symptom in the child with a sickle cell crisis?

THALASSEMIA

The thalassemia blood disorders are inherited mild to severe anemias in which the hemoglobin production is abnormal. Thalassemia major (Cooley's anemia) presents in childhood and is the most common. The disorder

■ **Figure 37-4** The mechanism of the formation of a blood clot is complex.

often occurs in people of Mediterranean descent, but may also be seen in other populations.

Clinical Manifestations

Anemia, fatigue, pallor, irritability, and anorexia are noted in children with thalassemia. Bone pain and fractures are seen. Many body systems can be affected, including enlargement of the spleen, overstimulation of bone marrow, and heart failure. The liver, gallbladder, and pancreas can also be involved. The skin may appear bronze-colored or jaundiced. Skeletal changes occur, including deformities of the face and skull. The upper teeth protrude, the nose is broad and flat, and the eyes are slanted.

Treatment and Nursing Care

Blood transfusions maintain the hemoglobin levels, diet and medications are used to prevent heart failure, and splenectomy or bone marrow transplants may be necessary. Frequent transfusions can lead to complications and additional concerns for the child, including the possibility of iron overload. For these children, iron-chelating drugs such as deferoxamine mesylate (Desferal) may be given. Slowed growth and delayed sexual maturation may cause the child to feel self-conscious. Child and family support is important because of the chronic nature, long-term treatment, and poor outcome of the disease. Even with treatment, the prognosis is poor, and the child often dies of cardiac failure.

HEMOPHILIA

Hemophilia is one of the oldest known hereditary diseases. Recent research has demonstrated that hemophilia is a syndrome of several distinct inborn errors of metabolism; all result in the delayed coagulation of blood. Defects in protein synthesis lead to deficiencies in any of the factors in the blood plasma needed for thromboplastic activity. The principal factors involved are factors VIII, IX, and XI.

Mechanism of Clot Formation

The mechanism of clot formation is complex. In a simplified form, it can best be described as occurring in three stages:

1. Prothrombin is formed through plasma–platelet interaction.
2. Prothrombin is converted to thrombin.
3. Fibrinogen is converted into fibrin by thrombin.

Fibrin forms a mesh that traps RBCs and WBCs and platelets into a clot, closing the defect in the injured vessel. A deficiency in one of the thromboplastin precursors may lead to hemophilia. This progression of events is shown in Figure 37-4

Refer to a specialized text on the circulatory system for a detailed discussion of the clot-forming mechanism.

Common Types of Hemophilia

The two most common types of hemophilia are factor VIII deficiency and factor IX deficiency. These two types are briefly presented in this chapter.

Factor VIII Deficiency

Factor VIII deficiency includes hemophilia A, antihemophilic globulin deficiency, and classic hemophilia. Classic hemophilia is inherited as a sex-linked recessive Mendelian trait, with transmission to affected males by carrier females. Hemophilia A (classic hemophilia), the most common type, occurs in about 1 in 10,000 people and is also the most severe. It is caused by a deficiency of antihemophilic globulin C, which is the factor VIII necessary for blood clotting.

Factor IX Deficiency

Factor IX deficiency includes hemophilia B, plasma thromboplastin component deficiency, and Christmas disease. Christmas disease was named after a 5-year-old boy who was one of the first patients diagnosed with a deficiency of factor IX. This deficiency constitutes about

15% of the hemophilias. It is a sex-linked recessive trait appearing in male offspring of carrier females and is caused by a deficiency of one of the necessary thromboplastin precursors: factor IX, the plasma thromboplastin component. Hemophilia B is indistinguishable from classic hemophilia in its clinical manifestations, particularly in its severe form. It also may exist in a mild form, probably more commonly than in hemophilia A. In either hemophilia A or B, 25% or more of the affected people can trace no family history of the disease; it is assumed that spontaneous mutations have occurred in some cases.

Clinical Manifestations

All types of hemophilia are characterized by prolonged bleeding, with frequent hemorrhages externally and into the skin, the joint spaces, and the intramuscular tissues. Bleeding from tooth extractions, brain hemorrhages, and crippling disabilities are serious complications. Death during infancy or early childhood is not unusual in severe hemophilia and results from a great loss of blood, intracranial bleeding, or respiratory obstruction caused by bleeding into the neck tissues.

An infant with hemophilia who is beginning to creep or walk bruises easily, and serious hemorrhages may result from minor lacerations. Bleeding often occurs from lip biting or from sharp objects put in the mouth. Tooth eruption seldom causes bleeding, but extractions require specialized handling and should be avoided by preventive care, if possible. However, family caregivers must avoid overprotecting the child. The preschooler is active and plays hard, and injuries are practically unavoidable. Clinical manifestations in any type of hemophilia are similar and are treated by administration of the deficient factor and by measures to prevent or treat complications. In severe bleeding, the quantities of fresh blood or frozen plasma needed may easily overload the circulatory system. Administration of factor VIII concentrate eliminates this problem.

Diagnosis

A careful examination of the family history and the type of bleeding present is conducted. Abnormal bleeding beginning in infancy when combined with a positive family history suggests hemophilia. A markedly prolonged clotting time is characteristic of severe factor VIII or IX deficiency, but mild conditions may have only a slightly prolonged clotting time. The partial prothrombin time is the test that most clearly demonstrates that factor VIII is low.

Treatment

For many years, the only treatment for bleeding in hemophilia was the use of fresh blood or plasma. When fresh-frozen plasma came into use, it became the mainstay in hemophilia management. It has been particularly helpful in emergencies. Frozen plasma, however, does have several shortcomings. One major problem has been the large volumes needed to control bleeding. Another is the danger that injections of large amounts of plasma may lead to CHF. In addition, plasma must be given within 30 minutes because factor VIII loses its potency at room temperature.

Commercial preparations are now available that supply higher-potency factor VIII than previous preparations. These concentrates are supplied in dried form together with diluent for reconstitution. Directions for mixing and administration are included with the package. The preparations can be stored for a long time but have the disadvantage of exposing the recipient to a large number of donors. A synthetic preparation, DDAVP (1-deamino-8-D-arginine vasopressin), is used in mild factor VIII deficiencies and von Willebrand disease. Von Willebrand disease (vascular hemophilia; pseudohemophilia) is classified with the hemophilias. It is a Mendelian-dominant trait present in both sexes and is characterized by prolonged bleeding times.

One of the serious problems with using blood products of any kind has been the risk of exposure to hepatitis B and human immunodeficiency virus (HIV), the causative organism of acquired immunodeficiency syndrome (AIDS). Currently, blood is screened thoroughly for viral contamination, which greatly diminishes the danger of HIV transmission. However, large numbers of hemophiliacs treated before the late 1980s were exposed to HIV and now test positive for HIV antibodies. Researchers continue to explore new ways to replace the missing factor while protecting the recipient from the threat of contracting an unknown illness.

Nursing Process for the Child With Hemophilia

Assessment

Begin the nursing data collection by reviewing the child's history with the caregiver. Include previous episodes of bleeding, the usual treatment, medications the child takes, and the current episode of bleeding. Include the child in the interview if he or she is old enough to answer questions. Carefully observe the child for any signs of bleeding. Inspect the mucous membranes, examine the joints for tenderness and swelling, and check the skin for evidence of bruising. Question the child or caregiver about hematuria, hematemesis, headache, or black tarry stools.

Selected Nursing Diagnoses

- Acute Pain related to joint swelling and limitations secondary to hemarthrosis
- Impaired Physical Mobility related to pain and tenderness of joints
- Risk for Injury related to hemorrhage secondary to trauma
- Deficient Knowledge related to condition, treatments, and hazards
- Compromised Family Coping related to treatment and care of the child

Outcome Identification and Planning

Use the information gathered to set goals with the cooperation and input of the caregiver and the child. The major goals for the child include stopping the bleeding, decreasing pain, increasing mobility, and preventing injury. The family caregiver goals include increasing knowledge about the child's condition and care and helping the family learn to cope with the disease condition.

Implementation

Relieving Pain

Bleeding into the joint cavities often occurs after some slight injury and seems nearly unavoidable if the child is allowed to lead a normal life. Extreme pain is caused by the pressure of the confined fluid in the narrow joint spaces and requires the use of sedatives or narcotics. Promptly immobilize the involved extremity to prevent contractures of soft tissues and the destruction of the bone and joint tissues. Immobilization helps to relieve pain and decrease bleeding. A bivalve plaster cast may be applied in the hospital to immobilize the affected part.

Although aspirin and most nonsteroidal anti-inflammatory drugs (NSAIDs) are not given to children with hemophilia, ibuprofen, also an NSAID, has been proven safe for these children. Use of cold packs to stop bleeding is acceptable. The affected limb may be elevated above the level of the heart to slow blood flow. Use age-appropriate diversionary activities to help the child deal with the pain. Handle the affected joints carefully to prevent additional pain.

Here's a pharmacology fact.
Do not administer aspirin (or drugs containing aspirin) or other NSAIDs, such as indomethacin, to the child with hemophilia because of the danger of prolonging bleeding.

Preventing Joint Contractures

Passive range-of-motion exercises help prevent the development of joint contractures. Do not use them, however, after an acute episode because stretching of the joint capsule may cause bleeding. Encourage the child to do active range-of-motion exercises because he or she can recognize his or her own pain tolerance. Many patients who have had repeated episodes of **hemarthrosis** (bleeding into the joints) develop functional impairment of the joints, despite careful treatment. Use splints and devices to position the limb in a functional position. Physical therapy is helpful after the bleeding episode is under control. Joint contractures are a serious risk, so make every effort to avoid them.

Preventing Injury

The child with hemophilia is continuously at risk for additional injury. Protect the child from trauma caused by necessary procedures. Limit invasive procedures as much as possible; if possible, collect blood samples by a finger stick. Avoid intramuscular injections. When an invasive procedure must be done, compress the site for 5 minutes or longer after the procedure and apply cold compresses.

Remove any sharp objects from the child's environment. If the child is young, pad the crib sides to prevent bumping and bruising. Examine toys for sharp edges and hard surfaces. Soft toys are best for the young child. For mouth care, use a soft toothbrush or sponge-type brush to decrease the danger of bleeding gums. During daily hygiene, trim the nails to prevent scratching and give adequate skin care to prevent irritation.

Providing Family Teaching

Provide the family with a thorough explanation of hemophilia or reinforce information they already have. Review the family's knowledge about the disease and give additional information when needed. A child with hemophilia is healthy between bleeding episodes, but the fact that bleeding may occur as the result of slight trauma or often without any known injury causes considerable anxiety. For an unknown reason, bleeding episodes are more common in the spring and fall. Some evidence indicates that emotional stress can initiate bleeding episodes.

Topical fluoride applications to the teeth are particularly important in these children. Pay particular attention to proper oral hygiene, a well-balanced diet, and proper dental treatment, and teach the family about these considerations. Advise the family to select a dentist who understands the problems presented and who will set up an appropriate program of preventive dentistry.

Discuss safety measures for the home and the child's lifestyle. When possible, carpeting in the home helps to soften the falls of a toddler just learning to walk. An older child may need to wear protective devices when playing outdoors. Playground areas can be treacherous for these children, but the child can participate in normal play activities, within reason.

This advice could be a lifesaver.
A young child with hemophilia may need a protective helmet and elbow and knee pads for everyday wear, especially when first becoming mobile.

Instruct the family about medications, range-of-motion exercises, emergency measures to stop or limit bleeding, and all aspects of the child's care. Emergency splints should be kept in the home of every person with hemophilia. Ice packs also should be available for instant use. If possible, the bleeding area can be raised above the level of the heart. Before leaving for the health care facility, the caregiver should apply a splint and cold packs and give factor replacement according to the protocol established with the child's physician.

The family experiences continuous anxiety over how much activity to allow their child, how to keep from overprotecting him or her, and how to help the child achieve a healthy mental attitude, while preventing mishaps that may cause serious bleeding episodes. Teach the family that it is essential to guide the child toward autonomy and independence within the framework of necessary limitations. At times, the emotional effects of social deprivation and restrained activity must be weighed against possible physical harm.

The financial strain on the family is considerable, as it is with most families with a child who has a chronic condition. Children who have had several episodes of hemarthrosis may be disabled to the extent of needing crutches and braces or wheelchairs. Measures toward rehabilitation require hospitalization, with possible surgery, casts, and other orthopedic appliances.

A hemophiliac child usually misses a lot of school. Any child who must frequently interrupt schooling, for whatever reason, experiences a considerable setback. Each child should be considered individually and provided with as normal an environment as possible.

Promoting Family Coping

Both the child and family must accept the limitations and yet realize the importance of having normal social experiences. School, health, and community agencies can offer the family counseling and encouragement and can help them raise the affected child in a healthy manner, both emotionally and physically. The National Hemophilia Foundation is a resource for services and publications (Web site: www.hemophilia.org). Give the family information about other available support systems.

Review all these concerns with the family. Through discussion, questions, and demonstrations, confirm that the family understands the information provided. Counseling may be required for the family to learn to cope with the child's needs. Encourage family members to express their feelings about the effect the disease has on their lifestyle. The family may fear that the child will die of hemorrhaging. Guilt may play an important part in the family's reactions to the child. Recognizing and validating these feelings are important aspects of active listening. During hospitalization, involve the family in the child's care so they can learn how to help the child without causing additional pain.

Evaluation: Goals and Expected Outcomes

Goal: The child will experience diminished pain.
Expected Outcome:

- The child rests quietly with minimal pain as evidenced by the child using a pain scale to report decreased pain.

Goal: The child will move freely with minimal pain.
Expected Outcomes: The child

- is free from evidence of new joint contractures.
- maintains range of motion.

Goal: The child will be protected from any new injuries.
Expected Outcome:

- The child is free from injuries or bleeding episodes caused as a result of procedures, treatments, or unsafe environment.

A Personal Glimpse

My 6-year-old son Samuel has hemophilia. When he had a circumcision after he was born, he just kept bleeding. They asked us if anyone in our family had a bleeding disorder; we told them we didn't think so. We found out later my grandfather did have a bleeding problem, we just had never known that. When Sam was little, he had bruises a lot, and finally they told us he had hemophilia. I felt so guilty because it came from my side of the family. We were so afraid and tried to protect him from any little accident, but he was such an active boy, it was so hard. I would get so nervous and upset whenever he got any kind of cut or even a little scratch. Now that he is a little older, he understands better, but he is disappointed when he has to be more careful when he plays or can't ride a bike like his friends do. We had to learn all about how to stop the bleeding and giving him factor VIII. I still always worry that he could get AIDS—they say it would be unlikely, but I know it has happened. Sam's sister is only 2 years older than he is; she loves her little brother so much and always tries to protect him. I have learned to relax a little more, and he really handles it well, but every day, I still worry that some day he will have something serious happen to him and we won't be able to stop the bleeding.

Theresa

Learning Opportunity: What are some resources and information you could offer to this mother? What would you say in response to the mother's statement regarding her child getting AIDS?

Goal: The family caregivers will verbalize an understanding of the disease, injury prevention, and care of the child.
Expected Outcomes: The family caregivers

- list five safety measures to decrease the possibilities of injury to the child.
- explain the disease and the child's home care and ask and answer appropriate questions.

Goal: The family caregivers will develop appropriate coping mechanisms.
Expected Outcome:

- The family members express their feelings and demonstrate good coping mechanisms, such as seeking help from appropriate support systems.

Test Yourself

✔ Give examples of where bleeding might be seen in the child with hemophilia.

✔ Discuss how hemophilia is treated.

✔ What areas should be covered when teaching a family who has a child with hemophilia?

IDIOPATHIC THROMBOCYTOPENIC PURPURA

Purpura is a blood disorder associated with a deficit of platelets in the circulatory system causing hemorrhages into the skin or mucous membranes. The most common type of purpura is idiopathic thrombocytopenic purpura (ITP). Purpura is preceded by a viral infection in about half the diagnosed cases.

Clinical Manifestations and Diagnosis

The onset of ITP is often acute. Bruising and a generalized rash occur. In severe cases, hemorrhage may occur in the mucous membranes; hematuria or difficult-to-control epistaxis may be present. Rarely, the serious complication of intracranial hemorrhage occurs. In most cases, symptoms disappear in a few weeks without serious hemorrhage. A few cases may continue in a chronic form of the disease.

In ITP, the platelet count may be 20,000/mm^3 (normal, 150,000–300,000/mm^3) or lower. The bleeding time is prolonged, and the clot retraction time is abnormal. The WBC count remains normal, and anemia is not present unless excessive bleeding has occurred.

Treatment and Nursing Care

Corticosteroids are useful in reducing the severity and shortening the duration of the disease in some, but not all, cases of ITP. Intravenous immunoglobulin has been used to increase the production of platelets until recovery occurs spontaneously. If the platelet count is >20,000/mm^3, treatment may be delayed to see if a spontaneous remission will occur.

Nursing care consists of protecting the child from falls and trauma, observing for signs of external or internal bleeding, and providing a regular diet and general supportive care.

ACUTE LEUKEMIA

Leukemia, the most common type of cancer in children, accounts for about 30% of all childhood cancers. Acute lymphoblastic leukemia (ALL) is responsible for about 70% to 75% of the childhood leukemias and acute myelogenous leukemia (AML) is responsible for almost all the rest. Fortunately, ALL is also the most curable of all major forms of leukemia. The cure rate for AML is about 40%. The incidence of ALL is greatest between the ages of 2 and 6 years and is higher in boys; ALL is more common in white children than in African American children. This discussion focuses on ALL.

Pathophysiology

Leukemia is the uncontrolled reproduction of deformed WBCs. Despite intensive research, its cause is unknown. Mature leukocytes (WBCs) are made up of three types of cells:

- **Monocytes** (5% to 10% of WBCs) defend the body against infection.

- **Granulocytes** are divided into eosinophils, basophils, and neutrophils. Neutrophils (60% of the WBCs) can pass through capillary walls to surround and destroy bacteria.
- **Lymphocytes** (30% of WBCs) are divided into T cells, which attack and destroy virus-infected cells, foreign tissue, cancer cells, and B cells, which produce antibodies (proteins that help destroy foreign matter). An immature lymphocyte is called a **lymphoblast**.

Leukemia occurs when lymphocytes reproduce so quickly that they are mostly in the blast, or immature, stage. This rapid increase in lymphocytes causes crowding, which in turn decreases the production of red blood cells and platelets. The decrease in RBCs, platelets, and normal WBCs causes the child to become easily fatigued and susceptible to infection and increased bleeding.

Clinical Manifestations

Clinical manifestations of leukemia appear with surprising abruptness in many affected children with few, if any, warning signs. The symptoms result from the proliferation of lymphoblasts. Presenting manifestations are often fatigue, pallor, and low-grade fever caused by anemia. Other early or presenting symptoms are bone and joint pain caused by invasion of the periosteum by lymphocytes, widespread **petechiae** (pinpoint hemorrhages beneath the skin), and purpura (hemorrhages into the skin or mucous membranes) as a result of a low thrombocyte count. The lymph nodes often are enlarged.

Although they are seldom presenting signs, anorexia, nausea and vomiting, headache, diarrhea, and abdominal pain often occur during the course of the disease, as a result of enlargement of the liver and spleen. Easy bruising is a constant problem. Ulceration of the gums and throat develops as a result of bacterial invasion and contributes to anorexia. Intracranial hemorrhages are not uncommon. Anemia becomes increasingly severe.

Diagnosis

In addition to the history, symptoms, and laboratory blood studies, a bone marrow aspiration must be done to confirm the diagnosis of leukemia. Radiographs of the long bones demonstrate changes caused by the invasion of the lymphoblasts.

> **This is important to know.**
> The preferred site for bone marrow aspiration in children is the iliac crest.

Treatment

The advances in the treatment of ALL have dramatically improved long-term survival. In children whose initial prognosis is good, about 90% have long-term survival. For children who have a relapse, survival rates are greatly reduced. Each succeeding relapse reduces the probability of survival.

Intensive chemotherapy is initially divided into three phases:

- Induction—geared to achieving a complete remission with no leukemia cells
- Sanctuary—preventing invasion of the central nervous system by leukemia cells (no sanctuary is given to the leukemia cells)
- Maintenance—maintaining the remission

A combination of drugs is used during the induction phase to bring about remission; among the drugs used are vincristine, prednisone, and asparaginase. During the sanctuary phase, **intrathecal administration** (drugs injected into the cerebrospinal fluid by lumbar puncture) of methotrexate is used to eradicate leukemia cells in the central nervous system. The maintenance phase may last 2 or 3 years and includes treatment with methotrexate, vincristine, prednisone, and 6-mercaptopurine. The drugs are often administered through a double-lumen catheter (Broviac) placed in the subclavian vein.

Two additional phases are instituted for children who experience relapse:

- Reinduction—administration of the drugs previously used, plus additional drugs
- Bone marrow transplant—usually recommended after the second remission in children with ALL

Nursing Process for the Child With Leukemia

Assessment

The process of collecting data on the child with leukemia varies according to the stage of the illness. Conduct the admission interview with both the family caregiver and the child. Do not allow the caregiver to monopolize the interview; give the child an opportunity to express feelings and fears and answer the questions. The physical examination should include observing for **adenopathy** (enlarged lymph glands), abnormal vital signs (especially a low-grade fever), signs of bruising, petechiae, bleeding from or ulcerations of mucous membranes, abdominal pain or tenderness, and bone or joint pain. Observe the child for lethargic behavior, and question the caregiver about this. Note signs of local infection, including edema, redness, and swelling, or any indication of systemic infection. The diagnosis of leukemia is devastating. Observe and note the child and family's emotional states so that the nursing care plan can include helping them to discuss and resolve their feelings and fears.

Selected Nursing Diagnoses

- Risk for Infection related to increased susceptibility secondary to leukemic process and side effects of chemotherapy
- Risk for Injury related to bleeding tendencies

- Acute Pain related to the effects of chemotherapy and the disease process
- Fatigue related to disease, decreased energy, and anxiety
- Delayed Growth and Development related to impaired ability to achieve developmental tasks secondary to limitations of disease and treatment
- Disturbed Body Image related to alopecia and weight loss
- Grieving by the family related to the prognosis

Outcome Identification And Planning

Goals for the child with leukemia vary depending on individual circumstances. Preventing infection, preventing injury, relieving pain, and reducing fatigue are major goals. Other important goals for the child may be promoting normal growth and development and improving body image. The goal for the family may be to verbalize feelings and to increase coping abilities.

Implementation

Preventing Infection

The immune system is weakened by the uncontrolled growth of lymphoblasts that overpower the normal production of granulocytes (particularly neutrophils) and monocytes. In addition, the chemotherapy necessary to inhibit this proliferation of lymphoblasts causes immunosuppression. Thus, these children are susceptible to infection, especially during chemotherapy. Infections, such as meningitis, septicemia, and pneumonia, are the most common causes of death. The organism most often responsible is *Pseudomonas*. Other organisms that can be dangerous for the child are *Escherichia coli*, *Staphylococcus aureus*, *Klebsiella*, *Pneumocystis carinii*, and *Candida albicans*. These infectious organisms can threaten the child's life. To protect the child from infectious organisms, follow standard guidelines for protective isolation. Carefully screen staff, family, and visitors to eliminate any known infection. Enforce hand washing, gowning, and masking. The social isolation that this imposes on the child can be difficult for the child to understand and tolerate, so spend additional time with the child beyond that necessary for direct care. Playing games, coloring, reading stories, and doing puzzles are all good activities the child will enjoy. This also provides a much-needed break for the caregiver staying with the child.

Preventing Bleeding and Injury

The mucous membranes bleed easily, so be gentle when doing oral hygiene. Use a soft, sponge-type brush, or gauze strips wrapped around your finger. Mouthwash composed of one part hydrogen peroxide to four parts saline solution or normal saline solution may be used. Epistaxis (nosebleed) is a common problem that can usually be handled by applying external pressure to the nose. Apply pressure to sites of injections or venipunctures to prevent excessive bleeding. At least every 4 hours, monitor the child for other signs of bleeding such as pe-techiae, ecchymosis, hematemesis (bloody emesis), tarry stools, and swelling and tenderness of the joints. Protect the child from injury by external forces to prevent the possibility of hemorrhage from the injury. Take extra caution when the child's platelet count is especially low.

Reducing Pain

Pain from the invasion of lymphoblasts into the perios-teum and bleeding into the joints can be excruciating. Use gentle handling: Place sheepskin pads under bony prominences and position the child to help relieve dis-comfort and skin breakdown. Many times painful pro-cedures must be done that add to the child's discomfort. Explain to the child that these procedures are necessary to help and are not in any way a form of punishment. Provide a pain scale to help the child rate the pain and communicate its intensity. The numeric and the faces pain rating scales are useful with children 3 years of age and older (see Fig. 29-8, Chapter 29). Administer anal-gesics as ordered to achieve maximum comfort.

Promoting Energy Conservation and Relieving Anxiety

As a result of anemia, the child is fatigued. Pace proce-dures so that the child has as much uninterrupted rest as possible. Stress adds to the child's feelings of exhaustion; to decrease fatigue, help the child deal with the stress caused by the illness and treatments. To help relieve anx-iety, encourage the child to talk about feelings and ac-knowledge the child's feelings as valid.

Promoting Normal Growth and Development

During treatment, the child frequently may be prevented from participating in normal activity. The social isola-tion that accompanies reverse isolation often interferes with normal development. Physical activities often are limited simply because of the child's lack of energy. Knowledge of nor-mal growth and de-velopment expecta-tions is important to consider when plan-ning developmental activities. Stimulate growth and devel-opment within the child's physical ca-pabilities.

> **Think about this.**
> Even when working with the sick child, always stress positive devel-opmental tasks; for example, the school-age child can practice or improve reading skills and learn or increase computer skills.

Encourage the family to help the child return to nor-mal activities, as much as possible during the treatment's maintenance phase, when the child has been discharged from the hospital.

Promoting a Positive Body Image

The drugs administered in chemotherapy cause **alopecia** (loss of hair) (Fig. 37-5). Prepare the child and the fam-

■ **Figure 37-5** The child with alopecia needs support and encouragement.

ily psychologically for this change in appearance. The child may want to wear a wig, especially when returning to school. Encourage the family to choose the wig before chemotherapy is started so that it matches the child's hair and the child has time to get used to it. A cap or scarf often is appealing to a child, particularly if it car-ries a special meaning for him or her. Reassure the child and family that the hair will grow back in about 3 to 6 months. Wash the scalp regularly to avoid scaling. Pred-nisone therapy may cause the child to have a moon-faced appearance, which may be upsetting to the child or the family. Reassure them that this is temporary and will disappear when the drug is no longer needed. The child may be hesitant for peers to see these changes. Encourage visits from peers be-fore discharge, if possible, so that the child can be prepared to handle their reac-tions and questions.

> **Acceptance is not as hard as you think.**
> A schoolteacher can be invaluable in preparing classmates to wel-come the child with leukemia back to school, with minimal reaction to the child's physical changes.

Encourage the family to enlist the assistance of the child's teacher, school nurse, and pediatrician to ease the transition. Meeting other children who are undergoing chemotherapy and are in various stages of recovery of-ten is helpful to the child and helps to relieve the feeling that no one else has ever looked like this. Provide the child and the family opportunities to express their feel-ings and apprehensions.

Promoting Family Coping

Family members often are devastated when they first learn that their child has leukemia. Provide support from the moment of the first diagnosis, through the hospital-ization, and continuing through the maintenance phase. Family members live one day at a time, hoping that the remission will not end and that their child will be one who does not have a relapse and is finally considered cured. Provide opportunities for family members to freely express their feelings about the illness and treatment. The family will find comfort and stability in having one nurse caring for the child consistently. Involve the caregivers in the care of the child during hospitalization, and give them complete information about what to expect when caring for the child at home during the maintenance phase. Identify a contact person for the family to call to answer questions during this phase. Help the family work through feelings of overprotectiveness toward the child so that the child can lead as normal a life as possible. Encourage the family to consider how siblings can fit into the child's return home. Siblings may have many questions about the seriousness of the illness and about the possible death of their brother or sister. Provide support for families to deal with these concerns. Most hospitals that provide care for pediatric oncology patients have caregiver support groups that meet regularly. Candlelighters is a national organization for parents of young cancer patients (Web site: www.candlelighters.org).

Evaluation: Goals and Expected Outcomes

Goal: The child will remain free of signs and symptoms of infection.
Expected Outcomes: The child

- maintains a temperature that does not exceed 100°F (37.9°C).
- is free from inflammation, drainage, or other signs of infection.

Goal: The child will remain free from injury related to bleeding.
Expected Outcome:

- The child has no signs of petechiae, ecchymosis, hematemesis, tarry stools, or swelling and tenderness of the joints.

Goal: The child will show signs of being comfortable.
Expected Outcomes: The child

- rests quietly.
- uses a pain scale to indicate that the pain is at a tolerable level.

Goal: The child's energy level will be maintained or will increase.
Expected Outcomes: The child

- participates in activities and procedures paced so that the child has adequate rest periods.
- expresses anxieties and feelings of stress related to illness.

Goal: The child will accomplish appropriate growth and development milestones within the limits of the condition.
Expected Outcome:

- The child is involved in age-appropriate activities provided by staff and family.

Goal: The child will accept changes in physical appearance.
Expected Outcomes: The child

- shows pride and adjustment in changes in body image.
- shares feelings about body image changes.

Goal: The family will verbalize feelings and develop coping mechanisms.
Expected Outcomes: The family

- expresses feelings and fears about the child's prognosis.
- accepts counseling and support as needed.

Test Yourself

✔ What symptoms are usually seen in the child with leukemia?

✔ Give some examples of how infection can be prevented in the child with leukemia.

✔ Define alopecia and discuss ways you can support the child who has alopecia.

Key Points

➤ The cardiovascular system carries needed chemicals to and from the cells in the body, so they can function properly. The major organ is the heart. The hematologic system includes the blood and blood-forming tissues. The cardiovascular and hematologic systems work together to remove the waste products from the cells, so they can be excreted from the body.

➤ By the time a child is a few months of age, the left ventricle is about two times the size of the right, about the same proportion as an adult. The infant's

heart rate is higher than the older child's or adult's. By the time the child is 5 years old, the heart has matured, developed, and functions just as the adult's.

➤ The signs and symptoms seen in the child with CHF often include fatigue; feeding problems; failure to gain weight; pale, mottled, or cyanotic color; tachycardia; rapid respiration; dyspnea; flaring of the nares; and use of accessory muscles with retractions. Such children may also have edema, heart enlargement, and liver enlargement.

➤ Treatment includes improving the cardiac function, removing excess fluids, decreasing the workload on the heart, and improving tissue oxygenation. Nursing care is focused on improving cardiac output and oxygenation, relieving inadequate respirations, maintaining adequate nutritional intake, and conserving energy.

➤ Group A beta-hemolytic streptococcus is the bacterium usually responsible for rheumatic fever. Major manifestations include carditis (inflammation of the heart), polyarthritis (migratory arthritis), and chorea (disorder characterized by emotional instability, purposeless movements, and muscular weakness).

➤ Nursing care for the child with rheumatic fever is focused on reducing pain, providing diversional activities and sensory stimulation, conserving energy, and preventing injury. In addition, teach the caregiver to comply with drug therapy and the long-term care of the child.

➤ Kawasaki disease is an acute, febrile disease. The disease appears to be caused by an infectious agent. Intravenous immunoglobulin therapy is given to relieve the symptoms and prevent coronary artery abnormalities. Aspirin is used to control inflammation and fever. The most serious concern for a child with Kawasaki disease is development of cardiac involvement, which may not be seen for a period of time after the child's recovery.

➤ Iron deficiency anemia is a common nutritional deficiency in children. It is difficult to get enough iron from food the child eats, and if the iron intake is inadequate, anemia quickly results.

➤ If the sickle cell trait is inherited from one parent, a child can inherit the trait and carry the sickle cell trait. If both parents carry the trait, the child can inherit the trait from each parent and have sickle cell disease.

➤ In sickle cell anemia, the abnormal hemoglobin causes the red blood cells to assume a sickle shape. When sickling occurs, the affected red blood cells become crescent-shaped and the blood viscosity increases (blood becomes thicker), causing slowdown and sludging of the red blood cells. The impaired circulation results in tissue damage and infarction.

➤ Nursing care for the child with sickle cell anemia is focused on maintaining comfort and relieving pain, increasing fluid intake, conserving energy, improving physical mobility, and maintaining skin integrity.

➤ Work closely with the caregivers to decrease anxiety and increase their knowledge about the causes of crisis episodes.

➤ Common complications of thalassemia include enlargement of the spleen, overstimulation of bone marrow, and heart failure. Prognosis remains poor and the child often dies of cardiac failure despite treatment with blood transfusions (to maintain the hemoglobin levels), diet and medications (to prevent heart failure), and splenectomy or bone marrow transplants.

➤ The most common types of hemophilia are factor VIII deficiency and factor IX deficiency, which are inherited as a sex-linked recessive trait, with transmission to male offspring by carrier females.

➤ Hemophilia used to be treated by the use of fresh blood or plasma, but newer commercial preparations are now available that supply higher-potency factor VIII, including a synthetic preparation, DDAVP (1-deamino-8-D-arginine vasopressin), which is used in mild factor VIII deficiencies. Nursing care is focused on stopping the bleeding, decreasing pain, increasing mobility, and preventing injury. Work with the caregiver to increase knowledge about the child's condition and care and to help the family learn to cope.

➤ Symptoms of idiopathic thrombocytopenic purpura include bruising, a generalized rash and, in severe cases, hemorrhage in the mucous membranes, hematuria, or difficult-to-control epistaxis. Rarely the serious complication of intracranial hemorrhage is seen.

➤ The child with leukemia often has fatigue, pallor, low-grade fever, bone and joint pain, petechiae (pinpoint hemorrhages beneath the skin), and purpura (hemorrhages into the skin or mucous membranes). The lymph nodes may be enlarged and bruising is a constant problem.

➤ Four drugs commonly used in the treatment of acute lymphatic leukemia are methotrexate, vincristine, prednisone, and 6-mercaptopurine. Nursing care is focused on preventing infection, preventing injury, relieving pain, and reducing fatigue. Work with the child to help promote normal growth and development and improve body image. Encourage caregivers to verbalize feelings and help them to increase their coping abilities.

INTERNET RESOURCES

Sickle Cell Disease
www.sicklecelldisease.org

Hemophilia
www.hemophilia.org

Kawasaki Disease
www.kdfoundation.org

Leukemia
www.leukemiafoundation.org

Workbook

▪ NCLEX-STYLE REVIEW QUESTIONS

1. A child with rheumatic fever will *most* likely have a history of which of the following?

    a. A sibling diagnosed with the disease

    b. A recent strep throat infection

    c. Bruising easily

    d. Increased urinary output

2. When developing a plan of care for a child with sickle cell disease, which of the following nursing interventions would be *most* important to include?

    a. Provide support for family caregivers.

    b. Observe skin for any breakdown.

    c. Move the extremities gently.

    d. Administer analgesics promptly.

3. After discussing measures used to stop bleeding with the caregiver of a child diagnosed with hemophilia, the caregiver makes the following statements. Which of these statements indicates a need for further teaching?

    a. "I always have ice and cold packs in our freezer."

    b. "Keeping pressure on an injury usually helps stop the bleeding."

    c. "Whenever my child gets hurt, I have him sit up with his head elevated and his feet down."

    d. "I know how to keep his arm from moving by using splints."

4. A nurse admits a child with a diagnosis of possible leukemia. Of the following signs and symptoms, which would *most* likely be seen in the child with leukemia?

    a. Low-grade fever, bone and joint pain

    b. High fever, sore throat

    c. Swelling around eyes, ankles, and abdomen

    d. Upward and outward slanted eyes

5. In planning care for a child with leukemia, which of the following goals would be *most* important for this child?

    a. The child will remain free of signs and symptoms of infection.

    b. The child will participate in age-appropriate activities.

    c. The child will eat at least 60% of each meal.

    d. The child will share feelings about changes in body image.

6. The nurse is caring for a client who has leukemia. Which of the following nursing interventions should the nurse implement to decrease the likelihood of bleeding or injury? Select all that apply:

    a. Use a soft, sponge-type brush or gauze strips to give oral care.

    b. Maintain reverse isolation.

    c. Use mouthwash composed of hydrogen peroxide and saline solution.

    d. Wear gloves when delivering the client's meal tray.

    e. Have the child wear a cap or scarf.

    f. Apply pressure to sites of injections or venipunctures.

▪ STUDY ACTIVITIES

1. Using the table below, make a list of safety measures to help protect the child with hemophilia. Include measures to be taken at home, school, and in the hospital settings. Explain the reasons that these measures are important.

Setting	Safety Measure	Reasons Measures Are Important
Home		
School		
Hospital		

2. Missy is a 6-year-old girl with leukemia. Her single mother is unable to be away from her job to stay with Missy. Because of Missy's increased risk for infection, she has been placed in protective isolation. Create an age-appropriate game or list of activities that could be used in caring for Missy.

3. Go to the following Internet site: http://www.scinfo.org/. This is a site for the Sickle Cell Information Center. Go to section "How May We Serve You." Click on "Patients and Families Online Resources."

    a. What are some of the topics available that you might share with your peers?

    b. What are some of the topics available that you might suggest to a family who has a child with sickle cell anemia?

■ CRITICAL THINKING: WHAT WOULD YOU DO?

1. The family of Sean, a 3-year-old boy with hemophilia, is concerned that Sean might get AIDS from his treatments.

   a. What is the likelihood of Sean being HIV positive or of contracting AIDS from his treatments?

   b. What explanation will you give this family to re-assure them?

   c. What are your thoughts and feelings about children who are HIV positive because of a transfusion they received?

2. Andrew is an 18-month-old boy who has been admitted in a sickle cell crisis. His mother Jessica is 4 months pregnant with the family's second child. Tyrone, Andrew's father, tells you that they don't know much about sickle cell anemia, but they have heard their second child may also have the disease.

   a. What information would you share about sickle cell disease?

   b. What would you teach this family about the genetic factors related to sickle cell anemia?

   c. What is the likelihood that their second child will also have the disease?

   d. What organizations would you refer this family to?

3. Dosage calculation: The nurse is caring for a newborn who has symptoms of congestive heart failure and is being treated with Digoxin. The child weighs 6.5 lb. The usual dosage range of this medication is 4 to 8 μg/kg/day in divided doses, every 12 hours. Answer the following:

   a. How many micrograms (mcg) are in a milligram (mg)?

   b. How many kilograms (kg) does the child weigh?

   c. What is the lowest dose of Digoxin (in mcg) that this child could be given in a 24-hour time period?

   d. What is the highest dose of Digoxin (in mcg) that this child could be given in a 24-hour time period?

   e. How many doses will the child receive in a day?

4. Dosage calculation: A 5-year-old boy with a diagnosis of Kawasaki disease is being treated with aspirin. His initial dose is 90 mg/kg in divided doses every 6 hours. After his symptoms have subsided, he will be given a dose of 5 mg/kg a day for the antiplatelet effect of the drug. The child weighs 39 lb. The medication comes in 80-mg tablets. Answer the following:

   a. How many kilograms (kg) does the child weigh?

   b. How many milligrams (mg) per day will be given for the initial dose?

   c. How many milligrams (mg) per dose will be given for the initial dose?

   d. How many tablets will be given for each of the initial doses?

   e. How many milligrams (mg) per day will be given for the antiplatelet dose?

38

The Child With a Gastrointestinal/Endocrine Disorder

KEY TERMS

anthelmintic
chelating agent
colic
craniotabes
currant jelly stools
diabetic ketoacidosis
encephalopathy
gastroenteritis
insulin reaction
invagination
Kussmaul breathing
kwashiorkor
lactose
lactose intolerance
marasmus
pica
polydipsia
polyphagia
polyuria
pruritus
steatorrhea
urticaria

LEARNING OBJECTIVES

On completion of this chapter, you should be able to:

1. Discuss ways the child's gastrointestinal system differs from the adult's system.
2. Discuss ways the child's endocrine system differs from the adult's system.
3. Describe conditions related to nutritional deficiencies and food allergies and discuss nursing care.
4. Explain the diagnosis of celiac syndrome.
5. Discuss the diagnosis of gastroesophageal reflux including the cause, symptoms, treatment, and nursing care.
6. Describe the symptoms noted in the child with colic.
7. Discuss the symptoms, treatment, and nursing care for the child with diarrhea or gastroenteritis.
8. Identify the symptoms, treatment, and nursing care of pyloric stenosis.
9. State another name for congenital megacolon and discuss the diagnosis, including symptoms, treatment, and nursing care.
10. Describe the diagnosis and treatment of intussusception.
11. List the symptoms, treatment, and nursing care of appendicitis; differentiate symptoms of the older and the younger child.
12. Identify intestinal parasites common to children and state the route of entry, symptoms, and treatment for each.
13. Discuss ingestion of toxic substances in children.
14. List seven sources of lead that may cause chronic lead poisoning, and describe the symptoms, diagnosis, treatment, and prognosis.
15. Describe the treatment of a child who has swallowed a foreign object.
16. Discuss type 1 diabetes mellitus including symptoms, diagnosis, treatment, nursing care, and teaching.
17. Explain type 2 diabetes mellitus.

THE GASTROINTESTINAL (GI) system is responsible for taking in and processing nutrients that nourish all parts of the body. As a result, any problem of the GI system, whether a lack of nutrients, an infectious disease, or a congenital disorder, can quickly affect other parts of the body and ultimately affect general health, growth, and development. The endocrine system consists of a number of ductless glands throughout the body that secrete hormones. All of the body systems overlap with the working of the endocrine glands.

GROWTH AND DEVELOPMENT OF THE GASTROINTESTINAL AND ENDOCRINE SYSTEMS

Gastrointestinal System

The main organs of the gastrointestinal (GI) or digestive system are the mouth, pharynx (throat), esophagus, stomach, small intestine, large intestine, rectum, and anal canal. Other organs, called accessory organs, include structures that aid in the digestive process, as well as glands that secrete substances that further aid in digestion. These accessory organs include the teeth, tongue, gallbladder, appendix, the salivary glands, liver, and pancreas. Each of these organs and accessory organs plays a part in the process of digestion (Fig. 38-1).

The child takes in food and fluids through the GI tract, where they are broken down and absorbed to promote growth and maintain life. Food enters the mouth and the digestive process begins. Digestion takes place by mechanical and chemical mechanisms. Chewing, muscular action, and peristalsis are physical or mechanical actions that break down food. Chemicals secreted along the GI tract by accessory organs further help the breakdown of food so that absorption can take place. As food is processed, nutrients are absorbed and distributed to the body cells. The large intestine is the organ of elimination that collects wastes and pushes them to the anus so the waste materials can be excreted.

The functioning of the GI system begins at birth. The GI tract of the newborn works in the same manner as that of the adult but with some limitations. For example, the enzymes secreted by the liver and pancreas are reduced. Thus, the infant cannot break down and use complex carbohydrates. As a result, the newborn diet must be adjusted to allow for this immaturity. By the age of 4 to 6 months, the needed enzymes are usually sufficient in amount.

The smaller capacity of the infant's stomach and the increased speed at which food moves through the GI tract require feeding smaller amounts at more frequent intervals. In addition, the small capacity of the colon leads to a bowel movement after each feeding. Reflexes are present in infants that allow for swallowing and prevention of aspiration when swallowing. The cardiac sphincter at the end of the esophagus may be lax in the infant, and food may be regurgitated from the stomach back into the esophagus. As the child grows, the muscles of the sphincter work more effectively and prevent food from going back into the esophagus. With continued growth, the GI tract matures and the capacity of the GI tract increases, but the digestive functioning throughout childhood into adulthood is the same.

Disorders and disruptions in the GI tract can cause a change in the functioning of the system. Most of these disorders stem from congenital defects, diseases, or infections in the GI tract. If any of these occur and the body does not get the needed nutrients to the cells, health and normal growth and development can be altered in children.

Endocrine System and Hormonal Function

The hormones secreted by the endocrine system are circulated through the bloodstream to control and regulate most of the activities and functions in the body. Regulating metabolism, growth, development, and reproduction are all functions of hormones. The endocrine system of the infant is adequately developed, although the functions are immature. As the child grows, the endocrine system matures in function.

Various disorders are caused by decreases, increases, or the absence of hormone secretions by the endocrine glands. The pancreas is the gland that secretes the hormone insulin. Type 1 diabetes mellitus occurs in children when an insufficient amount of insulin is produced.

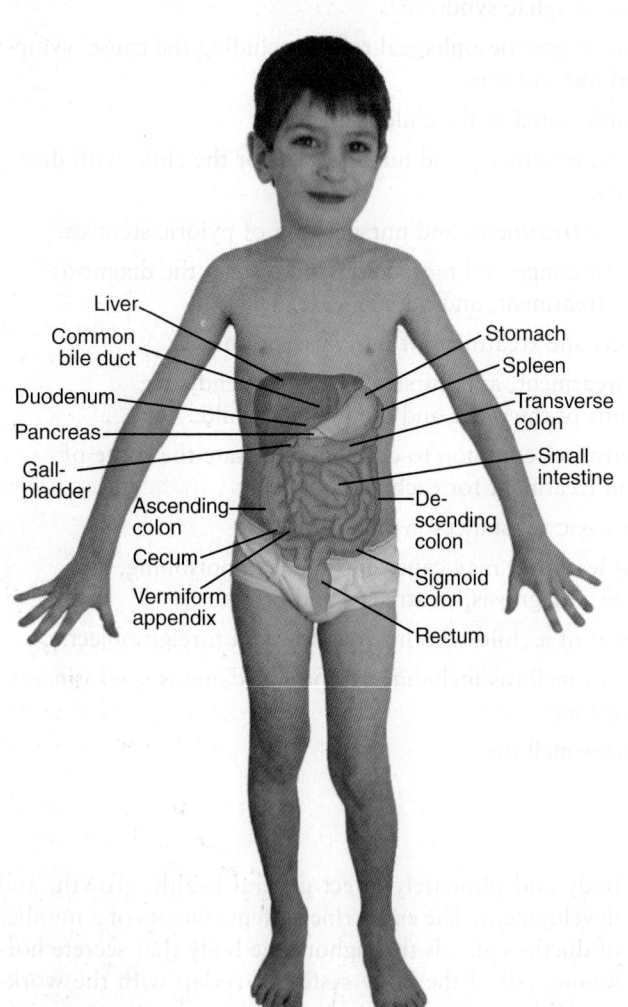

Liver
Common bile duct
Duodenum
Pancreas
Gall-bladder
Ascending colon
Cecum
Vermiform appendix
Stomach
Spleen
Transverse colon
Small intestine
Descending colon
Sigmoid colon
Rectum

■ **Figure 38-1** Anatomy of a child's gastrointestinal system.

GASTROINTESTINAL DISORDERS
MALNUTRITION AND NUTRITIONAL PROBLEMS

The World Health Organization has widely publicized the malnutrition and hunger that affect more than half the world's population. In the United States, malnutrition contributes to the high death rate of the children of migrant workers and Native Americans. Malnourished children grow at a slower rate, have a higher rate of illness and infection, and have more difficulty concentrating and achieving in school. Appendix D lists foods that are good sources of the nutrients that a child needs for healthy growth.

Protein Malnutrition

Protein malnutrition results from an insufficient intake of high-quality protein or from conditions in which protein absorption is impaired or a loss of protein increases. Clinical evidence of protein malnutrition may not be apparent until the condition is well advanced.

Kwashiorkor

Kwashiorkor results from severe deficiency of protein with an adequate caloric intake. It accounts for most of the malnutrition in the world's children today. The highest incidence is in children 4 months to 5 years of age. The affected child develops a swollen abdomen, edema, and GI changes; the hair is thin and dry with patchy alopecia; and the child becomes apathetic and irritable and has retarded growth with muscle wasting. In untreated patients, mortality rates are 30% or higher. Although strenuous efforts are being made around the world to prevent this condition, its causes are complex.

Traditionally, these babies have been breast-fed until the age of 2 or 3 years. The child is weaned abruptly when the next child in the family is born. The older child then receives the regular family diet, which consists mostly of starchy foods with little meat or vegetable protein. Cow's milk generally is unavailable; in many places where goats are kept, their milk is not considered fit for human consumption (Fig. 38-2).

Did you know?
The term kwashiorkor means "the sickness the older baby gets when the new baby comes."

Marasmus

Marasmus is a deficiency in calories as well as protein. The child with marasmus is seriously ill. The condition is common in children in Third World countries because of severe drought conditions. Not enough food is avail-

■ Figure 38-2 A child with kwashiorkor often has been abruptly weaned and may have a distended abdomen and muscle wasting.

able to supply everyone in these countries, and the children are not fed until adults are fed. The child is severely malnourished and highly susceptible to disease. This syndrome may be seen in the child with nonorganic failure to thrive.

Vitamin Deficiency Diseases
Vitamin D Deficiency

Rickets, a disease affecting the growth and calcification of bones, is caused by a lack of vitamin D. The absorption of calcium and phosphorus is diminished because of the lack of vitamin D, which is needed to regulate the use of these minerals. Early manifestations include **craniotabes** (softening of the occipital bones) and delayed closure of the fontanelles. There is delayed dentition, with defects in tooth enamel and a tendency to develop caries. As the disease advances, thoracic deformities, softening of the shafts of long bones, and spinal and pelvic bone deformities develop. The muscles are poorly developed and lacking in tone, so standing and walking are delayed. Deformities occur during periods of rapid growth. Although rickets itself is not a fatal disease, complications such as tetany, pneumonia, and enteritis are more likely to cause death in children with rickets than in healthy children.

Infants and children require an estimated 400 U of vitamin D daily to prevent rickets. Because a child living in a temperate climate may not receive sufficient exposure to ultraviolet light, vitamin D is administered orally in the form of fish liver oil or synthetic vitamin. Whole milk and evaporated milk fortified with 400 U of vitamin D per quart are available throughout the United States. Breast-fed infants should receive vitamin D supplements, especially if the mother's intake of vitamin D is poor.

Vitamin C Deficiency

Scurvy is caused by inadequate dietary intake of vitamin C (ascorbic acid). Early inclusion of vitamin C in the diet, in the form of orange or tomato juice or a vitamin preparation, prevents the development of this disease. Febrile diseases seem to increase the need for vitamin C. A variety of fresh vegetables and fruits supplies vitamin C for the older infant and child. Because much of the vitamin C content is destroyed by boiling or by exposure to air for long periods, the family caregivers should be taught to cook vegetables with minimal water in a covered pot and to store juices in a tightly covered opaque container. Vegetables cooked in a microwave oven retain more vitamin C because little water is added in the cooking process.

Early clinical manifestations of scurvy are irritability, loss of appetite, and digestive disturbances. A general tenderness in the legs severe enough to cause a pseudoparalysis develops. The child is apprehensive about being handled and assumes a frog position, with the hips and knees semiflexed and the feet rotated outward. The gums become red and swollen, and hemorrhage occurs in various tissues. Characteristic hemorrhages in the long bones are subperiosteal, especially at the ends of the femur and tibia.

Recovery is rapid with adequate treatment, but death may occur from malnutrition or exhaustion in untreated cases. Treatment consists of therapeutic daily doses of ascorbic acid.

Thiamine Deficiency

Thiamine is one of the major components of the vitamin B complex. Children whose diets are deficient in thiamine exhibit irritability, listlessness, loss of appetite, and vomiting. A severe lack of thiamine in the diet causes beriberi, a disease characterized by cardiac and neurologic symptoms. Beriberi does not occur when balanced diets that include whole grains are eaten.

Riboflavin Deficiency

Riboflavin deficiency usually occurs in association with thiamine and niacin deficiencies. A deficiency in riboflavin is mainly manifested by skin lesions. The primary source of riboflavin is milk. Riboflavin is destroyed by ultraviolet light; thus, opaque milk cartons are best for storage. Whole grains are also a good source of riboflavin.

Niacin Insufficiency

Niacin insufficiency in the diet causes a disease known as pellagra, which presents with GI and neurologic symptoms. Pellagra does not occur in children who ingest adequate whole milk or who eat a well-balanced diet.

Mineral Insufficiencies

Iron deficiency results in anemia. This condition is the most common cause of nutritional deficiency in children older than 4 to 6 months of age whose diets lack iron-rich foods. In the United States, anemia is often found in children younger than 6 years of age who are from low-income families. Iron deficiency anemia is discussed in more detail in Chapter 37.

Calcium is necessary for bone and tooth formation and is also needed for proper nerve and muscle function. Hypocalcemia (insufficient calcium) causes neurologic damage, including mental retardation. Rich sources of calcium include milk and milk products. Children with milk allergies are at an increased risk for hypocalcemia.

Food Allergies

The symptoms of food allergies vary from one child to another. Common symptoms are **urticaria** (hives), **pruritus** (itching), stomach pains, and respiratory symptoms. Some of the symptoms may appear quickly after the child has eaten the offending food, but other foods may cause a delayed reaction. Thus, the investigation to find the cause can be frustrating.

Foods should be introduced to the child one at a time, with an interval of 4 or 5 days between each new food. If any GI or respiratory reaction occurs, the food should be eliminated. Among the foods most likely to cause allergic reactions are milk, eggs, wheat, corn, legumes (including peanuts and soybeans), oranges, strawberries, and chocolate (Table 38-1). If a food has been eliminated because of a suspected allergy or reaction, it can be reintroduced at a later time in small amounts to test again for the child's response. This testing should be done in a carefully controlled manner to avoid serious or life-threatening reactions. Many allergies disappear as the child's GI tract matures.

Milk Allergy

Milk allergy is the most common food allergy in the young child. Symptoms that may indicate an allergy to milk are diarrhea, vomiting, colic, irritability, respiratory symptoms, or eczema. Infants who are breast-fed for the first 6 months or more may avoid developing milk allergies entirely unless a strong family history of allergies exists. Children with severe allergic reactions to milk are given commercial formulas that are soybean- or meat-based and formulated to be similar in nutrients to other infant formulas.

Lactose Intolerance

Children with **lactose intolerance** cannot digest **lactose**, the primary carbohydrate in milk, because of an inborn deficiency of the enzyme lactase. Congenital lactose intolerance is seen in some children of African American, Native American, Eskimo, Asian, and Mediterranean heritage. Symptoms include   cramping,

Here's a teaching tip for you.

If the child has a severe milk allergy, the caregiver must learn to carefully read the labels on prepared foods to avoid lactose or lactic acid ingredients.

Table 38-1 ▌ SOME FOODS THAT MAY CAUSE ALLERGIES AND POSSIBLE SOURCES

Food	Sources
Milk	Yogurt, cheese, ice cream, puddings, butter, hot dogs, foods made with nonfat dry milk, lunch meat, chocolate candies
Eggs	Baked goods, ice cream, puddings, meringues, candies, mayonnaise, salad dressings, custards
Wheat	Breads, baked goods, hot dogs, lunch meats, cereals, cream soups. Oat, rye, and cornmeal products may have wheat added.
Corn	Products made with cornstarch, corn syrup, or vegetable starch; many children's juices, popcorn, cornbreads or muffins, tortillas
Legumes	Soybean products, peanut butter, and peanut products
Citrus fruits	Oranges, lemons, limes, grapefruit, gelatins, children's juices, some pediatric suspensions (medications)
Strawberries	Gelatins, some pediatric suspensions
Chocolate	Cocoa, candies, chocolate drinks or desserts, colas

abdominal distention, flatus, and diarrhea after ingesting milk. Commercially available formulas such as Isomil, Nursoy, Nutramigen, and ProSobee are made from soybean, meat-based, or protein mixtures and contain no lactose. The child needs supplemental vitamin D. Yogurt is tolerated by these children.

Nursing Process for the Child With Malnutrition and Nutritional Problems

Assessment

Carefully interview the family caregiver to determine the underlying cause. If the difficulty lies in the caregiver's inability to give proper care, try to determine if this can be attributed to lack of information, financial problems, indifference, or other reasons. Do not make assumptions. Cases of malnutrition have been reported in children of families who believed it was better for their child to eat vegetables only; this severely limits fat intake, which the child needs. If food allergies are suspected as the cause of malnourishment, include a careful history of food intake. Obtain a history of stools and voiding from the caregiver.

The physical exam of the child includes observing skin turgor and skin condition, the anterior fontanelle, signs of emaciation, weight, temperature, apical pulse, respirations, responsiveness, listlessness, and irritability.

Selected Nursing Diagnoses

- Imbalanced Nutrition: Less Than Body Requirements related to inadequate intake of nutrients secondary to poor sucking ability, lack of interest in food, lack of adequate food sources, or lack of knowledge of caregiver
- Deficient Fluid Volume related to insufficient fluid intake
- Constipation related to insufficient fluid intake
- Impaired Skin Integrity related to malnourishment
- Deficient Knowledge of caregivers related to understanding of the child's nutritional requirements

Outcome Identification and Planning

The major nursing goals for the nutritionally deprived child focus on increasing nutritional intake, improving hydration, monitoring elimination, and maintaining skin integrity. Other goals concentrate on improving caregiver knowledge and understanding of nutrition and facilitating the infant's ability to suck. Even with focused and individualized goals, developing a plan of care for the malnourished child may be challenging. It may be necessary to try a variety of tactics to feed the child successfully. Include the family caregiver in the plan of care because this is in the best interest of both the child and the caregiver.

Implementation

Promoting Adequate Nutrition

One primary nursing care problem may be persuading the child to take more nourishment than he or she wants. Do not become discouraged if you find it difficult to persuade the uninterested child to take formula or food. Sometimes you can unknowingly communicate your insecurity and uncertainty to the child through impatience and a hurried attitude, and this will affect the amount of food you can persuade the child to eat. Instead, try wrapping and holding the infant snuggly while rocking the infant gently to promote relaxation and encourage a little more feeding. Also, you will find that as you and the child become accustomed to each other, you will both relax and feeding will become easier. Ask for help if the need to attend to other feedings causes tension. Never prop the bottle in the crib.

In addition to having a lack of interest, the child often is weak and debilitated with little strength to suck. It is important for the child to develop an interest in food and in the process of sucking. A hard or small-holed nipple may completely discourage the child. This situation can frustrate a weak child, who then no longer attempts to nurse. The nipple should be soft with holes large enough to allow the formula to drip without pressure. However, it should not be so soft that it offers no resistance and collapses when sucked on. The holes should not be so large that milk pours out, causing the child to choke. Gavage feedings or intravenous (IV) fluids may be needed to improve the child's nutritional status.

Scheduling feedings every 2 or 3 hours is best because most weak babies can handle frequent, small feedings better than feedings every 4 hours. With more frequent feedings, promptness is important. Feedings should be limited to 20 to 30 minutes so that the child does not tire. Demand schedules are not wise because the child has probably lost the power to regulate the supply-and-demand schedule.

Improving Fluid Intake

Improved nutritional status is evidenced by improved hydration, which is noted by monitoring skin turgor, fontanelle tension, and intake and output. Check the fontanelles each shift, and weigh the child daily in the early morning. Oral mucous membranes should be moist and pink. IV fluids may be needed, initially, to build up the child's energy so that he or she can take more oral nourishment to correct the fluid and electrolyte imbalance. During IV therapy, restraints should be adequate but kept to a minimum. Accurately document intake and output. At least every 2 hours, monitor the IV infusion placement, its patency, and the injection site for redness and induration. Report any unusual signs immediately.

Monitoring Elimination Patterns

Carefully document intake and output, as well as the character, frequency, and amount of stools. Report any unusual characteristics of the stools or urine at once.

Promoting Skin Integrity

Closely observe the skin condition. Use A+D Ointment or lanolin for dry or reddened skin, and promptly change soiled diapers to prevent skin breakdown in the weakened child.

Providing Family Teaching

If malnutrition is related to economic factors or inadequate caregiver knowledge of the child's needs, teach the family caregivers the essential facts of infant and child nutrition and make referrals for social services. Be alert to the possibility that the caregiver cannot read or understand English, and be certain that the teaching materials used are understood. Simply asking the family caregivers if they have questions is not sufficient to determine if the material has been understood.

Family caregivers may need information regarding assistance in obtaining nutritious food for the child. Infant formulas and baby food can be expensive, and economic factors may be the actual cause of the child's malnutrition. A referral to social services or the Women, Infant, and Children program may be appropriate (see Chapter 23).

Evaluation: Goals and Expected Outcomes

Goal: The child's nutritional intake will be adequate for normal growth.
Expected Outcomes: The child

- gains 0.75 to 1 oz (22–30 g) per day if younger than 6 months of age.
- gains 0.5 to 0.75 oz (13–22 g) per day if older than 6 months of age.

Goal: The child will show interest in feedings.
Expected Outcomes: The child

- shows evidence of adequate sucking.
- demonstrates ability to extend the amount of time feeding without showing signs of tiring.
- eats meals and snacks (older child).

Goal: The child's fluid intake will improve.
Expected Outcomes: The child's

- fontanelles are of normal tension.
- skin turgor is good.
- mucous membranes are pink and moist.

Goal: The child's urine and bowel outputs will be normal for age.
Expected Outcomes: The child's

- hourly urine output is 2 to 3 mL/kg.
- stool is soft and of normal character.

Goal: The child's skin will remain intact.
Expected Outcomes: The child's

- skin shows no signs of redness or breakdown.
- skin at the IV infusion site shows no signs of redness or induration.

Goal: The family caregivers will verbalize a beginning knowledge of appropriate nutrition for a growing child.
Expected Outcome:

- The family caregivers state essential facts about child nutrition.

CELIAC SYNDROME

The term **celiac syndrome** is used to designate the complex malabsorptive disorders. Intestinal malabsorption with **steatorrhea** (fatty stools) is a condition brought about by various causes, the most common being cystic fibrosis and gluten-induced enteropathy, the so-called idiopathic celiac disease. Cystic fibrosis is described in Chapter 36. Gluten-induced enteropathy is presented here.

Idiopathic celiac disease is a basic defect of metabolism precipitated by the ingestion of wheat gluten or rye gluten, which leads to impaired fat absorption. The exact cause is not known; the most acceptable theory is that of an inborn error of metabolism with an allergic reaction to the gliadin fraction of gluten (a protein factor in wheat) as a contributing or possibly the sole factor.

■ **Figure 38-3** A child with celiac disease. Notice the protruding abdomen and wasted buttocks.

Severe manifestations of the disorder have become rare in the United States and in Western Europe. Mild disturbances in intestinal absorption of rye, wheat, and sometimes oat gluten are common, however, occurring in about 1 in 2,000 children in the United States.

Clinical Manifestations

Signs generally do not appear before the age of 6 months and may be delayed until age 1 year or later. Manifestations include chronic diarrhea with foul, bulky, greasy stools and progressive malnutrition. Anorexia and a fretful, unhappy disposition are typical. The onset is generally insidious, with failure to thrive, bouts of diarrhea, and frequent respiratory infections. If the condition becomes severe, the effects of malnutrition are prominent. Retarded growth and development; a distended abdomen; and thin, wasted buttocks and legs are characteristic signs (Fig. 38-3).

The chronic course of this disease may be interrupted by a celiac crisis, an emergency situation. Frequently, this is triggered by an upper respiratory infection. The child vomits copious amounts, has large, watery stools, and becomes severely dehydrated. As the child becomes irritable and listless, an acute medical emergency develops. Parenteral fluid therapy is essential to combat acidosis and to achieve normal fluid balance.

Diagnosis

One way to determine if a small child's failure to thrive is caused by celiac disease is to initiate a trial gluten-free diet and observe the results. Improvement in the nature of the stools and general well-being with a gain in weight should follow, although several weeks may elapse before clear-cut manifestations can be confirmed. Conclusive diagnosis can be made by a biopsy of the jejunum through endoscopy that shows changes in the villi. Serum screening of immunoglobin G and immunoglobin A antigliadin antibodies shows the presence of the condition and also aids in monitoring the progress of therapy.

Treatment

The young child is usually started on a gluten-free, low-fat diet. If the condition is severe, this diet consists of skim milk, glucose, and banana flakes. Bananas contain invert sugar and are usually well tolerated. Lean meats, puréed vegetables, and fruits are gradually added to the diet. Eventually fats may be added, and the child can be maintained on a regular diet with the exception of all wheat, rye, and oat products.

The forbidden list of foods include wheat products; malted milk drinks; some candies; many baby foods; and breads, cakes, pastries, and biscuits, unless they are made from corn flour or

Watch out.
Commercially canned creamed soups, cold cuts, frankfurters, and pudding mixes generally contain wheat products.

cornmeal. Vitamins A and D in water-miscible (able to be mixed with water) solutions are needed in double amounts to supplement the deficient diet.

Although probably no cure can be expected, response to a diet from which rye, wheat, and oats are excluded is generally good, but dietary indiscretions or respiratory infections may bring relapses. The omission of wheat products in particular should continue through adolescence because the ingestion of wheat appears to inhibit growth in these children.

Nursing Care

The primary focus of nursing care is to help caregivers maintain a restrictive diet for the child. Family teaching should include information regarding the disease and the need for long-term management, as well as guidelines for a gluten-free diet. Caregivers must learn to read the list of ingredients on packaged foods carefully before purchasing anything. The diet of the young child may be monitored fairly easily, but when the child goes to school, monitoring becomes a much greater challenge. As the child grows, caregivers and children might need

Test Yourself

✔ Give some examples of vitamin and mineral deficiencies that can cause malnutrition in children.

✔ What are some common symptoms of food and milk allergies?

✔ List foods that may cause allergies and name some sources of these foods.

✔ How is celiac disease diagnosed and treated?

additional nursing support to help them make dietary modifications.

GASTROESOPHAGEAL REFLUX

Gastroesophageal reflux (GER) occurs when the sphincter in the lower portion of the esophagus, which leads into the stomach, is relaxed and allows gastric contents to be regurgitated back into the esophagus. GER is usually noted within the first week of the infant's life and is resolved within the first 18 months. The condition may correct itself as the esophageal sphincter matures, the child eats solid foods, and the child is more often in a sitting or standing position. Premature infants and children with neurologic conditions frequently have diagnoses of GER.

Clinical Manifestations

Almost immediately after feeding, the child vomits the contents of the stomach. The vomiting is effortless, not projectile in nature. The child with GER is irritable and hungry. Aspiration after vomiting may lead to respiratory concerns, such as apnea and pneumonia. Although the child may take in adequate nutrition because of the vomiting, failure to thrive and lack of normal weight gain occurs.

Diagnosis and Treatment

A complete history will offer information regarding feeding, vomiting, and weight patterns. An endoscopy will confirm the relaxed esophageal sphincter. Correcting the nutritional status of the child includes giving formula thickened with rice cereal, placing the child in an upright position during and after feeding, and nasogastric (NG) or gastrostomy feedings, if necessary. A histamine-2 (H2) receptor antagonist, such as ranitidine (Zantac), may be given to reduce the acid secretion, which lessens the complications gastric acid may have on the esophageal tissue. Other medications, such as omeprazole (Prilosec), may also be given to reduce the gastric acid. In severe cases, a surgical procedure known as Nissen fundoplication may be done. In this procedure, a part of the upper portion of the stomach is wrapped around the lower part of the esophagus to create a valvelike structure to prevent the regurgitation of stomach contents (Fig. 38-4).

Nursing Care

For the child with GER, thicken feedings with rice cereal to decrease the likelihood of aspiration. Immediately report any signs of respiratory distress. Offer small, frequent feedings and burp the child frequently. Positioning after feedings is a topic of debate. In the past, an infant car seat was used to keep the child positioned after feedings, but studies now suggest keeping the child in a prone position with the head elevated after daytime feedings and for several hours before the child goes to sleep at night may lessen the reflux of stomach acids. The child is then usually put in a side lying or supine position for sleeping. Monitor and document intake and output, daily weight, and emesis for amount and character. If a

■ Figure 38-4 In the Nissen fundoplication procedure, the upper portion of the stomach is wrapped around the lower part of the esophagus.

NG or gastrostomy tube is inserted, provide good skin care to help maintain skin integrity. It is important that you work with the family caregivers to teach them regarding feeding, positioning, and medication administration in order to decrease their anxiety.

The prone positioning of the child with GER is an exception to the recommendation that children be placed in the supine position for day and nighttime sleeping. This may create concern for the family caregiver and explanations need to be offered.

COLIC

Colic consists of recurrent paroxysmal bouts of abdominal pain and is fairly common in young infants. Although many theories have been proposed, none has been accepted as the causative factor.

Clinical Manifestations and Diagnosis

Attacks occur suddenly, usually late in the day or evening. The infant cries loudly and continuously. The infant appears to be in considerable pain but otherwise seems healthy, breast-feeds or takes formula well, and gains weight as expected. The baby may be momentarily soothed only by rocking or holding but eventually falls asleep, exhausted from crying. The infant with colic is often considered a "difficult" baby.

Differential diagnosis should be made to rule out an allergic reaction to milk or certain foods. Changing to a nonallergenic formula helps determine if there is an allergic factor or if the infant has lactose intolerance. If the baby is breast-fed, the mother's diet should be studied to determine if anything she is eating might be affecting the baby. Intestinal obstruction or infection also must be ruled out.

A little sensitivity is in order.

Colic often disappears around the age of 3 months, but this is small comfort to the caregiver vainly trying to soothe a colicky infant.

Treatment and Nursing Care

No single treatment is consistently successful. A number of measures may be employed, one or more of which might work. Medications such as sedatives, antispasmodics, and antiflatulents are sometimes prescribed, but their effectiveness is inconsistent. The family must remember that the condition will pass, even though at the time it seems it will last forever. Family caregivers need to be reassured that their parenting skills are not inadequate. You can support the family and promote coping skills by providing family teaching. See Family Teaching Tips: Colic.

DIARRHEA AND GASTROENTERITIS

Diarrhea in children is a fairly common symptom of a variety of conditions. It may be mild, accompanied by slight dehydration, or it may be extremely severe, requiring prompt and effective treatment. Simple diarrhea that does not respond to treatment can quickly turn into severe, life-threatening diarrhea.

Chronically malnourished children with diarrheal symptoms are a common problem in many areas of the world. This condition is prevalent in areas lacking adequate clean water and sanitary facilities. Certain metabolic diseases, such as cystic fibrosis, have diarrhea as a symptom. Diarrhea also may be caused by antibiotic therapy.

Some conditions that cause diarrhea require readjustment of the child's diet. Allergic reactions to food are not uncommon and can be controlled by avoiding the offending food. Adjusting the child's diet, adding less sugar to formula, or reducing bulk or fat in the diet may be necessary.

Did you know?
Overfeeding, underfeeding, or an unbalanced diet may be the cause of diarrhea in a child.

Many diarrheal disturbances in children are caused by contaminated food or human or animal fecal waste through the oral–fecal route. Infectious diarrhea is commonly referred to as **gastroenteritis.** The infectious organisms may be salmonella, *Escherichia coli*, dysentery bacilli, and various viruses, most notably rotaviruses. It is difficult to determine the causative factor in many instances. Because of the seriousness of infectious diarrhea in children and the danger of spreading diarrhea, the child with moderate or severe diarrhea is often isolated until the causative factor has been proved to be noninfectious.

Clinical Manifestations

Mild diarrhea may present as little more than loose stools; the frequency of defecation may be 2 to 12 per day. The child may be irritable and have a loss of appetite. Vomiting and gastric distention are not significant factors and dehydration is minimal.

Family Teaching Tips

COLIC

- Pick up and rock the baby in a rocker or, with baby's tummy down across your knees, swing your legs side to side. (Be sure baby's head is supported.)
- Walk around the room while rocking baby in your arms or in a front carrier. Hum or sing to baby.
- Try a bottle, but don't overfeed. Give a pacifier if baby has eaten well within 2 hours.
- Baby may like the rhythmic movements of a baby swing.
- Try taking baby outside or for a car ride.
- When feeding baby, try methods to decrease gas formation: frequent burping, giving smaller feedings more frequently; position baby in infant seat after eating.
- Try doing something to entertain but not overexcite baby.
- Gently rub baby's abdomen if it is rigid.
- Sit with baby resting on your lap with legs toward you; gently move baby's legs in pumping motion.
- Try putting baby down to sleep in a darkened room.
- Keep remembering that it's temporary. Try to stay as calm and relaxed as possible.

Cultural Snapshot

Diarrhea, constipation, and vomiting are symptoms that may be embarrassing to the child and family. In some cultures, the embarrassment of discussing these symptoms may lead to attempts to control or manage the symptom by using home remedies. Sometimes serious concerns may be missed or ignored. Exploration of these symptoms with the family caregiver and child during the interview and ongoing assessment process is necessary.

Mild or moderate diarrhea can quickly become severe diarrhea in a child. Vomiting usually accompanies the diarrhea; together, they cause large losses of body water and electrolytes.

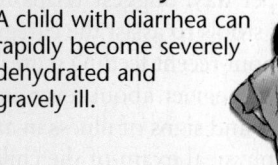

Watch closely.
A child with diarrhea can rapidly become severely dehydrated and gravely ill.

The skin becomes extremely dry and loses its turgor. The fontanelle becomes sunken, and the pulse is weak and rapid. The stools become greenish liquid and may be tinged with blood.

Diagnosis

Stool specimens may be collected for culture and sensitivity testing to determine the causative infectious organism, if there is one. Subsequently, effective antibiotics can be prescribed as indicated.

Treatment

Treatment to stop the diarrhea must be initiated immediately. Establishing normal fluid and electrolyte balance is the primary concern in treating gastroenteritis. The child with acute dehydration may be given oral feedings of commercial electrolyte solutions, such as Pedialyte, Rehydralyte, and Infalyte, unless there is shock or severe dehydration. This treatment is called oral rehydration therapy. As the diarrhea clears, food may be offered. Once commonly used, the BRAT diet (ripe banana, rice cereal, applesauce, and toast) has become somewhat controversial because it is high in calories, low in energy and protein, and does not provide adequate nutrition. Salty broths should be avoided. Infants can return to breast-feeding if they have been NPO; formula-fed infants are given their formula. Foods can be added as the child's condition improves, returning to a regular diet. Early return to the usual diet has been shown to reduce the number of stools and to decrease weight loss and the length of the illness.

In severe diarrhea with shock and severe dehydration, oral feedings are discontinued completely. Fluids to be given IV must be carefully calculated to replace the lost electrolytes. Frequent laboratory determinations of the child's blood chemistries are necessary to guide the physician in this replacement therapy. For the child who has had a serious bout of diarrhea, the care provider may prescribe soybean formula for a few weeks to avoid a possible reaction to milk proteins.

Nursing Process for the Child With Diarrhea and Gastroenteritis

Assessment

In addition to basic information about the child, the interview with the family caregiver must include specific information about the history of bowel patterns and the onset of diarrheal stools, with details on number and type of stools per day. Suggest terms to describe the color and odor of stools to assist the caregiver with descriptions. Inquire about recent feeding patterns, nausea, and vomiting. Ask the caregiver about fever and other signs of illness in the child and signs of illness in any other family members.

The physical exam of the child includes observation of skin turgor and condition, including excoriated diaper area, temperature, anterior fontanelle (depressed, normal, or bulging), apical pulse rate (observing for weak pulse), stools (character, frequency, amount, color, and presence of blood), irritability, lethargy, vomiting, urine (amount and concentration), lips and mucous membranes of the mouth (dry, cracked), eyes (bright, glassy, sunken, dark circles), and any other notable physical signs.

Selected Nursing Diagnoses

A primary nursing diagnosis is "Diarrhea related to (whatever the cause is)." Other nursing diagnoses vary with the intensity of the diarrhea (mild or severe), as determined by the physical exam and caregiver interview and may include the following:

- Risk for Infection related to inadequate secondary defenses or insufficient knowledge to avoid exposure to pathogens
- Impaired Skin Integrity related to constant presence of diarrheal stools
- Deficient Fluid Volume related to diarrheal stools
- Imbalanced Nutrition: Less Than Body Requirements related to malabsorption of nutrients
- Hyperthermia related to dehydration
- Risk for Delayed Development related to decreased sucking when infant is NPO
- Compromised Family Coping related to the seriousness of the child's illness
- Deficient Knowledge of caregivers related to understanding of treatment for diarrhea

Outcome Identification and Planning

The major goal for the ill child is to control and stop the diarrhea while minimizing the risk for infection transmission. Other important goals for the ill child include maintaining good skin condition, improving hydration and nutritional intake, and satisfying sucking needs in the infant. A major goal for the family with a child who has diarrhea or gastroenteritis is eliminating the risk of infection transmission. The family should also be supported and educated regarding the disease and treatment for the child. Plan individualized nursing care according to these goals.

Implementation

Controlling Diarrhea and Reducing the Risk of Infection Transmission

Institute measures to control and stop the diarrhea as ordered. To prevent the spread of possibly infectious organisms to other pediatric patients, follow standard precautions issued by the Centers for Disease Control and Prevention. All caregivers must wear gowns. Gloves are used when handling articles contaminated with feces, but masks are unnecessary. Place contaminated linens and clothing in specially marked containers to be processed according to the policy of the health care facility. Place disposable diapers and other disposable items in specially marked bags and dispose of them according to policy. Visitors are limited to family only.

Teach the family caregivers the principles of aseptic technique and observe them to ensure understanding and compliance. Good hand washing must be carried out and taught to the family caregivers. Stress that gloves are needed for added protection, but careful hand washing is also necessary.

Promoting Skin Integrity

To reduce irritation and excoriation of the buttocks and genital area, cleanse those areas frequently and apply a soothing protective preparation, such as lanolin or A+D Ointment. Change diapers as quickly as possible after soiling. Some infants may be sensitive to disposable diapers, and others may be sensitive to cloth diapers, so it may be necessary to try both types. Leaving the diaper off and exposing the buttocks and genital area to the air is often helpful. Placing disposable pads under the infant can facilitate easy and frequent changing. Teach caregivers that waterproof diaper covers hold moisture in and do not allow air circulation, which increases irritation and excoriation of the diaper area.

Preventing Dehydration

A child can dehydrate quickly and can get into serious trouble after <3 days of diarrhea. Carefully count diapers and weigh them to determine the infant's output accurately. Measure each voiding in the older child. Closely observe all stools. Document the number and character of the stools, as well as the amount and character of any vomitus.

Maintaining Adequate Nutrition

Weigh the child daily on the same scale. Take measurements in the early morning before the morning feeding if the child is on oral feedings. Maintain precautions to prevent contamination of equipment while weighing the child. Monitor intake and output strictly.

In severe dehydration, IV fluids are given to rest the GI tract, restore hydration, and maintain nutritional requirements. Monitor the placement, patency, and site of the IV infusion at least every 2 hours. The use of restraints, with relevant nursing interventions, may be necessary. Good mouth care is essential while the child is NPO.

When oral fluids are started, the child is given oral replacement solutions, such as those listed earlier. After the infant tolerates these solutions, half-strength formula may be introduced. After the infant tolerates this formula for several days, full-strength formula is given (possibly lactose-free or soy formula to avoid disaccharide intolerance or reaction to milk proteins). The breast-fed infant can continue breast-feeding. Give the mother of a breast-fed infant access to a breast pump if her infant is NPO. Breast milk may be frozen for later use, if desired. The infant who is NPO needs to have his or her sucking needs fulfilled. To accomplish this, offer the infant a pacifier.

Maintaining Body Temperature

Monitor vital signs at least every 2 hours if there is fever. Do not take the temperature rectally because insertion of a thermometer into the rectum can cause stimulation of stools, as well as trauma and tissue injury to sensitive mucosa. Follow the appropriate procedures for fever reduction, and administer antipyretics and antibiotics as prescribed. Take the temperature with a thermometer that is used only for that child.

Supporting Family Coping

Being the family caregiver of a child who has become so ill in such a short time is frightening. Meeting the child's emotional needs is difficult but very important. Suggest to the caregiver ways that the child might be consoled without interfering with care. Soothing, gentle stroking of the head, and speaking softly help the child bear the frustrations of the illness and its treatment. The child can be picked up and rocked, as long as this can be done without jeopardizing the IV infusion site. Threading a needle into the small veins of a dehydrated child is difficult, and replacement may be nearly impossible. The child's life may depend on receiving the proper parenteral fluids. Help fulfill the child's emotional needs, and encourage the family caregiver to have some time away from the child's room without feeling guilty about leaving.

Promoting Family Teaching

Explain to the family caregivers the importance of GI rest for the child. The family caregivers may not understand the necessity for NPO status. Cooperation of the caregiver is improved with increased understanding. See Family Teaching Tips: Diarrhea and Family Teaching Tips: Vomiting.

Evaluation: Goals and Expected Outcomes

Goal: The child's bowel elimination will return to preillness pattern.
Expected Outcomes: The child

- passes stool with decreasing frequency.
- has stool that is soft and consistency is appropriate for age.

Goal: The family caregivers will follow infection control measures.
Expected Outcomes: The family caregivers

- verbalize standard precautions for infection control.
- follow measures for standard precautions for infection control.

Goal: The child's skin integrity will be maintained.
Expected Outcomes: The child's

- diaper area shows no evidence of redness or excoriation (infant).
- skin is clean and dry with no redness or irritation.

Goal: The child will be well hydrated.
Expected Outcomes: The child's

Family Teaching Tips

DIARRHEA

The danger in diarrhea is dehydration (drying out). If the child becomes dehydrated, he or she can become very sick. Increasing the amount of liquid the child drinks is helpful. Solid foods may need to be decreased so the child will drink more.

SUGGESTIONS

- Give liquids in small amounts (3 or 4 tbsp) about every half hour. If this goes well, increase the amount a little each half hour. Don't force the child to drink, because he or she may vomit.
- Give solid foods in small amounts. Do not give milk for a day or two, because this can make diarrhea worse.
- Give only nonsalty soups or broths.
- Liquids recommended for vomiting also may be given for diarrhea.
- Soft foods to give in small amounts: applesauce, fine chopped or scraped apple without peel, bananas, toast, rice cereal, plain unsalted crackers or cookies, any meats.

CALL THE CARE PROVIDER IF

- Child develops sudden high fever.
- Stomach pain becomes severe.
- Diarrhea becomes bloody (more than a streak of blood).
- Diarrhea becomes more frequent or severe.
- Child becomes dehydrated (dried out).

SIGNS OF DEHYDRATION

- Child has not urinated for 6 hours or more.
- Child has no tears when crying.
- Child's mouth is dry or sticky to touch.
- Child's eyes are sunken.
- Child is less active than usual.
- Child has dark circles under eyes.

WARNING

Do not use medicines to stop diarrhea for children younger than 6 years of age unless specifically directed by the care provider. These medicines can be dangerous if not used properly.

DIAPER AREA SKIN CARE

- Change diaper as soon as it is soiled.
- Wash area with mild soap, rinse, and dry well.
- Use soothing, protective lotion recommended by your care provider.
- Do not use waterproof diapers or diaper covers; they increase diaper area irritation.
- Wash hands with soap and water after changing diapers or wiping the child.

Family Teaching Tips

VOMITING

Vomiting will usually stop in a couple days and can be treated at home as long as the child is getting some fluids.

WARNING

Some medications used to stop vomiting in older children or adults are dangerous in infants or young children. DO NOT use any medicine unless your physician has told you to use it for this child.

Give child clear liquids to drink in small amounts.

SUGGESTIONS

- Pedialyte, Lytren, Rehydralyte, Infalyte
- Flat soda (no fizz). Use caffeine-free type; do not use diet soda.
- Jell–O water—double the amount of water, let stand to room temperature.
- Ice popsicles
- Gatorade
- Tea
- Solid Jell-O
- Broth (not salty)

HOW TO GIVE

Give small amounts often. One tbsp every 20 minutes for the first few hours is a good rule of thumb. If this is kept down without vomiting, increase to 2 tbsp every 20 minutes for the next couple of hours. If there is no vomiting, increase the amount the child may have. If the child vomits, wait for 1 hour before offering more liquids.

- intake is sufficient to produce hourly urine output of 2 to 3 mL/kg.
- skin turgor is good.
- mucous membranes are moist and pink.
- fontanelles in the infant exhibit normal tension.

Goal: The child will consume adequate caloric intake.
Expected Outcome:

- The child consumes an age-appropriate amount of full-strength formula, breast milk, or other fluids 3 days after therapy with oral replacement solution.

Goal: The infant will satisfy nonnutritive sucking needs.
Expected Outcome:

- The infant uses a pacifier to satisfy sucking needs.

Goal: The child will maintain a temperature within normal limits.
Expected Outcome:

- The child's temperature is 98.6°F to 100°F (37°C–37.8°C).

Goal: The family caregivers' anxiety will be reduced.
Expected Outcome:

- The family caregivers participate in the care and soothing of the child.

Goal: The family caregivers will verbalize an understanding of the child's treatment.
Expected Outcomes: The family caregivers

- describe methods to increase hydration.
- list the warning signs of dehydration.

Test Yourself

✔ What is the major concern in the child who has diarrhea and vomiting?

✔ How is the child with diarrhea treated? What is this treatment called?

✔ What do the health care providers do when caring for a child with diarrhea to prevent the spread of infection from one child to another?

PYLORIC STENOSIS

The pylorus is the muscle that controls the flow of food from the stomach to the duodenum. Pyloric stenosis is characterized by hypertrophy of the circular muscle fibers of the pylorus, with a severe narrowing of its lumen. The pylorus is thickened to as much as twice its size, is elongated, and has a consistency resembling cartilage. As a result of this obstruction at the distal end of the stomach, the stomach becomes dilated (Fig. 38-5A).

■ **Figure 38-5 (A)** Hypertrophied pylorus muscle and narrowed stomach outlet. **(B)** In pyloromyotomy, the pylorus is incised, thus increasing the diameter of the pyloric outlet.

Pyloric stenosis is rarely symptomatic during the first days of life. It has occasionally been recognized shortly after birth, but the average affected infant does not show symptoms until about the third week of life. Symptoms rarely appear after the second month. Although symptoms appear late, pyloric stenosis is classified as a congenital defect. Its cause is unknown, but it occurs more frequently in white males and has a familial tendency.

Clinical Manifestations

During the first weeks of life, the infant with pyloric stenosis often eats well, gains weight, and then starts vomiting occasionally after meals. Within a few days, the vomiting increases in frequency and force, becoming projectile. The vomited material is sour, undigested food; it may contain mucus but never bile because it has not progressed beyond the stomach.

Because the obstruction is a mechanical one, the baby does not feel ill, is ravenously hungry, and is eager to try again and again, but the food invariably comes back. As the condition progresses, the baby becomes irritable, loses weight rapidly, and becomes dehydrated. Alkalosis develops from the loss of potassium and hydrochloric acid, and the baby becomes seriously ill.

Constipation becomes progressive because little food gets into the intestine, and urine is scanty. Gastric peristaltic waves passing from left to right across the abdomen usually can be seen during or after feedings.

Diagnosis

Diagnosis is usually made on the clinical evidence. The nature, type, and times of vomiting are documented. When the infant drinks, gastric peristaltic waves are observed. The infant may have a history of weight loss with hunger and irritability.

Ultrasonographic or radiographic studies with barium swallow show an abnormal retention of barium in the stomach and increased peristalsis.

Treatment

A surgical procedure called a pyloromyotomy (also known as a Fredet-Ramstedt operation) is the treatment of choice. This procedure simply splits the hypertrophic pyloric muscle down to the submucosa, allowing the pylorus to expand so that food may pass. Prognosis is excellent if surgery is performed before the infant is severely dehydrated (Fig. 38-5B).

Nursing Process for the Child With Pyloric Stenosis

Assessment

When the infant of 1 or 2 months of age has a history of projectile vomiting, pyloric stenosis is suspected. Carefully interview the family caregivers. Ask when the vomiting started and determine the character of the vomiting (undigested formula with no bile, vomitus progressively more projectile). The caregiver will relate a story of a baby who is an eager eater but cannot retain food. Ask the caregiver about constipation and scanty urine.

Physical exam reveals an infant who may show signs of dehydration. Obtain the infant's weight and observe skin turgor and skin condition (including diaper area), anterior fontanelle (depressed, normal, or bulging), temperature, apical pulse rate (observing for weak pulse and tachy-cardia), irritability, lethargy, urine (amount and concentration), lips and mucous membranes of the mouth (dry, cracked), and eyes (bright, glassy, sunken, dark circles). Observe for visible gastric peristalsis when the infant is eating. Document and report signs of severe dehydration to help determine the need for fluid and electrolyte replacement.

Do you know the why of it?

An experienced practitioner often can feel an olive-sized mass through deep palpation in the infant with pyloric stenosis.

Selected Nursing Diagnoses: Preoperative Phase

- Imbalanced Nutrition: Less Than Body Requirements related to inability to retain food
- Deficient Fluid Volume related to frequent vomiting
- Impaired Oral Mucous Membrane related to NPO status
- Risk for Impaired Skin Integrity related to fluid and nutritional deficit
- Compromised Family Coping related to seriousness of illness and impending surgery

Outcome Identification and Planning: Preoperative Phase

Before surgery, the major goals for the infant with pyloric stenosis include improving nutrition and hydration, maintaining mouth and skin integrity, and relieving family anxiety. Plan individualized nursing care according to these goals, including interventions to prepare the infant for surgery.

Implementation: Preoperative Phase

Maintaining Adequate Nutrition and Fluid Intake

Hypertrophy of the pylorus narrows the passage from the stomach into the duodenum. As a result, food (breast milk or formula) cannot pass. The infant loses weight and becomes dehydrated. If the infant is severely dehydrated and malnourished, rehydration with IV fluids and electrolytes is necessary to correct hypokalemia and alkalosis and prepare the infant for surgery. Carefully monitor the IV site for redness and induration. Improved skin turgor, weight gain, correction of hypokalemia and alkalosis, adequate intake of fluids, and no evidence of gastric distention are signs of improved nutrition and hydration.

Feedings of formula thickened with infant cereal and fed through a large-holed nipple may be given to improve nutrition before surgery. A smooth muscle relaxant may be ordered before feedings. Feed the infant slowly while he or she is sitting in an infant seat or being held upright. During the feeding, burp the infant frequently to avoid gastric distention. Document the feeding given and the approximate amount retained. Also, record the frequency and type of emesis.

In preparation for surgery, fluid and electrolyte balance must be restored and the stomach must be empty. Typically, oral fluids are omitted for a specified time before the procedure, and the infant receives IV fluids. After the infant undergoes a barium swallow x-ray for diagnosis, the physician may order placement of a NG tube with saline lavage to empty the stomach. The NG tube is left in place when the infant goes to surgery.

Providing Mouth Care

The infant needs good mouth care as the mucous membranes of the mouth may be dry because of dehydration and the omission of oral fluids before surgery. A pacifier can satisfy the baby's need for sucking because of the interruption in normal feeding and sucking habits.

Promoting Skin Integrity

Depending on the severity of dehydration, the skin may easily crack or break down and become irritated. The infant is repositioned, the diaper is changed, and lanolin or A+D Ointment is applied to dry skin areas. IV therapy may also affect skin integrity. Monitor the IV insertion site for redness and inflammation. Closely observe and document the infant's skin condition.

Promoting Family Coping

The family caregivers are anxious because their infant is obviously seriously ill, and when they learn that the infant is to undergo surgery, their apprehensions increase. Include the caregivers in the preparation for surgery and explain:

- The importance of added IV fluids preoperatively to improve electrolyte balance and rehydrate the infant.
- The reason for ultrasonographic or barium swallow examination.
- The function of the NG tube and saline lavage.

Explain the location of the pylorus (at the distal end of the stomach) and what happens when the circular muscle fibers hypertrophy. You can compare it to a doughnut that thickens, so that the opening closes and very little food gets through. Describe the surgical procedure to be performed. During the procedure, the muscle is simply split down to, but not through, the submucosa, allowing it to balloon and let food pass.

Direct the family caregivers to the appropriate waiting area during surgery so that the surgeon can find them immediately after surgery. Explain to the caregivers what to expect and about how long the operation will last.

Describe the procedure for the postanesthesia care unit so that the caregivers know the infant will be under close observation after surgery until fully recovered.

Evaluation: Goals and Expected Outcomes—Preoperative Phase

Goal: The infant's nutritional status will be adequate for normal growth.

Expected Outcome:

- The infant maintains weight.

Goal: The infant will be hydrated.

Expected Outcomes: The infant's

- skin turgor improves.
- mucous membranes are moist and pink.
- hourly urine output is 2 to 3 mL/kg.

Goal: The infant's IV infusion site will remain intact.

Expected Outcome:

- The infant's skin shows no signs of redness or induration.

Goal: The infant's oral mucous membranes will remain intact.

Expected Outcomes: The infant

- has mucous membranes that are moist and pink and saliva is sufficient, as evidenced by typical drooling.
- uses a pacifier sufficiently to meet sucking needs.

Goal: The infant's skin integrity will be maintained.

Expected Outcome:

- The infant shows no signs of skin irritation or breakdown.

Goal: The family caregivers' anxiety will be reduced.

Expected Outcomes: The family caregivers

- verbalize an understanding of the procedures and treatments.
- cooperate with the nursing staff.
- ask appropriate questions.
- express confidence in the treatment plan.

Selected Nursing Diagnoses: Postoperative Phase

- Risk for Aspiration related to postoperative vomiting
- Acute Pain related to surgical trauma
- Imbalanced Nutrition: Less Than Body Requirements related to postoperative condition
- Risk for Impaired Skin Integrity related to surgical incision
- Compromised Family Coping related to postoperative condition

Outcome Identification and Planning: Postoperative Phase

After surgery, the major goals for the infant include keeping the airway clear, maintaining comfort, improving nutrition status, preserving skin integrity, and reducing family anxiety. Individualize the nursing plan of care according to these goals.

Implementation: Postoperative Phase

Maintaining a Patent Airway

After surgery, position the infant on his or her side and prevent aspiration of mucus or vomitus, particularly during the anesthesia recovery period. After fully waking from surgery, the infant may be held by a family caregiver. Help the caregiver find a position that does not interfere with IV infusions and that is comforting to both the caregiver and child.

Promoting Comfort

Observe the infant's behavior to evaluate discomfort and pain. Excessive crying, restlessness, listlessness, resistance to being held and cuddled, rigidity, and increased pulse and respiratory rates can indicate pain. Administer analgesics, as ordered. Nursing interventions that may provide comfort include rocking, holding, cuddling, and offering a pacifier. Include the family caregivers in helping to comfort the infant.

Providing Nutrition

The first feeding, given 4 to 6 hours after surgery, is usually an electrolyte replacement solution, such as Lytren or Pedialyte. Give feedings slowly, in small amounts, with frequent burping. IV fluid is necessary until the infant is taking sufficient oral feedings. Continue to use all nursing measures for IV care that were followed before surgery. Accurate intake, output, and daily weight determinations are required.

Promoting Skin Integrity

Closely observe the surgical site for blood, drainage, and secretions. Make observations at least every 4 hours. Record and report any odor. Care for the incision and dressings as ordered by the physician.

Promoting Family Coping

The family caregivers will be anxious if the infant vomits after surgery, but reassure them that this is not uncommon during the first 24 hours after surgery. The caregivers should be involved in postoperative care. Reassure them that the care they gave at home did not cause the condition. Offer them support and understanding and encourage them in feeding and providing for the infant's needs. They can be told that the likelihood of a satisfactory recovery in a few weeks, with steady progression to complete recovery, is excellent. The operative fatality rate under these conditions has become <1%.

Evaluation: Goals and Expected Outcomes—Postoperative Phase

Goal: The infant will not aspirate vomitus or mucus.

Expected Outcome:

- The infant rests quietly in a side-lying position without choking or coughing.

Goal: The infant will show signs of being comfortable.
Expected Outcomes: The infant

- sleeps and rests in a relaxed manner.
- cuddles with caregivers and nurses.
- does not cry excessively.

Goal: The infant's nutrition status and fluid intake will improve.
Expected Outcomes: The infant's

- daily weight gain is 0.75 to 1 oz (22–30 g).
- oral fluids are retained with minimal vomiting.
- hourly urine output is 2 to 3 mL/kg.

Goal: The infant's skin integrity will be maintained.
Expected Outcome:

- The infant's surgical site shows no signs of infection, as evidenced by absence of redness, foul odor, or drainage.

Goal: The family caregivers' anxiety will be reduced.
Expected Outcomes: The family caregivers

- are involved in the postoperative feeding of the infant.
- demonstrate an understanding of feeding technique.

Test Yourself

✔ What type of vomiting is seen in the child with pyloric stenosis?

✔ What is done to treat a child with pyloric stenosis?

✔ Explain the reason it is important to monitor accurate intake and output in the child with pyloric stenosis.

CONGENITAL AGANGLIONIC MEGACOLON

Congenital aganglionic megacolon, also called Hirschsprung disease, is characterized by persistent constipation resulting from partial or complete intestinal obstruction of mechanical origin. In some cases, the condition may be severe enough to be recognized during the neonatal period; in other cases, the blockage may not be diagnosed until later infancy or early childhood.

Parasympathetic nerve cells regulate peristalsis in the intestine. The name aganglionic megacolon actually describes the condition because there is an absence of parasympathetic ganglion cells within the muscular wall of the distal colon and the rectum. As a result, the affected portion of the lower bowel has no peristaltic action. Thus, it narrows, and the portion directly proximal to (above) the affected area becomes greatly dilated and filled with feces and gas (Fig. 38-6).

Distended sigmoid colon
Aganglionic Portion
Rectum

■ **Figure 38-6** Enlarged megacolon of Hirschsprung's disease.

Clinical Manifestations

Accurate reporting of the first meconium stool in the newborn is vital. Failure of the newborn to have a stool in the first 24 hours may indicate a number of conditions, one of which is megacolon.

> **This is critical to remember.**
> If a newborn does not have a stool within the first 24 hours, this must be documented and reported.

Other neonatal symptoms are suggestive of complete or partial intestinal obstruction, such as bile-stained emesis and generalized abdominal distention. Gastroenteritis with diarrheal stools may be present, and ulceration of the colon may occur.

The affected older infant or child has obstinate, severe constipation dating back to early infancy. Stools are ribbonlike or consist of hard pellets. Formed bowel movements do not occur, except with the use of enemas, and soiling does not occur. The rectum is usually empty because the impaction occurs above the aganglionic segment.

As the child grows older, the abdomen becomes progressively enlarged and hard. General debilitation and chronic anemia are usually present. Differentiation must be made between this condition and psychogenic megacolon because of coercive toileting or other emotional problems. The child with aganglionic megacolon does not withhold stools or defecate in inappropriate places and no soiling occurs.

Diagnosis

In the newborn, the absence of a meconium stool within the first 24 hours requires evaluation; in the older infant or child, a history of obstinate, severe constipation may indicate the need for further evaluation. Definitive diagnosis is made through barium studies and must be confirmed by rectal biopsy.

Treatment

Treatment involves surgery with the ultimate resection of the aganglionic portion of the bowel. A colostomy is often performed to relieve the obstruction. This allows the child to regain any weight lost and also gives the bowel a period of rest to return to a more normal state. Resection is deferred until later in infancy.

Nursing Process for the Child Undergoing Surgery for Congenital Aganglionic Megacolon

Assessment

Carefully gather a history from the family caregivers, noting especially the history of stooling. Ask about the onset of constipation; the character and odor of stools; the frequency of bowel movements; and the presence of poor feeding habits, anorexia, and irritability.

During the physical exam, observe for a distended abdomen and signs of poor nutrition (see Nursing Process for the Child With Nutritional Problems earlier in this chapter). Record the child's weight and vital signs. Observe the child for developmental milestones.

Selected Nursing Diagnoses: Preoperative Phase

- Constipation related to decreased bowel motility
- Imbalanced Nutrition: Less Than Body Requirements related to anorexia
- Fear (in the older child) related to impending surgery
- Compromised Family Coping related to the serious condition of the child and lack of knowledge about impending surgery

Outcome Identification and Planning: Preoperative Phase

The preoperative goals for the child undergoing surgery for congenital aganglionic megacolon include preventing constipation, improving nutritional status, and relieving fear (in the older child). The major goal for the family is reducing anxiety. Base the preoperative nursing plan of care on these goals. Plan interventions that prepare the child for surgery.

Implementation: Preoperative Phase

Preventing Constipation

Decreased bowel motility may lead to constipation, which in turn may result in injury. Enemas may be given to achieve bowel elimination. They also may be ordered before diagnostic and surgical procedures are performed. Administer colonic irrigations with saline solutions. Neomycin or other antibiotic solutions are used to cleanse the bowel and prepare the GI tract.

> **Don't!**
> Never administer soap suds or tap water enemas to a child with Hirschsprung disease. The lack of peristaltic action causes the enemas to be retained and absorbed into the tissues, causing water intoxication. This could cause syncope, shock, or even death after only one or two irrigations.

Maintaining Adequate Nutrition

Parenteral nutrition may be needed to improve nutritional status because the constipation and distended abdomen cause loss of appetite. IV fluid therapy may be necessary. The child does not want to eat and has a poor nutritional status. In older children, a low residue diet is given.

Reducing Fear

Children who are preschool-aged or older are more aware of the approaching surgery and have a number of fears reflective of their developmental stage. Preschoolers are still in the age of magical thinking. They may overhear a word or two that they misinterpret and exaggerate; this can lead to imagined pain and danger. Careful explanations must be provided for the preschooler to reduce any fears about mutilation. Talk about the surgery; reassure the child that their "insides won't come out," and answer questions seriously and sincerely. Encourage family caregivers to stay with the child, if possible, to increase the child's feelings of security.

The older school-aged child may have a more realistic view of what is going to happen but may still fear the impending surgery. Peer contact may help comfort the school-aged child. For more information on reducing preoperative fears and anxiety, see Chapter 29.

Promoting Family Coping

Family caregivers are apprehensive about the preliminary procedures and the impending surgery. Explain all aspects of the preoperative care, including examinations, colonic irrigations, and IV fluid therapy. As with other surgical procedures, inform the caregivers about the waiting area, the postanesthesia care unit, and the approximate length of the operation and answer any questions. Building good rapport before surgery is an essential aspect of good nursing care. Answer the family caregivers' questions about the later resection of the aganglionic portion. With successful surgery, these children will grow and develop normally.

Evaluation: Goals and Expected Outcomes— Preoperative Phase

Goal: The child will have adequate bowel elimination with episodes of constipation.
Expected Outcomes: The child's

- bowel eliminations occur daily.
- colon is clean and well prepared for surgery.

Goal: The child's nutritional status will be maintained preoperatively.
Expected Outcome:

- The child ingests diet adequate to maintain weight and promote growth.

Goal: The older child will display minimal fear of bodily injury.
Expected Outcomes: The older child

- realistically describes what will happen in surgery.

■ interacts with family, peers, and nursing staff in a positive manner.

Goal: The family caregivers will demonstrate an understanding of preoperative procedures.

Expected Outcomes: The family caregivers

■ cooperate with care.
■ ask relevant questions.
■ accurately explain procedures when asked to repeat information.

Selected Nursing Diagnoses: Postoperative Phase

■ Risk for Impaired Skin Integrity related to irritation from the colostomy
■ Acute Pain related to the surgical procedure
■ Deficient Fluid Volume related to postoperative condition
■ Impaired Oral and Nasal Mucous Membranes related to NPO status and irritation from NG tube
■ Deficient Knowledge of caregivers related to understanding of postoperative care of the colostomy

Outcome Identification and Planning: Postoperative Phase

The major postoperative goals for the child include maintaining skin integrity; promoting comfort; maintaining fluid balance; and maintaining moist, clean nasal and oral mucous membranes. Goals for the family include reducing caregiver anxiety and preparing for home care of the child. Develop the individualized nursing plan of care according to these goals.

Implementation: Postoperative Phase

Promoting Skin Integrity

Maintaining skin integrity of the surgical site, especially around the colostomy stoma, is very important. When performing routine colostomy care, give careful attention to the area around the colostomy. Record and report redness, irritation, and rashy appearances of the skin around the stoma. Prepare the skin with skin-toughening preparations that strengthen it and provide better adhesion of the appliance.

Promoting Comfort

The child may have abdominal pain after surgery. Observe for signs of pain such as crying, pulse and respiration rate increases, restlessness, guarding of the abdomen, or drawing up the legs. Administer analgesics promptly, as ordered. Additional nursing measures that can be used are changing the child's position, holding the child when possible, stroking, cuddling, and engaging in age-appropriate activities. Observe for abdominal distention, which must be documented and reported promptly.

Maintaining Fluid Balance

The NG tube is left in place after surgery, and IV fluids are given until bowel function is established. Accurate intake and output determinations and reporting the character, amount, and consistency of stools help determine when the child may have oral feedings. To monitor fluid loss, record and report the drainage from the NG tube every 8 hours. Immediately report any unusual drainage, such as bright-red bleeding.

Providing Oral and Nasal Care

Perform good mouth care at least every 4 hours. At the same time, gently clean the nares to relieve any irritation from the NG tube. If the child is young, sucking needs can be satisfied with a pacifier.

Providing Family Teaching

Show the family caregiver how to care for the colostomy at home. If available, a wound, ostomy and continence, nurse (WOCN) may be consulted to help teach the family caregivers. Discuss topics such as devices and their use, daily irrigation, and skin care. The caregivers should demonstrate their understanding by caring for the colostomy under the supervision of nursing personnel several days before discharge. Family caregivers also need referrals to support personnel.

 A Personal Glimpse

When our son was born my wife and I were thrilled; we were so happy to be parents. My wife was breast-feeding, and I would get up at night and bring him to her so she could feed him; it was just like we had thought it would be. He started growing and getting bigger, so at first we weren't worried about his big belly. It was my job to change the "dirty" diapers when I was home. We started noticing the baby seemed constipated at times and had little hard stools but then had diarrhea. The pediatrician used the word "obstruction," and that was hard for us to really understand. They did a barium test and other tests; we felt so bad for our baby. My wife was so upset, she cried all the time. He had to have IVs and TPN, and then they told us he would have to have surgery and a colostomy. Seeing him with all those tubes and bags after surgery was heartbreaking. We took him home with the colostomy, and my job was still the "diaper" duty, but now it was taking care of the colostomy. I have gotten so good, now I can change the colostomy bag pretty fast. We know he has to go back for more surgery, but for now we are just glad we can take care of him at home and love and enjoy him.

David

Learning Opportunity: In what ways do you think this father was supportive of his wife and his son? What would be important to teach these parents about care of the colostomy? What community support might be available for this family?

Evaluation: Goals and Expected Outcomes— Postoperative Phase

Goal: The child's skin integrity will be maintained.

Expected Outcomes: The child

- has no skin irritation at the colostomy site.
- has no redness, foul odor, or purulent drainage at the surgical site.

Goal: The child's behavior will indicate minimal pain.

Expected Outcomes: The child

- rests quietly without signs of restlessness.
- verbalizes comfort if old enough to communicate verbally.

Goal: The child's fluid intake will be adequate.

Expected Outcome:

- The child's hourly urine output is 2 to 3 mL/kg, indicating adequate hydration.

Goal: The child's oral and nasal mucous membranes will remain intact.

Expected Outcomes:

- The child's oral and nasal mucous membranes are moist and pink.
- The infant uses a pacifier to meet sucking needs.

Goal: The family caregivers will demonstrate skill and knowledge in caring for the colostomy.

Expected Outcome:

- The family caregivers irrigate the colostomy and clean the surrounding skin under the supervision of nursing personnel.

INTUSSUSCEPTION

Intussusception is the **invagination,** or telescoping, of one portion of the bowel into a distal portion. It occurs most commonly at the juncture of the ileum and the colon, although it can appear elsewhere in the intestinal tract. The invagination is from above downward, the upper portion slipping over the lower portion and pulling the mesentery along with it (Fig. 38-7).

This condition occurs more often in boys than in girls and is the most common cause of intestinal obstruction in childhood. The highest incidence occurs in infants between the ages of 4 and 10 months. The condition

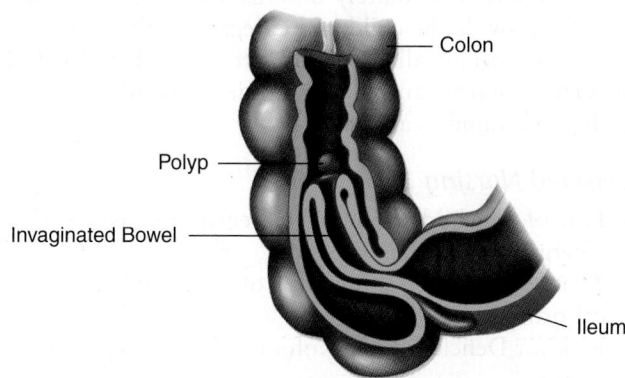

■ **Figure 38-7** In this drawing of intussusception, note the telescoping of a portion of the bowel into the distal portion.

usually appears in healthy babies without any demonstrable cause. Possible contributing factors may be the hyperperistalsis and unusual mobility of the cecum and ileum normally present in early life. Occasionally a lesion such as Meckel's diverticulum or a polyp is present.

Clinical Manifestations

The infant who previously appeared healthy and happy suddenly becomes pale, cries out sharply, and draws up the legs in a severe colicky spasm of pain. This spasm may last for several minutes, after which the infant relaxes and appears well until the next episode, which may occur 5, 10, or 20 minutes later.

Most of these infants start vomiting early. Vomiting becomes progressively more severe and eventually is bile-stained. The infant strains with each paroxysm, emptying the bowels of fecal contents. The stools consist of blood and mucus, thereby earning the name **currant jelly stools.**

> **Observation skills are critical.**
> Currant jelly stools are an important clue in the child with intussusception.

Signs of shock appear quickly and characteristically include a rapid, weak pulse; increased temperature; shallow, grunting respirations; pallor; and marked sweating. Shock, vomiting, and currant jelly stools are the cardinal symptoms of this condition. Because these signs coupled with the paroxysmal pain are quite severe, professional health care is often initiated early.

As a nurse, you will find that you are often consulted by neighbors, friends, and relatives when things go wrong; therefore, you need to be informed and alert. Be aware that on rare occasions a more chronic form of the condition appears, particularly during an episode of severe diarrheal disturbance. The onset is more gradual, and the infant may not show all the classic symptoms, but the danger of sudden, complete strangulation of the bowel is present. Such an infant should already be in the care of a physician because of the diarrhea.

Diagnosis

The care provider usually can make a diagnosis from the clinical symptoms, rectal examination, and palpation of the abdomen during a calm interval when it is soft. A baby is often unwilling to tolerate this palpation, and sedation may be ordered. A sausage-shaped mass can often be felt through the abdominal wall.

Treatment and Nursing Care

Unlike pyloric stenosis, this condition is an emergency in the sense that prolonged delay is dangerous. The telescoped bowel rapidly becomes gangrenous, thus markedly reducing the possibility of a simple reduction.

Adequate treatment during the first 12 to 24 hours should have a good outcome with complete recovery. The outcome becomes more uncertain as the bowel deteriorates, making resection necessary.

Immediate treatment consists of IV fluids, NPO status, and a diagnostic barium enema. The barium enema can often reduce the invagination, simply by the pressure of the barium fluid pushing against the telescoped portion. The barium enema should not be done if signs of bowel perforation or peritonitis are evident. Abdominal surgery is performed if the barium enema does not correct the problem. Surgery may consist of manual reduction of the invagination, resection with anastomosis, or possible colostomy if the intestine is gangrenous.

If the invagination was reduced, the infant is returned to normal feedings within 24 hours and discharged in about 48 hours. Carefully observe for recurrence during this period. If surgery is necessary, many of the same preoperative and postoperative nursing diagnoses used for congenital aganglionic megacolon also can be used when surgery is required for this condition.

Test Yourself

✔ Explain what happens in the GI tract of the child who has congenital aganglionic megacolon (Hirschsprung disease).

✔ Explain the cause of intussusception and describe the symptoms seen in the child with the diagnosis.

APPENDICITIS

Appendicitis refers to an inflammation of the appendix. The appendix is a blind pouch located in the cecum near the ileocecal junction. Obstruction of the lumen of the appendix is the primary cause of appendicitis. The obstruction usually is caused by hardened fecal matter or a foreign body. This obstruction causes circulation to be slowed or interrupted, resulting in pain and necrosis of the appendix. The necrotic area can rupture, causing escape of fecal matter and bacteria into the peritoneal cavity and resulting in the complication of peritonitis. Most cases of appendicitis in childhood occur in the school-aged child.

Clinical Manifestations

In young children, the symptoms may be difficult to evaluate. Symptoms in the older child may be the same as in an adult: Pain and tenderness in the right-lower quadrant of the abdomen, nausea and vomiting, fever,

Do you know the why of it?

When appendicitis is suspected, laxatives and enemas are contraindicated because they increase peristalsis, which increases the possibility of rupturing an inflamed appendix.

and constipation. However, these symptoms are uncommon in young children; many children already have a ruptured appendix when first seen by the physician. The young child has difficulty localizing the pain, may act restless and irritable, and may have a slight fever, a flushed face, and a rapid pulse. Usually, the white blood cell count is slightly elevated. It may take several hours to rule out other conditions and make a positive diagnosis.

Treatment

Surgical removal of the appendix is necessary and should be performed as soon as possible after diagnosis. If the appendix has not ruptured before surgery, the operative risk is nearly negligible. Even after perforation has occurred, the mortality rate is <1%.

Food and fluids by mouth are withheld before surgery. If the child is dehydrated, IV fluids are ordered. If fever is present, the temperature should be reduced to below 102°F (38.9°C).

Recovery is rapid and usually uneventful. The child is ambulated early and can leave the hospital a few days after surgery. If peritonitis or a localized abscess occurs, gastric suction, parenteral fluids, and antibiotics may be ordered.

Nursing Process for the Child With Appendicitis

Assessment

When a child is admitted with a diagnosis of possible appendicitis, an emergency situation exists. The family caregiver who brings the child to the hospital often is upset and anxious. The admission examination and assessment must be performed quickly and skillfully. Obtain information about the child's condition for the last several days to formulate a picture of how the condition has developed. Emphasize GI complaints, appetite, bowel movements for the last few days, and general activity level. During the physical exam, include vital signs, especially noting any elevation of temperature, presence of bowel sounds, abdominal guarding, and nausea or vomiting. Report immediately diminished or absent bowel sounds. Provide the child and caregiver with careful explanations about all procedures to be performed. Use special empathy and understanding to alleviate the child's and family's anxieties.

Selected Nursing Diagnoses

- Fear of the child and family caregiver related to emergency surgery
- Acute Pain related to necrosis of appendix and surgical procedure
- Risk for Deficient Fluid Volume related to decreased intake
- Deficient Knowledge of caregiver related to postoperative and home care needs

Outcome Identification and Planning

Because of the urgent nature of the child's admission and preparation for surgery, great efforts must be taken to provide calm reassuring care to both the child and the caregivers. A major goal for both the child and the caregivers is relieving fear. Additional goals for the child are relieving pain and maintaining fluid balance. Another goal for the family is increasing knowledge of the postoperative and home care needs of the child.

Implementation

Reducing Fear

Although procedures must be performed quickly, consider both the child's and the family's fear. The child may be extremely frightened by the sudden change of events and also may be in considerable pain. The family caregiver may be apprehensive about impending surgery. Introduce various health care team members by name and title as they come into the child's room to perform procedures. Explain to the child and the family what is happening and why. Explain the postanesthesia care unit (recovery room) to the child and the family. Encourage the family and child to verbalize fears and try to allay these fears as much as possible. Let family members know where to wait during surgery, how long the surgery will last, where dining facilities are located, and where the surgeon will expect to find them after surgery. Throughout the preoperative care, be sensitive to verbalized or nonverbalized fears and provide understanding care.

What a difference this can make. Before the child goes to surgery, if possible, demonstrate deep breathing, coughing, and abdominal splinting to the child and have her or him practice it.

Promoting Comfort

Analgesics are not given before surgery because they may conceal signs of tenderness that are important for diagnosis. Provide comfort through positioning and gentle care while performing preoperative procedures. Heat to the abdomen is contraindicated because of the danger of rupture of the appendix. After surgery, observe the child hourly for indications of pain and administer analgesics as ordered. Provide quiet activities to help divert the child's attention from the pain. The child may fear postoperative ambulation because of pain. Many children are worried that the stitches will pull out. Reassure the child that this worry is understood, but that the sutures (or staples) are intended to withstand the strain of walking and moving. Activity is essential to the child's recovery but should be as pain free as possible. Help the child understand that as activity increases, the pain will decrease. The child whose appendix ruptured before surgery may also have pain related to the NG tube, abdominal distention, or constipation.

Monitoring Fluid Balance

Dehydration can be a concern, especially if the child has had preoperative nausea and vomiting. On admission to the hospital, the child is maintained NPO until after surgery. Accurately measure and record intake and output. IV fluids are administered as ordered. After surgery, check dressings to detect evidence of excessive drainage or bleeding that indicates loss of fluids. Clear oral fluids are usually ordered soon after surgery. After the child takes and retains fluids successfully, a progressive diet is ordered. Monitor, record, and report bowel sounds at least every 4 hours because the physician may use this as a gauge to determine when the child can have solid food.

Providing Family Teaching

The child who has had an uncomplicated appendectomy usually convalesces quickly and can return to school within 1 or 2 weeks. Teach the caregiver to keep the incision clean and dry. Activities are limited according to the physician's recommendations. The child whose appendix ruptured may be hospitalized for as long as a week and is more limited in activities after surgery. Instruct the family to observe for signs and symptoms of postoperative complications, including fever, abdominal distention, and pain. Emphasize the need for making and keeping follow-up appointments.

Evaluation: Goals and Expected Outcomes

Goal: The child and family caregivers will have reduced or alleviated fear.
Expected Outcomes: The child and family

- verbalize fears.
- ask questions before surgery.
- cooperate with health care personnel.

Goal: The child's pain will be controlled.
Expected Outcome:

- The child's pain is at an acceptable level, as evidenced by the child's verbalization of pain according to a pain scale.

Goal: The child will have adequate fluid intake.
Expected Outcomes: The child's

- skin turgor is good.
- vital signs are within normal limits.
- hourly urine output is at least 30 to 40 mL.

Goal: The family caregivers will verbalize an understanding of postoperative and home care needs of the child.
Expected Outcomes: The family caregivers

- discuss recovery expectations.
- demonstrate wound care as needed.
- list signs and symptoms to report.

INTESTINAL PARASITES

A few intestinal parasites are common in the United States, especially in young and school-aged children. Hand-to-mouth practices contribute to infestations.

Enterobiasis (Pinworm Infection)

The pinworm (*Enterobius vermicularis*) is a white threadlike worm that invades the cecum and may enter the appendix. Articles contaminated with pinworm eggs spread pinworms from person to person. The infestation is common in children and occurs when a child unknowingly swallows the pinworm eggs. The eggs hatch in the intestinal tract and grow to maturity in the cecum. The female worm, when ready to lay her eggs, crawls out of the anus and lays the eggs on the perineum.

Itching around the anus causes the child to scratch and trap new eggs under the fingernails, which often causes reinfection when the child's fingers go into the mouth. Clothing, bedding, food, toilet seats, and other articles become infected, and the infestation spreads to other members of the family. Pinworm eggs also can float in the air and be inhaled.

The life cycle of these worms is 6 to 8 weeks, after which reinfestation commonly occurs without treatment. The incidence is highest in school-aged children and next highest in preschoolers. All members of the family are susceptible.

Clinical Manifestations and Diagnosis

Intense perianal itching is the primary symptom of pinworms. Young children who cannot clearly verbalize their feelings may be restless, sleep poorly, or have episodes of bed-wetting.

The usual method of diagnosis is to use cellophane tape to capture the eggs from around the anus and to examine them under a microscope. Adult worms also may be seen as they emerge from the anus when the child is lying quietly or sleeping. The cellophane tape test for identifying worms is performed in the early morning, just before or as soon as the child wakens. The test is performed in the following manner:

1. Wind clear cellophane tape around the end of a tongue blade, sticky side outward.
2. Spread the child's buttocks and press the tape against the anus, rolling the tape from side to side.
3. Transfer the tape to a microscope slide and cover with a clean slide to send to the laboratory. If the caregiver does not have slides or a commercially prepared kit, the caregiver should place the tongue blade in a plastic bag and bring it to the health care facility.

The tape then is examined microscopically for eggs in the laboratory.

Treatment and Nursing Care

Treatment consists of the use of an **anthelmintic** (or vermifugal, a medication that expels intestinal worms). Mebendazole (Vermox) is the most commonly used product. The medication should be repeated in 2 or 3 weeks to eliminate any parasites that hatch after the initial treatment. Because pinworms are easily transmitted, encourage all family members to be treated.

It is often disturbing to children and caregivers for the child to be found to have pinworms. Reassure them that pinworm infestation is as common as an infection or a cold. This support is important when caring for a child with any type of intestinal parasite.

As a preventive measure, teach the child to wash his or her hands after bowel movements and before eating. Encourage the child to observe other hygiene measures, such as regular bathing and daily change of underclothing. Teach caregivers to keep the child's fingernails short and clean. Caregivers also need to know that bedding should be changed frequently to avoid reinfestation. All bedding and clothing, especially underclothing, should be washed in hot water.

Roundworms

Ascaris lumbricoides is a large intestinal worm found only in humans. Infestation occurs through contact with the feces of people with infestation. It is usually found in areas where sanitary facilities are lacking and human excreta are deposited on the ground.

The adult worm is pink and 9 to 12 in long. The eggs hatch in the intestinal tract, and the larvae migrate to the liver and lungs. The larvae reaching the lungs ascend up through the bronchi, get swallowed, and reach the intestine, where they grow to maturity and mate. Eggs are then discharged into the feces. Full development requires about 2 months. In tropical countries where infestation may be heavy, bowel obstructions may present serious problems.

Generally, no symptoms are present in ordinary infestations. Identification is made by means of microscopic examination of feces for eggs. Pyrantel pamoate (Antiminth) is the medication commonly used. Caregivers require education about improved hygiene practices with sanitary disposal of feces, including diapers, as necessary to prevent infestation.

Hookworms

The hookworm lives in the human intestinal tract, where it attaches itself to the wall of the small intestine. Eggs are discharged in the feces of the host. These parasites are prevalent in areas where infected human excreta are deposited on the ground and where the soil, moisture, and temperature are favorable for the development of infective larvae of the worm. In the southeastern United States and tropical West Africa, the prevailing species is *Necator americanus*.

Clinical Manifestations and Diagnosis

After feces containing eggs are deposited on the ground, larvae hatch. They can survive there as long as 6 weeks and usually penetrate the skin of barefoot people. They produce an itching dermatitis on the feet (ground itch). The larvae pass through the bloodstream to the lungs and into the pharynx, where they are swallowed and reach the small intestine. In the small intestine, they attach themselves to the intestinal wall, where they feed on blood. Heavy infestation may cause anemia through loss of blood. Chronic infestation produces listlessness, fatigue, and malnutrition. Identification is made by examination of the stool under the microscope.

Treatment and Nursing Care

Pyrantel pamoate or mebendazole may be used in the treatment of hookworms. Stress the need for the affected child to receive a well-balanced diet with additional protein and iron. Transfusions are rarely necessary. To prevent hookworm infestation, instruct caregivers to keep children from running barefoot where there is any possibility of ground contamination with feces.

Giardiasis

Giardiasis is not caused by a worm, but by the protozoan parasite *Giardia lamblia*. It is a common cause of diarrhea in world travelers and is also prevalent in children who attend day care centers and other types of residential facilities; it may be found in contaminated mountain streams or pools frequented by diapered infants. The child ingests the cyst containing the protozoa. The cyst is activated by stomach acid and passes into the duodenum where it matures and causes signs and symptoms.

Clinical Manifestations and Treatment

Maturation of the cyst leads to diarrhea, weight loss, and abdominal cramps. Identification and diagnosis are made through examination of stool under the microscope. Metronidazole (Flagyl) or quinacrine (Atabrine) is effective in treating the infestation.

Nursing Care

Alert the caregiver that quinacrine causes a yellow discoloration of the skin. To prevent infestations, stress to caregivers the importance of careful handling of soiled diapers, especially in a childcare facility. Hand washing, avoiding pools and streams used by diapered infants, and avoiding contact with infected persons are also important.

Test Yourself

✔ What is the appendix and where is it located?
✔ What is contraindicated if a diagnosis of appendicitis is suspected?
✔ What are common ways pinworm infections are spread?

INGESTION OF TOXIC SUBSTANCES

One way in which toddlers find out about their environment is to taste the world around them. Toddlers and preschoolers are developing autonomy and initiative and

refining their gross and fine motor skills, which add to their tendency to examine their environment on their own. Because their senses of taste and smell are not yet refined, these age groups are prime targets for ingestion of poisonous substances.

The ordinary household has an abundance of poisonous substances in almost every room. The kitchen, bathroom, bedroom, and garage are the most common sites harboring substances that are poisonous when ingested. Although most poisonings occur in the child's home, grandparents' homes offer many temptations to the young child as well. Grandparents tend to be less concerned about placing dangerous substances out of children's reach simply because the children are not part of the household, or the grandparents may place supplies where they are convenient, while never considering the young grandchild's developmental stage and exploratory nature (see Family Teaching Tips: Poison Prevention in the Home).

Be careful.
Young children ingest substances with tastes or smells that would repel an adult.

Family Teaching Tips

POISON PREVENTION IN THE HOME

- Keep harmful products locked up and out of child's sight and reach.
- Use safety latches or locks on drawers and cabinets.
- Read labels with care before using any product.
- Replace child-resistant closures and safety caps immediately after using product.
- Never leave alcohol within a child's reach.
- Keep products in their original containers; never put nonfood products in food or drink containers.
- Teach children not to drink or eat anything unless it is given by an adult.
- Do not take medicine in front of small children; children tend to copy adult behavior.
- Do not refer to medicines as candy; call medicine by its correct name.
- Check your home often for old medications and get rid of them by flushing them down the toilet.
- Post the Poison Help Line (formerly called the Poison Control Center) number near each telephone: (800) 222–1222.
- Seek help if your child swallows a substance that is not food and call the Poison Help Line. Don't make your child vomit.

Adapted from the American Academy of Pediatrics. *Protect your child … Prevent poisoning.* Retrieved October 22, 2006, from http://www.aap.org/family/poistipp.htm.

When a child is found with a container whose contents he or she has obviously sampled, action should be taken immediately. When a child manifests symptoms that are difficult to pinpoint or that do not appear to relate specifically to any known cause, the possibility of poisoning should be suspected. Ingestion of a poisonous substance can produce symptoms that simulate an attack of an acute disease: vomiting, abdominal pain, diarrhea, shock, cyanosis, coma, and convulsions. If evidence of such a disease is lacking, acute poisoning should be suspected.

In instances of apparent poisoning where the substance is unknown, family caregivers are asked to consider all medications in their home. Is it possible that any medication could have been available to the child, or did an older child or other person possibly give the child the container to play with? Is it possible that a parent inadvertently gave a wrong dose or wrong medication to a child? All such possibilities need to be considered. In the meantime, the most important priority is treatment for the child who shows symptoms of poisoning.

The rate of deaths caused by poisoning has dramatically decreased because of the use of child-resistant closures, safer products, education, public awareness, poison control centers, and antidotes available.

Emergency Treatment

If the child has collapsed or is not breathing, 911 should be called for emergency help. In cases in which the child is conscious and alert and the caregiver suspects poison ingestion, the Poison Help Line (formerly called the Poison Control Center) should be called. The universal telephone number in the United States is (800) 222-1222. All homes with young children should have the Poison Help Line number posted by every telephone for quick reference. The caregiver should remove any obvious poison from the child's mouth before calling. The poison control center evaluates the situation and tells the caller whether the child can be treated at home or needs to be transported to a hospital or treatment center.

Except when corrosive or highly irritant poisons have been swallowed, the accepted treatment for many years has been to induce vomiting. The American Academy of Pediatrics (AAP) now believes that inducing vomiting has not been shown to prevent poisoning and should no longer be recommended. In addition, the AAP recommends that syrup of ipecac, recommended for many years to be kept in the home in case of poisoning, should no longer be used in the home for treatment of poisoning. The AAP further suggests that, because of the potential of misuse, existing ipecac in homes should be disposed of safely (AAP, 2003).

In the emergency care setting, gastric lavage may be used to empty the stomach of the toxic substances. Activated charcoal, which absorbs many types of materials, may be used to reduce the dangers of ingested substances. The charcoal is a black, fine powder that is mixed with water. A dose of 5 to 10 g per gram of in-

gested poison is given by mouth in 6 to 8 oz of water or may be given through a NG tube, if necessary.

If the substance the child has swallowed is known, the ingredients can be found on the label and the Poison Help Line can suggest an antidote. If the substance is a prescription drug, the pharmacist who filled the prescription or who is familiar with the drug also can be contacted for information. In some instances, it is necessary to analyze the stomach contents.

Specific antidotes are available for certain poisons, but not for all. Some antidotes react chemically with the poison to render it harmless, whereas others prevent absorption of the poison.

Treatment Steps in Order of Importance

The treatment steps in order of importance are as follows:

1. Remove the obvious remnants of the poison.
2. Call 911 for emergency help if child has collapsed or stopped breathing.
3. Call the Poison Help Line if child is conscious and alert. The universal poison control number is (800) 222-1222.
4. Follow instructions given by the Poison Help Line personnel.
5. Administer appropriate antidote if recommended.
6. Administer general supportive and symptomatic care.

Further specific treatment is given according to the kind and amount of the toxic substance ingested.

Common types of poisoning and general treatment are described in Table 38-2. Complete listings of poisonous substances with the specific treatment for each are available from the Poison Control Center, clinics, and pharmacies.

LEAD POISONING (PLUMBISM)

Chronic lead poisoning has been a serious problem among children for many years. It is responsible for neurologic handicaps, including mental retardation, because of its effect on the central nervous system. Infants and toddlers are potential victims because of their tendency to put any object within their reach into their mouths. In some children, this habit leads to **pica** (the ingestion of nonfood substances such as laundry starch, clay, paper, and paint). The unborn fetus of a pregnant mother who is exposed to lead (such as lead dust from renovation of an older home) also can be affected by lead contamination. Screening for lead poisoning is part of a complete well-child checkup between ages 6 months and 6 years.

Sources of Chronic Lead Poisoning

The most common sources of lead poisoning are:

- Lead-containing paint used on the outside or the inside of older houses
- Furniture and toys painted with lead-containing paint; vinyl mini blinds
- Drinking water contaminated by lead pipes or copper pipes with lead-soldered joints

Table 38-2 ▮ COMMONLY INGESTED TOXIC SUBSTANCES

Agent	Symptoms	Treatment
acetaminophen	Under 6 y—vomiting is the earliest sign Adolescents—vomiting, diaphoresis, general malaise. Liver damage can result in 48–96 h if not treated.	Gastric lavage may be necessary. Administer acetylcysteine (Mucomyst) diluted with cola, fruit juice, or water if plasma level elevated. Mucomyst may be administered by gavage, especially because its odor of rotten eggs makes it objectionable.
acetylsalicyclic acid (aspirin)	Hyperpnea (abnormal increase in depth and rate of breathing), metabolic acidosis, hyperventilation, tinnitus, and vertigo are initial symptoms. Dehydration, coma, convulsions, and death follow untreated heavy dosage.	Gastric lavage may be necessary. Activated charcoal may be administered. IV fluids, sodium bicarbonate to combat acidosis, and dialysis for renal failure may be necessary when large amounts are ingested.
ibuprofen (Motrin, Advil)	Similar to aspirin; metabolic acidosis, GI bleeding, renal damage	Activated charcoal is administered in emergency department. Observe for and treat GI bleeding. Electrolyte determination is done to detect acidosis. IV fluids are given.
ferrous sulfate (iron)	Vomiting, lethargy, diarrhea, weak rapid pulse, hypotension are common symptoms. Massive dose may produce shock; erosion of small intestine; black, tarry stools; bronchial pneumonia.	Deferoxamine, a chelating agent that combines with iron, may be used when child has ingested a toxic dose.
barbiturates	Respiratory, circulatory, and renal depression may occur. Child may become comatose.	Establish airway; administer oxygen if needed; perform gastric lavage. Close observation of level of consciousness is needed.
corrosives alkali: lye, bleaches acid: drain cleaners, toilet bowl cleaners, iodine, silver nitrate	Intense burning and pain with first mouthful; severe burns of mouth and esophageal tract; shock, possible death.	*Never have child vomit.* Alkali corrosives are treated initially with quantities of water, diluted acid fruit juices, or diluted vinegar. Acid corrosives are treated with alkaline drinks such as milk, olive oil, mineral oil, or egg white. *Lavage or emetics are never used.* Continuing treatment includes antidotes, gastrostomy or IV feedings, and specialized care. A tracheostomy may be needed.
hydrocarbons kerosene, gasoline, furniture polish, lighter fluid, turpentine	Damage to the respiratory system is the primary concern. Vomiting often occurs spontaneously, possibly causing additional damage to the respiratory system. Pneumonia, bronchopneumonia, or lipoid pneumonia may occur.	Emergency treatment and assessment are necessary. Vital signs are monitored; oxygen is administered as needed. Gastric lavage is performed only if the ingested substance contains other toxic chemicals that may threaten another body system such as the liver, kidneys, or cardiovascular system.

▪ Dust containing lead salts from lead paint; emission from lead smelters

▪ Storage of fruit juices or other food in improperly glazed earthenware

▪ Inhalation of fumes from engines containing lead or from burning batteries

▪ Exposure to industrial areas with smelteries or chemical plants

▪ Exposure to hobby materials containing lead (e.g., stained glass, solder, fishing sinkers, bullets)

Lead poisoning has other causes, but the most common cause has been the lead in paint. Children tend to nibble on fallen plaster, painted wooden furniture (including cribs), and painted toys because they have a sweet taste. Fine dust that results from removing lead paint in remodeling also can cause harm to the children in the household, without parents being aware of exposure. When the danger of lead poisoning became apparent, attempts were made to control the sale of lead-based paint. In 1973, federal regulations banned the sale of paint containing more than 0.5% lead for interior residential use or use on toys. However, this has not eliminated the problem because many homes built before the 1960s were painted with lead-based paint, and they still exist in inner-city areas, as well as small towns and suburbs. Older mansions where upper-income families may live also may have lead paint because of the building's age. Only contractors experienced in lead-based paint removal should do renovations.

Clinical Manifestations

The onset of chronic lead poisoning is insidious. Some early indications may be irritability, hyperactivity, aggression, impulsiveness, or disinterest in play. Short attention span, lethargy, learning difficulties, and distractibility are also are signs of poisoning.

The condition may progress to **encephalopathy** (degenerative disease of the brain) because of intracranial pressure. Manifestations may include convulsions, mental retardation, blindness, paralysis, coma, and death. Acute episodes sometimes develop sporadically and early in the condition.

Diagnosis

The nonspecific nature of the presenting symptoms makes it important to examine the child's environmental history. Testing blood lead levels is used as a screening method. Target screening is done in areas where the risk of lead poisoning is high. Fingersticks, or heelsticks for infants, can be used to collect samples for lead level screening. In 1997, the Centers for Disease Control and Prevention (CDC) in Atlanta modified the guidelines related to lead screening. The CDC continues to define elevated blood levels of lead as ≥10 mcg/dL. The CDC's emphasis is on primary prevention and screening.

Treatment and Nursing Care

The most important aspect of treatment of a child with lead poisoning is to remove the lead from the child's system and environment. The use of a **chelating agent** (an agent that binds with metal) increases the urinary excretion of lead. Several chelating agents are available; individual circumstances and the physician's choice determine the particular drug used. Edetate calcium disodium, known as EDTA, is usually given intravenously because intramuscular administration is painful. Renal failure can occur with inappropriate dosage. Dimercaprol, also known as BAL, causes excretion of lead through bile and urine; it may be administered intramuscularly. Because of its peanut oil base, BAL should not be used in children allergic to peanuts. These two drugs may be used together in children with extremely high levels of lead.

The oral drug penicillamine can be used to treat children with blood lead levels <45 mcg/dL. The capsules can be opened and sprinkled on food or mixed in liquid for administration. This drug should not be administered to children who are allergic to penicillin. The drug succimer (Chemet) is an oral drug used for treating children with blood lead levels >45 mcg/dL. Succimer comes in capsules that can be opened and mixed with applesauce, or other soft foods, or can be taken from a spoon, followed by a flavored beverage.

All the chelating drugs may have toxic side effects, and children being treated must be carefully monitored with frequent urinalysis, blood cell counts, and renal function tests. Any child receiving chelation therapy should be under the care of an experienced health care team.

Prognosis

The prognosis after lead poisoning is uncertain. Early detection of the condition and removal of the child from the lead-containing surroundings offer the best hope. Follow-up should include routine examinations to prevent recurrence and to observe for signs of any residual brain damage not immediately apparent.

Although the incidence of lead poisoning has decreased, it is still prevalent. Measures to educate the public on the importance of preventing this disorder are essential if the problem is to be eliminated. Education of the family caregivers is an essential aspect of the treatment (see Family Teaching Tips: Preventing Lead Poisoning). The National Lead Information Center (1-800-424-LEAD) is another resource for information regarding lead poisoning.

Family Teaching Tips

PREVENTING LEAD POISONING

- If you live in an older home, make sure your child does not have access to any chips of paint or chew any surface painted with lead-based paint. Look for paint dust on window sills, and clean with a high-phosphate sodium cleaner (the phosphate content of automatic dishwashing detergent is usually high enough).
- Wet-mop hard-surfaced floors and woodwork with cleaner at least once a week. Vacuuming hard surfaces scatters dust.
- Wash child's hands and face before eating.
- Wash toys and pacifiers frequently.
- Prevent child from playing in dust near an old lead-painted house.
- Prevent child from playing in soil or dust near a major highway.
- If your water supply has a high lead content, fully flush faucets before using for cooking, drinking, or making formula.
- Avoid contamination from hobbies or work.
- Make sure your child eats regular meals. Food slows absorption of lead.
- Encourage your child to eat foods high in iron and calcium.

From Centers for Disease Control and Prevention. (2005). *Preventing lead poisoning in young children: a statement by The Centers for Disease Control.* Atlanta, 2002. Retrieved May 15, 2008 from http://www.cdc.gov/nceh/lead/Publications/PrevleadPoisoning.pdf

INGESTION OF FOREIGN OBJECTS

Young children are apt to put any small objects into their mouths; they often swallow these objects. Normally many of these objects pass smoothly through the digestive tract and are expelled in the feces. Occasionally, however, something such as an open safety pin, a coin, a button, or a marble may lodge in the esophagus and need to be extracted. Foods such as hot dogs, peanuts, carrots, popcorn kernels, apple pieces, grapes, and round candy are frequent offenders.

Unless symptoms of choking, gagging, or pain are present, waiting and watching the feces carefully for 3 or 4 days is usually safe. Any object, however, may pass safely through the esophagus and stomach only to become fixed in one of the curves of the intestine, causing an obstruction or fever due to infection. Sharp objects also present the danger of perforation somewhere in the digestive tract.

Diagnosis of a swallowed solid object is often, but not always, made from the history. If a foreign object in the digestive tract is suspected, fluoroscopic and radiographic studies may be required.

Treatment and Nursing Care

If a caregiver has seen a child swallow an object and begin choking, the caregiver should hold the child along the rescuer's forearm with the child's head lower than his chest and give the child several back blows. After delivering the back blows, the caregiver should support the child's back and head and turn the child over onto the opposite thigh. The caregiver should deliver as many as five quick downward chest thrusts and remove the foreign body if visualized. A child older than age 1 year can be encouraged to continue to cough, as long as the cough remains forceful. If the cough becomes ineffective (no sound with cough) or respirations become more difficult and stridor is present, the caregiver can attempt the Heimlich maneuver (Fig. 38-8).

If the child is not having respiratory problems but coughing has not expelled the object, the child needs to be transported to an emergency department to be assessed by a physician. Objects in the esophagus are removed by direct vision through an esophagoscope. Attempts to push the object down into the stomach or to extract it blindly can be dangerous. Some objects may need to be removed surgically. If the object is small and the physician believes

■ **Figure 38-8 (A)** Back blows (*top*) and chest thrusts (*bottom*) to relieve foreign-body airway obstruction in infant. Hold infant over arm as illustrated, supporting head by firmly holding jaw. Deliver up to five back blows. Turn infant over while supporting head, neck, jaw, and chest with one hand and back with other hand. Keep head lower than trunk. Give five quick chest thrusts with one finger below the intermammary line. If the foreign body is not removed and the airway remains obstructed, attempt rescue breathing. Repeat these 2 steps, until successful. **(B)** Abdominal thrusts with the child standing or sitting can be performed when the child is conscious. Standing behind the child, place the thumb side of one fist against the child's abdomen in midline, slightly above navel and well below the xiphoid process. Grab your fist with the other hand and deliver five quick upward thrusts. Continue until successful or the child loses consciousness. **(C)** Abdominal thrusts with the child lying can be performed on a conscious or unconscious child. Place heel of your hand on the child's abdomen, slightly above the navel and below the xiphoid process and rib cage. Place your other hand on top of first hand. Deliver five separate, distinct thrusts. Open airway and attempt rescue breathing if object is not removed. Repeat until successful. **(D)** Combined jaw thrust–spine stabilization maneuver for a child trauma victim with possible head or neck injury. To protect from damage to cervical spine, the neck is maintained in a neutral position and traction on or movement of neck is avoided.

there is little danger to the GI tract, the caregiver may be advised to take the child home and watch the child's bowel movements over the next several days to confirm that the object has passed through the system.

Increasing respiratory difficulties indicate that the object has been aspirated rather than swallowed. Foreign objects aspirated into the larynx or bronchial tree may become lodged in the trachea or larynx. Back blows and chest thrusts or the Heimlich maneuver should be delivered, as described. The child's airway should be opened and rescue breathing attempted. If the child's chest does not rise, the child should be repositioned and rescue breathing tried again. If the airway is still obstructed, these steps should be repeated until the object is removed and respirations are established. The child should be transported to the emergency department as quickly as possible. The caregiver should get emergency assistance while continuing to try to remove the offending object.

Adults must be aware of the power of example. A child who sees an adult holding pins or nails in his or her mouth may follow this example with disastrous, and often fatal, results.

Test Yourself

✔ What are the steps that should be taken if a child has ingested a toxic substance?

✔ What are some indications that a child may have lead poisoning?

✔ How is lead poisoning treated?

ENDOCRINE DISORDERS

Diabetes mellitus is classified into two major types: type 1, formerly called insulin-dependent diabetes mellitus (IDDM) or juvenile diabetes, and type 2, formerly called noninsulin-dependent diabetes mellitus (Table 38-3). Type 1 diabetes mellitus is the most significant endocrine disorder that affects children. However, in recent years, type 2 diabetes mellitus, previously seen primarily in adults, has been seen more commonly in children.

Other endocrine conditions that may affect children are disorders of the pituitary gland, which alter growth, and diabetes insipidus. The incidence of these latter conditions is low.

TYPE 1 DIABETES MELLITUS

At least 15 million Americans have been diagnosed with diabetes. A significant number of them are children: Type 1 diabetes mellitus is estimated to affect about 1 in 600 children between the ages of 5 and 15 years. The incidence of this condition continues to increase.

Diabetes is often considered an adult disease, but at least 5% of cases begin in childhood, usually at about 6 years of age or around the time of puberty. Management of diabetes in children is different from that in adults and requires conscientious care geared to the child's developmental stage.

Pathogenesis

The exact pathophysiology of diabetes is not completely understood; however, it is known to result from

---

Table 38-3 ▮ **COMPARISON OF TYPE 1 AND TYPE 2 DIABETES**

Assessment	Type 1 Diabetes	Type 2 Diabetes
Age at onset	5–7 y or at puberty	Increasingly occuring in younger children
Type of onset	Abrupt	Gradual
Weight changes	Marked weight loss is often initial sign	Associated with obesity
Other symptoms	Polydipsia	Polydipsia
	Polyuria (often begins as bed-wetting)	Polyuria
	Fatigue (marks fall in school)	Fatigue
	Blurred vision (marks fall in school)	Blurred vision
	Glycosuria	Glycosuria
	Polyphagia	Pruritus
	Pruritus	Mood changes
	Mood changes (may cause behavior problems in school)	
Therapy	Hypoglycemic agents never effective; insulin needed	Managed by diet, oral hypoglycemic agents, or insulin
	Diet only moderately restricted; no dietary foods used	Diet tends to be strict
	Common-sense foot care for growing children	Good skin and foot care necessary
Period of remission	Period of remission for 1–12 mo generally follows initial diagnosis	Not demonstrable

Adapted from Pillitteri, A. (2007). *Maternal and child health nursing* (5th ed). Philadelphia: Lippincott Williams & Wilkins.

dysfunction of the beta (insulin-secreting) cells of the islets of Langerhans in the pancreas. Some researchers believe that the presence of an acute infection during childhood may trigger a mechanism in genetically susceptible children, activating beta-cell dysfunction and disrupting insulin secretion. Other conditions that may contribute to type 1 diabetes are pancreatic tumors, pancreatitis, and long-term corticosteroid use.

Normally, the sugar derived from digestion and assimilation of foods is burned to provide energy for the body's activities. Excess sugar is converted into fat or glycogen and stored in the body tissues. Insulin, a hormone secreted by the pancreas, is responsible for the burning and storage of sugar. In diabetes, the secretion of insulin is inadequate or nonexistent, allowing sugar to accumulate in the bloodstream and spill over into the urine. In children, type 1 diabetes causes an abrupt pronounced decrease in insulin production, resulting in decreased ability to derive energy from the food eaten. Large amounts of protein and fat are used to supply the child's energy needs, causing loss of weight and slowed growth. This combination of failure to gain weight and lack of energy may be the initial reason the child is brought to the health care provider's attention. However, a health care provider may not see the child until symptoms of ketoacidosis are evident.

Clinical Manifestations

Classic symptoms of type 1 diabetes mellitus are **polyuria** (dramatic increase in urinary output, probably with enuresis), **polydipsia** (increased thirst), and **polyphagia** (increased hunger and food consumption). These symptoms are usually accompanied by weight loss or failure to gain weight and lack of energy, even though the child has increased food consumption. Symptoms of diabetes in children often have an abrupt onset.

If the child's symptoms are not noted and referred for diagnosis, the disorder is likely to progress to diabetic ketoacidosis. Because of inadequate insulin production, carbohydrates are not converted into fuel for energy production. Fats are then mobilized for energy, but are incompletely oxidized in the absence of glucose. Ketone bodies (acetone, diacetic acid, and oxybutyric acid) accumulate. They are readily excreted in the urine, but the acid-base balance of body fluids excreted is upset and results in acidosis.

Diabetic ketoacidosis is characterized by drowsiness, dry skin, flushed cheeks and cherry-red lips, acetone breath with a fruity smell, and **Kussmaul breathing** (abnormal increase in the depth and rate of the respiratory movements). Nausea and vomiting may occur. If untreated, the child lapses into coma and exhibits dehydration, electrolyte imbalance, rapid pulse, and subnormal temperature and blood pressure.

Diagnosis

Early detection and control are critical in postponing or minimizing later complications of diabetes. Observe carefully for any signs or symptoms in all members of a family with a history of diabetes. The family also should be taught to observe the children for frequent thirst, urination, and weight loss. All relatives of diabetics are considered a high-risk group and should have periodic testing.

At each visit to a health care provider, children with a family history of diabetes should be monitored for glucose, using a fingerstick glucose test, and for ketones in the urine, using a urine dipstick test. If the blood glucose level is elevated or ketonuria is present, a fasting blood sugar is performed. A fasting blood sugar result ≥200 mg/dL almost certainly is diagnostic for diabetes when other signs, such as polyuria and weight loss, despite polyphagia, are present.

Although glucose tolerance tests are performed in adults to confirm diabetes, they are not commonly used in children. The traditional oral glucose tolerance test is often unsuccessful in children because they may vomit the concentrated glucose that must be swallowed.

Treatment

Management of type 1 diabetes in children includes insulin therapy and a meal and exercise plan. Treatment of the diabetic child involves the family, child, and a number of health team members such as the nurse, the pediatrician, the nutritionist, and the diabetic nurse educator. After diabetes is diagnosed, the child may be hospitalized for a period of time. This allows the condition to be stabilized under supervision. This is a trying time, so you must plan care with an understanding of the emotional impact of the diagnosis. Inform those who supervise the child during daily activities of the diagnosis, including the child's teacher and the school nurse.

Insulin Therapy

Insulin therapy is an essential part of the treatment of diabetes in children. The dosage of insulin is adjusted according to blood glucose levels so that the levels are maintained near normal. Two kinds of insulin are often combined for the best results. Insulin can be grouped into rapid acting, short acting, intermediate acting, and long acting (Table 38-4).

An intermediate-acting and a short-acting insulin often are given together. Some preparations come in a premixed proportion of 70% intermediate-acting and 30% short-acting insulin, eliminating the need for mixing. Many children are prescribed an insulin regimen in which a dose containing a short-acting insulin and an intermediate-acting insulin are given at two times during the day: One before breakfast and the second before the evening meal. Children's insulin doses need to be individually regulated to keep their blood glucose levels as close to normal as possible.

Table 38-4 ▌ TYPES OF INSULIN: ONSET, PEAK, AND DURATION

Action	Preparation	Onset (hrs)	Peak (hrs)	Duration (hrs)
Rapid-acting	Lispro Humalog	0.25	0.5–1	3–4
Short-acting	Regular	0.5–1	2–4	5–7
Intermediate-acting	NPH	1.5–2	6–12	18–24
	Lente	1.5–2	6–12	18–24
Long-acting	Ultralente	4–6	18–24	36–48

*References may vary slightly on these figures.

The introduction of rapid-acting insulin, such as Lispro or Humalog, has greatly changed insulin administration in children. The onset of action of rapid-acting insulin is <15 minutes. Rapid-acting insulin can even be used after a meal in children with unpredictable eating habits (Plotnick, 2006).

Good news.
Lispro or Humalog insulin can be administered immediately *after* the child has eaten, so the amount of food eaten can be taken into consideration when determining the dosage.

Insulin Reaction

Insulin reaction (insulin shock, hypoglycemia) is caused by insulin overload, resulting in metabolism of the body's glucose that is too rapid. This may be attributable to a change in the body's requirement, carelessness in diet (such as failure to eat proper amounts of food), an error in insulin measurement, or excessive exercise. Because diabetes in children is very labile (unstable, fluctuating), the child is subject to insulin reactions.

Some symptoms of impending insulin reaction in children are any type of odd, unusual, or antisocial behavior; weakness; nervousness; lethargy; headache; blurred vision and dizziness; and undue fatigue or hunger. Other symptoms might include pallor, sweating, convulsions, and coma. Children often have hypoglycemic reactions in the early morning. Observe the child at least every 2 hours during the night. Note tossed bedding, which would indicate restlessness, and any excessive perspiration. If necessary, try to arouse the child. As the child becomes regulated and observes a careful diet at home, parents do not need to watch so closely, but should have a thorough understanding of all aspects of this condition. Blood glucose

This advice could be a lifesaver.
Treatment of an insulin reaction should be immediate.

monitoring often is scheduled for an early morning time, in an effort to detect abnormal glucose levels.

To treat an insulin reaction, give the child sugar, candy, orange juice, or one of the commercial products designed for this emergency. Repeated or impending reactions require consultation with the physician.

If the child cannot take a sugar source orally, glucagon should be administered subcutaneously to bring about a prompt increase in the blood glucose level. Every adult responsible for a diabetic child should clearly understand the procedure for administering this drug and should have easy access to it. Glucagon is a hormone produced by alpha cells of the pancreatic islets. An elevation in the blood glucose level results in insulin release in a normal person, but a decrease in the blood glucose level stimulates glucagon release. The released glucagon in the bloodstream acts on the liver to promote glycogen breakdown and glucose release. Glucagon is available as a pharmaceutical product and is packaged in prefilled syringes for immediate use. It is administered in the same manner as insulin.

Glucagon acts within minutes to restore consciousness, after which the child can take candy or sugar. This treatment prevents the long delay while waiting for a physician to administer IV glucose or for an ambulance to reach the child. However, it is not a substitute for proper medical supervision.

Insulin Regimen

Most children with newly diagnosed diabetes show a decreased need for insulin during the first weeks or months after control is established. This is often referred to as the "honeymoon period," and it should be explained to the family in advance to avoid false hope. As the child grows, the need for insulin increases and continues to do so until the child reaches full growth. Again, family caregivers need to know that this is normal and that the child's condition is not getting worse.

Insulin Administration Methods

Insulin often is administered subcutaneously at different times of the day, or it may be administered continuously via a pump.

The child may not be able to take over management of the insulin injection as early as blood glucose monitoring, but he or she can watch the preparation of the syringe and learn the technique for drawing up the dosage. It may be helpful to encourage the child to watch the process until it becomes routine. By 8 or 9 years of age, the child should be encouraged to talk with the caregiver about the dose and to practice working with the syringe. The child also may draw up the dose and prepare for self-administration. The age at which this is possible varies. No two children mature at the same rate; some may be able to do this much earlier than others. Automatic injection devices can help the child self-administer insulin at a younger age. The child should be encouraged to take over the management of the therapy when ready. If included in decision making, the child can learn the importance of the routine and accept the restrictions the disease imposes.

The insulin pump is a method of continuous insulin administration useful for some diabetics. The pump is about the size of a transistor radio and can be worn strapped to the waist or on a shoulder strap. It delivers a steady low dose of insulin through a syringe housed in the pump and connected by polyethylene tubing to a small-gauge subcutaneous needle implanted in the abdomen. Extra insulin is released at mealtimes and other times when needed by pressing a button. The pump does not sense the blood glucose level; therefore careful blood glucose monitoring at least four times a day is necessary to adjust the dosage as needed. The pump must be removed to bathe, swim, or shower. The child may want to wear loose clothing to hide the pump. The needle site must be regularly observed for redness and irritation. The site is changed every 24 to 48 hours using aseptic technique.

Unique Needs of the Adolescent

Adolescence is an extremely trying period for many diabetics, as it is for other young people. Diabetics, like healthy adolescents, must work from dependence to independence. Even when an adolescent has accepted responsibility for self-care, it is not unusual for him or her to rebel against the control that this condition demands, become impatient, and appear to ignore future health. The adolescent may skip meals, drop diet controls, or neglect glucose monitoring. Going barefoot and neglecting proper foot care also can cause problems for the diabetic adolescent. It can be a difficult time for both the family and the adolescent. The caregivers naturally become concerned and are apt to give the adolescent more controls to rebel against. Special care should be taken by the family, teachers, nurses, and physicians to see that these young people find enough maturing satisfaction in other areas and do not need to rebel in this vital area.

The adolescent who completely understands all aspects of the condition (especially if allowed to assume control of treatment previously) should be allowed to continue managing her or his own treatment. Should the adolescent run into difficulty, an adolescent clinic can be of great value. There, the adolescent can discuss problems with understanding people who respond with care and provide dignity and attentive listening.

Treatment of Diabetic Ketoacidosis

Treatment for ketoacidosis requires skilled nursing care, and the child may be admitted to a pediatric intensive care unit. Fluid depletion is corrected; blood and urine glucose levels and other blood studies are monitored closely to evaluate the degree of ketoacidosis and electrolyte imbalance. If the child cannot urinate, a catheter is inserted. Regular insulin is given intravenously along with IV electrolyte fluids.

Nursing Process for the Child With Type 1 Diabetes Mellitus

Assessment

When collecting data, ask the caregiver about the child's symptoms leading up to the present illness. Ask about the child's appetite, weight loss or gain, evidence of polyuria or enuresis in a previously toilet-trained child, polydipsia, dehydration (which may include constipation), irritability, and fatigue. Include the child in the interview and encourage him or her to contribute information. Observe for evidence of the child's developmental stage to help determine appropriate nursing diagnoses and plan effective care. If the child is first seen in diabetic ketoacidosis, adjust the initial nursing interview accordingly.

In the physical exam, measure the height and weight and examine the skin for evidence of dryness or slowly healing sores. Note signs of hyperglycemia, record vital signs, and collect a urine specimen. Perform a blood glucose level determination using a bedside glucose monitor.

Selected Nursing Diagnoses

- Imbalanced Nutrition: Less Than Body Requirements related to insufficient caloric intake to meet growth and development needs and the inability of the body to use nutrients
- Risk for Impaired Skin Integrity related to slow healing process and decreased circulation
- Risk for Infection related to elevated glucose levels
- Readiness for Enhanced Management of Therapeutic Regimen related to blood glucose levels
- Deficient Knowledge related to complications of hypoglycemia and hyperglycemia
- Deficient Knowledge related to insulin administration
- Deficient Knowledge related to appropriate exercise and activity
- Compromised Family Coping related to the effect of the disease on the child's and family's life
- Risk for Impaired Adjustment related to long-term management of chronic disease

Outcome Identification and Planning

The major goals for the child include maintaining adequate nutrition, promoting skin integrity, preventing infection, regulating glucose levels, and learning to adjust to having a chronic disease. Goals for the child and family include learning about and managing hypoglycemia and hyperglycemia, insulin administration, and exercise needs for the child. An additional goal is for family members to express their concerns about coping with the child's illness.

Implementation

Ensuring Adequate and Appropriate Nutrition

The child with diabetes needs a sound nutritional program that provides adequate nutrition for normal growth while it maintains the blood glucose at near-normal levels. The food plan should be well balanced with foods that accommodate the child's food preferences, cultural customs, and lifestyle (see Family Teaching Tips: Child's Diabetic Food Plan).

Help the child and caregiver to understand the importance of eating regularly scheduled meals. Special occa-

Family Teaching Tips

CHILD'S DIABETIC FOOD PLAN

- Plan well-balanced meals that are appealing to child.
- Be positive with child when talking about foods that he or she can eat; downplay the negatives.
- Space three meals and three snacks throughout the day. Daily caloric intake is divided to provide 20% at breakfast, 20% at lunch, 30% at dinner, and 10% at each of the snacks.
- Calories should be made up of 50% to 60% carbohydrates, 15% to 20% protein, and no more than 30% fat.
- Avoid concentrated sweets such as jelly, syrup, pie, candy bars, and soda pop.
- Artificial sweeteners may be used.
- Child must not skip meals. Make every effort to plan meals with foods that the child likes.
- Include foods that contain dietary fiber such as whole grains, cereals, fruits and vegetables, nuts, seeds, and legumes. Fiber helps prevent hyperglycemia.
- Dietetic food is expensive and unnecessary.
- Keep complex carbohydrates available to be eaten before exercise and sports activities to provide sustained carbohydrate energy sources.
- Teach child day by day about the food plan to encourage independence in food selections when at school or away from home.

sions can be planned so that the child does not feel left out of celebrations. If a particular meal is going to be late, the child should have a complex carbohydrate and protein snack. Children should be included in meal planning, when possible, to learn what is permissible and what is not. In this way, they can handle eating when they are on their own in school and in social situations.

Preventing Skin Breakdown

Skin breakdowns, such as blisters and minor cuts, can become major problems for the diabetic child. Teach the caregiver and child to inspect the skin daily and promptly treat even small breaks in the skin. Encourage daily bathing. Teach the child and caregiver to dry the skin well after bathing, and give careful attention to any area where skin touches skin, such as the groin, axilla, or other skin folds. Emphasize good foot care. This includes wearing well-fitting shoes, inspecting between toes for cracks, trimming nails straight across, wearing clean socks, and not going barefoot. Establishing these habits early helps the child prepare for lifelong care of diabetes.

Preventing Infection

Diabetic children may be more susceptible to urinary tract and upper respiratory infections. Teach the child and caregiver to be alert for signs of urinary tract infection, such as itching and burning on urination. Instruct them to report signs of urinary tract or upper respiratory infections to the care provider promptly.

Many children are subject to minor infections and illnesses during the school years, with little long-term effect. However, the diabetic child is more susceptible to long-term complications. When the diabetic child has an infection and fever, the temperature and metabolic rate increase and the body needs more sugar and, therefore, more insulin to make the sugar available to the body. Although the child may not be eating because of vomiting or anorexia, the body still needs insulin. Insulin should never be skipped during illness. Blood glucose levels should be checked every 2 to 4 hours during this time. Fluids need to be increased. Instruct the caregivers to contact the care provider when the child becomes ill, especially if the child is vomiting, cannot eat, or has diarrhea, so that close supervision can be maintained. Give the caregiver guidelines for care of an ill child with the initial diabetic instructions.

It is extremely important for the child to wear a MedicAlert identification medal or a bracelet with information about diabetic status. Identification cards, such as those carried by many adult diabetics, are seldom practical for a child.

Regulating Glucose Levels

The child who is seen in the health care facility with diabetes may have a new diagnosis or may be experiencing an unstable episode as a result of illness or changing

■ **Figure 38-9** The child uses an automatic lancet to get blood sample (*left*) and blood glucose monitor to determine blood glucose level (*right*).

needs. The child's blood glucose level must be monitored to maintain it within normal limits. Determine the blood glucose level at least twice a day, before breakfast and before the evening meal, by means of bedside glucose monitoring.

On initial diagnosis of diabetes, the blood glucose level should be checked as often as every 4 hours until some stability is achieved. Because regular monitoring of the blood glucose level is necessary, teach the child and the caregiver how to perform monitoring (Fig. 38-9).

Because this procedure involves a fingerstick, the child may object and resist it. Offer encouragement and support, helping the child to express fears and acknowledging that the fingerstick does hurt and it is acceptable to dislike it. Consider the child's developmental stage when performing the testing. Table 38-5 provides some guidelines for diabetic care and teaching, based on developmental stage. School-aged children can be involved in much of the process. Encourage the child to choose the finger to be used and clean it with soap and water. Automatic-release instruments make it easier for the child to do the fingerstick. Teach the child to read the results and learn the desired level. School-aged children, in the stage of industry versus inferiority, are usually interested in learning new information. Appeal to this developmental characteristic to gain the cooperation of a child this age.

Providing Child and Family Teaching in the Management of Hypoglycemia and Hyperglycemia

The child is monitored closely for signs of hypoglycemia or hyperglycemia. If the blood glucose level is >240 mg/dL, the urine may be tested for ketones. In addition, during an illness the urine ketones are monitored. Be aware of the most likely times for an increase or decrease in the blood glucose level in relation to the insulin the child is receiving. Teach the child and family to recognize the signs of both hypoglycemia and hyperglycemia (see Family Teaching Tips: Signs of Hypoglycemia and

Family Teaching Tips

SIGNS OF HYPOGLYCEMIA AND HYPERGLYCEMIA

HYPOGLYCEMIA

- Shaking
- Irritability
- Hunger
- Diaphoresis
- Dizziness
- Drowsiness
- Pallor
- Changed level of consciousness
- Feeling "strange"

HYPERGLYCEMIA

- Polyphagia (excessive hunger)
- Polyuria (excessive urination)
- Dry mucous membranes
- Poor skin turgor
- Lethargy
- Change in level of consciousness

Hyperglycemia) and how to be prepared to take the appropriate action if necessary. They must be alert to signs of hypoglycemia, especially when insulin is at peak action (see Table 38-4).

Teach them to treat blood glucose levels <60 mg/dL with juice, sugar, or nondiet soda. If the blood glucose level cannot be checked promptly, the child should still consume a simple carbohydrate if there are any signs of hypoglycemia.

If the child cannot swallow, glucagon or dextrose should be administered, following the physician's orders. Glucagon is commercially available and can be administered intramuscularly or subcutaneously. Teach the caregiver how to mix and administer it.

Instruct the child to get help immediately when signs of hypoglycemia occur and to carry and take sugar cubes, Lifesavers, gumdrops, or a small tube of cake frosting. The reaction should be followed with a snack of a complex carbohydrate, such as crackers, and a protein such as cheese, peanut butter, or half of a meat sandwich. The snack is needed to maintain the increase in blood glucose level created by the simple carbohydrates and to prevent another hypoglycemic reaction.

Reassure the caregiver and the child that hypoglycemia is much more likely to occur than hyperglycemia. If there is any doubt as to whether the child is having a hypoglycemic or a hyperglycemic reaction, treat it like hypoglycemia. Instruct caregivers to keep a record of the hypoglycemic reactions to determine if there is a pattern and if the insulin schedule or food plan needs to be adjusted.

Table 38-5 ▮ DEVELOPMENTAL GUIDELINES FOR DIABETIC CHILD RESPONSIBILITIES*

Issue	Age (yr)					
	Under 4	4–5	6–7	8–10	11–13	14+
Food	Teaching focuses on parents	Knows likes and dislikes	Can begin to tell sugar content of food and know foods he or she should not have	Has more ability to select foods according to criteria like exchange lists	Knows if foods fit own diet plan	Helps plan meals and snacks
Insulin	Parents take responsibility for care	Can tell where injection should be Can pinch the skin	Can begin to help with aspects of injections	Gives own injections with supervision	Can learn to measure insulin	Can mix two insulins
Testing		Can choose finger for fingerstick Can wash finger with soap and water Collects urine; should watch caregiver do testing; helps with recording	Can do own fingerstick using automatic puncture device. Can help with some aspects of blood test Can do own urine test and record results	Can do blood tests with supervision	Can see test results forming a pattern	Can begin to use test results to adjust insulin
Psychological		Identifies with being "bad" or "good"; these words should be avoided. A child this age may think he or she is bad if the test is said to be "bad."	Needs many reminders and supervision	Needs reminders and supervision Understands only immediate consequences, not long-term consequences, of diabetes control. "Scientific" mind developing; intrigued by tests	May be somewhat rebellious Concerned with being "different"	Understands long-term consequences of actions including diabetes control Independence and self-image are important. Rebellion continues and some supervision and continued support are still needed.

*These are only guidelines. Each child is an individual. Talk to your health care provider about any concerns you may have.

Providing Child and Family Teaching on Insulin Administration

Teach the family caregiver and the child the correct way to give insulin. Disposable syringes make caring for equipment relatively easy. A doll may be used to practice the actual administration until the caregiver (and child, if old enough) is comfortable and confident. Provide direct supervision until proficiency is demonstrated (Fig. 38-10).

Insulin administration is probably the most threatening aspect of the illness. Remember your feelings when you gave your first injection in nursing school. The child and family need a great deal of empathy and warm support. Increasing their confidence and skills of insulin administration will reduce their fear.

Give clear instructions concerning the importance of rotating injection sites. A site that is used too frequently is likely to become indurated and eventually fibrosed, which

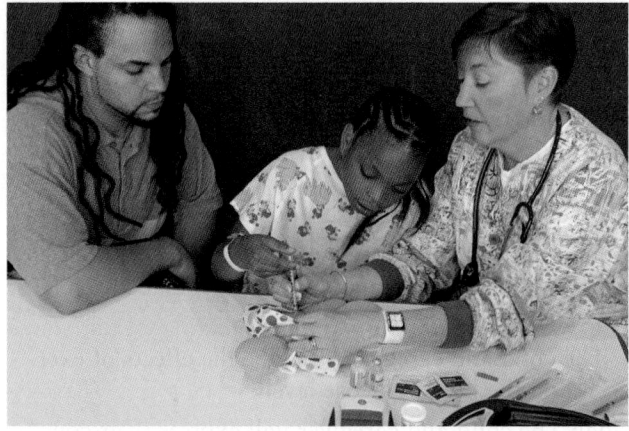

■ **Figure 38-10** The school-aged child may first practice insulin injections on a doll.

hinders proper insulin absorption. The atrophic hollows in the skin, or the lumps of hypertrophied tissue, are unsightly as well. Some people appear to have greater skin sensitivity than others. Areas on the upper arms, upper thighs, abdomen, and buttocks can be used (Fig. 38-11).

Use of a careful plan allows several weeks to elapse before a site is used again. Usually, four to six injections are given in one area before going on to the next area. Starting from the inner–upper corner of the area, each injection is given 0.5 in below the preceding one, going down in a vertical line. The next series of injections in this area would start 0.5 in outward at the upper level. If there is any sign of induration, the local site should be avoided for a few weeks until all signs of irritation have disappeared. A chart recording the sites used and the rotation schedule is recommended.

■ **Figure 38-11** Insulin injection sites.

Providing Child and Family Teaching About Exercise and Activity

Exercise decreases the blood glucose level because carbohydrates are being burned for energy. The therapeutic program should be adjusted to allow for this increase in energy requirements to avoid hypoglycemia. Adjustments also may be needed in the child's school schedule. For instance, physical education should never be scheduled right before lunch for a diabetic child. Also, the diabetic child should not be scheduled for a late lunch period.

Promoting Family Coping

When the diagnosis of diabetes is confirmed, the family caregiver may feel devastated. A young child will not understand the implications, but the school-aged or adolescent child will experience a great amount of fear and anxiety. The caregiver may have feelings of guilt, resentment, or denial. Other family members also may experience strong feelings about the illness. All these feelings and concerns must be recognized and resolved to work successfully with the diabetic child. Encourage the family to express these feelings and fears. To help him or her deal with feelings, involve the caregiver in the child's caring during hospitalization. Carefully listen to questions and answer them completely and honestly. Many written materials are available to give to the caregiver, but be sure the caregiver can read and understand them. Videos are also available that are helpful in educating the diabetic and the family. Recommend available community support groups. Cover home care in detail. Provide the family caregiver with a support person to contact when questions arise after discharge.

Because so much information must be absorbed in a brief time, the caregivers may seem forgetful or confused. Careful patient repetition of all aspects of diabetes and the child's care is necessary. When anxiety levels are high, information is often heard but not digested. Provide written material in an understandable form. Have caregivers repeat information, and question them to confirm that they understand. Demonstrate warmth and caring throughout the teaching to increase the family's comfort; this also develops their confidence in nursing responses to their questions and apprehensions.

Promoting Self-Care and Positive Self-Esteem

The school-aged or older child may experience some strong feelings of inadequacy or being "sick." These feelings must be expressed and handled. To help allay fear, teach the child as much as is appropriate for his or her age. Tell the child about athletes and other famous people who are diabetic. When possible, another child who is diabetic may visit so that the child does not feel so alone. Encourage the child to become active in helping with self-care. Answer questions about how diabetes will affect the child's activities. Summer camps for children with diabetes are available in many areas and can help develop the child's self-assurance.

The diabetic child can participate in normal activities. However, at least one friend should be told about the diabetic condition, and the child should not go swimming or hiking without a responsible person nearby who knows what to look for and what to do if the child has a reaction.

Some children are sensitive about their condition and fear they seem different from their friends. Even with the best instruction and preparation, they may feel this way and wish to keep their condition secret. They must understand that a teacher or some other adult in their environment must be acquainted with their condition. Classroom teachers need to know which of their students have such a condition and should understand the signs of an impending reaction.

Diabetic children with their glucose levels under good control do not need to be kept from activities such as camp-outs, overnight trips with the school band, or other similar activities away from home. Of course, these children must first be capable of measuring their insulin and giving their own injections. Some young people may find that a desire to participate in such an activity can be the factor that helps them overcome reluctance to measure and administer their own insulin.

Evaluation: Goals and Expected Outcomes

Goal: The child's caloric intake will be adequate to meet nutritional needs and to maintain appropriate growth.
Expected Outcomes: The child

- eats food at meals and snack times and maintains normal weight for age and height.
- demonstrates (along with caregiver) understanding of meal planning by making appropriate menu selections.

Goal: The child's skin integrity will be maintained.
Expected Outcomes: The child

- exhibits skin that is intact with no signs of breakdown.
- describes (along with caregiver) methods for skin inspection and care.

Goal: The child will be free from signs and symptoms of infection.
Expected Outcomes: The child

- shows no signs of infection.
- has temperature within normal range.
- discusses (along with caregiver) the importance of promptly reporting infections.

Goal: The child will maintain normal glucose levels.
Expected Outcomes: The child

- maintains blood glucose level of 60 to 100 mg/dL.
- has urine that is negative for ketones.
- does not show signs of hypoglycemia or hyperglycemia.

Goal: The child and caregiver will verbalize an understanding of the signs, symptoms, and management of hypoglycemia and hyperglycemia.
Expected Outcomes: The child and caregiver

- list the signs of hypoglycemia and hyperglycemia and discuss how to handle each.
- ask questions to clarify information.

Goal: The child and caregiver will verbalize an understanding of insulin administration.
Expected Outcomes: The child and caregiver

- demonstrate insulin injection.
- describe various types of insulin and their reaction and peak times.
- develop a site rotation schedule.

Goal: The child and caregiver will verbalize an understanding of exercise and activity for a diabetic child.
Expected Outcome:

- The child and caregiver describe the effects of exercise on the blood glucose levels.

Goal: The child and caregiver will express their concerns about coping with the child's illness.
Expected Outcomes:

- As appropriate for age, the child discusses necessary adjustments to the daily schedule and activities and names several people to inform about the diabetic condition.
- The caregiver demonstrates support of the child in managing daily and long-term care of diabetes.

Goal: The child will show adjustment and have a positive attitude about the condition.
Expected Outcomes: The child

- expresses feelings about having diabetes.
- participates in age-appropriate activities and realistic goal planning.

Test Yourself

✔ What do the terms polyuria, polydipsia, and polyphagia mean?
✔ What causes diabetic ketoacidosis to occur?
✔ How is type 1 diabetes in the child treated?
✔ Describe the symptoms of hypoglycemia and hyperglycemia.

TYPE 2 DIABETES MELLITUS

Type 2 diabetes mellitus, also referred to as noninsulin-dependent diabetes, is a condition in which the body does not use insulin properly. Previously, type 2 diabetes was primarily diagnosed only in adults, usually over 45 years of age and overweight. More recently, this type of diabetes has been diagnosed in children and adolescents. In particular, children who are overweight, have a family history of type 2 diabetes, or are from a race or ethnic group, such as American Indian, African American, Hispanic, or Asian, are at the greatest risk of developing type 2 diabetes.

Clinical Manifestations and Diagnosis

Many of the symptoms of type 2 diabetes are similar to those of type 1 diabetes—polydipsia, polyuria, and polyphagia (see Table 38-4 for a comparison between types 1 and 2 diabetes). The child is usually overweight or obese. Symptoms are often present for months before a diagnosis is made. Many times, type 2 diabetes is diagnosed when a urine screening test is performed for some other reason and glucosuria is found. In addition, these children have high blood glucose levels. Although diabetic ketoacidosis is not common in adults diagnosed with type 2 diabetes, the condition may be seen in children with the diagnosis.

Treatment

One goal of treatment is to achieve normal or close to normal blood glucose levels. A second goal of treatment is to prevent or decrease the occurrence of long-term complications such as neurologic, kidney, and eye conditions. If the child presents with diabetic ketoacidosis, initial treatment is insulin administration, but then oral hypoglycemic agents, such as metformin, are often effective for controlling blood glucose levels. Lifestyle changes, such as weight loss and increased exercise, are important aspects of treatment for the child.

Nursing Care

Recognizing the child who is at high risk for type 2 diabetes is critical in changing the lifestyle behaviors that increase the child's risk. Work with both the child and the family caregivers to change patterns. Promote lifestyle changes such as healthy eating habits and dietary modifications, and increased physical activity and exercise to help manage the disease. Monitoring blood glucose levels, insulin administration, treatment of hypoglycemia and hyperglycemia, diabetic food plans, and family teaching for type 2 diabetes are the same as with type 1 diabetes.

Key Points

➤ The GI tract of the newborn works in the same manner as that of the adult, but with some limitations. For example, the enzymes secreted by the liver and pancreas are reduced. The smaller capacity of the infant's stomach and the increased speed at which food moves through the GI tract require feeding smaller amounts at more frequent intervals. In addition, the small capacity of the colon leads to a bowel movement after each feeding.

➤ The endocrine system of the infant is adequately developed, although the functions are immature. As the child grows, the endocrine system matures in function.

➤ Nutritional deficiencies can cause children to grow at a slower rate, have a higher rate of illness and infection, and have more difficulty concentrating and achieving in school. Kwashiorkor is caused by a severe deficiency of protein. Marasmus is a deficiency of calories as well as protein. Rickets is caused by a lack of vitamin D. Scurvy is caused by inadequate intake of vitamin C. An iron deficiency may result in anemia and calcium deficiencies can cause bone, teeth, and neurologic concerns. Foods most likely to cause allergic reactions are milk, eggs, wheat, corn, legumes (including peanuts and soybeans), oranges, strawberries, and chocolate.

➤ Celiac syndrome is a malabsorptive disorder. Ingestion of wheat gluten or rye gluten leads to impaired fat absorption. It is often caused by an allergic reaction to the gliadin fraction of gluten (a protein factor in wheat). Treatment includes a restricted gluten-free diet.

➤ GER occurs when the sphincter in the lower portion of the esophagus, which leads into the stomach, is relaxed and allows gastric contents to be regurgitated back into the esophagus. After feeding, the child vomits the contents of the stomach. A histamine-2

(H2) receptor antagonist may be given to reduce the acid secretion. In severe cases, a surgical procedure known as Nissen fundoplication may be done.

➤ Colic consists of recurrent paroxysmal bouts of abdominal pain and is fairly common in young infants. Attacks occur suddenly, usually late in the day or evening. The infant cries loudly and continuously and appears to be in considerable pain but otherwise seems healthy.

➤ Mild diarrhea is loose stools, with the frequency of defecation 2 to 12 times per day. Severe diarrhea is usually accompanied by vomiting, and together they cause large losses of body water and electrolytes. The child is severely dehydrated and gravely ill. Infectious diarrhea is commonly referred to as gastroenteritis. Establishing normal fluid and electrolyte balance is the primary concern in treating gastroenteritis.

➤ The child with pyloric stenosis eats initially but then starts vomiting after meals. The vomiting increases in frequency and force, becoming projectile. The child is irritable, loses weight rapidly, and becomes dehydrated. A surgical procedure called a pyloromyotomy (also known as a Fredet-Ramstedt operation) is the treatment of choice.

➤ Congenital aganglionic megacolon is also called Hirschsprung disease. The common symptoms include failure of the newborn to have a stool in the first 24 hours, bile-stained emesis, and generalized abdominal distention. Gastroenteritis with diarrheal stools, ulceration of the colon, and severe constipation with ribbonlike or hard pellet stools are also seen. Treatment involves surgery with the resection of the aganglionic portion of the bowel.

➤ Intussusception is the invagination, or telescoping, of one portion of the bowel into a distal portion. It occurs most commonly at the juncture of the ileum and the colon. Immediate treatment consists of a barium enema to attempt to correct the telescoping or abdominal surgery if the barium enema does not correct the problem.

➤ Symptoms of appendicitis in the older child may be pain and tenderness in the right lower quadrant of the abdomen, nausea and vomiting, fever, and constipation. The young child has difficulty localizing the pain, may act restless and irritable, and may have a slight fever, a flushed face, and a rapid pulse. Usually the white blood cell count is slightly elevated. Surgical removal of the appendix is the treatment.

➤ Intestinal parasites common to the child include pinworm, roundworm, hookworm, and giardiasis. Pinworms invade the cecum and may enter the appendix. The infestation occurs when the pinworm eggs are swallowed. Roundworms are spread from the feces of infested people. It is usually found in areas where sanitary facilities are lacking and human excreta are deposited on the ground. The hookworm lives in the human intestinal tract and is prevalent in areas where infected human excreta is deposited on the ground; the hookworms penetrate the skin of barefoot people. Giardiasis is caused by the protozoan parasite *Giardia lamblia*. It is a common cause of diarrhea.

➤ The toddler and preschool-aged children often find out about their environment by tasting the world around them. Because their senses of taste and smell are not yet refined, young children ingest substances that would repel an adult because of their taste or smell and often are poisoned by the substance. Common substances children ingest include drugs such as acetaminophen, acetylsalicylic acid (aspirin), ibuprofen, ferrous sulfate, and barbiturates. They also ingest corrosives such as lye, bleach, and other cleaners and hydrocarbons, such as gasoline and kerosene.

➤ Chronic lead poisoning may be caused when children ingest lead from lead-containing paint, furniture, toys, and vinyl mini blinds. Drinking water contaminated by lead pipes; storage of food in improperly glazed earthenware; inhalation of engine fumes; and exposure to industrial areas and materials such as stained glass, solder, fishing sinkers, and bullets can also cause lead poisoning.

➤ Children with lead poisoning may have irritability, hyperactivity, aggression, impulsiveness, or disinterest in play. Short attention span, lethargy, learning difficulties, and distractibility also are signs of poisoning. Acute manifestations include convulsions, mental retardation, blindness, paralysis, coma, and death. Blood lead levels are used to diagnose lead poisoning; the best treatment for lead poisoning is to remove the lead from the child's system by using chelating agents. Early detection of the condition and removal of the child from the lead-containing surroundings offer the best prognosis.

➤ If a child who has swallowed a foreign object is having respiratory distress, the Heimlich maneuver should be used and cardiopulmonary resuscitation started, if necessary. If the child is not having respiratory problems and coughing has not resulted in removal of the object, the child should be taken to an emergency department to be assessed.

➤ In children, type 1 diabetes causes an abrupt pronounced decrease in insulin production, resulting in decreased ability to derive energy from the food eaten. Large amounts of protein and fat are used to supply the child's energy needs, causing loss of weight and slowed growth. Management of type 1 diabetes in children includes insulin therapy and a meal and exercise plan. Teaching for the child and family includes diet, skin concerns, preventing infection, regulating glucose levels, insulin administration, exercise, and learning to adjust to having a chronic disease.

➤ Type 2 diabetes mellitus is a condition in which the body does not use insulin properly. This type of diabetes has been diagnosed in children and adolescents. In particular, children who are overweight, have a family history of type 2 diabetes, or are from a race or ethnic group with high incidence of type 2 diabetes mellitus. Healthy eating habits, dietary modifications, physical activity, and exercise help with management of the disease.

INTERNET RESOURCES

Allergies
www.allergicchild.com

Celiac Disease
www.celiac.com

Diabetes
www.jdf.org
www.childrenwithdiabetes.com

Food Allergies
www.foodallergy.org

Workbook

▮ NCLEX-STYLE REVIEW QUESTIONS

1. If an infant has a diagnosis of pyloric stenosis, the child will likely have a history of which of the following?

   a. Iron deficiency
   b. Projectile vomiting
   c. Muscle spasms
   d. Nasal congestion

2. A nurse admits a child with a diagnosis of possible appendicitis. Of the following signs and symptoms, which would *most* likely be seen in the child with appendicitis?

   a. Sore throat, bone, and joint pain
   b. Itching, swelling around eyes and ankles
   c. Convulsions, weight gain or loss
   d. Fever, nausea, and vomiting

3. The nurse is teaching a group of parents of toddlers about what to do in cases of poisoning. If a toddler has swallowed an unknown substance, which of the following should be the *first* action of the caregiver? The caregiver should

   a. administer a recommended antidote.
   b. call the Poison Control Center.
   c. encourage the child to drink water.
   d. place the child on a flat surface.

4. The nurse is working with a 12-year-old child with type 1 diabetes mellitus. The child asks the nurse why she can't take pills instead of shots like her grandmother does. Which of the following would be the *best* response by the nurse?

   a. "The pills correct a different type of diabetes than you have."
   b. "When your blood glucose levels are better controlled, you can take the pills too."
   c. "Your body does not make its own insulin so the insulin injections help replace it."
   d. "The pills only work for adults who have diabetes. Maybe when you are older, you can take the pills."

5. A child with a diagnosis of failure to thrive because of malnutrition has had an inadequate intake of calories. In planning care, all of the following goals would be appropriate for this child. Which two goals would be the *highest* priority for the child?

   a. The child will maintain good mouth and skin integrity.
   b. The child will maintain current weight.
   c. The child will increase amount of daily exercise.
   d. The child will have decreased anxiety.
   e. The child will satisfy sucking needs.
   f. The child will increase daily fluid intake.
   g. The child will increase intake for appropriate weight gain.

▮ STUDY ACTIVITIES

1. Develop a teaching aid or poster to use in teaching diabetic children how to administer their own insulin injections. Include how you will help this child make an insulin site rotation chart. Present your project to your peers.

2. Survey your house (or a house you select) and list the hazards for ingestion of poisonous substances, drowning, and burns. Include all types of burns. After the hazards are identified, formulate a plan to correct or lessen the hazards.

3. Carmella has idiopathic celiac disease. Using the foods listed in the table below, identify the foods that would be recommended and those that would not be recommended in her meal plan. With the help of a nutrition text or by reading labels, state why each of those foods is either recommended or not recommended.

Food	Recommended	Not Recommended	Explanation of Why Food Would or Would Not Be Recommended
Ice cream			
Corn flakes			
Grits			
Rice pudding			
Whole-wheat bread			
Baked beans			
Hamburger			
Hot dog			
French fries			
Fresh vegetables			
Yogurt			

(continue on page 866)

Food	Recommended	Not Recommended	Explanation of Why Food Would or Would Not Be Recommended
Oatmeal			
Rice Krispies			
Orange juice			
Graham crackers			
Corn chips			
Peanut butter			
Baked potato			
Tuna salad			
Pizza			

4. Go to the Web site: www.diabetes.org/for-parents-and-kids/for-schools/diabetes-management.jsp
   After reading about diabetes management at school, answer the following:
   a. What does this site suggest as the three elements of a school plan?
   b. What would be important for the diabetic child to be allowed to do at school in order to follow his diabetic plan?
   c. What are some ideas suggested to prevent discrimination of a child with diabetes?

■ CRITICAL THINKING: WHAT WOULD YOU DO?

1. Five-year-old Malcolm has been sent home from kindergarten with a note advising of an outbreak of pinworms. There are five children between 2 and 8 years of age in the household where he lives, including cousins. Malcolm's aunt is the person who cares for the children.
   a. What would you explain to Malcolm's aunt when she asks you what pinworms are and how children get them?
   b. What symptoms will you teach her to observe for in the children?
   c. How will the diagnosis of pinworms be made?
   d. What is the treatment for pinworms?

2. Your next-door neighbor has found their 18-month-old child with an empty bottle of children's acetaminophen. She brings the child to your house.
   a. What immediate actions should you take?
   b. What is the specific antidote used in acetaminophen overdose? (Use a drug reference.)
   c. What organ can be damaged with an overdose of acetaminophen?

3. Nine-month-old Tina has severe diarrhea. She has been admitted to your unit and you have been assigned to be her nurse.
   a. What symptoms would you expect Tina to exhibit?
   b. What physical characteristics will you observe her for?
   c. What documentation is especially important in her care?

4. Dosage calculation: After an appendectomy, an 8-year-old child is being medicated with meperidine (Demerol) for postoperative pain. The dosage range for this child is 1.0 to 1.8 mg/kg. The child weighs 55 lb. The Demerol comes in a prefilled syringe with 50 mg/mL. Answer the following:
   a. How many kilograms (kg) does the child weigh?
   b. What is the low dose for this child?
   c. What is the high dose for this child?
   d. How many milliliters (mL) will be given for the low dose of the medication?
   e. How many milliliters (mL) will be given for the high dose of the medication?

39

The Child With a Genitourinary Disorder

KEY TERMS

amenorrhea
ascites
dysmenorrhea
enuresis
hyperlipidemia
intercurrent infections
leukopenia
menarche
mittelschmerz
oliguria
orchiopexy
premenstrual syndrome (PMS)
pyelonephritis
striae
vaginitis

LEARNING OBJECTIVES

On completion of this chapter, you should be able to:

1. Discuss ways the child's genitourinary system differs from the adult's system.
2. Identify the symptoms, treatment, and nursing care of the child with a urinary tract infection.
3. Explain enuresis, including the possible physiologic and psychological causes.
4. Discuss the diagnosis of acute glomerulonephritis including the cause, symptoms, treatment, and nursing care.
5. Discuss the diagnosis of nephrotic syndrome including the symptoms, treatment, and nursing care.
6. Compare acute glomerulonephritis with nephrotic syndrome.
7. Explain the diagnosis of Wilms' Tumor.
8. Describe the structural defects that occur with hydrocele and cryptorchidism.
9. Compare premenstrual syndrome, dysmenorrhea, and amenorrhea.

ADEQUATE functioning of the genitourinary (urinary and reproductive) system is affected by structural problems or defects, infections, disorders, and conditions. Although the symptoms seen in these conditions may be vague or seemingly not serious, they can be chronic, long term, or serious in their effect on the genitourinary system.

GROWTH AND DEVELOPMENT OF THE GENITOURINARY SYSTEM

The genitourinary system is made up of the kidneys, ureters, urinary bladder, and the urethra (Fig. 39-1). There are two kidneys and two ureters located on each side of the body, just above the waistline. Functions of the kidney include excreting excess water and waste products and maintaining a balance of electrolytes and acid–base. Other functions of the kidney are regulating blood pressure by making the enzyme renin and making erythropoietin, which helps stimulate the production of red blood cells. Waste products are removed from the blood and excreted from the body through the urinary system.

The urine formed in the kidneys travels down the ureters and collects in the urinary bladder. When the bladder fills, there is an urge to empty the bladder.

Urine passes through the urethra to be excreted from the body. In infants and children, emptying the bladder is a reflex action. Between ages 2 and 3 years, the child is able to hold the urine in the bladder and learns to urinate voluntarily, thus developing the control of urination.

In the newborn, the bladder empties when only about 15 mL of urine is present, so the newborn voids as many as 20 times a day. As the child gets older, the bladder has more capacity to hold larger amounts of urine before the child feels the urge to void. The child at different ages voids average amounts, depending on fluid intake and kidney health (Table 39-1). The urethra in females is much shorter than in males at all ages, making the female more susceptible to urinary tract infections.

The kidneys in children are located lower in relationship to the ribs than in adults. This placement and the fact that the child has less of a fat cushion around the kidneys cause the child to be at greater risk for trauma to the kidneys. As the child grows, the kidneys also grow, especially during the first 2 years of life. The kidneys reach their full size and function by the time the child is an adolescent.

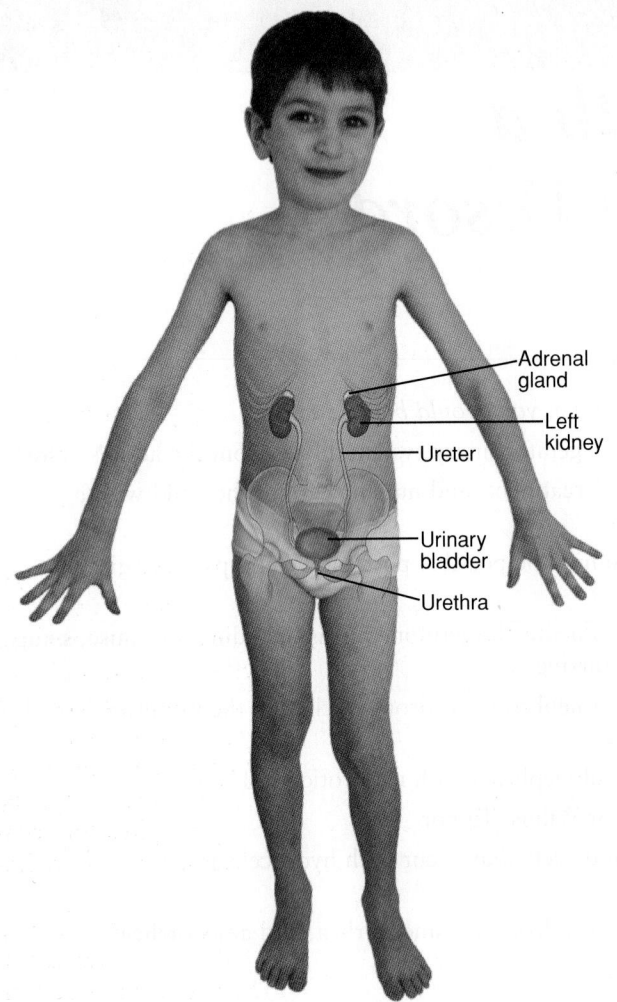

■ **Figure 39-1** The urinary tract.

The reproductive portion of the genitourinary system in males and females matures at the time of puberty. The systems are made up of organs with the primary function of producing cells necessary for reproduction. The organs also provide the mechanism for conception to occur. Males and females have different structures in the

Table 39-1 ■ CHILD'S AVERAGE URINE OUTPUT IN 24 HOURS	
Age	**Amount of Urine (mL)**
6 mo–2 yr	540–600
2–5 yr	500–780
5–8 yr	600–1,200
8–14 yr	1,000–1,500
>14 yr	1,500

From Pillitteri, A. (2007). *Maternal and child health nursing* (5th ed., p. 1454). Philadelphia: Lippincott Williams & Wilkins.

reproductive systems. In the male, the reproductive structures include the testes, located in the scrotum, which produce sperm; the ducts that aid in the passage of sperm; the glands that secrete necessary fluids; and the external genitalia, including the penis. In the female, the reproductive organs include the ovaries, fallopian tubes, uterus, vagina, and the external genitalia. The genitals gradually increase in size during childhood. The hormone changes in both males and females during puberty cause the reproductive system to more fully develop during adolescence.

URINARY TRACT INFECTIONS

Urinary tract infections (UTIs) are fairly common in the "diaper age," in infancy, and again between the ages of 2 and 6 years. The condition is more common in girls than in boys, except in the first 4 months of life, when it is more common in boys. Although many different bacteria may infect the urinary tract, intestinal bacteria, particularly *Escherichia coli*, account for about 80% of acute episodes. The female urethra is shorter and straighter than the male urethra, so it is more easily contaminated with feces. Inflammation may extend into the bladder, ureters, and kidney.

Clinical Manifestations

In children, the symptoms may be fever, nausea, vomiting, foul-smelling urine, weight loss, and increased urination. Occasionally there is little or no fever. Vomiting is common, and diarrhea may occur. The child is irritable. In acute **pyelonephritis** (inflammation of the kidney and renal pelvis), the onset is abrupt, with a high fever for 1 or 2 days. Convulsions may occur during the period of high fever. In younger children, bed-wetting may be a symptom.

Diagnosis

Diagnosis is based on the finding of pus in the urine under microscopic examination. The urine specimen must be fresh and uncontaminated. A "clean catch" voided urine, properly performed, is essential for microscopic examination (see Chapter 30). If a culture is needed, the child may be catheterized, but this is usually avoided if possible. A suprapubic aspiration also may be done to obtain a sterile specimen. In the cooperative, toilet-trained child, clean midstream urine may be used successfully.

Treatment

Simple UTIs may be treated with antibiotics (usually sulfisoxazole or ampicillin) at home. The child with acute pyelonephritis is hospitalized. Fluids are given freely. The symptoms usually subside within a few days after antibiotic therapy has been initiated, but this is not an indication that the infection is completely cleared. Medication must be continued after symptoms disappear. An intravenous pyelogram or ultrasonographic study may be performed to assess the possibility of structural defects if the child has recurring infections.

Nursing Process for the Child With a Urinary Tract Infection

Assessment

During the interview with the family caregiver, collect basic information about the child, such as feeding and sleeping patterns and history of other illnesses. Gather information about the current illness: When the fever started and its course thus far, signs of pain or discomfort on voiding, recent change in feeding pattern, presence of vomiting or diarrhea, irritability, lethargy, abdominal pain, unusual odor to urine, chronic diaper rash, and signs of febrile convulsions. If the child is toilet-trained, ask the caregivers about toileting habits (how does the child wipe? does the child wash the hands when toileting?). Also, ask about the use of bubble baths and the type of soap used, especially for girls.

Data to collect regarding the child includes temperature; pulse (be alert for tachycardia) and respiration rates; weight and height; observation of a wet diaper or the urine in an older child; inspection of the perineal area for rash; presence of irritability and lethargy; and general skin condition, color, and turgor. A urine specimen is needed on admission. A midstream urine collection method is desirable, and catheterization is avoided if possible. Record and report any indications of urinary burning, frequency, urgency, or pain.

In the child who has repeated UTIs, observe the interaction between the child and the family caregivers to detect any indications that the infection may be caused by sexual abuse. Look for possible indications of sexual abuse.

Pay attention.
Bruising, bleeding, or lacerations on the external genitalia, especially in the child who is extremely shy and frightened, may be a sign of child abuse and should be further explored.

Selected Nursing Diagnoses

- Hyperthermia related to infection
- Impaired Urinary Elimination related to pain and burning on urination and decreased fluid intake
- Deficient Knowledge of caregivers related to understanding of UTI

Outcome Identification and Planning

Major goals for the child with a UTI include reducing temperature, maintaining normal urinary elimination, and increasing fluid intake. An important family goal is improving knowledge about infection control to help prevent recurrent infections. Base the nursing plan of care on these goals, with adjustments appropriate for the child's age. To promote normal elimination, plan nursing care that helps relieve pain and increase fluid intake. Be sure to include family teaching that focuses on infection prevention at home.

Implementation

Maintaining Body Temperature

Monitor the child's temperature frequently, at least every 2 hours if it is higher than 101.3°F (38.5°C). If the child has a fever, follow the procedures to reduce elevated temperatures. Administer antibiotics as ordered and observe the child for signs of any reactions to the antibiotics. Antipyretic medications may be ordered. Increasing oral fluids also will help to reduce body temperature.

Promoting Normal Elimination

Because of pain and burning on urination, the toilet-trained child may try to hold urine and not void. Encourage the child to void every 3 or 4 hours to prevent recurrent infection. Observe the child for signs of burning and pain when urinating. In addition, observe the voiding pattern to note frequency of urination, trickling, or other signs that the bladder is not being emptied completely. Carefully monitor and measure urine output. An infant's diaper should be weighed for accuracy. Accurate intake and output measurements are important.

Increasing the child's fluid intake is necessary to help dilute the urine and flush the bladder. An increase in fluid intake also helps decrease the pain experienced on urination. Although getting the child to accept fluids often is difficult, frequent, small amounts of glucose water or liquid gelatin may be accepted. Enlisting the aid of family caregivers may be helpful, but if they are unsuccessful, you must persevere. Most infants and children like apple juice, which helps acidify the urine. Cranberry juice is a good choice for the older child, if he or she tolerates it. Administer analgesics and antispasmodics, as ordered.

Providing Family Teaching

The family caregivers are the key people in helping prevent recurring infections. See Family Teaching Tips: Urinary Tract Infection. Prepare the family caregivers and the child for any other procedures that may be ordered and give appropriate explanations.

Evaluation: Goals and Expected Outcomes

Goal: The child will maintain a temperature within normal limits.
Expected Outcome:

- The child's temperature is 98.6°F to 100°F (37°C–37.8°C).

Goal: The child's normal urinary elimination will be maintained.

Family Teaching Tips

URINARY TRACT INFECTION

- Change infant's diaper when soiled, and clean baby with mild soap and water. Dry completely.
- Teach girls to wipe from front to back.
- Teach child to wash hands before and after going to the toilet.
- Avoid using bubble baths, which create a climate that encourages bacteria to grow, especially in young girls.
- Teach young girls to take showers. Avoid using water softeners in tub baths.
- Encourage child to try to urinate every 3 or 4 hours and to empty the bladder.
- Have girls wear cotton underpants to provide air circulation to perineal area.
- Encourage child to drink fluids, especially cranberry juice.
- Have older girls avoid whirlpools or hot tubs.

Expected Outcomes: The child

- voids every 3 to 4 hours, emptying the bladder each time without apprehension.
- produces 2 to 3 mL/kg of urine per hour (infant).

Goal: The family caregivers will verbalize an understanding of the genitourinary system and good hygiene habits.

Expected Outcomes: The family caregivers

- list signs and symptoms of a UTI and methods to prevent a recurrence.
- state when to contact a health practitioner.

Test Yourself

✔ What bacterium is the most common cause of UTIs?

✔ How are UTIs detected and treated?

✔ Explain the reason a child with a UTI may try to hold his or her urine.

ENURESIS

Enuresis, or bed-wetting, is involuntary urination beyond the age when control of urination is commonly acquired. Many children do not acquire complete nighttime control before 5 to 7 years of age, and occasional bed-wetting may be seen in children as late as 9 or 10 years of age. Boys have more difficulty than do girls, and in some instances, enuresis may persist into the adult years.

Enuresis may have a physiologic or psychological cause and may indicate a need for additional exploration and treatment. Physiologic causes may include a small bladder capacity, UTI, and lack of awareness of the signal to empty the bladder because of sleeping too soundly. Persistent bed-wetting in a 5- or 6-year-old child may be a result of rigorous toilet training before the child was physically or psychologically ready. Enuresis in the older child may express resentment toward family caregivers or a desire to regress to an earlier level of development to receive more care and attention. Emotional stress can be a precipitating factor. The health care team also needs to consider the possibility that enuresis can be a symptom of sexual abuse.

If a physiologic cause has been ruled out, efforts should be made to discover possible psychological causes, including emotional stress. If the child is interested in achieving control, waking the child during the night to go to the toilet or limiting fluids before retiring may be helpful. However, these measures should not be used as a replacement for searching for the cause. Help from a pediatric mental health professional may be needed.

> **Here's a tip for you to share.**
> An upcoming event the child is excited about attending, such as going to camp or visiting friends overnight, might be a motivator in helping the child with enuresis to achieve bladder control.

The family caregiver may become extremely frustrated about having to deal with smelly wet bedding every morning. The child may go to great efforts to hide the fact that the bed is wet. Health care personnel must take a supportive understanding attitude toward the problems of the caregiver and the child, allowing each of them to ventilate feelings and providing a place where emotions can be freely expressed.

ACUTE GLOMERULONEPHRITIS

Acute glomerulonephritis is a condition that appears to be an allergic reaction to a specific infection, most often group A beta-hemolytic streptococcal infection, as in rheumatic fever. The antigen–antibody reaction causes a response that blocks the glomeruli, permitting red blood cells and protein to escape into the urine. Acute glomerulonephritis has a peak incidence in children 6 to 7 years of age and occurs twice as often in boys. The disease is similar in some ways to nephrotic syndrome, which is discussed later in this chapter and in Table 39-2. The prognosis is usually excellent, but a few children develop chronic nephritis.

Clinical Manifestations

Presenting symptoms appear 1 to 3 weeks after the onset of a streptococcal infection such as strep throat, otitis media, tonsillitis, or impetigo. Usually the presenting symptom is grossly bloody urine. The caregiver may

A Personal Glimpse

My 9-year-old daughter was potty trained when she was just barely 2 years old. I was so proud of her and happy that she was out of diapers and that she had so quickly been trained. When she was almost 4, I had her little brother. She occasionally had an accident and wet pants, but I wasn't concerned. I just thought she wanted some attention. It was quite upsetting to me when shortly after she started the second grade she started wetting the bed. At first she was wet a few times a week, then every night. One day I got a call from the school saying I needed to bring her some dry clothes because she had wet her pants at school. That is when the worst part began. Now at 9 years old, she wets her pants everyday. She takes dry clothes to school, but sometimes she just stays in her wet ones. She smells like urine all the time. It is so upsetting to me. I feel frustrated and sometimes angry. Most of all I just feel so bad for my daughter. Her friends make fun of her; she never wants to spend the night anywhere except at home, and now she doesn't even seem to care. About 3 weeks ago I started taking her to a counselor the school nurse recommended. I hope she can help my daughter and me understand and change what is going on for her. It is painful to watch this happen.

Angela

Learning Opportunity: What are some of the possible causes of this child's enuresis? What could you suggest to this mother to help her deal with her feelings regarding her child's situation?

describe the urine as smoky or bloody. Periorbital edema may accompany or precede hematuria. Fever may be 103°F to 104°F (39.4°C–40°C) at the onset of the condition but decreases in a few days to about 100°F (37.8°C). Slight headache and malaise are usual, and vomiting may occur. Hypertension appears in 60% to 70% of patients during the first 4 or 5 days. Both hematuria and hypertension disappear within 3 weeks.

Oliguria (production of a subnormal volume of urine) is usually present, and the urine has a high specific gravity and contains albumin, red and white blood cells, and casts. The blood urea nitrogen and serum creatinine levels and the sedimentation rates are elevated. Cerebral symptoms consisting mainly of headache, drowsiness, convulsions, and vomiting occur in connection with hypertension in a few cases. When the blood pressure is reduced, these symptoms disappear. Cardiovascular disturbance may be revealed in electrocardiogram tracings, but few children have clinical signs. In most children, this condition is short-term; in some children, it progresses to congestive heart failure.

Treatment

Although the child usually feels well in a few days, activities should be limited until the clinical manifestations subside, generally 2 to 4 weeks after the onset. Penicillin may be given during the acute stage to eradicate any existing infection; however, it does not affect the recovery from the disease because the condition is an immunologic response. The diet is generally not restricted, but additional salt may be limited if edema is excessive. Treatment of complications is symptomatic.

Table 39-2 ▌ COMPARISON OF FEATURES OF ACUTE GLOMERULONEPHRITIS AND NEPHROTIC SYNDROME

Assessment Factor	Acute Glomerulonephritis	Nephrotic Syndrome
Cause	Immune reaction to group A β-hemolytic streptococcal infection	Idiopathic; possibly a hypersensitivity reaction
Onset	Abrupt	Insidious
Hematuria	Grossly bloody	Rare
Edema	Mild	Extreme
Hypertension	Marked	Mild
Hyperlipidemia	Rare or mild	Marked
Peak age frequency	5–10 yr	2–3 yr
Interventions	Limited activity; antihypertensives as needed; symptomatic therapy if congestive heart failure occurs	Bed rest during edema stage Corticosteroid administration Possible cyclophosphamide administration
Diet	Normal for age; no added salt if child is hypertensive	High protein, low sodium
Prevention	Prevention through treatment of group A β-hemolytic streptococcal infections	None known

Adapted from Pillitteri, A. (2007). *Maternal and child health nursing* (5th ed.). Philadelphia: Lippincott Williams & Wilkins.

Nursing Care

Bed rest should be maintained until acute symptoms and gross hematuria disappear. The child must be protected from chilling and contact with people with infections. When the child is allowed out of bed, he or she must not become fatigued.

Fluid intake and urinary output should be carefully monitored and recorded. Special attention is needed to keep the intake within prescribed limits. The amount of fluid the child is allowed may be based on output, as well as on evidence of continued hypertension and oliguria. Blood pressure should be monitored regularly using the same arm and a properly fitting cuff. If hypertension develops, a diuretic may help reduce the blood pressure to normal levels. An antihypertensive drug may be added if the diastolic pressure ≥90 mm Hg.

> **Pay attention to the details.**
> Weigh the child with acute glomerulonephritis daily, at the same time, on the same scale, and in the same clothes.

The urine must be tested regularly for protein and hematuria, using dipstick tests. Traces of protein in the urine may persist for months after the acute symptoms disappear, and an elevated Addis count, indicating red blood cells in the urine persists as well. Family caregivers must learn to test for urinary protein routinely. If the urinary signs persist for more than 1 year, the disease has probably assumed a chronic form.

NEPHROTIC SYNDROME

Several different types of nephrosis have been identified in the nephrotic syndrome. The most common type in children is called lipoid nephrosis, idiopathic nephrotic syndrome, or minimal change nephrotic syndrome (MCNS). All forms of nephrosis have early characteristics of edema and proteinuria; therefore, definite clinical differentiation cannot be made early in the disease.

Nephrotic syndrome has an insidious onset in comparison to acute glomerupnephritis, which has an abrupt onset (see Table 39-2 for a comparison of the two disorders). Nephrotic syndrome has a course of remissions and exacerbations that usually lasts for months. The recovery rate generally is good with the use of intensive steroid therapy and protection against infection. The cause of MCNS is unknown. In rare cases, it is associated with other specific diseases. Nephrotic syndrome is present in as many as 7 per 100,000 children younger than 9 years of age. The average age of onset is 2.5 years, with most cases occurring between the ages of 2 and 6 years.

Clinical Manifestations

Edema is usually the presenting symptom, appearing first around the eyes and ankles (Fig. 39-2). As the

■ Figure 39-2 A child with nephrotic syndrome. Note the edema around the eyes.

swelling advances, the edema becomes generalized, with a pendulous abdomen full of fluid. Respiratory difficulty may be severe, and edema of the scrotum on the male is characteristic. The edema shifts when the child changes position when lying quietly or walking about. Anorexia, irritability, and loss of appetite develop. Malnutrition may become severe. However, the generalized edema masks the loss of body tissue, causing the child to present a chubby appearance and to double his or her weight. After diuresis, the malnutrition becomes quite apparent. These children are usually susceptible to infection, and repeated acute respiratory conditions are the usual pattern. The administration of prednisone causes immunosuppression that intensifies the susceptibility to infection.

Diagnosis

Laboratory findings include marked proteinuria, especially albumin, with large numbers of hyaline and granular casts in the urine. Hematuria is not usually present, although a few red blood cells may appear in the urine. The blood serum protein level is reduced, and there is an increase in the level of cholesterol in the blood (**hyperlipidemia**).

Treatment

The management of nephrotic syndrome is a long process with remissions and recurrence of symptoms common. In most cases, the use of corticosteroids has induced remissions and has reduced recurrences. Corticosteroid therapy usually produces diuresis in about 7 to 14 days, but use of the drug is continued until a remission occurs. Prednisone is the drug most commonly used. After the diuresis occurs, intermittent therapy is continued every other day or for 3 days a week. Daily urine testing for protein is continued whether the child is at home or in the hospital. It is important that accurate documentation be kept to track patterns of protein loss in the child.

Diuretics may not be necessary when diuresis can be induced with steroids. Diuretics have not been effective in reducing the edema of nephrotic syndrome, although a loop diuretic (e.g., furosemide) may be administered if the edema causes respiratory compromise.

Immunosuppressant therapy may be used to reduce symptoms and prevent further relapses in children who do not respond adequately to corticosteroids. Cyclophosphamide (Cytoxan) is the drug most commonly used. Because cyclophosphamide has serious side effects, the family caregivers must be fully informed before therapy is started. **Leukopenia** (leukocyte count $<5,000/mm^3$) can be expected, as well as the other common side effects of immunosuppressant therapy such as gastrointestinal symptoms, hematuria, and alopecia. The length of therapy is usually a brief period of 2 or 3 months.

A general diet is recommended that appeals to the child's poor appetite with frequent, small feedings if necessary. The addition of salt is discouraged, and sometimes the child is put on a low-sodium diet. In addition, the child may be placed on a high-protein diet. Family caregivers need encouragement and support for the long months ahead. Relapses usually become less frequent as the child gets older.

Nutrition news.

Including foods high in potassium, such as bananas, oranges, and raisins, in the diet of a child taking a loop diuretic is helpful in maintaining adequate potassium levels.

Nursing Process For The Child With Nephrotic Syndrome

Assessment

Observe for edema when performing the physical examination of the child with nephrotic syndrome. Weigh the child and record the abdominal measurements to serve as a baseline. Obtain vital signs, including blood pressure. Note any swelling about the eyes or the ankles and other dependent parts, and record the degree of pitting. Inspect the skin for pallor, irritation, or breakdown. Examine the scrotal area of the male child for swelling, redness, and irritation. Question the caregiver about the onset of symptoms, the child's appetite, urine output, and signs of fatigue or irritability.

Selected Nursing Diagnoses

- Excess Fluid Volume related to fluid accumulation in tissues and third spaces
- Risk for Imbalanced Nutrition: Less Than Body Requirements related to anorexia
- Risk for Impaired Skin Integrity related to edema

- Fatigue related to edema and disease process
- Risk for Infection related to immunosuppression
- Deficient Knowledge of the caregiver related to disease process, treatment, and home care
- Compromised Family Coping related to care of a child with chronic illness

Outcome Identification and Planning

The major goals for the child with nephrotic syndrome are relieving edema, improving nutritional status, maintaining skin integrity, conserving energy, and preventing infection. The family goals include learning about the disease and treatments, as well as learning ways to cope with the child's long-term care.

Implementation

Monitoring Fluid Intake and Output

Accurately monitor and document intake and output. Weigh the child at the same time every day on the same scale in the same clothing. Measure the child's abdomen daily at the level of the umbilicus, and make certain that all staff personnel measure at the same level. The abdomen may be greatly enlarged with **ascites** (edema in the peritoneal cavity). The abdomen can even become marked with **striae** (stretch marks).

This advice will be useful.

Note the desired location for measuring the abdomen of the child with nephrotic syndrome on the nursing care plan so that everyone follows the same practice.

Test the urine regularly for albumin and specific gravity. Albumin can be tested with reagent strips dipped into the urine and read by comparison with a color chart on the container.

Improving Nutritional Intake

Although the child may look plump, underneath the edema is a thin, possibly malnourished child. The child's appetite is poor for several reasons:

- The ascites diminishes the appetite because of the full feeling in the abdomen.
- The child may be lethargic, apathetic, and simply not interested in eating.
- A no-added-salt or low-salt diet may be unappealing to the child.
- Corticosteroid therapy may decrease the appetite.

Offer a visually appealing and nutritious diet. Consult the child and the family to learn which foods are appealing to the child. Cater to the child's wishes as much as possible to perk up a lagging appetite. A dietitian can help to plan appealing meals for the child. Serving six small meals may help increase the child's total intake better than the customary three meals a day.

Promoting Skin Integrity

The child's skin is stretched with edema and becomes thin and fragile. Inspect all skin surfaces regularly for breakdown. Because the child is lethargic, turn and position the child every 2 hours. Protect skin surfaces from pressure by means of pillows and padding. Protect overlapping skin surfaces from rubbing by careful placement of cotton gauze. Bathe the child regularly. Thoroughly wash the skin surfaces that touch each other with soap and water and dry them completely. A sheer dusting of cornstarch may be soothing. If the scrotum is edematous, use a soft cotton support to provide comfort.

Promoting Energy Conservation

Bed rest is common during the edema stage of the condition. The child rarely protests because of his or her fatigue. The sheer bulk of the edema makes movement difficult. When diuresis occurs several days after beginning prednisone, the child may be allowed more activity, but balance the activity with rest periods and encourage the child to rest when fatigued. Plan quiet, age-appropriate activities that interest the child. Most children love having someone read to them. Coloring books, dominoes, puzzles, and some kinds of computer and board games are quiet activities that many children enjoy. Involve the family in providing some of these activities. Avoid using television excessively as a diversion.

Preventing Infection

The child with nephrotic syndrome is especially at risk for respiratory infections because the edema and the corticosteroid therapy lower the body's defenses. Protect the child from anyone with an infection: staff, family, visitors, and other children. Hand washing and strict medical asepsis are essential. Monitor vital signs every 4 hours and observe for any early signs of infection.

Providing Family Teaching and Support

Children with nephrotic syndrome are usually hospitalized for diagnosis, thorough evaluation of their general health and specific condition, and institution of therapy. If the child has an infection, a course of antibiotic therapy may be given; unless unforeseen complications develop, the child is discharged with complete instructions for management. Provide a written plan to help family caregivers follow the program successfully. They must keep a careful record of home treatment for the health care provider to review at regular intervals. Teach the family caregivers about reactions that may occur with the use of steroids and the adverse effects of abruptly discontinuing use of these drugs. If the family understands these aspects well, the incidence of forgetting to give the medication or of neglecting to refill the prescription may be reduced or eliminated. Encourage the family caregivers to report promptly any symptoms that they think are caused by the medication. Teach the family that the necessary special care is important to keep the child in optimum health and that **intercurrent infections** (those occurring during the course of an already existing disease) must be reported promptly.

Also, teach the family that exacerbations are common and that they need to understand these will probably occur. Stress the information that they should report, including rapidly increasing weight, increased proteinuria, or signs of infections. Any of these may be a reason for altering the therapeutic regimen or changing the specific antibiotic agents used.

Provide the family caregivers with home care information appropriate for any chronically ill child. Bed rest is indicated during an intercurrent illness. Activity is restricted only by edema, which may slow the child down considerably; otherwise, normal activity is beneficial. Sufficient food intake may be a problem, as in other types of chronic illness. Fortunately, there are usually no food restrictions, and the appetite can be tempted by attractive, appealing foods. As the name implies, MCNS causes few changes in the kidneys; these children have a good prognosis. Complications from kidney damage alter the course of treatment. Failure to achieve satisfactory diuresis or the need to discontinue steroids because of adverse reactions requires a reevaluation of treatment. The presence of gross hematuria suggests renal damage. In a few children, the persistence of abnormal urinary findings after diuresis presents a less hopeful outlook. A child who has frequent relapses lasting into adolescence or adulthood may develop renal failure and eventually be a candidate for a kidney transplant.

> **Here's a hint.**
> Help the family caregivers of the child with nephrotic syndrome develop a method for keeping accurate records—charts or calendars might work well.

Evaluation: Goals and Expected Outcomes

Goal: The child's edema will be decreased.
Expected Outcome:

- The child has appropriate weight loss and decreased abdominal girth.

Goal: The child will have an adequate nutritional intake to meet normal growth needs.
Expected Outcome:

- The child eats 80% or more of his or her meals.

Goal: The child's skin integrity will be maintained.
Expected Outcome:

- The child's skin remains free of breakdown with no redness or irritation.

Goal: The child's energy will be conserved.
Expected Outcomes: The child

- rests as needed.
- engages in quiet diversional activities.

Goal: The child will be free from signs and symptoms of infection.

Expected Outcome:

- The child has normal vital signs with no respiratory or gastrointestinal symptoms.

Goal: The family caregivers will verbalize an understanding of the disease process, treatment, and the child's home care needs.

Expected Outcomes: The family

- explains nephrotic syndrome.
- describes aspects of medications given.
- states signs and symptoms of infection.
- discusses home care.
- asks and answers appropriate questions.

Goal: The family caregivers will verbalize feelings and concerns.

Expected Outcomes: The family

- verbalizes feelings and concerns related to caring for a child with a chronic illness.
- receives adequate support.

Test Yourself

✔ Give examples of physiologic and psychological causes of enuresis.

✔ Acute glomerulonephritis may be an allergic reaction to what bacterium?

✔ What is the presenting symptom in the child with nephrotic syndrome and where is this symptom noted?

✔ Why is the abdomen measured daily for the child with nephrotic syndrome? What might be detected with this measurement?

WILMS' TUMOR (NEPHROBLASTOMA)

Wilms' tumor, an adenosarcoma in the kidney region, is one of the most common abdominal neoplasms of early childhood. The tumor arises from bits of embryonic tissue that remain after birth. This tissue can spark rapid cancerous growth in the area of the kidney. The tumor is rarely discovered until it is large enough to be palpated through the abdominal wall. As the tumor grows, it invades the kidney or the renal vein and disseminates to other parts of the body. When the child is being evaluated and treated, a sign must be visibly posted stating that abdominal palpation should be avoided because cells may break loose and spread the tumor. Treatment consists of surgical removal as soon as possible after the growth is discovered, combined with radiation and chemotherapy.

Prognosis is best for the child younger than 2 years of age, but has improved markedly for others with im-

proved chemotherapy. Follow-up consists of regular evaluation for metastasis to the lungs or other sites. All long-term implications for chemotherapy apply to this child.

HYDROCELE

Hydrocele is a collection of peritoneal fluid that accumulates in the scrotum through a small passage called the processus vaginalis. This processus is a fingerlike projection in the inguinal canal through which the testes descend. Usually the processus closes soon after birth; if the processus does not close, fluid from the peritoneal cavity passes through, causing hydrocele. This is the same passage through which intestines may slip, causing an inguinal hernia. If the hydrocele remains by the end of the first year, corrective surgery is performed.

CRYPTORCHIDISM

Shortly before or soon after birth, the male gonads (testes) descend from the abdominal cavity into their normal position in the scrotum. Occasionally one or both of the testes do not descend, which is a condition called cryptorchidism. The testes are usually normal in size; the cause for failure to descend is not clearly understood.

In most infants with cryptorchidism, the testes descend by the time the infant is 1 year old. If one or both testes have not descended by this age, treatment is recommended. If both testes remain undescended, the male will be sterile.

A surgical procedure called **orchiopexy** is used to bring the testes down into the scrotum and anchor it there. Some physicians prefer to try medical treatment—injections of human chorionic gonadotropic hormone—before doing surgery. If this is unsuccessful in bringing the testes down, orchiopexy is performed. Surgery usually is performed when the child is 1 to 2 years of age. Prognosis for a normal functioning testicle is good when the surgery is performed at this young age and no degenerative action has taken place before treatment.

MENSTRUAL DISORDERS

The beginning of menstruation, called **menarche**, normally occurs between the ages of 9 and 16 years. For many girls, this is a joyous affirmation of their womanhood, but others may have negative feelings about the event, depending on how they have been prepared for menarche and for their roles as women. Irregular menstruation is common during the first year, until a regular cycle is established.

Some adolescent girls experience **mittelschmerz**, a dull, aching abdominal pain at the time of ovulation (hence the name, which means "midcycle"). The cause is not completely understood, but the discomfort usually lasts only a few hours and is relieved by analgesics, a heating pad, or a warm bath.

PREMENSTRUAL SYNDROME

Women of all ages are subject to the discomfort of **premenstrual syndrome (PMS)**, but the symptoms may be alarming to the adolescent. Symptoms include edema (resulting in weight gain), headache, increased anxiety, mild depression, and mood swings. The major cause of PMS is thought to be water retention after progesterone production after ovulation (see Figure 3-10 in Chapter 3).

Generally, the discomforts of PMS are minor and can be relieved by reducing salt intake during the week before menstruation, taking mild analgesics, and applying local heat. When symptoms are more severe, the physician may prescribe a mild diuretic to be taken the week before menstruation to relieve edema; occasionally oral contraceptive pills are prescribed to prevent ovulation.

DYSMENORRHEA

Dysmenorrhea (painful menstruation) is classified as primary or secondary. Many adolescent girls experience pain associated with menstruation, including cramping abdominal pain, leg pain, and backache. Primary dysmenorrhea occurs as part of the normal menstrual cycle without any associated pelvic disease. The increased secretion of prostaglandins, which occurs in the last few days of the menstrual cycle, is thought to be a contributing factor in primary dysmenorrhea. Nonsteroidal anti-inflammatory drugs, such as ibuprofen (Advil, Motrin), inhibit prostaglandins and are the treatment of choice for primary dysmenorrhea. These drugs are most effective when taken before cramps become too severe. Because nonsteroidal anti-inflammatory drugs are irritating to the gastric mucosa, they always should be taken with food and discontinued if epigastric burning occurs.

Secondary dysmenorrhea is the result of pelvic pathologic changes, most often pelvic inflammatory disease or endometriosis. The adolescent girl who has severe menstrual pain should be examined by a physician to determine if any pelvic pathologic changes are present. Treatment of the underlying condition helps relieve severe dysmenorrhea.

AMENORRHEA

The absence of menstruation, or **amenorrhea**, can be primary (no previous menstruation) or secondary (missing three or more periods after menstrual flow has begun). Primary amenorrhea after 16 years of age warrants a diagnostic survey for genetic abnormalities, tumors, or other problems. Secondary amenorrhea can be the result of discontinuing contraceptives, a sign of pregnancy, the result of physical or emotional stressors, or a symptom of an underlying medical condition. A complete physical examination, including gynecologic screening, is necessary to help determine the cause.

Table 39-3 ▮ INFECTIOUS CAUSES OF VAGINITIS

Organism/Incidence	Symptoms	Sexual Transmission	Treatment
Candida Albicans First episodes occur in adolescence, especially in sexually active girls	Severe itching, exacerbated just before menstruation Odor not present Milky "cottage cheese"–like discharge may be noted on examination	Normally present in vagina; most often results from glycosuria, antibiotic therapy, birth control pills, steroid therapy, or other factor that alters normal pH of vagina May result from oral–genital sex	Nystatin, miconazole (Monistat), or clotrimazole (Gyne-Lotrimin) vaginal suppositories or creams
Bacterial Vaginosis (multiple organisms) Common among adolescent girls; sexual partner will probably also be infected	About half of patients have no symptoms Fishy odor after intercourse Discharge, if present, grayish and thin	Sexually transmitted	Metronidazole (Flagyl)* or ampicillin; sexual partners may be treated
Trichomoniasis Most frequently diagnosed STI	Itching with severe infection, especially after menstruation Discharge has foul odor and may be frothy, gray or green	Sexually transmitted	Metronidazole (Flagyl)*, sexual partners also should be treated

*Flagyl is not ordered for the pregnant patient due to possible danger to fetus.

VAGINITIS

Vaginitis (inflammation of the vagina) can occur for a number of reasons, such as diaphragms or tampons left in place too long, irritating douches or sprays, estrogen changes caused by birth-control pills, and antibiotic therapy. These factors provide an opportunity for the infecting organisms to become active. The most common causes of vaginitis are *Candida albicans, Gardnerella vaginalis,* and the other organisms that cause bacterial vaginosis, and *Trichomonas. Trichomonas* is the only one of these organisms transmitted solely by sexual contact (Table 39-3).

Test Yourself

✔ If the testes remain undescended, what is the long-term complication for the male?

✔ How do premenstrual syndrome, dysmenorrhea, and amenorrhea differ?

Key Points

➤ The kidneys in children are located lower in relationship to the ribs than in adults. This placement and the fact that the child has less of a fat cushion around the kidneys cause the child to be at greater risk for trauma to the kidneys. In infants and children, emptying the bladder is a reflex action. Between ages 2 and 3 years, the child develops control of urination. The reproductive portion of the genitourinary system in males and females matures at the time of puberty.

➤ UTIs are usually treated with antibiotics such as ampicillin or sulfisoxazole. The entire course of the medication should be taken, even if the symptoms subside after a few days. Goals for the child with a UTI include reducing temperature, maintaining normal urinary elimination, and increasing fluid intake.

➤ Physiologic causes of enuresis may include a small bladder capacity, UTI, and lack of awareness of the signal to empty the bladder because of sleeping too soundly. If a physiologic cause has been ruled out, psychological causes, including emotional stress, may be the cause of the enuresis.

➤ Acute glomerulonephritis is a condition that appears to be an allergic reaction to a specific infection; most often group A beta-hemolytic streptococcal infection, as in rheumatic fever. Presenting symptoms of acute glomerulonephritis appear 1 to 3 weeks after the onset of a streptococcal infection, with the most common symptom being grossly bloody urine, which may be described as smoky or bloody. Periorbital edema may accompany or precede hematuria. Nursing care includes encouraging bed rest and preventing fatigue, protecting from infection, monitoring vital signs, intake and output, and urine for protein and hematuria.

➤ Edema is usually the presenting symptom in nephrotic syndrome, appearing first around the eyes and ankles. The edema becomes generalized with an abdomen full of fluid. Respiratory problems and edema of the scrotum on the male is characteristic. Anorexia, irritability, and loss of appetite develop. The goals for the child with nephrotic syndrome are relieving edema, improving nutritional status, maintaining skin integrity, conserving energy, and preventing infection.

➤ Acute glomerulonephritis has an abrupt onset and usually last for 2 to 3 weeks. Nephrotic syndrome has an insidious onset and a course of remissions and exacerbations that usually last for months.

➤ Wilms' tumor is one of the most common abdominal neoplasms of early childhood. The tumor arises from bits of embryonic tissue that causes cancerous growth in the area of the kidney. Abdominal palpation should be avoided because cells may break loose and spread the tumor.

➤ Hydrocele is a collection of peritoneal fluid that accumulates in the scrotum through a small fingerlike projection in the inguinal canal, through which the testes descend. Usually the processus closes soon after birth; if the processus does not close, fluid from the peritoneal cavity passes through, causing hydrocele.

➤ The condition called cryptorchidism occurs when the male gonads (testes) do not descend from the abdominal cavity into their normal position in the scrotum.

➤ PMS symptoms include edema (resulting in weight gain), headache, increased anxiety, mild depression, and mood swings. The major cause of PMS is thought to be water retention. Dysmenorrhea (painful menstruation) has symptoms of pain associated with menstruation, including cramping abdominal pain, leg pain, and backache. The absence of menstruation is called amenorrhea.

INTERNET RESOURCES

Kidney Disorders
www.kidney.org

Enuresis
www.enuresis.org

Glomerulonephritis and Nephrotic Syndrome
www.nephrologychannel.com

Workbook

■ NCLEX-STYLE REVIEW QUESTIONS

1. After discussing ways to lower a fever with the caregiver of an infant who has a urinary tract infection, the caregiver makes the following statements. Which statement requires further teaching?

   a. "I won't give my child baby aspirin when she has a fever."

   b. "I know I need to dress my baby lightly if she has a fever."

   c. "When my baby has a fever, I will sponge her in cool water for 20 minutes."

   d. "I need to recheck my baby's temperature until it is below 101°F."

2. In caring for a child with nephrotic syndrome, which of the following interventions will be included in the child's plan of care?

   a. Ambulating three to four times a day

   b. Weighing on the same scale each day

   c. Increasing fluid intake by 50 cc an hour

   d. Testing the urine for glucose levels regularly

3. A child diagnosed with acute glomerulonephritis will *most* likely have a history of which of the following?

   a. Sibling diagnosed with the same disease

   b. Recent illness, such as strep throat

   c. Hemorrhage or history of bruising easily

   d. Hearing loss with impaired speech development

4. The nurse is teaching the caregiver of a 5-year-old child diagnosed with nephrotic syndrome regarding the no-added-salt diet the child has been placed on. In addition to not adding salt to foods, the nurse has discussed with the caregiver that helping the child avoid foods high in sodium is also recommended. The caregiver marks the following foods on the child's menu selection for the next day. The nurse recognizes the caregiver needs further teaching when which of the following foods high in sodium were selected? Select all that apply.

   a. Cheddar cheese omelet

   b. Apple juice

   c. Blueberry muffin

   d. Hot dog in bun

   e. Fresh green beans

   f. Canned peaches

5. In caring for a child with a urinary tract infection, the nurse would do all of the following nursing interventions. Which two interventions would be the priority for the nurse?

   a. The nurse will collect a "clean catch" voided urine.

   b. The nurse will record and report any indications of urinary burning, frequency, or urgency.

   c. The nurse will observe for possible indications of sexual abuse.

   d. The nurse will instruct caregivers to avoid bubble baths, especially in young girls.

   e. The nurse will observe the child for signs of any reactions to the antibiotics.

   f. The nurse will teach girls to wipe from front to back.

■ STUDY ACTIVITIES

1. Create a poster to use as a teaching aid for a group of family caregivers of a child with nephrotic syndrome. Include information regarding the use of steroids and the adverse effects of abruptly discontinuing use of the drug, as well as symptoms that might be caused by the medication.

2. Develop a method to help the caregivers of a child with nephrotic syndrome record information to be shared with their provider. Include information such as the child's weight, protein in the urine, and signs of infection.

3. Go to the following Internet site: www.pediatricon-call.com

   Click on "Parent Corner," click on "Diseases." Under "Childhood Ailments," click on "Kidney Problems," and click on "Nephrotic Syndrome." After reading the questions and answers, answer the following:

   a. What organ is involved in nephrotic syndrome?

   b. How is the child with nephrotic syndrome monitored?

   c. What precautions should the caregivers of a child with nephrotic syndrome take for their child?

■ CRITICAL THINKING: WHAT WOULD YOU DO?

1. Bradley is a 6-year-old boy who is in a playgroup with your child. Bradley's mother is talking with you and tells you she is concerned about Bradley because he has been potty trained, but now he is wetting the bed every night and sometimes has accidents during the day. She asks you if you think she should take her child to see their pediatrician.

   a. What would you suggest to Bradley's mother about seeing his pediatrician?

   b. What questions do you think the pediatrician might ask Bradley's mother?

   c. What are the possible physiologic causes of enuresis in children?

   d. What are frequent psychological causes of enuresis in children?

IVAN

2. A classmate of yours has asked you to help give a presentation to a group of 12-year-old girls. The topic is human reproduction and sexuality. During the discussion, one of the girls tells you she has heard of PMS (premenstrual syndrome) but does not know what it means.

   a. What will you explain to this group of girls regarding what PMS is?

   b. What is the physiologic cause of PMS?

   c. What symptoms might be seen when a woman is experiencing PMS?

   d. What will you explain to this group regarding the treatments that may be done when a woman experiences PMS?

3. Dosage calculation: A preschool child with a diagnosis of nephrotic syndrome is being treated with Prednisolone. The child is being given a dose of 40 mg/day. The child weighs 44 lb. Answer the following:

   a. How many kilograms (kg) does the child's weigh?

   b. How many milligrams (mg) per kilogram is this child's dose?

   c. If the dose is decreased to 30 mg/day, how many milligrams per kilogram will this dose be?

40 The Child With a Musculoskeletal Disorder

KEY TERMS

ankylosis
compartment syndrome
halo traction
kyphosis
lordosis
metaphysis
scoliosis
skeletal traction
skin traction
synovitis
traction

LEARNING OBJECTIVES

On completion of this chapter, you should be able to:

1. Discuss ways the child's musculoskeletal system differs from the adult's system.
2. Discuss types of fractures seen in children and explain the treatment.
3. Describe the purpose of doing neurovascular checks in a child with a musculoskeletal disorder.
4. List and define the five Ps to observe, record, and report when caring for a child in a cast.
5. Identify and explain different types of traction.
6. Discuss osteomyelitis including the bacterium that usually causes it, the treatment, and nursing care.
7. Identify the most common form of muscular dystrophy and describe its characteristics.
8. Describe Legg-Calve-Perthes disease.
9. Identify the treatment for the child with osteosarcoma and Ewing sarcoma.
10. Discuss juvenile rheumatoid arthritis, including the drugs of choice used in the treatment.
11. Describe scoliosis and identify methods of correction and nursing care.

As CHILDREN explore the environment around them, they often cause injury to their musculoskeletal system. Physical activities including play and team sports create situations in which minor skeletal injuries, such as sprains and minor fractures, occur. However, some disorders of the musculoskeletal system can have lifelong effects.

GROWTH AND DEVELOPMENT OF THE MUSCULOSKELETAL SYSTEM

The musculoskeletal system provides the structure and framework to support, protect, and permit movement of the body. Bones are attached to each other by connecting links called joints, which allow for movement of the body parts. Skeletal muscles attach to the bones, with a moveable joint between them. Tendons and ligaments hold the muscles and bones together. Contraction of the muscles causes movement to take place. The heat produced as the muscles contract maintains the body temperature at a stable level. Minerals such as calcium, phosphorus, magnesium, and fluoride are stored in the bones. Blood cells are produced in the bone marrow.

The skeletal system is made up of four types of bone, each having a different function. Each of these types of bones has a specific shape—long, short, flat, irregular. During fetal life, tissue called cartilage, a type of connective tissue consisting of cells implanted in a gel-like substance, gradually calcifies and becomes bone. This calcification process develops the cartilage tissue into the major bones of the body.

Long bones grow from the long central shaft of the bone called the diaphysis to the rounded end of the bone called the epiphysis. Cartilage makes up the epiphyseal plate that is between the epiphysis

Think about this.
Bone growth takes place between birth and puberty, with most growth being complete by age 20 years.

and the diaphysis. As long as cartilage remains, the child's bones continue to grow. Bones grow in width at the same time they are growing in length. When the epiphyseal plate becomes an epiphyseal line and cartilage no longer is present, this marks the end of the growth of that bone in the child.

During childhood, the bones are more spongelike and can bend and break more easily than in adults. In addition, because the bones are still in the process of growing, breaks in the bone heal more quickly than do breaks in adults.

The bones of the skull give shape to the head. The areas where these bones meet are called suture lines. These suture lines do not ossify or harden into bone during fetal life. Because these suture lines are not fused, during delivery the bones of the skull can move and overlap, allowing for the head to pass through the birth canal. Within the first 2 years of life, these suture lines or fontanels fuse together.

The spine or vertebral column is made up of a series of separate bones connected in a way that allows for flexibility. There are four distinct curves in the adult spine. At birth, the spine is a continuous rounded convex curve. As the infant learns to hold up the head, the neck develops into a reverse curve. When the child begins to stand, another reverse curve is formed in the lower part of the back. The curves in the spine give support, strength, and balance to the body.

As the child grows, the muscles become stronger and the child has more muscle tone, strength, and coordination (Fig. 40-1).

FRACTURES

A fracture, a break in a bone that is usually accompanied by vascular and soft tissue damage, is characterized by pain, swelling, and tenderness. Children's fractures differ from those of adults in that generally they are less complicated, heal more quickly, and usually occur from different causes. The child has an urge to explore the environment but lacks the experience and judgment to recognize possible hazards. In some instances, caregivers may be negligent in their supervision, but often the child uses immature judgment or is simply too fast for them.

The bones most commonly fractured in childhood are the clavicle, femur, tibia, humerus, wrist, and fingers. The classification of a fracture reflects the kind of bone injury sustained (Fig. 40-2). If the fragments of fractured bone are separated, the fracture is said to be complete. If fragments remain partially joined, the fracture is termed incomplete. Greenstick fractures are one

Did you know?

When a child has a greenstick fracture, the bone bends and often just partially breaks, just as a green tree stick does when one tries to break it, thus the name "greenstick" fracture.

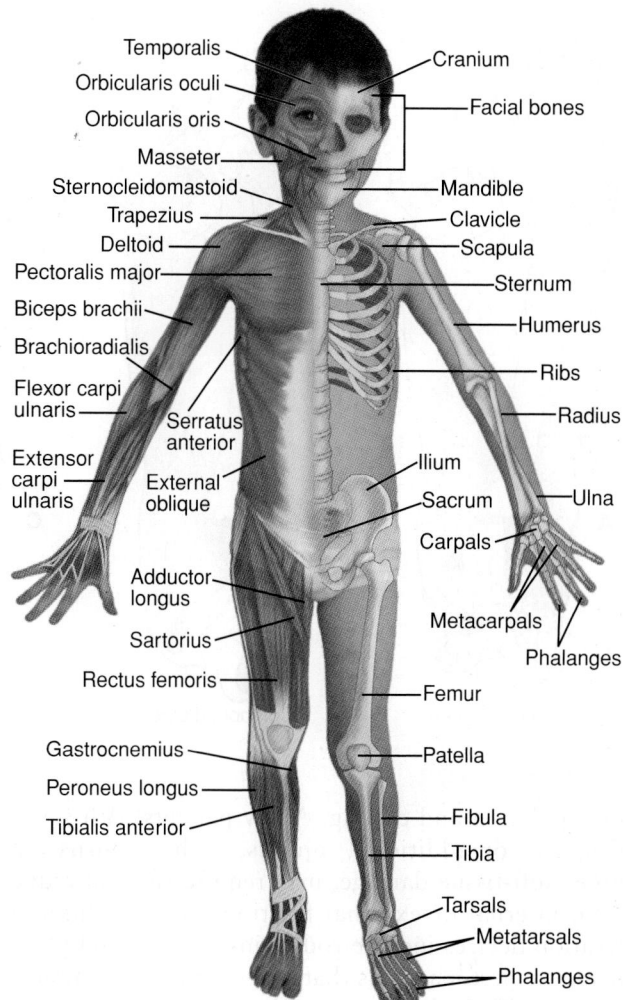

■ Figure 40-1 Bones and muscles of the body.

kind of incomplete fracture, caused by incomplete ossification, common in children.

When a broken bone penetrates the skin, the fracture is called compound, or open. A simple, or closed, fracture is a single break in the bone without penetration of the skin. Spiral fractures, which twist around the bone, are frequently associated with child abuse and are caused by a wrenching force. Fractures in the area of the epiphyseal plate (growth plate) can cause permanent damage and severely impair growth (Fig. 40-3).

Be aware.

Fractures occurring in the epiphyseal plate (growth plate) can cause permanent damage.

Treatment and Nursing Care

Most childhood fractures are treated by realignment and immobilization using either traction or closed

A Simple/Closed   B Compound/Open   C Spiral   D Greenstick

■ Figure 40-2 Types of fractures. All are examples of complete fractures except *D*, which is an incomplete fracture.

manipulation and casting. A few patients with severe fractures or additional injuries, such as burns and other soft-tissue damage, may require surgical reduction, internal or external fixation, or both. Internal fixation devices include rods, pins, screws, and plates made of inert materials that do not trigger an immune reaction. They allow early mobilization of the child to a wheelchair, crutches, or a walker.

External fixation devices are used primarily in complex fractures often with other injuries or complications.

■ Figure 40-3 One form of epiphyseal injury; a crushing injury (as might occur in a fall from a height) can destroy the layer of germinal cells of the epiphysis, resulting in disturbance of growth.

These devices are applied under sterile conditions in the operating room and may be augmented by soft dressings and elevated by means of an overhead traction rope. External fixation devices rarely are used on young children.

Casts

The kind of cast used is determined by the age of the child, the severity of the fracture, the type of bone involved, and the amount of weight the child is allowed to bear on the extremity. Most casts are formed from gauze strips impregnated with plaster of paris or other synthetic material, such as fiberglass or polyurethane resin, which is pliable when wet but hardens when dry. Synthetic materials are lighter in weight and present a cleaner appearance because they can be sponged with water when soiled.

Have some fun with this.

Casts made of synthetic material are available in many colors. Children enjoy choosing a favorite color, a school color, or a color associated with a specific holiday, such as red for Valentine's Day.

Synthetic casts dry more rapidly than do plaster of paris casts. The lightweight casts tend to be used as arm casts and hip spica casts that are used to treat infants with congenital hip conditions. The hip spica cast covers the lower part of the body, usually from the waist down, and either one or both legs while leaving the feet open. The cast maintains the legs in a froglike position. Usually, there is a bar placed between the legs to help support the cast.

■ **Figure 40-4** Encourage and support the child having a cast applied. Following cast application check the circulation in the extremity.

The child and the family should be taught what to expect after the cast is applied and how to care for the casted area. A stockinette is applied over the area to be casted, and the bony prominences are padded before the wet gauze-impregnated rolls are applied. Although the wet plaster of paris feels cool on the skin when applied, evaporation soon causes a temporary sensation of warmth. The cast feels heavy and cumbersome (Fig. 40-4).

A wet plaster cast should be handled only with open palms because fingertips can cause indentations and result in pressure points. If the cast has no protective edge, it should be petaled (Fig. 40-5) with adhesive tape strips. If the cast is near the genital area, plastic should be taped around the edge to prevent wetting and soiling of the cast.

After the fracture has been immobilized, any reports of pain signal possible complications, such as compartment syndrome, and should be recorded and reported immediately. **Compartment syndrome** is a serious neurovascular concern that occurs when increasing pressure within the muscle compartment causes decreased circulation. It is important that you monitor the child's neurovascular status frequently because of the risk of tissue and nerve damage.

Performing neurovascular checks is sometimes referred to as CMS (circulation, movement, sensation) checks and are done to assess for impaired neurovascular function. These include observing, documenting, and reporting the five Ps:

- Pain: Any sign of pain should be noted and the exact area determined.
- Pulse: If an upper extremity is involved, check brachial, radial, ulnar, and digital pulses. If a lower extremity is involved, monitor femoral, popliteal, posterior tibial, and dorsalis pedis pulses.
- Paresthesia: Check for any diminished or absent sensation or for numbness or tingling.
- Paralysis: Check hand function by having the child try to hyperextend the thumb or wrist, oppose the thumb and little finger, and adduct all fingers. Check function of the foot by having the child try to dorsiflex and plantarflex the ankles and flex and extend the toes.
- Pallor: Check the extremity and the nail beds distal to the site of the fracture for color. Pallor, discoloration, and coldness indicate circulatory impairment.

In addition to the five Ps, any foul odor or drainage on or under the cast; "hot spots" on the cast (areas warm to touch); looseness or tightness; or any elevation of temperature must be noted, documented, and reported. Family caregivers should be instructed to watch carefully for these same danger signals.

Children and caregivers should be cautioned not to put anything inside the cast, no matter how much the casted area itches. Small toys and sticks or sticklike objects should be kept out of reach until the cast has been removed. Ice packs applied over the cast may help decrease the itching.

When the fracture has healed, the cast is removed with a cast cutter. This can be frightening for the child unless the person using the cast cutter explains and demonstrates that the device will not cut flesh but only the hard surface of the cast. The child should be told that there will be vibration from the cast cutter, but it will not burn.

After cast removal, the casted area should be soaked in warm water to help remove the crusty layer of accumulated skin. Application of oil or lotion may prove

This is critical to remember.
Any complaint of pain in a child with a new cast or immobilized extremity needs to be explored and monitored closely for the possibility of compartment syndrome.

Here's a helpful hint.
Blowing cool air through a cast with a hair dryer set on a cool temperature or using a fan may help to relieve discomfort under a cast.

To petal a cast:

1. Cut several strips of adhesive tape or moleskin 3 to 4 inches in length. Use 1 inch tape for smaller areas (e.g., infant's foot) and 2 inch tape for larger areas (e.g., adolescent's waist).

2. Round one end of each strip to keep the corners from rolling.

3. Apply the first strip by tucking the straight end inside the cast and by bringing the rounded end over the cast edge to the outside.

4. Repeat the procedure, overlapping each additional strip, until all rough edges are completely covered.

■ **Figure 40-5** Petaling the cast.

A Personal Glimpse

One day I was jumping on my bed, trying to do a flip, but instead I fell on my arm. It hurt really bad and I cried. I told my mom, and she put ice on it. But then I went to soccer camp the next day, and I fell on it again. It hurt even worse. My mom took me to the doctor's office. I could wiggle my fingers, but it only kind of hurt at the doctor's. So they took an x-ray. It was fun to see the picture of my arm. The next day I fell again at soccer camp; I was standing on my ball. This time my mom was sure it was broken. We went to get a cast. I chose a blue cast. My arm felt better, but I felt bad because it was my big sister's birthday. Everyone signed it. I had my cast on for 4 weeks. I couldn't wait to get it off. I finally got my cast off. I was excited! The girl used a saw to take it off. I wasn't scared. My arm really smelled bad! They took another x-ray to make sure my arm was better. It was!! Then we left and my mom washed my arm and put sunscreen on it. After that everyone had trouble telling me and my twin apart.

Cassey, age 8

Learning Opportunity: What explanations would you give this child regarding the reason the x-rays were taken, the process of putting the cast on, and what to expect when the cast was removed? Which actions carried out by this mother would be important for the nurse to reinforce as appropriate actions for this situation?

comforting. Family caregivers and the child must be cautioned against scrubbing or scraping this area because the tender layer of new skin underneath the crust may bleed. Sunscreen should be applied to the previously casted area when the child will have sun exposure.

Traction

Traction is a pulling force applied to an extremity or other part of the body. A body part is pulled in one direction against a counter-pull or counter traction exerted in the opposite direction. A system of weights, ropes, and pulleys is used to realign and immobilize fractures, reduce or eliminate muscle spasm, and prevent fracture deformity and joint contractures.

Two basic types of traction are used: skin traction and skeletal traction. **Skin traction** applies pull on tape, rubber, or a plastic material attached to the skin, which indirectly exerts pull on the musculoskeletal system. Examples of skin traction are Bryant's traction, Buck's extension traction, and Russell traction. **Skeletal traction** exerts pull directly on skeletal structures by means of a pin, wire, tongs, or other device surgically inserted through a bone. Examples of skeletal traction are 90-degree traction and balanced suspension traction. Dunlop's traction, sometimes used for fractures of the humerus or the elbow, can be either skin or skeletal traction. It is skeletal traction if a pin is inserted into the bone to immobilize the extremity (Fig. 40-6).

Bryant's traction (Fig. 40-7) is often used for the treatment of a fractured femur in children younger than 2 years of age. These fractures are often transverse (crosswise to the long axis of the bone) or spiral fractures. The child's legs are wrapped with elastic bandages that should be removed at least daily to observe the skin and then rewrapped. Skin temperature and the color of the legs and feet must be checked frequently to detect any circulatory impairment. The use of Bryant's traction entails some risk of compromised circulation and may result in contractures of the foot and lower leg, particularly in an older child. Severe pain may indicate circulatory difficulty, and should be reported immediately. When a child is in Bryant's traction, the hips should not rest on the bed; a hand should be able to pass between the child's buttocks and the sheet.

Buck's extension traction, in which the child's body provides the countertraction to the weights, is used for short-term immobilization. It is used to correct contractures and bone deformities, such as Legg-Calvé-Perthes disease. For older children, Russell traction seems to be more effective.

However, a child in either type of traction tends to slide down until the weights rest on the bed or the floor. The child should be pulled up to keep the weights free, the ropes must be in alignment with the pulleys, and the alignment should be checked frequently. An older child may try to coax a roommate to remove the weights or the sandbags used as weights.

Children in any kind of traction must be carefully monitored to detect any signs of neurovascular complications. Skin temperature and color, presence or absence of edema, peripheral pulse, sensation, and motion must be monitored every hour for the first 24 hours after traction has been applied and every 4 hours after the first 24 hours, unless ordered otherwise. Skin care must be meticulous. Skin preparation (Skin-Prep) should be used to toughen the skin rather than lotions or oils, which soften the skin and contribute to tissue breakdown.

> **Pay attention to the details.**
> When a child is in traction, the weights must be hanging freely, not touching the bed or floor.

Children in skeletal traction require special attention to pin sites. Pin care should be performed every 8 hours. The provider may order that povidone-iodine or a hydrogen peroxide solution be used to clean the pin sites. Standard precautions and aseptic technique reduce the risk for infection. Any sign of infection (odor, local inflammation, or elevated temperature) must be recorded and reported at once (see the Nursing Care Plan 40–1: The Child in Traction).

■ **Figure 40-6** Types of traction. **(A)** Buck extension, skin traction. **(B)** Russell traction, skin traction. Two lines of traction (one horizontal and one vertical) allow for good bone alignment for healing. **(C)** 90°–90° (skeletal) traction; a wire pin is inserted into the distal femur. **(D)** Balanced suspension traction. **(E)** Dunlop's traction (skeletal).

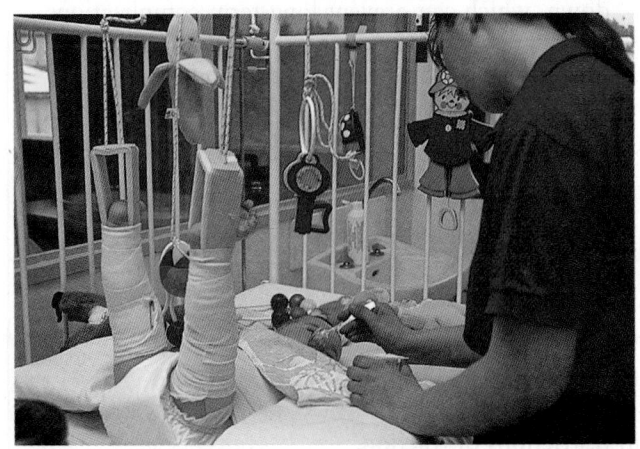

■ **Figure 40-7** An infant in Bryant's traction is being fed.

External Fixation Devices

In children who have severe fractures or conditions, such as having one extremity shorter than the other, external fixation devices are used to correct the condition (Fig. 40-8). When an external fixation device is used, special skin care at the pin sites is also necessary. The sites are left open to the air and should be inspected and cleansed every 8 hours. The appearance of the pins puncturing the skin and the unusual appearance of the device can be upsetting to the child, so be sensitive to any anxiety the child expresses.

As early as possible, the child (if old enough) or family caregivers should be taught to care for the pin sites. External fixation devices are sometimes left in place for as long as 1 year; therefore, it is important that the child accepts this temporary change in body image and learns to care for the affected site. Children with these devices probably will work with a physical therapist during the

Nursing Care Plan 40-1

THE CHILD IN TRACTION

TD is a 9-year-old boy who has been hospitalized following a serious bicycle accident in which he was struck by a motor vehicle. In the accident he sustained a fractured right femur and several cuts and abrasions. He has been placed in balanced suspension traction and will be in traction for several weeks before the extremity can be cast. He is in the 4th grade at school and plays soccer and basketball.

NURSING DIAGNOSIS
Risk for Peripheral Neurovascular Dysfunction related to fracture or effects of traction

GOAL: The child will maintain circulation and normal neurovascular status in extremities.

EXPECTED OUTCOMES:
- The child's pulse rate is within a normal range with adequate pulses and capillary refill in all extremities.
- The child has good skin color and temperature, appropriate movement and sensation in all extremities.

Nursing Interventions	*Rationale*
Maintain proper body alignment with traction weights and pulleys hanging free of bed and off the floor.	Body alignment must be maintained to prevent permanent injury or disalignment and decreased range of motion in effected extremity.
Monitor pulses in right leg and compare to pulses in other extremity.	Comparison helps to determine if circulation is adequate in affected extremity.
Monitor skin in extremities for color, temperature, sensation, and movement.	Any change in neurovascular status could indicate impaired nerve function.
Record and report any change in neurovascular status.	Immediate reporting leads to rapid treatment and decreases likelihood of long-term damage.

NURSING DIAGNOSIS
Impaired Skin Integrity related to abrasions
High Risk for Impaired Skin Integrity related to immobility

GOAL: The child will exhibit healed skin abrasions and no further skin breakdown.

EXPECTED OUTCOMES:
- The child's skin abrasions heal without signs or symptoms of infection.
- The child's skin remains intact without redness or irritation.

Nursing Interventions	*Rationale*
Wash and thoroughly dry skin every day.	Stimulates circulation and keeps skin clean
Inspect skin at least every 4 hours for evidence of redness or broken skin.	Allows early detection and treatment of skin breakdown, which can prevent long-term complications
Change position every 2 hours within restraints of traction.	Relieves pressure and decreases likelihood of skin breakdown and decreased circulation
Clean pin sites as ordered following standard precautions.	Decreases risk of infection
Observe for redness, drainage at pin sites, and elevated temperature.	Identifies signs and symptoms of possible infection

NURSING DIAGNOSIS
Activity Intolerance related to skeletal traction and bed rest

GOAL: The child will maintain adequate range of motion.

EXPECTED OUTCOMES:
- The child performs range of motion within limits of traction.
- The child does own self-care activities.
- The child participates in age-appropriate activities within restrictions of traction.

Nursing Care Plan 40-1 (continued)

THE CHILD IN TRACTION

Nursing Interventions	*Rationale*
Teach child active and passive range-of-motion exercises.	Maintains joint function and exercises circulation
Encourage child to become active in self-care.	Provides a feeling of control over hospitalization; increases use of parts of body not immobilized to allow normal muscle function

NURSING DIAGNOSIS
Deficient Diversional Activity related to lengthy hospitalization

GOAL: The child will achieve developmental tasks appropriate for age.

EXPECTED OUTCOMES:
* The child selects and participates in age-appropriate activities and play.
* The child shows enjoyment in participating in activities.
* The child communicates and interacts with peers.

Nursing Interventions	*Rationale*
Provide age-appropriate games, supplies, and activities that the child can do while in traction such as books, puzzles, and computer games.	Permits access to age-appropriate activities to help the child develop and achieve milestones of growth and development
Encourage child to communicate with peers by telephone, letter, computer.	Allows for normal growth and development opportunities
Move child's bed to hallway or playroom to enable participation in activities.	Increases interaction with other children; decreases boredom

■ **Figure 40-8 (A)** External fixation is required for complicated fractures. **(B)** The Ilizarov fixator is a circular apparatus usually used for complicated lower extremity fractures. The pins are smaller in diameter, more like wires, than those used in other fixators.

rehabilitation period and will have specific exercises to perform. Before discharge from the hospital, the child should feel comfortable moving about and should be able to recognize the signs of infection at the pin sites.

Crutches

Children with fractures of the lower extremities and other lower leg injuries often must learn to use crutches to avoid weight bearing on the injured area. Several types of crutches are available. The most common are axillary crutches, which are principally used for temporary situations. Forearm, or Canadian, crutches usually are recommended for children who need crutches permanently, such as paraplegic children with braces. Trough, or platform, crutches are more suitable for children with limited strength or limited function in the arms and hands.

The use of crutches is generally taught by a physical therapist, but it can be the responsibility of nurses. The type of crutch gait taught is determined by the amount of weight bearing permitted, the child's degree of stability, whether or not the knees can be flexed, and the specific treatment goal.

OSTEOMYELITIS

Osteomyelitis is an infection of the bone usually caused by *Staphylococcus aureus*. Acute osteomyelitis is twice as common in boys and results from a primary infection such as a staphylococcal skin infection (impetigo), burns, a furuncle (boil), a penetrating wound, or a fracture. The bacteria enter the bloodstream and are carried to the **metaphysis**, the growing portion of the bone, where an abscess forms, ruptures, and spreads the infection along the bone under the periosteum.

Clinical Manifestations and Diagnosis

Symptoms usually begin abruptly with fever, malaise, and pain and localized tenderness over the metaphysis of the affected bone. Joint motion is limited. Diagnosis is based on laboratory findings of leukocytosis (15,000–25,000 cells or more), an increased erythrocyte sedimentation rate, and positive blood cultures. Radiographic examination does not reveal the process until 5 to 10 days after the onset.

Treatment

Treatment for acute osteomyelitis must be immediate. Intravenous (IV) antibiotic therapy is started at once and continued for at least 6 weeks. Depending on the physician and the compliance of the child and family, a short course of IV antibiotics may be followed by administration of oral antibiotics to complete treatment. Surgical drainage of the involved metaphysis may be performed. If the abscess has ruptured into the subperiosteal space, chronic osteomyelitis follows.

If prompt specific antibiotic treatment is vigorously used, acute osteomyelitis may be brought under control rapidly and extensive bone destruction of chronic osteomyelitis is prevented. If extensive destruction of bone has occurred before treatment, surgical removal of necrotic bone becomes necessary.

Nursing Care

During the acute stage, nursing care includes reducing pain by positioning the affected limb, minimizing movement of the limb, and administering medication. The usual procedure for IV antibiotic therapy is followed, including careful observance of the venipuncture site and monitoring of the rate, dosage, and time of antibiotic administration. An intermittent infusion device or peripherally inserted central catheter may be used for long-term IV therapy.

Monitor oral nutrition and fluids because the child's appetite may be poor during the acute phase and may improve in later stages. Weight bearing on the affected limb must be avoided until healing has occurred because pathologic fractures occur very easily in the weakened stage. Physical therapy helps restore limb function.

MUSCULAR DYSTROPHY

Muscular dystrophy is a hereditary, progressive, degenerative disease of the muscles. The most common form of muscular dystrophy is Duchenne (pseudohypertrophic) muscular dystrophy. Duchenne muscular dystrophy, an X-linked recessive hereditary disease, occurs almost exclusively in males. Females usually are carriers of the disease. When muscular dystrophy has been diagnosed in a child, the mother and the siblings should be tested to see whether they have the disease or are carriers of the disease.

Clinical Manifestations and Diagnosis

The first signs are noted in infancy or childhood, usually within the first 3 to 4 years of life. The child has difficulty standing and walking and later trunk muscle weakness develops. Mild mental retardation often accompanies this disease. The child cannot rise easily to an upright position from a sitting or squatting position on the floor; instead, he or she develops Gower's sign, a method where the child rises from the floor by "walking up" the lower extremities with the hands (Fig. 40-9). Weakness of leg, arm, and shoulder muscles progresses gradually. Increasing abnormalities in gait and posture appear by school age, with **lordosis** (forward curvature of the lumbar spine or swayback), pelvic waddling, and frequent falling (Fig. 40-10). The child becomes progressively weaker, usually becoming wheelchair-bound by 10 to 12 years of age (middle school or junior high school age). The disease continues into adolescence and young adulthood, when the patient usually succumbs to respiratory or heart failure.

In addition to symptoms in the first 2 years of life, highly increased serum creatinine phosphokinase levels, as well as a decrease in muscle fibers seen in a muscle biopsy, can confirm the diagnosis.

Treatment and Nursing Care

No effective treatment for the disease has been found, but research is rapidly closing in on genetic identification,

■ **Figure 40-9** Gower's sign is used to rise from the floor: **(A)** First the child must roll onto his hands and knees. **(B)** Then he must bear weight by using his hands to support some of his weight, while raising his posterior. **(C-E)** The boy then uses his hands to "walk" up his legs to assume an upright position.

which promises exciting changes in treatment in the future. The child is encouraged to be as active as possible to delay muscle atrophy and contractures. To help keep the child active, promote physiotherapy, diet (to avoid obesity), and parental encouragement.

When a child becomes wheelchair-bound, **kyphosis** (hunchback) develops and causes a decrease in respiratory function and an increase in the incidence of infections. Breathing exercises are a daily necessity for these children.

■ **Figure 40-10** Characteristic posture of a child with Duchenne muscular dystrophy. Along with the typical toe gait, the child develops a lordotic posture as Duchenne dystrophy causes further deterioration.

Advise the family to keep the child's life as normal as possible, which may be difficult. This disease can drain the emotional and financial reserves of the entire family. Suggest assistance through the Muscular Dystrophy Association–USA (National Headquarters, 3300 E. Sunrise Drive, Tucson, AZ 85718; 800–344–4863; Web site: www.mdausa.org), through local chapters of this organization and by talking with other parents who face the same problem.

LEGG-CALVÉ-PERTHES DISEASE (COXA PLANA)

Legg-Calvé-Perthes disease is an aseptic necrosis of the head of the femur. It occurs 4 to 5 times more often in boys than in girls and 10 times more often in whites than in other ethnic groups. It can be caused by trauma to the hip, but generally the cause is unknown.

Clinical Manifestations and Diagnosis

Symptoms first noticed are pain in the hip or groin and a limp accompanied by muscle spasms and limitation of motion. These symptoms mimic **synovitis** (inflammation of a joint, which is most commonly the hip in children), which makes immediate diagnosis difficult. Radiographic examination may need to be repeated several weeks after the initial visit to demonstrate vascular necrosis for a definitive diagnosis.

There are three stages of the disease; each lasts 9 months to 1 year. In the first stage, radiographic studies show opacity of the epiphysis. In the second stage, the epiphysis becomes mottled and fragmented; during the third stage, reossification occurs.

Treatment and Nursing Care

In the past, immobilization of the hip through the use of braces and crutches and bed rest with traction or casting was considered essential for recovery without deformity. However, restricting a child's activity for 2 years or more was extremely difficult. Current treatment focuses on containing the femoral head within the acetabulum during the revascularization process so that the new femoral head will form to make a smoothly functioning joint. The method of containment varies with the portion of the head affected. Use of a brace that holds the necrotic portions of the head in place during healing is considered an effective method of containment. Reconstructive surgery is now possible, enabling the child to return to normal activities within 3 to 4 months.

The prognosis for complete recovery without difficulty later in life depends on the child's age at the time of onset, the amount of involvement, and the cooperation of the child and the family caregivers.

Nursing care focuses on helping the child and caregivers to manage the corrective device and the importance of compliance to promote healing and to avoid long-term disability.

OSTEOSARCOMA

Osteosarcoma is a malignant tumor seen in the long bones such as the femur, thigh, and humerus. It is more frequently seen in boys than in girls. Children who have had exposure to radiation or retinoblastoma are more prone to the malignancy.

Clinical Manifestations and Diagnosis

An injury, such as a sports injury, may draw attention to the pain and swelling at the sight of the tumor, but the injury itself did not cause the tumor. It is important to explain this to the child and caregiver to decrease their possible feelings of guilt. Pathologic fractures of the bone can occur.

A biopsy, as well as radiography, bone scan, computed tomography, and magnetic resonance imaging confirm the diagnosis. Metastasis to the lungs can occur.

Treatment and Nursing Care

Surgical removal of the bone or the limb followed by chemotherapy is the treatment for the tumor. A prosthesis is fitted, often soon after the surgery.

A cancer diagnosis is frightening to the child and family, and honest answers and support are helpful. After an amputation, phantom pain in the amputated extremity can be relentless. Learning to live with a prosthesis may be a long and challenging process. Support groups with other children living with a prosthetic device can be helpful. With early diagnosis and treatment, many children survive this diagnosis and live into adulthood.

EWING'S SARCOMA

Ewing's sarcoma is a malignant tumor found in the bone marrow of the long bones. It is often seen in older school-aged or adolescent boys.

Clinical Manifestations and Diagnosis

As with osteosarcoma, many times an injury draws attention to the pain at the site of the tumor. The pain may be sporadic for a period of time but continues and becomes severe enough to keep the child awake at night. Metastasis to the lung and other bones may already have taken place by the time of diagnosis. A biopsy, bone scan, and bone marrow aspiration are done to further diagnose the tumor.

Treatment and Nursing Care

The tumor is removed and radiation as well as chemotherapy is given. In many cases, the limb does not have to be amputated, although this may be part of the treatment.

About half of the children with Ewing's sarcoma achieve a 5-year survival rate, especially if there is no metastasis at the time of diagnosis. It is important that you offer support and encouragement while the child adjusts to the difficult course and effects of chemotherapy such as hair loss, nausea, and vomiting.

JUVENILE RHEUMATOID ARTHRITIS

Juvenile rheumatoid arthritis (JRA) is the most common connective tissue disease of childhood. Connective tissues are those that provide a supportive framework and protective covering for the body such as the musculoskeletal system, skin, and mucous membranes. The occurrence of JRA appears to peak at two age levels: 1 to 3 years and 8 to 12 years. This disease has a long duration, but 85% of children with JRA reach adulthood without serious disability (Cassidy, 2006).

Clinical Manifestations

Joint inflammation occurs first; if untreated, inflammation leads to irreversible changes in joint cartilage, ligaments, and menisci (the crescent-shaped fibrocartilage in the knee joints), eventually causing complete immobility. The inflammation can be subdivided into three different types: systemic; polyarticular, involving five or more joints; and oligoarthritis (pauciarticular), involving four or fewer joints, most often the knees and the ankles (Table 40-1).

Treatment and Nursing Care

The treatment goal is to maintain mobility and preserve joint function. Treatment can include drugs, physical therapy, and surgery. Early diagnosis and drug therapy to control inflammation and other systemic changes can reduce the need for other types of treatment.

Drug Therapy

Enteric-coated aspirin has long been the drug of choice for JRA, but because of the concern of aspirin therapy and Reye syndrome (see Chapter 35), nonsteroidal anti-inflammatory drugs (NSAIDs) are being used frequently to replace aspirin in treatment of JRA. Aspirin may still be used because it is an effective anti-inflammatory drug, is inexpensive, is easily administered, and has few side effects when carefully regulated. Both aspirin and NSAIDs,

Table 40-1 ▌ **CHARACTERISTICS OF DIFFERENT TYPES OF JUVENILE RHEUMATOID ARTHRITIS**

Sign/Symptom of Onset	Polyarthritis	Oligoarthritis (Pauciarticular)	Systemic
Frequency of cases	30%	60%	10%
Number of joints involved	5 or more	4 or fewer	Variable
Sex ratio (F:M)	3:1	5:1	1:1
Systemic involvement	Moderate	Not present	Prominent
Uveitis*	5%	5%–15%	Rare
Sensitivity			
Rheumatoid factors	10%	Rare	Rare
Antinuclear bodies	40%–50%	75%–85%	10%
Course	Systemic disease is generally mild; articular involvement may be unremitting	Systemic disease is absent; major cause of morbidity is uveitis	Systemic disease is often self-limited; arthritis is chronic and destructive in 50%
Prognosis	Guarded to moderately good	Excellent except for eyesight	Moderate to poor

*Uveitis—an inflammation of the middle (vascular) tunic of the eye: includes the iris, cilliary body, and choroide.
Adapted from Cassidy, J. T. (2006). Rheumatic disease of childhood. In *Oski's pediatrics: Principles and practice* (4th ed.). Philadelphia: Lippincott Williams & Wilkins.

such as naproxen and ibuprofen, may cause gastrointestinal irritation and bleeding.

Acetaminophen is not an appropriate substitute because it lacks anti-inflammatory properties. Teach family caregivers the importance of regular administration of the medications, even when the child is not experiencing pain. The primary purpose of aspirin or NSAIDs is not to relieve pain, but to decrease joint inflammation.

Here's a pharmacology fact.

Administer aspirin and NSAIDs with food or milk to decrease the side effects of gastrointestinal irritation and bleeding.

When aspirin or NSAIDs are no longer effective, gold preparations, steroids, D-penicillamine, or immunosuppressives may be used. All these are toxic, and their use must be closely monitored.

Physical Therapy

Physical therapy includes exercise, application of splints, and heat. Implementing this program at home requires the cooperation of the nurse, physical therapist, and care provider. Joints must be immobilized by splinting during active disease, but gentle daily exercise is necessary to prevent **ankylosis** (immobility of a joint). Stress to the caregivers the importance of encouraging the child to perform independent activities of daily living to maintain function and independence. The family caregiver must be patient, allowing the child time to accomplish necessary tasks.

Depending on the degree of disease, activity, range-of-motion exercises, isometric exercises, swimming, and riding a tricycle or bicycle may be part of the treatment plan. Inform caregivers that these exercises should not increase pain; if exercise does trigger increased pain, the amount of exercise should be decreased.

Test Yourself

✔ What is the cause of osteomyelitis, and how is it treated?

✔ What is the most common form of muscular dystrophy (MD), and what signs are usually noted in the child with MD?

✔ Why is it important to treat the joint inflammation in the child with juvenile rheumatoid arthritis (JRA)?

✔ Which medication is given for the child with JRA?

SCOLIOSIS

Scoliosis, a lateral curvature of the spine, occurs in two forms: structural and functional (postural). Structural scoliosis involves rotated and malformed vertebrae. Functional scoliosis, the more common type, can have several causes: poor posture, muscle spasm caused by trauma, or unequal length of legs. When the primary problem is corrected, elimination of the functional scoliosis begins.

Most cases of structural scoliosis are idiopathic (no cause is known); a few are caused by congenital deformities or infection. Idiopathic scoliosis is seen in school-age children at 10 years of age and older. Although mild curves occur as often in boys as in girls, idiopathic scoliosis requiring treatment occurs eight times more frequently in girls than in boys (Sponseller, 2006).

Diagnosis

Diagnosis is based on a screening examination. Many states require regular examination of students for scoliosis, beginning in the fifth or sixth grade. Scoliosis screening should last through at least eighth grade. Nurses play an important role in screening for this disorder. School nurses and others who work in health care settings with children aged 10 years and older should conduct or assist with screening programs. A school nurse often does the initial screening. Nurses in other health care settings are responsible for further screening of these children during regular well-child visits.

During examination, observe the undressed child from the back and note any lateral curvature of the spinal column; asymmetry of the shoulders, shoulder blades, or hips; and an unequal distance between the arms and waist (Fig. 40-11). The examiner then asks the child to bend at the hips (touch the toes) and observes for prominence of the scapula on one side and curvature of the spinal column (see Chapter 26).

Treatment

Treatment depends on many factors and is either nonsurgical or surgical. Treatment is long term and often lasts through the rest of the child's growth cycle.

Curvatures of less than 25 degrees are observed, but not treated. Electrical stimulation, a type of nonsurgical treatment, may be used for mild curvatures, but its effectiveness is unclear. Other nonsurgical treatment includes the use of braces or traction. Curvatures between 25 degrees and 40 degrees are usually corrected with a brace. More severe curvatures may be treated with traction.

Curvatures of more than 40 degrees are usually corrected surgically. Surgical treatment includes the use of rods, screws, hooks, and spinal fusion.

Electrical Stimulation

Electrical stimulation may be used as an alternative to bracing for the child with a mild to moderate curvature. Electrodes are applied to the skin or surgically implanted. Treatment occurs at night while the child is asleep. The leads are placed to stimulate muscles on the convex side of the curvature to contract as impulses are transmitted. This causes the spine to straighten. If external electrodes are used, the skin under the leads must be checked regularly for irritation. This treatment is the

■ **Figure 40-11** **(A)** Posterior view of child's back with lateral curvature. **(B)** View of child bending over with prominence of scapular area and asymmetry of flank demonstrated.

least disruptive to the child's life, but there is some controversy about its effectiveness.

Braces

The Milwaukee brace was the first type of brace used for scoliosis but is now more commonly used to treat kyphosis, an abnormal rounded curvature of the spine that is also called humpback. Either the Boston brace or the TLSO brace is more commonly used to treat scoliosis

(Fig. 40-12). The Boston brace and the TLSO brace are made of plastic and are customized to fit the child.

The brace should be worn constantly, except during bathing or swimming, to achieve the greatest benefit. It is worn over a T-shirt or undershirt to protect the skin. The fit of the device is monitored closely, and the child and caregiver should be taught to notify the health care provider if there is any rubbing. During the first couple weeks of wearing the brace, the child can be given a mild

■ **Figure 40-12** **(A)** Boston brace. **(B)** Milwaukee brace. **(C)** Nighttime bending brace.

■ **Figure 40-13** A 9-year-old girl in halo traction.

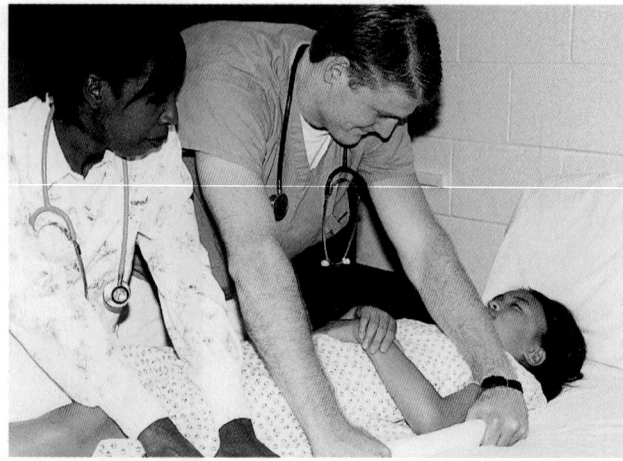

■ **Figure 40-14** Two nurses use a draw-sheet to logroll the child to a side-lying position.

analgesic for discomfort and aching. The child's provider may also prescribe certain exercises to be done several times a day. These are taught before the brace is applied, but are done while the brace is in place.

Traction

When a child has a severe spinal curvature or cervical instability, a form of traction known as **halo traction** (Fig. 40-13) may be used to reduce spinal curves and straighten the spine. Halo traction is achieved by using stainless steel pins inserted into the skull while counter-traction is applied by using pins inserted into the femur. Weights are increased gradually to promote correction. When the curvature has been corrected, spinal fusion is performed. In some cases, halo traction might be used after surgery if there is cervical instability.

The strange appearance of the halo traction apparatus magnifies the problems of body image; in addition, the head may need to be shaved. The child needs a thorough explanation of what will occur during the procedure and should be given the opportunity to talk about his or her feelings. Frequent shampooing, cleansing of the pin sites, and observation for signs of complications are critical for the child in halo traction.

Surgical Treatment

Various types of instruments, such as rods, screws, and hooks, may be placed along the spinal column to realign the spine and then spinal fusion is performed to maintain the corrected position. This procedure, which is done in cases of severe curvatures, is frightening to the child and family. It is major surgery, and the child and family must be well prepared for it. Because this is an elective procedure, thorough preoperative teaching can be carried out for the child and the family. The child can expect to have postoperative pain and will have to endure days of remaining flat in bed, being turned only in a logrolling fashion (Fig. 40-14). After surgery, the neurovascular status of the extremities is monitored closely. The child may be given a patient-controlled analgesia pump to control pain. An indwelling urinary (Foley) catheter is usually inserted because of the need for the patient to remain flat. The rods remain in place permanently. In some cases, the child may be placed in a body cast for a period of time to ensure fusion of the spine. About 6 months after surgery, the child can take part in most activities, except contact sports (such as tackle football, gymnastics, and wrestling). Because the bones are fused and rods are implanted, this procedure arrests the child's growth in height, which contributes to the emotional adjustment that the child and family must make.

Nursing Process For The Child With Scoliosis Requiring a Brace

Assessment

The child with scoliosis must be reassessed every 4 to 6 months. Document the degree of curvature and related impairments. Scoliosis often is diagnosed in late school age or early adolescence. This is a sensitive age for children, when privacy and the importance of being like everyone else are top priorities. Keep this in mind when interviewing and during examination of the child. Provide privacy and protect the child's modesty.

The child who is admitted to a health care facility for application of a brace or other instrumentation may be carrying a lot of unseen emotional baggage. Be sensitive to this emotional state. The family caregivers also may be upset but trying to hide it for the child's sake. In addition to routine observations, look for clues to the emotional state of both the child and family caregivers.

Selected Nursing Diagnoses

- Impaired Physical Mobility related to restricted movement
- Risk for Injury related to decreased mobility
- Risk for Impaired Skin Integrity related to irritation of brace
- Risk for Disturbed Body Image related to wearing a brace continuously
- Risk for Noncompliance related to long-term treatment

Outcome Identification and Planning

Consult the child and caregiver when establishing patient goals. Be especially sensitive to the child's needs. Goals for the child may include minimizing the disruption of activities, preventing injury, and maintaining skin integrity and self-image. Goals for the child and caregiver include complying with long-term care.

Implementation

Promoting Mobility

Prescribed exercises must be practiced and performed as directed. Encourage and support the child during these exercises. The child may need to be in traction for 1 or 2 weeks before the brace is applied. Encourage the child to perform exercises as directed. This can help to minimize the risks of immobility and promote self-esteem.

Preventing Injury

Evaluate the child's environment after the brace has been applied and take precautions to prevent injury. Help the child practice moving about safely: going up and down stairs; getting in and out of vehicles, chairs, and desks; and getting out of bed. Teach the child to avoid hazardous surfaces. Listen carefully to the child and the family caregiver to determine any other hazards in the home or school environment. Advise the family caregiver to contact school personnel to ensure that the child has comfortable, supportive seating at school and that adjustments are made in the physical education program.

Preventing Skin Irritation

When the brace is first applied, check the child regularly to confirm proper fit. Observe for any areas of rubbing, discomfort, or skin irritation and adjust the brace as necessary. Teach the child how to inspect all areas under the brace daily. Instruct the child and caregiver that reddened areas should be reported to the care provider so that adjustments can be made. Skin under the pads should be massaged daily. Daily bathing is essential, and clean cotton underwear or a T-shirt should be worn under the brace to provide protection.

Promoting Positive Body Image

The child should be involved in all aspects of care planning. Self-image and the need to be like others are very important at this age. Wearing a brace creates a distinct change in body image, especially in the older school-age child or adolescent, at a time when body consciousness is at an all-time high. Clothing choices are a challenge when wearing a brace.

Acceptance is important. Wearing clothing similar to what peers are wearing helps the child with scoliosis to feel more accepted.

The need to wear the brace and deal with the limitations it involves may cause anger; the change in body image can cause a grief reaction. Handling these feelings successfully requires understanding support from the nurse, family, and peers. It is important for the child to have an opportunity to talk about his or her feelings. Sometimes it is helpful for the patient in a brace to talk with other scoliosis patients and learn how they have coped. Understanding the disorder itself and the important benefits of treatment also can ease the adjustment.

Learning to be confident enough to handle the comments of peers can be difficult for the child. Give the child frequent opportunities to ventilate feelings about being different. Help the child select clothing that blends with current styles, but is loose enough to hide the brace. Encourage the child to find extracurricular activities with which the brace will not interfere. Active sports are not permitted, but many other activities are available. Help the child focus and enhance a positive attribute about characteristics, such as hair or complexion. Encourage the child and caregiver to discuss accommodations with school personnel together.

Promoting Compliance With Therapy

The child must wear the brace for years, until the spinal growth is completed. Then the child needs to be weaned from it gradually for another 1 or 2 years by wearing it only at night. During this period, the caregivers and the child need emotional support from health care personnel. Be certain that the child and caregivers have a complete understanding of the importance of wearing the brace continually. To encourage compliance, teach them about possible complications of spinal instability and possible further deformity if correction is unsuccessful. Inform the caregiver about the need to monitor the child for compliance. Help the caregiver understand the importance of being empathic to the child's need to be like others during this period of development. Offer ways in which the caregiver can help the child deal with adjustment to the therapy.

Evaluation: Goals and Expected Outcomes

Goal: The child will move effectively within the limits of the brace.

Expected Outcome: The child

- ambulates regularly.
- participates in daily activities.

Goal: The child will remain free from injury while in the brace.

Expected Outcome:

- The child demonstrates safe practices related to everyday activities at home and in the school environment.

Goal: The child's skin will remain intact.

Expected Outcome: The child

- uses methods to reduce skin irritation and bathes regularly.
- exhibits skin that is free from irritation and breakdown.

Goal: The child will exhibit positive coping behaviors.
Expected Outcome: The child

- demonstrates self-confidence.
- has an attractive well-groomed appearance.
- verbalizes feelings about the need to wear the brace.

Goal: The child will comply with therapy.
Expected Outcome:

- The child wears the brace as directed, and his or her condition shows evidence of compliance.
- Caregivers report compliance.

Test Yourself

✔ Explain the difference between structural and functional scoliosis.

✔ When should screening for scoliosis be started? What is the procedure for scoliosis screening?

✔ What are the ways scoliosis can be treated?

Key Points

➤ Bone growth takes place between birth and puberty. During childhood, the bones are more spongelike and can bend and break more easily than in adults. Because the bones are still in the process of growing, breaks in the bone heal more quickly than do breaks in adults.

➤ In a complete fracture, the fragments of the bone are separated. In an incomplete fracture, the fragments remain partially joined. The types of fractures seen in children are simple or closed; compound or open, where the bone penetrates the skin; spiral fractures, which twist around the bone; or greenstick fractures, another type of incomplete fracture. Most fractures are treated by realignment and immobilization using either traction or closed manipulation and casting.

➤ Neurovascular checks are done in a child with a musculoskeletal disorder to monitor the child's neurovascular status to detect and prevent tissue and nerve damage. Compartment syndrome is a serious neurovascular concern that occurs when increasing pressure within the muscle compartment causes decreased circulation.

➤ Monitoring the neurovascular status is sometimes referred to as CMS (circulation, movement, sensation) checks and includes observing, documenting, and reporting pain, pulses, paresthesia, paralysis, or pallor.

➤ The basic types of traction are skin traction and skeletal traction. Examples of skin traction are Bryant's traction, Buck's extension traction, and Russell traction. Examples of skeletal traction are 90-degree traction and balanced suspension traction. Dunlop's traction can be either skin or skeletal.

➤ Osteomyelitis is an infection of the bone usually caused by *Staphylococcus aureus*. IV antibiotics may be followed by administration of oral antibiotics for treatment. Nursing care includes reducing pain by positioning the affected limb, minimizing movement of the limb, and administering medication.

➤ The most common form of muscular dystrophy is Duchenne (pseudohypertrophic) muscular dystrophy. The characteristics include difficulty standing or walking, trunk muscle weakness, and mild mental retardation. Weakness of leg, arm, and shoulder muscles progresses gradually, with the child usually becoming wheelchair-bound.

➤ Legg-Calvé-Perthes disease is an aseptic necrosis of the head of the femur. The treatment includes use of a brace that holds the head of the femur in place or reconstructive surgery.

➤ The treatment for osteosarcoma is to remove the bone or the limb where the tumor is found. For Ewing's sarcoma, the tumor must be removed and radiation is done. In both disorders, chemotherapy is given.

➤ Juvenile rheumatoid arthritis (JRA) is a connective tissue disease. Enteric-coated aspirin has long been the drug of choice for JRA, but because of the concern of aspirin therapy and Reye syndrome, NSAIDs, such as naproxen and ibuprofen, are being used. The primary purpose of using these drugs is because of their anti-inflammatory effects. To decrease the side effects, the drugs should be administered with food or milk.

➤ Scoliosis is a lateral curvature of the spine, either structural or functional. Nonsurgical treatment includes electrical stimulation or the use of braces, such as the Boston brace or TLSO brace, or traction. Surgical treatment includes the use of rods, screws, hooks, and spinal fusion. Goals include minimizing the disruption of activities, preventing injury, and maintaining skin integrity and self-image.

INTERNET RESOURCES

Juvenile Rheumatoid Arthritis
www.arthritis.org

Muscular Dystrophy
www.mdausa.org

Scoliosis
www.scoliosis-assoc.org

Workbook

■ NCLEX-STYLE REVIEW QUESTIONS

1. The nurse is teaching a group of peers regarding different types of fractures. Which of the following best describes an open fracture?

   a. A fracture in which the fragments of the bone are separated.

   b. A fracture in which the broken bone penetrates the skin.

   c. A fracture in which there is a single break in the bone without penetration of the skin.

   d. A fracture in which the fragments of the bone remain partially joined.

2. In caring for a child in traction, of the following interventions, which is the *highest* priority for the nurse?

   a. The nurse should monitor for decreased circulation every 4 hours.

   b. The nurse should clean the pin sites at least once every 8 hours.

   c. The nurse should provide age-appropriate activities for the child.

   d. The nurse should record accurate intake and output.

3. The nurse is doing patient teaching with a child who has been placed in a brace to treat scoliosis. Which of the following statements made by the child indicates an understanding of the treatment?

   a. "I am so glad I can take this brace off for the school dance."

   b. "At least when I take a shower I have a few minutes out of this brace."

   c. "Wearing this brace only during the night won't be so embarrassing."

   d. "When I start feeling tired, I can just take my brace off for a few minutes."

4. The nurse is caring for a child after an accident in which the child fractured his arm. A cast has been applied to the child's right arm. Which of the following actions should the nurse implement? Select all that apply.

   a. Wear a protective gown when moving the child's arm.

   b. Document any signs of pain.

   c. Check radial pulse in both arms.

   d. Wear sterile gloves when removing or touching the cast.

   e. Monitor the color of the nail beds in the right hand.

■ STUDY ACTIVITIES

1. Using the table below, list the areas that must be checked and monitored when doing a neurovascular status check (CMS check) on a child with a fracture. Include the area to be monitored, the definition or explanation, observations, and documentation.

Area to Be Monitored (the 5 Ps)	Definition or Explanation	Observations (What Signs to Look for)	Documentation

2. Develop a list of games and activities that would be appropriate to use for a 10-year-old girl in skeletal traction. Keep in mind the child's age and stage of growth and development. Share your list with your peers.

3. Call the Muscular Dystrophy Association national headquarters or your local Muscular Dystrophy Association chapter. Ask what is available in your community to help and support children and families of children with muscular dystrophy.

4. Go to the following Internet site: www.arthritis.org/conditions

   Search this site for information on "Juvenile Arthritis." List the topics you found discussing the disorder. Share with your peers how you can use this information in working with children and families of children who have juvenile arthritis.

■ CRITICAL THINKING: WHAT WOULD YOU DO?

1. Twelve-year-old Carrie has scoliosis and must wear a TLSO brace. She says she thinks it is really ugly. Carrie tells you she does not want to go to school because she cannot wear clothes similar to those of her friends.

   a. What feelings do you think Carrie might be going through in this situation?

   b. What would you say in response to Carrie?

   c. What are some ideas you could share with Carrie regarding clothing she might wear?

2. You are caring for 2-year-old Cole, who has muscular dystrophy. Cole's family begins asking you questions about the disease. How would you answer the following questions?

   a. What caused Cole to have muscular dystrophy?

   b. What will happen to Cole physically as he gets older and the disease progresses?

c. What is the long-term prognosis for Cole?

d. Where can we find other families who have a child with muscular dystrophy?

3. Dosage calculation: After a course of IV antibiotics for treatment of osteomyelitis, a child has been prescribed a regimen of nafcillin (Unipen) by mouth. The child weighs 17.6 pounds. The usual dosage range of this medication is 6.25 mg to 12.5 mg/kg every 6 hours. Answer the following:

a. How many kilograms does the child weigh?

b. What is the low dose of nafcillin for this child every 6 hours?

c. What is the high dose of nafcillin for this child every 6 hours?

d. If the child is given the high dose, how much nafcillin will be given in a 24-hour period?

41

The Child With an Integumentary Disorder/ Communicable Disease

KEY TERMS

allergen
allograft
autograft
chancre
comedones
contractures
débridement
eschar
heterograft
homograft
hydrotherapy
hypervolemic
hyposensitization
impunity
sebum
tinea

LEARNING OBJECTIVES

On completion of this chapter, you should be able to:

1. Discuss ways the child's integumentary and immune systems differ from the adult's system.
2. Explain integumentary disorders including seborrheic dermatitis, miliaria rubra, diaper rash, Candidiasis, and impetigo.
3. Discuss acne vulgaris including the causes, treatment, and nursing care.
4. Explain fungal infections seen in children.
5. Describe pediculosis and scabies and discuss the treatment and nursing concerns when treating a child with this condition in the hospital.
6. Discuss allergic disorders and how allergens that produce a positive reaction on skin testing are commonly treated.
7. Describe the causes, manifestations, treatment, and nursing care of the child diagnosed with atopic dermatitis (infantile eczema).
8. Discuss how skin and plant allergies are treated.
9. Compare various types of bites often seen in children including animal, spider, tick, snake, and insect bites.
10. Differentiate between first-, second-, and third-degree burns.
11. Describe emergency treatment of a minor burn and of a moderate or severe burn.
12. State the three major causes of burns in small children and discuss the nursing care of the child with a burn.
13. List the organisms that cause gonorrhea, chlamydia, genital herpes, and syphilis, and the drug of choice to treat them.
14. Discuss acquired immunodeficiency syndrome including how the human immunodeficiency virus is transmitted, treatment, and nursing care.
15. Describe infectious mononucleosis.
16. Discuss communicable diseases including modes of transmission, ways to prevent, active, natural, and passive immunity; and nursing care.

GROWTH AND DEVELOPMENT OF THE INTEGUMENTARY AND IMMUNE SYSTEM

The skin is the major organ of the integumentary system and is the largest organ of the body. Accessory structures, such as the hair and nails, also make up the integumentary system. The major role of the skin is to protect the organs and structures of the body against bacteria, chemicals, and injury. The skin helps regulate the body temperature by heating and cooling. Excretion in the form of perspiration is also a function of the skin glands, called the sweat glands. Sebaceous glands in the skin secrete oils to lubricate the skin and hair. These oils help in preventing dryness of the skin. As a sensory organ, the skin has nerve endings that respond to pain, pressure, heat, and cold. When the skin is exposed to sunlight (ultraviolet light), synthesis of vitamin D occurs.

The integumentary system, including the accessory structures, is in place at birth but the system is immature. The newborn's skin is thin and has less subcutaneous fat between the layers of skin. Regulating temperature is more difficult in the newborn because of these factors. As the child grows, the sweat glands mature and increase the capability of the skin to help in the regulation of the temperature. The sebaceous secretions in the infant and young child are less than those in the older child and adult, causing the skin of children to dry and crack more easily. In addition, the infant is more susceptible to bacteria, which might cause infection, and to skin irritants. Injury and some disorders can cause bruising to the skin, especially in the child.

Protecting the body from attacks from microorganisms and helping the body get rid of or resist invasion by foreign materials are the major roles of the immune system. Unlike other systems in the body that are made up of organs, the immune system is made up of cells and tissues that work to protect the body. Protective barriers such as the skin and mucous membranes help to prevent pathogens from entering the body. When a pathogen enters the body, the immune system works to destroy the pathogen. This occurs when white blood cells known as macrophages surround, ingest, or neutralize the pathogen. The inflammatory process further helps to get rid of the foreign substances. Another process of the immune system occurs when substances called antibodies destroy antigens, which are foreign protein substances. When the body is exposed to certain bacteria or viruses, the immune system fights to destroy the substance. In addition, the body develops immunity to that disease, so if the person has an exposure in the future, the immune system immediately responds and symptoms do not occur. Immunizations work by creating an artificial exposure to a certain agent that helps the body create immunity to that agent.

During fetal life, the mother's antibodies cross the placenta, giving the fetus a temporary immunity against certain diseases. This immunity is present at birth and decreases during the first year of life. In the meantime, the infant begins developing antibodies to fight against pathogens and disease. In addition, during the first year of life immunizations are started to help the infant develop protection against certain diseases. As the child grows and develops, the immune system also develops. The antibodies in the child increase as the child progresses through childhood.

INTEGUMENTARY DISORDERS

Integumentary disorders occur often in children. These disorders can be mild and resolve quickly or chronic and severe and be difficult for the child and family caregivers to cope with.

SEBORRHEIC DERMATITIS

Seborrheic dermatitis is commonly known as cradle cap. Washing child's hair and scalp every day can usually prevent it. Characterized by yellowish, scaly, or crusted patches on the scalp, it occurs in newborns and older infants, possibly as a result of excessive sebaceous gland activity. Family caregivers may be afraid to wash vigorously over the "soft spot." However, they need to understand that this is where cradle cap often begins and that careful but vigorous washing of the area with a washcloth can prevent this disorder. Using a fine-toothed baby comb after shampooing is also a helpful preventive measure. These principles are stressed during teaching about care of the newborn.

Once the condition exists, daily application of mineral oil helps loosen the crust. However, no attempt should be made to loosen it all at once because the delicate skin on the scalp may break and bleed and can easily become infected.

MILIARIA RUBRA

Miliaria rubra, often called prickly heat, is common in children who are exposed to summer heat or are overdressed. It also may appear in febrile illnesses and may be mistaken for the rash of one of the communicable diseases.

Clinical Manifestations

The rash appears as pinhead-sized erythematous (reddened) papules. It is most noticeable in areas where sweat glands are concentrated such as folds of the skin, the chest, and around the neck. It usually causes itching, making the child uncomfortable and fretful.

Treatment and Nursing Care

Treatment should be primarily preventive. Family caregivers should be taught that a diaper might be all the child needs to wear.

Tepid baths without soap help control the itching. A small amount of baking soda may be added to the bath water to help relieve discomfort.

Here's a tip to share. Caregivers are often concerned that their baby is going to be cold; it is important they avoid bundling their child in layers of clothing in hot weather.

DIAPER RASH

Diaper rash is common in infancy, causing the baby discomfort and fretfulness. Some children seem to be more susceptible than others, possibly because of inherited sensitive skin.

Clinical Manifestations

Bacterial decomposition of urine produces ammonia, which is irritating to a child's tender skin. Diarrheal stools also produce a burning erythematous area in the anal region. Prolonged exposure to wet or soiled diapers, use of plastic or rubber pants, infrequently changed disposable diapers, inadequate cleansing of the diaper area (especially after bowel movements), sensitivity to some soaps or disposable diaper perfumes, and the use of strong laundry detergents without thorough rinsing are considered to be causes. Yeast infections, notably candidiasis, are also causative factors.

Treatment and Nursing Care

Caregivers should be taught that the primary treatment is prevention. Diapers must be changed frequently, without waiting for obvious leaking. Regular checking is necessary. Manufacturers of disposable diapers are constantly trying to improve the ability of disposable diapers to wick the wetness away from the child's skin. Diapers washed at commercial laundries are sterilized, preventing the growth of ammonia-forming bacteria. However, caregivers may be unable to afford disposable diapers or a commercial diaper service. Diapers washed at home should be presoaked (good commercial products are available), washed in hot water with a mild soap, and rinsed thoroughly with an antiseptic added to the final rinse. Drying diapers in the sun or in a dryer also helps destroy bacteria. Exposing the diaper area to the air helps clear up the dermatitis.

Cleaning the diaper area from front to back with warm water and drying thoroughly with each diaper change helps improve or prevent the condition. If soap is necessary when cleaning stool from the child's buttocks and rectal area, be certain that the soap is completely rinsed before diapering. The use of commercial wet wipes may aggravate the condition. If the area becomes excoriated and sore, the health care provider may prescribe an ointment. See Family Teaching Tips: Preventing and Treating Diaper Rash.

> ### Did you know.
> The use of baby powder when diapering is discouraged because caked powder helps create an environment in which organisms thrive.

CANDIDIASIS

Candidiasis is caused by *Candida albicans,* the organism responsible for thrush and some cases of diaper rash.

Clinical Manifestations

Newborns can be exposed to a candidiasis vaginal infection in the mother during delivery. Thrush appears in the child's mouth as a white coating that looks like milk curds. Poor hand-washing practices and inadequate washing of bottles and nipples are contributing factors. In addition, infants and toddlers may experience episodes of thrush or diaper rash after antibiotic therapy, which may upset the balance of normal intestinal flora, leading to candidal overgrowth.

Family Teaching Tips

PREVENTING AND TREATING DIAPER RASH

- Rinse all baby's clothes thoroughly to eliminate soap or detergent residue that may irritate baby's skin.
- Rinse cloth diapers in clear water. Do not use fabric softeners because they can cause a skin reaction.
- Use plastic or rubber diaper covers only when necessary. They hold moisture, which makes rash worse.
- Change diapers as soon as wet or soiled. Disposable diapers hold moisture the same as plastic or rubber covers.
- Avoid fastening diaper too tightly, which irritates baby's skin.
- Expose baby's bottom to air without diapers as much as possible to help rash heal.
- Do not overdress or overcover baby. Sweating makes rash worse.
- Wash baby's bottom with lukewarm water only, using wet cotton balls or pouring over bath basin or sink. Pat dry with soft cloth. Do not use commercial baby wipes. Do not rub rash.
- Use a cool, wet cloth placed over red diaper rash, which can be very soothing. Try this for 5 minutes three or four times a day.
- Use ointment only as recommended by health care provider. Apply very thin layer only. Wash off at each diaper change.
- Dry diaper area thoroughly before rediapering. A hair dryer on low warm setting used after patting dry may help.

Treatment and Nursing Care

Treatment for diaper rash caused by *Candida albicans* (Fig. 41-1) is the application of nystatin ointment or cream to the affected area. Application of nystatin (Mycostatin, Nilstat) to the oral lesions every 6 hours is an effective treatment. In all cases, good hygiene practices should be reinforced.

> ### Test Yourself
> ✔ How can seborrheic dermatitis (cradle cap) be prevented?
> ✔ What causes diaper rash?
> ✔ What is the causative agent for thrush? How might a newborn be exposed to this, and how is it treated?

■ **Figure 41-1** A bright red rash occurs with diaper rash caused by *Candida albicans*.

IMPETIGO

Impetigo is a superficial bacterial skin infection (Fig. 41-2). In the newborn, the primary causative organism is *Staphylococcus aureus*. In the older child, the most common causative organism is group A beta-hemolytic streptococci. Impetigo in the newborn is usually bullous (blisterlike); in the older child, the lesions are nonbullous.

Warning.
Impetigo is highly contagious and can spread quickly. Impetigo in the newborn nursery is cause for immediate concern.

Treatment

Medical treatment includes oral penicillin or erythromycin for 10 days. Daily washing of the crusts helps speed

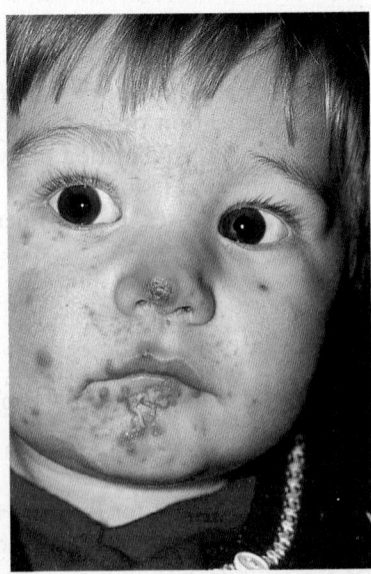

■ **Figure 41-2** Typical lesions of impetigo.

the healing process. Mupirocin (Bactroban) ointment may be used. Because impetigo is commonly a streptococcal infection in the older child, rheumatic fever or acute glomerulonephritis may follow. Family caregivers should be alerted to this rare possibility.

Nursing Care

When caring for a young child who has impetigo and is hospitalized, you must follow contact (skin and wound) precautions, including wearing a cover gown and gloves. The child should be segregated from other children to deter spread of the disease. Crusts can be soaked off with warm water, followed by an application of topical antibiotics, such as Bacitracin and Neosporin. Cover the child's hands or apply elbow restraints to prevent scratching of lesions. Careful hand washing by nursing personnel and family members is essential.

The older child with impetigo is treated at home. The family caregivers must be taught hygiene practices to prevent the spread of impetigo to other children in the household or other contacts of the child in the day care center, nursery school, or elementary school. Lesions occur primarily on the face, but may spread to any part of the body. The crusts and drainage are contagious. Because the lesions are pruritic (itchy), the child must learn to keep his or her fingers and hands away from the lesions. Nails should be trimmed to prevent scratching of lesions. Family members should be taught not to share towels and washcloths.

ACNE VULGARIS

Acne may be only a mild case of oily skin and a few blackheads, or it may be a severe type with ropelike cystic lesions that leave deep scars, both physical and emotional. To adolescents who want to be attractive and popular, even a mild case of acne (often called "zits") can cause great anxiety, shyness, and social withdrawal.

Clinical Manifestations

Characterized by the appearance of **comedones** (blackheads and whiteheads), papules, and pustules on the face and the back and the chest to some extent, acne is caused by a variety of factors, including:

- Increased hormonal levels, especially androgens
- Hereditary factors
- Irritation and irritating substances, such as vigorous scrubbing and cosmetics with a greasy base
- Growth of anaerobic bacteria

Each hair follicle has an associated sebaceous gland that in adolescents produces increased **sebum** (oily secretion). The sebum is blocked by epithelial cells and becomes trapped in the follicle. When anaerobic organisms infect this collection, inflammation occurs, which causes papules, pustules, and nodules (Fig. 41-3). Several types of acne lesions are often present at one time.

■ **Figure 41-3** Acne vulgaris.

Treatment and Nursing Care

The topical medications benzoyl peroxide (Clearasil, Benoxyl) and tretinoin (Retin-A) come in a variety of forms such as topical cleansers, lotions, creams, sticks, pads, gels, and bars. The usual treatment plan for mild acne is topical application of one of these medications once or twice a day. These medications should not be applied to normal skin or allowed to get into the eyes or nose or on other mucous membranes. Antibiotics, such as erythromycin and tetracycline, may be administered for inflammatory acne. Antibiotic therapy requires an extended treatment course of at least 6 to 12 months, followed by tapering of the dosage.

Isotretinoin (Accutane) may be used for severe inflammatory acne. This potent, effective oral medication is used for hard-to-treat cystic acne. Side effects are common but often diminish when the drug dosage is reduced. Warn the adolescent about some of the side effects, including dry lips and skin, eye irritation, temporary worsening of acne, epistaxis (nosebleed), bleeding and inflammation of the gums, itching, photosensitivity (sensitivity to the sun), and joint and muscle pain.

> **This is critical to remember.**
> Isotretinoin is a pregnancy category X drug; it must not be used at all during pregnancy because of serious risk of fetal abnormalities.

To rule out pregnancy, a urine test is done before treatment begins. For the sexually active adolescent girl, an effective form of contraception must be used for a month before beginning and during isotretinoin therapy. The risk to the fetus if pregnancy were to occur should be discussed with the girl, whether or not she is sexually active.

Although the adolescent's perception of the disfigurement caused by acne may seem out of proportion to the actual severity of the condition, acknowledge and accept his or her feelings. Teach the adolescent and the family caregiver to wash the lesions gently with soap and water; do not scrub vigorously. Comedones should be removed gently by following the physician's recommendations and using careful aseptic techniques. Careful removal produces no scarring—a goal for every teen.

Yours and the family caregiver's understanding and support are the most important aspects of caring for the adolescent with acne. Reassure the teen that eating chocolate and fatty foods does not cause acne, but a well-balanced, nutritious diet does promote healing.

FUNGAL INFECTIONS

Fungi that live in the outer (dead) layers of the skin, hair, and nails can develop into superficial infections. **Tinea** (ringworm) is the term commonly applied to these infections, which are further differentiated by the part of the body infected.

TINEA CAPITIS (RINGWORM OF THE SCALP)

Ringworm of the scalp is called tinea capitis or tinea tonsurans. The most common cause is infection with *Microsporum audouinii*, which is transmitted from person to person through combs, towels, hats, barber scissors, or direct contact. A less common type, *Microsporum canis*, is transmitted from animal to child.

Clinical Manifestations

Tinea capitis begins as a small papule on the scalp and spreads, leaving scaly patches of baldness. The hairs become brittle and break off easily.

Treatment and Nursing Care

Griseofulvin, an oral antifungal, is the medication of choice. Because treatment may be prolonged (3 months or more), compliance must be reinforced. Be sure that parents and children understand the medication therapy. Children who are properly treated may attend school. Advise the child and parents that hair loss is not permanent.

TINEA CORPORIS (RINGWORM OF THE BODY)

Tinea corporis is ringworm of the body that affects the epidermal skin layer. The child usually contracts tinea corporis from contact with an infected dog or cat.

The lesions appear as a scaly ring with clearing in the center, occurring on any part of the body. They resemble the lesions of scalp ringworm. Topical antifungal agents, such as clotrimazole, econazole nitrate, tolnaftate, and miconazole, are effective. Griseofulvin also is used to treat this condition.

TINEA PEDIS

Tinea pedis, ringworm of the feet, is more commonly known as athlete's foot. It is evidenced by the scaling or cracking of the skin between the toes. Transmission is by direct or indirect contact with skin lesions from infected people. Contaminated sidewalks, floors, pool decks, and shower stalls spread the condition to those who walk barefoot. Tinea pedis, usually found in adolescents and adults, is becoming more prevalent among school-age children because of the popularity of plastic shoes. Examination under a microscope of scrapings from the lesions is necessary for definite diagnosis.

Care includes washing the feet with soap and water and then gently removing scabs and crusts and applying a topical agent, such as tolnaftate. Griseofulvin by mouth is also useful. During the chronic phase, the use of ointment, scrupulous foot hygiene, frequent changing of white cotton socks, and avoidance of plastic footwear are helpful. Application of a topical agent for as long as 6 weeks is recommended.

TINEA CRURIS

Tinea cruris, more commonly known as jock itch or ringworm of the inner thighs and inguinal area, is caused by the same organisms that cause tinea corporis. It is more common in athletes and is uncommon in preadolescent children. Tinea cruris is pruritic and localized to the area. Treatment is the same as for tinea corporis. Sitz baths also may be soothing.

Test Yourself

✔ Why is impetigo a concern in the newborn nursery? What procedures should you follow when caring for a child with impetigo?

✔ Why should comedones, seen in acne vulgaris, be removed carefully?

✔ How is ringworm of the scalp, tinea capitis, usually transmitted?

✔ Which classification of medication is given to treat ringworm?

PARASITIC INFECTIONS

Parasites are organisms that live on or within another living organism from which they obtain their food supply. Lice and the scabies mite live by sucking the blood of the host.

PEDICULOSIS

Pediculosis (lice infestation) may be caused by *Pediculus humanus capitis* (head lice), *Pediculus humanus corporis* (body lice), or *Pthirus pubis* (pubic lice). Head lice are the most common infestation in children. Animal lice are not transferred to humans.

Head lice are passed from child to child by direct contact or indirectly by contact with combs, headgear, or bed linen.

Clinical Manifestations

Lice, which are rarely seen, lay their eggs, called nits, on the head where they attach to hair strands. The nits can be seen as tiny pearly white flecks attached to the hair shafts. They look much like dandruff, but dandruff flakes can be flicked off easily, whereas the nits are tightly attached and not easily removed. The nits hatch in about 1 week, and the lice become sexually mature in about 2 weeks.

> **Don't forget the importance of your observation skills.**
> Severe itching of the scalp is the most obvious symptom in cases of head lice.

Treatment and Nursing Care

Nonprescription medications are available to treat cases of head lice. Products such as Pronto, RID, and A-200 contain pyrethrins, which are extracts from the chrysanthemum flower. Permethrin (Nix) may also be used. These medications are safe and usually effective in killing the lice. A second treatment is suggested in 7 to 10 days to kill the nits after they have hatched. If over-the-counter preparations do not effectively kill the lice, prescription medications may be used. Malathion (Ovide) is effective in treating lice and nits. Few side effects have been reported, but if used on open sores, it may cause the skin to sting, so it should not be used if the head has been scratched. Lindane (Kwell) shampoo has been one of the most commonly used treatments for many years and is usually safe. Overuse, misuse, or accidentally swallowing of Lindane can be toxic to the brain and nervous system, so its use is suggested only in cases that do not respond to other treatments.

After the hair is wet with warm water, the medication is applied like any ordinary shampoo—about 1 oz is used. The head should be lathered for several minutes, following the directions on the label for each specific medication, and then rinsed thoroughly and dried. After the hair is dry, it should be combed with a combing tool, such as a LiceMeister or a fine-toothed comb dipped in warm white vinegar, to remove remaining nits and nit shells. Shampooing may be repeated in 2 weeks to remove any lice that may have been missed as nits and since hatched. Avoid getting medication into the eyes or on mucous membranes. When treating a child in the hospital for pediculosis, wear a disposable gown, gloves, and head cover for protection.

Family caregivers are often embarrassed when the school nurse sends word that the child has head lice. They can be reassured that lice infestation is common and can happen to any child; it is not a reflection on the caregiver's housekeeping. All family members should be inspected and treated, as needed. See Family Teaching

Family Teaching Tips

ELIMINATING PEDICULI INFESTATIONS

- Wash all child's bedding and clothing in hot water and dry in hot dryer.
- Vacuum carpets, car seats, mattresses, and upholstered furniture very thoroughly. Discard vacuum dust bag.
- Wash pillows, stuffed animals, and other washable items the same way clothing is washed.
- Dry clean nonwashable items.
- If items cannot be washed or dry cleaned, seal in plastic bag for 2 weeks to break the reproductive cycle of lice.
- Wash combs, brushes, and other hair items (rollers, curlers, barrettes, etc.) in shampoo and soak for 1 hour.
- If you discover the infestation, report to child's school or day care.
- Have school personnel disinfect headphones.

Tips: Eliminating Pediculi Infestations for other useful information.

SCABIES

Scabies is a skin infestation caused by the scabies mite *Sarcoptes scabiei.* The female mite burrows in areas between the fingers and toes and in warm folds of the body, such as the axilla and groin, to lay eggs.

Clinical Manifestations

Burrows are visible as dark lines, and the mite is seen as a black dot at the end of the burrow. Severe itching occurs, causing scratching with resulting secondary infection.

Treatment and Nursing Care

The body, except for the face, is treated with permethrin cream (Elimite) or lindane lotion. The directions for each medication should be followed closely. The body is first scrubbed with soap and water, and then the lotion is applied on all areas of the body except the face. Permethrin is the preferred treatment because of the decreased risk of neurologic problems. It is usually left on the skin for 8 to 14 hours. With lindane, the medication is left on for 8 to 12 hours and then completely washed off with warm water.

Caregivers should follow the tips recommended for pediculosis. All who had close contact with the child within a 30- to 60-day period should be treated. The rash and itch may continue for several weeks, even though the mites have been successfully eliminated.

Test Yourself
✔ Explain what pediculosis is and at what sites it is frequently found in children.
✔ How is pediculosis treated?
✔ Why is it important for the child with scabies to avoid scratching involved areas?

ALLERGIC DISORDERS

Millions of Americans have allergic diseases, most of which begin in childhood. Children with allergies are hampered because of poor appetites, poor sleep, and restricted physical activity in play and at school, all of which often result in altered physical and personality development. Children whose parents or grandparents have allergies are more likely to become allergic than are other children. An allergic condition is caused by sensitivity to a substance called an **allergen** (an antigen that causes an allergy). Thousands of allergens exist. Some of the most common allergens are:

- Pollen
- Mold
- Dust
- Animal dander
- Insect bites
- Tobacco smoke
- Nuts
- Chocolate
- Milk
- Fish
- Shellfish

Drugs, particularly aspirin and penicillin, can be allergens as well. Some plants and chemicals cause allergic reactions on the skin. Allergens may enter the body through various routes, the most common being the nose, throat, eyes, skin, digestive tract, and bronchial tissues in the lungs. The first time the child comes in contact with an allergen, no reaction may be evident, but an immune response is stimulated—helper lymphocytes stimulate B lymphocytes to make immunoglobulin E antibody. The immunoglobulin E antibody attaches to mast cells and macrophages. When contacted again, the allergen attaches to the immunoglobulin E receptor sites, and a response occurs in which certain substances, such as histamine, are released; these substances produce the symptoms known as allergy.

Diagnosis of an allergy requires a careful history and physical examination and possibly skin and blood tests, including a complete blood count, serum protein electrophoresis, and immunoelectrophoresis. Skin testing is generally done when removal of obvious allergens is impossible or has not brought relief. If a food allergy is suspected, an elimination diet may help identify the allergen.

Eliminating the food suspected is sometimes difficult because there are often "hidden" ingredients in food products.

When specific allergens have been identified, patients can either avoid them or, if this is impossible, undergo immunization therapy by injection. This process is called **hyposensitization** or immunotherapy.

Hyposensitization is performed for the allergens that produce a positive reaction on skin testing. The allergist sets up a schedule for injections in gradually increasing doses until a maintenance dose is reached. The patient should remain in the physician's office for 20 to 30 minutes after the injection in case any reaction occurs. Reactions are treated with epinephrine. Severe reactions in children are uncommon, and hyposensitization is considered a safe procedure with considerable benefit for some children.

Symptomatic relief in allergic reactions can be gained through antihistamine or steroid therapy, but the best treatment is prevention.

ATOPIC DERMATITIS (INFANTILE ECZEMA)

Atopic dermatitis or infantile eczema is considered, at least in part, an allergic reaction to an irritant. It is fairly common during the first year of life after the age of 3 months. It is uncommon in breast-fed babies before they are given additional foods.

Infantile eczema is characterized by three factors:

- Hereditary predisposition
- Hypersensitivity of the deeper layers of the skin to protein or proteinlike allergens
- Allergens to which the child is sensitive that may be inhaled, ingested, or absorbed through direct contact such as house dust, egg white, and wool

Infants who have eczema tend to have allergic rhinitis or asthma later in life.

Clinical Manifestations

Infantile eczema usually starts on the cheeks and spreads to the extensor surfaces of the arms and legs (Fig. 41-4). Eventually the entire trunk may become affected. The initial reddening of the skin is quickly followed by papule and vesicle formation. Itching is intense, and the child's scratching makes the skin weep and crust. The areas easily become infected by hemolytic streptococci or by staphylococci.

Diagnosis

The most common allergens involved in eczema are:

- Foods: egg white, cow's milk, wheat products, orange juice, tomato juice

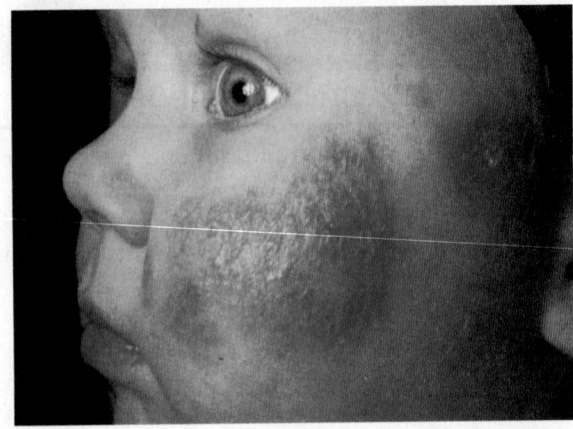

■ **Figure 41-4** Infant with infantile eczema (atopic dermatitis).

- Inhalants: house dust, pollens, animal dander
- Materials: wool, nylon, plastic

However, diagnosis is not simple. Often trial by elimination is as effective as any other diagnostic tool. Skin testing on a young child generally is not considered valid, so it is discouraged as a means of diagnosis.

An elimination diet may be helpful in ruling out offending foods. A hypoallergenic diet consisting of a milk substitute, such as soy formula; vitamin supplement; and other foods known to be hypoallergenic is given. If the skin condition shows improvement, other foods are added one at a time at an interval of about 1 week; the effects are noted and any foods that cause a reaction are eliminated. The protein of egg white is such a common offender that most pediatricians advise against feeding whole eggs to infants until late in the first year of life (see Chapter 38, Table 38-1 for a list of foods that may cause allergies).

Great care must be taken to prevent the child from becoming undernourished. An elimination program must always be initiated under the supervision of a competent pediatric nurse practitioner, dietitian, or physician.

Treatment

Smallpox vaccination is definitely contraindicated for the child with eczema. In fact, such a child must be kept away from anyone who has recently been vaccinated. A serious condition called eczema vaccinatum results when a child with eczema is vaccinated or is exposed to the vaccination of another person. The child becomes seriously ill, and mortality rates have been high. Fortunately, because smallpox vaccination is no longer required, this is not a major concern; the reaction could occur if the child is exposed to someone who has been vaccinated in preparation for travel.

Of greater current concern is protecting the child from anyone with a herpes simplex infection (cold sore). If the lesions become infected with herpes simplex, a generalized reaction may occur. In the child with severe eczema with many lesions, body fluid loss from oozing through the lesions can be serious. The child may have severe pain and be gravely ill with this complication.

Oral antibiotics may be ordered for a coexistent infection, such as a staphylococcal or streptococcal infection. Oral antihistamines and sedatives may help relieve the itching and allow rest. If no infection exists, topical hydrocortisone ointments may be used to relieve inflammation. Wet soaks or colloidal baths also may be prescribed for their soothing effects. The water should be tepid for further soothing, and soap may not be used because of its drying effect. Some physicians recommend the use of a mild soap, such as Dove or Neutrogena, or a soap substitute. Lubrication is essential to retain moisture and prevent evaporation after the bath. Emollients containing lanolin or petrolatum, such as Eucerin, may be prescribed.

Inhalant and contact allergens should be avoided as far as possible. In the child's bedroom, window drapes or curtains, dresser scarves, and rugs should be removed or made of washable fabric that can be frequently laundered. Furniture should be washed frequently. The crib mattress should have a nonallergenic covering and be washed frequently with careful cleaning along the binding. Feather pillows must be eliminated, and stuffed toys should be washable. It may be necessary to provide new homes for household pets. However, dander from the pets can remain in carpets, crevices, and overstuffed furniture for a long time. Carpets and area rugs may need to be removed. A home, especially an older one with a damp basement, may be harboring molds that shed allergenic spores. Bathrooms are also places for molds and mildews to hide, especially in warm, humid climates.

Nursing Process for the Child With Infantile Eczema

Assessment

The family caregivers of the child with eczema are often frustrated and exhausted. Although the caregiver can be assured that most cases of eczema clear up by the age of 2 years, this does little to relieve the current situation. Hospitalization is avoided, when possible, because these children are highly susceptible to infections. Sometimes, however, admission seems to be the only answer to provide therapy that is more intensive or to relieve an exhausted caregiver.

During the interview with the family caregivers, cover the history of the condition, including treatments that have been tried and foods that have been ruled out as allergens. Include a thorough review of the home environment. Evaluate the caregivers' knowledge of the condition.

The data collection about the child includes obtaining vital signs, observing general nutritional state, and doing a complete examination of all body parts with careful documentation of the eruptions and their location and size. Unaffected areas as well as those that are weeping and crusted should be indicated.

Selected Nursing Diagnoses

- Impaired Skin Integrity related to lesions and inflammatory process
- Acute Pain related to intense itching and irritation
- Disturbed Sleep Pattern related to itching and discomfort
- Imbalanced Nutrition: Less Than Body Requirements related to elimination diet
- Risk for Infection related to broken skin and lesions
- Deficient Knowledge of caregivers related to disease condition and treatment

Outcome Identification and Planning

The major goals for the child with infantile eczema are preserving skin integrity, maintaining comfort, improving sleep patterns, maintaining good nutrition (within the constraints of allergens), and preventing infection of skin lesions. A family goal is increasing knowledge about the disease process. Base the nursing plan of care on these goals.

Implementation

Maintaining Skin Integrity

Cover the lesions with light clothing. Especially appropriate are the one-piece, loose-fitting terry pajamas or one-piece cotton underwear known as "onesies."

The child's nails must be kept closely cut, and mittenlike hand coverings can be used. Use restraints only if necessary. Elbow restraints may sometimes be used. Remove restraints at least every 4 hours—more often, if feasible—but do not allow the child to rub or scratch while the restraints are off. If ointments or wet dressings must be kept in place on the child's face, a mask may be made by cutting holes into a cotton stockinette-type material to correspond to eyes, nose, and mouth. Wet dressings on the rest of the body can be kept in place by wrapping the child "mummy" fashion. Dressings may be left on for an extended period, but should not be allowed to dry, because that can create open areas when they are removed.

Check out this tip.

"Onesies," one-piece outfits for children, come in many colors, patterns, and designs and can be helpful in keeping a child from scratching.

Providing Comfort Measures

Plan soothing baths, such as a colloidal bath (Aveeno), just before naptime or bedtime. Time medications such as sedatives or antihistamines so that they will be effective immediately after the bath, when the child is most relaxed.

Maintaining Adequate Nutrition

Weigh the child on admission and daily thereafter. This procedure gives some indication of weight gain. If an elimination diet is being used, the diet should be carefully balanced within the framework of the foods permitted and supplemented with vitamin and mineral preparations as needed. Encourage the drinking of fluids to prevent dehydration.

Preventing Infection

As stated, usually these children are kept out of the health care facility because of the concern about infection. However, they can also become infected at home. Whether in the health care facility or at home, the child should be placed in a room alone or in a room where there is no other child with any type of infection. Administer antibiotics as ordered. For open lesions, aseptic techniques are necessary to prevent infection.

Providing Family Teaching

Help the family caregivers understand the condition and possible food, contact, or inhalant allergens. Teach them ways to soothe the child. They should avoid overdressing and overheating the child because perspiration causes itching. Explain that they should use a mild detergent to launder the child's clothing and bedding. Help them determine ways to encourage normal growth and development. Teach them to read labels of prepared foods, watching carefully for hidden allergens. Family caregivers may feel apprehensive or repulsed by this unsightly child. Support them in expressing their feelings, and help them view this as a distressing but temporary skin condition.

Children with eczema are frequently active and "behaviorally itchy." Assist caregivers in handling challenging behavior. Help caregivers develop a strong self-image in the child to protect against strangers' openly negative reactions.

Evaluation: Goals and Expected Outcomes

Goal: The child's skin integrity will be maintained or will improve.
Expected Outcomes: The child

- has decreased scratching.
- exhibits skin with fewer breakdowns.

Goal: The child will report less itching.
Expected Outcome:

- The child states itching is lessened.

Goal: The child's sleep pattern will not be disturbed.
Expected Outcome:

- The child sleeps an adequate amount for his or her age after comfort measures are provided.

Goal: The child's nutritional intake will meet the needs for growth and development.
Expected Outcomes: The child

- has no weight loss.
- has weight gain appropriate for age.

Goal: The child will be free of infected skin lesions.
Expected Outcomes: The child

- does not scratch lesions.
- shows no signs of infection related to lesions.

Goal: The family caregivers understand the disease and its treatment.
Expected Outcome:

- The family caregivers demonstrate an acceptance of the child and the condition by interacting in a positive fashion with the child.

SKIN ALLERGIES

Skin disorders of allergic origin include hives (urticaria), giant swellings (angioedema), and rashes caused by poison ivy, poison oak, and other plants or drug reactions. Skin rashes are common in children. Infectious diseases cause some, and allergies cause others.

Clinical Manifestations

Hives appear in different sizes on many different parts of the body and are usually caused by foods or drugs. They are bright red and itchy and can occur on the eyelids, tongue, mouth, hands, feet, or in the brain or stomach. When affecting the mouth or tongue, hives can cause difficulty in breathing. Hives in the stomach can cause swelling, which can produce pain, nausea, and vomiting. Swelling in brain tissue causes headache and other neurologic symptoms.

Foods such as chocolate, nuts, shellfish, berries or other raw fruit, fish, and highly seasoned foods are likely to cause hives. Possible drug allergens include aspirin and related drugs, laxatives, anti-inflammatory drugs, tranquilizers, and antibiotics (penicillin is the most common allergen of this group). Sometimes it is impossible to identify the cause.

Treatment

Treatment is aimed at reducing the swelling and relieving the itching. If the allergen can be identified, it can be removed from the child's environment and hyposensitization can be performed. If the allergen is a certain food, that food must be eliminated from the child's diet. Rashes, regardless of cause, are usually treated with cool soaks and topical preparations such as lotions, ointments, and greases. Antihistamines (topical or systemic) are used to relieve itching and reduce swelling. The itching must be relieved as much as possible because scratching can introduce additional pathogens to the affected area. Cool soaks also help to relieve itching. Fingernails should be kept short and clean. In severe cases, corticosteroids may be necessary.

PLANT ALLERGIES

Poison ivy, poison oak, and poison sumac are common causes of contact dermatitis. Of these, poison ivy is the

■ **Figure 41-5** Poison ivy on a child's arm. Note characteristic vesicular rash in linear formation.

worst offender, particularly during the summer (Fig. 41-5). The cause of the allergy is the extremely potent oil, urushiol, which is present in all parts of these plants.

Clinical Manifestations

Effects of plant allergies vary from slight inflammation and itching to severe extensive swelling that can virtually immobilize the child. This disorder causes intense itching (pruritus) and forms tiny blisters that weep and continue to spread the inflammation.

Treatment

Antihistamines or oral corticosteroids help to relieve itching and prevent scratching. Cool soaks, Aveeno baths, calamine lotion, or topical corticosteroids help minimize discomfort. The child should be taught to recognize and avoid the poisonous plants. The plants also should be removed from the environment, when possible.

BITES

Because children are active, inquisitive, and not completely inhibited in their actions, they commonly experience animal and human bites as well as insect stings and bites. Many of these are minor, particularly if the skin is not broken.

ANIMAL BITES

Children enjoy pets, but often they are not alert to possibly dangerous encounters with pets or wild animals. Dog bites are common. Fortunately, because of rabies vaccination programs for dogs, few dog bites cause rabies; in fact, cats are the domestic animal most likely to carry rabies.

Any pet that bites should be held until it can be determined if the animal has been vaccinated against rabies. If not, the child must undergo a series of injections to prevent this potentially fatal disease. The series consists of both active and passive immunizations. Active immunity is established with five injections of human diploid cell vaccine, beginning on the day of the bite and on days 3, 7, 14, and 28. Human rabies immunoglobulin is given on the first day, along with the diploid cell vaccine.

> **Pay attention.** Some bites can have life-threatening implications if proper care is not given.

All animal and human bites should be thoroughly washed with soap and water. An antiseptic, such as 70% alcohol or povidone-iodine, should be applied after the wound has been thoroughly rinsed. The wound must be observed for signs of infection until it is well healed. Animal bites should be promptly reported to the proper authorities.

Children should be taught at an early age about the danger of animal bites, particularly of strange or wild animals such as skunks, raccoons, bats, and squirrels.

SPIDER BITES

Spider bites can cause serious illness if untreated. Bites of black widow spiders, brown recluse spiders, and scorpions demand medical attention. Applying ice to the affected area until medical care is obtained can slow absorption of the poison.

TICK BITES

Wood ticks carried by chipmunks, ground squirrels, weasels, and wood rats can cause Rocky Mountain spotted fever. Most cases are found in the south Atlantic, south central, and southeastern United States. Dogs are often the carriers to humans. People living in areas where ticks are common can be immunized against this disease.

Deer ticks, carried by white-footed mice and white-tailed deer, can carry the organism that causes Lyme disease. Most cases of Lyme disease in the United States have been seen in northeastern, mid-Atlantic, and upper north central regions and in some northwestern counties of California. The first stage of the disease begins with a lesion at the site of the bite. The lesion appears as a macule with a clear center. The second stage occurs several weeks to months later if the patient is not treated. The symptoms of this stage may affect the central nervous system and the heart. If untreated, the third stage may occur months to years later, causing arthritis, neurologic disorders, and bone and joint disease.

Children and adults should wear long pants, long-sleeved shirts, and insect repellent when walking in the woods. Pant legs should be tucked into socks. If a tick is found on the body, alcohol may be applied and the tick carefully removed with tweezers. To prevent the release of pathogenic organisms, care should be taken not to crush the tick. A health care provider must be consulted if there is any suspicion that a deer tick has bitten a child or an adult.

SNAKE BITES

Snake bites demand immediate medical intervention. The wound should be washed, ice applied, and the involved body part immobilized. Prompt transport to the nearest medical facility is essential.

INSECT STINGS OR BITES

Insect stings or bites can prove fatal to children who are sensitized. Swelling may be localized or may include an entire extremity. Circulatory collapse, airway obstruction, and anaphylactic shock can cause death within 30 minutes if the child is untreated. Immediate treatment is necessary and may include injection of epinephrine, antihistamines, or steroids. These children should wear a MedicAlert bracelet and carry an anaphylaxis kit that includes a plastic syringe of epinephrine and an antihistamine. The teacher, school nurse, and anyone who cares for the child should be alerted to the child's allergy and should know where the anaphylaxis kit is and how to use it when necessary.

BURNS

Among the many accidents that occur in children's lives, burns are the most frightening. More than 70% of burn accidents happen to children younger than age 5 years. Nearly all childhood burns are preventable, and this causes considerable guilt for families and the child. Adult carelessness, the child's exploring and curious nature, and failure to supervise the child adequately all contribute to the high incidence of burns in children. In addition, burns are a common form of child abuse.

Burns may result from various causes including:

- Scalds from hot liquids, which are common in small children and result from a dangling electric coffee-maker cord, pans of hot liquid on the stove with handles turned out, cups of hot tea or coffee, bowls of soup or other hot liquids, or small children left alone in bathtubs. Dangerous, sometimes fatal, burns can occur from these conditions.
- Burns from fire are the second most common kind of burn, resulting from children playing with matches or being left alone in buildings that catch fire. Careless use of smoking materials is a common cause of house fires. Even if cigarette lighters contain a "child-safe" lighting mechanism, they should still be kept away from children.
- Electricity can cause severe facial or mouth burns in infants and toddlers who bite on electrical cords plugged into a socket; such burns may require extensive plastic surgery.

> **Caution!**
> Children are fascinated by fires and must be carefully supervised around fireplaces, campfires, room heaters, and outside barbecues.

These burns may be more serious than they first appear because of the damage to underlying tissues.

Types of Burns

Burns are divided into types according to the depth of tissue involvement: superficial, partial-thickness, or full-thickness (Fig. 41-6 and Table 41-1).

Epidermis — First-degree

Second-degree

Dermis —

Third-degree

Subcutaneous tissue —

Muscle —

■ **Figure 41-6** Cross-section of the skin showing the relative depths of the types of burn injuries.

Table 41-1 ▮ CHARACTERISTICS OF BURNS

Degree	Cause	Surface Appearance	Color	Pain Level	Histologic Depth	Healing Time
Superficial (first) All are considered minor unless under 18 mo, over 65 yrs, or with severe loss of fluids	Flash, flame, ultraviolet (sunburn)	Dry, no blisters, edema	Erythematous	Painful	Epidermal layers only	2 to 5 days with peeling, no scarring, may have discoloration
Partial-thickness (second) Minor—less than 15% in adults, less than 10% in children Moderate—15% to 30% in adults or less than 15% with involvement of face, hands, feet, or perineum; minor chemical or electrical; in children, 10% to 30% Severe—more than 30%	Contact with hot liquids or solids, flash flame to clothing, direct flame, chemical	Moist blebs, blisters	Mottled white to pink, cherry red	Very painful	Epidermis, papillary, and reticular layers of dermis; may include fat domes of subcutaneous layer	Superficial—5 to 21 days with no grafting Deep with no infection—21 to 35 days If infected, convert to full thickness.
Full-thickness (third) Minor—less than 2% Moderate—2% to 10%, any involvement of face, hands, feet, or perineum Severe—more than 10% and major chemical or electrical	Contact with hot liquids or solids, flame, chemical, electricity	Dry with leathery eschar until débridement; charred blood vessels visible under eschar	Mixed white (waxy or pearly), dark (khaki or mahogany), charred	Little or no pain; hair pulls out easily	Down to and including subcutaneous tissue; may include fascia, muscle, and bone	Large areas require grafting that may take many months. Small areas may heal from the edges after weeks.

Superficial or First-Degree Burns

The epidermis is injured, but there is no destruction of tissue or nerve endings. Thus, there is erythema, edema, and pain but prompt regeneration (Fig. 41-7).

Partial-Thickness or Second-Degree Burns

The epidermis and underlying dermis are both injured and devitalized or destroyed. Blistering usually occurs with an escape of body plasma, but regeneration of the skin occurs from the remaining viable epithelial cells in the dermis (Fig. 41-8).

Full-Thickness or Third-Degree Burns

The epidermis, dermis, and nerve endings are all destroyed (Fig. 41-9). Pain is minimal, and there is no longer any barrier to infection or any remaining viable epithelial cells. Fourth-, fifth-, and sixth-degree burns have been described that are extensions of full-thickness

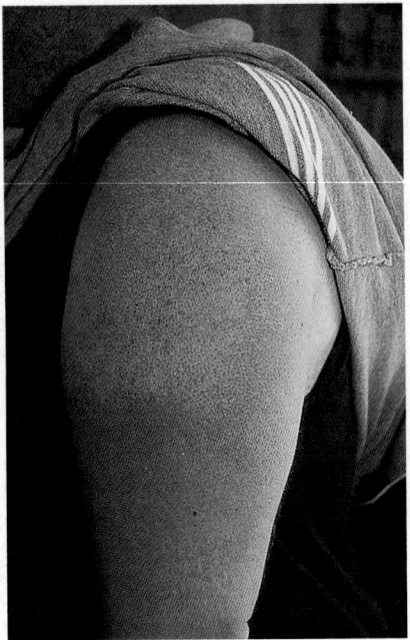

■ **Figure 41-7** Superficial burn—painful but without blisters.

burns with involvement of fat, muscle, and bone, respectively.

Emergency Treatment

Cool water is an excellent emergency treatment for burns involving small areas. The immediate application of cool compresses or cool water to burn areas appears to inhibit capillary permeability and thus suppress edema, blister formation, and tissue destruction. Ice water or ice packs must not be used because of the danger of increased tissue damage. Immersing a burned extremity in cool water alleviates pain and may prevent further thermal injury. This can be done after the airway, breathing, and circulation have been observed and restored if necessary. This action should not be done

■ **Figure 41-8** Partial-thickness burn—very painful, with blistering.

■ **Figure 41-9** Full-thickness burn of the foot.

when large areas are involved because of the danger of hypothermia.

In the case of a fire victim, special attention should be given to the airway to observe for signs of smoke inhalation and respiratory passage burns. Clothing should be removed to inspect the whole body for burned areas; in addition, clothing may retain heat, which can cause additional tissue damage. The child should be transported to a medical facility for assessment. If transported to a special burn unit, the child may be wrapped in a sterile sheet and the burn treated on arrival.

Superficial Burns

Superficial burns can usually be treated on an outpatient basis because they heal readily unless infected. The area is cleaned, an anesthetic ointment is applied, and the burn is covered with a sterile gauze bandage or dressing. An analgesic may be needed to relieve pain. Blisters should not be intentionally broken because of the risk of infection, but blisters that are already broken may be débrided (cut away). The child is seen again in 2 days to inspect for infection. The caregiver is instructed to keep the area clean and dry (no bathing the area) until the burn is healed, usually in about a week to 10 days.

Partial- and Full-Thickness Burns

Distinguishing between partial and full-thickness burns is not always possible. In the presence of infection, a partial-thickness burn may be converted into a full-thickness one, and with extensive burns, a greater amount of full-thickness burn often exists than had been estimated.

Full-thickness burns require the attention, skill, and conscientious care of a team of specialists. Children with mixed second- and third-degree burns or with third-degree burns involving 15% or more of the body surface require hospitalization. Burns are classified according to criteria of the American Burn Association (Table 41-2).

Table 41-2 ■ CLASSIFICATION OF BURNS

Classification	Description
Minor	First-degree burn or second degree <10% of body surface or third degree <2% of body surface; no area of the face, feet, hand, or genitalia is burned
Moderate	Second-degree burn 10% to 20% body surface or on the face, hands, feet, or genitalia, or third-degree burn <10% body surface or if smoke inhalation has occurred
Severe	Second-degree burn >20% body surface or third-degree burn >10% body surface

Treatment of Moderate to Severe Burns: First Phase—48 to 72 Hours

Hypovolemic shock is the major manifestation in the first 48 hours in massive burns. As extracellular fluid pours into the burned area, it collects in enormous quantities, which dehydrates the body. Edema becomes noticeable and symptoms of severe shock appear. Intense pain is seldom a major factor. Symptoms of shock are low blood pressure, rapid pulse, pallor, and considerable apprehension.

Airway

The adequacy of the airway must be determined in case an endotracheal tube needs to be inserted or (rarely) a tracheostomy performed. Inhalation injury is a leading cause of complications in burns. If there are burns around the face and neck or if the burns occurred in a small enclosed space, inhalation injury should be suspected. In fires, toxic substances and the heat produced can cause damage to the respiratory tract. All these possibilities must be considered and the child should be observed for them.

Intravenous Fluids

The primary concern is to replace body fluids that have been lost or immobilized at the burn areas. Because there is a distinct relationship between the extent of the surface area burned and the amount of fluid lost, the percentage of affected skin area, as well as the classification of the burns must be estimated to determine the medical treatment (Fig. 41-10). The extent and depth of the burn and the expertise available within the hospital determine whether the child is treated at the general hospital or immediately transported to a burn unit.

An intravenous (IV) infusion site must be selected and fluids started; most often lactated Ringer's solution, isotonic saline, or plasma is used with a large-bore catheter to administer replacement fluids and maintain total parenteral nutrition (TPN). Intravenous fluids for maintenance and replacement of lost body fluids are estimated for the first 24 hours, with half of this calculated requirement given during the first 8 hours.

However, the patient's needs may change rapidly, necessitating a change in the rate of flow or the amount or type of fluid. The patient's urinary output, vital signs, and general appearance are all part of the information that the physician needs to determine the fluid requirements. With TPN, fluids can be administered to provide needed amino acids, glucose, fats, vitamins, and minerals so that large amounts of food do not need to be consumed orally. This nutrition is essential for tissue repair and healing.

Oral Fluids

The administration of oral fluids should be omitted or minimized for 1 or 2 days. Delayed gastric emptying causing acute gastric dilatation is a common complication of burns and can become a serious problem resulting in vomiting and anorexia. A nasogastric tube may be inserted and attached to low suction to prevent vomiting. IV fluids should relieve the child's thirst, which is usually severe, and sips of water may be allowed.

Oral feedings can be started when bowel sounds are heard. Nasogastric feedings may be needed to supplement intake. The child's caloric and nutritional requirements are two or three times those needed for normal growth; thus, nutritional supplements will most likely be needed.

Urine Output and Diuresis

Urinary output, which may be decreased because of the decrease in blood volume, must be monitored closely. Renal shutdown may be a threat. An output of 1 to 2 mL/kg/hr for children weighing 30 kg (66 lb) or less, or 30 to 50 mL/hr for those weighing more than 30 kg is desirable. An indwelling catheter facilitates the accurate measurement of urine and specific gravity. After the first hour, the volume of urine should be relatively constant. Any change in volume or specific gravity should be reported.

After the initial fluid therapy brings the burn shock under control and compensates for the extracellular fluid deficit, the patient faces another hazard with the onset of the diuretic phase. This occurs within 24 to 96 hours after the accident. The plasmalike fluid is picked up and reabsorbed from the third space in the burn areas, and the patient may rapidly become **hypervolemic** (exhibit an abnormal increase in the blood volume in the circulatory system), even to the point of pulmonary edema. This is the principal reason for the extremely close check on all vital signs and for the close monitoring of IV fluids that must now be slowed or stopped entirely.

EXAMPLE

Calculating TBSA By Age
(Total Body Surface Area)

Color Code
Red - 3°
Blue - 2°

Area	Birth 1 yr	1-4 yrs	5-9 yrs	10-14 yrs	15 yrs	Adult	2	3	Total
Head	19	17	13	11	9	7	—	8	8.0
Neck	2	2	2	2	2	2	—	1	1.0
Ant. Trunk	13	13	13	13	13	13	1	12	13.0
Post. Trunk	13	13	13	13	13	13	—	—	—
R. Buttock	2 1/2	2 1/2	2 1/2	2 1/2	2 1/2	2 1/2	—	—	—
L. Buttock	2 1/2	2 1/2	2 1/2	2 1/2	2 1/2	2 1/2	—	—	—
Genitalia	1	1	1	1	1	1	—	—	—
R.U. Arm	4	4	4	4	4	4	—	3.5	3.5
L.U. Arm	4	4	4	4	4	4	1	2.5	3.5
R.L. Arm	3	3	3	3	3	3	—	3	3
L.L. Arm	3	3	3	3	3	3	—	3	3
R. Hand	2 1/2	2 1/2	2 1/2	2 1/2	2 1/2	2 1/2	—	2.5	2.5
L. Hand	2 1/2	2 1/2	2 1/2	2 1/2	2 1/2	2 1/2	—	2.5	2.5
R. Thigh	5 1/2	6 1/2	8	8 1/2	9	9 1/2	1	2	3
L. Thigh	5 1/2	6 1/2	8	8 1/2	9	9 1/2	—	2	2
R. Leg	5	5	5 1/2	6	6 1/2	7	—	—	—
L. Leg	5	5	5 1/2	6	6 1/2	7	—	—	—
R. Foot	3 1/2	3 1/2	3 1/2	3 1/2	3 1/2	3 1/2	—	—	—
L. Foot	3 1/2	3 1/2	3 1/2	3 1/2	3 1/2	3 1/2	—	—	—
Total							3%	42%	45%

■ **Figure 41-10** Calculate total body surface area (TBSA) affected by using the child's age and the area affected, as well as whether the burned area is second degree (partial thickness) or third degree (full thickness).

Notifying the physician immediately is necessary if any of the following signs of the onset of this phase occur:

- Rapid rise in urinary output; may increase to 250 mL/hr or higher.
- Tachypnea followed by dyspnea.
- Increase in pulse pressure; mean blood pressure also may increase. Central venous pressure, if measured, is elevated.

Infection Control

The child has lost a portion of the integumentary system, which is a primary defense against infection. For this reason, measures must be taken to protect the child from infection. Antibiotics are not considered very effective in controlling infection of this type, most likely because the injured capillaries cannot carry the antibiotic to the site. If used, antibiotics are usually added to the IV fluids. Tetanus antitoxin or toxoid should be ordered, according to the status of the child's previous immunization. If inoculations are up to date, a booster dose of tetanus toxoid is all that is required.

To protect the child from infection introduced into the burn, sterile equipment must be used in the child's care. Everyone who cares for the child must wear a gown, a mask, and a head cover. Visitors also are required to scrub, gown, and mask.

Burn units are designed to be self-contained with treatment and operating areas, hydrotherapy units, and patient care areas. In hospitals where there is no specific burn unit, a private room with a door that can be closed should be set up as a burn unit. The strictest aseptic technique must be observed.

Wound Care

Two types of burn care are generally used: the open method and the closed method. The open method of burn care is most often used for superficial burns, burns of the face, and burns of the perineum. In open burn care, the wound is not covered but antimicrobial ointment is applied topically. This type of care requires strict aseptic technique.

In the closed burn method of burn care, nonadherent gauze is used to cover the burn. The child can be moved more easily, and the danger of added injury or pain is decreased. However, in the closed method, dressing changes are very painful, and infection may occur under the dressings. Occlusive dressings help minimize pain because of the reduced exposure to air.

In both methods, daily **débridement** (removal of necrotic tissue) usually preceded by **hydrotherapy** (use of water in treatment) is performed. Débridement is extremely painful, and the child must have an analgesic administered before the therapy. The child is placed in the tub of water to soak the dressings; this helps to remove any sloughing tissue, **eschar** (hard crust or scab), exudate, and old medication. Often the tissue is trapped in the mesh gauze of the dressing, so soaking eases necrotic tissue removal. Loose tissue is trimmed before the burn is redressed. Hosing instead of tub soaking is used in some centers to reduce the risk of infection. Débridement is difficult emotionally for both you and the child (Fig. 41-11). Diversionary activities may be used to help distract the child. Researchers also have found that children who are encouraged to participate actively in their burn care, even to help change dressings, experience healthy control over their situation and often experience less anxiety than those who are completely dependent on the nurse. The child should never be scolded or reprimanded for uncooperative behavior.

Topical medications that may be used to reduce invading organisms are silver sulfadiazine (Silvadene), silver nitrate, mafenide acetate (Sulfamylon), Bacitracin, and povidone-iodine (Betadine). Each of these agents has advantages and disadvantages. The choice of agent is made by the physician and is determined, at least partially, by the organisms found in cultures of the burn area.

Grafting

Grafts may be **homografts, heterografts** (xenografts), or **autografts.** Homografts and heterografts are temporary

■ **Figure 41-11** The nurse gives support to the child during débridement.

grafts. A homograft consists of skin taken from another person, which is eventually rejected by the recipient tissue and sloughed off after 3 to 6 weeks. Skin from cadavers is often used in a procedure called an **allograft;** this skin can be stored and used up to several weeks, and permission for this use is seldom refused.

A heterograft is skin obtained from animals, usually pigs (porcine). Both homografts and heterografts provide a temporary dressing after débridement and have been proven to be lifesaving measures for children with extensive burns.

An autograft, consisting of skin taken from the child's own body, is the only kind of skin accepted permanently by recipient tissues, in addition to the skin from an identical twin. Obtaining enough healthy skin to cover a large area is usually impossible; therefore, homografts are of great value for immediate covering. If the donor site is kept free from infection and grafts of sufficient thinness are taken, the site should be ready for use again in 10 to 12 days. After grafting, the donor and the graft sites are kept covered with sterile dressings.

Complications

Curling's ulcer (also called a stress ulcer) is a gastric or duodenal ulcer that often occurs after serious skin burns. It can easily be overlooked when attention is directed toward the treatment of the burn area and the prevention of infection. Symptoms are those of any gastric ulcer but usually are vague, concerned with abdominal discomfort, with or without localization, or related to eating. Ulcers appear during the first 6 weeks. Blood in the stools combined with abdominal discomfort may be the basis for diagnosis. If desired, roentgenograms can confirm the diagnosis. Treatment consists of a bland diet and the use of antacids and antispasmodics.

Remember this.

Praise for cooperation should be used generously in the child who has to undergo débridement for a burn.

The health care team must guard carefully against the complication of **contractures**. If the burn extends over a movable body part, fibrous scarring that forms in the healing process can cause serious deformities and limit movement. Joints must be positioned, possibly in over-extension, so that maximal flexibility is maintained. Splinting, exercise, and pressure also are used to prevent contractures. When burns are severe, pressure garments may be used. These garments help decrease hypertrophy of scar tissue. However, they may need to be worn for 12 to 18 months. The child must wear these garments continuously, except when bathing.

Long-term Care

The rehabilitative phase of care for the child is often long and difficult. Even after discharge from the health care facility, the child needs to return for additional treatment or plastic surgery to release contractures and revise scar tissue. The emotional scars of the family and the child must be evaluated, and therapy must be initiated or continued. The impact of scarring and disfigurement may need to be resolved by both the child and members of the family. If the child is of school age, schoolwork and social interaction must be considered (see Nursing Care Plan 41-1: The Child With a Burn).

Nursing Process For The Child With A Burn

Assessment

Assessment of the child with a burn is complex and varies with the extent and depth of the burn, the stage of healing, and the age and general condition of the child. Initially, the primary concerns are the cardiac and respiratory state, the assessment of shock, and an evaluation of the burns.

After the first phase (the first 24 to 48 hours), the healing of the child's burns must be evaluated and the child's nutrition, signs of infection, and pain level must be monitored. The emotional conditions of the child and the family also must be evaluated.

Selected Nursing Diagnoses

- Risk for Infection related to the loss of the protective layer (skin) secondary to burn injury
- Imbalanced Nutrition: Less Than Body Requirements related to increased caloric needs secondary to burns and anorexia
- Acute Pain related to tissue destruction and painful procedures
- Risk for Impaired Physical Mobility related to pain and scarring
- Anxiety related to changes in body image caused by thermal injury
- Compromised Family Coping related to the effect of the injury on the child's and family's lives
- Deficient Knowledge of caregivers related to optimizing the child's healing process and to the long-term care required by the child

Outcome Identification and Planning

During the first phase of care, the major goals relate to cardiopulmonary stabilization, fluid and electrolyte balance, and infection control. After the first 72 hours in the phase, sometimes called the management or subacute phase, more long-term goals are developed. The child's goals are limited by his or her age and ability to communicate. Goals related to the child include preventing infection, maintaining adequate nutrition, reducing pain, increasing mobility, and relieving anxiety. The family caregiver's goals include concerns about stress on the family related to the child's injury. Other goals relate to optimizing healing and decreasing complications to minimize permanent disability and gaining an understanding of the long-term implications of care.

Implementation

Preventing Infection

The immaturity of the child's immune system, the destruction of the skin layer, and the presence of necrotic tissue (an ideal medium for bacterial growth) contribute to a significant danger of infection. Conscientious hand washing is necessary by anyone who has contact with the child. Observe rigid infection control precautions and use only sterile equipment and supplies. Monitor vital signs, including temperature, on a 1-, 2-, or 4-hour schedule. Screen all people who have any contact with the child, including visitors, family, or staff caregivers for any signs of upper respiratory or skin infection.

When caring for the burn, wear a sterile gown, mask, and cap. Wear sterile gloves or use a sterile tongue blade to apply ointment to the burn. Maintain the room temperature at around 80°F because water evaporates quickly through the denuded areas and even through the leathery burn eschar, with thermal loss resulting. Note and document all drainage. Report immediately and document any unusual odor. Cultures are done regularly, usually several times a week. Avoid injury to the eschar and the donor site. Hair on the tissue adjacent to the burn area is usually shaved.

Ensuring Adequate Nutrition

The child who has received extensive burns requires special attention regarding nutritional needs. The nutritional problem is much more complex than simply getting a seriously ill child to eat. The child is in negative caloric balance from a number of causes, including:

- Poor intake because of anorexia, ileus, Curling's ulcer, or diarrhea
- External loss caused by exudative losses of protein through the burn wound
- Hypermetabolism caused by fever, infection, and the state of toxicity

A bland diet high in protein (for healing and replacement) and calories is an essential component of therapy for the child with a burn. It is important to use every effort

Nursing Care Plan 41-1

THE CHILD WITH A BURN

Two-year-old JW was watching his mother fix dinner. She turned away from the stove where she had vegetables cooking. JW climbed on his chair and grabbed the handle of the pan. Before his mother could react, the boiling liquid from the vegetables poured down over his right arm, the right side of his torso, and his right groin and leg. He is now in the pediatric unit for care of second- and third-degree burns of his right arm, right torso and groin, and right leg.

NURSING DIAGNOSIS
Risk for Infection related to the loss of a protective layer secondary to burn injury

GOAL: The child will be free from signs and symptoms of infection.

EXPECTED OUTCOMES:
• The child's burns show no signs of foul-smelling drainage.
• The child's vital signs remain within normal limits: pulse ranging between 80 and 110 bpm, respirations 20–30/minute, and temperature ranging between 98.6° and 101°F (37°–38.4°C).

Nursing Interventions	*Rationale*
Carry out conscientious handwashing and follow other infection control precautions including the use of sterile equipment and supplies. Wear sterile gown, mask, and cap; use sterile gloves when giving direct care to the burned area.	Sterile technique decreases the introduction of microorganisms. Handwashing is the foundation of good medical asepsis. These procedures reduce the risk of infection.
Teach family and visitors handwashing and sterile techniques.	Infection control procedures must include all who enter the child's room in order to be effective.
Screen visitors for signs of upper respiratory or skin infections.	The child with severe burns may be easily susceptible to upper respiratory and skin infections.
Note and document all drainage and any unusual odor; take regular cultures as ordered.	Early detection and prompt treatment of infection are essential as severe infection places an additional burden on the child's already stressed system.

NURSING DIAGNOSIS
Imbalanced Nutrition: Less than Body Requirements related to increased caloric needs secondary to burns and anorexia

GOAL: The child's caloric intake will be adequate to meet needs for tissue repair and growth.

EXPECTED OUTCOMES:
• The child will consume at least 80% of diet high in calories and protein.
• The child will maintain his preburn weight or will have weight gain appropriate for age.

Nursing Interventions	*Rationale*
Offer a high-calorie, high-protein, bland diet.	Increased calories and high-protein diet are required to promote wound healing.
Plan appealing meals offered in small servings catering to the child's food likes and dislikes. Give choices when appropriate.	Small servings are more appealing to a child. Allowing JW to make choices gives him some feeling of control and encourages his cooperation.
Weigh daily in the morning with only underwear on.	Daily or weekly weights provide information to determine nutritional status.

NURSING DIAGNOSIS
Acute Pain related to tissue destruction and painful procedures

GOAL: The child will show signs of being comfortable and pain will be kept at an acceptable level.

(continues on page 918)

Nursing Care Plan 41-1 *(continued)*

THE CHILD WITH A BURN

EXPECTED OUTCOMES:
- The child rests quietly with pulse between 80 and 110 bpm and respirations 20–30/minute and regular.
- The child uses the faces pain rating scale to indicate his pain level as appropriate for age.
- Analgesics are administered before dressing changes and débridement procedures.

Nursing Interventions	*Rationale*
Monitor every 2 to 4 hours to determine the child's comfort level, vital signs, and if the child is restless.	Each individual reacts differently to pain and analgesics. Learning child's responses helps to effectively plan to reduce his pain.
Administer analgesics 20 to 30 minutes before dressing changes and débridement.	This gives the analgesics time to reach optimum effectiveness for pain relief during procedures.
Support and comfort during procedures. Plan a favorite activity after procedures to give child something pleasant to anticipate.	Acknowledging that the procedures are painful and his cooperation deserves a reward may help the child accept the inevitable.
Give opportunities to exercise some control when possible over timing, what gets done first, or other details.	A feeling of control over some aspects of his care and situation helps offset feelings of powerlessness.

NURSING DIAGNOSIS
Risk for Impaired Physical Mobility related to pain and scarring

GOAL: The child will have increased mobility and contractures will be minimal.

EXPECTED OUTCOMES:
- The child participates in range-of-motion activities and uses both arms and legs.
- The child's splints, pressure suit, and positions are maintained.
- The child has no evidence of contractures.
- The child participates in ambulatory activities.

Nursing Interventions	*Rationale*
Position so that no two skin surfaces touch; give special attention to right armpit, right elbow, wrist and hand, right groin, and right knee.	When any two skin surfaces touch, scarring will occur that results in contractures and limited movement.
Maintain splints and pressure dressings to hyperextend joints.	Hyperextension limits the formation of contractures.
Plan self-care activities that give the child some control and also will encourage movement of affected joints.	Encouraging child to do small activities to help himself promotes movement and decreases contractures.
Encourage active play and ambulation.	A child is more likely to cooperate in exercise and movement that is fun.

NURSING DIAGNOSIS
Deficient Knowledge of the Caregiver related to optimizing the child's healing process and to the long-term care required by the child

GOAL: The child's family caregivers will verbalize an understanding of the child's long-term home care.

EXPECTED OUTCOMES:
- Family caregivers demonstrate wound care and dressing changes.
- Family caregivers verbalize an understanding of the long-term management of child's care and needed treatment.
- The child's family secures the home care equipment needed for his care.
- The family caregivers plan for follow-up care and utilize social service assistance.

Nursing Care Plan 41-1 *(continued)*

THE CHILD WITH A BURN

Nursing Interventions	*Rationale*
Explain to mother and other family caregivers what you are doing and why as you give care and perform procedures for child.	Having a child with a burn is an overwhelming experience. Providing explanations as you give care helps the family to begin to grasp the care process.
Provide information to the child's mother and other family caregivers in small amounts, repeating information from one time to another. Allow ample opportunity for questions.	Family caregivers can absorb only so much information at a time. Repetition and patient, careful answering of questions helps the family to understand the long-term view.
Teach the child's family about the importance of diet, infection control, exercise, rest, activity, pressure suit, and all aspects of child's care.	The child's family needs to understand all aspects of care including how the pressure suit is worn, the care of the suit, and the need to change the suit as the child grows.
Teach signs and symptoms that are important to note and what may need to be reported promptly.	Learning what to observe for and which signs or symptoms need to be reported promptly gives the family caregivers confidence in their ability and improves the level of home care that they give.
Provide family with information and contacts for social services, which will help in the care for the child.	Long-term care is improved and aided by contact and interaction with appropriate social services.

possible to interest the child in foods essential for tissue building and repair. Do not serve large servings because the child often experiences anorexia. In addition, the child's physical condition often interferes with his or her ability to eat. Foods are of no value if the child refuses to eat them. Try using colorful trays, foods with eye appeal, and any special touches to spur a child's appetite. Allow the child to have some control to encourage cooperation.

> **A little nutrition news.**
> Foods high in protein and calories that may appeal to and encourage the child to eat are flavored milk, ice cream, milk shakes, high-protein drinks, milk and egg desserts, and puréed meats and vegetables.

Even with the best efforts of nurses, dietitians, and the child, the burn patient seldom can eat enough food to meet the increased needs. Total parenteral nutrition (TPN) or tube feedings often are necessary to supplement the oral intake. Commercial high-calorie formulas are available for tube feedings that meet the child's needs. Avoid using TPN or tube feedings as a threat to the child. Explain carefully to the child what is to be done and why, and make sure the child understands. Try demonstrating the feeding process with a doll to help the child grasp the idea.

Weigh the child daily at the same time and with the child wearing the same amount of clothing or covering. Carefully monitor intake and output.

Relieving Pain and Providing Comfort Measures

The pain of a thermal injury can be severe. As a result of the pain or the fear and anxiety that pain causes, the child may not sleep well, may experience anorexia, and may be apprehensive and uncooperative during treatments and care. Analgesics must be administered to provide the most relief possible. Administer analgesics at least 20 to 30 minutes before dressing changes and débridement. Avoid scheduling the administration of pain medications close to mealtimes; otherwise, the child may be too sedated to eat.

Monitor the child's physiologic response to the pain and analgesics. Document the child's pupil reaction, heart and respiratory rates, and behavior in response to pain and analgesics.

Provide support and comfort during painful procedures. Use diversionary activities to help the child focus on something other than the pain. Promising a favorite activity after a dreaded procedure is acceptable. Television may be helpful, but be cautious not to overuse it. The younger child may enjoy learning new songs, playing age-appropriate games, or listening to someone reading stories. The older child may enjoy video or computer games, tape recordings, books, and board or card games. The child should never be admonished for crying or behaving "like a baby." Acknowledge the child's pain, give the child as much control as possible, and work with the child and the family to minimize the pain and to bring about the greatest rewards for all involved.

Promoting Mobility and Preventing Contractures

Care must be taken to avoid contractures and scarring that limit movement. Never permit two burned body surfaces, such as fingers, to touch. If the neck is involved, the child may have to be kept with the neck hyperextended, the arms may need to be placed in a brace to prevent underarm contractures, and joints of the knee or elbow must be extended to prevent scar formation from causing contractures that limit movement. Pressure dressings and pressure suits may be used for this purpose and may need to be worn for more than a year. Physical therapy may be needed, and splints may be used to position the body part to prevent contractures. All these measures can add to the child's discomfort.

Encourage range-of-motion, early ambulation, and self-help activities as additional means of promoting mobility and preventing contractures. Use creativity to devise ways to involve the child in enjoyable activities that encourage movement of the affected part.

Reducing Anxiety

The child's age and level of understanding influence the amount of anxiety that he or she has about scarring and disability related to the burn. If the child is in a burn unit with other children, seeing others may cause unrealistic fears. Encourage the child to explore his or her feelings about changes, especially those involving body image. Use therapeutic play with puppets or dolls if possible. Encourage both the family and the nursing staff to provide the child with continuous support.

Promoting Family Coping

The family may feel guilty about the injury; one member may feel especially responsible. These feelings affect the family's coping abilities. Give both the family and the child opportunities to discuss and express their feelings. Suggest counseling if necessary to help family members handle their feelings. Put the family in touch with support groups, if available, to help the family work through problems. Explain the child's care to family members and involve them in the care when possible. Avoid saying anything that might add to the guilt or anxiety that the family members are feeling.

Providing Family Teaching

Provide the family caregivers with explanations about the whole process of burns, the care, the healing process, and the long-term implications. Give information to the family as they are ready for it; do not thrust it on them all at once. To prepare for home care, teach the family about wound care, dressing changes, signs and symptoms to observe and report, and the importance of diet, rest, and activity. Help the family to find resources for any necessary supplies and equipment. Make a referral to social services to assist them in home care planning.

Evaluation: Goals and Expected Outcomes

Goal: The child will be free from signs or symptoms of infection.

Expected Outcomes: The child

- exhibits pulse and respirations within normal limits for age.
- has temperature of 98.6°F to 101°F (37°C–38.4°C).
- is free from malodorous drainage.

Goal: The child's caloric intake will be adequate to meet his or her needs for tissue repair and growth.

Expected Outcomes: The child

- consumes at least 80% of diet high in calories and protein.
- maintains weight or has weight gain appropriate for age.

Goal: The child will show signs of being comfortable.

Expected Outcomes: The child

- rests quietly and does not cry or moan excessively.
- has pulse and respiratory rates that are regular and normal for age.

Goal: The child will have increased mobility and contractures will be minimal.

Expected Outcomes: The child

- participates in range-of-motion activities.
- maintains splints, pressure dressings and suits, and positions.
- shows no evidence of contractures.

Goal: The older child will express feelings related to changes associated with burns.

Expected Outcomes: The child

- expresses feelings and fears about body image.
- demonstrates a positive attitude of acceptance.

Goal: The family caregivers will verbalize feelings related to the child's injury and take steps to develop coping skills.

Expected Outcomes: The family caregivers

- verbalize fears, anxieties, and other feelings related to the child's injury.
- discuss the impact of the injury on the child and family's life.
- participate in counseling.
- become involved in support groups.

Goal: The family caregivers will verbalize an understanding of the child's long-term home care management.

Expected Outcomes: Family members

- demonstrate wound care and dressing changes.
- list signs and symptoms to observe for and report.
- secure needed home care equipment.
- use social service assistance if appropriate.

SEXUALLY TRANSMITTED INFECTIONS

The incidence of sexually transmitted infections (STIs) (sometimes referred to as sexually transmitted diseases [STDs]) is higher in adolescents than in any other age group. The diseases range from infections that can be easily treated to diseases that are life-threatening, such as infection with human immunodeficiency virus (HIV) (Table 41-3).

Infants infected with STIs usually are infected prenatally or during birth. Children infected after the neonatal period must be considered victims of sexual abuse until disproved. Severe or repeated cases of pelvic inflammatory disease (PID) or severe genital warts are warning signs that a girl should be tested for HIV.

Prevention is the most effective tool in the campaign against STIs. The only certain way to avoid contracting an STI is sexual abstinence. However, sexual activity in adolescents indicates that this is often not a practical solution. Condoms with spermicide (discussed in Chapter 4) provide protection, although they are not fail-safe. Adolescents must be educated about all aspects of the consequences of sexual activity.

GONORRHEA

Gonorrhea is one of the most commonly reported communicable diseases in the United States. Also called "the clap," "the drips," or "the dose," gonorrhea has mild primary symptoms, particularly in females, and often goes undetected and thus untreated until it progresses to a serious pelvic disorder. This disease can cause sterility in males.

Several drugs may be used to treat gonorrhea, but the current drug of choice is ceftriaxone (Rocephin) followed by a week of oral doxycycline (Vibramycin) to prevent an accompanying chlamydial infection. Adolescents are asked to name their sexual contacts so that they also may be treated. Penicillin-resistant strains of the organism have developed, so penicillin is no longer an effective method of treatment. Adolescents must learn that their bodies will not develop immunity to the organism and they might become infected again if they continue to expose themselves by engaging in sexual activity, especially high-risk sexual behavior.

CHLAMYDIAL INFECTION

Chlamydial infections have replaced gonorrhea as the most common and fastest spreading STI in the United States. Symptoms may be mild, causing a delay in diagnosis and treatment until serious complications and transmission to others has occurred.

Adolescents must be made aware of the seriousness of PID, a common result of a chlamydial infection. Pelvic inflammatory disease can cause sterility in the female, primarily by causing scarring in the fallopian tubes that prohibits the passage of the fertilized ovum into the uterus. A tubal pregnancy may be the consequence of a chlamydial infection. In the male, sterility may result from epididymitis caused by a chlamydial infection.

Doxycycline or azithromycin is used to treat chlamydial infection. In the pregnant adolescent, erythromycin or amoxicillin can be used to avoid the teratogenic effects of these drugs. All sexual partners must be treated.

GENITAL HERPES

Genital herpes has reached epidemic proportions in the United States. The disease begins as a vesicle that ruptures to form a painful ulcer on the genitalia. The initial ulcer lasts 10 to 12 days. Recurrent episodes occur intermittently and last 4 to 5 days. No cure is available, but acyclovir (Zovirax) is useful in relieving or suppressing the symptoms.

Genital herpes is associated with a much higher than average risk for cervical cancer; therefore, the female who has genital herpes should have an annual Pap smear. Genital herpes is not transmitted to the fetus in utero. However, if the mother has an active case of genital herpes at the time of delivery, cesarean birth is indicated to reduce the risk of infection as the fetus passes through the vagina. In newborns, the infection can become systemic and cause death.

SYPHILIS

Caused by the spirochete *Treponema pallidum*, syphilis is a destructive disease that can involve every part of the body. Untreated, it can have devastating long-term effects. Infected mothers are highly likely to transmit the infection to their unborn infants.

Syphilis is spread primarily by sexual contact. Symptoms of the primary stage usually appear about 3 weeks after exposure. If allowed to progress without treatment, syphilis has a secondary stage, a latent stage, and a tertiary stage.

Clinical Manifestations

The cardinal sign of the primary stage is the **chancre**, which is a hard, red, painless lesion at the point of entry of the spirochete. This lesion can appear on the penis, the vulva, or the cervix. It also can appear on the mouth, the lips, or the rectal area as a result of oral-genital or anal-genital contact. The secondary stage, marked by rash, sore throat, and fever, appears 2 to 6 months after

Table 41-3 ▌ MAJOR SEXUALLY TRANSMITTED INFECTIONS

Infection and Agent	Transmission	Symptoms	Possible Complications	Prevention
Gonorrhea— gonococcus: *Neisseria gonorrhoeae*	Sexual contact; mother to fetus during vaginal delivery	Yellow mucopurulent discharge of the genital area, painful or frequent urination, pain in the genital area; may be asymptomatic Frequent cause of pelvic inflammatory disease	Sterility, cystitis, arthritis, endocarditis	Public should be educated on safe sex practices; mother should be tested before delivery. Newborn's eyes should be treated with tetracycline ointment, erythromycin ointment, or silver nitrate. All contacts should be treated with antibiotics.
Chlamydia— bacteria: *Chlamydia trachomatis*	Sexual contact; mother to fetus during vaginal delivery	Mucopurulent genital discharge, genital pain, dysuria Frequent cause of pelvic inflammatory disease, often in combination with gonorrhea	Sterility	Public should be educated about safe sex practices. Sexual contact should be avoided when lesions are present. Infected mothers should have a cesarean delivery.
Genital herpes virus: herpes simplex type 2	Sexual contact; mother to fetus during vaginal delivery	Genital soreness, pruritus, and erythema; vesicles appear that usually last for about 10 days during which time transmission of virus is likely		Public should be educated about safe sex practices. Sexual contact should be avoided when lesions are present. Infected mother should have a cesarean delivery.
Syphilis—spirochete: *Treponema pallidum*	Sexual contact; mother to fetus via placenta; blood transfusions if undiagnosed donor is in early stage of disease	Primary stage: genital lesion, enlarged lymph nodes Secondary stage (6 weeks later): lesions of skin and mucous membrane with generalized symptoms of headache and fever	Tertiary stage: central nervous system and cardiovascular damage, paralysis, psychosis	Public should be educated about safe sex practices. Screen blood donors; do serologic testing before and during pregnancy. Contact with body secretions from infected patients should be avoided.
Acquired immunodeficiency syndrome (AIDS)— virus: human immunodeficiency virus	Sexual contact; exposure to blood or blood products; mother to fetus or infant	Primary infection: rash, fever, cough, malaise, lymphadenopathy Mildly symptomatic: HIV-positive, enlarged lymph nodes, liver, spleen, persistent upper respiratory infections, otitis media Moderately symptomatic: HIV positive, candidiasis, meningitis, pneumonia, sepsis, herpes infections Severely symptomatic: HIV positive, serious infections, opportunistic infections	Neurologic impairment	Public, especially high-risk groups, should be educated about safe sex practices. Blood or blood products used for transfusion should be carefully screened. Intravenous drug abusers should not share needles. Standard precautions should be used consistently in all health care settings. Measures to avoid needlesticks among health care workers should be instituted.

the original infection. Signs of both the first and second stages disappear without treatment, but the spirochete remains in the body. The latent period can persist for as long as 20 years without symptoms; however, blood tests are still positive. In the tertiary stage, syphilis causes severe neurologic and cardiovascular damage, mental illness, and gastrointestinal disorders.

Treatment

Syphilis responds to one intramuscular injection of penicillin G benzathine; if the child is sensitive to penicillin, oral doxycycline, tetracycline, or erythromycin can be administered as alternative treatment. If treatment is not obtained before the tertiary stage, the neurologic and cardiovascular complications can lead to death.

ACQUIRED IMMUNODEFICIENCY SYNDROME

Acquired immunodeficiency syndrome (AIDS) is caused by the human immunodeficiency virus (HIV), which attacks and destroys the T-helper lymphocytes (CD4+). The T-helper lymphocytes are cells that direct the immune response to viral, bacterial, and fungal infections and remove some malignant cells from the body.

Because not all persons who test positive for HIV develop AIDS immediately, the Centers for Disease Control and Prevention (CDC) have established criteria for a classification system for HIV infection and AIDS surveillance. The most significant of these criteria for children and adults is the CD4+ T-lymphocyte count. Normal CD4 cell counts vary in children, depending on the age of the child. As the disease progresses, the CD4 count drops and puts the child at risk for developing life-threatening infections. The CDC classifies HIV/AIDS in three categories:

- Category A: Mildly symptomatic: HIV positive as well as two or more symptoms, such as enlarged spleen, liver, or lymph nodes, frequent respiratory or ear infections
- Category B: Moderately symptomatic: HIV positive as well as illnesses such as candidiasis, bacterial pneumonia or meningitis, chronic diarrhea, herpes simplex virus or herpes zoster, persistent fever
- Category C: Severely symptomatic: HIV positive as well as serious bacterial infections, encephalopathy, lymphoma, tuberculosis, severe failure to thrive, or an opportunistic infection

Transmission of HIV occurs through contact with infected blood or blood products during transfusions or sharing of infected needles, exposure to infected body secretions through sexual contact, as well as from an HIV-positive woman to her unborn fetus or newborn infant. The virus cannot be transmitted through casual contact. The diagnosis of any STI increases the statistical risk of HIV infection by 300%.

Infants usually are infected through the placenta during prenatal life, in the birth process when contaminated by the mother's blood, or through breast-feeding. Children and teens also can be infected through sexual abuse. Adolescents are most often infected through intimate heterosexual or homosexual relations and through intravenous drug use. Hemophiliacs who received blood products before 1985 were infected in some cases, but safeguards are now in place, and the blood supply has become much safer.

Although most children with AIDS are between the ages of 1 and 4 years, the alarming increase occurring among adolescents is causing great concern in those who work with adolescents. African-American adolescents have a disproportionately high rate of AIDS. The numbers of adolescent girls with HIV continues to rise.

Teenagers' attitude of **impunity** (the belief that nothing can hurt them) and the increasing rate of sexual activity in this age group, often involving multiple partners, contribute to the fear that this group will experience widespread illness from HIV. The incubation period for HIV can vary from 3 to 10 years; thus many who contract the disease in adolescence will not have symptoms until they are in their 20s, when they are at their reproductive peak. The proper use of a condom with spermicide (see Chapter 24) during any type of sexual contact is essential to prevent the spread of HIV. Adolescent girls may have sexual experiences with older men who have had many previous sexual partners. This increases the risk for the girl and, in turn, can increase the risk for any adolescent boy with whom she is sexually intimate. Adolescent boys also are at increased risk if they engage in unprotected homosexual relations, use intravenous drugs, have multiple partners, or have sex with a prostitute.

About 20% to 30% of the infants born to HIV-infected mothers develop AIDS. Although the infants may test positive in the first year of life, testing is not reliable until 18 months of age because the infant may retain antibodies from the mother for this length of time. However, for affected infants younger than 1 year of age, the disease can move rapidly to AIDS and serious complications. Failure to thrive, *Pneumocystis carinii* pneumonia, recurrent bacterial infections, progressive encephalopathy, and malignancy often develop in affected

Cultural Snapshot

Cultural influences may play an important role in the spread of HIV. The adolescent girl often finds it difficult to insist that her partner use a condom. If the partner refuses and claims to be "safe" (uninfected) or protests that the condom decreases his pleasure, she might give in for fear of breaking up the relationship. In addition, in some cultures the more sexual conquests a boy has, the more manly he is considered.

infants. Some of these children progress quickly to terminal illness and death, but with aggressive chemotherapy some of them are living long enough to enter school.

Clinical Manifestations and Treatment

Children and adolescents manifest the symptoms of HIV in much the same way as adults. Females rarely have Kaposi sarcoma, a cancer often seen in homosexual men. Many women including adolescents present with a chronic infection of vaginitis caused by C. albicans that has not responded to local antifungal treatments. These infections may be controlled by oral systemic medications. The female who tests positive for HIV should have a pelvic examination every 6 months to detect early STIs and institute vigorous treatment as needed.

Nursing Process For The Child With AIDS
Assessment

When seeking data from the child with AIDS, gather a complete history, including chief complaint, presenting symptoms, past medical history, immunization status, family history, and social history. Interview the family caregiver if present, but be certain to provide the adolescent with a private interview. The adolescent may be extremely reluctant to reveal either social or sexual history, especially in the presence of a family member. Review carefully the teen girl's history of vaginal candidiasis, PID, and sexual activity. Review the teen boy's sexual activity, including partners who are of the same sex or who are intravenous drug users. The adolescent may have various emotions, including anger, denial, guilt, and rebelliousness; it is important that you accept all these emotions as legitimate reactions to the illness.

During the physical exam, maintain strict standard precautions. Include vital signs and especially observe for fever, which may indicate infection, and perform a thorough survey of all body systems. Observe for poor skin turgor, rashes or lesions, alopecia, mucous membrane lesions or thrush, weight loss, mental or neurologic changes, respiratory infections or signs of tuberculosis, diarrhea or abdominal pain, vaginal discharge, perineal lesions, or genital warts. Help prepare the child for diagnostic tests that must be performed.

Selected Nursing Diagnoses

- Risk for Infection related to increased susceptibility secondary to a compromised immune system
- Risk for Injury related to the possible transmission of the virus
- Risk for Impaired Skin Integrity related to perineal and anal tissue excoriation secondary to genital candidiasis or genital warts
- Acute Pain related to symptoms of the disease
- Imbalanced Nutrition: Less Than Body Requirements related to anorexia, oral or esophageal lesions, or diarrhea
- Social Isolation related to rejection by others secondary to the diagnosis of AIDS
- Hopelessness related to the diagnosis and prognosis
- Compromised Family Coping related to the diagnosis of AIDS

Outcome Identification and Planning

Planning the nursing care of a child with AIDS can be challenging. The child needs support to accept the diagnosis and move in a positive direction to follow the treatment plan to the best of his or her ability. You can play a critical role in helping the child understand the treatment and prognosis and their impact on his or her life. Major goals for the child include maintaining the highest level of wellness possible by preventing infection and the spread of the infection, maintaining skin integrity, minimizing pain, improving nutrition, alleviating social isolation, and diminishing a feeling of hopelessness. The primary goal for the family is improving coping skills and helping the teen cope with the illness.

Implementation
Preventing Infection

In the health care facility, strict adherence to appropriate infection control measures is extremely important. A primary goal is to teach the child to prevent infections. Teach good hand-washing technique; the patient should take care to wash between the fingers and under rings and should use a pump-type soap. Encourage the child to keep nails trimmed to avoid harboring microorganisms under the nails. Teach that skin care includes showering (not a tub bath) with a mild soap (no strong, perfumed soaps), using an emollient cream, and patting the skin dry while avoiding vigorous rubbing. Instruct the child to brush the teeth at least three times a day using a soft toothbrush and nonabrasive toothpaste. Routine dental care is vital.

A little nutrition news. To help decrease the possibility of infection, raw fruits and vegetables should be washed and peeled or cooked to avoid the danger of bacteria; meats must be well cooked. The child must avoid unpasteurized dairy products and foods grown in organic fertilizer.

The household where the child lives must be cleaned carefully and regularly. A household bleach solution of one part bleach to 10 parts of water is a good solution to use. Particular attention should be paid to the refrigerator, the stove, the oven, and the microwave to prevent contamination of foods during preparation or storage. Household items that may be contaminated should be discarded in double plastic bags to prevent spread to others. Laundry bleach should be used when washing the child's clothing, especially underwear.

Teach the child that someone else should care for pets. Cleaning an aquarium or birdcage or emptying a cat's litter box can expose the child to opportunistic organisms that will attack the compromised immune system. Help the child learn to avoid persons who have any infectious disease. Advise him or her that prompt attention to an apparently minor infection helps avoid more serious illness. The child with AIDS should not receive any live vaccine immunizations, but should continue to receive other immunizations as indicated.

Preventing Infection Transmission

The good hygienic practices necessary to protect the child from an acquired or opportunistic infection also help to prevent transmission of the virus to others. In addition, the adolescent needs counseling about sexual practices. One of the most emotionally difficult tasks for the adolescent may be to list sexual contacts. This is a delicate matter that must be approached in a nonjudgmental, sympathetic manner, but the teen needs to understand that anyone with whom he or she has been sexually intimate may be infected and must be identified. The teen may find that the sexual partner from whom he or she contracted the virus already knew that he or she was infected. Infection with HIV does not necessarily mean that the child was promiscuous. The adolescent may have been sexually intimate with only one person, and that person may have assured the teen that he or she was not infected. The adolescent may be extremely angry about exposure by a trusted person.

Teach the adolescent about safe sex practices. The adolescent needs to understand that he or she is protecting not only future sexual partners from contracting the disease, but also himself or herself from contracting other strains of the virus. Both boys and girls need to have complete instructions on the use of condoms and spermicide (see Chapter 4). The adolescent must not be sexually intimate with anyone without using a condom, no matter what kind of argument the other person uses. Also the teen needs to learn how HIV is transmitted, including vaginal intercourse, oral-genital contact, anal intercourse, or any contact with blood or body fluids, including menstrual discharge. The teen who practices oral-genital sex must learn to use a dental dam (a square of latex worn in the mouth to prevent contact of body fluids with mucous membranes of the mouth).

The adolescent girl needs to be counseled about pregnancy. The probability of transmitting the virus to her unborn child may be as high as 30%, and no way currently exists to determine if she will pass the virus to her child. She must consider that even if her child is not infected, there is a possibility that she may not live to see the child reach adulthood. All these considerations are overwhelming, and the adolescent needs continuous support to understand, accept, and deal with them.

A discussion of the use of illicit, injectable drugs is important. Counsel the child and adolescent about the importance of stopping drug use. However, the reality is that he or she may not quit, so explain how to sterilize needles using chlorine bleach. A mixture of one part bleach to five parts water should be drawn through the needle into the syringe, flushed two or three times, and finally rinsed with water.

> **This approach is important to remember.**
> The adolescent has the right to decide how to conduct his or her life; you must remain nonjudgmental through all contacts with the teen.

Promoting Skin Integrity

Skin lesions are common symptoms of many STIs. The child must report any new skin lesion to the health care provider for diagnosis and immediate treatment. The best preventive measure is to follow careful infection control measures, including careful hand washing and to protect skin integrity by using skin emollients to guard against dryness; avoiding harsh, perfumed soaps; and guarding against injury to the skin. In advanced disease, nursing measures are implemented to protect and pad pressure points and improve peripheral circulation.

Promoting Comfort

Pain is caused by several manifestations of AIDS. Skin and mucous membrane lesions may be very painful. Topical anesthetic solutions, such as viscous lidocaine, and meticulous mouth care can relieve pain caused by oral mucous membrane infections. Smoking, alcohol, and spicy or acidic foods irritate the oral mucous membranes and often cause additional pain. Pelvic inflammatory disease, a common complication of STIs, is usually accompanied by abdominal pain. The child with respiratory complications also has bouts of chest pain. Administer analgesics to relieve pain and use all appropriate nursing measures to help the child feel more comfortable. As the disease develops, the pain may be greater, so every effort must be made to provide comfort.

Improving Nutrition

Anorexia, or a poor appetite, is a common problem of the patient with AIDS. Dehydration, diarrhea, infection, malabsorption, oral candidiasis, and some drugs also can contribute to the child's poor state of nutrition. Malnutrition can cause additional problems with increased and more serious infections. The child's diet must be more nutritious and higher in calories than normal. Several small meals supplemented by high-calorie, high-protein snacks may be desirable. Dietary supplements, such as Ensure and Isocal, also may be useful. Explore the child's food likes and dislikes and develop a meal plan using this information. If malnutrition becomes severe, the child may need tube feedings or parenteral nutrition.

Easing Social Isolation and Hopelessness

The child may fear having others know about the illness because he or she anticipates a negative reaction from peers and family. Provide the child with supportive counseling and guidance to help him or her deal with these fears. The child may not feel that he or she can tell the family for fear of rejection. In fact, many families have rejected their children who have AIDS. Many others have risen to the challenge; although family members may tell the teenager they do not like his or her behavior, they continue to offer love and support. The child may need support to help tell social acquaintances as well. Refer the child or adolescent to an HIV support group if one is available through the hospital or community. Adolescents often find that adult support groups are not as helpful because the adults' needs are different from those of adolescents.

Because the child is facing life with a serious, chronic illness that requires frequent treatment and lifelong medication and has an unknown outcome, the child may feel a special sense of purpose to "spread the word" to others. The child needs support and guidance to set priorities. School officials may need to be told, but families have the legal right to decide whether or not they share the diagnosis with others. If the family is not supportive, the child needs even more support from health care providers.

Promoting Family Coping

The adolescent must be involved in telling family members about the diagnosis if they do not already know.

The sexual activity of adolescent children is a topic that many families find difficult to deal with, especially if the activity is homosexual or promiscuous.

The family caregivers usually need support as much as the child does. They often are devastated by the prospect of their child's illness. If the adolescent is pregnant or has a child, the family also must consider the future of that child. For the family who plays a supportive role in the child's life, the period after diagnosis is a difficult one.

Teach the family as much about the disease as possible. They must learn how to prevent the spread of the virus among family members, as well as how to prevent opportunistic infections in the child who is HIV positive. It is important to teach the family about treatments, medications, nutrition guidelines, and signs and symptoms of opportunistic infections. Stress the importance of reporting even minor complications to the health care provider, and suggest ways to help support the child. See Family Teaching Tips: Supporting the Child or Adolescent With HIV/AIDS.

A little sensitivity is in order.
When working with children and families of children diagnosed with HIV or AIDS, be aware of possible unspoken feelings and questions and carefully bring them into the discussion.

Family Teaching Tips

SUPPORTING THE CHILD OR ADOLESCENT WITH HIV/AIDS

- Assist in learning about and accepting diagnosis.
- Provide educational literature on HIV.
- Explain the difference between being HIV positive and having AIDS.
- Encourage him or her to verbalize feelings (anger, fear, hopelessness, etc.).
- Encourage participation in local support groups.
- Promote eating an adequate diet, exercising regularly, sleeping 8 to 10 hours/night.
- Encourage small, frequent meals or suggest nutritional supplements, such as Ensure, to prevent weight loss.
- Discuss prescribed drugs: indications, schedules, doses, and how to recognize and manage side effects.
- Make a schedule for medicines and daily eating times that will work for you and your child.
- Use reminders, such as a timer or a watch with an alarm, calendars, and a check-off list of when a dose is due or has been taken.

- Color-code the bottles of liquid medicines with matching oral syringes. This helps make giving the right dose easier. Put the same color for the medicine on the calendar or checklist.
- Explain how HIV is spread (by direct contact with infected body fluids, usually through sex, sharing needles, or blood transfusion).
- Talk about how to avoid transmitting the virus to others or contracting yet another strain.
- Discuss safer sex strategies, such as using condoms.
- Discuss why and how to notify sex partners of infection; explain that partners need counseling, testing, and, if HIV positive, referral for treatment; offer to help with the notification process if necessary.
- Discuss the importance of primary health care.
- Encourage adolescent girls to have regular gynecologic examinations and Pap smears.

Although teaching the child and the family all this information is necessary, remember that a person can absorb only so much detail at one time. To teach them successfully and to be sure they understand the information, do not present too much information at one time. Give the family and the child written materials that repeat the information, and review it verbally with them by asking questions and clarifying material until they show evidence of clear understanding of the concepts they need to know. It is important to provide the entire family with the best possible support and information.

Evaluation: Goals and Expected Outcomes

Goal: The child will experience minimal risk of infection.
Expected Outcomes: The child

- practices good hygiene measures.
- identifies ways to prevent infection and ways to protect his or her health at home.

Goal: The child will not spread the disease to others.
Expected Outcomes: The child

- practices infection control measures.
- identifies sexual partners and safer sexual practices.

Goal: The child's skin integrity will remain intact.
Expected Outcomes: The child

- protects the skin and mucous membranes.
- promptly reports skin lesions or infections.

Goal: The child will experience minimal pain from complications of the disease.
Expected Outcomes: The child

- learns to manage pain.
- rests comfortably with minimal discomfort.

Goal: The child's food intake will meet his or her nutritional needs.
Expected Outcomes: The child

- eats nutritionally sound meals.
- includes frequent small meals in the food plan.
- maintains his or her weight.

Goal: The child will not experience social isolation.
Expected Outcomes: The child

- voices fears about social isolation.
- makes and carries out plans to maintain relationships.

Goal: The adolescent will make adjustments to his or her future expectations.
Expected Outcomes: The child or adolescent

- expresses feelings about his or her future.
- seeks support from others.
- begins to make realistic future plans.

Goal: The family will show evidence of coping with the illness and supporting the child.
Expected Outcomes: The family

- expresses anxieties.
- voices understanding of the illness.
- supports the child in future plans.

INFECTIOUS MONONUCLEOSIS

Common in the adolescent population and sometimes called the "kissing disease," infectious mononucleosis ("mono") is caused by the Epstein-Barr virus, one of the herpes virus groups. The organism is transmitted through saliva. No immunization is available and treatment is symptomatic. Adolescents and young adults seem to be most susceptible to this disorder, although sometimes it also is seen in younger children.

Clinical Manifestations

Infectious mononucleosis can present a variety of symptoms, ranging from mild to severe and including symptoms that mimic hepatitis. Symptoms include fever; sore throat with enlarged tonsils; thick, white membrane covering the tonsils (Fig. 41-12); palatine petechiae (red spots on the soft palate); swollen lymph nodes; and enlargement of the spleen accompanied by extreme fatigue and lack of energy. In some instances, headache, abdominal pain, and epistaxis are also present.

Diagnosis

Diagnosis of infectious mononucleosis is based on clinical symptoms, laboratory evidence of lymphocytes in the peripheral blood (with 10% or more abnormal lymphocytes present in a peripheral blood smear), and a positive heterophil agglutination test. Monospot is a valuable diagnostic test—rapid, sensitive, inexpensive, and simple to perform. Mono-spot can detect significant agglutinins at lower levels, thus allowing earlier diagnosis. Infectious mononucleosis often is confused with streptococcal infections because of the fever and the appearance of the throat and tonsils.

∎ **Figure 41-12** Tonsils of an adolescent who has infectious mononucleosis; note the red, enlarged tonsils with the thick white covering.

Treatment and Nursing Care

No cure exists for infectious mononucleosis; treatment is based on symptoms. An analgesic-antipyretic, such as acetaminophen, usually is recommended for the fever and headaches. Fluids and a soft, bland diet are encouraged to reduce throat irritation. Corticosteroids sometimes are used to relieve the severe sore throat and fever. Bed rest is suggested to relieve fatigue, but is not imposed for a specific amount of time. If the spleen is enlarged, the child is cautioned to avoid contact sports that might cause a ruptured spleen. Because the immune system is weakened, the child must take precautions to avoid secondary infections.

The course of mononucleosis is usually uncomplicated. Fever and sore throat may last from 1 week to 10 days. Fatigue generally disappears 2 to 4 weeks after the appearance of acute symptoms, but may last as long as 1 year. The limitations that this disorder imposes on the teenager's school and social life may cause depression. However, in most instances the child can resume normal activities within 1 month after symptoms present.

Nursing care includes encouraging the child to express feelings about the interruptions the illness is causing in school, social, and work plans. Long-term effects rarely are seen.

Test Yourself

✔ List the most common sexually transmitted infections in adolescents and explain how each of these is treated.

✔ Discuss what you could talk to an adolescent about regarding sexually transmitted infections.

✔ How is mononucleosis treated?

COMMUNICABLE DISEASES OF CHILDHOOD

Half a century ago, growing up meant being able to survive measles, mumps, whooping cough, diphtheria, and often poliomyelitis. These diseases were expected almost as routinely as the loss of the deciduous teeth. Immunization has changed that outcome so drastically that some caregivers have become less conscientious about having their children immunized until the immunization is required for entrance to school. Nevertheless, the incidence of childhood diseases has decreased with only an occasional outbreak in certain communities where many children are not immunized.

Understanding the various communicable diseases and their prevention, symptoms, and treatment (Table 41-4) requires knowledge of specific terms (Box 41-1). Some

---

Box 41-1 ■ COMMON TERMS IN COMMUNICABLE DISEASE NURSING

Active immunity: stimulates development of antibodies to destroy infective agent without causing disease; occurs when vaccine is given

Antibody: a protective substance in the body produced in response to the introduction of an antigen

Antigen: a foreign protein that stimulates the formation of antibodies

Antitoxin: an antibody that unites with and neutralizes a specific toxin

Carrier: a person in apparently good health whose body harbors the specific organisms of a disease

Causative agent: pathogen that causes disease

Enanthem: an eruption on a mucous surface

Endemic: habitual presence of a disease within a given area

Epidemic: an outbreak in a community of a group of illnesses of similar nature in excess of the normal expectancy

Erythema: redness of the skin produced by congestion of the capillaries

Exanthem: an eruption appearing on the skin during an eruptive disease

Host: a human, animal, or plant that harbors or nourishes another organism

Incubation period: the time interval between the infection and the appearance of the first symptoms of the disease

Macule: a discolored skin spot not elevated above the surface

Mode of transmission: mechanism by which infectious agent is spread or transferred to humans

Natural immunity: resistance to pathogen or infection, genetically determined

Pandemic: a worldwide epidemic

Papule: a small, circumscribed, solid elevation of the skin

Passive immunity: antibodies obtained from an immune person, given to someone exposed to disease to prevent him or her from getting disease

Period of communicability: time that infectious agent can be transmitted or passed from an infected person or animal to another person

Pustule: a small elevation of epidermis filled with pus

Toxin: a poisonous substance produced by certain organisms, such as bacteria

Toxoid: a toxin that has been treated to destroy its toxicity but that retains its antigenic properties

Vaccine: a suspension of attenuated or killed microorganisms administered for the prevention of a specific infection

Table 41-4 ▌ COMMUNICABLE DISEASES OF CHILDHOOD

Disease	Period of Communicability When/How Long Contagious	Prevention Immunization Immunity	Clinical Manifestations	Treatment Nursing Care Implementation	Complications
Hepatitis B Causative agent: A *Hepadnavirus; hepatitis B virus* Mode of transmission: body fluids, transfusion of contaminated blood, use of contaminated needle, to fetus via mother Incubation period: average 60–90 days	End of incubation time and during acute stage	Use of standard precautions Vaccine for hepatitis B After exposure—HBIG (hepatitis B immune globulin)	Anorexia, abdominal discomfort, nausea, vomiting, jaundice	Rest, nutrition with good caloric intake	Possibly fatal, liver problems, in some cases possibly leading to chronic hepatitis
Diphtheria Causative agent: *Corynebacterium diphtheriae* Mode of transmission: droplet, direct contact with infected person, carrier, or contaminated article Incubation period: 2–7 days	2–4 weeks in untreated person 1–2 days with antibiotic therapy	Active immunity from diphtheria toxin in DTaP vaccine Passive immunity with diphtheria antitoxin	Mucous membranes of nose and throat covered by gray membrane; purulent nasal discharge; brassy cough; toxin from organism passes through bloodstream to heart and nervous system	Strict droplet precautions; intravenous antitoxin and antibiotics; bed rest; liquid to soft diet; analgesics for throat pain; immunization for nonimmunized contacts	Neuritis, carditis, heart failure, respiratory failure
Tetanus (lockjaw) Causative agent: *Clostridium tetani* Mode of transmission: direct or indirect contamination of a closed wound Incubation period: 3–21 days	None—not transmitted from person to person	Active immunity from tetanus toxoid in DTaP vaccine	Stiffness of neck and jaw, muscle rigidity of trunk and extremities, arched back, abdominal muscle stiffness, unusual facial appearance, pain due to muscle spasms	Quiet room, wound cleaning and débridement, penicillin G or erythromycin, muscle relaxants	Serious, fatal if untreated, possible respiratory complications
Pertussis (whooping cough) Causative agent: *Bordetella pertussis* Mode of transmission: droplet, direct contact with respiratory discharges Incubation period: 5–21 days	About 4–6 weeks, greatest in respiratory stage	Active immunity from pertussis vaccine in DTaP vaccine; Disease gives natural immunity	Begins with mild upper respiratory symptoms; in 2nd week progresses to severe paroxysmal cough with inspiratory whoop, sometimes followed by vomiting; especially dangerous for young infants, may last 4–6 weeks	Bed rest; infants hospitalized; oxygen therapy possible, observation for airway obstruction; provision of high humidity; protection from secondary infections, increased fluid intake; refeeding if vomiting occurs	Pneumonia (can cause death of infant); otitis media; hemorrhage; convulsions

(continues on page 930)

Table 41-4 ▮ **COMMUNICABLE DISEASES OF CHILDHOOD** *(continued)*

Disease	Period of Communicability When/How Long Contagious	Prevention Immunization Immunity	Clinical Manifestations	Treatment Nursing Care Implementation	Complications
Haemophilus influenzae type B Causative agent: *Coccobacilli H. influenzae bacteria* Mode of transmission: droplet, discharge from nose and throat Incubation period: 2–4 days	As long as organisms are present; noncommunicable after antibiotic therapy for 24–48 hours	Vaccine *haemophilus influenzae type b* (HIB)	Fever, vomiting, lethargy, meningeal irritation with bulging fontanel or stiff neck and back, stupor, coma	Antibiotics	Meningitis, epiglottitis, pneumonia
Poliomyelitis (infantile paralysis) Causative agent: *poliovirus* Mode of transmission: Direct and indirect contact, fecal-oral route Incubation period: 7–14 days	Greatest just before onset and just after onset of symptoms, when virus is present in throat and feces, 1–6 weeks	Inactivated polio vaccine (IPV) Disease causes active immunity against specific strain	Fever, headache, nausea, vomiting, abdominal pain; stiff neck, pain, and tenderness in lower extremities that proceeds to paralysis	Bed rest; moist hot packs to extremities; range-of-motion exercises; supportive care; long-term ventilation if respiratory muscles involved	Permanent paralysis; respiratory arrest
Rubeola (measles) Causative agent: *measles virus* Mode of transmission: Direct or indirect contact with droplets, nasal, and throat secretions Incubation period: 10–12 days	5th incubation day through first few days after rash erupts	Attenuated live vaccine (part of MMR vaccine) Disease gives lasting natural immunity	High fever, sore throat, coryza (runny nose), cough, enlarged lymph nodes (head and neck), Koplik spots (small red spots with blue-white centers on oral mucosa, specific to rubeola), conjunctivitis, photophobia, maculopapular rash starts at hairline and spreads to entire body	Antipyretics, comfort measures for rash including tepid baths, soothing lotion, maintenance of dry skin; dimly lighted room for comfort, fluids	Otitis media, pneumonia, encephalitis, airway obstruction
Parotitis (mumps) Causative agent: *Paramyxovirus* Mode of transmission: airborne, droplet, direct contact with saliva of infected person Incubation period: 14–21 days	Shortly before swelling appears until after it disappears	Attenuated live mumps vaccine (part of MMR vaccine) Disease gives natural immunity	Parotid glands swollen, unilaterally or bilaterally; may have fever, headache, malaise, and complain of earache before swelling appears; angle of jaw obliterated on affected side	Liquids and soft foods because chewing is painful; avoidance of sour foods, which cause discomfort; analgesics for pain; antipyretics for fever; local compresses of heat or cold	In males past puberty orchitis (inflammation of the testes); meninoencephalitis; possible severe hearing impairment (rare)

Table 41-4 ▮ COMMUNICABLE DISEASES OF CHILDHOOD *(continued)*

Disease	Period of Communicability When/How Long Contagious	Prevention Immunization Immunity	Clinical Manifestations	Treatment Nursing Care Implementation	Complications
Rubella (German measles) Causative agent: Rubella virus Mode of transmission: direct or indirect contact with droplets, nasopharyngeal secretions Incubation period: 14–21 days	5–7 days before until about 5 days after rash appears	Attenuated live vaccine (part of MMR vaccine) Disease gives lasting natural immunity Immune serum globulin may be given to pregnant women	Low-grade fever; headache, malaise, anorexia, sore throat, lymph glands of neck and head enlarged; pink-red rash begins on face, spreads downward, disappears in 3 days, may have joint pain	Comfort measures for rash, antipyretics for fever and joint pain	Severe birth defects possible if mother is exposed and nonimmunized (especially in 1st trimester)
Varicella (chickenpox) Causative agent: *Varicella zoster* virus Mode of transmission: airborne, direct or indirect contact with saliva or uncrusted vesicles Incubation period: 10–21 days	1 day before rash appears to about 5–6 days after it appears (until all vesicles crusted)	Attenuated live varicella virus vaccine gives active immunity Disease causes lasting natural immunity; may reactivate in adult as herpes zoster	Low-grade fever; malaise; successive crops of macules, papules, vesicles, and crusts, all present at the same time; itching is intense; scarring may occur when scabs are removed before ready to fall off	Antihistamines, soothing baths and lotions to reduce itching; prevention of scratching with short fingernails or use of mittens; acyclovir to shorten the course of the disease; **no aspirin** should be given	Reye syndrome possible if child has had aspirin during illness; secondary infection of lesions if scratched; pneumonia, encephalitis
Hepatitis A Causative agent: *A picornavirus; hepatitis A virus* Mode of transmission: Ingestion of fecal contaminated food or water or contaminated surfaces Incubation period: Average 25–30 days	Highest during 2 weeks before onset of symptoms	Good hand washing, sanitary disposal of feces Vaccine for hepatitis A After exposure—immune globulin	Fever, malaise, anorexia, nausea, abdominal discomfort, jaundice	Enteric precautions, rest, nutritious diet	
Erythema infectiosum (fifth disease) Causative agent: *Human parvovirus B19* Mode of transmission: droplet, contact with respiratory secretions Incubation period: 6–14 days	Uncertain, child may return to school when rash appears, no longer infectious at that point	No immunity	Fever, headache, malaise; a week later, red rash appears on face, called a "slapped face" rash; rash appears on extremities, then on trunk; rash can reappear with heat, sunlight, cold	Supportive treatment with antipyretics, analgesics, droplet precautions (when hospitalized)	Arthritis possible; dangerous for fetus (keep infected child away from pregnant women)

(continues on page 932)

Table 41-4 ■ COMMUNICABLE DISEASES OF CHILDHOOD (continued)

Disease	Period of Communicability When/How Long Contagious	Prevention Immunization Immunity	Clinical Manifestations	Treatment Nursing Care Implementation	Complications
Roseola (exanthema subitum) Causative agent: Human *herpesvirus* type 6 Mode of transmission: Unknown Incubation period: about 10 days	During febrile period	Contracting disease gives lasting immunity	High fever; irritability; anorexia; lymph nodes enlarged; decreased WBC; rash appears just after sharp decline in temperature; rash is rose-pink, mostly on trunk, lasts 1–2 days	Symptomatic for rash and fever; standard precautions (if hospitalized)	
Lyme disease Causative agent: *Borrelia burgdorferi* Mode of transmission: deer tick bite Incubation period: 3–30 days	Not communicable from one person to another	Avoid tick-infected areas; inspect skin after being in wooded areas Active immunity from Lyme disease vaccine	Starts as a red papule that spreads and becomes a large, round red ring; fever; malaise; headache; mild neck stiffness with rash; leads to systemic symptoms and chronic problems	Antibiotics	Cardiac, musculoskeletal and neurologic involvement
Scarlet Fever Causative agent: *Beta-hemolytic streptococci group A* Mode of transmission: direct contact, droplet Incubation period: 2–5 days	During acute respiratory phase, 1–7 days	Lasting immunity after having disease	Begins abruptly; fever; sore throat; headache; chills; malaise; red rash on skin and mucous membranes; tonsils inflamed; enlarged; white exudate; tongue—differentiates from other rashes, by day 4–5 "red strawberry" appearance	Soft or liquid diet, antipyretics, analgesics, comfort measures for itching rash; penicillin for streptococcal infection	Glomerulonephritis or rheumatic fever if untreated

communicable diseases require specific precautions to prevent spreading of the infection. Specific transmission precaution procedures can be found in the procedure manuals of individual institutions.

Prevention

The recommended schedule of childhood immunization is found in Appendix J. Parents of children whose immunizations are incomplete must be urged to have the immunizations brought up to date. For families of limited means, free immunizations are usually available at clinics.

Nursing Care

Many times the child who develops a communicable disease is at home. However, in some cases the child may develop the disease while hospitalized. For the child who develops a communicable disease and is hospitalized, explain to the child and the caregivers the reason for the transmission precautions. Precautions are done to protect the child from the threat of infection or to protect others from the infection the child has. Otherwise, the child may feel that the precautions are a form of punishment. Families are more likely to follow the correct procedures if they understand the need for them. Transmission precautions may intensify the normal loneliness of being ill, so the child needs extra attention and stimulation during this time.

A Personal Glimpse

One time last year when I was in kindergarten I felt so sick. I had a red spot on my face, and when I woke up my tummy was covered with spots. I was so hot, and I itched all over. My mom called the nurse at my doctor's office to see if she should take me and they said, "No way. She's got the chickenpox." It was like Halloween at school, but it was really called the Fall Fiesta. I was going to be Bruce the shark from Finding Nemo because I watch it all the time on DVD. My sister and all my friends walked to school in their costumes, but I couldn't go, and I itched a lot. I was so sad. To keep me from being sad my mom said I could draw pictures and I drew pictures of me making a soccer goal and of my slingshot. I decided when I was better I could use my costume to play Shark Attack. I would pretend I was swimming in the ocean and if I catch other people, they turn into friendly sharks. I was crying and I was so itchy and my mom put lotion on, but it didn't help. My mom said she could give me a bath in oatmeal and it would feel better. I was kind of grossed out because I don't usually take a bath in food, but she said we could put it in a special cloth instead of a bowl. She was right; I stopped itching a little. When my sister came home with candy and treats I felt a little better, but I still had the chickenpox.

Jocie, age 6

Learning Opportunity: What questions do you think the nurse in the pediatrician's office asked to determine this child should be cared for at home, rather than be seen in the office? For what reason would this mother give her child an "oatmeal" bath?

Key Points

➤ The integumentary system, including the accessory structures, are in place at birth and mature as the child grows. Protecting the body from attacks from microorganisms and helping the body get rid of or resist invasion by foreign materials are the major roles of the immune system. The immune system matures and develops as the child progresses through childhood.

➤ Seborrheic dermatitis is known as cradle cap. It appears as yellowish, scaly crusted patches on the scalp and can usually be prevented by daily washing of hair and scalp. In the child with Miliaria rubra, a rash appears as pinhead-sized erythematous (reddened) papules and usually causes itching. Treatment is primarily preventive by not overdressing, especially in warm weather. C. *albicans* is the causative agent for thrush and some cases of diaper rash. It appears as a white coating in the child's mouth and is treated with nystatin.

➤ Acne vulgaris is caused by a variety of factors, including increased hormonal levels, hereditary factors, irritation and irritating substances, and growth of anaerobic bacteria. Treatment for mild acne is

application of a topical medication, such as benzoyl peroxide (Clearasil, Benoxyl) and tretinoin (Retin-A), once or twice a day. Antibiotics, such as erythromycin and tetracycline, may be administered for inflammatory acne. Isotretinoin (Accutane) may be used for severe inflammatory acne.

➤ Tinea (ringworm) is the term commonly applied to fungal infections. These occur in various parts of the body and are treated by antifungal medications.

➤ Pediculosis of the scalp is treated using nonprescription medications such as Pronto, RID, A-200, and permethrin (Nix). After the hair is shampooed thoroughly and dried, it is combed with a fine-toothed comb dipped in warm white vinegar to remove remaining nits and nit shells. For protection when treating a child in the hospital, wear a disposable gown, gloves, and head cover. Scabies is a skin infestation and is treated with permethrin cream (Elimite) or lindane lotion.

➤ Hyposensitization is performed for the allergens that produce a positive reaction on skin testing. The allergist sets up a schedule for injections in gradually increasing doses until a maintenance dose is reached.

➤ Atopic dermatitis or infantile eczema is considered, at least in part, an allergic reaction to an irritant. Common allergens involved in eczema are foods, inhalants, and materials. Goals when caring for the child include preserving skin integrity, maintaining comfort, improving sleep patterns, maintaining good nutrition, and preventing infection of skin lesions.

➤ Skin and plant allergies resulting in rashes are usually treated with topical preparations, such as lotions or ointments; antihistamines; and cool soaks to reduce the itching and swelling. In severe cases, oral corticosteroids may be used. If the allergen can be identified, preventing the allergic reaction by avoiding or removing it from the child's environment is the best treatment.

➤ All animal and human bites should be thoroughly cleaned and observed for signs of infection. Spider bites can cause serious illness if untreated. Tick bites can be prevented by wearing long pants, long-sleeved shirts, and using insect repellent when walking in the woods. Snakebites demand immediate medical intervention. Insect stings or bites can prove fatal to children who are sensitized, so immediate treatment is required if a child with sensitivity is bitten.

➤ Superficial or first-degree burns occur when the epidermis is injured but there is no destruction of tissue or nerve endings. Partial-thickness or second-degree burns occur when the epidermis and underlying dermis are both injured and devitalized or destroyed. Blistering usually occurs, as does an escape of body plasma. With full-thickness or third-degree burns, the epidermis, dermis, and nerve endings are all destroyed. Pain is minimal, and there is no longer any barrier to infection or any remaining viable epithelial cells.

➤ Emergency treatment for burns involving small areas is the immediate application of cool compresses or cool water to burn areas to inhibit capillary permeability and thus suppress edema, blister formation, and tissue destruction. For moderate burns, immersing a burned extremity in cool water alleviates pain and may prevent additional thermal injury. In severe burns, the airway, breathing, and circulation must be observed and restored if necessary and the child transported to a medical facility for assessment. Hypovolemic shock is the major manifestation in the first 48 hours in massive burns. As extracellular fluid pours into the burned area, it collects in enormous quantities, which dehydrates the body and causes the symptoms of shock to occur.

➤ Major causes of burns in children include hot liquids, fire, and electricity.

Nursing care for the child with a burn focuses on preventing infection, maintaining adequate nutrition, reducing pain, increasing mobility, and relieving anxiety as well as optimizing healing and decreasing complications to minimize permanent disability.

➤ Gonorrhea is caused by the organism *Neisseria gonorrhoeae*. Chlamydia is caused by *Chlamydia trachomatis*. Genital herpes is caused by herpes simplex type 2. Syphilis is caused by *Treponema pallidum*.

➤ The drug of choice to treat gonorrhea is ceftriaxone (Rocephin) followed by a week of oral doxycycline (Vibramycin) to prevent an accompanying chlamydial infection. Doxycycline or azithromycin is used to treat chlamydial infection. Acyclovir (Zovirax) is useful in relieving or suppressing the symptoms of genital herpes. Syphilis responds to one intramuscular injection of penicillin G benzathine; if the individual is sensitive to penicillin, oral doxycycline, tetracycline, or erythromycin can be administered.

➤ The human immunodeficiency virus (HIV) is transmitted by contact with infected blood or sexual contact with an infected person. Nursing care focuses on maintaining the highest level of wellness possible by preventing infection and the spread of the infection, maintaining skin integrity, minimizing pain, improving nutrition, alleviating social isolation, and diminishing a feeling of hopelessness.

➤ Infectious mononucleosis ("mono") is caused by the Epstein-Barr virus, which is one of the herpes virus groups. The organism is transmitted through saliva and treatment is symptomatic.

➤ Modes of transmission of communicable diseases include droplet, direct or indirect contact with body fluids and discharges, and contaminated blood, food, or water. Many communicable diseases can be prevented by immunization with vaccinations and the use of standard precautions.

➤ Active immunity occurs when antibodies are formed after immunization with a vaccine. Natural immunity often is genetically determined and gives a person a resistance to a pathogen. Passive immunity occurs when a person who has been exposed to a certain disease is given antibodies that have been obtained from an immune person.

➤ Nursing interventions for the child with a communicable disease are usually supportive. Depending on the disease symptoms, the implementations might include providing rest, adequate nutrition and fluids, following standard precautions, giving medications as appropriate, and offering comfort measures.

INTERNET RESOURCES

Burns
www.ameriburn.org

Sexually Transmitted Infections
www.ashastd.org

Workbook

■ NCLEX-STYLE REVIEW QUESTIONS

1. In caring for a 3.5-year-old child admitted after being severely burned, the nurse collects the following data. Which of the following would be *most* important for the nurse to report immediately?

   a. The child's respiratory rate is 32 breaths a minute.
   b. The child's temperature is 38.4°C.
   c. The child's hourly urinary output is 150 cc.
   d. The child's pain level is an 8 on the pain scale.

2. The nurse is discussing sexually transmitted infections with a group of adolescents. If the adolescents make the following statements, which statement indicates a need for further teaching?

   a. "Even though guys don't like to use condoms, at least they protect a person from most STIs."
   b. "My girlfriend has never had sex with anyone except me, so I don't have to worry about STIs."
   c. "It is a relief to know that other than HIV, most STIs can be treated with antibiotics."
   d. "My girlfriend is pregnant, but since she does not have an STI, our baby most likely won't either."

3. In caring for a child with atopic dermatitis (infantile eczema), which of the following nursing interventions would be included in this child's care? Select all that apply.

   a. The nurse will keep child's fingernails cut short.
   b. The nurse will dress the child in several layers of clothing at all times.
   c. The nurse will monitor for symptoms of infection.
   d. The nurse will give soothing baths just before bedtime.
   e. The nurse will encourage the child to drink fluids frequently.
   f. The nurse will use a bleach solution to launder the child's clothing.

4. After an outbreak of pediculosis in the school, the nurse is doing teaching with a group of parents and teachers about ways to help prevent the spread of head lice in the classroom and at home. Which of the following actions would the nurse recommend to this group? Select all that apply.

   a. Wash all bedding and clothing in hot water and dry in a hot dryer.
   b. Apply medicated lotion to all areas of the body except the face.
   c. Wash combs and brushes in medicated shampoo and soak for at least an hour.
   d. Report any evidence of infestation immediately to the school officials.
   e. Vacuum carpets, car seats, mattresses, and upholstered furniture thoroughly.
   f. Wear gloves when preparing food or snacks.

■ STUDY ACTIVITIES

1. Using the table below, compare the five most common sexually transmitted infections (STIs) seen in adolescents. Describe the symptoms, treatment, and complications or long-term concerns seen with these diseases.

Sexually Transmitted Infection (STI)	Symptoms	Treatment	Complications or Long-term Concerns

2. Using the table below, make a list of substances that may cause allergies in infants and children. List some sources of these substances that may cause allergies.

Substance That May Cause Allergies	Sources of Substances That May Cause Allergies

3. Identify the relation between *Candida albicans* and some cases of diaper rash. Detail the teaching that you would provide for a mother about diaper rash.

4. Go to the following Internet site: www.cooltheburn.com

   Click on "Learn about burns." Click on "The Burn Center." Click on "Bandages."

   a. How could you use this site to help explain a dressing change to a child with a burn?

      Hit the back arrow two times and Click on "Stories"

   b. How could you use these stories in teaching children about burns?

■ CRITICAL THINKING: WHAT WOULD YOU DO?

1. Brian is HIV positive and lives with his family. The family is frightened that other members may get the virus.

   a. What will you tell the family to reassure them?
   b. What will you teach them in regard to prevention of the spread of the virus in their home?
   c. What guidelines will you give the family caregivers to help them protect Brian from infectious or opportunistic diseases?

2. Two-year-old Omar has partial- and full-thickness burns from a wood stove accident. You are helping develop a teaching plan covering the importance of infection control for Omar during his convalescence.

   a. What is the most important action that can be taken to prevent infection?

   b. Who should be included in teaching regarding infection control?
   c. What are signs that might indicate an infection?
   d. Why is it important to detect signs and symptoms of an infection early?

3. Dosage calculation: An adolescent with a diagnosis of gonorrhea is being treated with Rocephin. The dose to be given is 250 mg IM. The medication is available in a preparation of l g/10 mL. Answer the following:

   a. How many milligrams (mg) are in 1 g?
   b. How many milliliters will be given in this 250 mg dose to this adolescent?

After the administration of the Rocephin, the adolescent will be given doxycycline 100 mg BID by mouth for 7 days. Answer the following:

   c. How many milligrams (mg) will be given in a 24-hour period?
   d. How many total milligrams (mg) will be given in the 7 days?

42 The Child With a Psychosocial Disorder

KEY TERMS

anorexia nervosa
bulimia nervosa
dependence
echolalia
encopresis
gynecomastia
obesity
overweight
polyphagia
rumination
substance abuse
tolerance
withdrawal symptoms

LEARNING OBJECTIVES

On completion of this chapter, you should be able to:

1. Describe autism including the diagnosis, characteristics, goals of treatment, and nursing care.
2. Identify characteristics that may be seen in a child with attention deficit hyperactivity disorder (ADHD) and discuss the treatment of the disorder.
3. Differentiate enuresis and encopresis.
4. State the cause of the symptoms seen in children with school phobia.
5. Discuss the warning signs seen in children who are considering suicide.
6. List substances commonly abused by children.
7. State the negative effects of commonly abused substances.
8. Describe the characteristics, treatment, and nursing care of the child with nonorganic failure to thrive (NFTT).
9. Discuss the characteristics and signs and symptoms seen in the child with anorexia, and state goals of treatment for the hospitalized anorexic patient.
10. Describe the signs and symptoms and nursing care for the child with bulimia.
11. Discuss obesity and the goal of health care professionals who work with obese children.

AUTISM

Although often called infantile autism because it is thought to be present from birth, autism usually is not conclusively diagnosed until after 12 months of age. The word *autism* comes from the Greek word *auto* meaning "self" and was first used by Dr. Leo Kanner in 1943 to describe a group of behavioral symptoms in children. The term *pervasive developmental disorder* was introduced in 1980 when the American Psychiatric Association revised the terminology. Disorders in this category are characterized by severe behavioral disturbance that affects the practical use of language as a means of communication, interpersonal interaction, attention, perception, and motor activity. Autistic children are totally self-centered and unable to relate to others; they often exhibit bizarre behaviors and often are destructive to themselves and others.

Autism occurs in about 2 to 5 of 10,000 births and four times as often in males as in females. Several theories exist about its cause, as well as its treatment or management. Originally thought to result from an unsatisfactory early mother–child relationship (with emotionally cold, detached mothers sometimes described as "refrigerator mothers"), autism now appears to have organic and perhaps genetic causes instead. Researchers suggest that autism may result from a disturbance in language comprehension, a biochemical problem involving neurotransmitters or abnormalities in the central nervous system, and probably brain metabolism. These children score poorly on intelligence tests but may have good memories and good intellectual potential.

Because the cause of autism is not understood, treatment attempts have had limited success. Autistic children experience the normal health problems of childhood in addition to those that result from their behaviors. Therefore, it is important that you understand this unexplained disorder and how it affects children and families.

Clinical Manifestations

The characteristics of autism are divided into three categories: inability to relate to others, inability to communicate with others, and obviously limited activities and interests. Children with autism do not develop a

937

smiling response to others or an interest in being touched or cuddled. In fact, they can react violently to attempts to hold them. Their blank expressions and lack of response to verbal stimulation can suggest deafness. They do not show the normal fear of separation from parents that most toddlers exhibit. Often they seem not to notice when family caregivers are present.

During their second year, autistic children become completely absorbed in strange repetitive behaviors such as spinning an object, flipping an electrical switch on and off, or walking around the room feeling the walls. Their bodily movements are bizarre: rocking, twirling, flapping arms and hands, walking on tiptoe, and twisting and turning fingers. If these movements are interrupted or if objects in the environment are moved, a violent temper tantrum may result. These tantrums may include self-destructive acts, such as hand biting and head banging. Although infants and toddlers normally are self-centered, ritualistic, and prone to displays of temper, autistic children show these characteristics to an extreme degree coupled with an almost total lack of response to other people.

> **Think about this.**
> Although autistic children are self-centered, their speech indicates that they seem to have no sense of self because they are unlikely to use the pronouns "I" or "me."

The autistic child is slow to develop speech and any speech that develops is primitive and ineffective in its ability to communicate. **Echolalia** ("parrot speech") is typical of autistic children; they echo words they have heard, such as a television commercial, but offer no indication that they understand the words.

Standard intelligence tests that count on verbal ability usually indicate that these children test in the mentally retarded range of intelligence. However, many of these children also demonstrate unusual memory and mathematic, artistic, and musical abilities.

Diagnosis

To confirm a diagnosis of autism, at least 8 of 16 identified characteristics must be present, and all three categories of characteristics must be represented. The symptoms of autism can suggest other disorders such as lead poisoning, phenylketonuria, congenital rubella, and measles encephalitis. Therefore, a complete pediatric physical and neurologic examination is necessary, including vision and hearing testing, electroencephalography, radiographic studies of the skull, urine screening, and other laboratory studies. In addition, a complete prenatal, natal, and postnatal history, including development, nutrition, and family dynamics, is taken. Other members of the health team may be involved in the evaluation and treatment of the autistic child, including audiologists, psychiatrists, psychologists, special education teachers, speech and language therapists, and social workers.

Treatment

The treatment of an autistic child is extremely challenging. The child is mentally retarded, but may demonstrate exceptional talent in areas, such as factual memory and art or music. Treatment focuses on four goals:

- Promotion of normal development
- Specific language development
- Social interaction
- Learning

Behavioral modification, pharmacotherapeutics, and other techniques are used. These treatments must be individually planned and highly structured. Mixed results occur, and no one technique has met with resounding success. The family needs therapy to help relieve guilt and help them understand this puzzling child. The overall long-term prognosis for these children is not optimistic; however, the long-term outlook is better the earlier treatment is started. Facilitated communication involves helping autistic children express themselves in language through use of a computer keyboard. However, this method of promoting language development is controversial and is not totally supported by the American Psychological Association.

Nursing Care

Caring for the autistic child requires recognizing that autism creates great stresses for the entire family. The problems that cause family caregivers to seek diagnosis are difficult to live with; diagnosis itself is usually a lengthy and expensive process, and the hope for successful treatment is slight. Most caregivers of autistic children feel guilty, despite the fact that current theories accept organic, rather than psychological, causes for this disorder. The possibility of genetic factors adds to this guilt. Often other children in the family who are normal suffer from a lack of attention because the caregivers' energies are almost totally directed to solving the autistic child's problems.

Family caregivers are your most valuable source of information about the autistic child's habits and communication skills. To gain the child's cooperation, learn which techniques the caregivers use to communicate with the child. It is essential to establish a relationship of trust with the child. To provide consistency, this child should be cared for by a constant primary nurse.

In the hospital setting, a private or semiprivate room is generally preferred; visual and auditory stimulation should be minimized. Familiar toys or other valued objects from home reduce the child's anxiety about the strange environment.

> *Test Yourself*
> ✔ Into what three categories are the characteristics of autism divided?
> ✔ When a child with autism is said to have echolalia, what does this mean?
> ✔ Explain the goals in the treatment of autism.

ATTENTION DEFICIT HYPERACTIVITY DISORDER

Attention deficit hyperactivity disorder (ADHD), or attention deficit disorder (ADD), is a syndrome characterized by degrees of inattention, impulsive behavior, and hyperactivity. About 3% to 5% of all American school-aged children have ADHD; boys are more commonly affected than are girls. The cause of the disorder is unclear: Developmental lag, biochemical disorder, and food sensitivities are all theories under consideration. The disorder affects every part of the child's life.

Clinical Manifestations

The child with ADHD may have these characteristics:

- Impulsiveness
- Easy distractibility
- Frequent fidgeting or squirming
- Difficulty sitting still
- Problems following through on instructions, despite being able to understand them
- Inattentiveness when being spoken to
- Frequent losing of things
- Going from one uncompleted activity to another
- Difficulty taking turns
- Frequent excessive talking
- Engaging in dangerous activities without considering the consequences

These children also often demonstrate signs of clumsiness or poor coordination, such as the inability to use a pencil or scissors in a child who is older than 3 or 4 years of age. No one child has all these symptoms. Although it was believed that these symptoms were resolved by late adolescence, it is now apparent that they continue into adulthood, at least for some people.

Although these children may have poor success in the classroom because of their inability to pay attention, they are not intellectually impaired. The child's poor impulse control also contributes to disciplinary problems in the classroom. Some children with ADHD may have learning disorders, such as dyslexia and perceptual deficits. The child's self-confidence can suffer from feeling inferior to the other children in the class. Special arrangements can be made to provide an educational atmosphere that is supportive for the child without the need for the child to leave the classroom.

Diagnosis

Diagnosis can be made after the child is 3 years of age, but often is not made until the child reaches school age and has trouble settling into the routine of being in the classroom setting. Diagnosis can be difficult and also may be controversial because many of the symptoms are subjective and rely on the assessment of caregivers and teachers. Some authorities have expressed concern that teachers incorrectly label children as hyperactive. The symptoms may be a result of environmental factors that can include broken homes, stress, and nonsupportive caregivers.

The multidisciplinary approach is most effective for diagnosis, that is, one involving pediatric and education specialists, a psychologist, the classroom teacher, family caregivers, and others. A careful detailed history, including school and social functioning, psychological testing, and physical and neurologic examinations, can help in making the diagnosis.

Treatment and Nursing Care

Treatment is also multidisciplinary. Learning situations should be structured so that the child has minimal distractions and a supportive teacher. Home support is necessary and requires structured, consistent guidance from the caregivers. Medication is used for some children. Stimulant medications, such as methylphenidate (Ritalin, Concerta) and dextroamphetamine (Dexedrine), have often been used. When given in large amounts, these medications may suppress the appetite and affect the child's growth. Pemoline (Cylert) has been used but generally with less success than methylphenidate and dextroamphetamine. Using stimulants for a hyperactive child seems paradoxical, but these drugs apparently stimulate the area of the child's brain that aids in concentration, thus enabling the child to have better control.

Maintain a calm, patient attitude toward the child with ADHD. The child should be given only one simple instruction at a time. Limiting distractions, using consistency, and offering praise for accomplishments are invaluable methods of working with these children. The families of children with ADHD need a great deal of support. Primary family caregivers in particular can become frustrated and upset by the constant challenge of dealing with a child with ADHD. Building the child's self-esteem, confidence, and academic success must be the primary goal of all who work with these children.

 A Personal Glimpse

I don't really mind it. When I don't take my meds. I go crazy or bonkers (sometimes). I'm on my pills cause of my behavior. And also to control the ways I talk (like so I won't blurt out in class). I was taught to control my actions, don't let my actions control me.

Eddie, a 9-year-old who takes medication for ADHD.

Learning Opportunity: What feelings do you think this child experiences in those times when he is not able to control his behavior? What would you say to this child to encourage him to talk about his disorder and his feelings?

ENURESIS AND ENCOPRESIS

Enuresis, or bed-wetting, is involuntary urination beyond the age when control of urination commonly is acquired. Enuresis may have a physiologic or psychological cause and may indicate a need for further exploration and treatment (see Chapter 39 for further discussion).

Encopresis is chronic involuntary fecal soiling beyond the age when control is expected (about 3 years of age). Speech and learning disabilities may accompany this problem. If no organic causes (e.g., worms, megacolon) exist, encopresis indicates a serious emotional problem and a need for counseling for the child and the family caregivers. Some experts believe that over control or under control by a caregiver can cause encopresis. Recommendations for treatment differ; however, the most important goal is recognition of the problem and referral for treatment and counseling.

SCHOOL PHOBIA

School absenteeism is a national problem. Children are absent from school for a variety of reasons, one of which may be school phobia. Children who develop school phobia may be good students, with girls affected more often than boys. Teachers and nurses can help detect school phobia by paying close attention to absence patterns.

Clinical Manifestations

School-phobic children may have a strong attachment to one parent, usually the mother, and they fear separation from that parent, perhaps because of anxiety about losing her or him while away from home. School phobia may be the child's unconscious reaction to a seemingly overwhelming problem at school. The parent can unwittingly reinforce school phobia by permitting the child to stay home. The symptoms—vomiting, diarrhea, abdominal or other pain, and even a low-grade fever—are genuine and are caused by anxiety that may approach panic. They disappear with relief of the immediate anxiety after the child has been given permission to stay home.

Treatment and Nursing Care

Treatment includes a complete medical examination to rule out any organic cause for the symptoms and school–family conferences to help the child return to school. It is important to realize that these children are not delinquents; they really do want to go to school but for whatever reason cannot make themselves go. The school nurse and teacher along with other professionals, such as a social worker, psychologist, or psychiatrist, all may contribute to resolving the problem. If the child fears a specific factor at school, such as an overly critical teacher, the child may need to be moved to another class or school.

SUICIDE

Suicide is one of the leading causes of death in children 10 to 19 years of age, falling just short of the death rate for homicide. Because some deaths reported as accidents, particularly one-car accidents, are thought to be suicides, the rate actually may be higher. Adolescent males commit suicide four times more often than girls do, but girls attempt suicide five times more often than boys do. Boys use more violent means of committing suicide than girls do and thus are successful more often.

Children who have attempted suicide once have a high risk of attempting it again, perhaps more effectively. Attempted suicide rarely occurs without warning and usually is preceded by a long history of emotional problems, difficulty forming relationships, feelings of rejection, and low self-esteem. Loss of one or both parents through death or divorce, a family history that includes suicide of one or more members, and lack of success in academic or athletic performance are other common contributing factors. To this history is added one or more of the normal developmental crises of adolescence:

- Difficulty establishing independence
- Identity crisis
- Lack of intimate relationships
- Breakdown in family communication
- A sense of alienation
- A conflict that interferes with problem solving

The child's situation may be further complicated by an unwanted or unplanned pregnancy, alcohol or drug addiction, or physical or sexual abuse that leads to depression and a feeling of total hopelessness.

Clinical Manifestations

Health professionals involved with children and family caregivers must be aware of factors that place a child at risk for suicide, as well as hints that signal an impending suicide attempt (see Family Teaching Tips: Suicide Warning Signs for Caregivers). Some of these desperate young people will verbalize their hopelessness with statements such as "I won't be around much longer" or "After Monday, it won't matter anyhow." They may begin giving away prized possessions or appear suddenly elated after a long period of acting dejected.

Never, never!

Don't ignore behaviors or statements of hopelessness in children and teenagers. Make an effort to ensure the child's safety until counseling and treatment resources are in place.

Cultural Snapshot

Depression and other psychological concerns in some cultures may be disregarded or not expressed because of the fear of social stigma or shame. A confidential and compassionate approach by the nurse may encourage the child to express his or her feelings or the family to share the worry they have about symptoms in their child.

Family Teaching Tips

SUICIDE WARNING SIGNS FOR CAREGIVERS

WARNING SIGNS IN CHILDREN'S BEHAVIOR

- Previous suicide attempt
- Thoughts of wishing to kill self
- Plans for self-destructive acts
- Feeling "down in the dumps"
- Withdrawal from social activities
- Loss of pleasure in daily activities
- Change in activity—increase or decrease
- Poor concentration
- Complaints of headaches, upset stomach, joint pains, frequent colds
- Change in eating or sleeping patterns
- Strong feelings of guilt, inadequacy, hopelessness
- Preoccupation with thoughts of people dying, getting sick, or being injured
- Substance abuse
- Violence, truancy, stealing, or lying
- Lack of judgment
- Poor impulse control
- Rapid swing in appropriateness of expressed emotions, sudden lift in mood
- Pessimistic view of self and world
- Saying goodbye
- Giving things away

CHANGES IN CHILD'S INTERPERSONAL RELATIONSHIPS

- Conflicts with peers
- Loss of boyfriend or girlfriend
- School problems—behavioral or academic
- Feelings of great frustration, being misunderstood, or not being part of the group
- Lack of positive support from family, peers, or other
- Earlier suicide of family member, friend, or classmate
- Separations, deaths, births, moves, or serious illnesses in the family

During the initial interview with the child, include questions that draw out feelings of alienation, depression, and hopelessness. If any of these indications are present, report and document these findings immediately. Question the family caregiver about any such signs and follow through with seeking additional help for the child.

Treatment and Nursing Care

It is important that counseling and treatment resources be found to help these children. Strive to help the child understand that although suicide is an option in problem solving, it is a final option, and other options exist that are not so final. Be aware of the community resources such as hotlines and counselors that specialize in working with persons who are contemplating or have attempted suicide.

Test Yourself

- ✔ What characteristics are seen in the child with ADHD?
- ✔ How is ADHD treated?
- ✔ What warning signs are often seen in children who are contemplating committing suicide?

SUBSTANCE ABUSE

Substance abuse is the misuse of an addictive substance that changes the user's mental state. The addictive substances commonly abused are tobacco, alcohol, and controlled or illicit drugs. Children are influenced by peers and in some instances adults in their family use drugs and alcohol to avoid facing their problems, escape and forget the pain of life as they see it, add excitement to social events, or bow to peer pressure. Throughout history, people have used alcohol and other mood-altering drugs as a means of relieving the tensions and pressures of their lives. Many cultures still sanction use of some of these substances but object to their abuse (i.e., excessive use or use in a way that is medically, socially, or culturally unacceptable).

Unfortunately, frequent use or abuse of these substances can lead to addiction or **dependence** (a compulsive need to use a substance for its satisfying or pleasurable effects). Dependence may be psychological, physical, or both. Psychological dependence means that the substance is desired for the effects or sensations it produces: alertness, euphoria, relaxation, a sense of well-being, and a false sense of control over problems. Physical dependence results from drug-induced changes in body tissue functions that require the drug for normal activity. The magnitude of physical dependence determines the severity of **withdrawal symptoms** (physical and psychological symptoms that occur when the drug is no longer being used) such as vomiting, chills, tremors, and hallucinations. The symptoms vary with the amount, type, frequency, and duration of drug use. Continued use of an addictive substance can result in **tolerance** (the ability of body tissues to endure and adapt to continued or increased use of a substance); this dynamic means the drug user requires larger doses of the drug to produce the desired effect.

Four stages of use have been identified that help describe the progression of substance abuse (Table 42-1). Use the clues from these stages when you are working in any capacity with children in order to be more alert to signs of possible substance abuse.

The children at greatest risk of becoming substance abusers are those who:

- Have families in which alcohol or drug abuse is or has been present

Table 42-1 ▌ PROGRESSION OF SUBSTANCE ABUSE IN CHILDREN

Stage	Predisposition	Behavior	Family Reaction
Stage 1. Experimentation, Learning the Mood Swing			
Infrequent use of alcohol/ marijuana	Curiosity	Learning the mood	Often unaware
No consequences	Peer pressure	Feels good	Denial
Some fear of use	Attempt to assume adult role	Positive reinforcement	
Low tolerance		Can return to normal	
Stage 2. Seeking the Mood Swing			
Increasing frequency in use of various drugs	Impress others	Using to get high	Attempts at elimination
Minimal defensiveness	Social function	Pride in amount consumed	Blaming others
Tolerance	Modeling adult behavior	Using to relieve feelings (i.e., anxieties of dating)	
		Denial of problem	
Stage 3. Preoccupation With the Mood Swing			
Peer group activities revolve around use	Using to get loaded, not just high	Begins to violate values and rules	Conspiracy of silence
Steady supply		Use before and during school	Confrontation
Possible dealing		Use despite consequences	Reorganization with or without affected person
Few or no straight friends		Solitary use	
Consequences frequent		Trouble with school	
		Overdoses, "bad trips," blackouts	
		Promises to cut down or attempts to quit	
		Protection of supply, hides use from peers	
		Deterioration in physical condition	
Stage 4. Using to Feel Normal			
Continue to use despite adverse outcomes	Use to feel normal	Daily use	Frustration
Loss of control		Failure to meet expectations	Anger
Inability to stop		Loss of control	May give up
Compulsion		Paranoia	
		Suicide gestures, self-hate	
		Physical deterioration (poor eating and sleep habits)	

Adger, H. (1999). Adolescent drug abuse. In J. A. McMillan, C. D. DeAngelis, R. D. Feigin, & J. W. Warshaw (Eds.) *Oski's pediatrics: Principles and practice* (3rd ed.). Philadelphia: Lippincott Williams & Wilkins.

- Suffer from abuse, neglect, loss, or have no close relationships as a result of a dysfunctional family
- Have behavior problems, such as aggressiveness, or are excessively rebellious
- Are slow learners or have learning disabilities or attention deficit disorder
- Have problems with depression and low self-esteem

In some instances, early identification of these factors by family, teachers, counselors, or other caregivers and prompt referral for treatment can help avoid the potential tragedy of substance abuse.

Prevention and Treatment

The most effective and least expensive treatment for substance abuse is prevention, beginning with education in the early school years. Information about drugs and about how to cope with problems without using drugs should be provided.

Educational programs may have less impact if the child comes from a home where alcohol or other drugs are used by family caregivers.

When prevention is ineffective, emergency care and long-term treatment become necessary. An overdose or a "bad trip" may force the child to seek treatment. Emergency measures may even

Balance is the order of the day.

"Scare" techniques are completely ineffective in trying to persuade children to refrain from using substances. These techniques arouse disbelief and often add the tempting thrill of danger.

require artificial ventilation and oxygenation to restore normal respiration.

Long-term treatment involves many health professionals such as psychiatric nurses, psychologists or psychiatrists, social workers, drug rehabilitation counselors, and community health nurses. The child is an important member of the treatment team and must admit the problem and the need for help and be willing to take an active part in treatment. Both outpatient and inpatient treatment programs are available. Many of these programs are geared specifically to adolescents. The human services section of the local telephone directory provides specific listings. The earlier the child can be identified and treatment begun, the better the prognosis (see Family Teaching Tips: Resources for Information and Help With Drug and Alcohol Problems).

ALCOHOL ABUSE

In many parts of American culture, drinking alcoholic beverages is considered acceptable and desirable social behavior. Although the purchase of alcohol is legally restricted to adults 21 years of age and older in all states and the District of Columbia, alcohol is available in many homes and consequently is the first drug most children try. It is also the most commonly abused drug among children and adolescents. Alcohol abuse occurs when a person ingests a quantity sufficient to cause intoxication (drunkenness). Alcoholism (chronic alcohol abuse or dependence) has reached epidemic proportions in America.

Drinking often begins in the preadolescent years and increases in frequency throughout adolescence. Some children use alcohol in combination with marijuana and other drugs, potentiating the effects of both substances and increasing the probability of intoxication.

Alcoholism is costly in dollars and in damage to the lives of alcohol abusers and their families. During adolescence, alcohol abuse is closely linked to automobile accidents. A car is another symbol of adult status and a means to escape adult supervision. Drinking with friends before or while driving often has tragic results. Most states determine charges of driving under the influence using a standard of 0.1% blood alcohol content. However, many states have lowered the limit to 0.08%. Many children do not realize that fine motor control and judgment are affected at even lower levels, and driving ability may be decreased. Although the number of fatal alcohol-related accidents involving children has decreased because all states have set 21 years as the legal age for drinking, the fatality rate remains high.

Children and adolescents who receive treatment and counseling for problem drinking are more likely to recover than are adults who have been problem drinkers for a long time. However, children, especially adolescents, are difficult to treat because of their feelings of immortality and the rapid progression of the disease in adolescents.

Alcoholism is not a weakness of character but a major chronic, progressive, and potentially fatal disease

process that affects every organ of the body, mental health, and social competence. Alcoholism tendencies appear to be inherited, so children with a family history of alcoholism may be prone to problems with alcohol. Treatment is lengthy and expensive and has no chance of success until the alcoholic acknowledges the problem and his or her helplessness to deal with it.

Treatment begins with detoxification ("drying out") and management of withdrawal symptoms. After that, a well-balanced diet, high-potency vitamins (especially vitamin B), and plenty of rest help to eliminate the disease's harmful side effects.

Counseling to identify and address the problems that led to compulsive drinking is an essential part of treatment. Many counselors who work with alcoholic patients are people who are recovering from a drinking problem themselves. This experience gives the counselor additional insight and empathy for the problem and the victim and adds credibility to the counseling offered.

Alcoholics Anonymous (AA), the best known of all self-help groups, offers fellowship and understanding to the compulsive drinker (web site: www.aa.org). Chapters are available in every sizable community and many have special programs for children, as well as for families of alcoholics (Alateen, Al-Anon, ACA—Adult Children of Alcoholics). Anyone who has a desire to stop drinking is welcomed into AA and is helped to stay sober by taking it "one day at a time." Recovery from alcoholism is a lifetime matter. The earlier the problem is diagnosed, the better the person's chances to respond to treatment. Ongoing support from health professionals, peers, family, and community is essential to successful treatment.

TOBACCO ABUSE

Tobacco is a commonly abused drug among preadolescents and adolescents. Any use of tobacco is abuse. A high percentage of young people try tobacco, by smoking or chewing. Many children smoke because it gives them a feeling of maturity. Threats of long-term physical illnesses are far enough in the future that the child tends to ignore them. Many elementary and secondary schools have developed programs that warn children of the dangers of smoking, but the danger seems distant, and children believe that they can quit any time they want to quit. The more immediate result of smoking that may stir interest in adolescents is the fact that their hair, breath, and clothes smell bad.

Adolescents also have strong feelings of fairness and justice, so they may respond to the fact that children who are around persons who smoke are at increased risk for respiratory illness and cancer.

The use of "smokeless tobacco" (snuff or chewing tobacco) has increased steadily among adolescent males in the last several years. These children believe that they are not damaging their lungs. However, this type of tobacco use can cause mouth, lip, and throat cancers that are disfiguring and life threatening.

Children whose family caregivers smoke are at increased risk for smoking. They have difficulty accepting that they are seriously endangering themselves by smoking. Most hospitals, schools, and public buildings have adopted no-smoking policies. Perhaps the pressure of society will help deter smoking in the future. There is an effort at the federal level to discourage children and adolescents from beginning to smoke, but children do not seem to be responding to the warnings. This may be attributable in part to the previously mentioned attitude among adolescents that nothing can hurt them.

MARIJUANA ABUSE

The most frequently used illicit drug among adolescents is marijuana. The reported use of marijuana among children has decreased somewhat, but smoking marijuana at a younger age appears to be a current trend. Many children believe that marijuana smoking is not risky.

The effects of marijuana are mostly behavioral. It affects judgment, sense of time, and motivation. These effects make driving hazardous and may even cause hallucinations at higher doses. In addition, marijuana smoke is three to five times more carcinogenic than cigarette smoke. The marijuana available today may be three to five times more potent than that smoked in the 1960s. Because marijuana is illegal, no manufacturing control over it exists, and the user has no idea where it came from or what additives may have been used. As a nurse, you must make every effort to inform children about the dangers of marijuana and discourage them from using it.

COCAINE ABUSE

Although cocaine may not rank among the first three drugs most commonly used by children, it is an extremely dangerous drug. Use of cocaine and its derivative, "crack," can be found everywhere from inner cities to rural neighborhoods.

Cocaine is a fine, white, powdery substance that directly affects the brain cells and causes physical and psychological effects. It usually is inhaled or smoked and is absorbed through the mucous membranes into the bloodstream. The physical results are an increase in pulse, respirations, blood pressure, and temperature. The psychological effect is a feeling of euphoria and increased sociability. The high is reached in about 20 minutes and lasts 20 to 30 minutes. In contrast, crack enters the bloodstream in about 30 seconds with a fast and powerful but short high that lasts only about 5 minutes. As a result of the rapid, short high from crack, users tend to seek repeated highs over a short period, decreasing the time it takes to become addicted. Because of the rapid absorption of crack, immediate cardiac arrest can occur from its use. After smoking crack, the user may experience a "crash" that causes depression. To relieve this depression, crack users turn to alcohol and marijuana. This multiple use further complicates the drug's effects. Some cocaine users inject cocaine to obtain a faster high, which adds to their risk of contracting HIV from contaminated needles.

It is important to stress to children the danger of using cocaine and crack. School education programs should start at the elementary level. You can perform a community service by

This is important.
A drug education program should include activities that help the students increase their feeling of self-worth.

volunteering to present programs to local schoolchildren. Children and adolescents must be alerted to the dangers of these drugs and be taught ways to refuse offers of drugs.

NARCOTIC ABUSE

The most commonly abused narcotics are morphine and heroin. These drugs decrease anger, sex drive, and hunger by producing a dreamlike, euphoric state. Narcotics are highly addictive and extremely expensive, and narcotic abuse results in teenage prostitution, pushing (selling) drugs, and robbery as a means to support the drug habit. As mentioned, any drugs that are injected subject adolescents to the added risk of contracting HIV from using contaminated needles.

Although heroin use in actual numbers is lower than that of other illicit drugs, adolescents' use of heroin has increased because of several factors. In general, there is a decrease among children in the perceived danger of drug use. This trend seems to be evident across the entire scope of illicit drug use. Because heroin is now available in forms that can be smoked or snorted, the threat of HIV infection is no longer a deterrent.

OTHER ABUSED DRUGS

Other mood-altering drugs commonly abused by children include hallucinogens (psychedelic drugs), depressants, amphetamines, and analgesics. Anabolic steroids, although not mood altering, are also abused by adolescents.

Hallucinogens (psychedelic drugs), although not addictive in a physical sense, can create a psychological dependence from the resulting hallucinations. This category of drugs includes LSD, PCP ("angel dust"), psilocybin (derived from mushrooms), mescaline, DMT (derived from plants), and airplane glue. These drugs cause distortions in vision, smell, or hearing. Effects can include intoxication, "bad trips," and flashbacks, and overdoses are common.

The drug known as Ecstasy is similar to amphetamines in chemical makeup but has the effect of elevating mood and increasing tactile sensations similar to the use of hallucinogens. Use of Ecstasy has increased dramatically in the adolescent population. The drug releases large amounts of serotonin, the neurotransmitter that regulates mood and emotion. The drug is used in party and club settings, where the users dance and party for extended periods of time; the drug suppresses their needs to eat, drink, or sleep. The drug can cause increased heart rate and blood pressure, muscle tension, teeth clenching, nausea, blurred vision, chills, and sweating. The drug is harmful to the brain and can cause confusion, depression, and anxiety, even days and weeks after use.

Depressants, sometimes referred to as hypnotics, are as addictive as narcotics, and withdrawal from them must be carefully controlled to prevent delirium, seizures, or death. Barbiturates, glutethimide (Doriden), ethchlorvynol (Placidyl), and methaqualone (Quaalude) are the most commonly abused drugs in this group; they are sometimes used with alcohol, which increases the intoxicating effects such as sleepiness, slurred speech, and impaired cognitive and motor functions.

Amphetamines ("uppers" or "speed") produce increased alertness, wakefulness, reduced awareness of fatigue, and increased confidence and energy. Although not physically addicting, they encourage psychological dependence and are abused by millions of Americans, many of whom become trapped in a destructive cycle of uppers and "downers" (barbiturates). The amphetamines are often manufactured in methamphetamine ("meth") labs in people's homes, which increases the potential dangers to the child who uses these substances.

Children abuse analgesics, particularly those that are combinations of narcotic and nonnarcotics, such as Percocet and Darvon. Chronic abuse can result in blood and kidney disorders. These drugs may be prescribed to a family member, which makes them easy for the child to obtain.

Anabolic steroids are not mood-altering drugs, but their abuse among athletes is a cause for great concern. Adolescent athletes take anabolic steroids to build up muscle mass in the belief that the drug will increase their athletic ability. These athletes take megadoses of illegally obtained drugs. Other adolescents may take them to build muscles and to achieve a "manly" appearance that they believe will make them more attractive. The side effects of euphoria and decreased fatigue make these drugs even more inviting to adolescents. Some use also has been reported in high school female athletes.

The use of excessively large doses of steroids may cause **gynecomastia** (excessive development of mammary glands in the male) or premature fusion of the long bones, which stunts growth in the adolescent who has not yet completed growth. Liver damage, including liver tumors and cancer; predisposition to atherosclerosis; acne; hypertension; aggressiveness; and psychotic and manic symptoms also may result (National Institute of Drug Abuse Info-Facts: Steroids). School programs about drug abuse should include the topic of anabolic steroid abuse.

Test Yourself

✔ What are the reasons children use alcohol and other substances?

✔ Explain the difference between psychological and physical dependence in substance use.

✔ Name common substances children might use.

NONORGANIC FAILURE TO THRIVE

Four principal factors are necessary for human growth: food, rest and activity, adequate secretions of hormones, and a satisfactory relationship with a caregiver or nurturing person who provides consistent, loving human contact and stimulation. Growth is disturbed and development can be delayed when one of these four factors is missing, or when the infant has a major birth defect, such as congenital heart disease or a metabolic disorder.

Infants who fail to gain weight and who show signs of delayed development are classified as failure-to-thrive infants. Failure to thrive can be divided into two classifications: Organic failure to thrive, which is a result of a disease condition, and nonorganic failure to thrive (NFTT), which has no apparent physical cause. The section below discusses NFTT. Organic failure to thrive is covered under specific diseases, including congenital heart disease (Chapter 21), gastrointestinal reflux (Chapter 38), celiac syndrome (Chapter 38), and cystic fibrosis (Chapter 36).

Clinical Manifestations

Infants with NFTT often are listless and seriously below average weight and height, have poor muscle tone and a loss of subcutaneous fat, and are immobile for long periods of time (Fig. 42-1). They may be unresponsive to (or actually try to avoid) cuddling and vocalization. Examination of the child is likely to reveal no organic cause for this condition. However, examination of the family relationship, particularly the mother–child relationship, often provides important insights into the problem.

The family relationships of these children are often so disrupted that there is no warm, close relationship with a family caregiver. For some reason, proper attachment has not occurred. Often the father is absent or emotionally unavailable, adding to the mother's feelings of isolation and inadequacy and leading to an atmosphere of additional stress and conflict.

The problem is not with the caregiver alone or with the child but instead with their interaction and mutual lack of responsiveness. They are not in harmony. The caregiver does not stimulate the child; therefore, the child has no one to respond to and fails to do the "cute baby" things that would gain attention and stimulation. The child cannot accomplish the developmental task of establishing basic trust.

Children with NFTT often fall into the classification of "difficult" or irritable babies, but others may be listless and passive and do not seem to care about feedings. A common characteristic is **rumination** (voluntary regurgitation), perhaps as a means of self-satisfaction when the desired response is not received from the caregiver. When rumination occurs, a chain of events is activated that further strains the caregiver–child relationship. The child loses weight, sometimes becomes severely emaciated, grows listless and irritable, and smells "sour" because of frequent vomiting. None of this makes for an attractive baby to love, cuddle, and show off.

Diagnosis

The child must be thoroughly evaluated by the physician to rule out a systemic or congenital disorder. Signs of deprivation are important elements in the diagnosis. When the child begins to improve in a nurturing atmosphere, the diagnosis is confirmed.

Treatment

Treatment initially depends almost entirely on good nursing care. By teaching childcare skills, acting as a role model, and supporting caregiver–child interactions, you can help reverse the child's growth failure and begin an improved caregiver–child relationship.

Prognosis is uncertain; much depends on the support and counseling the family receives. Long-term care is almost certainly necessary and may require several members of the health care team such as a family therapist, clergy, social worker, and public health nurse. Avoid judgmental, stereotyped feelings when dealing with the family of such a child.

> **You can make a difference.**
> A positive, nonjudgmental attitude when working with family caregivers of children with failure to thrive can have a direct and lasting effect on the family's interaction with their child.

Figure 42-1 The child with failure to thrive is often seriously below average weight.

Nursing Process for the Child With Nonorganic Failure to Thrive

Assessment

Conduct a careful physical exam of the child, including observing skin turgor, anterior fontanel, signs of emaciation, weight, temperature, apical pulse, respirations, responsiveness, listlessness, and irritability. Observe for rumination or odor of vomitus.

When interviewing the family caregiver, carefully observe the interaction between the caregiver and the child and note the caregiver's responsiveness to the child's needs and the child's response to the caregiver. Listen carefully for underlying problems while talking with the family caregivers. Note if other supportive, involved people are present or if the caregiver is a single parent with no support system. Take a careful history of feeding and sleeping patterns or problems. Determine the caregiver's confidence in handling the child and note any apparent indication of feelings of stress or inadequacy.

Selected Nursing Diagnoses

- Disturbed Sensory Perception related to insufficient nurturing
- Imbalanced Nutrition: Less Than Body Requirements related to inadequate intake of calories
- Deficient Fluid Volume related to inadequate oral intake
- Impaired Urinary Elimination related to decreased fluid intake
- Constipation related to dehydration
- Risk for Impaired Skin Integrity related to malnourishment
- Impaired Parenting related to lack of knowledge and confidence in parenting skills

Outcome Identification and Planning

The major goals for the NFTT child focus on improving alertness and responsiveness, increasing caloric and oral fluid intake, maintaining normal urinary and bowel elimination, and maintaining skin integrity. Other goals for the child and family include improving parenting skills and building parental confidence. The caregiver's participation in the child's care is essential. Plan individualized nursing according to these goals.

Implementation
Providing Sensory Stimulation

You play a critical role in reversing the child's growth failure and improving the caregiver–child relationship. Providing sensory stimulation is vital in the care of the NFTT child. Attempt to cuddle the child and talk to him or her in a warm, soothing tone. Allow for play activities appropriate for the child's age. Family caregivers should be provided with information about normal growth and developmental activities appropriate for the child.

Maintaining Adequate Nutrition and Fluid Intake

Feed the child slowly and carefully in a quiet environment. During feeding, the child might be closely snug-

gled and gently rocked. It may be necessary to feed the child every 2 or 3 hours initially. Burp the child frequently during and at the end of each feeding, and then place him or her on the side with the head slightly elevated or held in a chest-to-chest position. Feed the child until good eating habits are established. Extra fluids of unsweetened juices are encouraged. If a family caregiver is present, encourage him or her to become involved in the child's feedings. Demonstrate the importance of talking encouragingly as the baby eats. An older child can sit at a low table facing the feeder while eating. Make the feeding time pleasant and comforting. Carefully document food intake with caloric intake and strict intake and output records.

Monitoring Elimination Patterns

As food and fluids are gradually increased and the child becomes hydrated, bowel activity and urine production return to normal. Daily stools are of a soft consistency, and the hourly urinary output is 2 to 3 mL/kg.

Promoting Skin Integrity

Protect the child's skin to prevent irritation. Lanolin or A+D Ointment can be used to lubricate dry skin. Apply the ointment at least once each shift and turn the child at least every 2 hours.

Providing Family Teaching

While caring for the child, point out to the caregiver the child's development and responsiveness, noting and praising any positive parenting behaviors the caregiver displays. The caregiver who has not had a close, warm childhood relationship may not understand the child's needs for cuddling and stimulation. Teaching about these needs must be done carefully and in a manner that does not further damage the caregiver's self-esteem. Many of these family caregivers are overly concerned about spoiling the child; it is important to dispel these fears. Explain the need for the child to develop trust, and teach the caregiver about the developmental tasks appropriate for children. Involve other health care team members as needed.

Evaluation: Goals and Expected Outcomes

Goal: The child will be more alert and responsive.
Expected Outcome:

- The child visually follows the caregiver around the room.

Goal: The child's caloric intake will be adequate for age.
Expected Outcome:

- The child's weight increases at a predetermined goal of 1 oz or more per day.

Goal: The child will have adequate fluid intake and urine output for age.

Expected Outcome:

■ The child's urine output will be 2 to 3 mL/kg/hr.

Goal: The child will have normal bowel elimination.

Expected Outcomes: The child

■ will have a bowel elimination pattern.
■ will have soft stools.

Goal: The child's skin integrity will be maintained.

Expected Outcome:

■ The child's skin shows no signs of redness or irritation and remains intact.

Goal: The family caregivers will demonstrate positive signs of good parenting.

Expected Outcomes: The family caregivers

■ feed the child successfully.
■ exhibit an appropriate response to the child.

EATING DISORDERS

ANOREXIA NERVOSA

Preoccupation with reducing diets and the quest for the "perfect" (i.e., thin) figure sometimes leads to **anorexia nervosa,** or self-inflicted starvation. This disorder occurs most commonly in adolescent white females, although there are reported cases among males and among African-American, Hispanic, and Asian adolescents. First described more than 100 years ago, anorexia has increased in incidence in recent years and is currently estimated to affect as many as 1% of adolescent girls. Anorexia is found in all the developed countries. The onset of the disorder may be seen in early adolescence and the greatest percentages of patients with the diagnosis are adolescent girls (Kreipe, 2006). Although considered a psychiatric problem, it causes severe physiologic damage and even death.

Characteristics

Anorexic children often are described as successful students who tend to be perfectionists and are always trying to please parents, teachers, and other adults. The families of these children characteristically show little emotion and display no evidence of conflict within the family. An adolescent in a controlled family environment, in which the parents do not freely express emotions, may try to establish independence and identity by controlling his or her own appetite and body weight. Depression is common in these adolescents. Anorexic persons deny weight loss and actually see themselves as fat, even when they look skeletal to others. They often adhere to a rigid program of exercise to further their efforts in weight reduction. They may make demands on themselves for cleanliness and order in their environment, or they may engage in rigid schedules for studying and other ritualistic

behavior. These adolescents deny hunger but often suffer from fatigue.

Clinical Manifestations and Diagnosis

Persons with anorexia are visibly emaciated, with an almost skeletonlike appearance. They appear sexually immature, have dry skin and brittle nails, and often have lanugo (downy hair) over their backs and extremities. Other symptoms include amenorrhea (absence of menstruation), constipation, hypothermia, bradycardia, low blood pressure, and anemia.

The American Psychiatric Association (2000) identifies the following criteria for the diagnosis of anorexia nervosa:

■ Weight loss leading to maintenance of body weight <85% of that expected for age and height; or failure to make expected weight gain during a period of growth, leading to body weight <85% of that expected
■ Intense fear of gaining weight or becoming fat even though underweight
■ Disturbance in how one's body weight or shape is experienced; undue influence of body weight or shape on self-evaluation; denial of seriousness of the current low body weight (e.g., feeling fat even when emaciated or, although underweight, perceiving one part of the body as being too fat)
■ Amenorrhea as evidenced by absence of three consecutive menstrual cycles

Treatment and Nursing Care

Children with anorexia nervosa may be hospitalized to achieve the two goals of treatment: correction of malnutrition and identification and treatment of the psychological cause. An approach involving several disciplines is necessary. Therapy is required to help the child gain insight into the problem. In addition, family therapy, nutritional therapy, and behavior modification are used. Affected children fear they will gain too much weight; therefore, a compromise between what the physician prefers and what the adolescent desires may be necessary.

Adolescents with anorexia have become experts in manipulating others and their environment. Once treatment begins, they may try to avoid gaining weight by ordering only low-calorie foods; by disposing of their meals in plants, trash, toilets, or dirty linen; or by exercising in the hall or jogging in place in their rooms. In some instances, nasogastric tube feedings or total parenteral nutrition (TPN) is necessary to provide nutritional support.

Treatment based on behavior modification may deprive the patient of all privileges, such as visitors, television, and telephone, until the child begins to gain weight. Privileges are then gradually restored. These techniques are effective only when the patient and the

■ **Figure 42-2** This anorexic teen, who is in the later stages of treatment, continues to meet with the counselor to discuss her food choices, exercise program, and overall well-being.

caregivers understand the program and its purpose and have agreed on individualized goals and rewards.

Group therapy may be used to provide peer support and the opportunity to associate with other patients with the same diagnosis in a nonthreatening setting.

The long-term outlook for the child with anorexia is unclear. Some children recover completely, others have eating problems into adulthood, and still others have problems with social adjustment that are not related to eating. Predicting the outcome is difficult; more studies are needed before a definitive answer is available (Fig. 42-2).

Warning.
Death may occur from suicide, infection, or the effects of starvation in the child with anorexia.

BULIMIA NERVOSA

Bulimia nervosa (usually referred to simply as bulimia) is characterized by binge eating followed by purging. The typical bulimic person is a white female in late adolescence. Most often, the bulimic person is of normal weight or slightly overweight. Those who are underweight usually fulfill the criteria for anorexia nervosa, although some anorexic persons periodically practice binging and purging. Bulimia nervosa is seen increasingly in young adult women as well.

The binging often occurs late in the day when the child is alone. Secrecy is an important aspect of the process. The child eats large quantities of food within 1 or 2 hours. This binging is followed by guilt, fear, shame, and self-condemnation. To avoid weight gain from the food eaten, the child follows the binging with purging by means of self-induced vomiting, laxatives, diuretics, and excessive exercise.

Clinical Manifestations and Diagnosis

The clues to bulimia nervosa may be few but include dental caries and erosion from frequent exposure to stomach acid, throat irritation, and endocrine and electrolyte imbalances that may cause cardiac irregularities and menstrual problems. Calluses or abrasions may be noted on the back of the hand from frequent contact with the teeth while inducing vomiting. Possible complications are esophageal tears and acute gastric dilation. Hypokalemia also may occur, especially if the child abuses diuretics to prevent weight gain. Other behavior problems seen in many bulimic persons include drug abuse, alcoholism, stealing (especially food), promiscuity, and other impulsive activities.

According to the American Psychiatric Association (2000), the diagnostic criteria for bulimia nervosa include:

- Recurrent episodes of binge eating
- A feeling of lack of control over behavior during binges
- Self-induced purging; use of laxatives or diuretics, enemas, or other medications; and strict dieting, fasting, or vigorous exercise to prevent weight gain
- Average of at least two binge-eating episodes a week during a 3-month period
- Obsessiveness regarding body weight and shape

Treatment

Treatment of bulimia nervosa is varied. Many aspects of the treatment are similar to treatment for the child with anorexia. Food diaries often are used as a tool to assess the child's eating patterns. In some instances, antidepressant drugs may be useful. You can refer the child to a support group that may prove helpful.

Nursing Process for the Child With Anorexia Nervosa or Bulimia Nervosa
Assessment

Data collection of the child with an eating disorder begins with a complete interview and history, including previous illnesses, allergies, a dietary history, and a description of eating habits. The child may not give an accurate dietary history or description of eating habits. Question the family caregiver in a separate interview to gain added information. In the physical exam, include height, weight, blood pressure, temperature, pulse, and respirations. Carefully inspect and observe the skin, mucous membranes, state of nutrition, and state of alertness and cooperation. Complete documentation of findings is necessary.

Selected Nursing Diagnoses

■ Imbalanced Nutrition: Less Than Body Requirements related to self-induced vomiting and use of laxatives or diuretics

■ Disturbed Body Image related to fear of obesity and potential rejection

■ Risk for Activity Intolerance related to fatigue secondary to malnutrition

■ Risk for Constipation related to decreased food and fluid intake

■ Risk for Diarrhea related to use of laxatives

■ Risk for Impaired Skin Integrity related to loss of subcutaneous fat and dry skin secondary to malnutrition

■ Noncompliance with treatment regimen related to unresolved conflicts over food and eating

■ Compromised Family Coping related to eating disorders, treatment regimen, and dangers associated with an eating disorder

Outcome Identification and Planning

The major goals for the child with an eating disorder relate to meeting nutritional needs and improving body image, self-concept, and self-esteem. Other goals include establishing appropriate activity levels, maintaining normal bowel activity, maintaining skin integrity, and complying with the treatment program. The goals for the family include understanding the condition, learning how to manage the condition and its treatment, and reinforcing the child's self-esteem.

Implementation

Improving Nutrition

The child with bulimia nervosa or anorexia nervosa does not receive the nutrients needed to achieve adequate growth during this period of development. Supervise food intake. Weigh the child at the same time each day but do not make an issue of weight fluctuation. Be observant when weighing the patient: The child may try to add weight by putting heavy objects in pockets, shoes, or other hiding places. While being weighed, the patient should wear minimal clothing (preferably a patient gown with no pockets) and have bare feet.

The care provider and a dietitian work with the child to devise a food plan to meet the child's nutrition requirements. The goal of the food plan is not a sudden weight gain, but a slow, steady gain with an established goal that has been agreed on by the health care team and the child. Often the child keeps a food diary that is reviewed daily with the health team.

Patients with eating disorders are often manipulative and deceptive. Observe the patient during and after eating to make certain the child eats the required food and does not get rid of it after apparently consuming it.

Contract agreements are often recommended for patients with eating disorders. These agreements, which are usually part of a behavioral modification plan, specify the child's and the staff's responsibilities for the diet, activity expectations for the child, and other aspects of the child's behavior. The contract also may spell out specific privileges that can be gained by meeting the contract goals. This places the child in greater control of the outcome.

In addition to daily weights, test urine for ketones and regularly evaluate the skin turgor and mucous membranes to gather further information about nutritional status. Report and document immediately any evidence of deteriorating physical condition. If weight loss continues, nasogastric tube feedings may need to be implemented. This possibility also can be included in the contract.

If the child's condition is at a critical stage with fluid and electrolyte deficiencies, parenteral fluids are necessary immediately to hydrate the patient before additional treatment can be implemented. Observe the child continuously to prevent any attempt to remove intravenous lines or otherwise disrupt the treatment. Closely monitor serum electrolytes, cardiac and respiratory status, and renal complications. During administration of parenteral fluids, continue to encourage the child to maintain an oral intake.

Reinforcing Positive Body Image and Self-Concept

Consistent assignment of the same nursing personnel to care for the child helps to establish a climate in which the child can relate to the nurse and begin to build a positive self-concept. It is important that you function as an active, nonjudgmental listener to the child. Report and document, without delay, any signs of depression. Also, report and document any negative feelings expressed by the child. Do not minimize or ignore these feelings. Reinforce positive behavior. Psychotherapy and counseling groups are necessary to help the child work through feelings of negative self-worth. Encourage the child to express fears, anger, and frustrations and help the patient recognize that everyone has these feelings from time to time. Never ridicule or belittle these feelings. Encourage the child to explore ways in which destructive feelings may be changed. These are feelings that can be dealt with in counseling sessions; therefore, report and document them carefully.

Balancing Rest and Activity

Exercise and activity are important parts of the contract negotiated with the child. Explain to the child that fatigue is a result of the extreme depletion of energy reserves related to nutritional deficits. Encourage the child to become involved in all activities of daily living.

Provide ample rest periods when the child's energy reserves are depleted. Discourage the child from pushing beyond endurance and closely observe for secretive excessive activity.

Monitoring Bowel Habits

Make a careful record of bowel movements. The child may not be reliable as a reporter of bowel habits, so devise methods to prevent the child from using the bathroom without supervision. Report, at once, and document constipation or diarrhea. Watch carefully to prevent the child from obtaining and taking a laxative. These patients may go to great lengths to obtain a laxative to purge themselves of food. Report immediately any evidence or suspicions of this type of behavior.

Promoting Skin Integrity

Good skin care is essential in the care of the child with a severely restricted nutritional intake. The skin may be dry and tend to break down easily because of the lack of a subcutaneous fat cushion. Inspect daily for redness, irritation, or signs of decubitus ulcer formation. Observe specifically the bony prominences. Encourage the child to be out of bed most of the day. When the child is in bed, encourage regular position changes so that no pressure areas develop.

Promoting Compliance

The long-term outcome for children with eating disorders is precarious. Children with severe eating disorders often have multiple inpatient admissions. During inpatient treatment, goals should be set and plans made for discharge. Specific consequences must be established for noncompliance. Counseling must continue after discharge. A support group referral may be helpful in encouraging compliance. Family involvement is necessary. The child must recognize that discharge from the health care facility does not mean that he or she is "cured."

Improving Family Coping

The family of the child needs counseling along with the child. Some families may deny that the child has a problem or that the problem is as severe as perceived by health care team members. Family therapy meets with varied success. Usually the earlier family therapy is initiated, the better the results. Family members must be able to identify behaviors of their own that contribute to the child's problem. Family members also must learn to cooperate with behavior modification programs and, with guidance, carry them out at home when necessary. Ongoing contact between the family, the child, and consistent health team members is essential (see Nursing Care Plan 42-1: The Child With Anorexia Nervosa).

Evaluation: Goals and Expected Outcomes

The evaluation of a child with anorexia nervosa or bulimia nervosa is an ongoing process that continues throughout the hospital stay as well as in outpatient settings. Goals and expected outcomes are as follows:

Goal: The child will gain a predetermined amount of weight per week.

Expected Outcomes: The child

- eats at least 80% of each meal.
- gains 1 to 2 lb (450–900 g) a week.
- keeps a food diary.
- signs a contract agreement.

Goal: The child will show evidence of improved self-esteem.

Expected Outcomes: The child

- verbally expresses positive attitudes.
- maintains peer relationships.
- improves grooming.

Goal: The child will pace activity to avoid fatigue.

Expected Outcomes: The child

- is involved in activity as prescribed in a contract.
- does not exhibit any signs of excessive activity.

Goal: The child's bowel elimination will be normal.

Expected Outcomes: The child

- experiences no episodes of diarrhea or constipation.
- does not attempt deceit to obtain laxatives.

Goal: The child's skin will show no evidence of breakdown.

Expected Outcomes: The child's

- skin is intact with no signs of redness, irritation, or excessive pressure.
- skin turgor is good.

Goal: The child will show signs of compliance.

Expected Outcomes: The child

- agrees to, signs, and adheres to a contract agreement.
- keeps counseling appointments.
- joins a support group.
- continues to gain or maintain weight as per contract agreement.

Goal: The family will show evidence of improved coping.

Expected Outcomes: The family

- attends counseling sessions.
- identifies behaviors that aggravate the child's condition.

Nursing Care Plan 42-1

THE CHILD WITH ANOREXIA NERVOSA

FW is a 15-year-old girl who has had a complete physical examination to determine why she has lost weight. After her examination and testing was completed, a diagnosis of anorexia nervosa was made. The child denies that she is underweight. She has been hospitalized to initiate treatment because her weight has dropped to 87 pounds (39.5 kg).

NURSING DIAGNOSIS
Imbalanced Nutrition: Less Than Body Requirements related to self-inflicted starvation and excessive exercise

GOAL: The child's nutritional status will improve, reaching a goal weight of 100 pounds, and an adequate fluid intake will be maintained.

EXPECTED OUTCOMES:
- The child gains at least 1.5 pounds (680 grams) per week.
- The child eats 80% of her meals.
- The child is involved in plans to improve her nutrition.
- The child does not interrupt parenteral fluid administration.
- The child's mucous membranes are moist; her skin turgor is good.
- The child's electrolytes, cardiac and respiratory status, and renal function are within normal limits.

Nursing Interventions	*Rationale*
Supervise intake by observing her during and after meals.	A child with an eating disorder may go to any length to avoid eating.
Weigh daily at the same time wearing the same type of clothes. Make certain nothing can be secreted in pockets or other hiding places that could add to her weight.	A child can be very innovative in finding ways to hide heavy objects on her to increase her weight gain.
Include the child with other health care providers to establish a mutually agreed upon, long-term weight goal and food plan that provide her with a slow, steady, weekly weight gain. Make a contract agreement to clearly state expectations and privileges that she can gain or lose.	The child is central to the planning process and cannot be made to meet goals set by others. Her participation and agreement to specific plans give her a feeling of more control of the overall outcome and encourage her to stick to the plan.
Observe continuously when parenteral fluids are being administered to prevent any attempts to disrupt the IV line. Also encourage her to take oral fluids at the same time.	The anorectic child may deprive herself so much that the fluid and electrolyte deficiencies become life-threatening. A balance must be restored before any further treatment can begin.
Test urine for ketones and regularly evaluate her skin turgor and mucous membranes.	These tests provide further indication of nutritional status.

NURSING DIAGNOSIS
Disturbed Body Image related to fear of obesity and potential rejection

GOAL: The child will express positive feelings about self.

EXPECTED OUTCOMES:
- The child verbally expresses positive attitudes about herself.
- The child expresses insight into reasons behind eating patterns and self-destructive behavior.
- The child expresses feelings about food, exercise, weight loss, and medical condition.

THE CHILD WITH ANOREXIA NERVOSA

Nursing Interventions	*Rationale*
Be a nonjudgmental, active listener; never minimize or ignore feelings expressed.	This is a first step in establishing and maintaining a climate of trust.
Report any negative feelings or any signs of depression expressed.	The child's negative feelings and expression of depression are important to the therapeutic treatment plan. All health care providers need to know about signs of depression to alert them to take appropriate precautions.
Maintain continuity of care throughout treatment.	The same person working with the child will help foster trust and a relationship will be developed.

NURSING DIAGNOSIS
Risk for Activity Intolerance related to fatigue secondary to malnutrition

GOAL: The child will balance rest and activity.

EXPECTED OUTCOMES:
• The child follows her contract for activity.
• The child is not excessively active.
• The child paces her activity to avoid fatigue.

Nursing Interventions	*Rationale*
Teach the child that a nutritional deficit depletes energy reserves and results in fatigue; encourage her to engage in activities of daily living, but provide for rest periods when her energy is low.	The child needs to understand that activity and rest are related to her nutritional status and that a healthy balance is crucial to overall health.
Discourage the child from pushing herself beyond her physical limits, and observe closely for secretive excessive exercise.	The child with an eating disorder may attempt to burn off excess calories with exercise.

NURSING DIAGNOSIS
Risk for Constipation related to decreased food and fluid intake
Risk for Diarrhea related to use of laxatives

GOAL: The child will maintain normal bowel habits.

EXPECTED OUTCOMES:
• The child has bowel movements every day or every other day.
• The child's stools are soft-formed.
• The child's fluid and electrolyte balances are maintained.

Nursing Interventions	*Rationale*
Observe the child's trips to the bathroom and keep a careful record of bowel habits; report and document any occurrence of diarrhea or constipation at once.	Typically the child may not be a reliable reporter of her bowel habits. A nurse observer is necessary to validate her stools.
Observe carefully to be certain that she does not have opportunity for purging or taking a laxative.	These children can be devious and will go to almost any length to prevent weight gain.
Monitor fluid intake and output and electrolyte levels.	Loss of fluids and electrolytes can cause long-term health conditions.

NURSING DIAGNOSIS
Risk for Impaired Skin Integrity related to loss of subcutaneous fat and dry skin secondary to malnutrition.

GOAL: The child's skin integrity will be maintained.

EXPECTED OUTCOMES:
• The child has no areas of red, dry, irritated skin.
• The child has no pressure ulcer formations.
• The child expresses feelings about body image and skin changes.

(continues on page 954)

Nursing Care Plan 42-1 (continued)

THE CHILD WITH ANOREXIA NERVOSA

Nursing Interventions	*Rationale*
Inspect skin daily for redness, irritation, or dryness. Provide good skin care.	Signs of redness, irritation, and dryness are preliminary signs for skin breakdown and formation of pressure ulcers.
Protect any bony prominences that may break down. Encourage position changes for child in bed to prevent decubiti formation.	Protection of pressure on bony surfaces and frequent changes of position improve circulation and prevent formation of pressure ulcers.

NURSING DIAGNOSIS

Noncompliance with treatment regimen related to unresolved conflicts over food and eating

GOAL: The child will comply with treatment regimen.

EXPECTED OUTCOMES:
* The child keeps counseling appointments.
* The child joins a support group.
* The child continues to gain weight as per her contract agreement.
* The child participates in decisions about care and treatment.

Nursing Interventions	*Rationale*
Make plans for discharge while she is still in the hospital. Include counseling plans in the contract.	Eating disorders are not cured with one hospitalization. Counseling is necessary to continue after discharge.
Encourage the child to make and maintain contact with a support group after discharge.	A support group may strengthen her desire to comply with the treatment regimen.
Make clear the established consequences for noncompliance with the program.	Consequences for noncompliance are important to reinforce the need to follow the program. Consequences set out a disciplinary action that will occur if the child fails to follow the program.
Encourage child to make decisions about care.	When the child makes decisions about care and treatment and complies with those plans, appropriate decision-making skills are fostered.

NURSING DIAGNOSIS

Compromised Family Coping related to eating disorders, treatment regimen, and dangers associated with an eating disorder

GOAL: The family's understanding of illness and treatment goals will improve.

EXPECTED OUTCOMES:
* The family attends counseling sessions.
* The family identifies behaviors that impact negatively on child behavior.

Nursing Interventions	*Rationale*
Provide for family counseling as well as counseling for the child.	It is important for the family to understand the dynamics of the problem and to face their possible contributions to the disorder.
Teach family members about the behavior modification program the child is using. Provide guidance on how to carry out the program at home.	Eating disorders are not cured simply because the child is discharged. Counseling, a continuation of the treatment program, and adherence to the signed contact agreement are essential. For these reasons, the family must become involved.

OBESITY

Obesity is a national problem in the United States, largely as a result of an overabundance of food and too little exercise. The thin figure, particularly for women, has become so idealized that being fat can handicap a person socially and professionally and severely damage self-esteem. **Obesity** generally is defined as an excessive accumulation of fat that increases body weight by 20% or more over ideal weight (see Appendix G). **Overweight**, although not necessarily signifying obesity, means that a person's weight is more than average for height and body build.

Clinical Manifestations and Diagnosis

Obesity often begins in childhood and, if not treated successfully, leads to chronic obesity in adult life. The obese child often feels isolated from the peer group that is normally a source of support and friendship. Because of the obesity, the child often is embarrassed to participate in sports, thus eliminating one method of burning excess calories. In addition, type 2 diabetes mellitus, which formerly was seen almost exclusively in adults and is associated with being overweight, is now being diagnosed in childhood with long-range health concerns.

Many children use food as a means of satisfying emotional needs, which establishes a vicious cycle. Children's eating habits include skipping meals, especially breakfast, and indulging in late-night eating. This behavior compounds the problem because calories consumed before a person goes to bed are not used for energy but are stored as fat. Snacking while watching television also contributes to the overindulgence in caloric intake.

Some children experience **polyphagia** (compulsive overeating). They lack control of their food intake, cannot postpone their urge to eat, hide food for later secret consumption, eat when not hungry or to escape from worries, and expend a great deal of energy thinking about securing and eating food. However, not all compulsive eaters are overweight, and in some ways, this disorder resembles anorexia nervosa.

Many factors, including genetic, social, cultural, metabolic, and psychological ones, contribute to the development of obesity. Children of obese parents are likely to share this problem not only because of some inherited predisposition toward obesity, but also because of family eating patterns and the emotional climate surrounding food. Certain cultures equate obesity with being loved and being prosperous. If these values carry over into a modern family, the child is torn between the standards of the peer group and those of the family.

Treatment

Obesity is difficult to treat in any age group, but is especially difficult in adolescence. Much of teenage life centers on food: after-school snacks, the ice cream shop, late-night diners, the pizza parlor, and fast-food restaurants serving high-fat, high-calorie foods with little nutritional value. Diets that emphasize nutritionally sound meals and reduced caloric intake produce results too slowly for impatient teenagers. Thus, the many quick weight-loss programs, diet pills, and diet books find a ready market among children.

Treatment must include a thorough exploration of the obese child's food attitudes. A team approach using the skills of a psychiatrist or psychologist, nutritionist, nurse, or other counselor is often useful in developing a complete treatment plan. Summer camps that center on weight reduction with nutritious, calorie-controlled food; exercise; and activity are successful for some children but are too costly for many families. In addition, many children may fall back into old habits after summer camp is over unless there is a continuing support system.

Caregivers who work with obese children should try to make them feel like worthwhile people, stressing that obesity does not automatically make them unacceptable. Finding the support of a caring adult who will help the child gain control of this aspect of his or her life can help give the necessary incentive to lose weight (see Family Teaching Tips: Tips for Caregivers of Obese Children).

Family Teaching Tips

TIPS FOR CAREGIVERS OF OBESE CHILDREN

- Have child keep a food diary for a week. Include food eaten, time eaten, what child was doing, and how child felt before and after eating; identify what stimulates urge to eat.
- Study diary with child to look for eating triggers.
- Set a reasonable goal of no more than 1 or 2 lbs of weight loss a week or perhaps maintaining weight with no gain.
- Advise child to eat only at specific, regular mealtimes.
- Recommend that child eat only at dining or kitchen table (not in front of TV or on the run).
- Have child use small plates to make amount of food seem larger.
- Teach child to eat slowly: Count and chew each bite (25 to 30 is a good goal).
- Suggest that the child try to leave a little on the plate when done.
- Have child survey home and get rid of tempting high-calorie foods.
- Stock up on low-calorie snacks: carrot sticks, celery sticks, and other raw vegetables.

- Help child get involved in an active project that occupies time and also helps burn calories: any active team sport; bicycling, walking, hiking, swimming, skating.
- Promote walking instead of riding whenever possible.
- Encourage the child to attend a support group or develop a buddy system for support.
- Weigh only once a week on the same scale at the same time of day in the same clothing.
- Make a chart to keep track of child weight.
- Help child to focus on a positive asset and make the most of it to help build self-concept.
- Encourage good grooming. A group could put on a "mini" fashion show, choosing with guidance clothes that help maximize best features, or simply using magazine illustrations if actual clothing is not available.
- Reward each small success with positive reinforcement.
- Enlist cooperation of all family members to support the child with encouragement and a positive atmosphere.

Key Points

> Autism is a severe behavioral disturbance that affects the practical use of language as a means of communication, interpersonal interaction, attention, perception, and motor activity. The characteristics of autism include a lack of development of a smiling response to others or an interest in being touched or cuddled, blank expressions, and lack of response to verbal stimulation. These children do not show the normal fear of separation from parents. Four goals in the treatment of autism include promotion of normal development, language development, social interaction, and learning. Supporting the family caregivers is a primary task, as they are the most valuable source of information about the autistic child's habits and communication skills.

> Characteristics seen in the child with ADHD include impulsive behavior, ease in being distracted, fidgeting or squirming, difficulty sitting still, problems following through on instructions despite being able to understand them, inattentiveness when spoken to, losing of things, going from one uncompleted activity to another, difficulty taking turns, and talking excessively.

The child often engages in dangerous activities without considering the consequences. Treatment is multidisciplinary and stimulant medications are often used.

> Enuresis, or bed-wetting, is involuntary urination beyond the age when control of urination commonly is acquired. Enuresis may have a physiologic or psychological cause. Encopresis is chronic involuntary fecal soiling beyond the age when control is expected. If no organic causes (e.g., worms, megacolon) exist, encopresis indicates a serious emotional problem.

> The symptoms seen in the child with school phobia are caused by anxiety that may approach panic.

> Children who are considering suicide often have previous suicide attempts, withdraw from or change participation in activities, have physical complaints and a preoccupation with dying, change moods, say goodbye, or give away personal items.

> Substances commonly abused by children include alcohol, tobacco, marijuana, cocaine, morphine, heroin, hallucinogens, depressants, amphetamines,

analgesics, anabolic steroids, hallucinogens, and Ecstasy.

➤ The use of substances can lead to addiction or dependence, which may be psychological, physical, or both. Tobacco or smokeless tobacco damages the lungs and can cause mouth, lip, and throat cancers. Marijuana affects judgment, sense of time, and motivation. The physical results of using cocaine are an increase in pulse, respirations, blood pressure, and temperature. Narcotics are highly addictive and extremely expensive, which can result in teenage prostitution, pushing (selling) drugs, and robbery as a means to support the drug habit. Hallucinogens (psychedelic drugs), although not addictive in a physical sense, can create a psychological dependence, as well as the effects of intoxication, "bad trips," and flashbacks, and often are associated with overdoses. Withdrawal from barbiturates must be carefully controlled to prevent delirium, seizures, or death.

➤ Children with NFTT are often listless and below average in weight and height; have poor muscle tone and a loss of subcutaneous fat; and are immobile for long periods of time. They may be unresponsive or try to avoid cuddling and vocalization. A common characteristic is rumination (voluntary regurgitation), perhaps as a means of self-satisfaction. Goals for the NFTT child focus on improving alertness and responsiveness, increasing caloric and oral fluid intake, maintaining normal urinary and bowel elimination, and maintaining skin integrity. Other goals for the child and family include improving parenting skills and building parental confidence.

➤ Anorexic children may be perfectionists, be depressed, deny weight loss, and actually see themselves as fat. Often they follow rigid programs of exercise. Persons with anorexia are visibly emaciated, with an almost skeletonlike appearance. Two goals of treatment for the hospitalized anorexic are correction of malnutrition and identification and treatment of the psychological cause.

➤ The child with bulimia may have dental caries and erosion from frequent exposure to stomach acid. She or he may also have throat irritation, endocrine and electrolyte imbalances, cardiac irregularities, and menstrual problems. Calluses or abrasions may be noted on the back of the hand from frequent contact with the teeth while inducing vomiting. Possible complications are esophageal tears, acute gastric dilation, and hypokalemia. Goals of treatment for the child with an eating disorder relate to meeting nutritional needs and improving body image, self-concept, and self-esteem.

➤ Professionals who work with obese children should try to make them feel like worthwhile persons, stressing that obesity does not automatically make them unacceptable. Finding the support of a caring adult who will help the child gain control of this aspect of his or her life can help give the necessary incentive to lose weight.

INTERNET RESOURCES

Alcohol
www.ncadd.org

ADHD
www.add.org

Suicide
www.suicidology.org

Substance Abuse
www.clubdrugs.org

Tobacco
www.tobaccofreekids.org

Workbook

■ NCLEX-STYLE REVIEW QUESTIONS

1. A nurse admits an adolescent girl with a diagnosis of possible anorexia nervosa. Of the following characteristics, which would *most* likely be seen in the adolescent with anorexia?

    a. The adolescent gets low grades in school.
    b. The adolescent has a sedentary lifestyle.
    c. The adolescent freely express emotions.
    d. The adolescent follows a strict routine.

2. The nurse is assisting with a physical exam on an adolescent with bulimia. Of the following signs and symptoms, which would *most* likely be seen in the adolescent with bulimia?

    a. Dry skin
    b. Dental caries
    c. Low body weight
    d. Amenorrhea

3. In planning care for an adolescent with an eating disorder, which of the following goals would be *most* important for the adolescent?

    a. The adolescent will verbally express positive attitudes and feelings.
    b. The adolescent will plan and participate in age-appropriate activities.
    c. The adolescent will maintain a fluid and electrolyte balance.
    d. The adolescent will have normal bowel and bladder patterns.

4. The nurse is discussing teenage depression and suicide with a group of caregivers of adolescent-aged children. If the caregivers make the following statements, which statement would require further data collection?

    a. "My child has so many ideas about how she can fix all the problems in the world."
    b. "She told me she is happy that she broke up with her long-time boyfriend."
    c. "My son enjoys spending all his time playing his CD player alone in his room."
    d. "My child eats all the time but never seems to want to go to sleep."

5. The nurse is caring for an infant with failure to thrive. The infant took in 2 oz of formula every 2 hours during the 12-hour shift, with the first 2 oz being at 0700 and the last feeding at 1900. She vomited three times: 20 cc the first time, 36 cc the second time, and 28 cc the third time. The infant had four wet diapers during the shift. After subtracting the dry weight of the diapers, the diapers weighed 20 g, 18 g, 25 g, and 22 g. She had one medium-sized stool during the shift. What was the infant's total intake and output during the 12-hour shift?

■ STUDY ACTIVITIES

1. A coworker says to you, "That Jeff in room 204 is bouncing off the walls." You are assigned to this child, who has a diagnosis of attention deficit hyperactivity disorder (ADHD). Make a list of behavior techniques to use with the child who has ADHD. Develop a plan of care you could use to care for Jeff.

2. Go to the following Internet site:
    www.dancesafe.org/parents
    Click on the section "Communicating With Your Teenagers About Drugs." Read down to and including the section "Communication Approaches."

    a. What are four important communication methods suggested for parents to use in communicating with their teens?
    b. List seven barriers that parents should be aware of when communicating with their teenage children.

■ CRITICAL THINKING: WHAT WOULD YOU DO?

1. Tanya, 16 years old, is 65 in (165 cm) tall and weighs 98 lb (44.5 kg). She moans about how fat her thighs are. You believe she is anorexic. A diagnosis of anorexia is confirmed and she is hospitalized.

    a. What symptoms will you observe for, in addition to her weight loss?
    b. What are the characteristics often seen in the anorexic child's personality?
    c. What will be included in Tanya's nursing care plan?

2. Your best friend shares with you that she thinks her teenage son might have a problem with alcohol and drugs. She tells you that her son has behaviors that make her think he is drinking every day and using drugs every weekend.

    a. Why do you think alcohol is the most commonly abused drug among adolescents?
    b. What factors do you think put adolescents at greatest risk of becoming substance abusers?
    c. What do you think could be helpful in reducing each of the above risk factors?

3. Dosage calculation: A child with a diagnosis of attention deficit hyperactivity disorder (ADHD) is being treated with methylphenidate (Ritalin). The child weighs 75 lb. The usual dosage of this medication is 0.3 mg/kg/dose to 2.0 mg/kg/day, not to exceed 60 mg/day. The medication is given two times a day (BID). Answer the following:

    a. How many kilograms (kg) does the child weigh?
    b. How many milligrams (mg) would be given for the low dose?
    c. How many milligrams (mg) would be given for the high dose?
    d. Would the high dose of the medication be an appropriate dose for this child? Explain your answer.

Use Standard Precautions, or the equivalent, for the care of all patients. *Category IB**

A. Hand washing

(1) Wash hands after touching blood, body fluids, secretions, excretions, and contaminated items, whether or not gloves are worn. Wash hands immediately after gloves are removed, between patient contacts, and when otherwise indicated to avoid transfer of microorganisms to other patients or environments. It may be necessary to wash hands between tasks and procedures on the same patient to prevent cross-contamination of different body sites. *Category IB*

(2) Use a plain (nonantimicrobial) soap for routine hand washing. *Category IB*

(3) Use an antimicrobial agent or a waterless antiseptic agent for specific circumstances (e.g., control of outbreaks or hyperendemic infections), as defined by the infection control program. *Category IB* (See Contact Precautions for additional recommendations on using antimicrobial and antiseptic agents.)

B. Gloves

Wear gloves (clean, nonsterile gloves are adequate) when touching blood, body fluids, secretions, excretions, and contaminated items. Put on clean gloves just before touching mucous membranes and nonintact skin. Change gloves between tasks and procedures on the same patient after contact with material that may contain a high concentration of microorganisms. Remove gloves promptly after use, before going to another patient or touching noncontaminated items and environmental surfaces, and wash hands immediately to avoid transfer of microorganisms to other patients or environments. *Category IB*

C. Mask, Eye Protection, Face Shield

Wear a mask and eye protection or a face shield to protect mucous membranes of the eyes, nose, and mouth during procedures and patient-care activities that are likely to generate splashes or sprays of blood, body fluids, secretions, and excretions. *Category IB*

D. Gown

Wear a gown (a clean, nonsterile gown is adequate) to protect skin and to prevent soiling of clothing during procedures and patient-care activities that are likely to generate splashes or sprays of blood, body fluids, secretions, or excretions. Select a gown that is appropriate for the activity and amount of fluid likely to be encountered. Remove a soiled gown as promptly as possible, and wash your hands to avoid transfer of microorganisms to other patients or environments. *Category IB*

E. Patient-Care Equipment

Handle used patient-care equipment soiled with blood, body fluids, secretions, and excretions in a manner that prevents skin and mucous membrane exposures, contamination of clothing, and transfer of microorganisms to other patients and environments. Ensure that reusable equipment is not used for the care of another patient until it has been cleaned and reprocessed appropriately. Ensure that single-use items are discarded properly. *Category IB*

F. Environmental Control

Ensure that the hospital has adequate procedures for the routine care, cleaning, and disinfection of environmental surfaces, beds, bedrails, bedside equipment, and other frequently touched surfaces, and ensure that these procedures are being followed. *Category IB*

G. Linen

Handle, transport, and process used linen soiled with blood, body fluids, secretions, and excretions in a manner that prevents skin and mucous membrane exposures and contamination of clothing and that avoids transfer of microorganisms to other patients and environments. *Category IB*

H. Occupational Health and Bloodborne Pathogens

(1) Take care to prevent injuries when using needles, scalpels, and other sharp instruments or devices; when handling sharp instruments after procedures; when cleaning used instruments; and when disposing of used needles. Never recap used needles, or otherwise, manipulate them using both hands, or use any other technique that involves directing the point of a needle toward any part of the body; rather, use either a one-handed "scoop" technique or a mechanical device designed for holding the needle sheath. Do not remove used needles from disposable syringes by hand, and do not bend, break, or otherwise manipulate used needles by hand. Place used disposable syringes and needles, scalpel blades, and other sharp items in appropriate puncture-resistant containers, which are located as close as practical to the area in which the items were used, and place

---

(From Recommendations for Isolation Precautions in Hospitals developed by the Centers for Disease Control and Prevention and the Hospital Control Practices Advisory Committee [HICPAC], February 18, 1997.)

*Category IB. Strongly recommended for all hospitals and reviewed as effective by experts in the field and a consensus of HICPAC members on the basis of strong rationale and suggestive evidence, even though definitive studies have not been done.

reusable syringes and needles in a puncture-resistant container for transport to the reprocessing area. *Category IB*

(2) Use mouthpieces, resuscitation bags, or other ventilation devices as an alternative to mouth-to-mouth resuscitation methods in areas where the need for resuscitation is predictable. *Category IB*

I. Patient Placement

Place a patient who contaminates the environment or who does not (or cannot be expected to) assist in maintaining appropriate hygiene or environmental control in a private room. If a private room is not available, consult with infection control professionals regarding patient placement or other alternatives. *Category IB*

J. Respiratory Hygiene/Cough Etiquette

Instruct symptomatic persons to cover mouth/nose when sneezing/coughing; use tissues and dispose in no-touch receptacle; observe hand hygiene after soiling of hands with respiratory secretions; wear surgical masks if tolerated or maintain spatial separation greater than 3 feet if possible. *Category IB.*[†]

[†]Guidelines for respiratory hygiene/cough etiquette have been added to the 2004 **DRAFT** CDC guidelines for isolation precautions: Preventing transmission of infectious agents in healthcare settings. 2004. https://www.cdc.gov/nicdod/hip/isoguide.htm

NANDA-APPROVED NURSING DIAGNOSES

This list represents the NANDA-approved nursing diagnoses for clinical use and testing.

DOMAIN 1: HEALTH PROMOTION

Description

The awareness of well-being or normality of function and the strategies used to maintain control of and enhance that well-being or normality of function

Approved Diagnoses

Effective Therapeutic Regimen Management
Ineffective Therapeutic Regimen Management
Ineffective Family Therapeutic Regimen Management
Ineffective Community Therapeutic Regimen Management
Health-Seeking Behaviors (specify)
Ineffective Health Maintenance
Impaired Home Maintenance
Readiness for Enhanced Immunization Status
Readiness for Enhanced Management of Therapeutic Regimen
Readiness for Enhanced Nutrition

DOMAIN 2: NUTRITION

Description

The activities of taking in, assimilating, and using nutrients for the purpose of tissue maintenance, tissue repair, and the production of energy

Approved Diagnoses

Ineffective Infant Feeding Pattern
Impaired Swallowing
Imbalanced Nutrition: Less Than Body Requirements
Imbalanced Nutrition: More Than Body Requirements
Risk for Imbalanced Nutrition: More Than Body Requirements
Deficient Fluid Volume
Risk for Deficient Fluid Volume
Excess Fluid Volume
Risk for Imbalanced Fluid Volume
Readiness for Enhanced Fluid Balance
Risk for Impaired Liver Function
Risk for Unstable Blood Glucose Level

DOMAIN 3: ELIMINATION

Description

Secretion and excretion of waste products from the body

Approved Diagnoses

Impaired Urinary Elimination
Urinary Retention
Total Urinary Incontinence
Functional Urinary Incontinence
Stress Urinary Incontinence
Urge Urinary Incontinence
Reflex Urinary Incontinence
Risk for Urge Urinary Incontinence
Readiness for Enhanced Urinary Elimination
Bowel Incontinence
Diarrhea
Constipation
Risk for Constipation
Perceived Constipation
Impaired Gas Exchange

DOMAIN 4: ACTIVITY/REST

Description

The production, conservation, expenditure, or balance of energy resources

Approved Diagnoses

Insomnia
Sleep Deprivation
Readiness for Enhanced Sleep
Sedentary Lifestyle
Risk for Disuse Syndrome
Impaired Physical Mobility
Impaired Bed Mobility
Impaired Wheelchair Mobility
Impaired Transfer Ability
Impaired Walking
Deficient Diversional Activity
Dressing/Grooming Self-Care Deficit
Bathing/Hygiene Self-Care Deficit
Feeding Self-Care Deficit
Toileting Self-Care Deficit
Readiness for Enhanced Self-care
Delayed Surgical Recovery
Disturbed Energy Field
Fatigue
Decreased Cardiac Output
Impaired Spontaneous Ventilation
Ineffective Breathing Pattern
Activity Intolerance
Risk for Activity Intolerance
Dysfunctional Ventilatory Weaning Response

Ineffective Tissue Perfusion (specify type: Renal, Cerebral, Cardiopulmonary, Gastrointestinal, Peripheral)

DOMAIN 5: PERCEPTION/COGNITION

Description

The human information-processing system, including attention, orientation, sensation, perception, cognition, and communication

Approved Diagnoses

Unilateral Neglect
Impaired Environmental Interpretation Syndrome
Wandering
Disturbed Sensory Perception (specify: Visual, Auditory, Kinesthetic, Gustatory, Tactile, Olfactory)
Deficient Knowledge (specify)
Readiness for Enhanced Knowledge
Acute Confusion
Chronic Confusion
Impaired Memory
Disturbed Thought Processes
Readiness for Enhanced Decision Making
Impaired Verbal Communication
Readiness for Enhanced Communication

DOMAIN 6: SELF-PERCEPTION

Description

Awareness about the self

Approved Diagnoses

Disturbed Personal Identity
Powerlessness
Risk for Powerlessness
Hopelessness
Risk for Loneliness
Readiness for Enhanced Self-Concept
Chronic Low Self-Esteem
Situational Low Self-Esteem
Risk for Situational Low Self-Esteem
Disturbed Body Image

DOMAIN 7: ROLE RELATIONSHIPS

Description

The positive and negative connections or associations between persons or groups of persons and the means by which those connections are demonstrated

Approved Diagnoses

Caregiver Role Strain
Risk for Caregiver Role Strain
Impaired Parenting
Risk for Impaired Parenting
Readiness for Enhanced Parenting
Interrupted Family Processes
Readiness for Enhanced Family Processes
Dysfunctional Family Processes: Alcoholism

Risk for Impaired Parent/Infant/Child Attachment
Effective Breast-feeding
Ineffective Breast-feeding
Interrupted Breast-feeding
Ineffective Role Performance
Parental Role Conflict
Impaired Social Interaction

DOMAIN 8: SEXUALITY

Description

Sexual identity, sexual function, and reproduction

Approved Diagnoses

Sexual Dysfunction
Ineffective Sexuality Patterns

DOMAIN 9: COPING/STRESS TOLERANCE

Description

Contending with life events/life processes

Approved Diagnoses

Relocation Stress Syndrome
Risk for Relocation Stress Syndrome
Rape-Trauma Syndrome
Rape-Trauma Syndrome: Silent Reaction
Rape-Trauma Syndrome: Compound Reaction
Post-Trauma Syndrome
Risk for Post-Trauma Syndrome
Fear
Anxiety
Death Anxiety
Chronic Sorrow
Ineffective Denial
Grieving
Complicated Grieving
Impaired Adjustment
Ineffective Coping
Disabled Family Coping
Compromised Family Coping
Defensive Coping
Ineffective Community Coping
Readiness for Enhanced Coping
Readiness for Enhanced Family Coping
Readiness for Enhanced Community Coping
Autonomic Dysreflexia
Risk for Autonomic Dysreflexia
Disorganized Infant Behavior
Risk for Disorganized Infant Behavior
Readiness for Enhanced Organized Infant Behavior
Decreased Intracranial Adaptive Capacity

DOMAIN 10: LIFE PRINCIPLES

Description

Principles underlying conduct, thought, and behavior about acts, customs, or institutions as being true or having intrinsic worth

Approved Diagnoses

Readiness for Enhanced Spiritual Well-Being
Spiritual Distress
Risk for Spiritual Distress
Decisional Conflict (specify)
Noncompliance (specify)

DOMAIN 11: SAFETY/PROTECTION
Description
Freedom from danger, physical injury, or immune
system damage; preservation from loss; and
protection of safety and security

Approved Diagnoses
Risk for Infection
Impaired Oral Mucous Membrane
Risk for Injury
Risk for Perioperative Positioning Injury
Risk for Falls
Risk for Trauma
Impaired Skin Integrity
Risk for Impaired Skin Integrity
Impaired Tissue Integrity
Impaired Dentition
Risk for Suffocation
Risk for Aspiration
Ineffective Airway Clearance
Risk for Peripheral Neurovascular Dysfunction
Ineffective Protection
Risk for Sudden Infant Death Syndrome
Risk for Self-Mutilation
Self-Mutilation
Risk for Other-Directed Violence
Risk for Self-Directed Violence
Risk for Suicide

Risk for Poisoning
Latex Allergy Response
Risk for Latex Allergy Response
Risk for Imbalanced Body Temperature
Ineffective Thermoregulation
Hypothermia
Hyperthermia

DOMAIN 12: COMFORT
Description
Sense of mental, physical, or social well-being or ease

Approved Diagnoses
Acute Pain
Chronic Pain
Nausea
Social Isolation

DOMAIN 13: GROWTH/DEVELOPMENT
Description
Age-appropriate increase in physical dimension, organ
systems, and/or attainment of developmental
milestones

Approved Diagnoses
Risk for Disproportionate Growth
Adult Failure to Thrive
Delayed Growth and Development
Risk for Delayed Development

Appendix C

THE JOINT COMMISSION'S "DO NOT USE" LIST OF ABBREVIATIONS, ACRONYMS, AND SYMBOLS

The Joint Commission and the Institute for Safe Medication Practices have listed the following abbreviations and symbols as dangerous, due to the potential of medication and other errors being made if these are used.

Abbreviation	Potential Problem	Use Instead
Official "Do Not Use" List*		
U (unit)	Mistaken as 0 (zero), 4 (four), or "cc"	Write "unit"
IU (international unit)	Mistaken as IV (intravenous) or 10 (ten)	Write "international unit"
Q.D., QD, q.d., qd (daily)	Mistaken for every other day	Write "daily"
Q.O.D., QOD, q.o.d, qod (every other day)	Mistaken for every other or daily The period after the "Q" can be mistaken for an "l" and the "O" can be mistaken for "l"	Write "every other day"
Trailing zero (X.O mg)†	Decimal point is missed	Write X mg
Lack of leading zero (.X mg)		Write O.X mg
MS	Can mean morphine sulfate or magnesium sulfate	Write "morphine sulfate" or "magnesium sulfate"
MSO_4 and $MgSO_4$	Confused for one another	Write "morphine sulfate" or "magnesium sulfate
Additional Abbreviations, Acronyms, and Symbols (For Possible Future Inclusion in the Official "Do Not Use" List)		
> (greater than)	Misinterpreted as the number "7" Confused with less than	Write "greater than"
< (less than)	Misinterpreted as the letter "L" Confused with greater than	Write "less than"
Abbreviations for drug names	Misinterpreted because of similar abbreviations for multiple drugs	Write drug names in full
Apothecary units	Unfamiliar to many practitioners; confused with metric units	Use metric units
@	Mistaken for the number "2" (two)	Write "at"
cc (cubic centimeter)	Mistaken for U (units) when poorly written	Write "mL" for milliliters
μg (microgram)	Mistaken for mg (milligrams), resulting in one thousand-fold overdose	Write "mcg" or "micrograms"

*Applies to all orders and medication-related documentation that is handwritten (including free-test computer entry) or on preprinted forms.
†Exception: A "trailing zero" may be used only where required to demonstrate the level of precision of the value being reported such as for laboratory results, imaging studies that report size of lesions, or catheter/tube sizes. It may not be used in medication orders or other medication-related documentation.
©Joint Commission Resources: *Official "Do Not Use" List-2006 National Patient Safety Goals*. Retrieved May 22, 2007, from http://www.jointcommission.org/PatientSafety/DoNotUseList/. Reprinted with permission.

GOOD SOURCES OF ESSENTIAL NUTRIENTS

Nutrient	Sources
Protein	Meat, poultry, fish, milk products, and eggs. Whole wheat grains, nuts, peanut butter, and legumes are also good sources of protein but need to be supplemented by some animal protein, such as meat, eggs, milk, cheese, cottage cheese, or yogurt.
Vitamin A	Green leafy vegetables, deep yellow vegetables and fruits, whole milk or whole milk products, egg yolk.
Vitamin B	
Thiamine	Meat, fish, poultry, eggs, whole grain, legumes, potatoes, green leafy vegetables.
Riboflavin	Milk (best source), meat, egg yolk, green vegetables.
Niacin	Meat, fish, poultry, peanut butter, wheat germ, brewer's yeast. Although the amount in milk is small, children whose intake of milk is adequate do not develop pellagra.
Vitamin C	Citrus fruits and tomatoes, fresh or frozen citrus fruit juices, strawberries, cantaloupe.
Vitamin D	Sunlight, fish liver oils, fortified milk, and synthetic vitamin D.
Minerals	
Calcium	Milk and milk products, squash, sweet potatoes, raisins, rhubarb, well-cooked dried beans, turnip greens, Swiss chard, mustard greens.
Iron	Green leafy vegetables, liver, meats and eggs, dried fruits, whole grain or enriched bread and cereals.
Iodine	Seafood, plants grown on soil near the sea, iodized salt.

Appendix E

BREAST-FEEDING AND MEDICATION USE

GENERAL CONSIDERATIONS

- Most medications are safe to use while breast-feeding; however, the woman should always check with the pediatrician, physician, or lactation specialist before taking any medications, including over-the-counter and herbal products.
- Inform the woman that she has the right to seek a second opinion if the physician does not perform a thoughtful risk-versus-benefit assessment before prescribing medications or advising against breast-feeding.
- Most medications pass from the woman's bloodstream into the breast milk. However, the amount is usually very small and unlikely to harm the baby.
- A preterm or other special needs neonate is more susceptible to the adverse effects of medications in breast milk. A woman who is taking medications and whose baby is in the neonatal intensive care unit or special care nursery should consult with the pediatrician or neonatologist before feeding her breast milk to the baby.
- If the woman is taking a prescribed medication, she should take the medication just after breast-feeding. This practice helps ensure that the lowest possible dose of medication reaches the baby through the breast milk.
- Some medications can cause changes in the amount of milk the woman produces. Teach the woman to report any changes in milk production.

LACTATION RISK CATEGORIES (LRC)

Lactation

Category	Risk	Rationale
L1	Safest	Clinical research or long-term observation of use in many breast-feeding women has not demonstrated risk to the infant.
L2	Safer	Limited clinical research has not demonstrated an increase in adverse effects in the infant.

Category	Risk	Rationale
L3	Moderately safe	There is possible risk to the infant; however, the risks are minimal or nonthreatening in nature. These medications should be given only when the potential benefit outweighs the risk to the infant.
L4	Possibly hazardous	There is positive evidence of risk to the infant; however, in life-threatening situations or for serious diseases, the benefit might outweigh the risk.
L5	Contraindicated	The risk of using the medication clearly outweighs any possible benefit from breast-feeding.

POTENTIAL EFFECTS OF SELECTED MEDICATION CATEGORIES ON THE BREAST-FED INFANT

Narcotic Analgesics

- Codeine and hydrocodone appear to be safe in moderate doses. Rarely the neonate may experience sedation and/or apnea. (LRC: L3)
- Meperidine (Demerol) can lead to sedation of the neonate. (LRC: L3)
- Low-to-moderate doses of morphine appear to be safe. (LRC: L2)
- Trace-to-negligible amounts of fentanyl are found in human milk. (LRC: L2)

Nonnarcotic Analgesics and NSAIDs

- Acetaminophen and ibuprofen are approved for use. (LRC: L1)
- Naproxen may cause neonatal hemorrhage and anemia if used for prolonged periods. (LRC: L3 for short-term use and L4 for long-term use)
- The newer COX2 inhibitors, such as celecoxib (Celebrex), appear to be safe for use. (LRC: L2)

Antibiotics

- Levels in breast milk are usually very low.
- The penicillins and cephalosporins are generally considered safe to use. (LRC: L1 and L2)
- Tetracyclines can be safely used for short periods but are not suitable for long-term therapy (e.g., for treatment of acne). (LRC: L2)
- Sulfonamides should not be used during the neonatal stage (the first month of life). (LRC: L3)

Antihypertensives

- A high degree of caution is advised when antihypertensives are used during breast-feeding.
- Some beta-blockers can be used.
- Hydralazine and methyldopa are considered to be safe. (LRC: L2)
- ACE inhibitors are not recommended in the early postpartum period.

Sedatives and Hypnotics

- Neonatal withdrawal can occur when antianxiety medications, such as lorazepam, are taken. Fortunately withdrawal is generally mild.
- Phenothiazines, such as Phenergan and Thorazine, may lead to sleep apnea and increase the risk for sudden infant death syndrome.

Antidepressants

- The risk to the baby often is higher if the woman is depressed and remains untreated, rather than taking the medication.
- The older tricyclics are considered to be safe; however, they cause many bothersome side effects, such as weight gain and dry mouth, which may lead to noncompliance on the part of the woman.
- The selective serotonin uptake inhibitors (SSRIs) also are considered to be safe and have a lower side effect profile, which makes them more palatable to the woman. (LRC: L2 and L3)

Mood Stabilizers (Antimanic Medication)

- Lithium is found in breast milk and is best not used in the breast-feeding woman. (LRC: L4)

- Valproic acid (Depakote) seems to be a more appropriate choice for the woman with bipolar disorder. The infant will need periodic lab studies to check platelets and liver function.

Corticosteroids

- Corticosteroids do not pass into the milk in large quantities.
- Inhaled steroids are safe to use because they don't accumulate in the bloodstream.

Thyroid Medication

- Thyroid medications, such as levothyroxine (Synthroid), can be taken while breast-feeding.
- Most are in LRC category L1.

MEDICATIONS THAT USUALLY ARE CONTRAINDICATED FOR THE BREAST-FEEDING WOMAN

- Amiodarone
- Antineoplastic agents
- Chloramphenicol
- Doxepin
- Ergotamine and other ergot derivatives
- Iodides
- Methotrexate and immunosuppressants
- Lithium
- Radiopharmaceuticals
- Ribavirin
- Tetracycline (prolonged use—more than 3 weeks)
- Pseudoephedrine (found in many over-the-counter medications)

Material in this Appendix was adapted from information found on the American Academy of Pediatrics Web site (www.aap.org) and from: Riordan, J. (2005). *Breastfeeding and human lactation* (3rd ed.). Jones and Bartlett Publishers: Boston; Hale, T. W. (2004). *Medications and mother's milk* (11th ed.). Amarillo, TX: Pharmasoft Publishing.

Appendix F

CERVICAL DILATION CHART

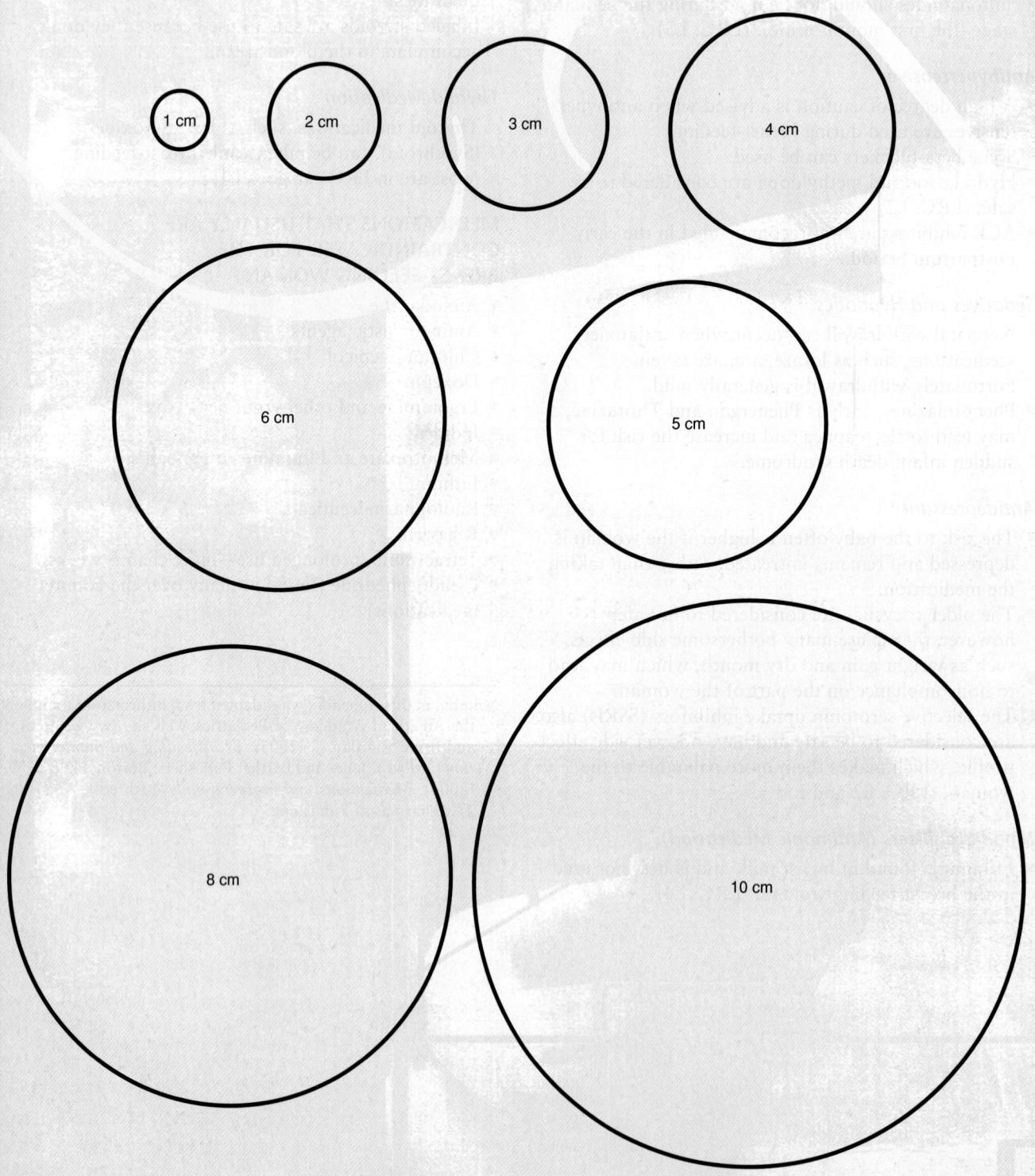

Birth to 36 months: Boys
Length-for-age and Weight-for-age percentiles

NAME _____

RECORD# _____

Published May 30, 2000 (modified 4/20/01).
SOURCE: Developed by the National Center for Health Statistics in collaboration with
the National Center for Chronic Disease Prevention and Health Promotion (2000).
http://www.cdc.gov/growthcharts

CDC
SAFER·HEALTHIER·PEOPLE™

Birth to 36 months: Boys
Head circumference-for-age and
Weight-for-length percentiles

NAME _____

RECORD# _____

Published May 30, 2000 (modified 10/16/00).
SOURCE: Developed by the National Center for Health Statistics in collaboration with
the National Center for Chronic Disease Prevention and Health Promotion (2000).
http://www.cdc.gov/growthcharts

SAFER • HEALTHIER • PEOPLE™

Birth to 36 months: Girls
Length-for-age and Weight-for-age percentiles

NAME _____

RECORD # _____

AGE (MONTHS)

Birth 3 6 9 **12** 15 18 21 **24** 27 30 33 **36**

LENGTH

WEIGHT

Mother's Stature _____

Father's Stature _____

Gestational Age: _____ Weeks

Comment

Date	Age	Weight	Length	Head Circ.
	Birth			

Birth 3 6 9

Published May 30, 2000 (modified 4/20/01).
SOURCE: Developed by the National Center for Health Statistics in collaboration with
the National Center for Chronic Disease Prevention and Health Promotion (2000).
http://www.cdc.gov/growthcharts

SAFER · HEALTHIER · PEOPLE™

Birth to 36 months: Girls
Head circumference-for-age and
Weight-for-length percentiles

NAME _____

RECORD# _____

Published May 30, 2000 (modified 10/16/00).
SOURCE: Developed by the National Center for Health Statistics in collaboration with
the National Center for Chronic Disease Prevention and Health Promotion (2000).
http://www.cdc.gov/growthcharts

SAFER · HEALTHIER · PEOPLE™

2 to 20 years: Boys
Stature-for-age and Weight-for-age percentiles

NAME _____

RECORD# _____

Mother's Stature		Father's Stature		
Date	Age	Weight	Stature	BMI*

***To Calculate BMI:** Weight (kg) ÷ Stature (cm) ÷ Stature (cm) x 10,000
or Weight (lb) ÷ Stature (in) ÷ Stature (in) x 703*

AGE (YEARS)

12 13 14 15 16 17 18 19 20

STATURE

95
90
75
50
25
10
5

cm — 190 — 185 — 180 — 175 — 170 — 165 — 160 — 155 — 150
in — 76 — 74 — 72 — 70 — 68 — 66 — 64 — 62 — 60

in / cm — 3 4 5 6 7 8 9 10 11

STATURE

in: 62 60 58 56 54 52 50 48 46 44 42 40 38 36 34 32 30
cm: 160 155 150 145 140 135 130 125 120 115 110 105 100 95 90 85 80

95
90
75
50
25
10
5

WEIGHT

cm — 105 — 100
in — 230 — 220 — 210 — 200 — 190 — 180 — 170 — 160 — 150 — 140 — 130 — 120

95
90
75
50
25
10
5

WEIGHT

lb: 80 70 60 50 40 30
kg: 35 30 25 20 15 10

AGE (YEARS)

kg — 55 50 45 40 35 30 25 20 15 10
lb — 120 110 100 90 80 70 60 50 40 30

2 3 4 5 6 7 8 9 10 11 12 13 14 15 16 17 18 19 20

Published May 30, 2000 (modified 11/21/00).
SOURCE: Developed by the National Center for Health Statistics in collaboration with
the National Center for Chronic Disease Prevention and Health Promotion (2000).
http://www.cdc.gov/growthcharts

SAFER · HEALTHIER · PEOPLE™

2 to 20 years: Girls
Stature-for-age and Weight-for-age percentiles

NAME _____

RECORD# _____

Date	Age	Weight	Stature	BMI*

Mother's Stature _____   Father's Stature _____

*To Calculate BMI: Weight (kg) ÷ Stature (cm) ÷ Stature (cm) x 10,000
or Weight (lb) ÷ Stature (in) ÷ Stature (in) x 703

AGE (YEARS)

STATURE

WEIGHT

Published May 30, 2000 (modified 11/21/00).
SOURCE: Developed by the National Center for Health Statistics in collaboration with
the National Center for Chronic Disease Prevention and Health Promotion (2000).
http://www.cdc.gov/growthcharts

SAFER · HEALTHIER · PEOPLE™

PULSE, RESPIRATION, AND BLOOD PRESSURE VALUES FOR CHILDREN

Normal Pulse Ranges in Children

Age	Normal Range	Average
0–24 hours	70–170 bpm	120 bpm
1–7 days	100–180 bpm	140 bpm
1 month	110–188 bpm	160 bpm
1 month–1 year	80–180 bpm	120–130 bpm
2 years	80–140 bpm	110 bpm
4 years	80–120 bpm	100 bpm
6 years	70–115 bpm	100 bpm
10 years	70–110 bpm	90 bpm
12–14 years	60–110 bpm	85–90 bpm
14–18 years	50–95 bpm	70–75 bpm

bpm: beats per minute.

Variations in Respirations With Age

Age	Rate per Minute
Newborn	40–90
1 year	20–40
2 years	20–30
3 years	20–30
5 years	20–25
10 years	17–22
15 years	15–20
20 years	15–20

Normal Blood Pressure Ranges

Age	Systolic (mm Hg)	Diastolic (mm Hg)
Newborn–12 hr (less than 1,000 g)	39–59	16–36
Newborn–12 hr (3,000 g)	50–70	24–45
Newborn–96 hr (3,000 g)	60–90	20–60
Infant	74–100	50–70
Toddler	80–112	50–80
Preschooler	82–110	50–78
School-Age	84–120	54–80
Adolescent	94–140	62–88

Appendix I

TEMPERATURE AND WEIGHT CONVERSION CHARTS

Conversion of Pounds to Kilograms

Pounds	0	1	2	3	4	5	6	7	8	9
0	—	0.45	0.90	1.36	1.81	2.26	2.72	3.17	3.62	4.08
10	4.53	4.98	5.44	5.89	6.35	6.80	7.25	7.71	8.16	8.61
20	9.07	9.52	9.97	10.43	10.88	11.34	11.79	12.24	12.70	13.15
30	13.60	14.06	14.51	14.96	15.42	15.87	16.32	16.78	17.23	17.69
40	18.14	18.59	19.05	19.50	19.95	20.41	20.86	21.31	21.77	22.22
50	22.68	23.13	23.58	24.04	24.49	24.94	25.40	25.85	26.30	26.76
60	27.21	27.66	28.12	28.57	29.03	29.48	29.93	30.39	30.84	31.29
70	31.75	32.20	32.65	33.11	33.56	34.02	34.47	34.92	35.38	35.83
80	36.28	36.74	37.19	37.64	38.10	38.55	39.00	39.46	39.91	40.37
90	40.82	41.27	41.73	42.18	42.63	43.09	43.54	43.99	44.45	44.90
100	45.36	45.81	46.26	46.72	47.17	47.62	48.08	48.53	48.98	49.44
110	49.89	50.34	50.80	51.25	51.71	52.16	52.61	53.07	53.52	53.97
120	54.43	54.88	55.33	55.79	56.24	56.70	57.15	57.60	58.06	58.51
130	58.96	59.42	59.87	60.32	60.78	61.23	61.68	62.14	62.59	63.05
140	63.50	63.95	64.41	64.86	65.31	65.77	66.22	66.67	67.13	67.58
150	68.04	68.49	68.94	69.40	69.85	70.30	70.76	71.21	71.66	72.12
160	72.57	73.02	73.48	73.93	74.39	74.84	75.29	75.75	76.20	76.65
170	77.11	77.56	78.01	78.47	78.92	79.38	79.83	80.28	80.74	81.19
180	81.64	82.10	82.55	83.00	83.46	83.91	84.36	84.82	85.27	85.73
190	86.18	86.68	87.09	87.54	87.99	88.45	88.90	89.35	89.81	90.26
200	90.72	91.17	91.62	92.08	92.53	92.98	93.44	93.89	94.34	94.80

Conversion of Pounds and Ounces to Grams for Newborn Weights

Pounds	Ounces															
	0	1	2	3	4	5	6	7	8	9	10	11	12	13	14	15
0	—	28	57	85	113	142	170	198	227	255	283	312	369	397	425	430
1	454	482	510	539	567	595	624	652	680	709	737	765	794	822	850	879
2	907	936	964	992	1,021	1,049	1,077	1,106	1,134	1,162	1,191	1,219	1,247	1,276	1,304	1,332
3	1,361	1,389	1,417	1,446	1,474	1,503	1,531	1,559	1,588	1,616	1,644	1,673	1,701	1,729	1,758	1,786
4	1,814	1,843	1,871	1,899	1,928	1,956	1,984	2,013	2,041	2,070	2,098	2,126	2,155	2,183	2,211	2,240
5	2,268	2,296	2,325	2,353	2,381	2,410	2,438	2,466	2,495	2,523	2,551	2,580	2,608	2,637	2,665	2,693
6	2,722	2,750	2,778	2,807	2,835	2,863	2,892	2,920	2,948	2,977	3,005	3,033	3,062	3,090	3,118	3,147
7	3,175	3,203	3,232	3,260	3,289	3,317	3,345	3,374	3,402	3,430	3,459	3,487	3,515	3,544	3,572	3,600
8	3,629	3,657	3,685	3,714	3,742	3,770	3,799	3,827	3,856	3,884	3,912	3,941	3,969	3,997	4,026	4,054
9	4,082	4,111	4,139	4,167	4,196	4,224	4,252	4,281	4,309	4,337	4,366	4,394	4,423	4,451	4,479	4,508
10	4,536	4,564	4,593	4,621	4,649	4,678	4,706	4,734	4,763	4,791	4,819	4,848	4,876	4,904	4,933	4,961
11	4,990	5,018	5,046	5,075	5,103	5,131	5,160	5,188	5,216	5,245	5,273	5,301	5,330	5,358	5,386	5,415
12	5,443	5,471	5,500	5,528	5,557	5,585	5,613	5,642	5,670	5,698	5,727	5,755	5,783	5,812	5,840	5,868
13	5,897	5,925	5,953	5,982	6,010	6,038	6,067	6,095	6,123	6,152	6,180	6,209	6,237	6,265	6,294	6,322
14	6,350	6,379	6,407	6,435	6,464	6,492	6,520	6,549	6,577	6,605	6,634	6,662	6,690	6,719	6,747	6,776
15	6,804	6,832	6,860	6,889	6,917	6,945	6,973	7,002	7,030	7,059	7,087	7,115	7,144	7,172	7,201	7,228

Conversion of Fahrenheit to Celsius

Celsius	Fahrenheit	Celsius	Fahrenheit	Celsius	Fahrenheit
34.0	93.2	37.0	98.6	40.0	104.0
34.2	93.6	37.2	99.0	40.2	101.4
34.4	93.9	37.4	99.3	40.4	104.7
34.6	94.3	37.6	99.7	40.6	105.2
34.8	94.6	37.8	100.0	40.8	105.4
35.0	95.0	38.0	100.4	41.0	105.9
35.2	95.4	38.2	100.8	41.2	106.1
35.4	95.7	38.4	101.1	41.4	106.5
35.6	96.1	38.6	101.5	41.6	106.8
35.8	96.4	38.8	101.8	41.8	107.2
36.0	96.8	39.0	102.2	42.0	107.6
36.2	97.2	39.2	102.6	42.2	108.0
36.4	97.5	39.4	102.9	42.4	108.3
36.6	97.9	39.6	103.3	42.6	108.7
36.8	98.2	39.8	103.6	42.8	109.0

$$(\text{°C}) \times (9/5) + 32 = \text{°F}$$
$$(\text{°F} - 32) \times (5/9) = \text{°C}$$

RECOMMENDED CHILDHOOD AND ADOLESCENT IMMUNIZATION SCHEDULES

Recommended Immunization Schedule for Persons Aged 0 Through 6 Years—United States • 2009
For those who fall behind or start late, see the catch-up schedule

Vaccine ▼ Age ▶	Birth	1 month	2 months	4 months	6 months	12 months	15 months	18 months	19–23 months	2–3 years	4–6 years
Hepatitis B[1]	HepB	HepB	see footnote 1		HepB						
Rotavirus[2]			RV	RV	RV[2]						
Diphtheria, Tetanus, Pertussis[3]			DTaP	DTaP	DTaP	see footnote 3	DTaP				DTaP
Haemophilus influenzae type b[4]			Hib	Hib	Hib[4]	Hib					
Pneumococcal[5]			PCV	PCV	PCV	PCV				PPSV	
Inactivated Poliovirus			IPV	IPV		IPV					IPV
Influenza[6]						Influenza (Yearly)					
Measles, Mumps, Rubella[7]						MMR		see footnote 7			MMR
Varicella[8]						Varicella		see footnote 8			Varicella
Hepatitis A[9]						HepA (2 doses)				HepA Series	
Meningococcal[10]										MCV	

Range of recommended ages

Certain high-risk groups

This schedule indicates the recommended ages for routine administration of currently licensed vaccines, as of December 1, 2008, for children aged 0 through 6 years. Any dose not administered at the recommended age should be administered at a subsequent visit, when indicated and feasible. Licensed combination vaccines may be used whenever any component of the combination is indicated and other components are not contraindicated and if approved by the Food and Drug Administration for that dose of the series. Providers should consult the relevant Advisory Committee on Immunization Practices statement for detailed recommendations, including high-risk conditions: http://www.cdc.gov/vaccines/pubs/acip-list.htm. Clinically significant adverse events that follow immunization should be reported to the Vaccine Adverse Event Reporting System (VAERS). Guidance about how to obtain and complete a VAERS form is available at http://www.vaers.hhs.gov or by telephone, 800-822-7967.

Recommended Immunization Schedule for Persons Aged 7 Through 18 Years—United States • 2009
For those who fall behind or start late, see the schedule below and the catch-up schedule

Vaccine ▼ Age ▶	7–10 years	11–12 years	13–18 years
Tetanus, Diphtheria, Pertussis[1]	see footnote 1	Tdap	Tdap
Human Papillomavirus[2]	see footnote 2	HPV (3 doses)	HPV Series
Meningococcal[3]	MCV	MCV	MCV
Influenza[4]		Influenza (Yearly)	
Pneumococcal[5]		PPSV	
Hepatitis A[6]		HepA Series	
Hepatitis B[7]		HepB Series	
Inactivated Poliovirus[8]		IPV Series	
Measles, Mumps, Rubella[9]		MMR Series	
Varicella[10]		Varicella Series	

Range of recommended ages

Catch-up immunization

Certain high-risk groups

This schedule indicates the recommended ages for routine administration of currently licensed vaccines, as of December 1, 2008, for children aged 7 through 18 years. Any dose not administered at the recommended age should be administered at a subsequent visit, when indicated and feasible. Licensed combination vaccines may be used whenever any component of the combination is indicated and other components are not contraindicated and if approved by the Food and Drug Administration for that dose of the series. Providers should consult the relevant Advisory Committee on Immunization Practices statement for detailed recommendations, including high-risk conditions: http://www.cdc.gov/vaccines/pubs/acip-list.htm. Clinically significant adverse events that follow immunization should be reported to the Vaccine Adverse Event Reporting System (VAERS). Guidance about how to obtain and complete a VAERS form is available at http://www.vaers.hhs.gov or by telephone, 800-822-7967.

abruptio placentae, or placental abruption the premature separation of a normally implanted placenta.

absence seizure seizure in which there is a sudden, brief loss of awareness, then a return to an alert state.

abstinence (as related to birth control); refraining from vaginal sexual intercourse.

abuse misuse, excessive use, rough or bad treatment; used to refer to misuse of alcohol or drugs (substance abuse) and mistreatment of children or family members (child abuse, domestic abuse).

accelerations spontaneous elevations of the fetal heart rate (FHR).

accommodation occurs when the pupils constrict in order to bring an object into focus. When a bright object is held at a distance and then quickly moved toward the face, the pupil will constrict.

achylia absence of pancreatic enzymes in gastric secretions.

acid–base balance state of equilibrium between the acidity and the alkalinity of body fluids.

acidosis excessive acidity of body fluids.

acrocyanosis cyanosis of the hands and feet seen periodically in the newborn.

actual nursing diagnoses diagnoses that identify existing health problems.

adenoids mass of lymphoid tissue in the nasal pharynx; extends from the roof of the nasal pharynx to the free edge of the soft palate.

adenopathy enlarged lymph glands.

akinetic seizure that causes a sudden, momentary loss of consciousness and muscle tone; also called atonic.

alcohol abuse drinking sufficient alcoholic beverages to induce intoxication.

alcoholism chronic alcohol abuse.

alkalosis excessive alkalinity of body fluids.

allergen antigen that causes an allergic reaction.

allograft skin graft taken from a genetically different person for temporary coverage during burn healing. Skin from a cadaver sometimes is used.

alopecia loss of hair.

amblyopia dimness of vision from disuse of the eye; sometimes called "lazy eye."

amenorrhea absence of menstruation.

amniocentesis a diagnostic procedure whereby a needle is inserted into the amniotic sac and a small amount of fluid is withdrawn and used for biochemical, chromosomal, and genetic studies.

amnioinfusion infusion of sterile fluid into the uterine cavity during labor

amnion a thick fibrous lining, made up of several layers, that helps to protect the fetus and forms the inner part of the sac in which the fetus grows.

amniotic fluid the specialized fluid that fills the amniotic cavity and serves to protect the fetus.

amniotomy artificial rupture of membranes (AROM).

analgesia the use of medication to reduce the sensation of pain.

android pelvis the typical male pelvis; in the woman, the heart shape of the android pelvis is not favorable to a vaginal delivery.

anesthesia the use of medication to partially or totally block all sensation to an area of the body.

ankylosis immobility of a joint.

anorexia nervosa eating disorder characterized by loss of appetite due to emotional causes (e.g., usually excessive fear of becoming [or being] fat).

anthelmintic medication that expels intestinal worms; vermifuge.

anthropoid pelvis woman's pelvis that is elongated in its dimensions and is sometimes referred to as apelike.

anticipatory grief preparatory grieving that often helps caregivers mourn the loss of their child when death actually comes.

antigen protein substance found on the surface of red blood cells capable of inducing a specific immune response and reacting with the products of that response.

antigen-antibody response response of the body to an antigen causing the formation of antibodies that protect the body from an invading antigen.

anuria absence of urine.

apnea temporary interruption of the breathing impulse.

appropriate for gestational age (AGA) a newborn whose weight, length, and/or head circumference falls between the 10th and 90th percentiles for gestational age

archetypes predetermined patterns of human development, which according to Carl Jung, replace instinctive behavior of other animals; prototype.

areola darkened area around the nipple.

arthralgia painful joints.

artificial nutrition infant formula.

ascites edema in the peritoneal cavity.

associative play being engaged in a common activity without any sense of belonging or fixed rules.

astigmatism error in light refraction on the retina caused by unequal curvature in the eye's cornea; light rays bend in different directions to produce a blurred image.

ataxia lack of coordination caused by disturbances in the kinesthetic and balance senses.

atonic seizure that causes a sudden, momentary loss of consciousness and muscle tone; also called akinetic.

atresia absence of a normal body opening or the abnormal closure of a body passage.

atrial septal defect is an abnormal opening between the right and left atria.

attachment the enduring emotional bond that develops between the parent and infant.

aura a sensation that signals an impending epileptic attack; may be visual, aromatic, or other sensation.

autistic totally self-centered and unable to relate to others, often exhibiting bizarre behaviors. Autistic children can sometimes be destructive to themselves and others.

autograft skin taken from an individual's own body. Except for the skin of an identical twin, autograft is the only kind of skin accepted permanently by recipient tissues.

autonomy ability to function in an independent manner.

autosomal dominant trait trait or condition appearing in a heterozygous person resulting from a dominant gene within a pair.

autosomal recessive trait trait or condition that is not expressed unless both parents carry the gene for that trait.

autosomes 22 pairs of chromosomes that are alike in the male and female. The sex chromosomes are not autosomes.

azotemia nitrogen-containing compounds in the blood.

Babinski reflex the flaring open of the infant's toes when the lateral plantar surface is stroked. Also called the plantar reflex, this reaction usually disappears by the end of the first year.

ballottement a probable sign of pregnancy that occurs when the examiner pushes up on the uterine wall during a pelvic examination, then feels the fetus bounce back against the examiner's fingers.

bilateral pertaining to both sides (e.g., bilateral cleft lip involves both sides of the lip).

binocular vision normal vision maintained through the muscular coordination of eye movements of both eyes. A single vision results.

biophysical profile (BPP) a method that uses a combination of factors to determine fetal well-being.

Bishop score one commonly used scoring method to determine cervical readiness that evaluates five factors: cervical consistency, position, dilation, effacement, and fetal station.

blastocyst the structure that forms about 5 days after fertilization when the dividing cell mass develops a hollow, fluid-filled core.

blended family both partners in a marriage bring children from a previous marriage into the household: his, hers, and theirs.

body surface area (BSA) formula used to calculate dosages. Using a West nomogram, the child's weight is marked on the right scale and the height is marked on the left scale. A straightedge is used to draw a line between the two marks. The point at which the line crosses the column labeled SA (surface area) is the BSA expressed in square meters (m^2).

body weight method for calculating dosages uses the child's weight as a basis for computing medication dosages.

boggy uterus a uterus that feels soft and spongy, rather than firm and well contracted.

bolus feeding an enteral feeding given intermittently

bonding development of a close emotional tie between the newborn and the parent or parents.

bottle mouth (nursing bottle) caries condition caused by the erosion of enamel on the infant's deciduous teeth from sugar in formula or sweetened juice that coats the teeth for long periods. This condition also can occur in infants who sleep with their mothers and nurse intermittently throughout the night.

brachycephaly shortness of the head.

bradycardia decreased pulse rate

Braxton Hicks contractions the painless, intermittent, "practice" contractions of pregnancy.

breakthrough pain pain that occurs when the basal dose of analgesia does not control the pain adequately.

bronchodilators medications used for quick relief of acute exacerbations of asthma symptoms.

brown fat a specialized form of heat-producing tissue found only in fetuses and newborns.

bulimia eating disorder characterized by episodes of binge eating, followed by purging by self-induced vomiting or use of laxatives.

capitation a method that managed care plans use to reduce costs by paying a fixed amount per person to the health care provider to provide services for enrollees.

caput succedaneum edematous swelling of the soft tissues of the scalp caused by prolonged pressure of the occiput against the cervix during labor and delivery. The edema disappears within a few days.

cardinal movements the turns and movements made during the journey of the fetus; referred to as the mechanisms of delivery.

carditis inflammation of the heart.

case management a systematic process to ensure that a client's health and service needs are met.

cataract development of opacity in the crystalline lens that prevents light rays from entering the eye.

cavernous hemangiomas congenital malformations that are subcutaneous collections of blood vessels with bluish overlying skin. Although these lesions are benign tumors, they may become so extensive as to interfere with the functions of the body part on which they appear.

celiac syndrome term used to designate the complex of malabsorptive disorders.

cephalhematoma collection of blood between the periosteum and the skull caused by excessive pressure on the head during birth.

cephalocaudal the pattern of growth of the child that follows an orderly pattern, starting with the head and moving downward.

cerclage procedure that involves placing a purse string type suture in the cervix to keep it from dilating.

cesarean birth the delivery of a fetus through abdominal and uterine incisions: laparotomy and hysterotomy, respectively. Cesarean comes from the Latin word "caedere," meaning "to cut."

Chadwick's sign the bluish-purplish color of the cervix, vagina, and perineum during pregnancy.

chancre hard, red, painless primary lesion of syphilis at the point of entry of the spirochete.

chelating agent agent that binds with metal.

chief complaint is the reason for the child's visit to the health care setting.

child abuse any intentional act of physical, emotional, or sexual abuse, including acts of negligence, committed by a person responsible for the care of the child.

child advocacy speaking or acting on behalf of a child to ensure that her or his needs are recognized.

child neglect failing to provide adequate hygiene, health care, nutrition, love, nurturing, and supervision as needed for a child's growth and development.

child-life program program to make hospitalization less threatening for children and their parents. These programs are usually under the direction of a child-life specialist whose background is in psychology and early childhood development.

chloasma or mask of pregnancy; brown blotchy areas on the forehead, cheeks, and nose of the pregnant woman.

chordee chord-like anomaly that extends from the scrotum to the penis; pulls the penis downward in an arc.

chorea continuous, rapid, jerky involuntary movements.

chorioamnionitis bacterial or viral infection of the amniotic fluid and membranes.

choriocarcinoma malignancy of the uterine lining.

chorion a second layer of thick fibrous tissue that surrounds the amnion.

chorionic villi finger-like projections that extend out from the chorion giving it a rough appearance.

chorionic villus sampling (CVS) a newer procedure that can provide chromosomal studies of fetal cells similar to that of amniocentesis.

chromosomes thread-like structures that occur in pairs and carry genetic information.

chronic illness condition that interferes with daily functioning, progresses slowly, and shows little change over a long duration of time.

circumcision surgical removal of all or part of the foreskin (prepuce) of the penis.

circumoral pallor a white area around the mouth.

classification ability to group objects by rank, grade, or class.

cleavage the process of mitotic division performed by the zygote.

client advocacy speaking or acting on behalf of others to help them gain greater independence and to make the health care delivery system more responsive and relevant to their needs.

climacteric the interlude surrounding menopause in which changes in reproductive functioning take place.

clonus rapid involuntary muscle contraction and relaxation.

clove hitch restraints restraints used to secure an arm or leg; used most often when a child is receiving an intravenous infusion. The restraint is made of soft cloth formed in a figure eight.

coarctation of the aorta is a constriction or narrowing of the aortic arch or the descending aorta usually adjacent to the ligamentum arteriosum.

codependent parent parent who supports, directly or indirectly, the other parent's addictive behavior.

cognitive development progressive change in the intellectual process, including perception, memory, and judgment.

cohabitation family a living situation in which a man and woman live together but are not legally married.

coitus interruptus or withdrawal; requires the man to pull the penis out of the vagina before ejaculation to avoid depositing sperm in or near the vagina.

cold stress exposure to temperatures cooler than normal body temperature so that the newborn must use energy to maintain heat.

colic recurrent paroxysmal bouts of abdominal pain that are fairly common among young infants and that usually disappear around the age of 3 months.

colostomy a surgical procedure in which a part of the colon is brought through the abdominal wall to create an outlet for elimination of fecal material.

colostrum thin, yellowish, milky fluid secreted by the woman's breasts during pregnancy or just after delivery (before the secretion of milk).

comedones collection of keratin and sebum in the hair follicle; blackhead; whitehead.

communal family alternative family in which members share responsibility for homemaking and child rearing. All children are the collective responsibility of adult members.

community-based nursing a type of nursing practice focused on wellness and a holistic approach to caring for the child in a community setting.

compartment syndrome a serious neurovascular concern that occurs when increasing pressure within the muscle compartment causes decreased circulation.

congenital hip dysplasia abnormal fetal development of the acetabulum that may or may not cause dislocation of the hip. If the malformed acetabulum permits dislocation, the head of the femur displaces upward and backward. This may be difficult to recognize in early infancy.

congestive heart failure (CHF) result of impaired pumping capability of the heart. It may appear in the first year of life in infants with conditions such as large ventricular septal defects, coarctation of the aorta, and other defects that place an increased workload on the ventricles.

conjunctivitis acute inflammation of the conjunctiva that may be caused by a virus, bacteria, allergy, or foreign body.

conservation ability to recognize that change in shape does not necessarily mean change in amount or mass.

contracture fibrous scarring that forms over a burned movable body part. This part of the healing process can cause serious deformities and limit movement.

cooperative play children play with each other, as in team sports.

cordocentesis or **percutaneous umbilical blood sampling (PUBS),** a procedure similar to amniocentesis whereby fetal blood is withdrawn from the umbilical cord.

corpus luteum a yellow body that forms after ovulation from the remnants of the follicle.

coryza runny nose.

couvade syndrome phenomenon in which some fathers actually experience some of the physical symptoms of pregnancy, such as nausea and vomiting, along with their partner.

cradle cap accumulation of oil and dirt that often forms on an infant's scalp; seborrheic dermatitis.

craniotabes softening of the occipital bones caused by a reduction of mineralization of the skull.

cretinism a congenital condition marked by stunted growth and mental retardation.

critical pathways standard plans of care used to organize and monitor the care provided.

croup general term that typically includes symptoms of a barking cough, hoarseness, and inspiratory stridor.

cultural competency the capacity of the nurse to work with people by integrating their cultural needs into their nursing care.

currant jelly stools stools that consist of blood and mucus.

cyanotic heart disease congenital heart disease that causes right-to-left shunting of blood in the heart; results in a depletion of oxygen to such an extent that the oxygen saturation of the peripheral arterial blood is 85% or less. Defects that permit right-to-left shunting may occur at the atrial, ventricular, or aortic level.

cystitis infection of the bladder.

dawdling wasting time; whiling away time; being idle.

débridement removal of necrotic tissue.

decentration ability to see several aspects of a problem at the same time and understand the relationships of various parts to the whole situation.

decidua the endometrium that has changed to support a pregnancy.

deciduous teeth primary teeth that usually erupt between 6 and 8 months of age.

deliriants inhalants that contain chemicals whose fumes can produce confusion, disorientation, excitement, and hallucinations.

denial defense mechanism in which the existence of unpleasant actions or ideas is unconsciously repressed; in the grieving process, one of the stages many people go through; also a type of response by caregivers when caring for chronically ill children in which the caregivers deny the condition's existence and encourage the child to overcompensate for any disabilities.

dependence compulsive need to use a substance for its satisfying or pleasurable effects.

dependent nursing actions nursing actions that the nurse performs as a result of a physician's orders, such as administering analgesics for pain.

deep vein thrombosis formation of a blood clot (thrombus) in the deeper veins of the calf, thigh, or pelvis.

dermatome an area on the body surface supplied by a particular sensory nerve.

development progressive change in the child's maturation.

developmental tasks basic achievements associated with each stage of development. Basic tasks must be mastered to move on to the next developmental stage. To achieve maturity, a person must successfully complete developmental tasks at each stage.

diabetic ketoacidosis characterized by drowsiness, dry skin, flushed cheeks, cherry-red lips, and acetone breath with a fruity smell as a result of excessive ketones in the blood in uncontrolled diabetes.

diabetogenic effect of pregnancy the normal state during pregnancy in which blood glucose levels are lower than normal (mild hypoglycemia) when fasting, blood glucose levels are higher than normal (mild hyperglycemia) after meals, and insulin levels are increased (hyperinsulinemia) after meals.

diagonal conjugate area that extends from the symphysis pubis to the sacral promontory, which is measured to provide an estimate of the size of the obstetric conjugate.

diastasis recti abdominis separation of the rectus abdominis muscle that supports the abdomen.

digitalization the use of large doses of digoxin, at the beginning of therapy, to build up the blood levels of the drug to a therapeutic level.

diplopia double vision.

discipline to train or instruct to produce self-control and a particular behavior pattern, especially moral or mental improvement.

dizygotic fraternal twins that develop from separate egg and sperm fertilizations.

doula Greek for servant; birth assistants who are trained to provide the highest quality emotional, physical, and educational support to women and their families during childbirth and the postpartum period.

dramatic play a type of play that allows a child to act out troubling situations and to control the solution to the problem.

ductus arteriosus prenatal blood vessel between the pulmonary artery and the aorta that closes functionally within the first 3 or 4 days of life.

ductus venosus prenatal blood vessel between the umbilical vein and the inferior vena cava; does not achieve complete closure until the end of the second month of life.

dysarthria poor speech articulation.

dysfunctional family family that cannot resolve routine stresses in a positive, socially acceptable manner.

dysmenorrhea painful menstruation.

dyspareunia painful intercourse.

dysphagia difficulty swallowing.

early adolescence begins at about age 10 years in girls and about age 12 years in boys with a dramatic growth spurt that signals the advent of puberty; preadolescence; pubescence.

early deceleration the dip in the fetal heart rate (FHR) tracing that occurs in conjunction with and mirrors a uterine contraction.

echolalia "parrot speech" typical of autistic children. They echo words they hear, such as a television commercial, but do not appear to understand the words.

eclampsia condition in which the woman with severe preeclampsia experiences a convulsion or a coma.

ectopic pregnancy a pregnancy that occurs outside of the uterus.

effacement softening and shortening of the cervix during labor.

effleurage a form of touch that involves light circular fingertip movements on the abdomen; a technique a woman can use in early labor.

ego in psychoanalytic theory, the conscious self that controls the pleasure principle of the id by delaying the instincts until an appropriate time.

egocentric concerned only with one's own activities or needs; unable to put oneself in another's place or to see another's point of view.

elbow restraints restraints made of muslin with two layers. Pockets wide enough to enclose tongue depressors are placed vertically along the width of the fabric. The restraints are wrapped around the arm to prevent the infant from bending the arm.

elective abortion an abortion performed at the woman's request that does not involve preservation of health.

elective induction induction of labor in which the physician and woman decide to end the pregnancy in the absence of a medical reason to do so.

electrolytes chemical compounds (minerals) that break down into ions when placed in water.

embryo the developing conceptus, from weeks 2 through 8.

emetic agent that causes vomiting.

en face position establishment of eye contact in the same plane between the caregiver and infant; extremely important to parent–infant bonding; also called mutual gazing.

encephalopathy degenerative disease of the brain.

encopresis chronic involuntary fecal soiling with no medical cause.

endometriosis a painful reproductive and immunologic disorder in which tissue implants resembling endometrium grow outside of the uterus.

endometritis an infection of the uterine lining.

endometrium the vascular mucosal inner layer of walls of the corpus and fundus that changes under hormonal influence every month in preparation for possible pregnancy.

engagement occurs when the presenting part of the fetus has settled into the true pelvis at the level of the ischial spines.

engorgement occurs when the milk comes in and the woman's body responds with increasing the blood supply to the breast tissues.

enteral tube feeding provides nourishment directly through a tube passed into the GI tract.

enuresis involuntary urination, especially at night; bedwetting beyond the usual age of control.

epididymis an intricate network of coiled ducts on the posterior portion of each testis that is approximately 6 m (20 ft) in length.

epiphyses growth centers at the ends of long bones and at the wrists.

episiotomy a surgical incision made into the perineum to enlarge the vaginal opening just before the baby is born.

episodic changes variations in the fetal heart rate not associated with uterine contractions.

epispadias condition in which the opening of the urinary meatus is located abnormally on the dorsal (upper) surface of the glans penis.

epistaxis nosebleed.

Epstein's pearls small white cysts found on the midline portion of the hard palate of some newborns.

Erb's palsy a facial paralysis resulting from injury to the cervical nerves.

erythema toxicum fine rash of the newborn that may appear over the trunk, back, abdomen, and buttocks. It appears about 24 hours after birth and disappears in several days.

erythroblastosis fetalis a condition in which the infant's red blood cells are broken down (hemolyzed) and destroyed, producing severe anemia and hyperbilirubinemia.

eschar hard crust or scab.

esotropia eye deviation toward the other eye.

estimated date of confinement (EDC) the estimated date that the baby will be born.

estimated date of delivery (EDD) the estimated date that the baby will be born.

exotropia eye deviation away from the other eye.

extended family consists of one or more nuclear families plus other relatives; often crosses generations to include grandparents, aunts, uncles, and cousins. The needs of individual members are subordinate to the needs of the group, and the children are considered an economic asset.

external version a process of manipulating the position of the fetus while in utero, to try to turn the fetus to a cephalic presentation.

extracellular fluid fluid situated outside a cell or cells.

extravasation escape of fluid into surrounding tissue.

extrusion reflex infant's way of taking food by thrusting the tongue forward as if to suck; has the effect of pushing solid food out of the mouth.

exudate drainage; fluid accumulation.

false pelvis the flared upper portion of the bony pelvis.

febrile seizure seizure occurring in infants and young children commonly associated with a fever of 102°F to 106°F (38.9°C–41.1°C).

fertilization process by which the male's sperm unites with the female's ovum.

fetal alcohol syndrome (FAS) syndrome seen in an infant born to a woman who abused alcohol during pregnancy, including shorter stature, lower birth weight, possible microcephaly, facial deformities, hearing disorders, poor coordination, minor joint and limb abnormalities, heart defects, delayed development, and mental retardation.

fetal attitude the relationship of the fetal parts to one another.

fetal fibronectin a protein found in fetal membranes and amniotic fluid.

fetal lie the long axis of the fetus in relation to the long axis of the pregnant woman.

fetal presentation the foremost part of the fetus that enters the pelvic inlet.

fetus term for the organism after it has reached the eighth week of life and acquires a human likeness.

fontanel "soft spot" covered by a tough membrane at the junctures of the six bones of a newborn's skull. At birth, two fontanels can be detected—the anterior fontanel at the junction of the frontal and parietal bones and the posterior fontanel at the junction of the parietal and occipital bones. They are ossified (filled in by bone) during the normal growth process.

foramen ovale opening between the left and right atria of the fetal heart that closes with the first breath.

forceps metal instruments with curved, blunted blades (somewhat like large hollowed-out spoons) that are placed around the head of the fetus by the birth attendant to facilitate delivery.

forceps marks noticeable marks on the infant's face that may occur if delivery was assisted with forceps; usually disappear within a day or two.

foremilk breast milk that is very watery and thin and may have a bluish tint. This is what the infant receives first during the breast-feeding session.

gag reflex reaction to any stimulation of the posterior pharynx by food, suction, or passage of a tube that causes elevation of the soft palate and a strong involuntary effort to vomit; continues throughout life.

galactosemia recessive hereditary metabolic disorder in which the enzyme necessary for converting galactose into glucose is missing. The infant generally appears normal at birth but experiences difficulties after the ingestion of milk.

gametes sex cells.

gametogenesis the formation and development of gametes or germ cells by the process of meiosis.

gastroenteritis infectious diarrhea caused by infectious organisms, including salmonella, *Escherichia coli,* dysentery bacilli, and various viruses, most notably rotaviruses.

gastrostomy tube tube surgically inserted through the abdominal wall into the stomach under general anesthesia. Used in children who have obstructions or surgical repairs in the mouth, pharynx, esophagus, or cardiac sphincter of the stomach or who are respirator dependent.

gavage feeding nourishment provided directly through a tube passed into the stomach.

genes units threaded along chromosomes that carry genetic instructions from one generation to another. Like chromosomes, genes also occur in pairs. There are thousands of genes in the chromosomes of each cell nucleus.

genetic counseling study of the family history and tissue analysis of both partners to determine chromosome patterns for couples concerned about transmitting a specific disease to their unborn children.

gestational age the length of time between fertilization of the egg and birth of the infant.

gestational diabetes mellitus (GDM) a type of diabetes mellitus (DM) that is unique to pregnancy but in many respects mimics type 2 DM.

gestational hypertension (formerly called pregnancy-induced hypertension or PIH) the current term used to describe elevated blood pressure (≥140/90 mm Hg) that develops for the first time during pregnancy without the presence of protein in the urine.

gestational surrogate or surrogate mother; a woman who donates the use of her uterus, or she may also donate her ovum and agree to be inseminated with the male partner's sperm.

glycosuria glucose in the urine.

goniotomy surgical opening into Schlemm's canal that allows drainage of aqueous humor; performed to relieve intraocular pressure in glaucoma.

Goodell's sign softening of the cervix during pregnancy.

gradual acceptance type of response by caregivers when caring for a chronically ill child in which caregivers adopt a common-sense approach to the child's condition and encourage the child to function within his or her capabilities.

grand multiparity five or more pregnancies.

granulocytes type of white blood cell; divided into eosinophils, basophils, and neutrophils.

gravida the number of pregnancies the woman has had (regardless of the outcome).

growth result of cell division and marked by an increase in size and weight; physical increase in body size and appearance caused by increasing numbers of new cells.

gynecoid pelvis categorized as a typical female pelvis (although only about half of all women have this type of pelvis); the rounded shape of the gynecoid inlet allows the fetus room to negotiate the dimensions of the bony passageway.

gynecomastia excessive growth of the mammary glands in the male.

halo traction metal ring attached to the skull that is added to a body cast using stainless steel pins inserted into the skull and into the femurs or iliac wings.

Harlequin sign or Harlequin coloring characterized by a clown-suit–like appearance of the newborn. The newborn's skin is dark red on one side of the body while the other side of the body is pale. The dark red color is caused by dilation of blood vessels, and the pallor is caused by contraction of blood vessels.

health maintenance organizations (HMOs) professional groups of physicians, laboratory service personnel, nurse practitioners, nurses, and consultants who care for the family's health on a continuing basis and are geared to health care and disease prevention. The family pays a set fee for total care; that fee covers any necessary hospitalization. The emphasis is on health and prevention.

Hegar's sign softening of the uterine isthmus during pregnancy.

hemarthrosis bleeding into the joints.

hematoma a clot of blood that collects within tissues and leads to concealed blood loss.

hemolysis destruction of red blood cells with the release of hemoglobin into the plasma.

hernia abnormal protrusion of part of an organ through a weak spot or other abnormal opening in a body wall.

heterograft graft of tissue obtained from an animal. For burn patients, pigskin (porcine) is often used.

heterosexual intimate relationship between two people of the opposite sex.

hierarchical arrangement grouping by some common system such as rank, grade, or class.

hind milk breast milk that is thicker and whiter. It contains a higher quantity of fat than foremilk and therefore has a higher caloric content than foremilk.

hip dysplasia see congenital hip dysplasia.

hirsutism abnormal body and facial hair growth.

homeostasis uniform state; signifies biologically the dynamic equilibrium of the healthy organism.

homograft graft of tissue, including organs, from a member of one's own species.

homosexual intimate relationship between two people of the same sex.

homozygous term used to describe a particular trait of an individual when any two members of a pair of genes carry the same genetic instructions for that trait.

hordeolum purulent infection of the follicle of an eyelash; generally caused by *Staphylococcus aureus*. Localized swelling, tenderness, and pain are present with a reddened lid edge; a stye.

hospice provides comforting and supportive care to terminally ill patients and their families. There are few hospice programs for children in the United States.

hyaline membrane disease also known as respiratory distress syndrome (RDS); occurs because of immature lungs that lack sufficient surfactant to decrease the surface tension of the alveoli; affects about half of all preterm newborns.

hydatidiform mole also referred to as a molar pregnancy and gestational trophoblastic disease; a condition characterized by benign growth of placental tissue.

hydramnios excessive amniotic fluid.

hydrotherapy use of water in a treatment.

hyperbilirubinemia high levels of unconjugated bilirubin in the bloodstream (serum levels of 4–6 mg/dL and greater).

hyperemesis gravidarum a disorder of early pregnancy that is characterized by severe nausea and vomiting.

hyperglycemia elevated blood glucose levels.

hyperinsulinemia increased insulin levels.

hyperlipidemia increase in the level of cholesterol in the blood.

hyperopia refractive condition in which the person can see objects better at a distance; farsightedness.

hyperpnea increase in depth and rate of breathing.

hyperthermia overheating.

hypervolemia increased volume of circulating plasma.

hypocholia diminished flow of pancreatic enzymes.

hypoglycemia low blood sugar levels.

hyposensitization immunization therapy by injection; immunotherapy.

hypospadias condition that occurs when the opening to the urethra is on the ventral (under) surface of the glans.

hypothermia low body temperature; may be a symptom of a disease or dysfunction of the temperature-regulating mechanism of the body, or it may be deliberately induced, such as during open-heart surgery, to reduce oxygen needs and provide a longer time for the surgeon to complete the operation without the patient experiencing brain damage. When caring for the newborn, it is important to remember that heat loss can lead to hypothermia because of the infant's immature temperature-regulating system.

hypovolemia decreased volume of circulating plasma.

hypovolemic shock condition characterized by a weak, thready, rapid pulse; drop in blood pressure; cool, clammy skin; and changes in level of consciousness.

id in psychoanalytic theory, part of the personality that controls physical needs and instincts of the body; dominated by the pleasure principle.

ileostomy a surgical procedure in which a part of the ileum is brought through the abdominal wall to create an outlet to drain fecal material.

immunologic properties properties from the woman that help protect the newborn from infections and strengthen the newborn's immune system.

imperforate anus congenital disorder in which the rectal pouch ends blindly above the anus and there is no anal orifice.

impunity belief, common among adolescents, that nothing can hurt them.

incest sexually arousing physical contact between family members not married to each other.

independent nursing actions nursing actions that may be performed based on the nurse's own clinical judgment.

induced abortion the purposeful interruption of pregnancy before 20 weeks' gestation.

induration hardness.

infant mortality rate the number of deaths during the first 12 months of life, which includes neonatal mortality.

infantile spasms a type of seizure activity that occurs in an infant between 3 and 12 months of age and usually indicates a cerebral defect with a poor prognosis.

infertility the inability to conceive after a year or more of regular and unprotected intercourse, or the inability to carry a pregnancy to term.

infiltration fluid leaking into the surrounding tissues.

inhalant substance that may be taken into the body through inhaling; substance whose volatile vapors can be abused.

insulin reaction excessively low blood sugar caused by insulin overload; results in too-rapid metabolism of the body's glucose; insulin shock; hypoglycemia.

intercurrent infection infection that occurs during the course of an already existing disease.

interdependent nursing actions nursing actions that the nurse must work with other health team members to accomplish, such as meal planning with a dietary therapist and teaching breathing exercises with a respiratory therapist.

intermittent infusion device a type of device that is used for administering medications by the intravenous route and can be left in place and used at intervals.

interstitial fluid also called intracellular or tissue fluid; has a composition similar to plasma but contains almost no protein. This reservoir of fluid outside the body cells decreases or increases easily in response to disease.

interstitial keratitis inflammation of the cornea; often caused by congenital syphilis and usually accompanied by lacrimation, photophobia, and opacity of the lens; may lead to blindness.

intracellular fluid fluid contained within the cell membranes; constitutes about two thirds of total body fluids.

intrathecal administration injection into the cerebrospinal fluid by lumbar puncture.

intrauterine growth restriction (IUGR) condition in which babies are small because of circumstances that occurred during the pregnancy, causing limited fetal growth.

intravascular fluid fluid situated within the blood vessels or blood plasma.

intraventricular hemorrhage (IVH) bleeding within a ventricle of the heart or brain.

invagination telescoping; infolding of one part of a structure into another.

involution the shrinking or returning to normal size of the uterus, cervix, and vagina.

isoimmunization development of antibodies against Rho (D) positive blood in the pregnant woman.

jacket restraint used to secure the child from climbing out of bed or a chair or to keep the child in a horizontal position; must be the correct size for the child.

jaundice a yellow staining of the skin that occurs when a large amount of unconjugated bilirubin is present (serum levels ≥4–6 mg/dL).

kangaroo care a way to maintain the newborn's temperature and promote early bonding; the nurse dries the newborn quickly, places a diaper or blanket over the genital area and a cap on the head, then places the newborn in skin-to-skin contact with the mother or father and covers them both with blankets.

kernicterus neurologic complication of unconjugated hyperbilirubinemia in the infant.

Kussmaul breathing abnormal increase in the depth and rate of the respiratory movements.

kwashiorkor syndrome occurring in infants and young children soon after weaning; results from severe deficiency of protein. Symptoms include a swollen abdomen, retarded growth with muscle wasting, edema, gastrointestinal changes, thin dry hair with patchy alopecia, apathy, and irritability.

kyphosis backward and lateral curvature of the cervical spine; hunchback.

labor dystocia an abnormal progression of labor.

lacrimation secretion of tears.

lactation consultant a nurse or layperson who has received special training to assist and support the breastfeeding woman.

lactose a sugar found in milk that, when hydrolyzed, yields glucose and galactose.

lactose intolerance inability to digest lactose because of an inborn deficiency of the enzyme lactase.

laminaria cervical dilators.

lanugo fine, downy hair that covers the skin of the fetus.

large for gestational age (LGA) an infant whose weight, length, and/or head circumference is above the 90th percentile for gestational age.

latchkey child child who comes home to an empty house after school each day because family caregivers are at work.

late decelerations decelerations that are offset from the labor contraction. Late decelerations begin late in the contraction and recover after the contraction has ended.

lecithin major component of surfactant.

leukemia uncontrolled reproduction of deformed white blood cells.

leukopenia leukocyte count <5,000 mm^3.

libido sexual drive.

linea nigra a darkened line that develops on the skin in the middle of the abdomen of pregnant women.

lochia vaginal discharge after birth.

lordosis forward curvature of the lumbar spine; swayback.

low birth weight (LBW) newborns that weigh <2,500 g.

lymphoblast lymphocyte that has been changed by antigenic stimulation to a structurally immature lymphocyte.

lymphocytes single-nucleus, nonphagocytic leukocytes that are instrumental in the body's immune response.

macroglossia abnormally large tongue.

macrosomia condition that is diagnosed if the birth weight exceeds 4,500 g (9.9 lb) or the birth weight is greater than the 90th percentile for gestational age.

magical thinking child's belief that thoughts are powerful and can cause something to happen (e.g., illness or death of a loved one occurs because the child wished it in a moment of anger).

malattachment emotional distancing in the maternal–infant relationship.

malocclusion the improper alignment of the teeth.

marasmus deficiency in calories as well as protein. The child suffers growth retardation and wasting of subcutaneous fat and muscle.

mastitis infection of the breast tissue.

maternal mortality rate the number of maternal deaths per 100,000 live births caused by a pregnancy-related complication that occurs during pregnancy or during the 42 days after pregnancy.

maturation completed growth and development.

meconium first stools of the newborn.

meconium aspiration occurs when the fetus inhales some meconium along with amniotic fluid.

menarche beginning of menstruation.

menorrhagia heavy or prolonged uterine bleeding.

metaphysic growing portion of the bone

metered-dose inhaler hand-held plastic device that delivers a premeasured dose of medicine.

metrorrhagia menstrual bleeding that is normal in amount but occurs at irregular intervals between menstrual periods.

microcephaly a very small cranium.

micrognathia abnormal smallness of the lower jaw.

milia pearly white cysts usually seen over the bridge of the nose, chin, and cheeks of a newborn. They are usually retention cysts of sebaceous glands or hair follicles and disappear within a few weeks without treatment.

mittelschmerz pain experienced midcycle in the menstrual cycle at the time of ovulation.

molding elongation of the fetal skull to accommodate the birth canal.

mongolian spots areas of bluish-black pigmentation resembling bruises; most often seen over the sacral or gluteal regions of infants of African, Mediterranean, Native American, or Asian descent; usually fade within 1 or 2 years.

monocytes 5% to 10% of white blood cells that defend the body against infection.

monozygotic identical twins that are derived from one zygote; one egg and one sperm divide into two zygotes shortly after fertilization.

mons pubis or mons; a rounded fatty pad located atop the symphysis pubis.

Montgomery's tubercles sebaceous glands on the areolas that produce secretions that lubricate the nipple. Montgomery's tubercles become more prominent during pregnancy.

morbidity the number of persons afflicted with the same disease condition per a certain number of population.

Moro reflex abduction of the arms and legs and flexion of the elbows in response to a sudden loud noise, jarring, or abrupt change in equilibrium: fingers flare, except the forefinger and thumb, which are clenched to form a C shape. Occurs in the normal newborn to the end of the fourth or fifth month.

morula the solid cell cluster that forms about 3 days after fertilization, when the total cell count has reached 32.

mottling a red and white lacy pattern sometimes seen on the skin of newborns who have fair complexions.

multigravida a woman who has had more than one pregnancy.

mummy restraint used to restrain an infant or small child during procedures that involve only the head or neck.

mutation fundamental change that takes place in the structure of a gene; results in the transmission of a trait different from that normally carried by that particular gene.

mutual gazing see *en face position.*

myoclonic seizure characterized by sudden jerking of a muscle or group of muscles often in the arms or legs. There is no loss of consciousness.

myometrium the muscular middle layer of the walls of the corpus and fundus that is responsible for the contractions of labor.

myopia ability to see objects clearly at close range but not at a distance; nearsightedness.

myringotomy incision of the eardrum performed to establish drainage and to insert tiny tubes into the tympanic membrane to facilitate drainage of serous or purulent fluid in the middle ear.

nadir the lowest point of the deceleration of the fetal heart rate (FHR).

Nagele's rule a formula used to determine the pregnancy due date by adding 7 days to the date of the first day of the last menstrual period (LMP), then subtracting 3 months.

nebulizer tube attached to a wall unit or cylinder that delivers moist air via a face mask.

necrotizing enterocolitis an acute inflammatory disease of the intestine.

negativism opposition to suggestion or advice; associated with the toddler age group because the toddler, in search of autonomy, frequently responds "no" to almost everything.

neonatal abstinence syndrome (NAS) symptoms seen in the newborn of the woman who has abused substances during pregnancy; withdrawal symptoms.

neonate term used to describe a newborn in the first 28 days of life.

nocturnal emissions involuntary discharge of semen during sleep; also known as wet dreams.

noncommunicative language egocentric speech exhibited by children who talk to themselves, toys, or pets without any purpose other than the pleasure of using words.

nuchal rigidity stiff neck.

nuclear family family structure that consists of only the father, the mother, and the children living in one household.

nulligravida a woman who has never been pregnant.

nursing process proven form of problem solving based on the scientific method. The nursing process consists of five components: assessment, nursing diagnosis, planning, implementation, and evaluation.

nutrition history information regarding the child's eating habits and preferences.

obesity excessive accumulation of fat that increases body weight by 20% or more over ideal weight.

objective data in the nursing assessment, the data gained by the nurse's direct observation.

obstetric conjugate the smallest diameter of the inlet through which the fetus must pass.

oliguria decreased production of urine, especially in relation to fluid intake.

onlooker play interest in the observation of an activity without participation.

open-glottis pushing method of expelling the fetus that is characterized by pushing with contractions using an open glottis so that air is released during the pushing effort.

opioids medications with opium-like properties (also known as narcotic analgesics); the most frequently administered medications to provide analgesia during labor.

opisthotonos arching of the back so that the head and the heels are bent backward and the body is forward.

ophthalmia neonatorum a severe eye infection contracted in the birth canal of a woman with gonorrhea or Chlamydia.

orchiopexy surgical procedure used to bring an undescended testis down into the scrotum and anchor it there.

orthodontia a type of dentistry dealing with prevention and correction of incorrectly positioned or aligned teeth.

orthoptics therapeutic exercises to improve the quality of vision.

outcomes goals that are specific, stated in measurable terms, and have a time frame for accomplishment.

overprotection type of response by caregivers when caring for chronically ill children in which the caregivers protect the child at all costs, prevent the child from achieving new skills by hovering, avoid the use of discipline, and use every means to prevent the child from suffering any frustration.

overriding aorta in tetralogy of Fallot; the aorta shifts to the right over the opening in the ventricular septum so that blood from both right and left ventricles is pumped into the aorta.

overweight more than 10% over ideal weight.

ovulation releasing the mature ovum into the abdominal cavity, which occurs on day 14 of a 28-day cycle.

palmar grasp reflex phenomenon that results when pressure is placed on the palm of the hand near the base of the digits causing flexion or curling of the fingers.

palpebral fissures opening between the eyes.

papoose board commercial restraint board for use with toddlers or preschool-age children that uses canvas strips to secure the child's body and extremities. One extremity can be released to allow treatment to be performed on that extremity.

parallel play one child plays alongside another child or children involved in the same type of activity, but the children do not interact with each other.

parity or para, communicates the outcome of previous pregnancies in the obstetric history.

partial seizure a type of seizure with manifestations that vary depending on the area of the brain where they arise.

patient-controlled analgesia (PCA) programmed intravenous infusion of narcotic analgesia that the patient can control within set limits.

pediatric nurse practitioner (PNP) professional nurse prepared at the postbaccalaureate level to give primary health care to children and families. These nurses use pediatricians or family physicians as consultants but offer day-to-day assessment and care.

pedodontist dentist who specializes in the care and treatment of children's teeth.

pelvic rest a physician's order requiring the woman to refrain from inserting anything into the vagina, such as tampons or the practitioner's fingers to perform a cervical examination; this order includes sexual abstinence.

percutaneous umbilical blood sampling (PUBS) or cordocentesis a procedure similar to amniocentesis whereby fetal blood is withdrawn from the umbilical cord.

perimenopause the time before menopause when vasomotor symptoms (hot flashes, night sweats) and irregular menses begin.

perimetrium the tough outer layer of the walls of the corpus and fundus, which is made of connective tissues and supports the uterus.

perinatologist a maternal–fetal medicine specialist.

periodic changes variations in the fetal heart rate (FHR) pattern that occur in conjunction with uterine contractions.

perioperative period the period of time encompassing the surgical procedure that has three phases: preoperative, intraoperative, and postoperative.

personal history data collected about a client's personal habits, such as hygiene, sleeping, and elimination patterns, as well as activities, exercise, special interests, and favorite objects (toys).

petechiae a small hemorrhage appearing as a nonraised, purplish-red spot of the skin, nail beds, or mucous membranes.

phenylketonuria (PKU) recessive hereditary defect of metabolism that results in a congenital disease caused by a defect in the enzyme that normally changes the essential amino acid, phenylalanine, into tyrosine. If untreated, PKU results in severe mental retardation.

philtrum vertical groove in the middle of the upper lip.

phimosis adherence of the foreskin to the glans penis.

photophobia intolerance to light.

photosensitivity sensitivity to sunlight.

physiologic jaundice icterus neonatorum; jaundice that occurs in a large number of newborns but has no medical significance; result of the breakdown of fetal red blood cells.

pica compulsive eating of nonfood substances.

pincer grasp using the thumb and index finger to pick up food or small objects.

pinna the upper, external, protruding part of the ear.

placenta previa a condition in which the placenta is implanted close to, or covers, the cervical os.

plantar grasp reflex phenomenon that results when pressure is placed on the sole of the foot at the base of the toes; causes the toes to curl downward.

platypelloid pelvis pelvis that is flat in its dimensions with a very narrow anterior-posterior diameter and a wide transverse diameter; this shape makes it extremely difficult for the fetus to pass through the bony pelvis.

play therapy technique of psychoanalysis that psychiatrists or psychiatric nurse clinicians use to uncover a disturbed child's underlying thoughts, feelings, and motivations, to better help him/her.

point of maximum impulse (PMI) the point over the heart on the chest wall where the heart beat can be heard the best using a stethoscope.

polyarthritis inflammation of several joints.

polycythemia excess number of red blood cells.

polydipsia abnormal thirst.

polyhydramnios excess levels of amniotic fluid that is associated with an increased incidence of fetal defects.

polyphagia increased food consumption.

polyuria dramatic increase in urinary output, often with enuresis.

postcoital test evaluates the interaction of the man's sperm with the woman's cervical mucus.

postpartum blues, sometimes called the "baby blues," a temporary depression that usually begins on the third day after delivery and lasts for 2 or 3 days, in which the woman may be tearful, have difficulty sleeping and eating, and feel generally let down.

Postterm, or postmature, a newborn born at 42 weeks' or more gestation.

precipitous labor labor that lasts <3 hours from the start of uterine contractions to birth.

preeclampsia a serious condition of pregnancy in which the blood pressure rises to 140/90 mm Hg or higher accompanied by proteinuria, the presence of protein in the urine.

pregestational diabetes condition in which a woman enters pregnancy with either type 1 or type 2 diabetes mellitus.

premenstrual syndrome (PMS) symptoms occurring before menstruation, including edema (resulting in weight gain), headache, increased anxiety, mild depression, or mood swings; premenstrual tension.

prepuce or foreskin; a layer of tissue that covers the glans of the penis.

preterm, or premature, a newborn born at 37 weeks' gestation or less; commonly called premature.

priapism prolonged, abnormal erection of the penis.

primary circular reactions a stage of development named by Piaget in which infants explore objects by touching or putting them in their mouths; the infant is unaware of actions that he or she can cause.

primary nursing system whereby one nurse plans the total care for a child and directs the efforts of nurses on the other shifts.

primary prevention limiting the spread of illness or disease by teaching, especially regarding safety, diet, rest, and exercise.

prospective payment system predetermined rates to be paid to the health care provider to care for patients with certain classifications of diseases.

proteinuria the presence of protein in the urine.

proximodistal pattern of growth in which growth starts in the center and progresses toward the periphery or outside.

pruritus itching.

pseudomenses (pseudomenstruation) false menstruation; a slight red-tinged vaginal discharge in female infants resulting from a decline in the hormonal level after birth compared with the higher concentration in the maternal hormone environment before birth.

pseudostrabismus the cross-eyed look found in infants caused by incomplete development of the nerves and muscles that control focusing and coordination; begins to disappear in the sixth month.

puberty period during which secondary sexual characteristics begin to develop and reproductive maturity is attained.

puerperal fever an illness marked by high fever caused by infection of the reproductive tract after the birth of a child.

puerperium the postpartum period.

pulmonary embolism the more serious manifestation of venous thromboembolism.

pulmonary stenosis narrowing of the opening between the right ventricle and the pulmonary artery that decreases blood flow to the lungs.

pulse oximeter photoelectric device used to measure oxygen saturation in an artery; can be attached to an infant's finger, toe, or heel.

punishment penalty given for wrongdoing.

purpura hemorrhages into the skin or mucous membranes.

purpuric rash rash consisting of ecchymoses (bruises) and petechiae caused by bleeding under the skin.

pyelonephritis infection of the kidneys.

pyrosis heartburn caused by acid reflux through the relaxed lower esophageal sphincter (LES).

recessive gene gene carrying different information for a trait within a pair that is not expressed (e.g., blue eyes versus brown eyes). A recessive gene is detectable only when present on both chromosomes.

refraction the way light rays bend as they pass through the lens of the eye to the retina.

regurgitation spitting up of small quantities of milk; occurs rather easily in the young infant.

rejection type of response by caregivers when caring for a chronically ill child in which the caregivers distance themselves emotionally from the child and, although they provide physical care, tend to scold and correct the child continuously.

respiratory distress syndrome (RDS) see *hyaline membrane disease*.

respite care care of the child by someone other than the usual caregiver so that the caregiver can get temporary relief and rest.

retinopathy of prematurity (ROP) a complication commonly associated with the preterm newborn that results from the growth of abnormal immature retinal blood vessels.

reversibility ability to think in either direction.

right ventricular hypertrophy increase in thickness of the myocardium of the right ventricle.

risk nursing diagnoses category of diagnoses that identifies health problems to which the patient is especially vulnerable.

ritual a routine; in labor, a repeated series of actions that the woman uses as an individualized way of dealing with the discomfort of labor.

ritualism practice employed by the young child to help develop security; consists of following a certain routine; makes rituals of simple tasks.

rooming-in arrangement in which the health care facility permits a family caregiver to stay with a child. A cot or sleeping chair is provided for the caregiver.

rooting reflex infant's response of turning the head when the cheek is stroked toward the stroked side.

ruddy dark red color seen in the palms of the hands and soles of the feet of the newborn.

rumination voluntary regurgitation.

runaway child child who is absent from home for overnight or longer without the permission of the caregiver.

salpingectomy removal of the fallopian tube.

salpingitis infection of the fallopian tube.

school history information regarding the child's grade level in school and his or her academic performance.

school phobia child's fear resulting in dread of a school situation or fear of leaving home; can be a combination of both.

scoliosis lateral curvature of the spine.

scurvy a disease that results from severe vitamin C deficiency and is characterized by spongy gums, loosened teeth, and bleeding into the skin and mucous membrane.

seborrhea a scalp condition characterized by yellow, crusty patches; also called cradle cap.

sebum oily secretion of the sebaceous glands.

secondary circular reactions a stage of development named by Piaget in which the infant realizes that his or her actions cause pleasurable sensations.

secondary prevention limiting the impact or reoccurrence of disease by focusing on early diagnosis and treatment.

seizure series of involuntary contractions of voluntary muscles; convulsion.

seminiferous tubules tiny coils of tissue in the lobes of the testis in which spermatogenesis occurs.

sexual abuse sexual contact between a child and someone in a caregiving position such as a parent, baby-sitter, or teacher.

sexual assault sexual contact made by someone who is not functioning in the role of the child's caregiver.

simian crease a single straight palmar crease; an abnormal finding that is associated with Down syndrome.

single-parent family household headed by one adult of either sex. There may be one or more children in the family.

skeletal traction pull exerted directly on skeletal structures by means of pins, wire, tongs, or another device surgically inserted through the bone.

skin traction pull on tape, rubber, or plastic materials attached to the skin that indirectly exerts pull on the musculoskeletal system.

small for gestational age (SGA) a newborn whose weight, length, and/or head circumference falls below the 10th percentile for gestational age.

smegma the cheese-like secretion of the sebaceous glands found under the foreskin.

social history information about the environment in which the child lives.

socialization process by which a child learns the rules of the society and culture in which the family lives, its language, values, ethics, and acceptable behaviors.

solitary independent play playing apart from others without making an effort to be part of the group or group activity.

sonogram a picture obtained with ultrasound.

spermatogenesis production of sperm.

spina bifida failure of the posterior lamina of the vertebrae to close; leaves an opening through which the spinal meninges and spinal cord may protrude.

spinnbarkeit an elastic quality of cervical mucus that allows it to be stretched 5 cm or more between the thumb and forefinger.

spontaneous abortion loss of a pregnancy before the age of viability (<20 weeks of gestation or fetal size <500 g). The common name for early pregnancy loss is miscarriage.

startle reflex follows any loud noise; similar to the Moro reflex, but the hands remain clenched. This reflex is never lost.

station the relationship of the presenting part of a fetus to the ischial spines.

status asthmaticus a potentially fatal complication of an acute asthma attack involving severe asthma symptoms that do not respond after 30 to 60 minutes of treatment.

status epilepticus an emergency complication of epilepsy whereby seizure activity continues for 30 minutes or more after treatment is initiated or when three or more seizures occur without full recovery between seizures.

steatorrhea fatty stools.

step reflex also called the dance reflex; tendency of infants to make stepping movements when held upright.

stepfamily consists of custodial parent, children, and a new spouse.

stigma negative perception of a person because he or she is believed to be different from the general population; may cause embarrassment or shame in the person being stigmatized.

strabismus failure of the two eyes to direct their gaze at the same object, simultaneously; squint; crossed eyes.

striae stretch marks.

stridor shrill, harsh respiratory sound, usually on inspiration.

subjective data in the nursing assessment, data spoken by the child or family.

sublimation process of directing a desire or impulse into more acceptable behaviors.

substance abuse the misuse of an addictive substance, such as alcohol or drugs, that changes the user's mental state.

sucking reflex infant's response of strong, vigorous sucking when a nipple, finger, or tongue blade is put in his or her mouth.

superego in psychoanalytic theory, the conscience or parental value system; acts primarily as a monitor over the ego.

supernumerary excessive in number (e.g., more than the usual number of teeth).

supine hypotensive syndrome condition that occurs during late pregnancy in which the gravid uterus can compress the woman's vena cava and aorta, causing the blood pressure to fall when the woman is in the supine position.

surfactant a substance found in the lungs of mature fetuses that keeps the alveoli from collapsing after they first expand.

suture narrow band of connective tissue that divides the six nonunited bones of a newborn's skull.

symmetry a balance in shape, size, and position from one side of the body to the other; a mirror image.

sympathetic ophthalmia inflammatory reaction of the uninjured eye. Symptoms can include photophobia, lacrimation, and some dimness of vision.

synovitis inflammation of a joint; most commonly the hip in children.

tachypnea rapid respirations.

talipes equinovarus clubfoot with plantar flexion.

temper tantrum behavior in children that springs from frustrations caused by their urge for independence; a violent display of temper. The child reacts with enthusiastic rebellion against the wishes of the caregiver.

temperament the combination of all of an individual's characteristics, the way the person thinks, behaves, and reacts.

teratogens from the Greek *terato,* meaning monster, and *genesis,* meaning birth; an agent or influence that causes a defect or disruption in the prenatal growth process. The effect of a teratogen depends on when it enters the fetal system and the stage of differentiation of the organs or organ systems at that time. Generally, the fetus is most vulnerable to teratogens during the first trimester.

term a newborn who is born between the beginning of week 38 and the end of week 41 of gestation.

tertiary prevention a focus on rehabilitation and teaching to prevent additional injury or illness.

tetralogy of Fallot is a grouping of heart defects (tetralogy denotes four abnormal conditions): (1) pulmonary stenosis, (2) ventricular septal defect, (3) overriding aorta, and (4) right ventricular hypertrophy.

thanatologist person, sometimes a nurse, trained especially to work with the dying and their families.

therapeutic abortion a pregnancy termination performed for reasons related to maternal or fetal health or disease.

therapeutic play play technique that may be used by play therapists, nurses, child-life specialists, and trained volunteers.

thermoneutral environment an environment in which heat is neither lost nor gained.

thermoregulation regulation of temperature.

throwaway child child (often a teenager) who has been forced to leave home and is not wanted back by the adults in the home.

thrush A fungal infection (caused by *Candida albicans*) in the oral cavity.

time out one part of the Universal Protocol developed to reduce the incidence of wrong site, wrong procedure, and wrong person surgery. Each member of the surgical team and the patient stop right before the procedure to confirm agreement that the right procedure is being performed on the right patient with documented informed consent.

tinea ringworm.

tissue perfusion circulation of blood through the capillaries carrying nutrients and oxygen to the cells.

tocolytic a substance that relaxes the uterine muscle.

tolerance in substance abuse, ability of body tissues to endure and adapt to continued or increased use of a substance.

tonic neck reflex also called the fencing reflex; seen when the infant lies on the back with the head turned to one side, the arm and leg on that side extended, and the opposite arm flexed as if in a fencing position.

tonic-clonic a type of seizure characterized by muscular contractions and rigidity changing to generalized jerking movements of the muscles followed by a state of relaxation.

tonsils two oval masses attached to the side walls of the back of the mouth between the anterior and posterior pillars (folds of mucous membranes at the sides of the passage from the mouth to the pharynx).

TORCH an acronym for a special group of infections that can be acquired during pregnancy and transmitted through the placenta to the fetus. The "T" stands for toxoplasmosis, the "O" for other infections (Hepatitis B, syphilis, varicella and herpes zoster), the "R" is for rubella, the "C" is for cytomegalovirus (CMV), and the "H" stands for herpes simplex virus (HSV).

total parenteral nutrition (TPN) the administration of dextrose, lipids, amino acids, electrolytes, vitamins, minerals, and trace elements into the circulatory system to meet the nutritional needs of the child whose needs cannot be met through the gastrointestinal tract.

tracheostomy surgical opening into the trachea to provide an open airway in emergency situations or when there is a blocked airway.

traction force applied to an extremity or other part of the body to maintain proper alignment and to facilitate healing of a fractured bone or dislocated joint.

transposition of the great arteries occurs when the aorta arises from the right ventricle instead of the left, and the pulmonary artery arises from the left ventricle instead of the right.

true pelvis the portion of the pelvis below the linea terminalis.

tympanic membrane sensor device used to determine the temperature of the tympanic membrane by rapidly sensing infrared radiation from the membrane. The tympanic thermometer offers the advantage of recording the temperature rapidly with little disturbance to the child.

unfinished business completing matters that will help ease the death of a loved one; saying the unsaid and doing the undone acts of love and caring that may seem difficult to express; recognizing time is limited and filling that time with the important issues that need to be taken care of.

unilateral one side (e.g., in cleft lip, only one side of the lip is cleft).

unoccupied behavior daydreaming; fingering clothing or a toy without any apparent purpose.

urge-to-push method method of expelling the fetus in which the woman bears down only when she feels the urge to do so using any technique that feels right for her.

urostomy a surgical opening created to help with the elimination of urine.

urticaria hives.

uterine atony inability of the uterus to contract effectively.

uterine subinvolution a condition in which the uterus returns to its prepregnancy shape and size at a rate that is slower than expected (usually the result of retained placental fragments or an infection).

uteroplacental insufficiency diminished or deficient blood flow to the uterus and placenta.

utilization review a systematic evaluation of services delivered by a health care provider to determine appropriateness and quality of care, as well as medical necessity of the services provided.

vaginitis inflammation of the vagina.

variability fluctuations in fetal heart rate (FHR).

variable deceleration a change in the FHR that may occur at any point during a contraction and has a jagged, erratic shape on the electronic fetal monitor (EFM) tracing.

vas deferens the muscular tube in which sperm begin their journey out of the man's body.

vascular nevus commonly known as a strawberry mark; a slightly raised, bright-red collection of hypertrophied skin capillaries that does not blanch completely on pressure.

vasectomy male sterilization.

vasospasm spasm of the arteries.

venous thromboembolism is the umbrella term for deep vein thrombosis (DVT) and pulmonary embolism.

ventricular septal defect abnormal opening in the septum of the heart between the ventricles; allows blood to pass directly from the left to the right side of the heart; the most common intracardiac defect.

ventriculoatrial shunting plastic tubing implanted into the cerebral ventricle passing under the skin to the cardiac atrium; provides drainage for excessive cerebrospinal fluid.

ventriculoperitoneal shunting plastic tubing implanted into the cerebral ventricle passing under the skin to the peritoneal cavity, providing drainage for excessive cerebrospinal fluid. Excessive tubing can be inserted to accommodate the child's growth.

vernix caseosa greasy, cheese-like substance that protects the skin during fetal life; consists of sebum and desquamated epithelial cells.

very low birth weight (VLBW) newborns weighing <1,500 g.

vestibule the area within the boundaries of the labia minora, which includes the urethral meatus, vaginal opening, and Bartholin glands.

viable able to live outside of the uterus (fetus).

vigorous pushing method of expelling the fetus in which the woman is told to take a deep breath, hold the breath, and push while counting to 10. She is encouraged to complete three "good" pushes in this manner with each contraction.

vulva the external genitalia of the female reproductive system.

wellness nursing diagnoses diagnoses that identify the potential of an individual, family, or community to move to a higher level of wellness.

West nomogram graph with several scales arranged so that when two values are known, the third can be plotted by drawing a line with a straightedge; commonly used to calculate body surface area (BSA).

Wharton's jelly a clear gelatinous substance that gives support to the cord and helps prevent compression of the cord, which could impair blood flow to the fetus.

wheezing sound of expired air being pushed through obstructed bronchioles.

withdrawal symptoms in substance abuse, physical and psychological symptoms that occur when the drug is no longer being used.

zygote or conceptus, results when an ovum and a spermatozoon unite. The zygote has the full complement of 46 chromosomes, arranged in 23 pairs.

English–Spanish Glossary

HELPFUL EXPLANATORY PHRASES

Both the tu (informal for younger people) and the usted (more formal for people, not known, older than one) forms are offered. In each case the informal is stated first.

Hello. My name is _____.	*Hola. Me llamo _____.*
I am your nurse.	*Soy tu enfermera.*
I don't understand much Spanish. When I ask you questions, please answer with one or two words.	*No entiendo mucho español. Por favor contesta con una o dos palabras.*
Please speak more slowly.	*Por favor conteste con una o dos palabras.*
	Habla más despacio, por favor.
	Hable más despacio, por favor.
I'm sorry, but I don't understand.	*Lo siento, pero no entiendo.*

OBSTETRIC PHRASES

Admission Questions

What is your name, including your last name?	*¿Cómo te llamas? Incluye tu apellido.*
	¿Cómo se llama? Incluya su apellido.
How many times have you been pregnant?	*¿Cuántas veces has estado embarazada?*
	¿Cuántas veces ha estado embarazada?
When did your contractions begin?	*¿Cuándo empezaron los dolores?*
Did your water bag break?	*¿Se te rompió la bolsa?*
	¿Se le rompió la bolsa?
Is the baby moving normally?	*¿Está moviéndose normalmente el bebé?*
Have you had any problems with this pregnancy?	*¿Has tenido problemas con este embarazo?*
	¿Ha tenido problemas con este embarazo?
Do you have any chronic illnesses, such as asthma, diabetes, tuberculosis, heart disease?	*¿Tienes alguna enfermedad crónica, como asma, diabetes, tuberculosis, enfermedades del corazón?*
	¿Tiene alguna enfermedad crónica, como asma, diabetes, tuberculosis, enfermedades del corazón?
Are you taking any medications?	*¿Estás tomando alguna medicina?*
	¿Está tomando usted alguna medicina?
How much alcohol do you drink?	*¿Tomas bebidas alcohólicas? ¿Cuánto tomas?*
	¿Toma bebidas alcohólicas? ¿Cuánto toma?
How many cigarettes do you smoke per day?	*¿Fumas cigarrillos? ¿Cuántos fumas por día?*
	¿Fuma cigarrillos? ¿Cuántos fuma por día?
What plans do you have for pain management?	*¿Qué planes tienes para manejar los dolores?*
	¿Qué planes tiene para manejar los dolores?
Do you want an epidural?	*¿Quieres una inyección epidural?*
	¿Quiere una inyección epidural?
Do you plan to breast-feed?	*¿Piensas dar pecho? ¿Piensas amamantar?*
	¿Piensa dar pecho? ¿Piensa amamantar?
Do you want the baby circumcised?	*¿Deseas circuncisión para el bebé?*
	¿Desea circuncisión para el bebé?

Admission Procedures

Please put on this gown.

Por favor, ponte esta bata.
Por favor, póngase esta bata.

Wipe with these, then urinate in this cup.

Límpiate con éstas. Luego orina en este vaso.
Límpiese con éstas. Luego orine en este vaso.

Press this button when you need the nurse.

Empuja este botón cuando necesitas a la enfermera.
Empuje este botón cuando necesite a la enfermera.

This is a fetal monitor.
This part monitors the contractions.
This part monitors the baby's heartbeat.

Esta máquina es para checar al bebé.
Esta parte es para checar los dolores.
Este es para checar el latido del corazón del bebé.

Intrapartum Procedures

I am going to check your labor progress.
Put your heels together and let your legs relax outward to each side.

Voy a checar como esta progresando el parto.
Pon juntos los talones y deja relajar las piernas hacia fuera para cada lado.
Ponga juntos los talones y deje relajar las piernas hacia fuera para cada lado.

Take a deep breath in, exhale, and then breathe with me

Respira profundo, exhala, y luego respira conmigo.
Respire profundo, exhale, y luego respire conmigo.

Please turn to your left (right) side.

Por favor, voltéate a tu lado izquierdo (derecho).
Por favor, voltéese a su lado izquierdo (derecho).

I am going to insert a catheter into your vein.

Voy a meterte una aguja a la vena.
Voy a meterle una aguja a la vena.

I am going to put a catheter into your bladder to drain the urine, and then I will remove the catheter.

Voy a meterte(le) un catéter (un tubo) en la vejiga para vaciarla (sacar la orina), y después voy a quitar el catéter.

Don't push. Blow out, like this.

No empujes. Sopla, así.
No empuje. Sople, así.

Push!

¡Empuja!
¡Empuje!

It's a boy (girl)!

¡Es varón!
¡Es mujer!

Congratulations!

¡Felicidades!

Cesarean Delivery

You need a cesarean section.

Usted necesita una sección cesariana

I am going to shave your abdomen and your upper thighs.

Voy a rasurar el abdomen (estomago) y los muslos.

I am going to put a catheter into your bladder. The urine will drain into the bag. The nurses will take the catheter out 24 hours after your surgery.

Voy a insertarte(le) un catéter en la vejiga. La orina va a drenarse en la bolsa. Las enfermeras te(le) sacaran el catéter unas veinticuatro horas después de tu(su) cirugía.

Hold the pillow over your incision, and then cough.

Pon (ponga) la almohada sobre la incisión (cortada) y luego tose (tosa).

What kind of pain do you have? Is it your incision? Is it cramping? Is it gas pains?

¿Qué clase de dolor tienes (tiene)?
¿Es tu (su) incisión (cortada)?
¿Son calambres (espasmos)?
¿Son dolores de gas?

Are you having any nausea?	*¿Tienes (tiene) nausea?*
Have you vomited?	*¿Has (Ha) vomitado?*
Are you passing gas?	*¿Estás (Está) pasando gas?*
Have you had a bowel movement?	*¿Has (Ha) defecado?*
	¿Has (Ha) hecho del baño?

PEDIATRIC PHRASES

Interviewing the Caregiver

What is your name, including your last name?	*¿Cómo te llamas? Incluye tu apellido.*
	¿Cómo se llama? Incluya su apellido.
What is your child's name?	*¿Cómo se llama tu niño? ¿niña?*
	¿Cómo se llama su niño? ¿niña?
How old is he/she?	*¿Cuántos años tiene?*
What is the reason your child is being seen today?	*¿Por qué lo/la han traído hoy?*
How long has he/she been sick?	*¿Por cuánto tiempo ha estado enfermo/enferma?*
Has he/she had	*¿Ha tenido . . . ?*
▪ fever	▪ *fiebre*
▪ diarrhea	▪ *diarrea*
▪ constipation	▪ *constipación*
▪ coughing	▪ *tos*
▪ sneezing	▪ *estornudos*
▪ nasal drainage	▪ *drenaje nasal*
▪ drooling	▪ *babas*
▪ trouble breathing	▪ *dificultades para respirar*
▪ pain	▪ *dolor*
▪ rash	▪ *erupciones, ronchas (hives), urticaria, comezón*
▪ bruising	▪ *morotones*
▪ convulsions	▪ *convulsions, ataques*
Has he/she vomited?	*¿Ha vomitado?*
Has he/she cried unusually?	*¿Ha llorado fuera de lo normal?*
When did these symptoms begin?	*¿Cuándo empezaron estos síntomas?*
Can you describe the symptoms?	*¿Puedes (puede) describir los síntomas?*
What have you done to treat these symptoms?	*¿Qué has (ha) hecho para tratar estos síntomas?*
Has he/she ever had these symptoms before?	*¿Ha tenido estos síntomas antes de ahora?*
Is anyone else in your family sick?	*¿Está enfermo cualquier otro miembro de tu (su) familia?*
Has he/she been around anyone who was sick?	*¿Ha estado alrededor de (cerca de) alguien que estaba enfermo?*
Is he/she allergic to any medications?	*¿Tiene alergias a cualquier medicina?*
What medications is he/she taking?	*¿Qué medicina está tomando?*
Is he/she breast-fed?	*¿Amamanta? Está criado(a) con pecho?*
Does he/she drink from a bottle?	*¿Bebe de una botella?*
What does your child eat? Drink?	*¿Qué come tu (su) niño? ¿Qué bebe?*
How often does he/she eat?	*¿Con qué frecuencia come?*
When was the last time he/she ate?	*¿Cuándo fue la última vez que comió?*
When was the last time he/she had something to drink?	*¿Cuándo fue la última vez que bebió algo?*
Is he/she allergic to any foods?	*¿Tiene alergias a alguna comida?*

Does he/she feed himself/herself?	*¿El mismo se da de comer?*
	¿Ella misma se da de comer?
	¿Come sin ayuda?
When was the last time he/she urinated?	*¿Cuándo fue la última vez que orino?*
How many wet diapers has he/she had today?	*¿Cuántos panales ha mojado hoy?*
When is the last time he/she had a bowel movement?	*¿Cuándo fue la última vez que defecó? (. . . que hizo del baño?)*
How often does he/she have a bowel movement?	*¿Con qué frecuencia defeca? (hace del baño?)*
Is he/she toilet trained?	*¿Puede usar el baño sin ayuda?*
What word does your child use to say he/she needs to urinate?	*¿Qué palabra usa tu (su) niño para decir que tiene que orinar?*
What word does your child use to say he/she needs to have a bowel movement?	*¿Qué palabra usa tu (su) niño para decir que tiene que ir al excusado?*
How long does your child sleep at night?	*¿Cuánto tiempo duerme tu (su) niño cada noche?*
Does he/she wake up during the night?	*¿Se despierta durante la noche?*
Does he/she take a nap?	*¿Toma una siesta?*
Have you noticed anything unusual about his/her sleeping?	*¿Has (Ha) notado algo raro de su dormir?*
Is he/she sleeping more than usual? Less than usual?	*¿Está durmiendo más de lo normal?*
	¿Menos de lo normal?
Has he/she had any unusual behavior?	*¿Se ha portado de una manera rara?*
Does your child suck his/her thumb?	*¿Se chupa el pulgar?*
Does your child bite his/her nails?	*¿Se come las uñas?*
Has he/she ever been hospitalized?	*¿Ha sido hospitalizado? ¿Lo han internado?*
Why was he/she hospitalized?	*¿Por qué fue hospitalizado?*
	¿Por qué lo internaron?

Working with the Child

What is your name?	*¿Cómo te llamas?*
How old are you?	*¿Cuántos años tienes?*
I am your nurse.	*Soy tu enfermera.*
I am going to	*Voy a*
■ take your temperature	■ *tomarte la temperatura*
■ take your blood pressure	■ *tomarte la presión de sangre*
■ listen to your heart	■ *escuchar el latido de tu corazón*
■ look in your ears	■ *mirarte en las orejas*
■ measure how tall you are	■ *medir qué tan alto eres*
■ measure how much you weigh	■ *medir cuánto pesas*
■ give you your medicine	■ *darte medicina*
This is going to hurt a little.	*Esto va a dolerte un poco.*
Point to where it hurts.	*Muéstrame donde te duele.*
Tell me how it feels.	*Dime cómo se siente.*
Are you hungry?	*¿Tienes hambre?*
Are you thirsty?	*¿Tienes sed?*
Do you feel tired?	*¿Te sientes cansado/cansada?*
Do you have trouble seeing? Hearing?	*¿Tienes dificultad de ver? ¿de oír?*
Do you wear glasses?	*¿Usas anteojos?*

References and Suggested Readings

CHAPTER 1

Alden, E. R. (2006). The field of pediatrics. In J. McMillan, R. Feigin, C. DeAngelis, & M. Jones, Jr. (Eds.), *Oski's pediatrics: Principles and practice* (4th ed.). Philadelphia: Lippincott Williams & Wilkins.

Brush, C. A., Kelly, M. M., Green, D., Gaffney, M., Kattwinkel, J., & French, M. (2005). Meeting the challenge: Using policy to improve children's health. *American Journal of Public Health, 95*(11), 1904–1909.

Callister, L. C. (2006). Perinatal ethics: State of the science. *Journal of Perinatal & Neonatal Nursing, 20*(1), 37–39.

Carr, I. (n.d.). Dying to have a baby: The history of childbirth. Retrieved January 20, 2007, from http://www.umanitoba.ca/outreach/manitoba_womens_health/hist1.htm

Centers for Disease Control (CDC). (1999). Healthier mothers and babies. *MMWR: Morbidity and Mortality Weekly Report, 48*(38), 849–856. Retrieved October 17, 2007, from http://www.cdc.gov/mmwr/PDF/wk/mm4838.pdf

Centers for Disease Control (CDC) (Eds.). (2001). The cover: Ignaz Philipp Semmelweis (1818–65). *Emerging Infectious Diseases, 7*(2), page unnumbered. Retrieved November 3, 2007, from http://www.cdc.gov/ncidod/eid/vol7no2/cover.htm

Centers for Disease Control (CDC). (2005). Racial/ethnic disparities in infant mortality—United States 1995 – 2002. *MMWR, 54*(22), 553–556. Retrieved October 17, 2007, from http://www.cdc.gov/mmwr/preview/mmwrhtml/mm5422a1.htm

Centers for Disease Control (CDC). (2006). Sudden, unexplained infant death initiative (SUIDI): Fetal and infant mortality information. Retrieved October 17, 2007, from http://www.cdc.gov/SIDS/mortality.htm

Colen, C. G., Geronimus, A. T., Bound, J., & James, S. A. (2006). Maternal upward socioeconomic mobility and black-white disparities in infant birthweight. *American Journal of Public Health, 96*, 2032–2039.

Cone, T. E. Jr. (1980). *History of American pediatrics*. Boston: Little Brown.

Centers for Medicare & Medicaid Services. (2005). Medicaid progam – General information: Technical summary. Retrieved January 13, 2007, from http://www.cms.hhs.gov/MedicaidGenInfo/03_Technical Summary.asp

DeLashmutt, M. B. (2007). JOGNN clinical issues: Students' experience of nursing presence with poor mothers. *Journal of Obstetric, Gynecologic, & Neonatal Nursing, 36*(2), 183–189.

Embassy of France in Canada Science and Technology Article. (Undated). Louis Pasteur. Retrieved January 20, 2007, from http://www.ambafrance-ca.org/HYPERLAB/PEOPLE/_pasteur.html

FNS/USDA. (2006). WIC program coverage: How many eligible individuals participated in the special supplemental nutrition program for women, infants, and children (WIC): 1994–2003? Food & Nutrition Services, Office of Analysis, Nutrition, and Evaluation (Eds.). Retrieved January 13, 2007, from http://www.fns.usda.gov/oane/MENU/Published/WIC/FILES/WICEligibles.pdf

Healthy People 2010, A Systematic Approach to Health Improvement. (2001). Retrieved October 17, 2007, from www.health.gov/healthy-people

Healthy People 2010, Midcourse Review. (2006). Retrieved January 13, 2007, from http://www.healthypeople.gov/data/midcourse/html/default.htm

Herrman, J. W. (2001). Updates & kidbits: Pediatric nursing and Healthy People 2010: A call to action. *Pediatric Nursing, 27*(1), 82–86.

Hoyert, D. L., Heron, M. P., Murphy, S. L., & Kung, H-C. (2006). Deaths: Final data for 2003. *National Vital Statistics Reports (NVSS), 54*(13). Retrieved January 14, 2007, from http://www.cdc.gov/nchs/data/nvsr/nvsr54/nvsr54_13.pdf

Kenner, C., Sugrue, N. M., & Finkelman, A. (2007). Poverty and neonatal outcomes: How nurses around the world can make a difference. *Nursing for Women's Health, 11*(5), 468–473.

Martell, L. K. (2006). Historical perspective in perinatal and neonatal nursing: From innovation to common practice: Perinatal nursing pre-1970 to 2005. *Journal of Perinatal and Neonatal Nursing, 20*(1), 8–16.

NANDA-I Nursing Diagnoses: Definitions and Classification 2007–2008. (2007) Philadelphia: NANDA International.

National Center for Health Statistics (NCHS). (2007). Deaths: Leading causes for 2003. Centers for Disease Control and Prevention (CDC) & NCHS. Retrieved January 14, 2007, from http://www.cdc.gov/nchs/products/pubs/pubd/hestats/leadingdeaths03/leadingdeaths03.htm

National Center for Health Statistics (NCHS). (2006). Overweight and obesity: Childhood overweigh: Overweight prevalence. Retrieved January 20, 2007, from http://www.cdc.gov/nccdphp/dnpa/obesity/childhood/prevalence.htm

The World Factbook. (2007). Infant mortality rate. Retrieved January 14, 2007, from http://www.bartleby.com/151 (click on "Index by Field," then "People," and "Infant Mortality Rate")

Wertz, R. W., & Wertz, D. C. (1989). *Lying-in: A history of childbirth in America, expanded edition.* Yale University Press: New Haven & London.

Wilkins, I. (2006). Perinatal mortality. *UpToDate(15.1).* Last updated December 20, 2006. Retrieved June 6, 2007. Available with an online subscription at http://patients.uptodate.com

Zindler, L. (2005). Ethical decision making in first trimester pregnancy screening. *Journal of Obstetric, Gynecologic & Neonatal Nursing, 19*(2), 122–131.

CHAPTER 2

Allender, J. A., Rector, C., Warner, K. D. (2010). *Community health nursing: Promoting & protecting the public's health.* (7th ed.). Philadelphia: Lippincott Williams & Wilkins.

Anderson, R. E., & Murphy, P. A. (1995). Outcomes of 11,788 planned home births attended by certified nurse-midwives: A retrospective descriptive study. *Journal of Nurse Midwifery, 40*(6), 468–473, 483–492.

Brucker, M. C., & Reedy, N. J. (2006). Nurse-midwifery state of the practice. *Journal of Perinatal & Neonatal Nursing, 20*(1), 91–92.

Child Welfare Information Gateway. (2003). *Openness in adoption: A fact sheet for families.* Retrieved October 21, 2007, from http://childwelfare.gov/pubs/f_openadopt.cfm

Dowdell, E. (2004). Grandmother caregivers and caregiver burden. *American Journal of Maternal/Child Nursing, 29*(5), 299–304.

Downs, A. C., & James, S. E. (2006). Gay, lesbian, and bisexual foster parents: Strengths and challenges for the child welfare system. *Child Welfare, 85*(2), 281–298.

Gardner, M. R., & Deatrick, J. A. (2006). Understanding interventions and outcomes in mothers of infants. *Issues in Comprehensive Pediatric Nursing, 29*, 25–44.

Groner, J., French, G., Ahijevych, K., & Wewers, M. E. (2005). Process evaluation of a nurse-delivered smoking relapse prevention program for new mothers. *Journal of Community Health Nursing, 22*(3), 157–167.

Hunt, R. (2004). *Introduction to community-based nursing* (3rd ed.). Philadelphia: Lippincott Williams & Wilkins.

Jack, S. M., DiCenso, A., & Lohfeld, L. (2005). A theory of maternal engagement with public health nurses and family visitors. *Journal of Advanced Nursing, 49*(2), 182–190.

Jeltova, I., & Fish, M. C. (2005). Creating school environments responsive to gay, lesbian, bisexual, and transgender families: Traditional and systemic approaches for consultation. *Journal of Educational and Psychological Consultation, 16*(1&2), 17–33.

Johnson, K. C., & Daviss, B. A. (2005). Outcomes of planned home births with certified professional midwives: Large prospective study in North America. *BMJ Online First,* 1–7. Retrieved January 28, 2007, from http://www.bmj.com/cgi/content/full/330/7505/1416?ehom

Kelly, N., Greaves, C., Buckland, L., & Rose, J. (2005). School nurses: Well placed to address challenging behaviour [abstract]. *Community Practitioner, 78*(3), 88–92.

Kotzer, A. M. (2005). Characteristics and role functions of advance practice nurses in a tertiary pediatric setting. *Journal for Specialists in Pediatric Nursing, 10*(1), 20–28.

Livermore, J., & Leach, B. (2006). *Strengthening partnership between service providers and families.* Retrieved October 21, 2007, from http://childwelfare.gov/calendar/cbconference/resourcebook/102.cfm

Miller, L. (2006). Adoption. In J. McMillan, R. Feigin, C. DeAngelis, & M. Jones, Jr. (Eds.), *Oski's pediatrics: Principles and practice* (4th ed.). Philadelphia: Lippincott Williams & Wilkins.

O'Gorman, S. (2006). Theoretical interfaces in the acute pediatric context: A psychotherapeutic understanding of the application of infant-directed singing. *American Journal of Psychotherapy, 60*(3), 271–283.

Pacey, S. (2005). Step change: The interplay of sexual and parenting problems when couples form stepfamilies. *Sexual and Relationship Therapy, 20*(3), 359–369.

Patterson, G. J. (1996). Lesbian and gay parenthood. *Handbook of parenting.* Hillsdale, NJ: Lawrence Erlbaum Associates.

Perks, J. (2006). Reaching out in women's health: A nurse practitioners perspective. *Australian Nursing Journal, 14*(4), 34.

Renaud, M. T. (2007). We are mothers too: Childbearing experiences of lesbian families. *Journal of Obstetric, Gynecologic, & Neonatal Nursing, 36*(2), 190–199.

Schim, S. M., Doorenbos, A. Z., & Borse, N. N. (2006). Cultural competence among hospice nurses. *Journal of Hospice & Palliative Nursing, 8*(5), 302–307.

Sealey, L. J., Burnett, M., & Johnson, G. (2006). Cultural competence of baccalaureate nursing faculty: Are we up to the task? *Journal of Cultural Diversity, 13*(3), 131–140.

Sherman, C. (2004). *Living with a single parent.* Retrieved October 21, 2007, from http://kidshealth.org/kid/feeling/home_family/single_parents.html

Stoeckle, M. L. (2005). Journey to Anna and Marie. *American Journal of Maternal/Child Nursing, 30*(3), 166–176.

United States Bureau of Census. (2007). *Statistical abstract of the United States: 2007.* Washington DC: Superintendent of Documents. Retrieved November 4, 2007, from http://www.census.gov/compendia/statab/2007edition.html

CHAPTER 3

Barclay, L., & Lie, D. (2006). AAP issues guidelines for menstrual cycle evaluation. *Medscape medical news.* Retrieved December 9, 2006, from http://www.medscape.com/viewarticle/547340

Barron, M. L., & Fehring, R. J. (2005). Basal body temperature assessment: Is it useful to couples seeking pregnancy? *American Journal of Maternal Child Nursing, 30*(5), 290–296.

Bielak, K. M., & Harris, G. S. (2006). Amenorrhea. In E. M. Alderman, M. L. Windle, W. Wolfram, P. D. Petry, & M. Strafford (Eds.), *eMedicine.* Retrieved December 24, 2006, from http://www.emedicine.com/ped/topic2779.htm

Cesario, S. K., & Hughes, L. A. (2007). Precocious puberty: A comprehensive review of literature. *JOGNN, 36*(3), 263–274.

Cunningham, F. G., Leveno, K. J., Bloom, S. L., Hauth, J. C., Gilstrap, L. C. III, & Wenstrom, K. D. (2005). Ch. 3. Implantation, embryogenesis, and placental development. In *Williams obstetrics* (22nd ed., pp. 40–51). New York: McGraw-Hill.

Cunningham, F. G., Leveno, K. J., Bloom, S. L., Hauth, J. C., Gilstrap, L. C. III, & Wenstrom, K. D. (2005). Maternal anatomy of the reproductive tract. In *Williams obstetrics* (22nd ed., pp.15–38). New York: McGraw-Hill.

Fehring, R. J., Schneider, M., & Raviele, K. (2006). Variability in the phases of the menstrual cycle. *Journal of Obstetric, Gynecologic, and Neonatal Nursing, 36*(3), 376–384.

Katz, A. (moderator). (2007). Sexuality and women: The experts speak. *Nursing for Women's Health, 11*(1), 36–43.

Kimball, J. W. (2005). Hormones of the reproductive system. *Kimball's biology pages: An online biology textbook.* Retrieved December 9, 2006, from http://users.rcn.com/jkimball.ma.ultranet/BiologyPages/S/SexHormones.html

CHAPTER 4

Aeby, T. C., & Hiraoka, M. K. (2006). Endometriosis. In E. M. Alderman, M. L. Windle, W. Wolfram, P. D. Petry, & M. Strafford (Eds.),

eMedicine. Retrieved December 25, 2006, from http://www.emedicine.com/ped/topic677.htm

Alan Guttmacher Institute (Eds.). (2006). Facts in brief: Contraceptive use. Retrieved December 29, 2006, from http://www.guttmacher.org/pubs/fb_contr_use.html

American Cancer Society (ACS). (2005). *Breast cancer facts & figures 2005 –2006.* Atlanta: American Cancer Society, Inc. Retrieved December 22, 2006, from http://www.cancer.org/downloads/STT/CAFF2005BrF.pdf

American Cancer Society (ACS). (2006). *Cancer facts & figures 2006.* Atlanta: American Cancer Society, Inc. Retrieved December 22, 2006, from http://www.cancer.org/downloads/STT/CAFF2006PWSecured.pdf

American College of Obstetricians and Gynecologists (ACOG) (Eds.). (2004). Revised cervical cancer screening guidelines require reeducation of women and physicians. *ACOG news release,* May 4, 2004. Retrieved December 23, 2006, from http://www.acog.org/from_home/publications/press_releases/nr05-04-04-1.cfm

Arias, R., & Wysocki, S. (2005). The spectrum of menstrual symptoms: Strategies for counseling and treatment. (Monograph). Dannemiller Memorial Educational Foundation, National Association of Nurse Practitioners in Women's Health and MedPro Communications, Inc., (publisher).

AWHONN Lifelines (Eds.). (2005). Conversations with colleagues: ACOG issues hormone therapy guidelines experts expand estrogen advice; renounce herbs for hot flashes. *AWHONN Lifelines, 9*(1): 39–42.

Barmat, L. I. (Undated). Peri-menopause and infertility: Treatments. *Abington Reproductive Medicine Online (Abington's former newsletter).* Retrieved December 9, 2006, from http://www.abington-repromed.com/academic_papers/content_layout2.cfm?pid=40

Barron, M. L., & Fehring, R. J. (2005). Basal body temperature assessment: Is it useful to couples seeking pregnancy? *American Journal of Maternal Child Nursing, 30*(5), 290–296.

Bates, J. (2006). Reflections: Age of innocence. *Nursing Standard, 20*(19), 28.

Behera, M., Whitman-Elia, G. F., Price, T. M., & Queenan, J. T. (2006). Dysfunctional uterine bleeding. In A. C. Sciscione, F. Talavera, A. D. Barnes, F. B. Gaupp, & L. P. Shulman (Eds.), *eMedicine.* Retrieved December 24, 2006, from http://www.emedicine.com/med/topic2353.htm

Calis, K. A., Popat, V., Nelson, L. M., & Kalantaridou, S. N. (2006). Dysmenorrhea. In A. C. Sciscione, F. Talavera, A. D. Barnes, F. B. Gaupp, & L. P. Shulman (Eds.), *eMedicine.* Retrieved December 24, 2006, from http://www.emedicine.com/med/topic606.htm

Casper, R. F. (2006). Clinical manifestations and diagnosis of menopause. *UpToDate(15.2).* Last updated on October 6, 2006. Retrieved from http://patients.uptodate.com

Chandran, L. (2006). Menstruation disorders. In E. Alderman, M. L. Windle, W. Wolfram, P. D. Petry, & M. Strafford (Eds.), *eMedicine.* Retrieved December 24, 2006, from http://www.emedicine.com/ped/topic2781.htm

Cockey, C. D. (Ed.). (2005). Pregnancy possible after UAE. In C. D. Cockey (Ed), *On the Edge, AWHONN Lifelines, 9*(1), 31–32.

Cottrell, B. H. (2006). Discussing the health risks of douching. *AWHONN Lifelines, 10*(2), 130–136.

Cunningham, F. G., Leveno, K. J., Gilstrap, L. C. III, Hauth, J. C., & Wenstrom, K. D. (2005). Contraception, Ch. 32. In *Williams obstetrics* (22nd ed., pp. 725–750). New York: McGraw-Hill.

Cunningham, F. G., Leveno, K. J., Gilstrap, L. C. III, Hauth, J. C., & Wenstrom, K. D. (2005). Sterilization, Ch. 33. In *Williams obstetrics* (22nd ed., pp. 751–757). New York: McGraw-Hill.

Curran, D., & Bachmann, G. (2006). Menopause. In R. K. Zurawin, F. Talavera, G. F. Whitman-Elia, F. B. Gaupp, & L. P. Shulman (Eds.), *eMedicine.* Retrieved December 30, 2006, from http://www.emedicine.com/med/topic3289.htm

Darney, P. D., & Arias, R. (2006). Advances in the use of intrauterine contraception. *Dialogues in Contraception, 10*(2), 1–4.

Dirubbo, N. (2006). Counsel your patients about contraceptive options. *Nurse Practitioner, 31*(4), 40–44.

Doskoch, P., Flaherty, M., & Gibb, T. (Eds.). (2005). Conference diary: Advances in uterine leiomyoma research. *Women's Health in Primary Care: Gynecology Edition, 5*(3), 134–136.

Edmundson, L. D., Erogul, M., Clark, A. D., Steele, T. (2006). Dysmenorrhea. In S. A. Conrad, F. Talavera, M. Zwanger, J. Halamka,

& P. Dyne (Eds.), *eMedicine*. Retrieved December 24, 2006, from http://www.emedicine.com/emerg/topic156.htm

Edwards, M. (2006). Preconception care. *Practice Nurse, 32*(2), 43–46.

Falcone, T. (2005). Endometriosis: Diagnosis and management. *Practical Strategies in Women's Health, 1*(1), 4–5.

Forbus, S. B. (2005). Age-related infertility: Tuning in to the 'ticking clock.' *AWHONN Lifelines, 9*(2), 126–132.

Garcia, A. A., Hamid, O., & El-Khoueiry, A. (2006). Cervical cancer. In J. J. Kavanagh, F. Talavera, A. D. Barnes, F. B. Gaupp, & L. P. Shulman (Eds.), *eMedicine*. Retrieved December 23, 2006, from http://www.emedicine.com/med/topic324.htm

Garcia, J. E., & Nelson, L. M. (2006). Infertility. In R. K. Zurawin, F. Talavera, A. D. Barnes, F. B. Gaupp, & L. P. Shulman (Eds.), *eMedicine*. Retrieved December 30, 2006, from http://www.emedicine.com/med/topic3535.htm

Gearhart, P. A., Randall, T. C., & Buckley, R. M. (2006). Gynecologic cryosurgery. In M. Nettleman, F. Talavera, R. A. Greenfiled, E. Mylonakis, & B. A. Cunha (Eds.), *eMedicine*. Retrieved December 23, 2006, from http://www.emedicine.com/med/topic1037.htm

Graham, L. (2006). CDC releases guidelines on improving preconception health care. *American Family Physician, 74*(11), 1967–1970.

Griffin, K. W., & Wilder, L. (2005). What is the appropriate diagnostic evaluation of fibroids? *Journal of Family Practice, 54*(5), 458–462.

Gupta, G. (2005). Microbicidal spermicide or spermicidal microbicide? *European Journal of Contraception and Reproductive Health, 10*(4), 212–218.

Harvard Women's Health Watch (Eds.). (2005). What to do about pelvic organ prolapse. *Harvard Women's Health Watch, 12*(10), 4–6.

Helm, C. W. (2005). Ovarian cysts. In S. H. Ural, F. Talavera, A. D. Barnes, F. B. Gaupp, & L. P. Shulman (Eds.), *eMedicine*. Retrieved December 27, 2006, from http://www.emedicine.com/med/topic1699.htm

Hesley, G. K., Felmlee, J. P., Gebhart, J. B., Dunagan, K. T., Gorny, K. R., Kesler, J. B., Brandt, K. R., Glantz, J. N., & Gostout, B. S. (2006). Noninvasive treatment of uterine fibroids: Early May Clinic experience with magnetic resonance imaging-guided focused ultrasound. *Mayo Clinic Proceedings, 81*(7), 936–942.

Hill, J. B., & Lockrow, E. (2005). Pelvic inflammatory disease. In R. Levine, F. Talavera, M. E. Rivlin, F. B. Gaupp, & L. P. Shulman (Eds.), *eMedicine*. Retrieved December 26, 2006, from http://www.emedicine.com/med/topic1774.htm

Hobar, C. (2005). Osteoporosis. In A. Davidson, F. Talavera, H. S. Diamond, A. J. Mechaber, & A. Weinstein (Eds.), *eMedicine*. Retrieved December 30, 2006, from http://www.emedicine.com/med/topic1693.htm

Huntington, A., & Gilmour, J. A. (2005). A life shaped by pain: Women and endometriosis. *Journal of Clinical Nursing, 14*, 1124–1132.

Istvan, N. (2005). Conization of cervix. In S. H. Ural, F. Talavera, M. E. Rivlin, F. B. Gaupp, & L. P. Shulman (Eds.), *eMedicine*. Retrieved December 23, 2006, from http://www.emedicine.com/med/topic3338.htm

Kaminski, P., Hoffman, M., & Payne, K. (2006). Benign cervical lesions. In J. G. Pritzker, F. Talavera, M. E. Rivlin, F. B. Gaupp, & L. P. Shulman (Eds.), *eMedicine*. Retrieved December 26, 2006, from http://www.emedicine.com/med/topic3297.htm

Kelley, R. (2005). Return of a silent killer. *Newsweek, 145*(8).

Kirkham, C., Harris, S., & Grzybowski, S. (2005). Evidence-based prenatal care: Part I. General prenatal care and counseling issues. *American Family Physician, 71*(7), 1307–1316, 1321–1322.

Lynch, E. (2006). Painful delays: A greater awareness of endometriosis is helping speed up diagnosis. *Nursing Standard, 20* (50), 21.

Moghissi, K. S. (2005). Medical treatment of endometriosis: Diagnosis and therapeutic options. *Women's Health in Primary Care Gynecology Edition, 5*(4), 207–212.

Moghissi, K. S. (2005). Additional options for the medical treatment of endometriosis: Danazol and Gn-RH agonists. *Women's Health in Primary Care Gynecology Edition, 5*(5), 260–265.

Moos, M. (2006). Preconception care: Every woman, every time. *AWHONN Lifelines, 10*(4), 332–334.

Moreno, M. A., Giesel, A. E., & Clark, L. R. (2006). Premenstrual syndrome. In E. M. Alderman, M. L. Windle, W. Wolfram, D. Rauch, & M. Strafford (Eds.), *eMedicine*. Retrieved December 24, 2006, from http://www.emedicine.com/ped/topic1890.htm

Mounsey, A. L., Wilgus, A., & Slawson, D. C. (2006). Diagnosis and management of endometriosis. *American Family Physician, 74*(4), 594–602.

National Cancer Institute (Eds.). (2006). Cervical cancer (PDQ®): Screening. U.S. National Institutes of Health: National Cancer Institute. Retrieved December 23, 2006, from http://www.cancer.gov/cancertopics/pdq/screening/cervical/healthprofessional/allpages

Nicita, G., Marzi, V. L., Filocamo, M. T., Dattolo, E., Marzocco, M., Paoletti, M. C., et al. (2005). Uterus-sparing vaginal surgery of genitourinary prolapse employing biocompatible material. *Urologia International, 75*, 314–318.

O'Dell, K. K., & Jacelon, C. S. (2005). Not the surgery for a young person: Women's experience with vaginal closure surgery for severe prolapse. *Urologic Nursing, 25*(5), 345–351.

Parviainen, K., & Gaba, N. D. (2006). Gynecologic cryosurgery. In S. H. Ural, F. Talavera, M. E. Rivlin, F. B. Gaupp, & L. P. Shulman (Eds.), *eMedicine*. Retrieved December 23, 2006, from http://www.emedicine.com/med/topic3337.htm

Pattan, C., Zuellig, A., Hong, B., Stewart, S., & Grossman, M. (2005). Colposcopy. In S. H. Ural, F. Talavera, M. E. Rivlin, F. B. Gaupp, & L. P. Shulman (Eds.), *eMedicine*. Retrieved December 23, 2006, from http://www.emedicine.com/med/topic3298.htm

Petrozza, J. C., & Styer, A. K. (2006). Assisted reproductive technology. In B. D. Cowan, F. Talavera, C. V. Smith, F. B. Gaupp, & L. P. Shulman (Eds.), *eMedicine*. Retrieved December 30, 2006, from http://www.emedicine.com/med/topic3288.htm

Pierzynski, P., Swiatecka, J., Oczeretko, E., Laudanski, P., Batra, S., & Laudanski, T. (2006). Effect of short-term, low-dose treatment with tamoxifen in patients with primary dysmenorrhea. *Gynecological Endocrinology, 22*(12), 698–703.

Planned Parenthood (Eds.). (2005). *Fertility awareness-based methods*. Retrieved December 30, 2006, from http://www.plannedparenthood.org/birth-control-pregnancy/birth-control/fertility-awareness-based-methods.htm

Pradhan, A., & Lim, C. (2006). Myths & management of PMS: Treating sometimes-misunderstood symptoms. *Women's Health in Primary Care, OB-GYN Edition, 6*(1), 39–45.

Rapkin, A. J. (2006). Premenstrual dysphoric disorder. *The Forum: A Working Group for Women's Healthcare, 4*(1), 2–6.

Reyes, I., & Abbuhl, S. (2006). Pelvic inflammatory disease. In D. S. Howes, F. Talavera, M. Zwanger, J. Halamka, & P. Dyne (Eds.), *eMedicine*. Retrieved December 26, 2006, from http://www.emedicine.com/emerg/topic410.htm

Rice, C., & Thompson, J. (2006). Selecting a hormonal contraceptive that suits your patient's needs. *Women's Health in Primary Care, OB-GYN Edition, 6*(6), 26–34.

Rubenstein, J., & Brannigan, R. E. (2005). Infertility, male. In D. B. Rukstalis, F. Talavera, M. J. Noble, J. S. Wolf, & S. W. Leslie (Eds.), *eMedicine*. Retrieved December 30, 2006, from http://www.emedicine.com/med/topic1167.htm

Salandy, D., & Brenner, B. (2005). Toxic shock syndrome. In T. Gaeta, F. Talavera, M. L. Plaster, J. Halamka, & C. V. Pollack (Eds.), *eMedicine*. Retrieved December 26, 2006, from http://www.emedicine.com/emerg/topic600.htm

Samra, O. M., & Wood, E. (2006). Contraception. In J. J. Kavanagh, F. Talavera, A. D. Barnes, F. B. Gaupp, & L. P. Shulman (Eds.), *eMedicine*. Retrieved December 29, 2006, from http://www.emedicine.com/med/topic3211.htm

Shaw, J. A., & Shaw, H. A. (2005). Menorrhagia. In T. M. Price, F. Talavera, A. D. Barnes, F. B. Gaupp, & L. P. Shulman (Eds.), *eMedicine*. Retrieved December 26, 2006, from http://www.emedicine.com/med/topic1449.htm

Shulman, L. P. (2006). Contraception today: Risks and benefits in scientific, clinical, and sociocultural context. *Medscape*. Retrieved December 29, 2006, from http://www.medscape.com/viewprogram/6049_pnt

Szarewski, A., & Hope, S. (2006). Contraception. *Primary Health Care, 16*(2), 42–50.

Theroux, R. (2005). The women's health initiative: Evaluating its impact. *AWHONN Lifelines, 9*(2), 140–145.

Thomason, P. (2005). Leiomyoma, uterus (fibroid). In C. L. Sistrom, B. D. Coombs, K. L. Reuter, R. M. Krasny, & E. C. Lin (Eds.), *eMedicine*. Retrieved December 26, 2006, from http://www.emedicine.com/radio/topic777.htm

Tolan, R. W., & Dhawan, V. K. (2006). Toxic shock syndrome. In D. Jaimovich, M. L. Windle, L. I. Lutwick, D. Rauch, & R. W. Steele (Eds.), *eMedicine*. Retrieved December 26, 2006, from http://www.emedicine.com/ped/topic2269.htm

Trupin, S. R. (2006). Abortion. In S. D. Spandorfer, F. Talavera, A. D. Barnes, F. B. Gaupp, & L. P. Shulman (Eds.), *eMedicine*. Retrieved December 30, 2006, from http://www.emedicine.com/med/topic5.htm

Vega, C. P. (2006). Dysfunctional uterine bleeding in *AAFP 2006 – Women's healthcare issues during the childbearing years*. Retrieved December 18, 2006, from http://www.medscape.com/viewarticle/549078

Welch-Carre, E. (2005). The neurodevelopmental consequences of prenatal alcohol exposure. *Advances in Neonatal Care, 5*(4), 217–229.

Workowski, K. A., & Berman, S. M. (2006). Sexually transmitted diseases treatment guidelines, 2006. *MMWR, 55*(RR11), 1–94.

Winer, S. A., & Rapkin, A. J. (2006). Premenstrual disorders: Prevalence, etiology, and impact. *Journal of Reproductive Medicine, 51*(4 Suppl), 339–370.

Xu, J., Bartoces, M., Neale, V. M., et al. (2005). Natural history of menopause symptoms in primary care patients: A metronet study. *Journal of American Board of Family Medicine, 18*(5), 374–382. Retrieved December 9, 2006, from http://www.medscape.com/viewarticle/512567

CHAPTER 5

Cunningham, F. G., Leveno, K. J., Bloom, S. L., Hauth, J. C., Gilstrap, L. C. III, & Wenstrom, K. D. (2005a). Fetal growth and development. In *Williams obstetrics* (22nd ed., pp. 91–120). New York: McGraw-Hill .

Cunningham, F. G., Leveno, K. J., Bloom, S. L., Hauth, J. C., Gilstrap, L. C. III, & Wenstrom, K. D. (2005b). Implantation, embryogenesis, and placental development. In *Williams obstetrics* (22nd ed., pp. 39–90). New York: McGraw-Hill.

Flanagan, M. F., Yeager, S. B., & Weindling, S. N. (2005). Cardiac disease. In M. G. MacDonald, M. D. Mullett, & M. M. K. Seshia (Eds.), *Avery's neonataology: Pathophysiology & management of the newborn* (6th ed., pp. 631–709). Philadelphia: Lippincott Williams & Wilkins.

March of Dimes. (Undated). Thalidomide. *Quick Reference: Fact Sheets, Professionals & Researchers*. Retrieved December 18, 2006, from http://www.marchofdimes.com/printableArticles/14332_1172.asp

Pridjian, G. (2005). Feto-maternal interactions: Placental physiology, the in utero environment, and fetal determinants of adult disease. In M. G. MacDonald, M. D. Mullett, & M. M. K. Seshia (Eds.), *Avery's neonataology: Pathophysiology & management of the newborn* (6th ed., pp. 149–165). Philadelphia: Lippincott Williams & Wilkins.

Robinson, J. N., & Abuhamad, A. Z. (2002). Determining chorionicity and amnionicity in multiple pregnancies. *Contemporary Ob/Gyn, 6*, 94–108. Retrieved December 18, 2006, from http://www.modernmedicine.com/modernmedicine/Ultrasound+Clinics/Determining-chorionicity-and-amnionicity-in-multip/ArticleStandard/Article/detail/139439

Sepilian, V, & Wood, E. (2005). Ectopic pregnancy. In R. K. Zurawin, F. Talavera, A. D. Barnes, F. B. Gaupp, & L. P. Shulman. (Eds.), *eMedicine*. Retrieved December 18, 2006, from http://www.emedicine.com/med/topic3212.htm

Zach, R., & Pramanik, A. (2006). Multiple births. In D. N. Sheftel, R. Konop, D. A. Clark, C. L. Wagner, & N. N. Finer. (Eds.), *eMedicine*. Retrieved December 18, 2006, from http://www.emedicine.com/ped/topic2599.htm

CHAPTER 6

Bastion, L. A. & Brown, H. L. (2006). Diagnosis and clinical manifestations of early pregnancy. *UpToDate*(15.2). Retrieved August 17, 2007, from http://patients.uptodate.com

Bermas, B. L. (2006). Pain related to the musculoskeletal system during pregnancy. *UpToDate*(15.2). Retrieved August 17, 2007, from http://patients.uptodate.com

Bianco, A. (2006). Maternal gastrointestinal tract adaptation to pregnancy. *UpToDate*(15.2). Retrieved August 17, 2007, from http://patients.uptodate.com

Cunningham, F. G., Leveno, K. J., Bloom, S. L., Hauth, J. C., Gilstrap, L. C. III, & Wenstrom, K. D. (2005). Maternal physiology. In *Williams obstetrics* (22nd ed., pp. 121–150). New York: McGraw-Hill.

Foley, M. R. (2007). Maternal cardiovascular and hemodynamic adaptation to pregnancy. *UpToDate(15.2)*. Retrieved August 17, 2007, from http://patients.uptodate.com

Funai, E. F., Gillen-Goldstein, J., & Roqué, H. (2006). Changes in the respiratory tract during pregnancy. *UpToDate(15.2)*. Retrieved August 17, 2007 from http://patients.uptodate.com

Funai, E. F., & Hayslett, J. P. (2007). Renal and urinary tract physiology in pregnant women. *UpToDate(15.2)*. Retrieved August 17, 2007, from http://patients.uptodate.com

Gillen-Goldstein, J., Funai, E. F., & Roqué, H. (2007). Nutrition in pregnancy. *UpToDate(15.2)*. Retrieved August 17, 2007, from http://patients.uptodate.com

Hofmeyr, G. J., Atallah, A. N., & Duley, L. (2006). Calcium supplementation during pregnancy for preventing hypertensive disorders and related problems. Cochrane Database of Systematic Reviews 2006, (Issue 3. Art. No.: CD001059. DOI: 10.1002/14651858.CD001059.pub2).

ICCIDD, (Eds.). (2007). Iodine requirements in pregnancy and infancy. *IDD Newsletter, 23*(1), 1–2. Retrieved October 7, 2007, from http://thyroid.org/professionals/education/documents/IDD_NL_Feb07.pdf

March of Dimes, (Eds.). (2006). Folic acid. *Professionals & Researchers Quick Reference and Fact Sheets*. Retrieved October 7, 2007, from http://www.marchofdimes.com/printableArticles/14332_1151.asp

March of Dimes, (Eds.). (Undated). Weigh to grow. *Pregnancy & newborn health education center*. Retrieved October 7, 2007, from http://www.marchofdimes.com/pnhec/159_153.asp

Marchiano, D., & Ural, S. H. (2005). Prenatal nutrition. In S. R. Trupin, F. Talavera, D. Chelmow, F. B. Gaupp, & L. P. Shulman (Eds.), *eMedicine*. Retrieved October 7, 2007, from http://www.emedicine.com/med/topic3234.htm

Mills, M. E. (2007). Craving more than food: The implications of pica in pregnancy. *Nursing for Women's Health, 11*(3), 266 – 273.

Paidas, M. J., Ku, D. W., & Arkel, Y. S. (2006). Hematologic changes in pregnancy. *UpToDate(15.2)*. Retrieved August 17, 2007, from http://patients.uptodate.com

Petroglia, F., & D'Antona, D. (2006). Maternal endocrine and metabolic adaptation to pregnancy. *UpToDate(15.2)*. Retrieved August 17, 2007, from http://patients.uptodate.com

Pomeranz, M. K. (2007). Physiologic changes of the skin, hair, nails, and mucous membranes during pregnancy. *UpToDate(15.2)*. Retrieved August 17, 2007, from http://patients.uptodate.com

Rumbold, A., Duley, L., Crowther, C., & Haslam, R. (2005). Antioxidants for preventing pre-eclampsia. *Cochrane Database of Systematic Reviews 2005*, Issue 4.

U.S. Department of Health & Human Services & USDA, (Eds.). (2005). Dietary guidelines for Americans 2005. Retrieved October 7, 2007, from www.healthierus.gov/dietaryguidelines

U.S. Food and Drug Administration (FDA), (Eds.). (2005). Food safety for moms-to-be. A publication of CFSAN/Office of Food Safety, Defense, and Outreach. Retrieved October 7, 2007, from http://www.cfsan.fda.gov/pregnant/pregnant.html

Weinberger, S. E. (2006). Dyspnea during pregnancy. *UpToDate(15.2)*. Retrieved August 17, 2007, from http://patients.uptodate.com

CHAPTER 7

American College of Obstetricians and Gynecologists (ACOG), (Eds.). (2002, January). Exercise during pregnancy and the postpartum period. *ACOG Committee Opinion, number 267*.

Artal, R. (2007). Recommendations for exercise during pregnancy and the postpartum period. *UpToDate(15.2)*. Retrieved August 17, 2007, from http://patients.uptodate.com

Badell, M. L., Ramin, S. M., & Smith, J. A. (2006). Treatment options for nausea and vomiting during pregnancy. *Pharmacotherapy, 26*(9), 1273–1287. Retrieved October 13, 2007, from http://www.medscape.com/viewarticle/545629

Baschat, A. A. (2006). Venous doppler for fetal assessment. *UpToDate(15.1)*. Retrieved June 16, 2007, from http://patients.uptodate.com

Beebe, K. R., & Lee, K. A. (2007). Sleep disturbance in late pregnancy and early labor. *Journal of Perinatal & Neonatal Nursing, 23*(2), 103–108.

Bing, E. (1994). *Six practical lessons for an easier childbirth* (3rd Rev. ed.). New York: Bantam Books.

Born, D., & Barron, M. L. (2005). Herb use in pregnancy: What nurses should know. *American Journal of Maternal/Child Nursing,* 30(3), 201–206.

Bradley, R. A. (1996). *The Bradley method of natural childbirth husband coached childbirth,* (4th ed.). New York: Bantam Books.

Cesario, S. K. (2007). Seat belt use in pregnancy: History, misconceptions, and the need for education. *Nursing for Women's Health,* 11(5), 474–481.

Chen, X., Stanton, B., Shankaran, S., & Li, X. (2006). Age of smoking onset as a predictor of smoking cessation during pregnancy. *American Journal of Health Behavior,* 30(3), 247–258.

Constantinou, A. (2005). Alcohol and pregnancy: Experts warn that inconsistent messages are causing harm. *Drugs and Alcohol Today,* 5(4), 41–44.

Cottrell, B. H. (2006). Discussing the health risks of douching. *AWHONN Lifelines,* 10(2), 130–136.

Edelman, A., Anderson, J. Lai, S., Braner, D. A. V., Tegtmeyer, K. (2007). Pelvic examination. *New England Journal of Medicine,* 356(26), e26.

Fowler, J. R., & Culpepper, L. (2007). Work and pregnancy. *UpToDate(15.2).* Retrieved August 17, 2007, from http://patients.uptodate.com

Ghidini, A., & McLaren, R. (2006). Chorionic villus sampling: Risks, complications, and techniques. *UpToDate(15.1).* Retrieved June 16, 2007, from http://patients.uptodate.com

Golde, M. P. (2007, April). Expectant mothers, expert care: Your guide to helping every mom-to-be have a healthy smile. *Modern Hygienist,* 20–23.

Hunter, L. P., & Young, R. E. (2007). Nausea and vomiting of pregnancy: Clinical management. *American Journal for Nurse Practitioners,* 11(8), 57–67.

Kelly, A. K. W. (2005). Practical exercise advice during pregnancy: Guidelines for active and inactive women. *Physician and Sportsmedicine,* 33(6), 24–30, 47–48.

Krulewitch, C. J. (2005). Alcohol consumption during pregnancy. *Annual Review of Nursing Research,* 2005(23), 101–134.

Kuczkowski, K. M. (2005). Peripartum care of the cocaine-abusing parturient: Are we ready? *Acta Obstetricia Et Gynecologica Scandinavica,* 84(2), 108–116.

Lockwood, C. J. (2007). The initial prenatal assessment and routine prenatal care. *UpToDate(15.2).* Retrieved August 17, 2007, from http://patients.uptodate.com

Lothian, J. A. (2006). Preparation for labor and childbirth. *UpToDate(15.1).* Retrieved June 16, 2007, from http://patients.uptodate.com

MacKenzie, A. P., Stephenson, C. D., & Funai, E. F. (2006). Prenatal assessment of gestational age and fetal weight. *UpToDate(15.1).* Retrieved June 16, 2007, from http://patients.uptodate.com

Maulik, D. (2005). Doppler ultrasound of the umbilical artery for fetal surveillance. *UpToDate(15.1).* Retrieved June 16, 2007, from http://patients.uptodate.com

March of Dimes, (Eds.). (2005, November). Caffeine in pregnancy. *Professionals & Researchers Quick Reference and Fact Sheets.* Retrieved October 13, 2007, from http://www.marchofdimes.com/printableArticles/14332_1148.asp

March of Dimes, (Eds.). (2006, November). Illicit drug use during pregnancy. *Professionals & Researchers Quick Reference and Fact Sheets.* Retrieved October 13, 2007, from http://www.marchofdimes.com/printableArticles/14332_1169.asp

March of Dimes, (Eds.). (2007, March). Fitness for two. *Professionals & Researchers Quick Reference and Fact Sheets.* Retrieved October 13, 2007, from http://www.marchofdimes.com/printableArticles/14332_1150.asp

McCarter-Spaulding, D. E. (2005). Medications in pregnancy and lactation. *American Journal of Maternal/Child Nursing,* 30(1), 10–17.

Monti, D. (2006). Heartburn in pregnancy – no, your baby won't have more hair! *International Journal of Childbirth Education,* 21(4), 32–33.

Natarajan, G., & Klein, M. D. (2006). The fetus as a patient: Prenatal diagnosis and fetal therapy. In D. Farmer, M. L. Windle, N. A. Shorter, H. B. Othersen, & H. Grewal (Eds.), *eMedicine.* Retrieved October 12, 2007, from http://www.emedicine.com/ped/topic2953.htm

National Center for Health Statistics, (Eds.). (2007). Prenatal care. *Fast Stats A to Z.* Retrieved October 11, 2007, from http://www.cdc.gov.mill1.sjlibrary.org/nchs/fastats/prenatal.htm

Okah, F. A., Cai, J., Dew, P. C., Hoff, G. L. (2005). Are fewer women smoking during pregnancy? *American Journal of Health Behavior,* 29(5), 456–461.

Pennick, V. E., & Young, G. (2007). Interventions for preventing and treating pelvic and back pain in pregnancy. Cochrane Database of Systematic Reviews 2007, Issue 2. Art. No.: CD001139. DOI: 10.1002/14651858.CD001139.pub2.

Richter, J. E. (2005). Review article: The management of hearburn in pregnancy. *Alimentary Pharmacology & Therapeutics,* 22(9), 749–757.

Shipp, T. D. (2006). Ultrasound examination in obstetrics and gynecology: Procedure. *UpToDate(15.1).* Available with an online subscription. Retrieved June 16, 2007, from http://patients.uptodate.com

Taylor, C. R., Alexander, G. R., & Hepworth, J. T. (2005). Clustering of U.S. women receiving no prenatal care: Differences in pregnancy outcomes and implications for targeting interventions. *Maternal and Child Health Journal,* 9(2), 125–133.

Trupin, S. R. (2006). Common pregnancy complaints and questions. In A. Whitlin, F. Talavera, R. S. Legro, F. B. Gaupp, & L. P. Shulman (Eds.), *eMedicine.* Retrieved October 13, 2007, from http://www.emedicine.com/med/topic3238.htm

Women's Health USA. (2005). Health status: Maternal health. Retrieved October 13, 2007, from http://mchb.hrsa.gov/whusa_05/pages/0424pc.htm

Wyatt, S. N., & Rhoads, S. J. (2006). A primer on antenatal testing for neonatal nurses: Part 2: Tests of fetal well-being. *Advances in Neonatal Care,* 6(5), 228–241.

Young, G. L., & Jewell, D. (2007). Interventions for leg cramps in pregnancy. (Cochrane Review). In *The Cochrane Library,* Issue 2, 2007. Oxford: Update Software.

Zindler, L. (2005). Ethical decision making in first trimester pregnancy screening. *Journal of Perinatal & Neonatal Nursing,* 19(2), 122–131.

CHAPTER 8

Cheng, Y. W., Caughey, A. B., Khan, F. O., & Razi, M. S. (2006). Normal labor and delivery. In B. A. Meyer, F. Talavera, D. Chelmow, F. B. Gaupp, & L. P. Shulman (Eds.), *eMedicine.* Retrieved October 23, 2007, from http://www.emedicine.com/med/topic3239.htm

Cunningham, F. G., Leveno, K. J., Bloom, S. L., Hauth, J. C., Gilstrap, L. C. III, & Wenstrom, K. D. (2005a). Maternal anatomy. In *Williams obstetrics* (22nd ed., pp. 15–38). New York: McGraw-Hill.

Cunningham, F. G., Leveno, K. J., Bloom, S. L., Hauth, J. C., Gilstrap, L. C. III, & Wenstrom, K. D. (2005b). Normal labor and delivery. In *Williams obstetrics* (22nd ed., pp. 409–441). New York: McGraw-Hill.

Cunningham, F. G., Leveno, K. J., Bloom, S. L., Hauth, J. C., Gilstrap, L. C. III, & Wenstrom, K. D. (2005c). Parturition. In *Williams obstetrics* (22nd ed., pp. 151–186). New York: McGraw-Hill.

Funai, E. F., & Norwitz, E. R. (2006). Mechanism of normal labor and delivery. *UpToDate(15.1).* Retrieved June 16, 2007, from http://patients.uptodate.com

Joy, S., & Lyon, D. (2005). Diagnosis of abnormal labor. In R. K. Zurawin, F. Talavera, R. S. Legro, F. B. Gaupp, & L. P. Shulman (Eds.), *eMedicine.* Retrieved October 23, 2007, from http://www.emedicine.com/med/topic3488.htm

Julien, S., & Galerneau, F. Face, brow, and compound presentations in labor. *UpToDate(15.1).* Retrieved June 16, 2007, from http://patients.uptodate.com

Lavender, T., O'Brien, P., & Hart, A. (2007). Effect of partogram use on outcomes for women in spontaneous labour at term (Protocol for Cochrane Review). In *The Cochrane Library,* Issue 2, 2007. Oxford: Update Software.

Low, L. K., & Moffat, A. (2006). Every labor is unique, but "call when your contractions are 3 minutes apart." *American Journal of Maternal/Child Nursing,* 31(5), 307–312.

Norwitz, E. R. (2006). Physiology of parturition. *UpToDate(15.1).* Retrieved June 16, 2007, from http://patients.uptodate.com

Ridley, R. T. (2007). Diagnosis and intervention for occiput posterior malposition. *Journal of Obstetric, Gynecologic, & Neonatal Nursing,* 36(2), 135–143.

Smith, J. R., & Brennan, B. G. (2006). Management of the third stage of labor. In B. D. Cowan, F. Talavera, D. Chelmow, F. B. Gaupp, & L. P. Shulman (Eds.), *eMedicine.* Retrieved October 23, 2007, from http://www.emedicine.com/med/topic3569.htm

Smith, R. (2007). Parturition. *New England Journal of Medicine, 356*(3), 271–283.

Tranmer, J. E., Hodnett, E. D., Hannah, M. E., & Stevens, B. J. (2005). The effect of unrestricted oral carbohydrate intake on labor progress. *Journal of Obstetric, Gynecologic, & Neonatal Nursing, 34*(3), 319–328.

Varney, H., Kriebs, J. M., & Gegor, C. L. (2004). Anatomy of the pelvis, pelvic types, evaluation of the bony pelvis, and clinical pelvimetry. In *Varney's Midwifery* (4th ed., pp. 1205–1216). Boston: Jones and Bartlett Publishers.

CHAPTER 9

American Academy of Pediatrics Committee on Fetus and Newborn, (Eds.). (2005). Underwater births. *Pediatrics, 115*(5), 1413–1414.

Anim-Somuah, M., Smyth, R., Howell, C. (2005). Epidural versus non-epidural or no analgesia in labour. Cochrane Database of Systematic Reviews 2005, Issue 4. Art. No.: CD000331. DOI: 10.1002/14651858.CD000331.pub2.

Barragán Loayza, I. M., & Gonzales, F. (2007). Biofeedback for pain during labour (Protocol for Cochrane Review). In *The Cochrane Library*, Issue 2, 2007.

Courtney, K. (2007). Maternal anesthesia: What are the effects on neonates? *Nursing for Women's Health, 11*(5), 499–502.

Cunningham, F. G., Leveno, K. J., Bloom, S. L., Hauth, J. C., Gilstrap, L. C. III, & Wenstrom, K. D. (2005a). Obstetrical anesthesia. In *Williams obstetrics* (22nd ed., pp. 473–494). New York: McGraw-Hill.

Grant, G. J. (2006a). Anesthesia for cesarean delivery. *UpToDate(15.2)*. Retrieved August 15, 2007, from http://patients.uptodate.com

Grant, G. J. (2006b). Pharmacologic management of pain during labor and delivery. *UpToDate(15.2)*. Retrieved August 15, 2007, from http://patients.uptodate.com

Grant, G. J. (2006c). Prevention and treatment of adverse effects of neuraxial anesthesia. *UpToDate(15.2)*. Retrieved August 15, 2007, from http://patients.uptodate.com

Prkachin, K. M., Solomon, P. E., & Ross, J. (2007). Underestimation of pain by health-care providers: Towards a model of the process of inferring pain in others. *Canadian Journal of Nursing Research, 39*(2), 88–106.

Simkin, P. & Klein, M. C. (2007). Nonpharmacological approaches to management of labor pain. *UpToDate(15.2)*. Retrieved September 15, 2007, from http://patients.uptodate.com

Stark, M. A., & Jones, M. (2006). Advanced preparation and positive labor support create an optimal experience for normal birth. *Journal of Perinatal Education, 15*(2), 4–7.

Stuebe, A. & Barbieri, R. L. (2005). Continuous intrapartum support. *UpToDate(15.1)*. Retrieved June 16, 2007, from http://patients.uptodate.com

Tillet, J. (2005). Epidural anaesthesia: A resource to use judiciously. *Journal of Perinatal & Neonatal Nursing, 19*(3), 207–209.

Waterbirth International, (Eds.). (Undated). Waterbirth FAQ. Retrieved November 6, 2007, from http://www.waterbirth.org/mc/page.do?sitePageId = 38564&orgId = wi

Zwelling, E., Johnson, K., & Allen, J. (2006). How to implement complementary therapies for laboring women. *American Journal of Maternal/Child Nursing, 31*(6), 364–370.

CHAPTER 10

Acker, D. (2007). Clinical pearls in application of electronic fetal heart rate monitoring. *UpToDate(15.3)*. Retrieved November 1, 2007, from http://patients.uptodate.com

Alfirevic, Z., Devane, D., Gyte, G. M. L. (2007). Continuous cardiotocography (CTG) as a form of electronic fetal monitoring (EFM) for fetal assessment during labour (Cochrane Review). In *The Cochrane Library*, 2, 2007.

Association of Women's Health, Obstetric and Neonatal Nurses (AWHONN). (2006). Course outline slides with script. *Advanced Fetal Monitoring Course Instructor Resource CD*: Dubuque, IA: Kendall/Hunt.

Association of Women's Health, Obstetric and Neonatal Nurses (AWHONN), (Eds.). (2005). Moving toward NICHD nomenclature: AWHONN fetal heart monitoring program transitioning to NICH terms. *AWHONN News & Views: AWHONN Lifelines, 9*(3), 258–259.

Bloom, S. L., Casey, B. M., Schaffer, J. L., McIntire, D. D., & Leveno, K. J. (2006a). A randomized trial of coached versus uncoached maternal pushing during the second stage of labor. *American Journal of Obstetrics & Gynecology, 194*(1), 10–13.

Bloom, S. L., Casey, B. M., Schaffer, J. L., McIntire, D. D., & Leveno, K. J. (2006b). Fetal pulse oximetry and cesarean delivery. *New England Journal of Medicine, 355*(21), 2195–2202.

Briggs, G. G., & Wan, S. R. (2006). Drug therapy during labor and delivery, part 2. *American Journal Health-System Pharmacology, 63*(12), 1131–1139. Retrieved November 6, 2007, from http://www.medscape.com/viewarticle/535774

Campbell, D. A., Lake, M. F., Falk, M., & Backstrand, J. R. (2006). A randomized control trial of continuous support in labor by a lay doula. *Journal of Obstetric, Gynecologic & Neonatal Nursing, 35*(4), 456–464.

Cunningham, F. G., Leveno, K. J., Bloom, S. L., Hauth, J. C., Gilstrap, L. C. III, & Wenstrom, K. D. (2005a). Intrapartum assessment. In *Williams obstetrics* (22nd ed., pp. 443–471). New York: McGraw-Hill.

Cunningham, F. G., Leveno, K. J., Bloom, S. L., Hauth, J. C., Gilstrap, L. C. III, & Wenstrom, K. D. (2005b). Normal labor and delivery. In *Williams obstetrics* (22nd ed., pp. 409–441). New York: McGraw-Hill.

Cunningham, F. G., Leveno, K. J., Bloom, S. L., Hauth, J. C., Gilstrap, L. C. III, & Wenstrom, K. D. (2005c). Parturition. In *Williams obstetrics* (22nd ed., pp. 151–186). New York: McGraw-Hill.

Funai, E. F., & Norwitz, E. R. (2006). Management of normal labor and delivery. *UpToDate(15.2)*. Retrieved August 17, 2007, from http://patients.uptodate.com

Gillen-Goldstein, J., & Young, B. K. (2006). Overview of fetal heart rate assessment. *UpToDate(15.2)*. Retrieved August 17, 2007, from http://patients.uptodate.com

Heffron, C. (2006). The honor of your presence. *AWHONN Lifelines, 10*(6), 532, 531.

Hottenstein, S. E. (2005). Creating optimal birth experiences through theory-driven nursing care: Continuous labor support. *AWHONN Lifelines, 9*(3), 242–247.

Low, L. K., & Moffat, A. (2006). Every labor is unique but "Call when your contractions are 3 minutes apart." *American Journal of Maternal/Child Nursing, 31*(5), 307–312.

NANDA, International (Eds.). (2007). *Nursing diagnoses: Definitions & classification 2007 – 2008*. Philadelphia: NANDA, International.

Parsons, M., Bidewell, J., & Griffiths, R. (2007). A comparative study of the effect of food consumption on labour and birth outcomes in Australia. *Midwifery, 23*(2), 131–138.

Price, S., Noseworthy, J., & Thornton, J. (2007). Women's experience with social presence during childbirth. *American Journal of Maternal/Child Nursing, 32*(3), 184–191.

Ruhl, C. (2006). Labor support: Exploring its role in modern and high-tech birthing practices. *AWHONN Lifelines, 10*(1), 58–65.

Sampselle, C. M., Miller, J. M., Luecha, Y., Fischer, K., & Rosten, L. (2005). Provider support of spontaneous pushing during the second stage of labor. *Journal of Obstetric, Gynecologic & Neonatal Nursing, 34*(6), 695–702.

Schaffer, J. I., Bloom, S. L., & Casey, B. M. (2005). A randomized trial of the effects of coached versus uncoached pushing during second stage of labor on postpartum pelvic floor structure and function. *American Journal of Obstetrics & Gynecology, 192*(5), 1692–1696.

Silverman, F. (2006). Management of the third stage of labor. *UpToDate(15.2)*. Retrieved August 17, 2007, from http://patients.uptodate.com

Simpson, K. R. (2005a). Intrauterine resuscitation during labor. *American Journal of Maternal/Child Nursing, 30*(5), 344.

Simpson, K. R. (2005b). The context & clinical evidence for common nursing practices during labor. *American Journal of Maternal/Child Nursing, 30*(6), 356–363.

Simpson, K. R., & James, D. C. (2005). Effects of immediate versus delayed pushing during second-stage labor on fetal well-being: A randomized clinical trial. *Nursing Research, 54*(3), 149–157.

Simpson, K. R., & Know, G. E. (2005). Essential criteria to promote safe care during labor and birth. *AWHONN Lifelines, 9*(6), 478–483.

Simpson, K. R. & Thorman, K. E. (2005). Obstetric "conveniences" elective induction of labor, cesarean birth on demand, and other potentially unnecessary interventions. *Journal of Perinatal & Neonatal Nursing, 19*(2), 134–144.

Sleutel, M., Schultz, S., & Wyble, K. (2007). Nurses' views of factors that help and hinder their intrapartum care. *Journal of Obstetric, Gynecologic, & Neonatal Nursing, 36*(3), 203–211.

Snelgrove-Clarke, E., & Scott-Findlay, S. (2005). Fetal health surveillance: The use of research evidence in practice. *AWHONN Lifelines, 9*(5), 400–403.

Stokowski, L. A. (2005). Reminder to stop using terms "fetal distress" and "birth asphyxia. Critical connections: Noteworthy professional news. *Advances in Neonatal Care, 5*(2), 62–63.

Stuebe, A., & Barbieri, R. L. (2005). Continuous intrapartum support. *UpToDate*(15.2). Retrieved August 17, 2007, from http//patients.uptodate.com

Tillet, J. (2005). Obstetric rituals: Is practice supported by evidence? *Journal of Perinatal & Neonatal Nursing, 19*(2), 91–93.

Tillett, J. (2007). Intermittent auscultation of the fetal heartbeat: Can nurses change the culture of technology? *Journal of Perinatal & Neonatal Nursing, 21*(2), 80–82.

Tranmer, J. E., Hodnett, E. D., Hannah, M. E.,& Stevens, B. J. (2005). The effect of unrestricted oral carbohydrate intake on labor progress. *Journal of Obstetric, Gynecologic, & Neonatal Nursing, 34*(3), 319–328.

Wenstrom, K. D. (2006). [Commentary on] A randomized trial of coached versus uncoached maternal pushing during the second stage of labor. *Obstetrical & Gynecological Survey 61*(5), 304–305.

Yeomans, E. R., & Ramin, S. M. (2006). Fetal acid-base physiology. *UpToDate*(15.3). Retrieved October 1, 2007, from http://patients.uptodate.com

Young, B. K. (2007). Intrapartum fetal heart rate assessment. *UpToDate*(15.2). Retrieved August 17, 2007, from http://patients.uptodate.com

CHAPTER 11

ACOG, (Eds.). (2006a, August). ACOG committee opinion. Episiotomy. Induction of labor for vaginal birth after cesarean delivery. Number 342. *Obstetrics & Gynecology, 108*(2), 465–467.

ACOG, (Eds.). (2006b, April). ACOG practice bulletin. Episiotomy. Clinical management guidelines for Obstetrician-Gynecologists. Number 71. *Obstetrics & Gynecology, 107*(4), 957–962.

ACOG, (Eds.). (2006c, August 31). Cesarean delivery associated with increased risk of maternal death from blood clots, infection, anesthesia. *ACOG News Release.*

ACOG, (Eds.). (2005, November 30). Vaginal birth not associated with incontinence later in life. *ACOG News Release:* ACOG Office of Communications.

The American Academy of Family Physicians (AAFP), (Eds.). (2005). Trial of labor after cesarean (TOLAC), formerly trial of labor versus elective repeat cesarean section of the woman with a previous cesarean section. *A Review of the Evidence and Recommendations by the American Academy of Family Physicians.* Retrieved December 28, 2007, from http://www.aafp.org/online/en/home/clinical/clinicalrecs/tolac.html

Briggs, G. G., & Wan, S. R. (2006, June 15). Drug therapy during labor and delivery, part 2. *American Journal of Health-System Pharmacology, 63,* 1131–1139.

Buhimschi, C. S., Buhimski, I. A., Patel, S., Malinow, A. M., & Weiner, C. P. (2005). Rupture of the uterine scar during term labour: Contractility or biochemistry? *BJOG: An International Journal of Obstetrics and Gynaecology, 112*(1), 38–42.

Cahill, A. G., & Macones, G. A. (2007). Vaginal birth after cesarean delivery: Evidence-based practice. *Clinical Obstetrics and Gynecology, 50*(2), 518–525.

Cahill, A. G., Stamilio, D. M., Obido, A. O., Peipert, J. F., Stevens, E. J., & Macones, G. A. (2007). Does a maximum dose of oxytocin affect risk for uterine rupture in candidates for vaginal birth after cesarean delivery? *American Journal of Obstetrics and Gynecology, 197*(5), 495e 1–5.

Cahill, A. G., Stamilio, D. M., Obido, A. O., Peipert, J. F., Ratcliffe, S. J., Stevens, E. J., Sammel, M. D., & Macones, G. A. (2006). Is vaginal birth after cesarean (VBAC) or elective repeat cesarean safer in women with a prior vaginal delivery? *American Journal of Obstetrics and Gynecology, 195*(4), 1143 – 1147.

Capeless, E., & Damron, D. (2007). Cesarean delivery. *UpToDate*(15.2). Retrieved August 17, 2007, from http://patients.uptodate.com

Caughey, A. B. (2006). Vaginal birth after cesarean delivery. In S. D. Spandorfer, F. Talavera, C. V. Smith, F. B. Gaupp, & L. P. Shulman (Eds.), *eMedicine.* Retrieved December 28, 2007, from http://www.emedicine.com/med/topic3434.htm

Crane, J. M. (2006). Factors predicting labor induction success: A critical analysis. *Clinical Obstetrics and Gynecology, 49*(3), 573–584.

Craver, P. E., Mertz, H. L., Beaver, B. W., Koontz, G., Martinez-Borges, A., Smith, J. G., & Merrill, D. (2007). Intrapartum predictors of uterine rupture. *American Journal of Perinatology, 24*(5), 317–321.

Crawford, P., & Kaufmann, L. (2006). How safe is vaginal birth after cesarean section for the mother and fetus? *Journal of Family Practice, 55*(2), 149–151. Retrieved December 28, 2007, from http://www.jfponline.com/Pages.asp?AID=3853&issue=February%202006&UID=

Crenshaw, J. T., & Winslow, E. H. (2006). Actual versus instructed fasting times and associated discomforts in women having scheduled cesarean birth. *Journal of Obstetric, Gynecologic, and Neonatal Nursing, 35*(2), 257–264.

Cunningham, F. G., Leveno, K. J., Bloom, S. L., Hauth, J. C., Gilstrap, L. C. III, & Wenstrom, K. D. (2005a). Cesarean delivery and peripartum hysterectomy. In *Williams obstetrics* (22nd ed., pp. 587–606). New York: McGraw-Hill Medical Publishing Division.

Cunningham, F. G., Leveno, K. J., Bloom, S. L., Hauth, J. C., Gilstrap, L. C. III, & Wenstrom, K. D. (2005b). Prior cesarean delivery. In *Williams obstetrics* (22nd ed., pp. 607–617). New York: McGraw-Hill.

Daskalakis, G., Thomakos, N., Hatziioannou, L., Mesogitis, S., Papantoniou, N., & Antsaklis, A. (2006). Sonographic cervical length measurement before labor induction in term nulliparous women. *Fetal Diagnosis & Therapy, 21*(2006), 34–38.

Declercq, E., Barger, M., Cabral, H. J., Evans, S. R., Kotelchuck, M., Simon, C., Weiss, J., & Heffner, L.J. (2007). Maternal outcomes associated with planned primary cesarean births compared with planned vaginal births. *Obstetrics and Gynecology, 109*(3), 669–677.

Ebell, M. H. (2007). Predicting the likelihood of successful vaginal birth after cesarean delivery. *American Family Physician, 76*(8), 1192–1194.

Emmett, C. L., Shaw, A. R. G., Montgomery, A. A., Murphy, D. J. (2006). Women's experience of decision making about mode of delivery after a previous caesarean section: The role of health professionals and information about health risks. *BJOG an International Journal of Obstetrics and Gynaecology, 113*(12), 1438–1445.

Greenberg, J. (2006). Procedure for vacuum assisted operative vaginal delivery. *UpToDate*(15.3). Retrieved November 15, 2007, from http://patients.uptodate.com

Hamilton, B. E., Martin, J. A., & Ventura, S. J. (2007). Births: Preliminary data for 2006. *National Vital Statistics Reports, 56*(7). Hyattsville, MD: Centers for Disease Control. Retrieved December 28, 2007, from http://www.cdc.gov/nchs/data/nvsr/nvsr56/nvsr56_07.pdf

Hastings-Tolsma, M., Vincent, D., Emeis, C., & Francisco, T. (2007). Getting though birth in one piece: Protecting the perineum. *American Journal of Maternal/Child Nursing, 32*(3), 158–164.

HRSA, (Eds.). (2006). Women's Health USA 2006. U.S. Department of Health and Human Services, Health Resources and Services Administration (HRSA). Rockville, Maryland: U.S. Department of Health and Human Services. Retrieved December 23, 2007, from ftp://ftp.hrsa.gov/mchb/whusa_06/w06ctocprg.pdf

Kripke, C. (2007). Repeat cesarean delivery vs. planned induction of labor. *American Family Physician, 76*(7), 971–972.

Kwee, A., Smink, M., Vanderlaar, R., Bruinse, H. W. (2007). Oucome of subsequent delivery after a previous early preterm cesarean section. *Journal of Maternal-Fetal and Neonatal Medicine, 20*(1): 33–37

Leeman, L. M., & Plante, L. A. (2006). Patient choice vaginal delivery? *Annals of family Medicine, 4*(3), 265–268.

Legal Eagle Eye Newsletter for the Nursing Profession, (Eds.). (2007). Pitocin, vaginal delivery post-cesarean: Nurse must watch for uterine hyperstimulation. *Legal Eagle Eye Newsletter for the Nursing Profession, 15*(9), 4.

Locatelli, A., Ghidini, A., Ciriello, E., Incerti, M., Bonardi, C., & Regalia, A. L. (2006). Induction of labor: Comparison of a cohort with uterine scar from previous cesarean section vs. a cohort with intact uterus. *Journal of Maternal-Fetal and Neonatal Medicine, 19*(8), 471–475.

Lowe, N. K. (2007). A review of factors associated with dystocia and cesarean section in nulliparous women. *Journal of Midwifery and Women's Health, 52*(3), 216–228. Retrieved November 6, 2007, from http://www.medscape.com/viewarticle/558115

Lui, S., Liston, R. M., Joseph, K. S., Hearman, M., Sauve, R., & Kramer, M. S. (2007). Maternal mortality and severe morbidity associated with low-risk planned cesarean delivery versus planned vaginal delivery at term. *Canadian Medical Association Journal*, 176(4), 455–460.

MacDorman, M. F., Declercq, E., Menacker, E., & Malloy, M. H. (2006). Infant and neonatal mortality for primary cesarean and vaginal births to women with "no indicated risk," United States, 1998–2001 birth cohorts. *Birth*, 33(3), 175–182.

Macones, G. A. et al. (2005). Maternal complication with vaginal birth after cesarean delivery: A multicenter study. *American Journal of Obstetrics and Gynecolog*, 193(5), 1656–1662.

Mahlmeister, L. R. (2005). Best practices in perinatal and neonatal nursing: Vacuum-assisted vaginal delivery. *Journal of Perinatal & Neonatal Nursing*, 19(1), 09–11.

Martin, J. A., Hamilton, B. E., Sutton, P. D., Ventura, S. J., Menacker, F., & Kirmeyer, S. (2007). Births: Final data for 2005. *National Vital Statistics Reports*, 56(6). Hyattsville, MD: Centers for Disease Control. Retrieved December 28, 2007, from http://www.cdc.gov/nchs/data/nvsr/nvsr56/nvsr56_06.pdf

McDonagh, M. S., Osterweil, P., & Guise, J. (2005). The benefits and risks of inducing labour in patients with prior caesarean delivery: A systematic review. *BJOG: an International Journal of Obstetrics and Gynaecology*, 112(8), 1007–1015.

National Institutes of Health, (Eds.). (2006). NIH state-of-the-science conference statement on caesarean delivery on maternal request. *NIH Consensus and State-of-the-Science Statements*, 23(1), 1–29. Retrieved July 22, 2007, from http://www.ahrq.gov/clinic/tp/cesar-reqtp.htm

Norwitz, E. R. (2007). Patient choice cesarean delivery. *UpTo-Date*(15.2). Retrieved August 17, 2007, from http://patients.uptodate.com

O'Mahony, F., Hofmeyr, G. J., & Menon, V. I. (2005). Instruments for assisted vaginal delivery. [Protocol] *Cochrane Database of Systematic Reviews 2005*, Issue 3. Art. No.: CD005455. DOI: 10.1002/14651858.CD005455

Pope, C. S., & O'Grady, J. P. (2006). Vacuum extraction. In S. R. Trupin, F. Talavera, R. S. Legro, F. B. Gaupp, & L. P. Shulman (Eds.), *eMedicine*. Retrieved December 22, 2007, from http://www.emedicine.com/med/TOPIC3389.htm

Rai, J., & Schreiber, J. R. (2007). Cervical ripening. In R. K. Zurawin, F. Talavera, R. S. Legro, F. B. Gaupp, & C. V. Smith (Eds.), *eMedicine*. Retrieved December 20, 2007, from http://www.emedicine.com/med/topic3282.htm

Richter, R., Bergmann, R. L., & Dudenhausen, J. W. (2007). Previous cesarean or vaginal delivery: Which mode is a greater risk of perinatal death at the second delivery? *European Journal of Obstetrics, Gynecology, and Reproductive Biology*, 132(1), 51–57.

Robinson, J. N. (2007). Approach to episiotomy. *UpToDate* (15.2). Retrieved August 17, 2007, from http://patients.uptodate.com

Ross, M. G., & Beall, M. H. (2007). Forceps delivery. In S. R. Trupin, F. Talavera, F. B. Gaupp, & D. Chelmow (Eds.), *eMedicine*. Retrieved December 22, 2007, from http://www.emedicine.com/med/TOPIC3284.HTM

Simpson, K. R. (2005). The context & clinical evidence for common nursing practices during labor. *American Journal of Maternal/Child Nursing*, 30(6), 356–363.

Simpson, K. R. (2006). Elective preterm birth. *American Journal of Maternal/Child Nursing*, 31(1), 68.

Simpson, K. R. (2007a). Assessing fetal well-being prior to cesarean birth. *American Journal of Maternal/Child Nursing*, 32(5), 328.

Simpson, K. R. (2007b). Emergent cesarean birth preparedness. *American Journal of Maternal/Child Nursing*, 32(4), 264.

Simpson, K. R. (2007c). Surgical safety: Minimizing risk of retained foreign bodies during cesarean birth. *American Journal of Maternal/Child Nursing*, 32(3), 200.

Simpson, K. R., & Thorman, K. E. (2005). Obstetric "conveniences:" Elective induction of labor, cesarean birth on demand, and other potentially unnecessary interventions. *Journal of Perinatal & Neonatal Nursing*, 19(2), 134–144.

Stamilio, D. M., DeFranco, E., Paré, E., Odibo, A. O., Peipert, J. F., Allsworth, J. E., Stevens, E., & Macones, G. A. (2007). Short interpregnancy interval: Risk of uterine rupture and complications of vaginal birth after cesarean delivery. *Obstetrics and Gynecology*, 110(5), 1075–1082.

Tan, P. C., Subramaniam, R. N., & Omar, S. Z. (2007). Labour and perinatal outcome in women at term with one previous lower-segment Caesarean: A review of 1000 consecutive cases. *Australian & New Zealand Journal of Obstetrics & Gynaecology*, 47(1), 31–36.

Tillett, J. (2005). Should elective cesarean birth be an accepted option for women? *Journal of Perinatal & Neonatal Nursing*, 19(1), 4–6.

Turner, M. J. A., Agnew, G., & Langan, H. (2006). Uterine rupture and labour after a previous low transverse caesarean section. *BJOG: An International Journal of Obstetrics and Gynaecology*, 113(6), 729–732.

Viswanathan, M., Hartmann, K., Palmieri, R., Lux, L., Swinson, T., Lohr, K. N., et al. (2005). The use of episiotomy in obstetrical care: A systematic review. *Evidence Report/Technology Assessment #112*. (Prepared by the RTI-UNC Evidence-based Practice Center, under Contract No. 290-02-0016.) AHRQ Publication No. 05-E009-2. Rockville, MD: Agency for Healthcare Research and Quality.

Wegner, E. K., & Bernstein, I. M. (2007). Operative vaginal delivery. *UpToDate*(15.2). Retrieved August 17, 2007, from http://patients.uptodate.com

Welischar, J., & Quirk, J. G. (2007). Vaginal birth after cesarean delivery. *UpToDate*(15.2). Retrieved August 17, 2007, from http://patients.uptodate.com

Whitehouse, J. D., & Sexton, D. J. (2007). Control measures to prevent surgical site infection. *UpToDate*(15.2). Retrieved August 17, 2007, from http://patients.uptodate.com

Williams, D. R. (2005). The top 10 reasons elective cesarean section should be on the decline. *AWHONN Lifelines*, 9(1), 23–24.

Wing, D. A. (2007a). Induction of labor. *UpToDate* (15.2). Retrieved August 17, 2007, from http://patients.uptodate.com

Wing, D. A. (2007b). Induction of labor in women with prior cesarean delivery. *UpToDate* (15.2). Retrieved August 17, 2007, from http://patients.uptodate.com

Wing, D. A. (2007c). Techniques for cervical ripening prior to labor induction. *UpToDate* (15.2). Retrieved August 17, 2007, from http://patients.uptodate.com

Witter, F., & Devoe, L. (2005). Update on successful induction of labor. *Johns Hopkins Advanced Studies in Medicine*, 5(9D), S888–901.

CHAPTER 12

Barclay, L. (2007, November 21). Postpartum women should be evaluated for fatigue, mental and physical symptoms. *Medscape Medical News*. Retrieved February 1, 2008, from http//www.medscape.com/viewarticle/566350_print

Berens, P. (2007). Overview of postpartum care. *UpToDate*(15.2). Retrieved April 10, 2007, from http://patients.uptodate.com.

Boggs, W. (2007). Graduated compression stockings reduce postpartum venous stasis. *Reuters Health Information 2007*. Retrieved March 2, 2008, from http://www.medscape.com/viewarticle/564022.

Cheng, C., Fowles, E. R., & Walker, L. O. (2006). Postpartum maternal health care in the United States: A critical review. *Journal of Perinatal Education*, 15(3), 34–42.

Choi, P., Henshaw, C., Baker, S., & Tree, J. (2005). Supermum, superwife, supereverything: Performing femininity in the transition to motherhood. *Journal of Reproductive and Infant Psychology*, 23(2), 167–180.

Corwin, E. J., & Arbour, M. (2007). Postpartum fatigue and evidence-based intervention. *American Journal of Maternal/Child Nursing*, 32(4), 215–220.

Cunningham, F. G., Leveno, K. J., Bloom, S. L., Hauth, J. C., Gilstrap, L. C. III, & Wenstrom, K. D. (2005). The puerperium. In *Williams obstetrics* (22nd ed., pp. 695–710). New York: McGraw-Hill.

Deglin, J. H., & Vallerand, A. H. (2006). Rh_o(D) Immune Globulin. In *Davis's drug guide for nurses* (10th ed.). Philadelphia: F. A. Davis Company.

Deneux-Tharaux, C., Carmona, E., Bouvier-Colle, M. H., & Breart, G. (2006). Postpartum maternal mortality and cesarean delivery. *Obstetrics and Gynecology*, 108(2 Pt 1), 541–548.

Fowles, E. R., & Horowitz, J. A. (2006). Clinical assessment of mothering during infancy. *Journal of Obstetric, Gynecologic & Neonatal Nursing*, 35(5), 662–670.

Gardner, M. R., & Deatrick, J. A. (2006). Understanding interventions and outcomes in mothers of infants. *Issues in Comprehensive Pediatric Nursing*, 29(1), 25–44.

George, L. (2005). Lack of preparedness. *American Journal of Maternal/Child Nursing, 30*(4), 251–255.

Hall, P. L., & Wittkowski, A. (2006). An exploration of negative thoughts as a normal phenomenon after childbirth. *Journal of Midwifery & Women's Health, 51*(5), 321–330. Retrieved December 18, 2006, from http://www.medscape.com/viewarticle/544983

Jeon, Y., Hwang, J., Kang, J., Han, S., Rhee, K., & Oh, Y. (2005). Effects of epidural naloxone on pruritus induced epidural morphine: A randomized controlled trial. *International Journal of Obstetric Anesthesia, 14*(1), 22–25.

Karlstrom, A., Engstrom-Olofsson, R., Norbergh, K., Sjoling, M., & Hildingsson, I. (2007). Postoperative pain after cesarean birth affects breastfeeding and infant care. *Journal of Obstetric, Gynecologic & Neonatal Nursing, 36*(5), 430–440.

Kennedy, H. P., Gardiner, A., Gay, C., & Lee, K. A. (2007). Negotiating sleep: A qualitative study of new mothers. *Journal of Perinatal & Neonatal Nursing, 21*(2), 114–122.

Kim, M. K., Nam, S. B., Cho, M. J., & Shin, Y. S. (2007). Epidural naloxone reduces postoperative nausea and vomiting in patients receiving epidural sufentanil for postoperative analgesia. *British Journal of Anaesthesia, 99*(2), 270–275.

Koniak-Griffin, D., Logsdon, M. C., Hines-Martin, V., & Turner, C. C. (2006). Contemporary mothering in a diverse society. *Journal of Obstetric, Gynecologic & Neonatal Nursing, 35*(5), 671–678.

Lee, S., & Lee, K. A. (2007). Early postpartum sleep and fatigue for mothers after cesarean delivery compared with vaginal delivery. *Journal of Perinatal & Neonatal Nursing, 21*(2), 109–113.

Lusskin, S. I., & Misri, S. (2007). Postpartum blues and depression. *UpToDate(15.2)*. Retrieved August 31, 2007, from http://patients.uptodate.com

McCoy, K. (2008, February 1). Rubella vaccine. *Health Library: Evidence-Based Information.*

Mercer, R. T. (2006). Nursing support of the process of becoming a mother. *Journal of Obstetric, Gynecologic & Neonatal Nursing, 35*(5), 649–651.

Mercer, R. T., & Walker, L. O. (2006). A review of nursing interventions to foster becoming a mother. *Journal of Obstetric, Gynecologic & Neonatal Nursing, 35*(5), 568–582.

Panke, E. S., & Donnenfeld, A. E. (2005). Parentage testing using DNA. *UpToDate(15.2)*. Retrieved August 17, 2007, from http://patients.uptodate.com

Rubin, R. (1984). *Maternal identity and the maternal experience.* New York: Springer.

Runquist, J. (2007). Persevering through postpartum fatigue. *Journal of Obstetric, Gynecologic & Neonatal Nursing, 36*(1), 28–37.

Salem, L., & Singer, K. R. (2007). Rh incompatibility. In A. J. Sayah, F. Talavera, M. Zwanger, J. Halamka, & P. L. Dyne (Eds.), *eMedicine.* Retrieved March 16, 2008, from http://www.emedicine.com/emerg/topic507.htm

Shin, H., Park, Y., & Kim, M. J. (2006). Predictors of maternal sensitivity during the early postpartum period. *Journal of Advanced Nursing, 55*(4), 425–434.

Weydert, J. A. & Benda. J. A. (2006). Subinvolution of the placental site as an anatomic cause of postpartum uterine bleeding. *Archives of Pathology & Laboratory Medicine, 130*(10), 1538–1542.

Witt, K. & Franzblau, N. (2006). Normal and abnormal puerperium. In R. Levine, F. Talavera, G. F. Whitman-Elia, F. B. Gaupp, & L. P. Shulman (Eds.), *eMedicine.* Retrieved January 5, 2008, from http://www.emedicine.com/med/topic3240.htm

CHAPTER 13

Askin, D. F. (2007). Physical assessment of the newborn part 1 of 2: Preparation through auscultation. *Nursing for Women's Health, 11*(3), 292–301.

Askin, D. F. (2007). Physical assessment of the newborn part 2 of 2: Inspection through palpation. *Nursing for Women's Health, 11*(3), 304–313.

The Brazelton Institute. (Undated). Understanding the baby's language. Retrieved April 5, 2008, from http://www.brazelton-institute.com

Cheffer, N. D. (2004). Adaptation to extrauterine life and immediate nursing care. In S. Mattson & J. E. Smith (Eds.), *Core Curriculum for Maternal–Newborn Nursing* (3rd ed., pp. 421–436). St. Louis: Elsevier Saunders.

Cheffer, N. D., & Rannalli, D. A. (2004). Newborn biologic/behavioral characteristics and psychosocial adaptations. In S. Mattson & J. E. Smith (Eds.), *Core Curriculum for Maternal–Newborn Nursing* (3rd ed., pp. 437–464). St. Louis: Elsevier Saunders.

Karlsen, K. (2006). *The S.T.A.B.L.E. program: Post-resuscitation/Pretransport stabilization care of sick infants guidelines for neonatal healthcare providers learner manual* (5th ed.). Park City, UT: S.T.A.B.L.E., Inc.

Mercer, J. S., Erickson-Owens, D. A., Graves, B., & Haley, M. M. (2007). Evidence-based practices for the fetal to newborn transition. *Journal of Midwifery & Women's Health, 52*(3), 262–272.

CHAPTER 14

Adcock, L. M., & Freysdottir, D. (2006). Screening the newborn for hearing loss. *UpToDate (15.1)*. Retrieved January 15, 2007, from http://patients.uptodate.com

American Academy of Pediatrics (AAP). (2005). Policy statement: AAP publications retired and reaffirmed. *Pediatrics, 116*(3), 796.

American Academy of Pediatrics NRP Steering Committee. (2006). Neonatal resuscitation program: Textbook of neonatal resuscitation (5th ed.). Elk Grave Village, IL: American Academy of Pediatrics.

American Academy of Pediatrics Task Force on Sudden Infant Death Syndrome. (2005). Policy statement: The changing concept of sudden infant death syndrome: Diagnostic and coding shifts, controversies regarding the sleeping environment, and new variables to consider in reducing risk. *Pediatrics, 116*(5), 1245 – 1255.

Baily, M. A., & Murray, T. H. (2008). Ethics, evidence, & cost in newborn screening. *Hastings Center Report, 38*(3), 23–31.

Burgess, A. W., Carr, K. E., Nahirny, C., & Rayburn, J. B. (2008). Nonfamily infant abuctions, 1983–2006: A comparison of cases from 1983–1992 with those from 1993–2006. *AJN, 108*(9), 32–38.

Centers for Disease Control & Prevention (CDC). (Eds.). (2007). Jaundice/Kernicterus - FAQs. Retrieved October 25, 2008, from http://www.cdc.gov/ncbddd/dd/kernichome.htm

Chizawsky, L. L. K., & Scott-Findlay, S. (2005). Tummy time! Preventing unwanted effects of the "back to sleep" campaign. *AWHONN Lifelines, 9*(5), 382–387.

Esposito, L., Hegyi, T., & Ostfeld, B. M. (2007). Educating parents about the risk factors of sudden infant death syndrome: The role of neonatal intensive care unit and well baby nursery nurses. *Journal of Perinatal & Neonatal Nursing, 21*(2), 158–164.

Folk, L. A. (2007). Guide to capillary heelstick blood sampling in infants [Foundation in newborn care]. *Advances in Neonatal Care, 7*(4), 171–178.

Forsythe, P. L., Maher, R., Kirchick, C., & Bieda, A. (2007). Family teaching toolbox: Infant safety at home. *Advances in Neonatal Care, 7*(2), 78–79.

Galligan, M. (2006). Proposed guidelines for skin-to-skin treatment of neonatal hypothermia. *American Journal of Maternal Child Nursing, 31*(5), 298–304.

Hummel, P., & Fortado, D. (2005). Impacting infant head shapes. *Advances in Neonatal Care, 5*(6), 329–340.

Hummel, P., & Fortado, D. (2005). Family teaching toolbox: A parents' guide to improving head shape. *Advances in Neonatal Care, 5*(6), 341–342.

Karlsen, K. (2006). *The S.T.A.B.L.E. program: Post-resuscitation/Pretransport stabilization care of sick infants guidelines for neonatal healthcare providers learner manual* (5th ed.). Park City, UT: S.T.A.B.L.E., Inc.

Krisberg, K. (2006). Newborn screening a success, but testing varies widely by state: Push to make tests universal nationwide. *American Public Health Association, 36*(9).

Moyer, V. A., Calonge, N., Teutsch, S. M., & Botkin, J. R. (2008). Expanding newborn screening: Process, policy, & priorities. *Hastings Center Report, 38*(3), 32–39.

Schwoebel, A., & Gennaro, S. (2006). Neonatal hyperbilirubinemia. *Journal of Perinatal & Neonatal Nursing, 20*(1), 103–107.

Shoemaker, C. (2007). Neonatal circumcision: Risks and benefits. *UpToDate (15.2)*. Retrieved October 15, 2007, fromhttp://patients.uptodate.com

Sielski, L. A. (2006). Initial routine management of the newborn. *UpToDate (15.1)*. Retrieved January 15, 2007, from http://patients.uptodate.com

Simpson, K. R. (2006). Circumcision pain management. *American Journal of Maternal Child Nursing, 31*(4), 276.

Spivak, L., & Sokol, H. (2005). Beyond newborn screening: Early diagnosis and management of hearing loss in infants. *Advances in Neonatal Care, 5*(2), 104–112.

Spivak, L., & Sokol, H. (2005). Family teaching toolbox: A parents' guide to further hearing testing. *Advances in Neonatal Care, 5*(2), 113–114.

Winberg, J. (2005). Research review: Mother and newborn baby: Mutual regulation of physiology and behavior—a selective review. *Developmental Psychobiology, 47*(3), 217–229.

Wong, R. J., & Stevenson, D. K. (2007). Patient information: Jaundice in newborn infants. *UpToDate (15.2)*. Retrieved October 15, 2007, from http://patients.uptodate.com

CHAPTER 15

Armstrong, M. L., Caliendo, C., & Roberts, A. E. (2006). Pregnancy, lactation, and nipple piercings. *AWHONN Lifelines, 10*(3), 212–217.

Blanchard, D. S. (2006). Omega-3 fatty acid supplementation in perinatal settings. *American Journal of Maternal Child Nursing, 31*(4), 250–256.

Butte, N. F. (2006). Maternal nutrition during lactation. *UpToDate (15.1)*. Retrieved June 15, 2007, from http://patients.uptodate.com

CDC. (2008). Breastfeeding-related maternity practices at hospitals and birth centers – United States, 2007. *Morbidity and Mortality Weekly Report, 57*(23), 621–625.

CDC. (2008). Breastfeeding among U.S. children born 1999–2005. *CDC National Immunization Survey*. Retrieved September 13, 2008, from http://www.cdc.gov/breastfeeding/data/NIS_data/2005/socio-demographic_any.htm

Chamblin, C. (2006). Breastfeeding after breast reduction: What nurses & moms need to know. *AWHONN Lifelines, 10*(1), 42–48.

Chang, K., & Spatz, D. L. (2006). The family & breastfeeding laws: What nurses need to know. *American Journal of Maternal Child Nursing, 31*(4), 224–230.

Click, E. R. (2006). Developing a worksite lactation program. *American Journal of Maternal Child Nursing, 31*(5), 313–317.

Clifford, J., & McIntyre, E. (2008). Who supports breastfeeding? *Breastfeeding Review, 16*(2), 9–19.

Cockey, C. D. (2006). Breastfeeding and diabetes risk: Increased duration has protective effect against developing diabetes. *AWHONN Lifelines, 9*(6), 443–444.

Dennis, C. E. (2006). Identifying predictors of breastfeeding self-efficacy in the immediate postpartum period. *Research in Nursing & Health, 29*, 256–268.

Doan, T., Gardiner, A., Gay, C. L., & Lee, K. A. (2007). Breast-feeding increases sleep duration of new parents. *Journal of Perinatal & Neonatal Nursing, 21*(3), 200–206.

Dornan, B. A., & Oermann, M. H. (2006). Evaluation of breastfeeding web sites for patient education. *American Journal of Maternal Child Nursing, 31*(1), 18–23.

Dumphy, D. (2008). The breastfeeding surgical patient. *AORN Journal, 87*(4), 759–766.

Glenn, L. L., & Quillin, S. I. M. (2007). Opposing effects of maternal and paternal socioeconomic status on neonatal feeding method, place of sleep, and maternal sleep time. *Journal of Perinatal & Neonatal Nursing, 21*(2), 165–172.

Gregory, K. (2005). Update on nutrition for preterm and full-term infants. *Journal of Obstetric, Gynecologic, & Neonatal Nursing, 34*(1), 98–108.

Gribble, K. D. (2008). Long-term breastfeeding; Changing attitudes and overcoming challenges. *Breastfeeding Review, 16*(1), 5–15.

Groer, M. W., & Davis, M. W. (2006). Cytokines, infections, stress, and dysphoric moods in breastfeeders and formula feeders. *Journal of Obstetric, Gynecologic, & Neonatal Nursing, 35*(5), 599–607.

Hahn, J. (2005). Building a breastfeeding center of excellence: A community hospital's experience with baby-friendly. *AWHONN Lifelines, 9*(4), 306–311.

Helliwig, J. P. (2007). Which drugs affect breastfeeding? Database offers quick info. *Nursing for Women's Health, 11*(1), 92–94.

Hernandez, I. F. (2006). Promoting exclusive breastfeeding for Hispanic women. *American Journal of Maternal/Child Nursing, 31*(5), 318–324.

Hill, P. D., & Aldag, J. C. (2007). Predictors of term infant feeding at week 12 postpartum. *Journal of Perinatal & Neonatal Nursing, 21*(3), 250–255.

Hopkinson, J., & Schanler, R. J. (2005). Common problems of breastfeeding in the postpartum period. *UpToDate (15.2)*. Retrieved October 17, 2007, from http://patients.uptodate.com

Hopkinson, J., & Schanler, R. J. (2005). Physiology of lactation. *UpToDate (15.1)*. Retrieved June 15, 2007, from http://patients.uptodate.com

Hopkinson, J., & Schanler, R. J. (2006). Breastfeeding in the perinatal period. *UpToDate (15.2)*. Retrieved October 17, 2007, from http://patients.uptodate.com

Johnson, T. S., Mulder, P. J., & Strube, K. (2007). Mother-infant breastfeeding progress tool: A guide for education and support of the breastfeeding dyad. *Journal of Obstetrics, Gynecologic & Neonatal Nursing, 36*(4), 319–327.

Johnston, M. L. & Esposito, N. (2007). Barriers and facilitators for breastfeeding among working women in the United States. *Journal of Obstetrics, Gynecologic & Neonatal Nursing, 36*(1), 9–20.

Komara, C., Simpson, D., Teasdale, C., Whalen, G., Bell, S., & Giovanetto, L. (2007). Intervening to promote early initiation of breastfeeding in the LDR. *Journal of Maternal/Child Nursing, 32*(2), 117–121.

Keister, D., Roberts, K. T., & Werner, S. L. (2008). Strategies for breastfeeding success. *American Family Physician, 78*(2), 225–232.

Lusskin, S. I., & Misri, S. (2007). Use of psychotropic medications in breastfeeding women. *UpToDate (15.2)*. Retrieved October 17, 2007, from http://patients.uptodate.com

McCarter-Spaulding, D. E. (2005). Medication in pregnancy and lactation. *Journal of Maternal/Child Nursing, 30*(1), 10–17.

Miller, L. C., Cook, J. T., Brooks, C. W., Heine, A. G., & Curtis, T. K. (2007). Breastfeeding education: Empowering future health care providers. *Nursing for Women's Health, 11*(4), 374–380.

Mofenson, L. M. (2007). Transmission of HIV through breastfeeding: Risk factors and prevention. *UpToDate (15.2)*. Retrieved October 17, 2007, from http://patients.uptodate.com

Morin, K. (2006). Update on what and how much infants and toddlers eat. *Journal of Maternal/Child Nursing, 31*(4), 269.

Morin, K. (2006). Infant nutrition and genetics: Inextricably related. *Journal of Maternal/Child Nursing, 31*(3), 198.

Morin, K. (2005). Information parents need about preparing formula. *Journal of Maternal/Child Nursing, 30*(5), 334.

Powers, D. (2008). Understanding the physics behind correctly positioning a baby at the breast. *IJCE, 23*(2), 18–19.

Rosenberg, K. D., Eastham, M. S., Kasehagen, L. J., & Sandoval, A. P. (2008). Marketing infant formula through hospitals: The impact of commercial hospital discharge packs on breastfeeding. *American Journal of Public Health, 98*(2), 290–295.

Schanler, R. J. (2006). Benefits of breastfeeding. *UpToDate (15.1)*. Retrieved June 15, 2007, from http://patients.uptodate.com

Schanler, R. J. (2005). Nutritional composition of human milk for full-term infants. *UpToDate (15.1)*. Retrieved June 15, 2007, from http://patients.uptodate.com

Shealy, K. R., Li, R., Benton-Davis, S., & Grummer-Strawn L. M. (2005). *The CDC guide to breastfeeding interventions*. Atlanta: U.S. Department of Health and Human Services, Centers for Disease Control and Prevention. Retrieved September 13, 2008, from http://www.cdc.gov/breastfeeding/pdf/breastfeeding_interventions.pdf

Simmie, E. (2006). Breastfeeding: Different ethnic background, different perceptions? *British Journal of Midwifery, 14*(1), 20–26.

Spear, H. J. (2006). Breastfeeding behaviours and experiences of adolescent mothers. *Journal of Maternal/Child Nursing, 31*(2), 106–113.

Stuebe, A., Fiumara, K., & Lee, K. G. (2007). Principles of medication use during lactation. *UpToDate (15.2)*. Retrieved October 17, 2007, from http://patients.uptodate.com

Tofteland, L. (2006). Conceiving care: How the desires of nursing mothers transformed the delivery of our care. *AWHONN Lifelines, 10*(4), 312–319.

Tully, M. R. (2005). Working & breastfeeding: Helping moms and employers figure it out. *AWHONN Lifelines, 9*(3), 198–203.

Wagner, C. L., Graham, E. M., Hope, W. W., & Hughes, N. (2006). Counseling the breastfeeding mother. In G. Cassady, M. L. Windle, B. S. Carter, P. D. Petry, & T. Rosenkrantz (Eds.), *eMedicine*. Retrieved September 14, 2008, from http://www.emedicine.com/PED/topic2594.htm

Walker, M. (2007). Breastfeeding: Good starts, good outcomes. *Journal of Perinatal & Neonatal Nursing, 21*(3), 191–197.

Wilhem, S. L., Stepans, M. B., Hertzog, M., Rodehorst, T. K., & Gardner, P. (2006). Motivational interviewing to promote sustained breastfeeding. *JOGNN, 35*(3), 340–348.

CHAPTER 16

ACOG (Eds.). (2005). Pregestational diabetes mellitus. *ACOG Practice Bulletin, 60*, 675–684.

AHRQ (Eds.). (2005). Prenatal screening and treatment are needed to identify pregnant women with asymptomatic chlamydial infections. *AHRQ Research Activities, 299*(July 2005), 10.

Alter, S. (2007). Herpes simplex virus infection. In L. R. Krilov, M. L. Windle, M. R. Schleiss, R. W. Tolan, & R. W. Steele (Eds.), *eMedicine*. Retrieved August 13, 2007, from http://www.emedicine.com/ped/topic995.htm

Artal, R. (2007). Recommendations for exercise during pregnancy and the postpartum period. *UpToDate (15.1)*. Retrieved from http://patients.uptodate.com

AWHONN Lifelines (Eds.). (2005). Treating asthma in pregnant women revised federal guidelines address new medications & emerging science. *AWHONN Lifelines, 9*(2), 123–124.

Barclay, L. (2007). CDC issues new treatment recommendations for gonorrhea. *Medscape Medical News*. Retrieved August 17, 2007, from http://www.medscape.com/viewarticle/555228

Barclay, L., & Vega, C. (2007). Recommendations for treating asthma in pregnancy. *Medscape medical news*. Retrieved August 04, 2007, from http://www.medscape.com/viewarticle/556184

Barss, V. A., & Blatman, R. N. (2006). Obstetrical management of pregnancy complicated by diabetes mellitus. *UpToDate (15.1)*. Retrieved from http://patients.uptodate.com

Bartlett, J. G. (2006). The stages and natural history of HIV infection. *UpToDate (15.2)*. Retrieved August 17, 2007, from http://patients.uptodate.com

Bartlett, J. G. (2007a). Initial antiretroviral therapy for HIV infection. *UpToDate (15.2)*. Retrieved August 18, 2007, from http://patients.uptodate.com

Bartlett, J. G. (2007b). Techniques and interpretation of measurement of the CD4 cell count in HIV-infected patients. *UpToDate (15.2)*. Retrieved August 17, 2007, from http://patients.uptodate.com

Breen, E., & Bleday, R. (2007). Condylomata acuminate (anogenital warts). *UpToDate (15.2)*. Retrieved from http://patients.uptodate.com

Bryant, K. D. (2006). Update on adolescent pregnancy in the black community. *ABNF Journal, 17*(4), 133–136.

Carolan, M. (2007). Health literacy and the information needs and dilemmas of first-time mothers over 35 years. *Journal of Clinical Nursing, 16*(6), 1162–1172.

Caughey, A. B. (2005). Seizure disorders in pregnancy. S. R. Trupin, F. Talavera, D. Chelmow, F. B. Gaupp, & L. P. Shulman (Eds.), *eMedicine*. Retrieved August 5, 2007, from http://www.emedicine.com/med/topic3433.htm

Centers for Disease Control and Prevention (CDC). (2005). Information about CMV for clinicians and others in healthcare settings. Retrieved August 13, 2007, from http://www.cdc.gov/cmv/clinicians.htm

Centers for Disease Control and Prevention (CDC). (2006). About CMV. *CDC Fact Sheet*. Retrieved August 13, 2007, from http://www.cdc.gov/cmv/facts.htm

Centers for Disease Control and Prevention (CDC). (2007a). HIV/AIDS among African Americans. *CDC HIV/AIDS Fact Sheet*. Retrieved August 18, 2007, from http://www.cdc.gov/hiv/topics/aa/resources/factsheets/pdf/aa.pdf

Centers for Disease Control and Prevention (CDC). (2007b). Increases in gonorrhea – eight western states, 2000–2005. *Morbidity and Mortality Weekly Report, 56*(10), 222–225.

Centers for Disease Control and Prevention (CDC). (2007c). Pink book's chapter on rubella. Epidemiology & prevention of vaccine-preventable diseases textbook. Retrieved August 13, 2007, from http://www.cdc.gov/vaccines/pubs/pinkbook/downloads/rubella.pdf

Centers for Disease Control and Prevention (CDC). (2007d). Recommended immunization schedule for persons aged 0–6 years—United States, 2007. Approved by the Advisory Committee on Immunization Practices, the American Academy of Pediatrics, and the American Academy of Family Physicians. Retrieved August 13, 2007, from http://www.cdc.gov/vaccines/recs/schedules/downloads/child/2007/child-schedule-color-print.pdf

Centers for Disease Control and Prevention (CDC). (2007e). Teen pregnancy. *Adolescent Reproductive Health* (Home page). Retrieved August 19, 2007, from http://www.cdc.gov/reproductivehealth/AdolescentReproHealth/

Chacko, M. R., (2006). Pregnancy in adolescents. *UpToDate (15.2)*. Retrieved August 18, 2007, from http://patients.uptodate.com

Colson, A. E., & Sax, P. E. (2007). Primary HIV-1 infection: Diagnosis and treatment. *UpToDate (15.2)*. Retrieved August 17, 2007, from http://patients.uptodate.com

Cunningham, F. G., Leveno, K. J., Bloom, S. L., Hauth, J. C., Gilstrap, L. C. III, & Wenstrom, K. D. (2005a). *Williams obstetrics* (22nd ed.). New York: McGraw-Hill.

Curran, C. A. (2006). The effects of rhinitis, asthma, and acute respiratory distress syndrome as acute or chronic pulmonary conditions during pregnancy. *Journal of Perinatal & Neonatal Nursing, 20*(2), 147–154.

Curran, D., & Poggi, S. H. (2007). Hematologic disease and pregnancy. In G. S. Letterie, F. Talavera, C. V. Smith, F. B. Gaupp, & L. P. Shulman (Eds.), *eMedicine*. Retrieved August 03, 2007, from http://www.emedicine.com/med/topic3254.htm

DeCara, J. M., Jacobs, A. G., & Lang, R. M. (2006). Management of heart failure in pregnancy. *UpToDate (15.1)*. Retrieved from http://patients.uptodate.com

Demmler, G. J. (2006). Cytomegalovirus infection and disease in newborns, infants, children, and adolescents. *UpToDate (15.2)*. Retrieved August 13, 2007, from http://patients.uptodate.com.

Dobbenga-Rhodes, Y. A., & Prive, A. M. (2006). Assessment and evaluation of the woman with cardiac disease during pregnancy. *Journal of Perinatal and Neonatal Nursing, 20*(4), 295–302.

Endo, S., Maeda, K., Suto, M., Kaji, T., Morine, M., Kinoshita, T., Yasui, T., & Irahara, M. (2006). Differences in insulin sensitivity in pregnant women with overweight and gestational diabetes mellitus. *Gynecological Endocrinology, 22*(6), 343–349.

Erikson, E. H. (1963). *Childhood and society* (2nd ed.). New York: Norton.

Fanta, C. H. (2007). Treatment of acute exacerbations of asthma in adults. *UpToDate (15.2)*. Retrieved from http://patients.uptodate.com

Finegold, B. (2006). Data points: Pregnant with implications. *Scientific American, 295*(3).

Fischer, R. (2006). Genital herpes in pregnancy. In A. Witlin, F. Talavera, R. S. Legro, F. B. Gaupp, & L. P. Shulman (Eds.), *eMedicine*. Retrieved August 13, 2007, from http://www.emedicine.com/med/topic3554.htm

Fletcher, J., & Ball, G. (2006). Chlamydia screening in pregnancy: A missed opportunity? *British Journal of Midwifery, 14*(7), 390–392.

Freij, B. J., & Sever, J. L. (2005). Viral and protozoal infections. In M. G. MacDonald, M. D. Mullett, & M. K. Seshia (Eds.), *Avery's Neonatology Pathophysiology & Management of the Newborn*, (6th ed., pp. 1274–1356). Philadelphia: Lippincott Williams & Wilkins.

Fretts, R. C. (2007). Effect of advanced age on fertility and pregnancy in women. *UpToDate (15.2)*. Retrieved August 18, 2007, from http://patients.uptodate.com

Fox, P. A., & Tung, M-Y. (2005). Human papillomavirus burden of illness and treatment cost considerations. *American Journal of Clinical Dermatology, 6*(16), 365–381.

Furniss, K., McCaffrey, M., Parnell, V., & Rovi, S. (2007). Nurses and barriers to screening for intimate partner violence. *American Journal of Maternal/Child Nursing, 32*(4), 238–243.

Garofalo, R. (2006). Adolescent sexuality. *UpToDate (15.2)*. Retrieved August 19, 2007, from http://patients.uptodate.com

Gray, J. R. (2007). HPV vaccination should it be mandatory for entry into public school? *Nursing for Women's Health, 11*(2), 133–138.

Gray, R. H., Li, X., Kigozi, K., Serwadda, D., Brahmbhatt, H., Wabwire-Mangen, F., et al. (2005). Increased risk of incident HIV during pregnancy in Rakai, Uganda: A prospective study. *Lancet 366*(9492), 1182–1188.

Hall, D. A., Wadwa, R. P., Goldenberg, N. A., & Norris, J. M. (2006). Maternal risk factors for term neonatal seizures: Population-based study in Colorado, 1989–2003. *Journal of Child Neurology, 21*(9), 795–798.

Hamilton, B. E., Martin, J. A., & Ventura, S. J. (2007). Births: Preliminary data for 2006. *National Vital Statistics Reports, 56*(7). Retrieved December 28, 2007, from http://www.cdc.gov/nchs/data/nvsr/nvsr56/nvsr56_07.pdf

Hawkins, D., Blott, M., Clayden, P., Ruiter, A., Foster, G., Gilling-Smith, C., et al. (2005). Guidelines for the management of HIV infection in pregnant women and the prevention of mother-to-child transmission of HIV. *HIV Medicine, 6*(Supplement 2), 107–148.

Hoffman, M. C., et. al. (2007). Pregnancy at or beyond 40 years is associated with an increased risk of fetal death and other adverse outcomes [Abstract]. *American Journal of Obstetrics & Gynecology, 196*(5), e11-3

Hofmanova, I. (2006). Pre-conception care and support of women with diabetes. *British Journal of Nursing, 15*(2), 90–94.

Homko, C. J., & Reece, E. A. (2006). Insulins and oral hypoglycemic agents in pregnancy. *Journal of Maternal-Fetal and Neonatal Medicine, 19*(11), 679–686.

Johnson, K. E. (2006). Overview of TORCH infections. *UpToDate (15.2).* Retrieved from http://patients.uptodate.com

Jovanovic, L. (2007a). Glycemic control in women with type 1 and type 2 diabetes mellitus during pregnancy. *UpToDate (15.2).* Retrieved from http://patients.uptodate.com

Jovanovic, L. (2007b). Prepregnancy counseling and evaluation of women with diabetes mellitus. *UpToDate (15.2).* Retrieved from http://patients.uptodate.com

Jovanovic, L. (2007c). Screening and diagnosis of gestational diabetes mellitus. *UpToDate (15.2).* Retrieved from http://patients.uptodate.com

Jovanovic, L. (2007d). Treatment and course of gestational diabetes mellitus. *UpToDate (15.2).* Retrieved from http://patients.uptodate.com

Jovanovic, L., & Nakai, Y. (2006). Successful pregnancy in women with type 1 diabetes: From preconception through postpartum care. *Endocrinology Metabolism Clinics of North America, 35*(2006), 79–97.

Kilpatrick, K., & Purden, M. (2007). Using reflective nursing practice to improve care of women with congenital heart disease considering pregnancy. *Journal of Maternal/Child Nursing, 32*(3), 140–147.

Klein, J. D. (2005). Adolescent pregnancy: Current trends and issues. *Pediatrics, 116*(1), 281–286.

Koenig, L. J., Whitaker, D. J., Royce, R. A., Wilson, T. E., Ethier, K., & Fernandez, M. I. (2006). Physical and sexual violence during pregnancy and after delivery: A prospective multistate study of women with or at risk for HIV infection. *American Journal of Public Health, 96*(6), 1052–1058.

Kriebs, J. M. (2006). Changing the paradigm HIV in pregnancy. *Journal of Perinatal & Neonatal Nursing, 20*(1), 71–73.

Laartz, B., & Gompf, S. G. (2006) Viral infections and pregnancy. In S. R. Trupin, F. Talavera, D. Chelmow, F. B. Gaupp, & L. P. Shulman (Eds.), *eMedicine.* Retrieved August 13, 2007, from http://www.emedicine.com/med/topic3270.htm

Lachat, M. F., & Relf, M. V. (2006). HIV and pregnancy: Considerations for nursing practice. *American Journal of Maternal/Child Nursing, 31*(4), 233–240.

Lazaro, N. (2006). Sexual health update: Chlamydia. *Pulse, 66*(37), 44–47.

Liu, P., & Euerle, B. (2006). Syphilis. In D. R. Lucey, F. Talavera, J. L. Brusch, E. Mylonakis, & B. A. Cunha (Eds.), *eMedicine.* Retrieved August 13, 2007, from http://www.emedicine.com/med/topic2224.htm

Lockwood, C. J. (2007). The initial prenatal assessment and routine prenatal care. *UpToDate (15.2).* Retrieved from http://patients.uptodate.com

Lutwick, L. I., & Seenivasan, M. (2006). Herpes simplex. In T. J. Marrie, F. Talavera, C. V. Sanders, E. Mylonakis, & B. A. Cunha (Eds.), *eMedicine.* Retrieved August 13, 2007, from http://www.emedicine.com/med/topic1006.htm

Lutz, K. F. (2005). Abused pregnant women's interactions with health care providers during the childbearing year. *Journal of Obstetric, Gynecologic, and Neonatal Nursing, 34*(2), 151–162.

MacMullen, N. J., & Tymkow, C. (2006). Adverse maternal outcomes in women with asthma: Differences by race. *American Journal of Maternal/Child Nursing, (31)*4, 263–268.

Majeroni, B. A., & Ukkadam, S. (2007). Screening and treatment for sexually transmitted infections in pregnancy. *American Family Physician, 76*(2), 265–270.

Malamitsi-Puchner, A., & Boutsikou, T. (2006). Adolescent pregnancy and perinatal outcome [Abstract]. *Pediatric Endocrinology Reviews, 3*(Supplement 1), 170–171.

Martin, J. A., Hamilton, B. E., Sutton, P. D., Ventura, S. J., Menacker, F., & Kirmeyer, S. (2007). Births: Final data for 2005. *National Vital Statistics Reports, 56*(6). Retrieved December 28, 2007, from http://www.cdc.gov/nchs/data/nvsr/nvsr56/nvsr56_06.pdf

Metcalf-Wilson, K. (2002). Confidentiality, communication and compliance: The three 'C's' of female adolescent care. *AWHONN Lifelines, 6*(4), 344–348.

Mofenson, L. M. (2007). Antiretroviral treatment during pregnancy. *UpToDate (15.2).* Retrieved August 18, 2007, from http://patients.uptodate.com

Montan, S. (2007). Increased risk in the elderly parturient [Abstract]. *Current Opinion in Obstetrics and Gynecology, 19*(2), 110–112.

Moore, T. R., & Warshak, C. (2005). Diabetes mellitus and pregnancy. In R. K. Zurawin, F. Talavera, C. V. Smith, M. Cooper, & L. P. Shulman (Eds.), *eMedicine.* Retrieved July 29, 2007, from http://www.emedicine.com/med/topic3249.htm

Moscicki, A. B., Dempsey, A., & Humiston, S. G. (2006). Pediatricians at the forefront of preventing cervical cancer: What you need to know about HPV. *Medscape CME Activity.* Retrieved August 17, 2007, from http://www.medscape.com/viewprogram/6281_pnt

National Society for Epilepsy (Eds.). (2007). Information on epilepsy: Pregnancy and parenting. Retrieved August 5, 2007, from http://www.epilepsynse.org.uk/pages/info/leaflets/preg.cfm

Nelson, J. C., Sherin, K. M., & Garland, E. (2006). Telltale signs of intimate partner violence among adolescents: Screening, reporting, and creating and exit plan. *CME Activity from Medscape.* Retrieved August 19, 2007, from http://www.medscape.com/viewprogram/6108_pnt

Norwitz, E. R. (2006). Syphilis in pregnancy. *UpToDate (15.2).* Retrieved August 12, 2007, from http://patients.uptodate.com

O'Donovan, D. J. (2007). Hepatitis viruses and the newborn: Clinical manifestations and treatment. *UpToDate (15.2).* Retrieved August 13, 2007, from http://patients.uptodate.com

Ogata, E. S. (2005). Carbohydrate homeostasis. In M. G. McDonald, M. D. Mullett, & M. M. K. Seshia (Eds.), *Avery's neonatology pathophysiology & management of the newborn* (6th ed., pp. 881–888). Philadelphia: Lippincott Williams & Wilkins.

Perinatal HIV Guidelines Working Group. (2006, October 12). Public Health Service Task Force recommendations for use of antiretroviral drugs in pregnant HIV-1 infected women for maternal health and interventions to reduce perinatal HIV-1 transmission in the United States, 1–65. Retrieved August 18, 2007, from http://aidsinfo.nih.gov/ContentFiles/PerinatalGL.pdf

Perloff, J. K., & Waksmonski, C. A. (2006a). Pregnancy in women with congenital heart disease: General principles. *UpToDate (15.1).* Retrieved from http://patients.uptodate.com

Perloff, J. K., & Waksmonski, C. A. (2006b). Pregnancy in women with congenital heart disease: Specific lesions. *UpToDate (15.1).* Retrieved from http://patients.uptodate.com

Petraglia, F., & D'Antona, D. (2006). Maternal endocrine and metabolic adaptation to pregnancy. *UpToDate (15.1).* Retrieved from http://patients.uptodate.com

Pyrosopoulos, N. T., & Reddy, K. R. (2007). Hepatitis B. In G. Wu, F. Talavera, O. S. Brann, A. J. Mechaber, & J. Katz (Eds.), *eMedicine.* Retrieved August 13, 2007, from http://www.emedicine.com/med/topic992.htm

Ravin, C. R. (2007). Preventing STIs ask the questions. *Nursing for Women's Health, 11*(1), 88–91.

Reddy, U. M., Ko, C., & Willinger, M. (2006). Maternal age and the risk of stillbirth throughout pregnancy in the United States [Abstract]. *American Journal of Obstetrics & Gynecology, 195*(3), 764–770.

Reece, E. A., & Homko, C. J. (2006). Pregnancy in women with diabetic nephropathy. *UpToDate (15.1).* Retrieved from http://patients.uptodate.com

Reichman, R. (2006a). Clinical presentation and diagnosis of human papillomavirus infections. *UpToDate (15.2).* Retrieved August 17, 2007, from http://patients.uptodate.com

Reichman, R. (2006b). Treatment and prevention of human papillomavirus infections. *UpToDate (15.2).* Retrieved August 17, 2007, from http://patients.uptodate.com

Riley, L. E. (2006a). Rubella in pregnancy. *UpToDate (15.2).* Retrieved August 13, 2007, from http://patients.uptodate.com

Riley, L. E. (2006b). Varicella-zoster virus infection in pregnancy. *UpToDate (15.2).* Retrieved from http://patients.uptodate.com

Riley, L. E. (2007). Genital herpes simplex virus infection and pregnancy. *UpToDate (15.2).* n. Retrieved August 12, 2007, from http://patients.uptodate.com

Santelli, J. S., Lindberg, L. D., Finer, L. B., & Singh, S. (2007). Explaining recent declines in adolescent pregnancy in the United States: The contribution of abstinence and improved contraceptive use. *Contemporary Sexuality, 41*(7), 8–12.

Schachter, S. C. (2006). Management of epilepsy and pregnancy. *UpToDate (15.2)*. Retrieved from http://patients.uptodate.com

Schachter, S. C. (2007a). Overview of the management of epilepsy in adults. *UpToDate (15.2)*. Retrieved from http://patients.uptodate.com

Schachter, S. C. (2007b). Risks associated with epilepsy and pregnancy. *UpToDate (15.2)*. Retrieved from http://patients.uptodate.com

Schatz, M. (2006). Recognition and management of allergic disease during pregnancy. *UpToDate (15.2)*. Retrieved from http://patients.uptodate.com

Schatz, M. & Weinberger, S. E. (2007). Management of asthma during pregnancy. *UpToDate (15.2)*. Retrieved from http://patients.uptodate.com

Schelonka, R. L., Freij, B. J., & McCracken, G. H. (2005). Bacterial and fungal infections. In M. G. MacDonald, M. D. Mullett, & M. M. K. Seshia (Eds.), *Avery's Neonatology Pathophysiology & Management of the Newborn* (6th ed., pp. 1235–1273). Philadelphia: Lippincott Williams & Wilkins.

Schmidt, J. V. (2007). HPV vaccine implications for nurses and patients. *Nursing for Women's Health 11*(1), 83–87.

Schuklenk, U., & Kleinsmidt, A. (2007). Rethinking mandatory HIV testing during pregnancy in areas with high prevalence rates: Ethical and policy issues. *American Journal of Public Health, 97*(7), 1179–1183.

Schwarzwald, H. (2007). Diagnostic testing for HIV infection in infants and young children. *UpToDate (15.2)*. Retrieved August 18, 2007, from http://patients.uptodate.com

Scollan-Koliopoulos, M., Guadagna, S., & Walker, E. A. (2006). Gestational diabetes management: Guidelines to a healthy pregnancy. *Nurse Practitioner, 31*(6), 14–23.

Secco, M. L., Profit, S., Kennedy, E., Walsh, A., Letourneau, N., & Stewart, M. (2007). Factors affecting postpartum depressive symptoms of adolescent mothers. *Journal of Obstetric, Gynecologic & Neonatal Nursing, 36*(1), 47–54.

Sharma, S. (2006). Pulmonary disease and pregnancy. In S. P. Peters, F. Talavera, G. F. Whitman-Elia, T. D. Rice, & Z. Mosenifar (Eds.), *eMedicine*. Retrieved August 04, 2007, from http://www.emedicine.com/med/topic3252.htm

Sillman, J. S. (2005). Diagnosing, screening and counseling for domestic violence. *UpToDate (15.2)*. Retrieved August 18, 2007, from http://patients.uptodate.com

Simpson, K. R. (2006). Prevention of perinatal transmission of HIV. *American Journal of Maternal/Child Nursing, 31*(6), 396.

Stang, J., Story, M., & Feldman, S. (2005). Nutrition in adolescent pregnancy. *International Journal of Childbirth Education, 20*(2), 4–11.

Stecker, M. M. (2006). Status epilepticus in adults. *UpToDate (15.2)*. Retrieved from http://patients.uptodate.com

Swygard, H., Seña, A. C., & Cohen, M. S. (2007). Neisseria gonorrhoeae infections in women. *UpToDate (15.2)*. Retrieved August 13, 2007, from http://patients.uptodate.com

Teo, E., & Lok, A. S. F. (2007) Epidemiology, transmission and prevention of hepatitis B virus infection. *UpToDate (15.2)*. Retrieved August 13, 2007, from http://patients.uptodate.com

Tettenborn, B. (2006). Management of epilepsy in women of childbearing age practical recommendations. *CNS Drugs, 20*(5), 373–387.

Tough, S., Benzies, K., Newburn-Cook, C., Tofflemire, K., et al. (2006). What do women know about the risks of delayed childbearing? *Canadian Journal of Public Health, 97*(4), 330–334.

Tremblay, C. (2006). Cytomegalovirus infection in pregnancy. *UpToDate (15.2)*. Retrieved August 13, 2007, from http://patients.uptodate.com

U.S. Preventive Services Task Force (Eds.). (2005). Screening for gonorrhea: Recommendation statement. *American Family Physician, 72*(9), 1783–1786.

Venkatesh, M. P., & Hammerschlag, M. R. (2006). Chlamydia trachomatis infections in the newborn. *UpToDate (15.2)*. Retrieved from http://patients.uptodate.com

Watts, D. H. (2006). Treating HIV during pregnancy an update on safety issues. *Drug Safety, 29*(6), 467–490.

Watts, D. H., & Mofenson, L. M. (2006). Cotrimoxazole prophylaxis in HIV-infected women: only a first step. *Journal of Infectious Diseases, 194*(11), 1478–1480, 1510–1518.

Weinberger, S. E., & Schatz, M. (2006). Physiology and clinical course of asthma during pregnancy. *UpToDate (15.2)*. Retrieved from http://patients.uptodate.com

Wenner, C., & Nashelsky, J. (2005). FPIN's clinical inquires. Antiviral agents for pregnant women with genital herpes. *American Family Physician, 72*(9), 1807–1808.

Williams, K. (2007). Toxoplasmosis and pregnancy. *UpToDate (15.2)*. Retrieved from http://patients.uptodate.com

Wills, T., & Goodrich, J. M. (2006). Cytomegalovirus. In D. A. Drevets, F. Talavera, J. W. King, E. Mylonakis, & B. A. Cunha (Eds.), *eMedicine*. Retrieved August 13, 2007, from http://www.emedicine.com/med/topic504.htm

Witcher, P. M., & Harvey, C. J. (2006). Modifying labor routines for the woman with cardiac disease. *Journal of Perinatal and Neonatal Nursing, 20*(4), 303–310.

Workowski, K. A., & Berman, S. M. (2006). Sexually transmitted diseases treatment guidelines, 2006. *MMWR Recommendations and Reports, 55*(RR11), 1–94.

Zenilman, J. M. (2007). Genital chlamydia trachomatis infections in women. *UpToDate (15.2)*. Retrieved from http://patients.uptodate.com.

CHAPTER 17

Abalos, E., Duley, L., Steyn, D. W., & Henderson-Smart, D. J. (2007). Antihypertensive drug therapy for mild to moderate hypertension during pregnancy. *Cochrane Database of Systematic Reviews 2007*, Issue 1. Art. No.: CD002252. DOI: 10.1002/14651858.CD002252.pub2.

Allahyar, J. (2008). Surgical management of ectopic pregnancy. In J. J. Kavanagh, F. Talavera, F. Gaupp, & M. E. Rivlin (Eds.), *eMedicine*. Retrieved November 04, 2008, from http://www.emedicine.com/med/topic3316.htm

Ananth, C. V., & Cnattingius, S. (2007). Influence of maternal smoking on placental abruption in successive pregnancies: A population-based prospective cohort study in Sweden. *American Journal of Epidemiology, 166*(3), 289–295.

Anderson, C. M. (2007). Preeclampsia: Exposing future cardiovascular risk in mothers and their children. *JOGNN, 36*(1), 3–8.

Arafeh, J. M. (2006). Preeclampsia: Pieces of the puzzle revealed. *Journal of Perinatal and Neonatal Nursing, 20*(1), 85–87.

August, P., & Sibai, B. (2007). Clinical features, diagnosis, and long-term prognosis of preeclampsia. *UpToDate (15.2)*. Retrieved November 20, 2007, from http://patients.uptodate.com

Berkman, N.D., et al. (2000). Management of preterm labor. (AHRQ Publication No. 01-E021). Rockville, MD: Agency for Healthcare Research and Quality.

Bess, K. A., & Wood, T. L. (2006). Understanding gestational trophoblastic disease: How nurses can help those dealing with a diagnosis. *AWHONN Lifelines, 10*(4), 320–326.

Black, K. D. (2007). Stress, symptoms, self-monitoring, confidence, well-being, and social support in the progression of preeclampsia/gestational hypertension. *JOGNN, 36*(5), 419–429.

Briggs, G. G., & Wan, S. R. (2006). Drug therapy during labor and delivery, Part 2. *American Journal of Health-System Pharmacists, 63*(12), 1131–1139.

Bryan, E. (2006). Multiple children and their families: What nurses need to know. *AWHONN Lifelines, 10*(2), 138–144.

Campbell, D. E., & Jenkins, M. B. (2006). Preeclampsia. In T. Rosenkrantz, M. L. Windle, B. S. Carter, D. Rauch, & M. Stafford (Eds.), *eMedicine*. Retrieved November 09, 2008, from http://www.emedicine.com/med/topic3316.htm

Cedergren, M., Brynhildsen, J., Josefsson, A., Sydsjo, A, & Sydsjo, G. (2008). Hyperemesis gravidarum that requires hospitalization and the use of antiemetic drugs in relation to maternal body composition. *American Journal of Obstetrics & Gynecology, 198*(4), 412.e1 – 412.e5.

Chiang, J. W., & Berek, J. S. (2007). Epidemiology, clinical manifestations and diagnosis of gestational trophoblastic disease. *UpToDate (15.2)*. Retrieved November 20, 2007, from http://patients.uptodate.com

Cockey, C. D. (2005). Predicting preeclampsia: Substance in urine signals likelihood of high-risk development. *AWHONN Lifelines, 9*(1), 25–26.

Cunningham, F. G., Leveno, K. J., Bloom, S. L., Hauth, J. C., Gilstrap, L. C. III, & Wenstrom, K. D. (2005). *Williams obstetrics* (22nd ed.). New York: McGraw-Hill Medical Publishing Division.

Deering, S. H. (2007). Abruptio placentae. In B. A. Meyer, F. Talavera, A. V. Sison, F. B. Gaupp, & L. P. Shulman (Eds.), *eMedicine*. Retrieved November 09, 2008, from http://www.emedicine.com/med/topic6.htm

Dorigo, O., & Berek, J. S. (2006). Pathology of gestational trophoblastic disease. *UpToDate (15.2)*. Retrieved November 20, 2007, from http://patients.uptodate.com.

Duley, L., Henderson-Smart, D. J., Meher, S., & King, J. F. (2007). Antiplatelet agents for preventing preeclampsia and its complications. *Cochrane Database of Systematic Reviews 2007*, Issue 2, Article No.: CD004659. DOI:10.1002/14651858.CD004659.pub2.

Funai, E. F. (2006). Hyperemesis gravidarum. *UpToDate (15.1)*. Retrieved January 15, 2007, from http://patients.uptodate.com

Fugate, S. R., & Chow, G. E. (2005). Eclampsia. In B. A. Meyer, F. Talavera, A. V. Sison, F. B. Gaupp, & L. P. Shulman (Eds.), *eMedicine*. Retrieved November 9, 2008, from http://www.emedicine.com/med/topic633.htm

Garner, E. (2007a). Management of hydatidiform mole. *UpToDate (15.2)*. Retrieved November 20, 2007, from http://patients.uptodate.com

Garner, E. (2007b). Staging and treatment of malignant gestational trophoblastic disease. *UpToDate (15.2)*. Retrieved November 20, 2007, from http://patients.uptodate.com

Gaufberg, S. V. (2006a). Abortion, septic. In R. Alson, M. Zwanger, J. Halamka, & P. Dyne (Eds.), *eMedicine*. Retrieved November 04, 2008, from http://www.emedicine.com/emerg/topic10.htm

Gaufberg, S. V. (2006b). Abortion, threatened. In R. Alson, M. Zwanger, J. Halamka, & P. Dyne (Eds.), *eMedicine*. Retrieved November 04, 2008, from http://www.emedicine.com/emerg/topic11.htm

Gaufberg, S. V. (2006c). Abruptio placentae. In R. Alson, F. Talavera, M. Zwanger, J. Halamka, & P. L. Dyne (Eds.), *eMedicine*. Retrieved November 09, 2008, from http://www.emedicine.com/emerg/topic12.htm

Gibson, P., and Carson, M. P. (2007). Hypertension and pregnancy. In G. S. Letterie, F. Talavera, F. B. Gaupp, & C. V. Smith (Eds.), *eMedicine*. Retrieved November 09, 2008, from http://www.emedicine.com/emerg/topic12.htm

Gillen-Goldstein, J. (2007). Clinical features and diagnosis of abruptio placentae. *UpToDate (15.2)*. Retrieved November 20, 2007, from http://patients.uptodate.com

Gillen-Goldstein, J. (2006). Management and outcome of abruptio placentae. *UpToDate (15.2)*. Retrieved November 20, 2007, from http://patients.uptodate.com

Hajenius, P. J., Mol, F., Mol, B. W. J., Bossuyt, P. M. M., Ankum, W. M., Van der Veen, F. (2007). Interventions for tubal ectopic pregnancy. *Cochrane Database of Systematic Reviews 2007*, Issue 1. Art. No.: CD000324. DOI: 10.1002/14651858.CD000324.pub2.

Hayslett, J. P. (2006). Evaluation of proteinuria in pregnant women. *UpToDate (15.2)*. Retrieved November 20, 2007, from http://patients.uptodate.com

Hernandez, E. (2008). Gestational trophoblastic neoplasia. In R. C. Shepard, F. Talavera, R. McKenna, & D. Chelmow (Eds.), *eMedicine*. Retrieved November 09, 2008, from http://www.emedicine.com/med/topic866.htm

Johnson, J. R., & Iams, J. D. (2006). Cervical insufficiency. *UpToDate (15.1)*. Retrieved January 15, 2007, from http://patients.uptodate.com

Joy, S., & Lyon, D. (2008). Placenta previa. In R. Levine, F. Talavera, R. S. Legro, F. B. Gaupp, & C. V. Smith (Eds.), *eMedicine*. Retrieved November 09, 2008, from http://www.emedicine.com/med/topic3271.htm

Jung, D. C., & Erogul, M. (2007). Pregnancy, preeclampsia. In A. J. Sayah, F. Talavera, M. Zwanger, J. Halamka, & P. Dyne (Eds.), *eMedicine*. Retrieved November 11, 2008, from http://www.emedicine.com/emerg/topic480.htm

Karumanchi, S. A., Lim, K-H., Sukhatme, V. P., & August, P. (2007). Pathogenesis of preeclampsia. *UpToDate (15.2)*. Retrieved November 20, 2007, from http://patients.uptodate.com

Kim, C., Brawarsky, P., Jackson, R. A., Fuentes-Afflick, E., & Haas, J. (2005). Changes in health status experienced by women with gestational diabetes and pregnancy-induced hypertensive discords. *Journal of Women's Health, 14*(8), 729–736.

Ko, P., & Yoon, Y. (2007). Placenta previa. In J. J. Sachter, F. Talavera, M. Zwanger, J. Halamka, & P. L. Dyne (Eds.), *eMedicine*. Retrieved November 09, 2008, from http://www.emedicine.com/emerg/topic427.htm

Kremer, J. M. (2006). Major side effects of methotrexate. *UpToDate (15.2)*. Retrieved November 20, 2007, from http://patients.uptodate.com

Lindsey, J. L., & Rivera, V. R. (2008). Missed abortion. In S. R. Trupin, F. Talavera, R. S. Legro, F. Gaupp, & M. E. Rivlin (Eds.), *eMedicine*. Retrieved November 04, 2008, from http://www.emedicine.com/med/topic3309.htm

Magloire, L., & Funai, E. F. (2006). Gestational hypertension. *UpToDate (15.2)*. Retrieved November 20, 2007, from http://patients.uptodate.com

Mandy, G. T. (2006). Multiple births. *UpToDate (15.1)*. Retrieved January 15, 2007, from http://patients.uptodate.com

March of Dimes (Eds.). (2004). High blood pressure during pregnancy. Retrieved February 17, 2007, from http://www.marchofdimes.com/professionals/681_1222.asp

Marrinan, G., & Stein, M. (2008). Placenta previa. In C. L. Sistrom, B. D. Coombs, K. L. Reuter, R. M. Krasny, & E. C. Lin (Eds.), *eMedicine*. Retrieved November 09, 2008, from http://www.emedicine.com/radio/topic559.htm

Molinaro, T. A., & Barnhart, K. T. (2007). Abdominal pregnancy, cesarean scar pregnancy, and heterotopic pregnancy. *UpToDate (15.2)*. Retrieved November 20, 2007, from http://patients.uptodate.com

Montgomery, K. S., Cubera, S., Belcher, C., Patrick, D., Funderburk, H., Melton, C., et al. (2005). Childbirth education for multiple pregnancy: Part 1: Prenatal considerations. *Journal of Perinatal Education, 14*(2), 26–35.

Moore, L. E., & Hernandez, E. (2008). Hydatidiform mole. In J. G. Pritzker, F. Talavera, A. D. Barnes, F. B. Gaupp, & D. Chelmo (Eds.), *eMedicine*. Retrieved November 8, 2008, from http://www.emedicine.com/med/topic1047.htm

Mulrow C. D., Chiquette E., Ferrer R. L., et al. (2000). Management of chronic hypertension during pregnancy (AHRQ Publication No. 00-E011). Rockville, MD: Agency for Healthcare Research and Quality.

Nanda, K., Peloggia, A., Grimes, D., Lopez, L., & Nanda, G. (2006). Expectant care versus surgical treatment for miscarriage. *Cochrane Database of Systematic Reviews 2006*, Issue 2. Art. No.: CD003518. DOI: 10.1002/14651858.CD003518.pub2.

Ness, R. B., Zhang, J., Bass, D., & Kelbanoff, M. A. (2008). Interactions between smoking and weight in pregnancies complicated by preeclampsia and small-for-gestational-age birth. *American Journal of Epidemiology 168*(4), 427–433.

Nilsen, R. M., Vollset, S. E., Rasmussen, S. A., Ueland, P. M., & Daltveit, A. K. (2008). Folic acid and multivitamin supplement use and risk of placental abruption: A population-based registry study. *American Journal of Epidemiology, 167*(7), 867–874.

Norwitz, E. R. (2007). Predicting preeclampsia. *UpToDate (15.2)*. Retrieved November 20, 2007, from http://patients.uptodate.com

Norwitz, E. R. (2006). Eclampsia. *UpToDate (15.2)*. Retrieved November 20, 2007, from http://patients.uptodate.com

Norwitz, E. R., & Funai, E. F. (2007). Expectant management of severe preeclampsia. *UpToDate (15.2)*. Retrieved November 20, 2007, from http://patients.uptodate.com

Peters, R. M. (2008). High blood pressure in pregnancy. *Nursing for Women's Health, 12*(5), 410–422.

Puscheck, E., & Pradhan, A. (2006). First trimester pregnancy loss. In S. R. Trupin, R. S. Legro, F. Gaupp, & M. E. Rivlin (Eds.), *eMedicine*. Retrieved November 04, 2008, from http://www.emedicine.com/med/topic3310.htm

Rumbold, A. R., Crowther, C. A., Haslam, R. R., Dekker, G. A., & Robinson, J. S. (2006). Vitamins C and E and the risks of preeclampsia and perinatal complications. *New England Journal of Medicine, 2006*(354), 1796–1806.

Sepilian, V. P., & Wood, E. (2007). Ectopic pregnancy. In R. K. Zurawin, F. Talavera, A. D. Barnes, F. B, Gaupp, & L. P. Shulman (Eds.), *eMedicine*. Retrieved November 04, 2008, from http://www.emedicine.com/med/topic3312.htm

Shah, A. K. (2007). Preeclampsia and eclampsia. In J. F. Hulihan, F. Talavera, J. E. Cavazos, S. R. Benbadis, & N. Lorenzo (Eds.) *eMedicine*. Retrieved November 13, 2008, from http://www.emedicine.com/neuro/topic323.htm

Shen, T. T., DeFrance, E. A., Stamilio, D. M., Chang, J. J., & Muglia, L. J. (2008). A population-based study of race-specific risk for placental abruption. *BMC Pregnancy Childbirth*. Retrieved November 9, 2008, from http://www.medscape.com/viewarticle/582136

Simpson, K. R. (2005). The context & clinical evidence for common nursing practices during labor. *American Journal of Maternal/Child Nursing, 30*(6), 356–363.

Stella, C. L., & Sibai, B. M. (2006). Preeclampsia: Diagnosis and management of the atypical presentation. *Journal of Maternal-Fetal and Neonatal Medicine, 19*(7), 381–386.

Stevens, E., & Gilbert-Cohen, J. (2007). Surgical considerations in early pregnancy: Ectopic pregnancy and ovarian torsion. *Journal of Perinatal and Neonatal Nursing, 21*(1), 22–29.

Tanaka, M., Jaamaa, G., Kaiser, M., Hills, E., Soim, A., Zhu, M., et al. (2007). Racial disparity in hypertensive disorders of pregnancy in New York state: A 10-year longitudinal population-based study. *American Journal of Public Health, 97*(1), 163–170.

Theroux, R. (2007). Preventing pre-eclampsia: Do multivitamins work? *Nursing for Women's Health, 11*(1), 77–79.

Tulandi, T. (2007a). Cervical pregnancy. *UpToDate (15.2)*. Retrieved November 20, 2007, from http://patients.uptodate.com

Tulandi, T. (2007b). Clinical manifestations, diagnosis, and management of ectopic pregnancy. *UpToDate (15.2)*. Retrieved November 20, 2007, from http://patients.uptodate.com

Tulandi, T. (2007c). Methotrexate therapy of ectopic pregnancy. *UpToDate (15.2)*. Retrieved November 20, 2007, from http://patients.uptodate.com

Tulandi, T. (2007d). Surgical treatment of ectopic pregnancy and prognosis for subsequent fertility. *UpToDate (15.2)*. Retrieved November 20, 2007, from http://patients.uptodate.com

Tulandi, T., & Al-Fozan, H. M. (2007a). Evaluation and management of couples with recurrent pregnancy loss. *UpToDate (15.2)*. Retrieved November 20, 2007, from http://patients.uptodate.com

Tulandi, T., & Al-Fozan, H. M. (2007b). Incidence and etiology of recurrent pregnancy loss. *UpToDate (15.2)*. Retrieved November 20, 2007, from http://patients.uptodate.com

Tulandi, T., & Al-Fozan, H. M. (2007c). Spontaneous abortion: Risk factors, etiology, clinical manifestations, and diagnostic evaluation. *UpToDate (15.2)*. Retrieved November 20, 2007, from http://patients.uptodate.com

Tulandi, T. (2006). Expectant management of ectopic pregnancy. *UpToDate (15.2)*. Retrieved November 20, 2007, from http://patients.uptodate.com

Turner, M. (2007). Hyperemesis gravidarum: Providing woman-centered care. *British Journal of Midwifery, 15*(9), 540–544.

Wilcox, S. R., Edelman, A., & Logan, J. R. (2006). Pregnancy, hyperemesis gravidarum. In A. J. Sayah, F. Talavera, M. Zwanger, J. D. Halamka, & P. L. Dyne (Eds.), *eMedicine*. Retrieved November 02, 2008, from http://www.emedicine.com/emerg/topic479.htm

Yang, Q., Wen, S. W., Oppenheimer, L., Chen, X. K., Black, D., Gao, J., & Walker, M. C. (2007). Association of caesarean delivery for first birth with placenta praevia and placental abruption in second pregnancy. *BJOG, 2007*(114), 609–613.

Zach, T., Pramanik, A. K., & Ford, S. P. (2007). Multiple births. In D. N. Sheftel, M. Windle, D. A. Clark, C. L. Wagner, & T. Rosenkrantz (Eds.), *eMedicine*. Retrieved November 13, 2008, from http://www.emedicine.com/ped/topic2599.htm

CHAPTER 18

ACOG (Eds.). (2005). Progesterone treatment decreases preterm birth rate. *ACOG News Release*. Retrieved March 10, 2007, from http://www.acog.org/from_home/publications/press_releases/nr01-31-05-1.cfm

Belogolovkin, V., Bush, M., & Eddleman, K. (2005). Umbilical cord prolapse. *UpToDate (15.2)*. Retrieved August 17, 2007, from http://patients.uptodate.com.

Briggs, G. G., & Wan, S. R. (2006). Drug therapy during labor and delivery, part 2. *American Journal of Health-System Pharmacology, 63*(June 15, 2006), 1131–1139.

Butler, J. R., & Wilkes, P. T. (2006). Postterm pregnancy. In B. D. Cowan, F. Talavera, R. S. Legro, F. B. Gaupp, & L. P. Shulman (Eds.), *eMedicine*. Retrieved March 10, 2007, from http://www.emedicine.com/med/topic3248.htm

Callister, L. C. (2006). Perinatal loss: A family perspective. *Journal of Perinatal and Neonataly Nursing, 20*(3), 227–234.

Camune, B., & Brucker, M. C. (2007). An overview of shoulder dystocia: The nurse's role. *Nursing for Women's Health, 11*(5), 488–497.

Capitulo, K. L. (2005). Evidence for healing interventions with perinatal bereavement. *American Journal of Maternal/Child Nursing, 30*(6), 389–396.

Cunningham, F. G., Leveno, K. J., Bloom, S. L., Hauth, J. C., Gilstrap, L. C. III, & Wenstrom, K. D. (2005). *Williams obstetrics* (22nd ed.). New York: McGraw-Hill Medical Publishing Division.

Cypher, R. (2007). Gestiva for preventing prematurity: A new view of an old therapy. *Nursing for Women's Health, 11*(3), 322–325.

Dare, M. R., Middleton, P., Crowther, C. A., Flenady, V. J., & Varatharaju, B. (2006). Planned early birth versus expectant management (waiting) for prelabour rupture of membranes at term (37 weeks or more). *Cochrane Database of Systematic Reviews* 2006, Issue 1. Art. No.: CD005302. DOI:10.1002/14651858.CD005302.pub2.

Duff, P. (2006). Preterm premature rupture of membranes. *UpToDate (15.2)*. Retrieved August 20, 2007, from http://patients.uptodate.com.

Fischer, R. (2006). Breech presentation. In A. Witlin, F. Talavera, R. S. Legro, F. B. Gaupp, & L. P. Shulman (Eds.), *eMedicine*. Retrieved December 1, 2007, from http://www.emedicine.com/med/topic3272.htm

Fonseca, E. B., Celik, E., Parra, M., Singh, M., & Nicolaides, K. H. (2007). Progesterone and the risk of preterm birth among women with a short cervix. *New England Journal of Medicine (NEJM), 357*(9), 462–469.

Fraser, W. D., Hofmeyr, J., Lede, R., Faron, G., Alexander, S., Goffinet, F., et al. (2005). Amnioinfusion for the prevention of the meconium aspiration syndrome. *New England Journal of Medicine (NEJM), 353*(9), 909–917.

Giarratano, G. (2006). Genetic influences on preterm birth. *American Journal of Maternal/Child Nursing, 31*(3), 169–175.

Gray, B. A. (2006). A ticking uterus: How nurses can identify, treat and prevent preterm labor. *AWHONN Lifelines, 10*(5), 380–389.

Hofmeyr, G. J. (2007). Amnioinfusion for potential or suspected umbilical cord compression in labour. *Cochrane Database of Systematic Reviews, 2007*(4).

Husslein, P., Roura, L. C., Dudenhausen, J. W., Helmer, H., Frydman, R., Rizzo, N., et al. (2007). Atosiban versus usual care for the management of preterm labor. *Journal of Perinatal Medicine, 35*(4), 305–313.

Institute of Medicine (Eds.). (2006). Preterm birth: Causes, consequences, and prevention. *Report Brief, July 2006*. Retrieved February 11, 2007, from http://www.iom.edu/Object.File/Master/35/975/pretermbirth.pdf

Jazayeri, A., & Galan, H. (2006). Premature rupture of membranes. In S. R. Trupin, F. Talavera, G. F. Whitman-Elia, F. B. Gaupp, & L. P. Shulman (Eds.), *eMedicine*. Retrieved February 11, 2007, from http://www.emedicine.com/med/topic3246.htm

Jeavons, W. (2005). Sterile speculum exams & fFN collection. *AWHONN Lifelines, 9*(3), 237–240.

Lindsey, J. L., & Azad, S. (2007). Evaluation of fetal death. In A. Witlin, F. Talavera, C. V. Smith, F. B. Gaupp, & L. P. Shulman (Eds.), *eMedicine*. Retrieved March 10, 2007, from http://www.emedicine.com/med/topic3235.htm

Lyndon, A. (2006). Preterm labor and birth: Where are we now? *Journal of Perinatal & Neonatal Nursing, 20*(1), 82–84.

Lyndrup, J., & Lamont, R. F. (2007). The choice of tocolytic for the treatment of preterm labor: A critical evaluation of nifedipine versus atosiban. *Expert Opinion on Investigational Drugs, 16*(6), 843–853.

Medina, T. M., & Hill, D. A. (2006). Preterm premature rupture of membranes: Diagnosis and management. *American Family Physician, 73*(4), 659–666.

Moore, L. E., & Ware, D. (2005). Amniotic fluid embolism. In J. J. Kavanagh, F. Talavera, A. D. Barnes, F. B. Gaupp, & L. P. Shulman (Eds.), *eMedicine*. Retrieved March 10, 2007, from http://www.emedicine.com/med/topic122.htm

Morgan, B. L. G., & Ross, M. G. (2006). Umbilical cord complications. In R. Levine, F. Talavera, G. F. Whitman-Elia, F. B. Gaupp, & L. P. Shulman (Eds.), *eMedicine*. Retrieved January 2, 2007, from http://www.emedicine.com/med/topic3276.htm

Nahum, G. G., & Pham, K. Q. (2006). Uterine rupture in pregnancy. In B. D. Cowan, F. Talavera, R. S. Legro, F. B. Gaupp, & L. P. Shulman (Eds.), *eMedicine*. Retrieved July 14, 2007, from http://www.emedicine.com/med/topic3746.htm

Nardin, J. M., Carroli, G., & Alfirevic, Z. (2007). Combination of tocolytic agents for inhibiting preterm labour. In *The Cochrane Library*, Issue 2, 2007.

Norwitz, E. R. (2006). Postterm pregnancy. *UpToDate (15.2)*. Retrieved August 20, 2007, from http://patients.uptodate.com.

Rideout, S. L. (2005). Tocolytics for pre-term labor: What nurses need to know. *AWHONN Lifelines, 9*(1), 56–61.

Ridley, R. T. (2007). Diagnosis and intervention for occiput posterior malposition. *Journal of Obstetric, Gynecologic, & Neonatal Nursing, 36*(2), 135–143.

Rodis, J. F. (2006a). Diagnosis and management of pregnancies at risk for shoulder dystocia. *UpToDate (15.2)*. Retrieved August 20, 2007, from http://patients.uptodate.com.

Rodis, J. F. (2006b). Intrapartum management of shoulder dystocia. *UpToDate (15.2)*. Retrieved August 20, 2007, from http://patients.uptodate.com.

Saju, J., & Lyon, D. (2005). Diagnosis of abnormal labor. In R. K. Zurawin, F. Talavera, R. S. Legro, F. B. Gaupp, & L. P. Shulman (Eds.), *eMedicine*. Retrieved March 17, 2007, from http://www.emedicine.com/med/topic3488.htm

Satin, A. J. (2007). Abnormal labor: Protraction and arrest disorders. *UpToDate (15.3)*. Retrieved October 20, 2007, from http://patients.uptodate.com.

Schoening, A. (2007). Amniotic fluid embolism: Recognizing trouble. *Nursing 2007, 37*(1), 64cc1–64cc3.

Schoening, A. (2006). Amniotic fluid embolism: Historical perspectives & new possibilities. *American Journal of Maternal/Child Nursing, 31*(2), 78–83.

Shim, J. Y., Park, Y. W., Yoon, B. H., Cho, Y. K., Yang, H. J., Lee, Y., et al. (2006). Multicentre, parallel group, randomized, single-blind study of the safety and efficacy of atosiban versus ritodrine in the treatment of acute preterm labour in Korean women. *BJOG: An International Journal of Obstetrics & Gynaecology, 113*(11), 1228–1234.

Simhan, H. N., & Caritis, S. N. (2007). Prevention of preterm delivery. *The New England Journal of Medicine (NEJM), 357*(3), 477–487.

Spong, C., & Ross, M. G. (2006). Amnioinfusion: Indications and outcome. *UpToDate* (15.2). Retrieved August 17, 2007, from http://patients.uptodate.com.

Stokowski, L. A. (Ed.). (2007). Transdermal nitroglycerin for preterm labor. Noteworthy professional news. In *Advances in Neonatal Care, 7*(4), 169–170.

Swadpanich, U., Lumbiganon, P., Prasertcharoensook, W., & Laopaiboon, M. (2007). Antenatal lower genital tract infection screening and treatment programs for preventing preterm delivery (Protocol for Cochrane Review). In *The Cochrane Library*, Issue 2, 2007.

Wyatt, S. N., & Rhoads, S. J. (2006). A primer on antenatal testing for neonatal nurses: Part 1. Tests used to predict preterm labor. *Advances in Neonatal Care, 6*(4), 175–180.

CHAPTER 19

Anderson, J. M., & Etches, D. (2007). Prevention and management of postpartum hemorrhage. *American Family Physician, 75*(6), 875–882.

Aurbach, R. D., & Lockwood, C. J. (2006). Overview of prevention of venous thrombosis in pregnant and postpartum women. *UpToDate* (15.1). Retrieved July 12, 2007, from http://patients.uptodate.com

Baskett, T. F. (2007). Uterine compression sutures for postpartum hemorrhage: Efficacy, morbidity, and subsequent pregnancy. *Obstetrics & Gynecology, 110*(1), 68–71.

Beck, C. T. (2008a). State of the science on postpartum depression: What nurse researchers have contributed – Part 1. *American Journal of Maternal/Child Nursing, 33*(2), 121–127.

Beck, C. T. (2008b). State of the science on postpartum depression: What nurse researchers have contributed – Part 2. *American Journal of Maternal/Child Nursing, 33*(3), 151–157.

Beck, C. T., Records, K., & Rice, M. (2006). Further development of the postpartum depression predictors inventory-revised. *JOGNN, 35*(6), 735–745.

Bernstein, I. H., Rush, A. J., Yonkers, K., Carmody, T. J., Woo, A., McConnell, K., et al. (2008). Symptom features of postpartum depression: Are they distinct? *Depression & Anxiety, 25*(1), 20–26.

Betzold, C. M. (2007). An update on the recognition and management of lactational breast inflammation. *Journal of Midwifery and Women's Health, 52*(6), 595–605.

Bose, P., Regan, F., & Paterson-Brown, S. (2006). Improving the accuracy of estimated blood loss at obstetric haemorrhage using clinical reconstructions. *BJOG, 2006, 113*, 919–924.

Bouwmeester, F. W., Bolte, A. C., & van Geijn, H. P. (2005). Pharmacological and surgical therapy for primary postpartum hemorrhage. *Current Pharmaceutical Design, 11*(6), 759–773.

Chen, K. T. (2007). Postpartum endometritis. *UpToDate (15.2)*. Retrieved November 20, 2007, from http://patients.uptodate.com

Cunningham, F. G., Leveno, K. J., Bloom, S. L., Hauth, J. C., Gilstrap, L. C. III, & Wenstrom, K. D. (2005a). Obstetrical hemorrhage. In *Williams obstetrics* (22nd ed., pp. 809–854). New York: McGraw-Hill Medical Publishing Division.

Cunningham, F. G., Leveno, K. J., Bloom, S. L., Hauth, J. C., Gilstrap, L. C. III, & Wenstrom, K. D. (2005b). Puerperal infection. In *Williams obstetrics* (22nd ed., pp. 711–724). New York: McGraw-Hill.

Cunningham, F. G., Leveno, K. J., Bloom, S. L., Hauth, J. C., Gilstrap, L. C. III, & Wenstrom, K. D. (2005c). Thromboembolic disorders. In *Williams obstetrics* (22nd ed., pp. 1073–1091). New York: McGraw-Hill.

Dennis, C. L., & Ross, L. (2006). Women's perceptions of partner support and conflict in the development of postpartum depressive symptoms. *Journal of Advanced Nursing, 56*(6), 588–599.

Dresang, L. T., Fontaine, P., Leeman, L., & King, V. J. (2008). Venous thromboembolism during pregnancy. *American Family Physician, 77*(12), 1709–1716.

Driscoll, J. W. (2006a). Postpartum depression: How nurses can identify and care for women grappling with this disorder. *AWHONN Lifelines, 10*(5), 400–409.

Driscoll, J. W. (2006b). Postpartum depression: The state of the science. *Journal of Perinatal & Neonatal Nursing, 20*(1), 40–42.

Edhborg, M., Matthiesen, A. S., Lundh, W., & Widstrom, A. M. (2005). Some early indicators for depressive symptoms and bonding 2 months postpartum: A study of new mothers and fathers. *Archives of Women's Mental Health, 8*, 221–231.

Engqvist, I., Nilsson, A., Nilsson, K., & Sjostrom, B. (2007). Strategies in caring for women with postpartum psychosis: An interview study with psychiatric nurses. *Journal of Clinical Nursing, 16*(7), 1333–1342.

Goldbort, J. (2006). Transcultural analysis of postpartum depression. *American Journal of Maternal/Child Nursing, 31*(2), 121–126.

Goyal, D., & Lee, K. A. (2007). Patterns of sleep disruption and depressive symptoms in new mothers. *Journal of Perinatal & Neonatal Nursing, 21*(2), 123–129.

Honikman, J. I. (2006). The role of postpartum support international in helping perinatal families. *JOGNN, 35*(5), 659–661.

Horowitz, J. A., & Goodman, J. H. (2005). Identifying and treating postpartum depression. *JOGNN, 34*(2), 264–273.

Isaac, C., & Schlife, J. (2007). More than the blues: Perinatal depression. *Nebraska Nurse, 2007 (September, October, November)*, 8–13.

Jacobs, A. J. (2007a). Causes and treatment of postpartum hemorrhage. *UpToDate (15.2)*. Retrieved November 20, 2007, from http://patients.uptodate.com

Jacobs, A. J. (2007b). Peripartum hysterectomy. *UpToDate (15.2)*. Retrieved November 20, 2007, from http://patients.uptodate.com

Jolley, S. N., & Betrus, P. (2007). Comparing postpartum depression and major depressive disorder: Issues in assessment. *Issues in Mental Health Nursing, 28*(7), 765–780.

Jones, I. (2006). Why do women experience mood disorders following childbirth? *British Journal of Midwifery, 14*(11), 654–657.

Kammerer, M., Taylor, A., & Glover, V. (2006). The HPA axis and perinatal depression: A hypothesis. *Archives of Women's Mental Health, 2006*(9), 187–196.

Keifer, D., & Roman, A. S. (2007). Management of hematomas incurred as a result of obstetrical delivery. *UpToDate (15.2)*. Retrieved November 20, 2007, from http://patients.uptodate.com

Kennedy, E. S. (2007). Pregnancy, postpartum infections. In A. J. Sayah, F. Talavera, M. Zwanger, J. Halamka, & P. L. Dyne's (Eds.), *eMedicine*. Retrieved November 21, 2008, from http://www.emedicine.com/emerg/topic482.htm

Leung, S., Arthur, D. G., & Martinson, I. (2005). Stress in women with postpartum depression: A phenomenological study. *Journal of Advanced Nursing, 51*(4), 353–360.

Lindahl, V., Pearson, J. L., & Colpe, L. (2005). Prevalence of suicidality during pregnancy and the postpartum. *Archives of Women's Mental Health, 8*, 77–87.

Logsdon, M. C., Wisner, K. L., & Pinto-Foltz, M. D. (2006). The impact of postpartum depression on mothering. *JOGNN, 35*(5), 652–658.

MacMullen, N. J., Dulski, L. A., & Meagher, B. (2005). Red alert: Perinatal hemorrhage. *American Journal of Maternal/Child Nursing, 30*(1), 46–51.

Marchant, S., Alexander, J., Thomas, P., Garcia, J., Brocklehurst, P., & Keene, J. (2006). Risk factors for hospital admission related to excessive and/or prolonged postpartum vaginal blood loss after the first 24 hours following childbirth. *Paediatric and Perinatal Epidemiology, 20,* 392–402.

Maughan, K. L., Heim, S. W., & Galazka, S. S. (2006). Preventing postpartum hemorrhage: Managing the third stage of labor. *American Family Physician, 73*(6), 1025–1028.

Mayberry, L. J., Horowitz, J. A., & Declercq, E. (2007). Depression symptom prevalence and demographic risk factors among U.S. women during the first 2 years postpartum. *JOGNN, 36*(6), 542–549.

Milne, L. C., Greenway, P., & Hansen, L. (2007). Predictors of postnatal depression in a community sample. *Neonatal, Paediatric and Child Health Nursing, 10*(1), 20–26.

Morrissey, M. V. (2007). Suffer no more silence: Challenging the myths women's mental health in childbearing. *International Journal of Psychiatric Nursing Research, 12*(2), 1429–1438.

Ng, C., Jahanfar, S., & Teng, C. L. (2007). Antibiotics for mastitis in breastfeeding women (Protocol for Cochrane Review). In *The Cochrane Library,* Issue 2, 2007.

Nonacs, R. M. (2007). Postpartum depression. In S. R. Trupin, F. Talavera, F. B. Gaupp, & D. Chelmow (Eds.), *eMedicine.* Retrieved November 21, 2008, from http://www.emedicine.com/med/TOPIC3408.HTM

O'Grady, J. P. (2008). Malposition of the uterus. In G. S. Letterie, F. Talavera, R. S. Legro, F. B. Gaupp, & M. E. Rivlin (Eds.), *eMedicine.* Retrieved November 15, 2008, from http://www.emedicine.com/med/TOPIC3473.HTM

Patnaik, M. M., Haddad, T., & Morton, C. T. (2007). Pregnancy and thrombophilia. *Expert Review Cardiovascular Therapy, 5*(4), 753–765.

Pearlstein, T. (2008). Perinatal depression: Treatment options and dilemmas. *Journal of Psychiatry & Neurosciences, 33*(4), 302–318.

Pippins, J. R., Brawarsky, P., Jackson, R. A., Fuentes-Afflick, E., & Haas, J. S. (2006). Association of breastfeeding with maternal depressive symptoms. *Journal of Women's Health, 15*(6), 754–762.

Priest, S. R., Austin, M., & Sullivan, E. (2007). Antenatal psychosocial screening for prevention of antenatal and postnatal anxiety and depression (Protocol for Cochrane Review). In *The Cochrane Library,* Issue 2, 2007.

Registered Nurses' Association of Ontario (Eds.). (2005). Interventions for postpartum depression. *Nursing Best Practice Guideline.* Toronto, Canada: Registered Nurses' Association of Ontario.

Ross, L. E., Murray, B. J., & Steiner, M. (2005). Sleep and perinatal mood disorders: A critical review. *Journal of Psychiatry & Neurosciences, 30*(4), 247–256.

Schwartz, D. R., Malhotra, A., & Weinberger, S. E. (2005). Deep vein thrombosis and pulmonary embolism in pregnancy. *UpToDate (15.2).* Retrieved November 20, 2007, from http://patients.uptodate.com

Secco, M. L., Profit, S., Kennedy, E., Walsh, A., Letourneau, N., & Stewart, M. (2007). Factors affecting postpartum depressive symptoms of adolescent mothers. *Journal of Obstetric, Gynecologic & Neonatal Nursing, 36*(1), 47–54.

Sharma, S. (2006). Shock and pregnancy. In S. D. Spandorfer, F. Talavera, D. Chelmow, T. D. Rice, & L. P. Shulman (Eds.), *eMedicine.* Retrieved November 15, 2008, from http://www.emedicine.com/med/TOPIC3285.HTM

Sharp, D. (2008). Postnatal depression. *Pulse, 68*(35), 26–27.

Simmons, G. T. (2007). Endometritis. In A. C. Sciscione, F. Talavera, A. V. Sison, F. B. Gaupp, & M. E. Rivlin (Eds.), *eMedicine.* Retrieved November 21, 2008, from http://www.emedicine.com/med/topic676.htm

Simpson, K. R. (2006). Venous thromboembolism during pregnancy and postpartum: An inherited risk. *American Journal of Maternal/Child Nursing, 31*(3), 208.

Singhal, H., & Kaur, K. (2008). Wound infection. In B. J. Daley, F. Talavera, A. L. Friedman, M. E. Zevitz, & J. Geibel (Eds.), *eMedicine.* Retrieved November 22, 2008, from http://www.emedicine.com/MED/topic2422.htm

Smith, J. R., & Brennan, B. G. (2006). Postpartum hemorrhage. In S. H. Ural, F. Talavera, M. E. Rivlin, F. B. Gaupp, & L. P. Shulman (Eds.), *eMedicine.* Retrieved November 15, 2008, from http://www.emedicine.com/med/topic3568.htm

St. Pierre, C. M. (2007). The taboo of motherhood: Postpartum depression. *International Journal for Human Caring, 11*(2), 22–31.

Strayer, D. A. (2007a). Postpartum depression: Assessment and screening. *Evidence-Based Care Sheet,* D. Pravikoff (Ed.). Cinahl Information Systems.

Strayer, D. A. (2007b). Postpartum depression in fathers. *Evidence-Based Care Sheet,* D. Pravikoff (Ed.). Last updated November 16, 2007. Cinahl Information Systems.

Turner, J. H., & Ray, C. E. (2008). Embolization, hemorrhage. In A. Watkinson, B. D. Coombs, R. M. Krasny, & K. J. Cho (Eds.), *eMedicine.* Retrieved November 15, 2008, from http://www.emedicine.com/radio/TOPIC760.HTM

Wainscott, M. P. (2006). Pregnancy, postpartum hemorrhage. In A. J. Sayah, F. Talavera, M. Zwanger, J. Halamka, & P. Dyne (Eds.), *eMedicine.* Retrieved November 15, 2008, from http://www.emedicine.com/emerg/topic481.htm

Weydert, J. A., & Benda, J. A. (2006). Subinvolution of the placental site as an anatomic cause of postpartum uterine bleeding. *Archives of Pathological Laboratory Medicin, 130*(10), 1538–1542.

Wilen, J. M., & Mounts, K. O. (2006). Women with depressions: "You can't tell by looking." *Maternal Child Health Journal, 2006*(10), S183–S186.

Wilde, S. (2005). Obstetric heamorrhage in the perioperative environment. *BJPN, 15*(7), 292–301.

Wisner, K. L., Hanusa, B. H., Perel, J. M., Peindl, K. S., Piontek, C. M., Sit, D. K., et al. (2006). Postpartum depression: A randomized trial of sertraline versus nortriptyline. *Journal of Clinical Psychopharmacology, 26*(4), 353.

Zauderer, C. R. (2008). A case study of postpartum depression & altered maternal-newborn attachment. *American Journal of Maternal/Child Nursing, 33*(3), 173–179.

CHAPTER 20

Ambalavanan, N. (2008). Fluid, electrolyte, and nutrition management of the newborn. In S. MacGilvray, M. L. Windle, B. S. Carter, C. L. Wagner, & T. Rosenkrantz, *eMedicine.* Retrieved December 13, 2008, from http://www.emedicine.com/ped/topic2554.htm

Ballard, J. L., Khoury, J. C., Wedig, K., Wang, L., EilersWalsman, B. L., & Lipp, R. (1991). New Ballard score expanded to include extremely premature infants. *Journal of Pediatrics, 119*(3), 417–423.

Barnes-Powell, L. L. (2007). The effects of hyperglycemia on the fetus and neonate. *Neonatal Network, 26*(5), 283–290.

Beal, J. A. (2005). Evidence for best practices in the neonatal period. *American Journal of Maternal Child Nursing, 30*(6), 397–403.

Berger, K. S. (2006). The developing person through childhood and adolescence (7th ed.). New York: Worth Publishers.

Callen, J., Pinelli, J., Atkinson, S., & Saigal, S. (2005). Qualitative analysis of barriers to breastfeeding in very-low-birthweight infants in the hospital and postdischarge. *Advances in Neonatal Care, 5*(2), 93–103.

Callen, J., & Pinelli, J. (2005). A review of the literature examining the benefits and challenges, incidence and duration, and barriers to breastfeeding in preterm infants. *Advances in Neonatal Care, 5*(2), 72–88.

Campbell, S. H., & Gutman, C. (2006). A case study: Challenges of breastfeeding preterm infants. *AWHONN Lifelines, 10*(5), 490–497.

Carroll, J. L., Slobodzian, R., Steward, D. K. (2005). Extremely low birthweight infants: Issues related to growth. *American Journal of Maternal/Child Nursing, 30*(5), 312–320.

Carroll, J. L., & Laughlin, G. M. (2006). Sudden infant death syndrome. In J. McMillan, R. Feigin, C. DeAngelis, & M. Jones, Jr. (Eds.), *Oski's pediatrics: Principles and practice* (4th ed.). Philadelphia: Lippincott Williams & Wilkins.

Carter, B. M. (2007). Treatment outcomes of necrotizing enterocolitis for preterm infants. *Journal of Obstetric, Gynecologic, and Neonatal Nursing, 36*(4), 377–385.

Coe, K. (2007). Nursing update on retinopathy of prematurity. *Journal of Obstetric, Gynecologic, and Neonatal Nursing, 36*(3), 288–292.

Cohen, D. W. (2006). Hemolytic disease of the newborn: RBC alloantibodies in pregnancy and associated serologic issues. *UpToDate (15.1).* Retrieved June 1, 2008, from http://patients.uptodate.com

Dabrowski, G. A. (2007). Skin-to-skin contact: Giving birth back to mothers and babies. *Nursing for Women's Health, 11*(1), 64–71.

Divon, M. Y., & Ferber, A. (2007). Fetal growth restriction: Etiology. *UpToDate* (15.2). Retrieved November 15, 2007, from http://patients.uptodate.com

Fink, J. L. W. (2006). Diabetes in pregnancy. *RN, 69*(5), 26–30.

Furdon, S. A., & Clark, D. A. (2006). Prematurity. In T. Rosenkrantz, M. L. Windle, A. K. Pramanik, C. L. Wagner (Eds.), *eMedicine*. Retrieved December 3, 2008, from http://www.emedicine.com/ped/TOPIC1889.HTM

Gregory, K. (2005). Update on nutrition for preterm and full-term infants. *Journal of Obstetric, Gynecologic and Neonatal Nursing, 34*(1), 98–108.

Griffin, T. (2006). Family-centered care in the NICU. *Journal of Perinatal and Neonatal Nursing, 20*(1), 98–102.

Gross, I. (2006). Causes of respiratory distress in the newborn. In *Oski's pediatrics: Principles and practice* (4th ed.). Philadelphia: Lippincott Williams & Wilkins.

Hamdan, A. H. (2008). Neonatal abstinence syndrome. In S. MacGilvray, M. L. Windle, B. S. Carter, C. L. Wagner, & T. Rosenkrantz (Eds.), *eMedicine*. Retrieved November 26, 2008, from http://www.emedicine.com/ped/topic2760.htm

Hockenberry, M. J., & Wilson, D. (2007). *Wong's nursing care of infants and children* (8th ed.). St. Louis, MO: Mosby Elsevier.

Howarth, C., Gazis, A., & James, D. (2007). Associations of type 1 diabetes mellitus, maternal vascular disease, and complications of pregnancy. *Diabetic Medicine, 24*(11), 1229–1234.

Hurst, N. M. (2007). The 3 m's of breast-feeding the preterm infant. *Journal of Perinatal and Neonatal Nursing, 21*(3), 234–239.

Kirkby, S., Greenspan, J. S., Kornhauser, M., & Schneiderman, R. (2007). Clinical outcomes and cost of the moderately preterm infant. *Advances in Neonatal Care, 7*(2), 80–87.

Kriebs, J. M. (2008). Infectious diseases in pregnancy: Issues of screening, prevention, and treatment. *Journal of Perinatal and Neonatal Nursing, 22*(3), 214–220.

Lawrence, E. J. (2007). A matter of size: Part 2: Evaluating the large-for-gestational age neonate [focus on the physical]. *Advances in Neonatal Care, 7*(4), 187–197.

Lawrence, E. J. (2006). Part 1: A matter of size: Evaluating the growth-restricted neonate. *Advances in Neonatal Care, 6*(6), 313–322.

Lott, J. W. (2006). State of the science: Neonatal bacterial infection in the early 21st century. *Journal of Perinatal and Neonatal Nursing, 20*(1), 62–70.

Lusskin, S. I., & Misri, S. (2007). Infants with antenatal exposure to serotonin reuptake inhibitors. *UpToDate (15.1)*. Retrieved June 1, 2008, from http://patients.uptodate.com

Mandy, G. T. (2007). Small for gestational age infant. *UpToDate (15.2)*. Retrieved November 15, 2007, from http://patients.uptodate.com

Mandy, G. T. (2006a). Large for gestational age newborn. *UpToDate* (15.1). Retrieved April 1, 2007, from http://patients.uptodate.com

Mandy, G. T. (2006b). Prematurity. *UpToDate* (15.1). Retrieved April 1, 2007, from http://patients.uptodate.com

McGrath, J. M. (2005). Partnerships with families: A foundation to support them in difficult times. *Journal of Perinatal and Neonatal Nursing, 19*(2), 94–96.

Medhoff-Cooper, B. (2005). Nutritive sucking research: From clinical questions to research answers. *Journal of Perinatal and Neonatal Nursing, 19*(3), 265–272.

Minkes, R. K., Chen, L. E., Palit, T. K., & Bloss, R. S. (2008). Necrotizing enterocolitis: Surgical perspective. In D. Farmer, M. L. Windle, A. Hebra, H. B. Othersen, & P. Glick (Eds.), *eMedicine*. Retrieved December 07, 2008, from http://www.emedicine.com/ped/TOPIC2981.HTM

Mohamed, I. S., Piwko, J. G., Caty, M. G., & Ryan, R. M. (2006). Neonatology considerations for the pediatric surgeon. In M. L. Hilfiker, M. L. Windle, M. G. Caty, H. B. Othersen, & M. Reynolds (Eds.), *eMedicine*. Retrieved November 30, 2008, from http://www.emedicine.com/ped/TOPIC2982.HTM

Moise, K. J. (2006). Diagnosis and management of Rhesus (Rh) alloimmunization. *UpToDate* (15.1). Retrieved June 1, 2008, from http://patients.uptodate.com

Moylett, E. H., & Shearer, W. T. (2006). Pediatric human immunodeficiency virus infection. In *Oski's pediatrics: Principles and practice* (4th ed.). Philadelphia: Lippincott Williams & Wilkins.

Narayanan, S. K., & Ossiani, M. (2006). Streptococcus group B infections. In P. H. Chandrasekar, F. Talavera, J. L. Brusch, E. Mylonakis, & B. A. Cunha (Eds.), *eMedicine*. Retrieved December 17, 2008, from http://www.emedicine.com/med/TOPIC2185.HTM

Nimavat, D. J., Sherman, M. P., Santin, R. L., & Porat, R. (2007). Apnea of prematurity. In S. M. Donn, M. L. Windle, A. K. Pramanik, C. L. Wagner, & T. Rosenkarntz (Eds.), *eMedicine*. Retrieved December 7, 2008, from http://www.emedicine.com/ped/TOPIC1157.HTM

North American Nursing Diagnosis Association (NANDA). (2001). NANDA nursing diagnoses: Definitions and classification 2001–2002. Philadelphia: Author.

Oepkes, D., Seaward, P. G., Vandenbussche, F. P., Windrim, R., Kingdom, J., Beyene, J., et al. (2006). Doppler ultrasonography versus amniocentesis to predict fetal anemia. *New England Journal of Medicine, 355*(2), 156–164.

Peterec, S. M., & Warshaw, J. B. (2006). The premature newborn. In *Oski's pediatrics: Principles and practice* (4th ed.). Philadelphia: Lippincott Williams & Wilkins.

Pillitteri, A. (2007). *Material and child health nursing: Care of the childbearing and childrearing family* (5th ed.). Philadelphia: Lippincott Williams & Wilkins.

Potter, C. F., & Kicklighter, S. D. (2006). Infant of diabetic mother. In G. Cassady, M. L. Windle, B. S. Carter, C. L. Wagner, & T. Rosenkrantz (Eds.), *eMedicine*. Retrieved November 30, 2008, from http://www.emedicine.com/ped/TOPIC845.HTM

Pramanik, A. K. (2006). Respiratory distress syndrome. In S. M. Donn, M. L. Windle, D. A. Clark, C. L. Wagner, & T. Rosenkrantz (Eds.), *eMedicine*. Retrieved December 03, 2008, from http://www.emedicine.com/ped/topic1993.htm

Primji, S. S. (2005). Enteral feeding for high-risk neonates: A digest for nurses into putative risk and benefits to ensure safe and comfortable care. *Journal of Perinatal and Neonatal Nursing, 19*(1), 59–71.

Ralph, S. S., & Taylor, C. M. (2005). *Nursing diagnosis reference manual* (6th ed.). Philadelphia: Lippincott Williams & Wilkins.

Ricci, S. S. (2007). *Essentials of maternity, newborn, and women's health nursing*. Philadelphia: Lippincott Williams & Wilkins.

Salem, L., & Singer, K. R. (2008). Rh incompatibility. In A. J. Sayah, M. Zwanger, J. D. Halamka, & P. L. Dyne (Eds.), *eMedicine*. Retrieved November 26, 2008, from http://www.emedicine.com/emerg/TOPIC507.htm

Schanler, R. J. (2006). Approach to enteral nutrition in the premature infant. *UpToDate (15.1)*. Retrieved June 1, 2008, from http://patients.uptodate.com

Shaker, C. S., & Woida, A. M. (2007). *Neonatal Network, 26*(2), 77–83.

Sielski. L. A. (2007). Neonatal opioid withdrawal. *UpToDate (15.1)*. Retrieved June 1, 2008, from http://patients.uptodate.com

Sielski. L. A. (2006). Infants of mothers with substance abuse. *UpToDate (15.1)*. Retrieved June 1, 2008, from http://patients.uptodate.com

Springer, S. C., & Annibale, D. J. (2008). Necrotizing enterocolitis. In O. Itani, M. L. Windle, D. A. Clark, C. L. Wagner, & T. Rosenkrantz (Eds.), *eMedicine*. Retrieved December 07, 2008, from http://www.emedicine.com/ped/TOPIC2601.HTM

Stichler, J. F. (2007). When birth is not as planned: Joy and fear interwoven. *Nursing for Women's Health, 11*(2), 220, 217–219.

Stokowski, L. A. (2005). A primer on apnea of prematurity. *Advances in Neonatal Care, 5*(3), 155–170.

Subramanian, K. S., Bahri, M., Vicente, G., & Higgins, R. D. (2008). Retinopathy of prematurity. In O. Itani, M. L. Windle, A. K. Pramanik, C. L. Wagner, & T. Rosenkrantz (Eds.), *eMedicine*. Retrieved December 6, 2008, from http://www.emedicine.com/ped/TOPIC1998.HTM

Thomas, K. A. (2003). Infant weight and gestational age effects on thermoneutrality in the home environment. *Journal of Obstetric, Gynecologic and Neonatal Nursing, 32*(6), 745–752.

Thompson, A. M., & Bizzarro, M. J. (2008). Necrotizing enterocolitis in newborns: Pathogenesis, prevention and management. *Drugs, 68*(9), 1227–1238.

Thoya, S. M., Shaker, C. S., & Pridham, K. F. (2005). The early feeding skills assessment for preterm infants. *Neonatal Network, 24*(3), 7–16.

Wagle, S., & Deshpande, P. G. (2008). Hemolytic disease of the newborn. In O. Itani, M. L. Windle, D. A. Clark, C. L. Wagner, & T. Rosenkrantz (Eds.), *eMedicine*. Retrieved November 26, 2008, from http://www.emedicine.com/ped/topic959.htm

Wang, M. (2008). Perinatal drug abuse and neonatal drug withdrawal. In D. N. Sheftel, M. L. Windle, B. S. Carter, C. L. Wagner, & T. Rosenkrantz (Eds.), *eMedicine*. Last updated Retrieved November 26, 2008, from http://www.emedicine.com/ped/topic2631.htm

White-Traut, R. C., Berbaum, M. L., Lessen, B., McFarlin, B., & Cardenas, L. (2005). Feeding readiness in preterm infants: The relationship between preterm behavioral state and feeding readiness behaviors and efficiency during transition from gavage to oral feeding. *American Journal of Maternal/Child Nursing, 30*(1), 52–59.

Wong, D. L., Perry, S., Hockenberry, M., Lowdermilk, D. L., & Wilson, D. (2006). *Maternal child nursing care* (3rd ed.). St. Louis. MO: Mosby.

Yeo, S. L. (2006). NICU update: State of the science of NEC. *Journal of Perinatal and Neonatal Nursing, 20*(1), 46–50.

Zukowsky, K. (2007). Breast-fed low-birth-weight premature neonates: Developmental assessment and nutritional intake in the first 6 months of life. *Journal of Perinatal and Neonatal Nursing, 21*(3), 242–249.

CHAPTER 21

Fishman, M. A. (2006). Developmental defects. In J. McMillan, R. Feigin, C. DeAngelis, & M. Jones, Jr. (Eds.), *Oski's pediatrics: Principles and practice* (4th ed.). Philadelphia: Lippincott Williams & Wilkins.

Gorlin, R. J. (2006). Craniofacial defects. In J. McMillan, R. Feigin, C. DeAngelis, & M. Jones, Jr. (Eds.), *Oski's pediatrics: Principles and practice* (4th ed.). Philadelphia: Lippincott Williams & Wilkins.

Hockenberry, M. J., & Wilson, D. (2007). *Wong's nursing care of infants and children* (8th ed.). St. Louis, MO: Mosby Elsevier.

Holmes, L. B. (2006). Congenital malformations. In J. McMillan, R. Feigin, C. DeAngelis, & M. Jones, Jr. (Eds.), *Oski's pediatrics: Principles and practice* (4th ed.). Philadelphia: Lippincott Williams & Wilkins.

Kyle, T. (2008). *Essentials of pediatric nursing.* Philadelphia: Lippincott Williams & Wilkins.

Lewanda, A. F., & Jabs, E. W. (2006). Dysmorphology: Genetic syndromes and associations. In J. McMillan, R. Feigin, C. DeAngelis, & M. Jones, Jr. (Eds.), *Oski's pediatrics: Principles and practice* (4th ed.). Philadelphia: Lippincott Williams & Wilkins.

NANDA-I nursing diagnoses: Definitions and classification 2007–2008. (2007). Philadelphia: NANDA International.

Pillitteri, A. (2007). *Maternal and child health nursing: Care of the childbearing and childrearing family* (5th ed.). Philadelphia: Lippincott Williams & Wilkins.

Ralph, S. S., & Taylor, C. M. (2005). *Nursing diagnosis reference manual* (6th ed.). Philadelphia: Lippincott Williams & Wilkins.

Ricci, S. S. (2007). *Essentials of maternity, newborn, and women's health nursing.* Philadelphia: Lippincott Williams & Wilkins.

Upham, M., & Medoff-Cooper, B. (2005). What are the responses and needs of mothers of infants diagnosed with congenital heart disease?. *American Journal of Maternal/Child Nursing, 30*(1), 24-29.

Wong, D. L., Perry, S., Hockenberry, M., Lowdermilk, D. L., & Wilson, D. (2006). *Maternal child nursing care* (3rd ed.). St. Louis, MO: Mosby.

CHAPTER 22

Berger, K. S. (2005). *The developing person through the life span* (6th ed.). New York: Worth Publishers.

Berger, K. S. (2006). *The developing person through childhood and adolescence* (7th ed.). New York: Worth Publishers.

Bowlby, J. (1969). *Attachment.* New York: Basic Books.

Brazelton, T. B., & Greenspan, S. (2001). *The irreducible needs of children: What every child must have to grow, learn, and flourish.* Cambridge, MA: Perseus Publishing.

Dudek, S. G. (2006). *Nutrition essentials for nursing practice* (5th ed.). Philadelphia: Lippincott Williams & Wilkins.

Erikson, E. H. (1963). *Childhood and society* (2nd ed.). New York: Norton.

Erikson, E. H., & Senn, M. J. E. (1958). *Symposium on the healthy personality.* New York: Macy Foundation.

French L, Howell, G., Haven, J., & Britten, P. (2006) Designing MyPyramid for kids materials to help children eat right, exercise, have fun. *Journal of Nutrition Education and Behavior,* 38, S158-S159.

Gilligan, C. (1982). *In a different voice.* Cambridge, MA: Howard University Press.

Hockenberry, M. J., & Wilson, D. (2007). *Wong's nursing care of infants and children* (8th ed.). St. Louis, MO: Mosby Elsevier.

McEvoy, M. (2003). Culture and spirituality as an integrated concept in pediatric care. *American Journal of Maternal Child Nursing, 28*(1), 39–43.

National Institute of Child Health and Human Development. (Undated). *Biobehavioral development: From cells to selves.* Retrieved September 22, 2007, from http:// www.nichd.nih.gov/publications/

Piaget, J. (1967). *The language and thought of the child.* Cleveland, OH: World Publishing.

Pillitteri, A. (2007). *Maternal and child health nursing: Care of the childbearing and childrearing family* (5th ed.). Philadelphia: Lippincott Williams & Wilkins.

Shives, L. (2007). *Basic concepts of psychiatric–mental health nursing* (7th ed.). Philadelphia: Lippincott Williams & Wilkins.

Traboulsi, E. I. (2006). Pediatric ophthalmology. In J. McMillan, R. Feigin, C. DeAngelis, & M. Jones, Jr. (Eds.), *Oski's pediatrics: Principles and practices* (4th ed.). Philadelphia: Lippincott Williams & Wilkins.

Wadsworth, B. J. (1984). *Piaget's theory of cognitive and affective development.* New York: Longman.

Wong, D. L., Perry, S., Hockenberry, M., Lowdermilk, D. L., & Wilson, D. (2006). *Maternal child nursing care* (3rd ed.). St. Louis, MO: Mosby.

CHAPTER 23

Berger, K. S. (2006). *The developing person through child-hood and adolescence* (7th ed.). New York: Worth Publishers.

Dudek, S. G. (2006). *Nutrition essentials for nursing practice* (5th ed.). Philadelphia: Lippincott Williams & Wilkins.

Falconer, J. (2006). Practical management of infant food allergies. *Nursing Times, 102*(30), 54–56.

Finberg, L. (2006). Feeding the healthy child. In J. McMillan, R. Feigin, C. DeAngelis, & M. Jones, Jr. (Eds.), *Oski's pediatrics: Principles and practice* (4th ed.). Philadelphia: Lippincott Williams & Wilkins.

Halsey, N. A. (2006). Immunization. In J. McMillan, R. Feigin, C. DeAngelis, & M. Jones, Jr. (Eds.), *Oski's pediatrics: Principles and practice* (4th ed.). Philadelphia: Lippincott Williams & Wilkins.

Hockenberry, M. J., & Wilson, D. (2007). *Wong's nursing care of infants and children* (8th ed.). St. Louis, MO: Mosby Elsevier.

Keefe, M. R., et al. (2005). An intervention program for families with irritable infants. *American Journal of Maternal/Child Nursing, 30*(4), 230–236.

Morin, K. (2004). Current thoughts on healthy term infant nutrition: The first twelve months. *American Journal of Maternal/Child Nursing, 29*(5), 312–318.

Morin, K. (2005). Infant nutrition: Preparing baby food at home safely. *American Journal of Maternal/Child Nursing, 30*(l), 67.

Morin, K. (2005). Infant nutrition: Water-soluble vitamins. *American Journal of Maternal/Child Nursing, 30*(4), 271.

North American Nursing Diagnosis Association (NANDA). (2003). *NANDA nursing diagnoses: Definitions and classification 2003–2004.* Philadelphia: Author.

Pillitteri, A. (2007). *Material and child health nursing: Care of the childbearing and childrearing family* (5th ed.). Philadelphia: Lippincott Williams & Wilkins.

Ralph, S. S., & Taylor, C. M. (2005). *Nursing diagnosis reference manual* (6th ed.). Philadelphia: Lippincott Williams & Wilkins.

Richter, S. B., et al. (2006). Normal infant and childhood development. In J. McMillan, R. Feigin, C. DeAngelis, & M. Jones, Jr. (Eds.), *Oski's pediatrics: Principles and practice* (4th ed.). Philadelphia: Lippincott Williams & Wilkins.

Smeltzer, S. C., Bare, B. G., Hinkle, J. L., & Cheever, K. H. (2008). *Brunner and Suddarth's textbook of medical-surgical nursing* (11th ed.). Philadelphia: Lippincott Williams & Wilkins.

Spock, B. (2004). *Dr. Spock's baby and child care* (8th ed.). New York: Pocket Books.

Wong, D. L., Perry, S., Hockenberry, M., Lowdermilk, D. L., & Wilson, D. (2006). *Maternal child nursing care* (3rd ed.). St. Louis, MO: Mosby.

CHAPTER 24

Berger, K. S. (2006). *The developing person through childhood and adolescence* (7th ed.). New York: Worth Publishers.

Dudek, S. G. (2006). *Nutrition essentials for nursing practice* (5th ed). Philadelphia: Lippincott Williams & Wilkins.

Finberg, L. (2006). Feeding the healthy child. In J. McMillan, R. Feigin, C. DeAngelis, & M. Jones, Jr. (Eds.), *Oski's pediatrics: Principles and practice* (4th ed.). Philadelphia: Lippincott Williams & Wilkins.

Hockenberry, M. J., & Wilson, D. (2007). *Wong's nursing care of infants and children* (8th ed.). St. Louis, MO: Mosby Elsevier.

French L., Howell, G., Haven, J., & Britten, P. (2006) Designing MyPyramid for kids materials to help children eat right, exercise, have fun. *Journal of Nutrition Education and Behavior, 38,* S158–S159.

Kyle, T. (2008). *Essentials of pediatric nursing.* Philadelphia: Lippincott Williams & Wilkins.

NANDA-I Nursing diagnoses: definitions and classification 2007–2008. (2007). Philadelphia: NANDA International.

Pillitteri, A. (2007). *Maternal and child health nursing: Care of the childbearing and childrearing family* (5th ed.). Philadelphia: Lippincott Williams & Wilkins.

Ralph, S. S., & Taylor, C. M. (2005). *Nursing diagnosis reference manual* (6th ed.). Philadelphia: Lippincott Williams & Wilkins.

Richter, S. B., et al. (2006). Normal infant and child-hood development. In J. McMillan, R. Feigin, C. DeAngelis, & M. Jones, Jr. (Eds.), *Oski's pediatrics: Principles and practice* (4th ed.). Philadelphia: Lippincott Williams & Wilkins.

Simpson, T., & Ivey, J. (2006). A well child visit. *Pediatric Nursing, 32*(2), 144.

Smeltzer, S. C., Bare, B. G., Hinkle, J. L., & Cheever, K. H. (2008). *Brunner and Suddarth's textbook of medical-surgical nursing* (11th ed.). Philadelphia: Lippincott Williams & Wilkins.

Wong, D. L., Perry, S., Hockenberry, M., Lowdermilk, D. L., & Wilson, D. (2006). *Maternal child nursing care* (3rd ed.). St. Louis, MO: Mosby.

CHAPTER 25

Berger, K. S. (2006). *The developing person through childhood and adolescence* (7th ed.). New York: Worth Publishers.

Dudek, S. G. (2006). *Nutrition essentials for nursing practice* (5th ed.). Philadelphia: Lippincott Williams & Wilkins.

French L., Howell, G., Haven, J., & Britten, P. (2006) Designing MyPyramid for kids materials to help children eat right, exercise, have fun. *Journal of Nutrition Education and Behavior, 38,* S158–S159.

Finberg, L. (2006). Feeding the healthy child. In J. McMillan, R. Feigin, C. DeAngelis, & M. Jones, Jr. (Eds.), *Oski's pediatrics: Principles and practice* (4th ed.). Philadelphia: Lippincott Williams & Wilkins.

Hockenberry, M. J., & Wilson, D. (2007). *Wong's nursing care of infants and children* (8th ed.). St. Louis, MO: Mosby Elsevier.

Kass, L. J. (2006). Sleep problems. *Pediatric Review, 27*(12), 455–462.

Kyle, T. (2008). *Essentials of pediatric nursing.* Philadelphia: Lippincott Williams & Wilkins.

NANDA-I Nursing Diagnoses: Definitions and Classification 2007–2008. (2007) Philadelphia: NANDA International.

Pillitteri, A. (2007). *Maternal and child health nursing: Care of the childbearing and childrearing family* (5th ed.). Philadelphia: Lippincott Williams & Wilkins.

Ralph, S. S., & Taylor, C. M. (2005). *Nursing diagnosis reference manual* (6th ed.). Philadelphia: Lippincott Williams & Wilkins.

Richter, S. B., et al. (2006). Normal infant and childhood development. In J. McMillan, R. Feigin, C. DeAngelis, & M. Jones, Jr. (Eds.), *Oski's pediatrics: Principles and practice* (4th ed.). Philadelphia: Lippincott Williams & Wilkins.

Smeltzer, S. C., Bare, B. G., Hinkle, J. L., & Cheever, K. H. (2008). *Brunner and Suddarth's textbook of medical-surgical nursing* (11th ed.). Philadelphia: Lippincott Williams & Wilkins.

Wong, D. L., Perry, S., Hockenberry, M., Lowdermilk, D. L., & Wilson, D. (2006). *Maternal child nursing care* (3rd ed.). St. Louis, MO: Mosby.

CHAPTER 26

Berger, K. S. (2006). *The developing person through childhood and adolescence* (7th ed.). New York: Worth Publishers.

Dudek, S. G. (2006). *Nutrition essentials for nursing practice* (5th ed). Philadelphia: Lippincott Williams & Wilkins.

Finberg, L. (2006). Feeding the healthy child. In J. McMillan, R. Feigin, C. DeAngelis, & M. Jones, Jr. (Eds.), *Oski's pediatrics: Principles and practice* (4th ed.). Philadelphia: Lippincott Williams & Wilkins.

Hockenberry, M. J., & Wilson, D. (2007). *Wong's nursing care of infants and children* (8th ed.). St. Louis, MO: Mosby Elsevier.

NANDA-I Nursing Diagnoses: Definitions and Classification 2007–2008. (2007) Philadelphia: NANDA International.

Pence, C., & McErlane, K. (2005). Tooth avulsion. *Nursing 2005, 35*(12), 88.

Pillitteri, A. (2007). *Maternal and child health nursing: Care of the childbearing and childrearing family* (5th ed.). Philadelphia: Lippincott Williams & Wilkins.

Ralph, S. S., & Taylor, C. M. (2005). *Nursing diagnosis reference manual* (6th ed.). Philadelphia: Lippincott Williams & Wilkins.

Richter, S. B., et al. (2006). Normal infant and childhood development. In *Oski's pediatrics: Principles and practice* (4th ed.). Philadelphia: Lippincott Williams & Wilkins.

Smeltzer, S. C., Bare, B.G., Hinkle, J.L., & Cheever, K.H. (2008). *Brunner and Suddarth's textbook of medical-surgical nursing* (11th ed.). Philadelphia: Lippincott Williams & Wilkins.

Wong, D. L., Perry, S., Hockenberry, M., Lowdermilk, D. L., & Wilson, D. (2006). *Maternal child nursing care* (3rd ed.). St. Louis, MO: Mosby.

CHAPTER 27

Armstrong, M. L. (2004). Caring for the patient with piercings. *RN, 67*(6), 46–53.

Berger, K. S. (2006). *The developing person through childhood and adolescence* (7th ed.). New York: Worth Publishers.

Dudek, S. G. (2006). *Nutrition essentials for nursing practice* (5th ed.). Philadelphia: Lippincott Williams & Wilkins.

Finberg, L. (2006). Feeding the healthy child. In J. McMillan, R. Feigin, C. DeAngelis, & M. Jones, Jr. (Eds.), *Oski's pediatrics: Principles and practice* (4th ed.). Philadelphia: Lippincott Williams & Wilkins.

Hernandez, G., & Nester, C. (2006). Educating teens about vaccines. *Journal of Pediatric Health Care, 20*(5), 342–349.

Heyman, R. B. (2006). Adolescent substance abuse and other high-risk behaviors. In J. McMillan, R. Feigin, C. DeAngelis, & M. Jones, Jr. (Eds.), *Oski's pediatrics: Principles and practice* (4th ed.). Philadelphia: Lippincott Williams & Wilkins.

Hockenberry, M. J., & Wilson, D. (2007). *Wong's nursing care of infants and children* (8th ed.). St. Louis, MO: Mosby Elsevier.

Joffe, A. (2006). Introduction to adolescent medicine. In J. McMillan, R. Feigin, C. DeAngelis, & M. Jones, Jr. (Eds.), *Oski's pediatrics: Principles and practice* (4th ed.). Philadelphia: Lippincott Williams & Wilkins.

NANDA-I Nursing Diagnoses: Definitions and Classification 2007–2008. (2007) Philadelphia: NANDA International.

Pillitteri, A. (2007). *Maternal and child health nursing: Care of the childbearing and childrearing family* (5th ed.). Philadelphia: Lippincott Williams & Wilkins.

Ralph, S. S., & Taylor, C. M. (2005). *Nursing Diagnosis Reference Manual* (6th ed.). Philadelphia: Lippincott Williams & Wilkins.

Richter, S. B., et al. (2006). Normal infant and childhood development. In J. McMillan, R. Feigin, C. DeAngelis, & M. Jones, Jr. (Eds.), *Oski's pediatrics: Principles and practice* (4th ed.). Philadelphia: Lippincott Williams & Wilkins.

Smeltzer, S. C., Bare, B. G., Hinkle, J. L., & Cheever, K. H. (2008). *Brunner and Suddarth's textbook of medical-surgical nursing* (11th ed.). Philadelphia: Lippincott Williams & Wilkins.

Wong, D. L., Perry, S., Hockenberry, M., Lowdermilk, D. L., & Wilson, D. (2006). *Maternal child nursing care* (3rd ed.). St. Louis, MO: Mosby.

CHAPTER 28

Barone, M. A. (2006). Pediatric procedures. In J. McMillan, R. Feigin, C. DeAngelis, & M. Jones, Jr. (Eds.), *Oski's pediatrics: Principles and practice* (4th ed.). Philadelphia: Lippincott Williams & Wilkins.

Barness, L. A. (2006). Pediatric history and physical examination. In J. McMillan, R. Feigin, C. DeAngelis, & M. Jones, Jr. (Eds.), *Oski's pediatrics: Principles and practice* (4th ed.). Philadelphia: Lippincott Williams & Wilkins.

Berger, K. S. (2006). *The developing person through childhood and adolescence* (7th ed.). New York: Worth Publishers.

Fife, P. (2006). The eyes of the pediatric nurse. *American Journal of Nursing, 106*(7), 15.

Hockenberry, M. J., & Wilson, D. (2007). *Wong's nursing care of infants and children* (8th ed.). St. Louis, MO: Mosby Elsevier.

Kyle, T. (2008). *Essentials of pediatric nursing.* Philadelphia: Lippincott Williams & Wilkins.

NANDA-I Nursing Diagnoses: Definitions and Classification 2007–2008. (2007) Philadelphia: NANDA International.

Pillitteri, A. (2007). *Maternal and child health nursing: Care of the childbearing and childrearing family* (5th ed.). Philadelphia: Lippincott Williams & Wilkins.

Ralph, S. S., & Taylor, C. M. (2005). *Nursing diagnosis reference manual* (6th ed.). Philadelphia: Lippincott Williams & Wilkins.

Smeltzer, S. C., Bare, B. G., Hinkle, J. L., & Cheever, K. H. (2008). *Brunner and Suddarth's textbook of medical-surgical nursing* (11th ed.). Philadelphia: Lippincott Williams & Wilkins.

Wong, D. L., Perry, S., Hockenberry, M., Lowdermilk, D. L., & Wilson, D. (2006). *Maternal child nursing care* (3rd ed.). St. Louis, MO: Mosby.

CHAPTER 29

Berger, K. S. (2006). The developing person through childhood and adolescence (7th ed.). New York: Worth Publishers.

Dlugosz, C. K., et al. (2006). Appropriate use of nonprescription analgesics in pediatric patients. *Journal of Pediatric Health Care, 20*(5), 316–325.

Dunn, D. (2005). Preventing perioperative complications in special populations. *Nursing 2005, 35*(11), 36–45.

Hockenberry, M. J., Wilson, D., & Barrera, P. (2006). Implementing evidence-based nursing practice in a pediatric hospital. *Pediatric Nursing, 32*(4), 371–377.

Hockenberry, M. J., & Wilson, D. (2007). *Wong's nursing care of infants and children* (8th ed.). St. Louis, MO: Mosby Elsevier.

Kyle, T. (2008). *Essentials of pediatric nursing.* Philadelphia: Lippincott Williams & Wilkins.

Little, K., & Cutcliffe, S. (2006). The safe use of children's toys within the healthcare setting. *Nursing Times, 102*(38), 34–37.

NANDA-I Nursing Diagnoses: Definitions and Classification 2007–2008. (2007) Philadelphia: NANDA International.

Pillitteri, A. (2007). *Maternal and child health nursing: Care of the childbearing and childrearing family* (5th ed.). Philadelphia: Lippincott Williams & Wilkins.

Ralph, S. S., & Taylor, C. M. (2005). *Nursing diagnosis reference manual* (6th ed.). Philadelphia: Lippincott Williams & Wilkins.

Smeltzer, S. C., Bare, B. G., Hinkle, J. L., & Cheever, K. H. (2008). *Brunner and Suddarth's textbook of medical-surgical nursing* (11th ed.). Philadelphia: Lippincott Williams & Wilkins.

Van Dijk, M., Peters, J. W., Van Deventer, P., & Tibboel, D. (2005). Pain control: The COMFORT behavior scale. *American Journal of Nursing, 105*(1), 33–37.

Van Hulle Vincent, C. (2005). Nurses' knowledge, attitudes and practices regarding children's pain. *American Journal of Maternal/Child Nursing, 30*(3), 177–183.

Wong, D. L., Perry, S., Hockenberry, M., Lowdermilk, D. L., & Wilson, D. (2006). *Maternal child nursing care* (3rd ed.). St. Louis, MO: Mosby.

Zengerle-Levy, K. (2006). Nursing the child who is alone in the hospital. *Pediatric Nursing, 32*(3), 226–231, 237.

CHAPTER 30

Barness, L. A. (2006). Pediatric history and physical examination. In J. McMillan, R. Feigin, C. DeAngelis, & M. Jones, Jr. (Eds.), *Oski's pediatrics: Principles and practice* (4th ed.). Philadelphia: Lippincott Williams & Wilkins.

Berger, K. S. (2006). The developing person through childhood and adolescence (7th ed.). New York: Worth Publishers.

Bowden, V. R., & Greenberg, C.S. (2008). *Pediatric Nursing Procedures.* Philadelphia: Lippincott Williams & Wilkins.

Hockenberry, M. J., & Wilson, D. (2007). *Wong's nursing care of infants and children* (8th ed.). St. Louis, MO: Mosby Elsevier.

Kyle, T. (2008). *Essentials of pediatric nursing.* Philadelphia: Lippincott Williams & Wilkins.

Little, K., & Cutcliffe, S. (2006). The safe use of children's toys within the healthcare setting. *Nursing Times, 102*(38), 34–37.

NANDA-I Nursing Diagnoses: Definitions and Classification 2007–2008. (2007) Philadelphia: NANDA International.

Pillitteri, A. (2007). *Maternal and child health nursing: Care of the childbearing and childrearing family* (5th ed.). Philadelphia: Lippincott Williams & Wilkins.

Ralph, S. S., & Taylor, C. M. (2005). *Nursing diagnosis reference manual* (6th ed.) Philadelphia: Lippincott Williams & Wilkins.

Schell, K. (2006). Evidence-based practice: Noninvasive blood pressure measurement in children. *Pediatric Nursing, 32*(3), 263–267.

Smeltzer, S. C., Bare, B. G., Hinkle, J. L., & Cheever, K. H. (2008). *Brunner and Suddarth's textbook of medical-surgical nursing* (11th ed.). Philadelphia: Lippincott Williams & Wilkins.

Westhus, N. (2004) Methods to test feeding tube placement in children. *American Journal of Maternal/Child Nursing, 29*(5), 282–287.

Wong, D. L., Perry, S., Hockenberry, M., Lowdermilk, D. L., & Wilson, D. (2006). *Maternal child nursing care* (3rd ed.). St. Louis, MO: Mosby.

CHAPTER 31

Berger, K. S. (2006). The developing person through childhood and adolescence (7th ed.). New York: Worth Publishers.

Doellman, D. (2005). Ease a child's anxiety during PICC insertion—without sedation. *Nursing 2005, 35*(3), 68.

Hockenberry, M. J., & Wilson, D. (2007). *Wong's nursing care of infants and children* (8th ed.). St. Louis, MO: Mosby Elsevier.

Kyle, T. (2008). *Essentials of pediatric nursing.* Philadelphia: Lippincott Williams & Wilkins.

NANDA-I Nursing Diagnoses: Definitions and Classification 2007–2008. (2007) Philadelphia: NANDA International.

Pillitteri, A. (2007). *Maternal and child health nursing: Care of the childbearing and childrearing family* (5th ed.). Philadelphia: Lippincott Williams & Wilkins.

Ralph, S. S., & Taylor, C. M. (2005). *Nursing diagnosis reference manual* (6th ed.). Philadelphia: Lippincott Williams & Wilkins.

Rodgers, G. C., Jr., & Matyunas, N. J. (2006). Pharmacologic principles of drug therapy. In J. McMillan, R. Feigin, C. DeAngelis, & M. Jones, Jr. (Eds.), *Oski's pediatrics: Principles and practice* (4th ed.). Philadelphia: Lippincott Williams & Wilkins.

Smeltzer, S. C., Bare, B. G., Hinkle, J. L., & Cheever, K. H. (2008). *Brunner and Suddarth's textbook of medical-surgical nursing* (11th ed.). Philadelphia: Lippincott Williams & Wilkins.

Springhouse nurse's drug guide 2008. (9th ed.). (2008). Springhouse, PA: Lippincott Williams & Wilkins.

Wong, D. L., Perry, S., Hockenberry, M., Lowdermilk, D. L., & Wilson, D. (2006). *Maternal child nursing care* (3rd ed.). St. Louis, MO: Mosby.

CHAPTER 32

Berger, K. S. (2006). The developing person through childhood and adolescence (7th ed.). New York: Worth Publishers.

Blann, L. E. (2005). Early intervention for children and families with special needs. *American Journal of Maternal/Child Nursing, 30*(4), 263–269.

Clayton, J. (2006). Helping children cope with a debilitating disorder: Interview by Clare Lomas. *Nursing Times, 102*(35), 20–21.

Hockenberry, M. J., & Wilson, D. (2007). *Wong's nursing care of infants and children* (8th ed.). St. Louis, MO: Mosby Elsevier.

Immelt, S. (2006). Psychological adjustment in young children with chronic medical conditions. *Journal of Pediatric Nursing, 21*(5), 362–377.

Kyle, T. (2008). *Essentials of pediatric nursing.* Philadelphia: Lippincott Williams & Wilkins.

NANDA-I Nursing Diagnoses: Definitions and Classification 2007–2008. (2007) Philadelphia: NANDA International.

Pillitteri, A. (2007). *Maternal and child health nursing: Care of the childbearing and childrearing family* (5th ed.). Philadelphia: Lippincott Williams & Wilkins.

Ralph, S. S., & Taylor, C. M. (2005). *Nursing diagnosis reference manual* (6th ed.). Philadelphia: Lippincott Williams & Wilkins.

Wong, D. L., Perry, S., Hockenberry, M., Lowdermilk, D. L., & Wilson, D. (2006). *Maternal child nursing care* (3rd ed.). St. Louis, MO: Mosby.

CHAPTER 33

Berger, K. S. (2006). *The developing person through childhood and adolescence* (7th ed.). New York: Worth Publishers.

Child Abuse Prevention and Treatment Act as Amended by the Keeping Children and Families Safe Act of 2003. 42 U.S.C. 5106g. Sec. 111. Definitions. Available from the US Department of Health and Human Services at http://www.acf.hhs.gov/programs/cb/laws_policies/cblaws/capta03/sec_I_111.htm

Hockenberry, M. J., & Wilson, D. (2007). *Wong's nursing care of infants and children* (8th ed.). St. Louis, MO: Mosby Elsevier.

Karch, A. M. (2008). *2008 Lippincott's nursing drug guide.* Philadelphia: Lippincott Williams & Wilkins.

Kyle, T. (2008). *Essentials of pediatric nursing.* Philadelphia: Lippincott Williams & Wilkins.

NANDA-I Nursing Diagnoses: Definitions and Classification 2007–2008. (2007) Philadelphia: NANDA International.

Pillitteri, A. (2007). *Material and child health nursing: Care of the childbearing and childrearing family* (5th ed.). Philadelphia: Lippincott Williams & Wilkins.

Ralph, S. S., & Taylor, C. M. (2005). *Nursing diagnosis reference manual* (6th ed.). Philadelphia: Lippincott Williams & Wilkins.

Reece, R. M. (2006). Child maltreatment. In J. McMillan, R. Feigin, C. DeAngelis, & M. Jones, Jr. (Eds.), *Oski's pediatrics: Principles and practice* (4th ed.). Philadelphia: Lippincott Williams & Wilkins.

Smeltzer, S. C., Bare, B. G., Hinkle, J. L., & Cheever, K. H. (2008). *Brunner and Suddarth's textbook of medical-surgical nursing* (11th ed.). Philadelphia: Lippincott Williams & Wilkins.

Wong, D. L., Perry, S., Hockenberry, M., Lowdermilk, D. L., & Wilson, D. (2006). *Maternal child nursing care* (3rd ed.). St. Louis, MO: Mosby.

CHAPTER 34

Anonymous. (1970). American Journal of Nursing, 70(2), 335.

Berg, S. (2006). In their own voices: Families discuss end-of-life decision making. *Pediatric Nursing, 32(3),* 238–242.

Berger, K. S. (2006). *The developing person through childhood and adolescence* (7th ed.). New York: Worth Publishers.

Clements, P., & Bradley, J. (2005). When a young patient dies. *RN, 68(4),* 40.

Hockenberry, M. J., & Wilson, D. (2007). *Wong's nursing care of infants and children* (8th ed.). St. Louis, MO: Mosby Elsevier.

Hufton, E. (2006). Parting gifts: The spiritual needs of children. *Journal of Child Health Care, 10(3),* 240–250.

NANDA-I Nursing Diagnoses: Definitions and Classification 2007–2008. (2007) Philadelphia: NANDA International.

Pillitteri, A. (2007). *Maternal and child health nursing: Care of the childbearing and childrearing family* (5th ed.). Philadelphia: Lippincott Williams & Wilkins.

Kyle, T. (2008). *Essentials of pediatric nursing.* Philadelphia: Lippincott Williams & Wilkins.

Ralph, S. S., & Taylor, C. M. (2005). *Nursing diagnosis reference manual* (6th ed.). Philadelphia: Lippincott Williams & Wilkins.

Wong, D. L., Perry, S., Hockenberry, M., Lowdermilk, D. L., & Wilson, D. (2006). *Maternal child nursing care* (3rd ed.). St. Louis, MO: Mosby.

CHAPTER 35

Accardo, P. J., et al. (2006). Mental retardation. In J. McMillan, R. Feigin, C. DeAngelis, & M. Jones, Jr. (Eds.), *Oski's pediatrics: Principles and practice* (4th ed.). Philadelphia: Lippincott Williams & Wilkins.

American Psychiatric Association. (2000). *Diagnostic and statistical manual of mental disorders* (4th ed., text revision). Washington, DC: Author.

Blann, L. E. (2005). Early intervention for children and families with special needs. *American Journal of Maternal/Child Nursing, 30(4),* 263–269.

Boyd-Monk, H. (2005). Bringing common eye emergencies into focus. *Nursing 2005, 35(12),* 46–51.

Gambrell, M., & Flynn, N. (2004). Seizures 101. *Nursing 2004, 34(8),* 36–42.

Hockenberry, M. J., & Wilson, D. (2007). *Wong's nursing care of infants and children* (8th ed.). St. Louis, MO: Mosby Elsevier.

Kamienski, M. C. (2003). Reye syndrome. *American Journal of Nursing, 103(7),* 54–57.

Kyle, T. (2008). *Essentials of pediatric nursing.* Philadelphia: Lippincott Williams & Wilkins.

Marin, S. (2005) The impact of epilepsy on the adolescent. *American Journal of Maternal/Child Nursing, 30(5),* 321-326

NANDA-I Nursing Diagnoses: Definitions and Classification 2007–2008. (2007) Philadelphia: NANDA International.

O'Reilly, R. C. (2006). *What's hearing loss?* Retrieved November 2, 2006, from http://kidshealth.org/kid/health_problems/sight/hearing_impairment.html

Pillitteri, A. (2007). *Material and child health nursing: Care of the childbearing and childrearing family* (5th ed.). Philadelphia: Lippincott Williams & Wilkins.

Ralph, S. S., & Taylor, C. M. (2005). *Nursing diagnosis reference manual* (6th ed.). Philadelphia: Lippincott Williams & Wilkins.

Schwarzwald, H., & Kline, M. K. (2006). Otitis media. In J. McMillan, R. Feigin, C. DeAngelis, & M. Jones, Jr. (Eds.), *Oski's pediatrics: Principles and practices* (4th ed.). Philadelphia: Lippincott Williams & Wilkins.

Smeltzer, S. C., Bare, B. G., Hinkle, J. L., & Cheever, K. H. (2008). *Brunner and Suddarth's textbook of medical-surgical nursing* (11th ed.). Philadelphia: Lippincott Williams & Wilkins. Ross, J. L. (2005). Summer injuries: Near drowning. *RN, 68(7),* 36–42.

Wong, D. L., Perry, S., Hockenberry, M., Lowdermilk, D. L., & Wilson, D. (2006). *Maternal child nursing care* (3rd ed.). St. Louis, MO: Mosby.

CHAPTER 36

Carpenter, D. R., & Narsavage, G. L. (2004). One breath at a time: Living with cystic fibrosis. *Journal of Pediatric Nursing, 19(1),* 25–32.

Hockenberry, M. J., & Wilson, D. (2007). *Wong's nursing care of infants and children* (8th ed.). St. Louis, MO: Mosby Elsevier.

Karch, A. M. (2008). *2008 Lippincott's nursing drug guide.* Philadelphia: Lippincott Williams & Wilkins.

Kumar, C., et al. (2005). Children with asthma: A concern for the family. *American Journal of Maternal/Child Nursing, 30(5),* 305–311

Lauts, N. M. (2005). RSV: Protecting the littlest patients. *RN, 68(12),* 46–52.

NANDA-I Nursing Diagnoses: Definitions and Classification 2007–2008. (2007) Philadelphia: NANDA International.

Pruitt, B. (2005). Keeping respiratory syncytial virus at bay. *Nursing 2005, 35(11),* 62–64.

Pruitt, B. and Jacobs, M. (2005) Caring for a patient with asthma. *Nursing 2005, 35(2),* 48–51.

Pruitt, W. (2005) Teaching your patient to use a peak flow meter. *Nursing2005, 35(3)*54–55.

Pillitteri, A. (2007). *Maternal and child health nursing: Care of the childbearing and childrearing family* (5th ed.). Philadelphia: Lippincott Williams & Wilkins.

Ralph, S. S., & Taylor, C. M. (2005). *Nursing diagnosis reference manual* (6th ed.). Philadelphia: Lippincott Williams & Wilkins.

Smeltzer, S. C., Bare, B. G., Hinkle, J. L., & Cheever, K. H. (2008). *Brunner and Suddarth's textbook of medical-surgical nursing* (11th ed.). Philadelphia: Lippincott Williams & Wilkins.

Starke, J. R. (2006). Tuberculosis. In J. McMillan, R. Feigin, C. DeAngelis, & M. Jones, Jr. (Eds.), *Oski's pediatrics: Principles and practice* (4th ed.). Philadelphia: Lippincott Williams & Wilkins.

Wong, D. L., Perry, S., Hockenberry, M., Lowdermilk, D. L., & Wilson, D. (2006). *Maternal child nursing care* (3rd ed.). St. Louis, MO: Mosby.

CHAPTER 37

Cassidy, J. T. (2006). Rheumatic diseases of childhood. In J. McMillan, R. Feigin, C. DeAngelis, & M. Jones, Jr. (Eds.), *Oski's pediatrics: Principles and practice* (4th ed.). Philadelphia: Lippincott Williams & Wilkins.Dorman, K. (2005). Sickle cell crisis! Managing the pain. *RN, 68(12),* 33–37.

French L, Howell, G., Haven, J., & Britten, P. (2006) Designing MyPyramid for kids materials to help children eat right, exercise, have fun. *Journal of Nutrition Education and Behavior, 38,* S158–S159.

Hockenberry, M. J., & Wilson, D. (2007). *Wong's nursing care of infants and children* (8th ed.). St. Louis, MO: Mosby Elsevier.

Kyle, T. (2008). *Essentials of pediatric nursing.* Philadelphia: Lippincott Williams & Wilkins.

Metules, T., & Bauer, J. (2006) Be on the lookout for this seasonal ailment. *RN, 69(2),* 26–32.

NANDA-I Nursing Diagnoses: Definitions and Classification 2007–2008. (2007) Philadelphia: NANDA International.

Pillitteri, A. (2007). *Maternal and child health nursing* (5th ed.). Philadelphia: Lippincott Williams & Wilkins.

Ralph, S. S., & Taylor, C. M. (2005). *Nursing diagnosis reference manual* (6th ed.). Philadelphia: Lippincott Williams & Wilkins.

Wong, D. L., Perry, S., Hockenberry, M., Lowdermilk, D. L., & Wilson, D. (2006). *Maternal child nursing care* (3rd ed.). St. Louis, MO: Mosby.

CHAPTER 38

American Academy of Pediatrics, Committee on Injury, Violence, and Poison Prevention. (2007). Poison treatment in the home. *Pediatrics, 119*(5), 1031. Retrieved June 19, 2008, from http://aappolicy.aappublications.org/cgi/content/full/pediatrics;112/5/1182

Broderick, M. (2004). Pediatric poisoning. *RN, 67*(9), 37–43.

Centers for Disease Control and Prevention. (2005). *Preventing lead poisoning in young children: A statement by the Centers for Disease Control and Prevention Atlanta.* Retrieved June 19, 2008, from http://www.cdc.gov/nceh/lead/publications/prevleadpoisoning.pdf

Karch, A. M. (2008). *2008 Lippincott's nursing drug guide.* Philadelphia: Lippincott Williams & Wilkins.

Kyle, T. (2008). *Essentials of pediatric nursing.* Philadelphia: Lippincott Williams & Wilkins.

Lifschitz, C. H. (2006). Celiac disease. In J. McMillan, R. Feigin, C. DeAngelis, & M. Jones, Jr. (Eds.), *Oski's pediatrics: Principles and practice* (3rd ed.). Philadelphia: Lippincott Williams & Wilkins.

Metules, T., & Bauer, J. (2006). Be on the lookout for this seasonal ailment. *RN, 69*(2), 26–32.

NANDA-I Nursing Diagnoses: Definitions and Classification 2007–2008. (2007) Philadelphia: NANDA International.

Needleman, H. L. (2006). Lead poisoning. In J. McMillan, R. Feigin, C. DeAngelis, & M. Jones, Jr. (Eds.), *Oski's pediatrics: Principles and practice* (4th ed.). Philadelphia: Lippincott Williams & Wilkins.

Pillitteri, A. (2007). *Material and child health nursing: Care of the childbearing and childrearing family* (5th ed.). Philadelphia: Lippincott Williams & Wilkins.

Plotnick, L. P. (2006). Type 1 (insulin dependent) diabetes mellitus. In J. McMillan, R. Feigin, C. DeAngelis, & M. Jones, Jr. (Eds.), *Oski's pediatrics: Principles and practice* (4th ed.). Philadelphia: Lippincott Williams & Wilkins.

Ralph, S. S., & Taylor, C. M. (2005). *Nursing diagnosis reference manual* (6th ed.). Philadelphia: Lippincott Williams & Wilkins.

Sullivan-Bolyai, S., Rosenberg, R., & Bayard, M. (2006). Fathers' reflections on parenting young children with type I diabetes. *American Journal of Maternal/Child Nursing, 31*(1), 24–31.

Wong, D. L., Perry, S., Hockenberry, M., & Lowdermilk, D. L., Wilson, D. (2006). *Maternal child nursing care* (3rd ed.). St. Louis, MO: Mosby.

CHAPTER 39

Berry, A. K. (2006). Helping children with nocturnal enuresis. *American Journal of Nursing, 106*(I8), 56–64.

Hockenberry, M. J., & Wilson, D. (2007). *Wong's nursing care of infants and children* (8th ed.). St. Louis, MO: Mosby Elsevier.

Karch, A. M. (2008). *2008 Lippincott's nursing drug guide.* Philadelphia: Lippincott Williams & Wilkins.

Kyle, T. (2008). *Essentials of pediatric nursing.* Philadelphia: Lippincott Williams & Wilkins.

McEvoy, M., Chang, J., & Coupey, S. (2004). Common menstrual disorders in adolescence: Nursing interventions. *American Journal of Maternal/Child Nursing, 29*, 41–49.

NANDA-I Nursing Diagnoses: Definitions and Classification 2007–2008. (2007) Philadelphia: NANDA International.

Pillitteri, A. (2007). *Material and child health nursing: Care of the childbearing and childrearing family* (5th ed.). Philadelphia: Lippincott Williams & Wilkins.

Ralph, S. S., & Taylor, C. M. (2005). *Nursing diagnosis reference manual* (6th ed.). Philadelphia: Lippincott Williams & Wilkins.

Wong, D. L., Perry, S., Hockenberry, M., &Lowdermilk, D. L., Wilson, D. (2006). *Maternal \child nursing care* (3rd ed.). St. Louis, MO: Mosby.

CHAPTER 40

Connelley, T. W. (2005). Family functioning and hope in children with juvenile rheumatoid arthritis. *American Journal of Maternal/Child Nursing, 30*(4), 245–250.

NANDA-I Nursing Diagnoses: Definitions and Classification 2007–2008. (2007) Philadelphia: NANDA International.

Karch, A. M. (2008). *2008 Lippincott's nursing drug guide.* Philadelphia: Lippincott Williams & Wilkins.

Kyle, T. (2008). *Essentials of pediatric nursing.* Philadelphia: Lippincott Williams & Wilkins.

Sponseller, P. D. (2006). Bone, joint, and muscle problems. In J. McMillan, R. Feigin, C. DeAngelis, & M. Jones, Jr. (Eds.), *Oski's pediatrics: Principles and practice* (4th ed.). Philadelphia: Lippincott Williams & Wilkins.

CHAPTER 41

Chiocca, E, (2006). Pertussis. *Nursing 2006, 36*(7), 72.

Cibulka, N. J. (2006). Mother-to-child transmission of HIV in the United States. *American Journal of Nursing, 106*(7), 56–64.

Gardner, J. (2006). What you need to know about genital herpes. *Nursing 2006, 36*(10), 26–27.

Goldrick, B. (2005). Emerging infections pertussis on the rise. *American Journal of Nursing, 105*(1), 69–71.

Karch, A. M. (2008). *2008 Lippincott's nursing drug guide.* Philadelphia: Lippincott Williams & Wilkins.

Kelly, P. J., Lesser, J., & Smoots, A. (2005). Tailoring STI and HIV prevention programs for teens. *American Journal of Maternal/ Child Nursing, 30*(4), 237–244.

Kyle, T. (2008). *Essentials of pediatric nursing.* Philadelphia: Lippincott Williams & Wilkins.

Laskowski-Jones, L. (2006). First aid for bee, wasp and hornet stings. *Nursing-2006, 36*(7), 58–59.

NANDA-I Nursing Diagnoses: Definitions and Classification 2007–2008. (2007) Philadelphia: NANDA International.

Nowlin, A. (2006). The delicate business of burn care. *RN, 69*(l), 52–63.

Orr, D. P., & Blythe, M. J. (2006). Sexually transmitted diseases. In J. McMillan, R. Feigin, C. DeAngelis, & M. Jones, Jr. (Eds.), *Oski's pediatrics: Principles and practice* (4th ed.). Philadelphia: Lippincott Williams & Wilkins.

Schweon, S. (2005). Whooping cough makes its return. *RN, 68*(2), 32–37.

Snow, M. (2006). Mumps makes a comeback. *Nursing 2006, 36*(10), 18–19.

Starke, J. R. (2006). Tuberculosis. In J. McMillan, R. Feigin, C. DeAngelis, & M. Jones, Jr. (Eds.), *Oski's pediatrics: Principles and practice* (4th ed.). Philadelphia: Lippincott Williams & Wilkins.

Stringer, M., Ratcliffe, S. J., & Gross, R. (2006). Acceptance of hepatitis b vaccination by pregnant adolescents. *American Journal of Maternal/Child Nursing, 31*(1), 54–60.

Wong, D. L., Perry, S., Hockenberry, M., Lowdermilk, D. L., & Wilson, D. (2006). *Maternal child nursing care* (3rd ed.). St. Louis, MO: Mosby.

CHAPTER 42

American Psychiatric Association. (2000). *Diagnostic and statistical manual of mental disorders* (4th ed., text revision). Washington, DC: Author.

Aschenbrenner, D. S. (2005). The use of antidepressants in children and adolescents. *American Journal of Nursing, 105*(2), 79–81.

Fox Quillen, T. (2005). Putting the brakes on attention-deficit/hyperactivity disorder. *Nursing 2005, 35*(2), 12–13

Harris, J.C. (2006). Depression in childhood and adolescence. In J. McMillan, R. Feigin, C. DeAngelis, & M. Jones, Jr. (Eds.), *Oski's pediatrics: Principles and practice* (4th ed.). Philadelphia: Lippincott Williams & Wilkins.

Harris, J.C. (2006). Suicide. In J. McMillan, R. Feigin, C. DeAngelis, & M. Jones, Jr. (Eds.), *Oski's pediatrics: Principles and practice* (4th ed.). Philadelphia: Lippincott Williams & Wilkins.

Hess, D., & DeBoer, S. (2002). Emergency: Ecstasy. *American Journal of Nursing, 102*(4), 45.

Heyman, R. B. (2006). Adolescent substance abuse and other high-risk behaviors. In J. McMillan, R. Feigin, C. DeAngelis, & M. Jones, Jr.

(Eds.), *Oski's pediatrics: Principles and practice* (4th ed.). Philadelphia: Lippincott Williams & Wilkins.

Hockenberry, M. J., & Wilson, D. (2007). *Wong's nursing care of infants and children* (8th ed.). St. Louis, MO: Mosby Elsevier.

Karch, A. M. (2008). *2008 Lippincott's nursing drug guide*. Philadelphia: Lippincott Williams & Wilkins.

Kirkland, R. T. (2006). Failure to thrive. In J. McMillan, R. Feigin, C. DeAngelis, & M. Jones, Jr. (Eds.), *Oski's pediatrics: Principles and practice* (4th ed.). Philadelphia: Lippincott Williams & Wilkins.

Kreipe, R. E. (2006) Eating disorders. In J. McMillan, R. Feigin, C. DeAngelis, & M. Jones, Jr. (Eds.), *Oski's pediatrics: Principles and practice* (4th ed.). Philadelphia: Lippincott Williams & Wilkins.

Kyle, T. (2008). *Essentials of pediatric nursing*. Philadelphia: Lippincott Williams & Wilkins.

Murphy, K. (2005). How you can help prevent teen suicide. *Nursing 2005, 35*(12), 43–45.

NANDA-I Nursing Diagnoses: Definitions and Classification 2007–2008. (2007) Philadelphia: NANDA International.

National Institute of Drug Abuse for Teens. (n.d.). Facts on Drugs: Anabolic Steroids. Retrieved June 23, 2008, from http://teens.drugabuse.gov/facts/facts_ster2.asp

Pillitteri, A. (2007). *Material and child health nursing: Care of the childbearing and childrearing family* (5th ed.). Philadelphia: Lippincott Williams & Wilkins.

Ralph, S. S., & Taylor, C. M. (2005). *Nursing diagnosis reference manual* (6th ed.). Philadelphia: Lippincott Williams & Wilkins.

Sand-Loud, N., & Rappaport, L.A. (2006). Enuresis. In J. McMillan, R. Feigin, C. DeAngelis, & M. Jones, Jr. (Eds.), *Oski's pediatrics: Principles and practice* (4th ed.). Philadelphia: Lippincott Williams & Wilkins.

Schonwald, A., & Rappaport, L.A. (2006). Encopresis. In J. McMillan, R. Feigin, C. DeAngelis, & M. Jones, Jr. (Eds.), *Oski's pediatrics: Principles and practice* (4th ed.). Philadelphia: Lippincott Williams & Wilkins.

Wong, D. L., Perry, S., Hockenberry, M., & Lowdermilk, D. L., Wilson, D. (2006). *Maternal child nursing care* (3rd ed.). St. Louis, MO: Mosby.

Index

A

A Balloon Story, 725–726, 726f
Abbreviations, Joint Commission's "Do Not Use" list of, 964
Abdomen assessment, newborn, 297
Abdominal incisions, for cesarean birth, 245, 246f
Abdominal thrusts, 853–854, 853f
Abduction, infant, 310, 310b, 313
ABO incompatibility, 405, 470
Abortion
  complete, 385t
  controversy over, 3
  habitual (recurrent), 385t
  incomplete, 385t
  induced, 72, 86–87, 86t
  inevitable, 385t
  missed, 385t
  spontaneous, 384–387
    causes of, 384–385
    clinical manifestations and types of, 385–386, 385t
    definition and epidemiology of, 384
    nursing care for, 386–387
    self-care after, 386
    treatment of, 385t, 386
  therapeutic, 86, 86t
  threatened, 385t
Abruptio placentae, 244, 390–392, 391f
Absence seizures, 756
Abstinence, 72
Abuse, in family, 711–719. See also specific types
  child, 711–717 (See also Child abuse)
  domestic violence, 718
  dysfunctional family in, 711
  nursing process for child in, 716–717, 716t
  signs of, 716t
  substance abuse, parental, 718–719
Accelerations, fetal heart rate, 214
Acceptance, gradual, 700
Accident prevention
  in adolescents, 616–617
  in infants, 552–553
  in preschoolers, 583–584, 583f
  in school-aged children, 598, 598f
  in toddlers, 567–569
    burns, 568
    drowning, 567–568
    motor vehicle, 567–568, 567f
    toxic ingestions, 568–569
Acetaminophen, on breast-fed infant, 966
Achylia, 793
Acid–base balance, 690–691
Acidosis, 691
Acne, 172, 174f
Acne vulgaris, 902–903, 903f
Acquired disorders, 467–475. See also specific disorders
  hemolytic disease of newborn, 469–471 (See also Hemolytic disease of newborn)

newborn of diabetic mother, 471–472
newborn of mother with substance abuse
  fetal alcohol syndrome, 472–473
  neonatal substance withdrawal, 473, 473f
  overview, 472
newborn with congenitally acquired infection, 473, 474t–475t
respiratory, 467–469
  meconium aspiration syndrome, 468
  sudden infant death syndrome, 468–469, 469f
  transient tachypnea of the newborn, 467–468
Acquired immunodeficiency syndrome (AIDS). See AIDS
Acrocyanosis, in newborn, 292
Acronyms, Joint Commission's "Do Not Use" list of, 964
Active immunity, 928b
Active phase (active labor)
  definition and overview of, 178, 178t
  nursing care in, 220–223
    evaluation, 223
    fetal status assessment, 221
    implementation, 222–223, 223f
    labor progress assessment, 220–221
    maternal status assessment, 221, 221b, 221f
    nursing diagnoses, 221–222
    outcome identification and planning, 222
Actual nursing diagnoses, 21
Acupressure, for labor/birth pain, 187t, 190
Acupuncture, for labor/birth pain, 187t, 190
Acute lymphoblastic leukemia (ALL), 820–823, 822f
Acute myelogenous leukemia (AML), 820–823, 822f
Acyclovir
  for genital herpes, 921
  for herpes simplex virus in pregnancy, 364
Adaptation, physiologic, of newborn, 284–288. See also Physiologic adaptation, of newborn
Adenoidectomy, 777–778
Adenoiditis, 777–778
Adenoids, 777
Adenopathy, 821
Admission, in labor and birth, 203–208
  additional assessments in, 205–208
    labor and birth preferences, 208
    labor status, 205–208, 206f
    maternal health history and physical, 205, 205b, 206f
  immediate assessments in, 203–205
    birth imminence, 203, 204f
    fetal status, 203–204
    maternal status, 204–205
    risk assessment, 204
  routine admission orders in, 208, 208t

Adolescence
  early, 605
  growth and development in, 604–605 (See also Growth and development, 11-18 years)
  preparation for, 606
Adolescent development, 605–609
  developmental tasks in, 606, 607t
  physical, 606
  psychosocial, 606–609
    body image in, 608–609
    overview of, 606–607, 608f
    personality in, 608, 608f
Adolescent health status, 15–16, 16t
Adolescents
  client interview of, 625
  communication with, 533
  death and dying in, understanding of, 725
  pregnancy in, 375–377
Adoption
  open, 28
  placing newborn for, grief from, 445–446
Adoptive family, 28
Afterpains, 271–272
Age-related concerns in pregnancy, 375–378
  adolescent pregnancy, 375–377
  pregnancy in later life, 377–378
Aggression, in preschoolers, 579
AIDS, in children, 922t, 923–927
  cause and classification of, 923
  clinical manifestations of, 922t, 924
  epidemiology of, 923
  in infants, 923–924
  nursing process for, 924–927
    assessment, 924
    evaluation, 927
    implementation, 924–927
    nursing diagnoses, 924
    outcome identification and planning, 924
  prevention of, 923
  transmission of, 922t, 923–924
  treatment of, 924
AIDS, in pregnancy, 366–372
  clinical manifestations of, 366–367, 367b
  diagnosis of, 367
  epidemiology of, 366
  nursing care for, 368
  nursing process for, 368–372
    assessment, 368–370, 369b–370b
    evaluation, 371–372
    implementation, 370–371
    nursing diagnoses, 370
    outcome identification and planning, 370
  treatment of, 367–368
Airplane glue, 945
Airway clearance, newborn
  nursing care for, 305, 305f, 310
  parent teaching on, 318

Airways, newborn, 305, 305f
Akinetic seizures, 756
Albuterol sulfate, for asthma, 784, 785t
Alcohol abuse (alcoholism)
    in adolescents, 617
    in children, 943–944
    resources on, 943
Alcohol consumption
    fetal alcohol syndrome from, 472–473
    preconception, 70–71
    on pregnancy, 155
Alcoholics Anonymous (AA), 943
Alkalosis, 691
Allergen, 905
Allergic disorders, 905–909
    atopic dermatitis, 906–908, 906f
    diagnosis of, 905
    epidemiology and etiology of, 905
    hyposensitization in, 906
    plant allergies, 908–909, 909f
    skin allergies, 908
Allergic rhinitis, 777, 777f
"Allergic salute," 777, 777f
Allografts, 915
Alopecia, 822
Alpha-fetoprotein, in spina bifida, 480
Alternative delivery systems, 10
Ambiguous genitalia, 500–501
Amblyopia, 748
Ambulatory payment classifications
        (APC), 10
Amenorrhea, 63, 876
    breast-feeding, 333
    causes of, 117
    lactational, 74
    in pregnancy, 117
Amniocentesis, 142–143, 142f, 143b
Amnioinfusion, 215, 418
Amnion, 104, 107, 107f
Amniotic cavity, 104
Amniotic fluid, 107
Amniotic fluid embolism (AFE), 419–420
Amniotic sac, 142
Amniotomy, 241
Amoxicillin, for Chlamydia in pregnancy,
        364
Amphetamine abuse, 946
Anabolic steroids, 945
Anal atresia, 498, 498f
Analgesia. See also specific types
Analgesics. See also specific analgesics
    abuse of, 945
Anal stage, 526
Android pelvis, 168, 168f
Anemia
    Cooley's, 815–816
    hypochromic, microcytic, 812
    iron-deficiency
        in children, 812–813
        in pregnancy, 355–356
    macrocytic, 355
    microcytic, 355
    in pregnancy, 355–356
    sickle cell
        in children, 813–815, 813f
        in pregnancy, 355–356
Anesthesia, for labor/birth pain, 191–196
    development of, 5
    general, 193t, 196
    regional, 191–195, 192t–193t
        complications with, 195–196
        epidural, 192t, 193–195, 194f

intrathecal, 193, 193t, 194f, 195
    overview, 191
    paracervical block, 192t, 193
    pudendal block, 191–193
Angel dust, 945
Angioedema, 908
Angiotensin-converting enzyme (ACE)
        inhibitors
    on breast-fed infant, 967
    for congestive heart failure, 806
    in pregnancy, 353
Angiotensin II receptor blockers, in
        pregnancy, 353
Animal bites, 909
Ankle edema, prenatal care for, 149t
Ankylosis, 892
Anorexia nervosa, 948–955
    in adolescents, 608–609, 949f
    in children, 948–949
    nursing care plan for, 952–954
    nursing process for, 949–951
Anthelmintic, 848
Anthropoid pelvis, 167–168, 168f
Antibiotics. See also specific agents;
        specific disorders
    10-day course of, 777
    on breast-fed infant, 967
Antibodies
    in children, 900
    in preterm newborn, 457
Antibody screen
    definition of, 928b
    in first prenatal visit, 138
Anticipatory grief, 728
Anticoagulant therapy, 442
Anticonvulsant agents, 758t
Antidepressants. See also specific agents
        and disorders
    on breast-fed infant, 967
Anti-D immunoglobulin, 140, 404–405
Antiepileptic drugs (AEDs)
    in pregnancy, 358–359
    for seizure disorders, 758t
Antigen, 928b
Antihypertensives. See also specific agents
    on breast-fed infant, 967
Antioxidants. See also specific agents
    in pregnancy, 130
Antitoxin, 928b
Anuria in children, postoperative, 653
Anus, imperforate, 498, 498f
Anxiety reduction
    in labor, 219
    in labor, first stage, 222
    prenatal care for, 146–147
Apgar score, 288, 289t
Apnea, in preterm newborn, 456,
        460–461
Apnea monitor
    in children, 634, 635f
    home, 469, 469f
Appearance
    general, in children, 628–629
    of newborn, 290
Appendicitis, 846–847
Appropriate for gestational age (AGA),
        451
Arm recoil, 453t
ART, 359t
Arthralgia, 808
Artificial nutrition, 335. See also
        Formula-feeding

Artificial rupture of membranes, 241
Ascaris lumbricoides, 848
Ascites, 873
Ascorbic acid. See Vitamin C
Asphyxia, fetal, biophysical profile of,
        145
Aspiration, in preterm newborn, 462
Aspirin
    food with, 892
    for juvenile rheumatoid arthritis,
        891–892
    for Kawasaki disease, 812
    signs of toxicity with, 810
Assault, sexual, 715
Assessment, 21, 21f. See also specific
        disorders
Assisted/advanced reproductive therapy
        (ART), 90, 90b
Assisted delivery, 241–244
    complications of, 244
    episiotomy, 241–242, 242b, 242f
    forceps-assisted, 243–244, 243f
    induction of labor, 238–241 (See also
        Labor, induction of)
    nursing care in, 244
    vacuum-assisted, 242, 243f
Associative play, 579
Asthma, 781–788
    causes of, 781
    clinical manifestations of, 782
    definition of, 781
    diagnosis of, 782
    epidemiology and types of, 781–782
    nursing process for
        assessment, 785–786
        evaluation, 787–788
        implementation, 786–787
        nursing diagnoses, 786
        outcome identification and planning,
            786
    pathophysiology of, 782, 782f
    in pregnancy, 356–358
    treatment of, 782–785
        chest physiotherapy, 784–785
        goals, 783
        medications, 784, 785t
        metered-dose inhaler, 784, 785f
        nebulizer, 784, 785f
        peak flow meter, 782–783, 782f
        stepwise approach, 784t
Astigmatism, 745
Ataxia, 762
Athlete's foot, 903–904
Atonic seizures, 756
Atopic dermatitis, 906–908, 906f
Atresia
    anal, 498, 498f
    definition of, 496
    esophageal, 496–498, 497f
Attachment, 265–267, 266b, 266f, 267f,
        446
    lack of, 446–447
    vs. malattachment, 447t
    maternal–newborn, 270, 270b
    parent–newborn, 232–233, 233f, 274
    poor, 270, 270b
Attention deficit disorder (ADD), 939
Attention deficit hyperactivity disorder
        (ADHD), 939
Attention focusing, for labor/birth pain,
        186–188, 187t
Attitude, fetal, 170–171, 171f

Atypical uterine bleeding, 63
Auditory Brainstem Response, 318
Aura, 756
Autism, 937–938
Autografts, 915
Autonomy
    in growth and develoment, 527t, 528,
        528f
    in toddlers, 558
Axillary temperature
    of children, 632–633, 633f
    of newborn, 290, 290f, 290t, 305
Azithromycin, for chlamydia, 921
Azotemia, 692

B
Babinski's sign, 298–299
Baby blues, 443–444, 444b
Baby bottle syndrome, 338–339
Baby care classes, 159, 159b
Backaches, prenatal care for, 148t, 150
Back assessment, newborn, 298
Back blows, 853–854, 853f
Back labor, 185
Back pain, in pregnancy, 122, 122f
Back to Sleep campaign, 17
Balanced suspension traction, 884, 885f
Ballard scoring system, 451, 452f, 453t
Balloon Story, A, 725–726, 726f
Ballottement, 118
Barbiturates. *See also specific agents*
    abuse of, 946
    for labor and birth pain, 190, 192t
Barlow's sign, 298–299, 502
Barrier methods, contraceptive, 76–79
    cervical cap, 79
    condom
        female, 77–78, 78f
        male, 76–77
    diaphragm, 78–79, 78f
    spermicidal agents, 76
Basal body temperature (BBT) method,
        74–75
Basic life support, for infants and
        children, 769t, 770f
Bathing
    first bath in, 311–312, 313f
    of infants, 550–551, 551f
    of preschooler, 582
    Sitz bath in, 271–272
    of toddlers, 563
Beckwith-Wiedemann syndrome, 455
Beclomethasone, for asthma, 784, 785t
Bed-wetting, 870, 940
Behavior
    in children, 629–630, 629t
    parental, 29–30, 29f
    unoccupied, 579
Behavioral adaptation, newborn, 288
Behavioral assessment, of newborn,
        299–300
Benzoyl peroxide, for acne, 903
Beriberi, 830
Beta-blockers, on breast-fed infant, 967
Beta-carotene, 129
Beta-hemolytic streptococci group A, 932t
Bettelheim, Bruno, 531
Bicycle helmets, 583, 583f, 598, 598f
Bilateral, 491
Bilirubin, in newborn, 287–288
Bimanual examination, in first prenatal
        visit, 137–138, 138f

Binocular vision, 747–748
Bioethical issues, in prenatal testing, 8–9
Biology, children's concept of, 599t
Biophysical profile, 145
Birth, 178t, 179. *See also* Labor
    in asthmatic, 357
    cesarean (*See* Cesarean birth)
    children's concept of, 599t
    communicating expectations about,
        155–156
    nursing care during (*See* Labor and
        birth nursing care)
    pain management in (*See* Pain
        management, labor and birth)
    preparing patient for, 155–160
        childbirth education classes in, 156,
            158b, 159b
        choosing support person in, 156
        communicating expectations in,
            155–156, 157b
        packing for hospital/birthing center
            in, 155, 156b
        pregnancy and postpartum exercise
            classes in, 156, 159
    vaginal canal in, 169
Birth center, packing for, 155, 156b
Birth control pills, for dysmenorrhea, 64
Birth defects. *See* Congenital
        malformations; *specific defects*
Birth imminence, on admission for
        labor/birth, 203, 204f
Birth marks, in newborn, 292
Birth nursing care. *See* Labor and birth
        nursing care
Birth plan, 156, 157b
    on admission for labor/birth, 208
    in transition phase, 224
Birth preferences, on admission for
        labor/birth, 208
Birth rate, 14b
Birth settings, 32–33, 32f
Birth weight
    high, 126
    low, 125–126
Bishop score, 239, 239t
Bites
    animal, 909
    insect, 910
    snake, 910
    spider, 909
    tick, 909–910
Black eye, 748
Blackheads, 902
Black widow spiders, 909
Bladder exstrophy, 500, 500f
Blastocyst, 102–103, 103f
Bleeding disorders of pregnancy, 383–394
    abruptio placentae, 390–392, 391f
    cervical insufficiency, 387
    early pregnancy loss, 384–387 (*See also*
        Spontaneous abortion)
    ectopic pregnancy, 112–113, 383–384,
        383f
    nursing process for, 392–394
    overview, 383
    placenta previa, 389–391, 389f
Blended family, 28
Blindness, 745
Blocks, for labor/birth pain
    paracervical, 192t, 193
    pudendal, 191–193
    spinal, 193–195, 193t, 194f

Blood-borne pathogens. *See also specific
        disorders and pathogens*
    occupational health and, 959–960
Blood clot formation, 816, 816f
Blood clotting factors, in pregnancy, 121
Blood collection, in children, 674, 674f
Blood glucose. *See* Glucose, blood
Blood incompatibilities
    ABO, 405
    Rh, 404–405
Blood plasma, in pregnancy, 121
Blood pressure
    in children, 635–636, 635f, 635t, 975
    in infants, 540
    in newborn, 290, 290t
    in pregnancy, 121–122, 122f
    prenatal assessment of, 139, 139f
Blood supply, for pelvic organs, female,
        53, 53f
Blood typing, in first prenatal visit, 138
Blood volume, in pregnancy, 121
Body image, in adolescents, 608–609
Body lice, 904–905
Body mass index (BMI)
    high (*See* Obesity)
    in pregnancy, 125
Body piercings, 611
Body proportions
    of children, 518, 518f
    of newborn, 290
Body surface area (BSA) method,
        683–684, 684f
Body temperature. *See* Temperature, body
Body weight method, 683
Boggy uterus, 262
Bolus feeding, 667
Bonding, 265–267, 266b, 266f, 267f. *See
        also* Attachment
    maternal–newborn, 270, 270b
    parent–newborn, 232–233, 233f, 274
    poor, 270, 270b
Bone age, 539
Bone marrow, 880. *See also*
        Musculoskeletal disorders
Bone marrow aspiration, in children, 820
Bones, 880–881, 882f. *See also*
        Musculoskeletal disorders
Bony pelvis, 167, 168f
Books about death, for children,
        725–726, 726f, 727t
Bordetella pertussis, 929t
Borrelia burgdorferi, 932t
Boston brace, 893–894, 893f
Bottle feeding
    bottle preparation in, 337–338
    vs. breast-feeding, 324–325
    of preterm newborn, 462–463
Bottle-mouth caries, 338–339
Bowel sounds, in newborn, 297
Bowlby, John, 531
Braces, for scoliosis, 893–894, 893f
Brachial pulse assessment, newborn, 297,
        298f
Brachycephaly, 508
Bradley method, 158b, 186
Bradycardia
    in children, 806
    fetal, in labor/birth, 213
BRAT
    for cystic fibrosis, 794
    for diabetes mellitus in pregnancy, 349
BRAT diet, 836

Braxton Hicks contractions, 118, 120
    at onset of labor, 175
    spontaneous, in contraction stress test,
        145
Breakthrough pain, after cesarean, 276
Breast anatomy, 327, 328f
Breast budding, 53
Breast cancer screening, 60–61, 60f
Breast care
    during formula-feeding, 338
    postpartum, 278
    in pregnancy, 152–153
Breast examination
    in first prenatal visit, 137
    self, 60, 613f–614f
Breast-feeding, 325–335
    advantages of, 326
    amenorrhea in, 333
    assessing readiness for, 329
    vs. bottle feeding, 324–325
    breast milk composition in, 328–329
    classes on, 159
    contraception during, 334, 334t
    contraceptive protection from, 74
    contraindications to, 326
    disadvantages of, 326–327
    Healthy People 2010 on, 326, 326t
    lactation consultants for, 329, 333
    medications contraindicated in, 967
    medication use in, 966–967
    misperceptions or perceived barriers to,
        326–327
    nutritional needs of mother in, 329
    physiology of
        breast in, 327, 328f
        lactation in, 327–328, 328f
        newborn facial anatomy in, 327
        rooting and sucking reflex in, 327
    pumping and storing milk in, 334–335,
        334f
    recommendations for, 325–326, 326t
    return to work during, 335
Breast-feeding, nursing care of mother in,
    329–335
    amenorrhea in, 334
    assisting with technique in, 329–332
        assessing session in, 331–332
        beginning breast-feeding session in,
            329–330
        ending session in, 332
        latching on in, 331, 331f
    available resources for mother in, 333
    breast-feeding readiness in, 329
    contraception in, 334, 334t
    growth spurts in, 333
    newborn fluid intake in, 332
    newborn not feeding well in, 333
    positioning newborn in, 330, 331f
    pumping and storing milk in, 334–335,
        334f, 335t
    returning to work in, 335
    supplements for newborn in, 333
    teaching in
        on engorgement, 332–333
        on mastitis, 333
        on plugged milk ducts, 333
        on sore nipples, 332
Breast-Friendly Workplace initiative, 17
Breast milk
    composition of, 328–329
    nutrition in, 324
    for preterm newborn, 463
    pumping of, 334, 334f
    storing of, 334–335, 335t
Breasts
    of newborn, 297
    postpartum, 263
    postpartum pain in, 271
    in pregnancy, 121
    tenderness of, prenatal care for, 148t
Breast self-examination (BSE), 60,
        613f–614f
Breath, shortness of
    in pregnancy, 122
    prenatal care for, 147–149, 148t
Breathing
    in children, 776
    in pregnancy, 122
Breathing patterns
    in labor, first stage, 221, 222, 223f
    in labor, transition phase, 224
    for labor and birth pain, 186, 187t,
        188t
Breech presentation, 170, 171f, 411–412,
        412f
Broad ligament, 52, 52f
Bronchiolitis, acute, 781
Bronchodilators. See also specific agents
    for asthma, 784, 785t
Brown fat, in newborn, 287
Brown recluse spiders, 909
Brow presentation, 171, 171f
Bruises, 712–713, 713f–715f
    from child abuse, 712, 714f, 716t
    facial, in newborn, 294
Bryant's traction, 884, 885f
Buck's extension traction, 884, 885f
Bulbourethral glands, 48, 48f
Bulimia nervosa, 949–951, 955
Burns, 910–920
    from child abuse, 712, 715f, 716t
    classification of, 912, 913t
    epidemiology of, 910
    etiology of, 910
    nursing process for
        assessment, 916
        evaluation, 920
        implementation, 916, 919–920
        nursing care plan, 917–919
        nursing diagnoses, 916
        outcome identification and planning,
            916
    in toddlers, 568
    treatment of
        48-72 hours, 913–916
        airway in, 913
        complications in, 915–916
        emergency, 912–913
        grafting in, 915
        infection control in, 914–915
        IV fluids in, 913, 914f
        long-term care in, 916
        oral fluids in, 913
        total body surface area in, 913, 914f
        urine output and diuresis in,
            913–914
        wound care in, 915, 915f
    types of
        full-thickness or third-degree, 910f,
            911–912, 911t, 912f
        partial-thickness or second-degree,
            910f, 911, 911t, 912f
        superficial or first-degree, 910f, 911,
            911t, 912f

C
Caffeine, on pregnancy, 155
CAL, 852
Calciferol. See Vitamin D
Calcium
    for calcium absorption in pregnancy,
        127, 128t
    good sources of, 965
    for premenstrual syndrome, 65
Calcium deficiency, in lactose-intolerant
        pregnant woman, 132
Calendar method, 74, 74b
Calluses, sucking, 295
Caloric intake
    first trimester, 147
    in pregnancy, 126
Camps, health care at, 35, 35f
Canadian crutches, 887
Candida albicans, fetal (thrush), 296
Candidiasis
    in children, 901, 902f
    in pregnant diabetics, 351
Capitation, 10
Captopril, for congestive heart failure, 806
Caput succedaneum (caput), 180, 294, 295f
Carbamazepine, 758t
Cardiac catheterization, for congenital
        heart defects, 490
Cardiac decompensation, in pregnancy,
        353, 354–355
Cardiac output, in pregnancy, 121–122,
        122f
Cardinal ligaments, 52
Cardinal movements, 176, 177f
Cardiopulmonary resuscitation (CPR), for
        infants and children, 769t, 770f
Cardiovascular adaptation, in newborn,
        285–286
Cardiovascular changes, in pregnancy,
        121–122, 122f
Cardiovascular disease, in pregnancy,
        352–356
    classification of, 352–353, 352t
    clinical manifestations and diagnosis
        of, 353, 353b
    epidemiology of, 352
    nursing care for, 354–355
    physiology of, 352
    treatment of, 353–354
Cardiovascular disorders, 805–812
    congestive heart failure, 805–807
    Kawasaki disease, 811–812
    rheumatic fever, 807–811 (See also
        Rheumatic fever)
Cardiovascular system
    in child vs. adult, 805, 805f
    growth and development of, 804–805
    postpartum, 263
Cardiovascular system defects, congenital,
        485–490
    atrial septal defects, 486, 487f
    classification of, 486
    clinical manifestations of, 489
    coarctation of the aorta, 487–488, 488f
    cyanotic heart disease, 486
    heart development and, 485–486, 485f
    overview, 485
    patent ductus arteriosus, 486–487, 487f
    right-to-left shunting, 486
    risk factors for, 489
    tetralogy of Fallot, 488–489, 488f
    transposition of the great arteries, 489

treatment and nursing care for, 489–490
ventricular septal defect, 486, 486f
Cardiovascular transition, newborn
nursing care for, 305, 305f
Carditis, 807–808
Caregiver, communication with, 533–534,
534f
Caregiver–infant interactions, positive,
541, 545t
Caregiver participation, in pediatric
hospitalization, 647–649, 647f
Caregiver–preschooler interactions, 579,
580t
Caries, bottle-mouth, 338–339
Carpopedal spasms, 221, 221f
Carrier, 928b
Car seats
educating parents on, 321
for toddlers, 567, 567f
Cartilage, 880–881. See also
Musculoskeletal disorders
Case management, 10–11, 37
Casts
for fractures in children, 882–884, 883f
orthopedic, infant care with, 505–506
Cataracts, 747
Cat bites, 909
Catheterization
cardiac, for congenital heart defects, 490
for urine collection in children, 674
Causative agent, 928b
Cavernous bodies, 46, 47f
CD4-positive T-cell (CD4) counts, 359t
Ceftriaxone
for gonorrhea, 921
for gonorrhea in pregnancy, 365
Celecoxib, on breast-fed infant, 966
Celiac syndrome, 832–834, 833f
Cell division, 99–101, 100f
Cell types, 99
Cellular reproduction, 102
Central auditory dysfunction, 750
Central intravenous access, 692
Central nervous system defects,
congenital, 479–485. See also
specific defects
hydrocephalus, 479f, 482–485
spina bifida, 479–482, 479f
Cephalhematoma, 294, 295f
Cephalic presentation, 170
Cephalocaudal, 517
Cephalopelvic disproportion (CPD), 244,
410
Cephalosporin, on breast-fed infant, 967
Cerclage, 387
Cerebral palsy (CP), 761–764, 762f
causes of, 761–762
clinical manifestations and types of,
762, 762f
diagnosis of, 762
nursing care for, 763–764
prevention of, 762
treatment and special aids for, 762–764
orthopedic, 763, 763f
physical therapy, 762f, 763
technological aids for daily living,
763, 764f
Cervical cap, 73f, 79
Cervical dilation chart, 968
Cervical dilators, 240
Cervical insufficiency, 387
Cervical mucus, in menstruation, 55

Cervical mucus method, 75, 75f
Cervical polyps, 67
Cervical readiness, 239, 239t
Cervical ripening, 240–241
Cervix, 51, 51f, 52f
effacement and dilation of, 169, 169f
in passageway, 169, 169f
postpartum, 262, 263f
in pregnancy, 120
Cesarean birth, 244–255
definition of, 244
fetal complications of, 245
incidence of, 244, 245b
incision types in
abdominal, 245, 246f
uterine, 245–247, 246f
indications for, 244
maternal complications of, 245
nursing care for, 250–254
family teaching in planned cesarean,
250–251
immediate recovery phase, 253–254
preoperative, 250–251, 251f
support in unplanned/emergency
cesarean, 251–253
postpartum nursing process in, 274–277
assessment, 275
evaluation, 277
implementation, 275–276
nursing diagnoses, 275
outcome identification and planning,
275
risks in, 245
steps of, 247–250
intraoperative phase, 247–250,
248f–249f
overview, 247
postoperative phase, 250, 250f
preoperative phase, 247, 247f
Chadwick's sign, 118, 120, 121, 137
Chancre, 921
Checkups, routine
for infants, 549
for preschoolers, 581–582
for school-aged children, 594–595, 595f
for toddlers, 563
Chelating agent, 852
Chest, of newborn
assessment of, 297
circumference of, 291–292, 292f, 292t
Chest physiotherapy
for asthma, 784–785
for cystic fibrosis, 796, 796f–797f
Chest thrust, 853–854, 853f
Chewing tobacco, 944
Chickenpox
characteristics of, 931t
in pregnancy, 361–362
Chief complaint, in children, 627
Chignon, 244, 294
Child abuse, 711–717
on child and family, 715
definition and history of, 711
emotional, 713, 716t
epidemiology of, 711–712
history and definition of, 711
laws on, 712
Munchausen syndrome by proxy, 713
neglect, 713–714, 716t
nursing process for, 716–717, 716t
parents in, 712
physical, 712–713, 713f–715f, 716t

bruises and misc., 712, 714f, 716t
burns, 712, 715f, 716t
fractures, 712
sites, 712, 713f
sexual, 714–715, 716t
shaken baby syndrome, 713
signs of, 716t
Child assessment, 623–639
objective data collection in, 628–639
(See also Data collection in
children, objective)
subjective data collection in, 623–628
(See also Data collection in
children, subjective)
Childbirth. See Birth; Labor
Childbirth education classes, 156, 158b,
159b
Child health status, 15–16, 16t
Child-life program, 644
Child neglect, 713–714, 716t
Child with psychosocial disorder, 937–958
Children's Hospice International, 731–732
Chlamydia
newborn infection with, 474t
in pregnancy, 364, 368–372 (See also
Sexually transmitted infections
(STIs), nursing process for)
Chloasma, 123
Cholestasis, in pregnancy, 123
Chordee, 500
Chorea, 808
Chorioamnionitis, 239, 413
Chorion, 107, 107f
Chorionic villi, 107
Chorionic villus sampling (CVS),
143–144, 143b
Christmas disease, 816–817
Chromosomal abnormalities, 508–510
Down syndrome, 508–509, 508f,
509f
Klinefelter syndrome, 510
Turner syndrome, 509–510
Chromosomes, 99
Chronic health problem, in children,
699–707
causes of, 699
effects on family of, 699–702
child, 701
parents, 700
siblings, 701–702, 702b
family in, parents, 700f
nurse role in, 703
assessment, 702
evaluation, 707
implementation, 703–704, 703f
nursing care plan, 705–707
nursing diagnoses, 702–703
outcome identification and planning,
703
Cigarette burns, in child abuse, 712,
713f–715f
Cigarette smoking. See Smoking
Circulation
cold therapy for, 672
fetal, 108, 109, 110f, 485, 485f
heat therapy for, 671–672
newborn, 485, 485f
in newborn, 286
placental, 109
Circulation therapies
cold, 667, 672
heat, 671–672

Circulatory system, in infants, 540, 540f
Circumcision, 314
　advantages and disadvantages of,
　　315b
　assisting with, 315–316, 316f
　family teaching on, 317
Circumcision board, 316, 316f
Circumoral, 788
Classification, 593
Clavicle assessment, newborn, 296–297
Clean catch urine specimen, 674
Cleavage, 102, 103f
Cleft lip and cleft palate, 491–496
　clinical manifestations of, 491, 491f
　diagnosis of, 491
　epidemiology of, 491
　etiology of, 491
　nursing process for, 492–496
　　assessment, 492
　　evaluation
　　　postoperative, 496
　　　preoperative, 495–496
　　nursing diagnoses, 492
　　outcome identification and planning
　　　postoperative, 494–495, 495f
　　　preoperative, 492–494, 493c
　treatment of, 491–492
Client advocacy
　in community-based nursing, 37, 37f
　definition of, 37
Climacteric, 55, 91
Clitoris, 49f, 50
Clitoris assessment, newborn, 297
Clomiphene citrate
　challenge test for, 89
　multifetal pregnancy from, 113
Clomipramine, for premenstrual
　　syndrome, 65
Clonazepam, 758t
Clonus
　in children, 762
　in preeclampsia-eclampsia, 396, 397f,
　　400
Closed fracture, 882f
Clostridium tetani, 929t
Clot, 443
Clot formation, 816, 816f
Clothing, in pregnancy, 153
Clot prevention, with cardiovascular
　　disease in pregnancy, 354
Clotrimazole, for tinea corporis, 903
Clotting factors, in newborn, 288
Clove hitch restraint, 664, 665f
Clubfoot, 481
　congenital, 501–502, 501f, 502f
　in newborn, 298
Cobalamine. See Vitamin B₁₂
Cocaine
　childhood abuse of, 944
　on pregnancy, 155
Coccobacilli H. influenzae, 930t
Codeine, on breast-fed infant, 966
Codependent parent, 718
Cohabitation family, 28
Coitus interruptus, 72–74
Cold, common, 776–777
Cold stress, 286, 289, 306
Cold therapy, 672
Colic, 834–835
Collection bag, for urine specimen,
　　673–674, 673f
Colostomy, 672

Colostrum, 121, 263, 328–329
Combination oral contraceptives (COCs),
　　73f, 79–80, 80b, 80f, 81b
Combined jaw thrust-spine stabilization
　　maneuver, 853f
Comedones, 902
Comfort measures, for labor/birth pain,
　　186, 219
Common cold, 776–777
Communal family, 28
Communicability, period of, 928b
Communicable diseases, 920–933
　of childhood, 927–933, 929t–932t (See
　　also specific diseases)
　glossary for, 928b
　infectious mononucleosis, 927–928, 927f
　sexually transmitted infections
　　AIDS, 922t, 923–927 (See also AIDS)
　　chlamydial, 921, 922t
　　definition and overview, 921, 922t
　　genital herpes, 921, 922t
　　gonorrhea, 921, 922t
　　syphilis, 921–923, 922t (See also
　　　Syphilis)
Communicable diseases, in pregnancy,
　　359–372. See also Infectious
　　diseases, in pregnancy
Communication, 531–534
　with adolescents, 533
　with caregivers, 533–534, 534f
　in community-based nursing, 36
　with infants, 532
　principles of, 531–532
　with school-aged children, 533
　settings for, 531
　with young children, 532, 532f
Community-based nursing, 31–39
　advantages of, 31–32
　challenge of, 37–38
　for children, 34–36, 35f
　　community centers, parishes, and
　　　intervention programs, 35–36
　　home health care, 34–35, 35f
　　outpatient, 34
　　residential programs, 36
　　schools and camps, 35, 35f
　definition and overview of, 31
　issues in, 38
　for maternal client
　　birth settings, 32–33, 32f
　　prenatal and postpartum home
　　　health care, 32, 32f
　nursing skills for, 36–37
　poverty in, 38
　prenatal and postpartum, 32, 32f
　prevention in, 31, 39
　rewards of, 38–39
　shift to, 31
　unique aspects of, 38
Community centers, health care at, 35–36
Compartment syndrome, 883
Complete abortion, 385t
Complete breech presentation, 412
Compound fracture, 882f
Concentration, for labor/birth pain,
　　186–188, 187t
Conception, 101–102
Conceptus, 102
Concrete operations, 529
Condom, 614
　female, 73f, 77–78, 78f
　male, 73f, 76–77

Conductive hearing loss, 750
Conductive heat loss, 286, 286f
Condylomata acuminata, 365
Congenital aganglionic megacolon,
　　842–845
　clinical manifestations of, 842
　diagnosis of, 842
　nursing process for, 843–845
　pathophysiology of, 842, 842f
　treatment of, 842–843
Congenital anomalies. See Congenital
　　malformations
Congenital disorders, 478–514
Congenital hip dysplasia, 502–504, 502f,
　　503f
Congenital hypothyroidism, 507–508, 507f
Congenital malformations, 479–504. See
　　also specific defects
　cardiovascular system, 485–490 (See
　　also Cardiovascular system
　　defects, congenital)
　central nervous system, 479–485
　　hydrocephalus, 479f, 482–485
　　spina bifida, 479–482, 479f
　etiology of, 479
　gastrointestinal system, 491–499
　genitourinary tract, 500–501
　grief from, 445–446
　skeletal system, 501–504
Congenital talipes equinovarus, 501–502,
　　501f, 502f
Congestive heart failure (CHF),
　　805–807
Conjugated estriol, in fetal well-being
　　assessment, 142
Conjunctivitis, 749
Conservation, 590
Constipation
　postpartum, 280
　prenatal care for, 149t, 150
Continuous fetal monitoring
　electronic, 209, 210t
　external electronic, 210t, 211–212
　internal electronic, 210t, 211–212, 213f
Continuous labor support, for labor/birth
　　pain, 186, 187t
Continuous uterine contraction
　　monitoring
　external, 209, 210t
　internal, 210t, 211
Contraception, 72–86
　barrier methods of, 76–79
　　cervical cap, 79
　　condom, female, 77–78, 78f
　　condom, male, 76–77
　　diaphragm, 78–79, 78f
　　spermicidal agents, 76
　during breast-feeding, 334, 334t
　choice of, assisting with, 84–86
　emergency, 83–84
　hormonal methods of, 79–83
　　combination oral contraceptives,
　　　79–80, 80b, 80f
　　combined monthly injection, 81
　　depot medroxyprogesterone acetate,
　　　81
　　implants, 81–82
　　intrauterine device, 82–83, 82f, 83b
　　overview, 79
　　progestin-only pills, 80–81
　　transdermal patch, 80f, 82
　　vaginal ring, 80f, 82

natural methods of, 72–76
  abstinence, 72
  coitus interruptus, 72–74
  fertility awareness methods, 74–76
    (See also Fertility awareness
    methods (FAMs))
  lactational amenorrhea, 74
sterilization for, 83
Contraceptives. See also specific agents
  comparative guide to, 73f
  oral
    combination, 73f, 79–80, 80b, 80f,
      81b
    for dysmenorrhea, 64
    for endometriosis, 66
    for uterine cysts, 68
Contractions, labor, 172–173, 174f
  in active labor, 178, 178t
  on admission for labor/birth, 205
  in birth, 178t, 179
  in early labor, 177–178, 178t
  at onset of labor, 174–175
  oxytocin in, 185
  pain from, 184–185 (See also Pain
    management, labor and birth)
  in transition, 178–179, 178t
  in true vs. false labor, 175–176
Contraction stress test (CST), 145
Contractures, burn, 916
Convection, heat loss via, 286, 286f,
  306
Conventional level, 530
Conversion charts
  Fahrenheit to Celsius, 978
  pounds and ounces to grams, 977
  pounds to kilograms, 683, 976
Cooley's anemia, 815–816
Cooling devices, 667, 672
Cooperative play, 579
Coping strategies in labor, first stage,
  222
Copper, in pregnancy, 128t
Copper intrauterine device
  for contraception, 73f, 82–83, 82f, 83b
  for emergency contraception, 84
Cord compression, on fetal heart rate,
  214–215, 215f
Cordocentesis, 144
Cord prolapse, 421–422, 422f
Corpus, of uterus, 51, 52f
Corpus cavernosa, 46, 47f, 48f
Corpus luteum, 55, 120
Corpus spongiosum, 46, 47f, 48f
Corticosteroids. See also specific agents
  for asthma, 784, 785t
  on breast-fed infant, 967
  for rheumatic fever, 809
Corynebacterium diphtheriae, 929t
Coryza, 779
Cost containment, 9–11
  definition of, 9
  inefficiencies in, 9–10
  nursing contribution to, 10–11, 11t
  nursing process in, 11, 11t
  strategies for, 10
Cost sharing, 10
Cost shifting, 10
Cotyledons, of placenta, 108
Cough, whooping, 929t
Cough etiquette, 960
Couvade syndrome, 125
Cowper's glands, 48, 48f

COX-2 inhibitors. See also specific agents
  on breast-fed infant, 966
Coxa plana, 890
Crackles, 504, 505t
Cradle cap, 900
Cradle hold, 330, 331f
Cramps, prenatal leg, 149t, 150
Cranial sutures, in infants, 539
Craniostenosis, 294–295
Craniotubes, 829
C-reactive protein, 809
Cremaster muscle, 46–47
Crepitus, in newborn, 297
Cretinism, 127
Crib top restraint, 664, 665f
Critical pathways, 10–11, 11t
Critical thinking, in maternal–child health
  care, 20
Cromolyn, for asthma, 784, 785t
Crossed eyes, 295
Croup, 779
Croupette, oxygen, 670–671, 670t
Croup syndromes
  definition of, 779
  epiglottitis, 780, 780f
  laryngotracheobronchitis, acute, 780
  spasmodic laryngitis, 779–780
Crowning, 227, 227f, 230f
Crutches, 887
Crying, newborn
  educating parents on, 319
  in healthy newborn, 285, 305
Crying signal, newborn, 300
Cryptorchidism, 297, 500, 875
Cultural competency, 30
Culture, 30, 30f
Curling's ulcer, 915
Currant jelly stools, 845
CycleBeads, 75–76, 76f
Cycle of violence, 372–373, 373f
Cystic fibrosis (CF), 793–799, 832
  clinical manifestations of, 793–794,
    793f
  diagnosis of, 794
  etiology and pathophysiology of,
    793
  nursing process for
    assessment, 795
    evaluation, 798–799
    implementation, 797–798
    nursing diagnoses, 795, 797
    outcome identification and planning,
      797
  treatment of
    dietary, 794
    overview, 794
    pulmonary, 794–795, 796f–797f
Cystocele, 68–70, 69f
Cysts, ovarian, 68
Cytomegalovirus (CMV), in pregnancy
  and neonates, 363

D

Danazol, for endometriosis, 66
Danger signs, of pregnancy, 146b, 155
Data collection in children, objective,
  628–639
  general appearance, 628–629
  head circumference, 631, 631f
  height and weight, 630–631, 630f,
    631f
  overview, 628

physical examination, 636–639
  abdomen, 637
  back and extremities, 638
  chest and lungs, 637
  ears, 637
  eyes, 636–637
  genitalia and rectum, 637–638
  head and neck, 636
  heart, 637, 638f
  neurologic, 638, 639f
  nose, mouth, and throat, 637, 637f
psychological status and behavior,
  629–630, 629t
vital signs, 631–636
  apnea monitor, 634, 635f
  blood pressure, 635–636, 635f,
    635t
  pulse, 633, 633t, 638f
  pulse oximetry, 634, 634f
  respirations, 633–634, 634f
  temperature, 632–633, 633f
Data collection in children, subjective,
  623–628
  client and family caregiver interview in,
    623–624, 624f
  client history in, 624–628
    allergies, medications, and substance
      abuse, 628
    biographic data, 624–627,
      625f–626f
    chief complaint, 627
    developmental level, 628
    family health history, 627
    health history, 627
    lifestyle, 628
    review of systems, 627, 627f
Date rape drug, 615–616
Dawdling, 560
Daycare, 30, 580
DDAVP, for hemophilia, 817
Dead space, 492c
Deafness, 749–752
Death and dying, in children, 722–736
  books for children about, 725–726,
    726f, 727t
  care settings for, 730–732
    home care, 731–732
    hospice care, 730–731
    hospital care, 732, 732f
  children's understanding of, 599t,
    724–728
    in adolescents, 725
    experience with death and loss in,
      725–726, 726f, 727t
    in infants and toddlers, 724
    in preschool children, 724
    in school-aged children, 724–725,
      724f
  child's reaction to, 729–730
    experience of death and loss in,
      725–726, 726f
    impending, awareness of, 726–728
  epidemiology of, 722
  family's reaction to, 728–730
    caregivers, sudden or unexpected
      death, 729
    caregivers, terminal illness, 728
    child, 729–730
    siblings, 730, 731b
  fetal, 14b, 418
    grief from, 14b, 418
    intrauterine, 418–419

Death and dying, in children, *(continued)*
　helping children cope with, 730, 731b
　impending, awareness of, 726–728
　infant, 14b
　newborn, grief from, 445–446
　nurse role in, 732–733
　nurse's reaction to, 722–724, 723b
　nursing care plan for, 734–736
　nursing process for, 732–733
　patient care in, 723–724
　self-examination on, 722–724, 723b
　talking to children about, 725b
Death rate, 14, 14b
Debridement, 915, 915f
Decelerations, fetal heart rate, 215f
　early, 214, 215f, 216, 216f
　late, 215–216, 215f, 216f
　variable, 214–215, 215f
Decentration, 593
Decidua, 103
Deciduous teeth eruption, 539–540,
　　540f
Decrement, 172, 174f
Deep vein thrombosis (DVT),
　　postpartum, 441–442
Deer ticks, 909, 932t
Dehiscence, wound, 480f
Dehydration, in children, 690
Deliriants, inhaled, 597, 597b
Delirium, postoperative, 481c
Delivery. *See also* Labor
　assisted (*See* Assisted delivery;
　　Cesarean birth)
　in diabetic mothers, 349
　nurse responsibilities in, 227, 229b
　pain management in (*See* Pain
　　management, labor and birth)
　of placenta, 178t, 179
　positions for, 226, 228t–229t
　sequence of, 227, 230f
　spontaneous vaginal, 176, 177f
Delivery, assisted, 241–244
　complications of, 244
　episiotomy, 241–242, 242b, 242f
　forceps-assisted, 243–244, 243f
　induction of labor, 238–241 (*See also*
　　Labor, induction of)
　nursing care in, 244
　vacuum-assisted, 242, 243f
Deltoid muscle, intramuscular injection
　　via, 688t
Demographic trends, 9
Denial, 647, 700
Denis Browne splint, 501–502, 502f
Dental braces, 612
Dental care
　for infants, 552
　for preschooler, 582
　for toddlers, 564–565, 565f
Dental hygiene
　in pregnancy, 151–152
　in school-aged children, 595, 596f
Dental malocclusion, 611–612
Dentition
　in preschoolers, 575, 575f
　in school-aged children, 589, 589f
Dependence, 941
Dependent nursing actions, 22
Depot medroxyprogesterone acetate
　　(DMPA, Depo-Provera), 81
Depressants, 946
Depression, postpartum, 443–444, 444b

Dermatitis
　atopic, 906–908, 906f
　seborrheic, 900
Dermatome, 362
Descent, 176, 177f
Despair, 529, 647
Detached retina, 748
Development. *See also* Growth and
　　development
　definition of, 517
　level of, in children, 627
　problems with, 16
　standards of, 518
Development, physical. *See also* Growth
　　and development; Physical
　　development
Developmental tasks (milestones), 517
　in preschoolers, 576t
　in school-aged children, 591t
Dextroamphetamine, for ADHD, 939
Diabetes, gestational, 121
Diabetes mellitus (DM)
　definition of, 346
　newborn of mother with, 471–472
Diabetes mellitus (DM), in pregnancy,
　　346–352
　classification of, 346
　epidemiology of, 346
　evaluation of, 352
　fetal surveillance in, 349
　gestational, 346–347, 347b
　nursing process for
　　assessment in, 350
　　fetal status monitoring in, 351
　　fetal weight estimation in, 351
　　infection monitoring and prevention
　　　in, 351
　　injury prevention in, 350–351,
　　　351b
　　nursing diagnoses in, 350
　　outcome identification and planning
　　　in, 350
　　therapeutic regimen monitoring in,
　　　350
　pregestational, 346
　specialists for, 346
　timing of delivery in, 349
　treatment of
　　diet therapy in, 349
　　exercise in, 349
　　maintaining glycemic control in,
　　　348–349, 348f
　　monitoring glycemic control in,
　　　347–348
　　oral hypoglycemic agents in, 349
　　overview of, 348, 348f
　　pre-pregnancy care in, 347
Diabetes mellitus (DM) type 1
　in children, 828, 854–862
　child responsibilities in, developmental
　　guidelines for, 860t
　clinical manifestations of, 855
　diagnosis of, 855
　epidemiology of, 854
　food plan for, child's, 858
　nursing process for, 857–862
　　assessment, 857
　　evaluation, 862
　　implementation, 858–862
　　nursing diagnoses, 857
　　outcome identification and planning,
　　　858

　　pathogenesis of, 854–855
　　treatment of, 855–857
　　　diabetic ketoacidosis in, 857
　　　insulin administration methods in,
　　　　856–857
　　　insulin reaction in, 856
　　　insulin regimen in, 856
　　　insulin therapy in, 855–856, 856t
　　　vs. type 2, 854t
Diabetes mellitus (DM) type 2, 862–863
　vs. type 1, 854t
Diabetic ketoacidosis (DKA)
　in children, 855, 857
　in pregnancy, 350, 351b
Diabetogenic effect of pregnancy, 347,
　　347b
Diagnosis, nursing, 21, 21f. *See also*
　　specific disorders
Diagnosis-related groups (DRGs), 10
Diagnostic tests and studies, 675–676.
　　See also specific disorders
Diagonal conjugate, 169
Diamniotic-dichorionic twins, 113
Diamniotic-monochorionic twins, 113
Diaper area care, in infants, 551–552, 552f
Diaper rash, 900–901
Diaphragm, contraceptive, 73f, 78–79, 78f
Diaphragmatic hernia, 498
Diarrhea, 835–839
　causes of, 835
　clinical manifestations of, 835–836
　diagnosis of, 836
　epidemiology of, 835
　in formula-fed newborn, 338–339
　nursing process for
　　assessment, 836
　　evaluation, 837–839
　　implementation, 836–837
　　nursing diagnoses, 836
　　outcome identification and planning,
　　　836
　treatment of, 836
Diastasis recti abdominis, 122, 122f, 264
Dick-Read method, 158b
Diet. *See also specific disorders*
　BRAT, 836
　for diabetes mellitus in pregnancy, 349
　fad, in adolescents, 610
　in growth and development, 11-18
　　years, 610, 610t
　in pregnancy, 130 (*See also*
　　Supplements for mother)
Diffusion, 486
Digitalization, 806
Digoxin, for congestive heart failure, 806
Dilatation and curettage (D&C), 86t
Dilatation and evacuation (D&E), 86t
Dilation, 177–179, 178t
　active labor, 178, 178t
　cervical, 169, 169f, 175
　early labor, 177–178, 178t
　transition, 178–179, 178t
Dilators, cervical, 240
Dimercaprol, 852
Dinoprostone, for cervical ripening, 240
Diphtheria, 929t
Diplopia, 748
Disadvantaged child, preschool, 580
Disbelief, postpartum, 445
Discipline
　for preschoolers, 579–580, 579f, 580t
　for toddlers, 561

Discrimination, against chronically ill child, 701
Disseminated intravascular coagulation (DIC), 388
Distressed fetus, signs of, 216b
Diuretics. *See also specific agents*
  for congestive heart failure, 806
  for premenstrual syndrome, 65
Divorce, 30, 523–524, 523f
Dizygotic twins, 113, 113f, 403–404
DMT, 945
Documentation, 21, 21f
Dog bites, 909
"Doll's eye," 295
Domestic violence, 718
Doppler flow studies (velocimetry), in prenatal care, 141
Dorsal recumbent position, modified, 228t
Dorsogluteal intramuscular injection, 689t
Dosage calculation, pediatric, 681–684
  body surface area method in, 683–684, 684f
  body weight method of, 683
  converting pounds to kilograms in, 683
Doubt, 528
Doula, 156, 186, 187t
Downers, 946
Down's syndrome, 508–509, 508f, 509f
  simian crease in, 297
  ultrasonography of, 141
Doxycycline
  for chlamydia, 921
  for gonorrhea, 921
  for syphilis, 923
Drainage, postural, 796, 796f–797f
Dramatic play, 579
Dressing
  of infants, 552
  of preschooler, 582
  of toddlers, 563–564
Drop attacks, 756
Drowning, 769–771, 769t, 770f
  in newborns, 321
  in toddlers, 567–568
Drug abuse. *See* Substance abuse
Dry heat, 672
Duchenne muscular dystrophy, 701, 888–890, 889f, 890f
Ductus arteriosus, 109, 110f, 485
Ductus venosus, 109, 110f, 286, 485
Due date estimation, 138–139
Duncan's mechanism, 179, 231
Dunlop's traction, 884, 885f
Duration, of labor contractions, 172, 174f
Dysarthria, 762
Dysfunctional family, 711
Dysfunctional labor, 409–411, 410t
Dysmenorrhea, 63–64, 876
Dyspareunia, 65, 263
Dysphagia, 780
Dystocia, 409–411, 410t
  labor, 244
  shoulder, 420–421, 421f

E

Ear alignment, newborn, 296, 296f
Ear assessment, newborn, 296, 296f
Early adolescence, 605
Early Childhood Intervention (ECI) program, 13–14
Early decelerations, fetal heart rate, 214, 215f, 216, 216f

Early labor. *See* Latent phase (early labor)
Early postpartum hemorrhage, 427. *See also* Hemorrhage, postpartum
Early pregnancy loss, 384–387
  causes of, 384–385
  clinical manifestations and types of, 385–386, 385t
  definition and epidemiology of, 384
  nursing care for, 386–387
  self-care after, 386
  treatment of, 385t, 386
Ears, 744, 745f
Easter Seals Early Childhood Intervention (ECI) program, 13–14
Eating. *See also specific disorders*
  family teaching on, 520c
Eating disorders, 948–955
  anorexia nervosa, 608–609, 948–955, 949f (*See also* Anorexia nervosa)
  bulimia nervosa, 949–951
  nursing care plan for, 952–954
  nursing process for, 949–951
Ecchymosis, 748
Echolalia, 938
Eclampsia, 394–403. *See also* Preeclampsia-eclampsia
Econazole nitrate, for tinea corporis, 903
Ecstasy, 945
Ectoderm, embryonic, 104, 104t
Ectopic pregnancy, 112–113, 383–384, 383f
Eczema, infantile, 906–908, 906f
Edema, ankle, prenatal care for, 149t
Edetate calcium disodium (EDTA), 852
Education, childbirth, 156, 158b, 159b
Effacement, cervical, 169, 169f, 175
Effleurage, for labor/birth pain, 187t, 188, 190f
Eggs, 45, 52–53
Eggs genesis, 100–101, 100f
Ego integrity, 529
Egophony, 504
Ejaculation, 46, 102
Ejaculatory ducts, 48, 48f
Elbow restraint, 664, 665f
Elective induction, 238
Electrical stimulation, for scoliosis, 892–893
Electrolytes, 690
Electronic fetal monitoring (EFM)
  continuous, 209
  continuous external, 210t, 211–212
  continuous internal, 210t, 211–212, 213f
Elimination procedures
  enema administration, 672
  ostomy care, 672
Elixir, 684
Embolus (embolism)
  amniotic fluid, 419–420
  postpartum
    pulmonary, 443
    venous thromboembolism, 441–443
Embryo, 103
Embryonic stage, 101f, 103–104, 104t, 105b
Emergency contraception, 83–84
Emesis, after formula-feeding, 338
Emetic, 779
Emotional abuse, of children, 713, 716t
Emotional support, in family-centered care, 26

Employment, in pregnancy, 153
Enanthem, 928b
Encephalopathy, 852
Encopresis, 940
Endemic, 928b
Endocrine changes, in pregnancy, 121
Endocrine disorders, 854–863. *See also specific disorders*
  diabetes mellitus type 1, 854–862
  diabetes mellitus type 2, 862–863
Endocrine system growth and development, 828
Endoderm, embryonic, 104, 104t
Endometriosis, 65–66
Endometritis, 433–435
Endometrium, uterine, 51, 52f
Endoscopic procedures, lung
  bronchoscopy, 510f
  thoracentesis, 513c–514c
  thoracoscopy, 511f
Endovaginal ultrasound, in prenatal care, 141
Enema administration, 672
Energy conservation, in preterm newborn, 464
Energy requirements
  of newborn, 324
  in pregnancy, 125
En face, 265–266
Engagement, 176, 177f
Engorgement, 332–333
Enteral feeding
  of preterm newborn, 462
  tube, 667–669
Enterobiasis, 848
Enterobius vermicularis, 848
Enterocele, 68–70, 69f
Entertainment, for children, 522
Enuresis, 870, 940
Environment, on growth and development, 522
Environmental control, 959
Epidemic, 928b
Epididymis, 47
Epidural anesthesia, for labor/birth pain, 192t, 193–195, 194f
Epiglottis, 488, 488f
Epiglottitis, 780, 780f
Epilepsy, pregnancy with, 357–359
Episiotomy, 241–242, 242b, 242f
Episodic changes, in fetal heart rate, 214
Epispadias, 297, 500
Epistaxis
  in pregnancy, 122
  prenatal care of, 147, 148t
Epstein-Barr virus, infectious mononucleosis from, 927
Epstein's pearls, 296
Erb palsy, 455
Erection, of penis, 46
Erickson, Erik, 526t, 527–529, 527t, 528f
Erythema infectiosum, 931t
Erythema toxicum, 293b, 928b
Erythroblastosis fetalis, 469–471
Erythromycin
  for acne, 903
  for chlamydia in pregnancy, 364
  for impetigo, 902
  for syphilis, 923
Eschar, 915
Esophageal atresia (EA), 496–498, 497f
Esotropia, 748, 748f

Essential nutrients, good sources of, 965
Essure Permanent Birth Control System, 73f, 83
Estimated date of confinement (EDC), 138
Estimated date of delivery (EDD), 138
Estriol, conjugated, in fetal well-being assessment, 142
Estrogen
    in menstrual cycle, 54f, 55
    placental, 108
Ethchlorvynol abuse, 946
Ethosuximide, 758t
Euglycemia, 347
Eupnea, 502t
Eustachian tube, 744, 745f, 752
Evaluation, 21f, 22. See also specific disorders
Evaporative heat loss, 286, 286f
Evisceration, wound, 480f
Ewing's sarcoma, 891
Exaggerated caput, 244
Exanthem, 928b
Exanthema subitum, 932t
Excitement, sexual, 55–56
Exercise
    for blood sugar control, in pregnancy, 349
    family teaching on, 520c
    preconception, 70
    in pregnancy, 152, 152b
Exercise classes, pregnancy and postpartum, 156, 159
Exotropia, 748, 748f
Expulsion, in delivery, 176, 177f
Exstrophy of the bladder, 500, 500f
Extended family, 27
Extension, in delivery, 176, 177f
External fixation, 882
External fixation devices, 885–887, 887f
External rotation, in delivery, 176, 177f
External version, 412, 412f
Extinction, 561
Extracellular fluid, 690, 690f
Extravasation, 692
Extremely low birth weight (ELBW), 451
Extremy assessment, newborn, 297–298, 298f
Extrusion reflex, 546, 546f
Exudate, 435
Eye assessment, newborn, 295
Eye conditions, 747–749
    cataracts, 747
    glaucoma, 747
    infections, 749
    injury and foreign objects, 748
    strabismus, 747–748, 748f
    surgery for, nursing care for, 749, 749f
Eyeglasses, 748
Eye movements, of newborns, 295
Eye protection, 959
Eyes, 744, 744f
Eye surgery, nursing care for child with, 749, 749f

F

Face assessment, newborn, 294–295
Face presentation, 171, 171f
Face shield, 959
Facial movements, newborn, 295
Facial paralysis, from forceps delivery, 295
Factor IX deficiency hemophilia, 816–817
Factor VIII, for hemophilia, 817

Factor VIII deficiency hemophilia, 816
Fad diets, in adolescents, 610
Fahrenheit to Celsius conversion charts, 978
Failure to thrive (FTT), nonorganic, 945–948, 946f
Faintness, prenatal care for, 147, 148t
Fallopian tubes, 51f, 52, 52f
Fall prevention, early postpartum, 273
False labor, 120, 175
False pelvis, 167, 168f
Family, as social unit, 26–27
Family-centered care, 6, 8f, 25–30
    culture in, 30, 30f
    divorce in, 30
    emotional support in, 26
    family size in, 29, 29f
    family structure in
        adoptive family, 28
        blended family, 28
        cohabitation family, 28
        communal family, 28
        extended family, 27
        gay or lesbian family, 28
        nuclear family, 27, 27f
        single-parent family, 28
        stepfamily, 28
    gender in, 29
    intellectual stimulation in, 26
    overview of, 25–26
    parental behavior in, 29–30, 29f
    physical sustenance in, 26
    sibling order in, 29
    socialization in, 26–27
    spirituality in, 27
Family planning, 70–86
    pregnancy planning in, 70–72, 71b
    pregnancy prevention in, 72–86 (See also Contraception)
Family size, 29, 29f
Farsightedness, 744–745
Fascia, of penis, 46, 47f
Fat, brown, in newborn, 287
Fatigue
    after delivery, 234
    effective pushing and, 226
    prenatal care for, 148t
Febrile seizures, 754
Fecal soiling, chronic involuntary, 940
Federally funded health services, 12–13, 13f
Feeding and nutrition, in children, 667–670. See also Nutrition
    bolus, 667
    in first year of life, 545–549
    gastrostomy, 667, 669–670, 669f
    gavage, 667–669
    intake and output measurements in, 667
    of newborn
        educating parents on, 319
        preterm, 462–463
    in toddlers, 562–563, 562t
Feeding schedule, in first year of life, 547t–548t
Fee-for-service, 10
Feet assessment, newborn, 298
Female sterilization, 73f, 83
Femoral pulse assessment, newborn, 297, 298f
Femoral venipuncture, 674, 674f
Fentanyl
    on breast-fed infant, 966
    for labor and birth pain, 190, 192t

Fertility awareness methods (FAMs), 73f, 74–76
    basal body temperature, 74–75
    calendar, 74, 74b
    cervical mucus, 75, 75f
    fertility window calculation in, 74, 74b
    overview and components of, 74
    Ovulation Predictor Test, 76
    standard days, 75–76, 76f
    symptothermal, 75
Fertility window, calculation of, 74, 74b
Fertilization, 101–102, 103f
Fertilization age, 101, 101t
Fetal alcohol syndrome (FAS), 70, 472–473
Fetal attitude, 170–171, 171f, 206–207
Fetal circulation, 108, 109, 110f, 485, 485f
Fetal death, 14b, 418–419
Fetal development, 99–113
    cellular processes in
        cellular division in, 99–101, 100f
        types of cells in, 99
    circulation in, fetal, 109, 110f
    ectopic pregnancy and, 112–113, 383–384, 383f
    stages of, 101–104
        embryonic, 101f, 103–104, 104t, 105b
        fetal, 101f, 104, 105b–106f
        gestational age and fertilization age in, 101, 101t
        overview, 101
        pre-embryonic, 101–103, 101f–103f
    of supportive structures, 104–109
        fetal membranes, 104, 107, 107f
        placenta, 107–108, 107f
        umbilical cord, 108–109
    teratogens on fetus in, 111–112, 111t
Fetal fibronectin, 239
Fetal fibronectin test, 415, 415b
Fetal growth restriction, 451–455. See also Small-for-gestational-age (SGA) newborn
Fetal heart rate (FHR)
    first stage
        active phase, 221
        transition phase of labor, 224
    second stage, during birth, 225–226
    variability definitions for, 213, 213b
Fetal heart rate (FHR) monitoring, in labor and birth, 211–217
    continuous EFM, 209, 210t
        external, 210t, 211–212
        internal, 210t, 211–212, 213f
    intermittent fetal heart rate auscultation, 210t, 211, 218b–219b
    pattern evaluation, 213–216
        baseline FHR, 213, 213f
        conditions influencing, 213–214, 214t
        deviations from, 213, 213b
    periodic changes, 214–216
        appearance and causes of, 125f, 214
        benign, 214, 215f
        nonreassuring, 214–216, 215f, 216b, 216f
        nonreassuring, clarifying, 216–217
        reassuring, 214
        variability definitions, 213, 213b
    tocodynamometer, 209, 210t

Fetal heart rate (FHR) monitoring, prenatal, 139, 139f
Fetal heart tones, Doppler assessment of, 146f
Fetal kick counts, 140
Fetal lie, 205–206, 207b
Fetal malposition, 410–411
Fetal malpresentation, 411–412
Fetal membranes, 104, 107, 107f
Fetal position, 171–172, 172b, 172t, 173f, 206–207
Fetal presentation, 170, 171f, 206–207
Fetal scalp pH, 180, 180t
Fetal scalp pulse oximetry, 210t, 217
Fetal scalp sampling, 210t, 217
Fetal skull, 170, 170f
Fetal stage, 101f, 104, 105b–106f
Fetal station, 172, 173f
Fetal status, on admission for labor/birth, 203–204
Fetal stimulation, for clarifying nonreassuring FHR patterns, 216
Fetal surveillance, in diabetic mothers, 349
Fetus, 104, 105b–106b, 285t
Fever, 666–667, 667b
Fibrinogen
  postpartum, 263
  in pregnancy, 121
Fibroids, uterine, 67–68
Fibronectin, fetal, 239, 415, 415b
Fifth disease, 931t
Fingers
  clubbing of, 499f
  of newborn, assessment of, 297
Fingersticks, in diabetic children, 858–859, 859f
Fistula, tracheoesophageal, 496–498, 497f
Flatulence, prenatal care for, 149t
Flexion, in delivery, 176, 177f
Fluid and electrolyte balance, in children, 689–691
  acid–base balance in, 690–691
  electrolytes in, 690
  extracellular fluid in, 690, 690f
  intracellular fluid in, 690, 690f
  regulation of, 691
  water in, 689–690
Fluid imbalance prevention, newborn, 308–309, 308f
Fluid intake assessment, newborn, 332
Folic acid (folacin, folate, Vitamin B₉)
  for diabetic mothers, 347
  preconception, 70
  in pregnancy, 128t, 129
Follicles, in pregnancy, 120
Follicle-stimulating hormone (FSH)
  on male reproduction, 49t
  in menstrual cycle, 54, 54f
Follicular phase, 54–55, 54f
Fontanels
  in infants, 539
  in newborn, 295
Food allergies, 830–831, 831t
Food jags, 562
Food pyramid, for children, 520, 521f, 562, 580
Foods, solid, in first year of life, 546–549
  infant feeding of, 546, 546f
  preparation of, 546, 546f, 548
  self-feeding of, 548–549, 548f
Food safety, in pregnancy, 131
Football hold, 330, 331f, 665, 666f

Footling breech presentation, 412
Foramen ovale, 109, 110f, 485
Forceps, 243, 243f
Forceps-assisted delivery, 243–244, 243f
Forceps mark, on newborn face/cheek, 294
Forearm crutches, 887
Foreign bodies
  in ear or nose, 752–753
  in eye, 748
  ingestion of, 853–854, 853f
Foremilk, 328–329
Foreskin, 46, 48f
Formal operations, 529
Formula
  comparison of, 336, 336t
  composition of, 336, 336t
  forms of, 336
  preparation of, 337–338
Formula feeding, 335–339
  advantages of, 335
  vs. breast-feeding, 324–325
  disadvantages of, 335–336
  formulas in
    comparison of, 336, 336t
    composition of, 336, 336t
  nursing care of mother in, 336–339
    adding supplements in, 338
    assessing mother and newborn in, 337
    assisting with technique in, 337, 337f
    bottle preparation in, 337–338
    common newborn problems in, 338–339, 339t
    maternal breast care in, 338
    overview of, 336–337
Fornix, posterior, 51
Fourchette, 49f, 50
Fractures, 882–887
  definition and types of, 882, 883f
  treatment and nursing care for, 882–887
    casts, 882–884, 883f
    crutches, 887
    external fixation, 882
    external fixation devices, 885–887, 887f
    internal fixation, 882
    overview, 882–883
    traction, 884, 885f, 886–887
Frank breech presentation, 412
Fraternal twins, 113, 113f
Fredet-Ramstedt operation, 839, 839f
Fremitus, tactile, 503f
Frequency, of labor contractions, 172, 174f
Fresh-frozen plasma (FFP), for hemophilia, 817
Freud, Sigmund, 525–527, 526t
Fruitarian, pregnancy in, 131
Fundal height measurement, 139, 139f
Fundal massage, 268–269, 278, 428
Fundal palpation, 268–269
Fundus, uterine, 107f, 120
Fungal infections
  tinea capitis, 903
  tinea corporis, 903
  tinea cruris, 904
  tinea pedis, 903–904
Furosemide, for congestive heart failure, 806

G

Gag reflex, 295–296, 462
Galactosemia, 326, 507

Gamete intrafallopian transfer (GIFT), 90
Gametes, 45, 99
Gametogenesis, 100–101, 100f
Ganciclovir, for congenital cytomegalovirus infection, 363
Gases, partial pressure of, 493c, 493f
Gas exchange, 492–494
  oxyhemoglobin dissociation curve, 494c
  partial pressure of gases, 493c, 493f
Gastric emptying, in pregnancy, 123
Gastroenteritis, 835–839. See also Diarrhea
Gastroesophageal reflux (GER), 834, 834f
Gastrointestinal changes, in pregnancy, 123
Gastrointestinal disorders, 829–854
  appendicitis, 846–847
  celiac syndrome, 832–834, 833f
  colic, 834–835
  congenital aganglionic megacolon, 842–845 (See also Congenital aganglionic megacolon)
  diarrhea and gastroenteritis, 835–839 (See also Diarrhea)
  foreign object ingestion, 853–854, 853f
  gastroesophageal reflux, 834, 834f
  intestinal parasites, 848–849
  intussusception, 845–846, 845f
  lead poisoning, 850–852
  malnutrition and nutritional problems, 829–832
    food allergies, 830–831, 831t
    kwashiorkor, 829, 829f
    marasmus, 829
    mineral insufficiencies, 830
    niacin insufficiency, 830
    nursing process for, 831–832
    riboflavin deficiency, 830
    thiamine deficiency, 830
    vitamin C deficiency, 830
    vitamin D deficiency, 829
  pyloric stenosis, 839–842 (See also Pyloric stenosis)
  toxic ingestion, 849–850, 850t
Gastrointestinal system
  anatomy of, 828, 828f
  growth and development of, 828
  postpartum, 264
Gastrointestinal system defects, congenital, 491–499. See also specific disorders
  cleft lip and cleft palate, 491–496
  esophageal atresia and tracheoesophageal fistula, 496–498, 497f
  hernias, 498–499
  imperforate anus, 498, 498f
Gastrostomy button, 669, 669f
Gastrostomy feeding, 462–463, 667–670, 669f
Gastrostomy tube, 667–670, 669, 669f
Gavage feeding, 462–463, 463f, 667–669
Gay family, 28
Gender identity, 29
General anesthesia, for labor/birth pain, 193t, 196
General appearance
  of children, 628–629
  of newborn, 290
Generalized seizures, 756–757
Generativity, 529
Gene therapy, 8
Genetic analysis, of fetus, 9

Genetic counseling, preconception, 70
Genetics, on growth and development, 519–520
Genetic testing, in first prenatal visit, 137, 137t
Genitalia, ambiguous, 500–501
Genital stage, 526–527, 526f
Genital warts, 365
Genitourinary disorders, 864–877. *See also specific disorders*
  cryptorchidism, 875
  enuresis, 870
  glomerulonephritis, acute, 870–872, 871t
  hydrocele, 875
  menstrual disorders, 875–876
  nephrotic syndrome, 872–875
  urinary tract infections, 868–870
  vaginitis, 876t, 877
  Wilms' tumor, 875
Genitourinary system
  anatomy of, 863–864, 864f
  growth and development of, 863–864
Genitourinary tract assessment, newborn, 297
Genitourinary tract defects, congenital
  ambiguous genitalia, 500–501
  exstrophy of the bladder, 500, 500f
  hypospadias and epispadias, 500
German measles, 931t
Germ cells, 99, 103, 103t
Germ layers, 104, 104t
Germ theory, 4–5
Gessell, Arnold, 530
Gestational age, 101, 101t
  assessment of, 300, 451, 452f, 453t
  classification of variations in, 451
  definition of, 451
  variations in, 451
Gestational diabetes mellitus (GDM), 121, 346–347, 347b. *See also Diabetes mellitus (DM), in pregnancy*
  newborn of mother with, 471–472
Gestational disorders, 451–467. *See also specific disorders*
  epidemiology of, 450
  size and gestational age variations, 451–467
    classification of, 451
    in large-for-gestational-age newborn, 455
    nursing care for, 467
    in postterm newborn, 466–467
    in preterm newborn, 451, 456–466 (*See also* Preterm newborn)
    in small-for-gestational-age newborn, 451–455 (*See also* Small-for-gestational-age (SGA) newborn)
Gestational hypertension, 394
Gestational surrogate, 91
Gestational trophoblastic disease, 387–389
Gestational trophoblastic neoplasia, 387
Giardia lamblia, 849
Giardiasis, 849
Gilligan, Carol, 531
Ginger, for morning sickness, 147, 382
Gingival hyperplasia, 757
Glans penis, 45–46, 46f
Glans penis assessment, newborn, 297
Glaucoma, 747
Glomerular filtration rate, in pregnancy, 123

Glomerulonephritis, acute, 870–872, 871t
  clinical manifestations of, 870–871
  vs. nephrotic syndrome, 871
  nursing care for, 872
  treatment of, 871
Glossary, 981–995
Gloves, 959
Glucagon, for insulin reaction, 856
Glucose, blood
  in diabetic children, 858–859, 859f
  in gestational diabetes mellitus, 346–347, 347b
  in pregestational diabetes mellitus, 346
Glucose testing
  of newborns, 287, 287b, 289
  oral glucose tolerance test for, 347, 347b
Glue sniffing, 945
Gluten-induced enteropathy, 832
Glutethimide abuse, 946
Glyburide, in pregnancy, 349
Glycemic control, in pregnancy
  maintaining, 348–349, 348f
  monitoring, 347–348
Glycosylated hemoglobin (HbA$_1$C), in pregnancy, 347
Glysouria, in pregnancy, 123
Gonadotropin-releasing hormone (GnRH) agonists
  for endometriosis, 66
  for uterine fibroids, 68
Goniotomy, 747
Gonorrhea
  newborn infection with, 474t
  in pregnancy, 364–365, 368–372 (*See also* Sexually transmitted infections (STIs), nursing process for)
Goodell's sign, 118, 120
Goserelin, for endometriosis, 66
Gower's sign, 888, 889f
Gown, 959
Gradual acceptance, 700
Grafts, skin, 915
Grand mal seizures, 756
Grand multiparity, 262
Granulocytes, 820
Gravida, 136, 136b
Green, Patricia, 531
Greenstick fracture, 882f
Grief
  anticipatory, 728
  postpartum, 445–446
Griseofulvin, for tinea, 903–904
Group B streptococcus (GBS), newborn infection with, 474t
Group homes, children's health care at, 36
Growth
  definition of, 517
  patterns of, 518
  standards of, 518
Growth and development, 517–534
  in communication, 531–534 (*See also* Communication)
  definition of, 517
  influences on, 519–525
    divorce, 523–524, 523f
    environment, 522
    genetics, 519–520
    homelessness, 522
    latchkey child, 524–525, 524f
    nutrition, 520–522, 521f
    runaway child, 525

nurse's role related to, 534
  overview of, 517
  patterns of growth in, 518
  standards of development in, 518
  standards of growth in, 518
  theories of, 525–531
    Arnold Gessell, 530
    Bruno Bettelheim, 531
    Carl Jung, 530–531
    Carol Gilligan, 531
    Erik Erickson, 526t, 527–529, 527t, 528f
    Jean Piaget, 526t, 529, 529f
    John Bowlby, 531
    Lawrence Kohlberg, 526t, 530
    Patricia Green, 531
    Sigmund Freud, 525–527, 526t
Growth and development, 1-3 years, 557–570, 559t
  autonomy in, 558
  in health care facility, 569–570, 569f, 570f
  health promotion and maintenance in, 563–569
    accident prevention, 567–569
      burns, 568
      drowning, 567–568
      motor vehicle, 567–568, 567f
      toxic ingestions, 568–569
    family teaching, 563–567
      bathing, 563
      dental care, 564–565, 565f
      dressing, 563–564
      sleep, 567
      toilet training, 565–567, 565f
    guidelines, 564t
    routine checkups, 563
  injury prevention in, 557
  nutrition in, 562–563, 562t
  physical development in, 558, 558f, 559t
  psychosocial development in, 558–562
    dawdling, 560
    discipline, 561
    negativism, 558
    play, 560–561, 560f
    ritualism, 558–560
    sharing with new baby, 561–562, 562f
    temper tantrums, 560
Growth and development, 3-6 years, 574–584
  in health care facility, 584, 584f
  health promotion and maintenance in, 581–584
    accident prevention, 583–584, 583f
    family teaching
      bathing, 582
      dental care, 582
      dressing, 582
      sleep, 583
      toileting, 582–583
    infection prevention, 583–584
    routine checkups, 581–582
  milestones for, 576t
  nutrition in, 580–581
    daily nutritional needs, 581, 581t
    eating skills, 581, 582f
    snacks, 581, 581b
  physical development in, 575, 576t
  psychosocial development in, 576–580
    aggression, 579
    disadvantaged child, 580
    discipline, 579–580, 579f, 580t
    imagination, 577

language, 576–577, 577t
nursery school or day care
  experience, 580
play, 578–579, 578f
sexual development, 578
Growth and development, 6-10 years,
  588–600
developmental milestones for, 591t
in health care facility, 598–600, 599t,
  600f
health promotion and maintenance in,
  594–596
  family teaching, 595–598
    accident prevention, 598, 598f
    dental hygiene, 595, 596f
    sex education, 596
    substance abuse education,
      596–597, 597b
    routine checkups, 594–595, 595f
nutrition in, 593–594, 594t
physical development in, 589–591,
  591t
  dentition, 589, 589f
  overview, 588–589
  skeletal growth, 589–590, 590f
  weight and height, 589
psychosocial development in, 590–593
  6-7 years, 591–592
  7-10 years, 592–593, 593f
Growth and development, 11-18 years,
  604–617
adolescent development in, 605–609
  developmental tasks, 606, 607t
  physical development, 606
  psychosocial development, 606–609
    body image, 608–609
    overview, 606–607, 608f
    personality, 608, 608f
  in health care facility, 617
health promotion and maintenance in,
  610–617
  accident prevention, 616–617
  dental checkups, 611–612
  family teaching, 612
  health education and counseling
    breast self-examination, 613f–614f
    sexuality, 612–614
    sexual responsibility, 614–616
    substance abuse, 616
    testicular self-examination, 615f
  mental health, 616
  routine checkups, 611, 612f
norms for, 605t
nutrition in, 609–610
  culture on, 609–610
  daily nutritional needs in, 609, 609t
  food fads and diets in, 610, 610t
  junk foods in, 609, 609f
  nutrients deficient in, 609, 610t
preadolescent development in, 604–605
self-identity in, 605, 605f
Growth and development, 28 days to 1
  year, 538–554
caregiver–infant interactions in,
  positive, 541, 545t
family teaching on, 541
in health care facility, 553–554, 554f
health promotion and maintenance in,
  549–553
  family teaching, 550–553
    accident prevention, 552–553
    bathing the infant, 550–551, 551f
    dental care, 552

diaper area care, 551–552, 552f
dressing, 552
sleep promotion, 552
immunizations, 549–550, 978
routine checkups, 549
norms for, 542t–543t, 544f
nutrition in, 545–549
  feeding schedule, 547t–548t
  first 4-6 months, 545–546
  solid foods, 546–549
    food preparation, 546, 546f, 548
    infant feeding, 546, 546f
    self-feeding, 548–549, 548f
  weaning, 549
  Women, Infants, and Children Food
    Program, 549
physical development in, 538–541
  circulatory system, 540, 540f
  fontanels and cranial sutures, 539
  head circumference, 539
  neuromuscular development,
    540–541
  norms, 542t–543t, 544f
  overview, 538–539
  respiratory rate, 540
  skeletal growth and maturation, 539
  tooth eruption, 539–540, 540f
  weight and height, 539, 539f
psychosocial development in, 541, 545
  hand movements in, 541, 545f
  norms for, 542t–543t
  positive caregiver–infant interactions
    in, 541, 545t
Growth charts, 518
2-20 years: stature-for-age and weight-
  for-age percentiles
  boys, 973
  girls, 973
birth to 36 months: boys
  head circumference-for-age and
    weight-for-length percentiles, 970
  length-for-age and weight-for-age
    percentiles, 969
birth to 36 months: girls
  head circumference-for-age and
    weight-for-length percentiles, 972
  length-for-age and weight-for-age
    percentiles, 971
Growth rate, in preschoolers, 575, 575f
Growth spurts, newborn, on breast-
  feeding, 333
GTPAL, 136b
Guilt, 528
Gums
  in pregnancy, 123
  prenatal care for bleeding of, 148t
Gynecoid pelvis, 167, 168f
Gynecomastia, 945

H
H. influenzae pneumonia, 788
HAART, 359t
Habitual abortion, 385t
Haemophilus influenzae meningitis, 675f,
  759–761
Haemophilus influenzae type B, 930t
Hair, 899–900
Hair assessment, newborn, 292
Hallucinogens, 945
Halo traction, 894, 894f
Hand assessment, newborn, 297
Hands and knees position, 229t
Handwashing, 310–311, 959

Harlequin coloring, 292
Harlequin sign, 292
Hay fever, 777, 777f
Headaches, from epidural anesthesia,
  195–196
Head assessment, newborn, 294–295,
  294f, 295f
Head circumference
  in children, 631, 631f
  in infants, 539
  in newborn, 291–292, 292f, 292t
Head compression, on fetal heart rate,
  214, 215f, 216f
Head injuries, in children, 768–769
Head lag assessment, newborn, 296, 296f
Head lice, 904–905
Head presentation, 170
Head sparing, 453
Head-to-toe assessment, newborn, 292–298
  abdomen, 297
  back and rectum, 298
  chest, 297
  ears, 296, 296f
  extremities, 297–298, 298f
  eyes, 295
  genitourinary, 297
  head and face, 294–295, 294f, 295f
  mouth, 295–296
  neck, 296–297, 296f
  nose, 295
  skin, hair, and nails, 292–294, 293b
Health, children's concept of, 599t
Health care facility
  adolescent in, 617
  infant in, 553–554, 554f
  preschooler in, 584, 584f
  school-aged child in, 598–600, 599t, 600f
  toddler in, 569–570, 569f, 570f
Health education. See also specific topics
  in community-based nursing, 36–37
  at schools and camps, 35
  for wellness, 20
Health maintenance. See also specific
  topics
  newborn, educating parents on, 319
Health maintenance organizations
  (HMOs), 12, 12b
Health promotion and maintenance, 10,
  59. See also under Growth and
  development; specific disorders
  in adolescents, 610–617 (See also
    Growth and development, 11-
    18 years)
  in infants, 549–553
  in newborns, 549–553
  in preschoolers, 581–584
  in school-aged children, 594–596 (See
    also Growth and development,
    6-10 years)
  in toddlers, 563–569
Health status
  on admission for labor/birth
    fetal, 203–204
    maternal, 204–205
  in adolescents, 15–16, 16t
  in children, 15–16, 16t
  maternal–infant, 14–15, 14b, 15f
Healthy living habits, in children, 16
Healthy People 2010, 18, 19b
  on breast-feeding, 326, 326b
  preterm labor goals in, 414
Hearing, 744, 745f
Hearing aids, 751

Hearing impairment, 749–752
  central auditory dysfunction, 750
  clinical manifestations of, 750
  conductive hearing loss, 750
  diagnosis of, 750–751
  epidemiology of, 749
  levels of, 749, 750t
  mixed hearing loss, 750
  nursing care for, 752
  sensorineural hearing loss, 750
  treatment and education for, 751–752,
      751f
Hearing screening, newborn, 17, 296,
    317–318
Heart
  anatomy of, 805, 805f
  development of, 485–486, 485f
  in pregnancy, 121–122, 122f
Heartbeat, fetal, 118
Heartburn
  in pregnancy, 123
  prenatal care for, 148t, 149–150
Heart failure, in pregnancy, 353
Heart murmurs, in newborn, 290, 290t
Heart rate
  fetal, prenatal assessment of, 139, 139f
  of infant, 540, 540f
  of newborn, 290, 290t, 305
Heart rhythm, of newborn, 290, 290t
Heart tones, fetal, Doppler assessment of,
    146, 146f
Heat loss, in neonates, 286–287, 286f
Heat therapy, 671–672
Heel stick, newborn, 307
Hegar's sign, 118, 120, 138
Height
  of children, 518, 630–631, 630f, 631f
  of infants, 539, 539f
  of newborn, 291–292, 292t
  of school-aged children, 589
Heimlich maneuver, 853–854, 853f
HELLP syndrome, 398
Helmets, bicycle, 583, 583f, 598, 598f
Hemarthrosis, 818
Hematologic changes, in pregnancy, 121
Hematologic disorders, 812–823
  hemophilia, 816–819 (See also
      Hemophilia)
  idiopathic thrombocytopenic purpura,
      820
  iron-deficiency anemia, 812–813
  leukemia, acute, 820–823 (See also
      Leukemia, acute)
  sickle cell disease, 813–815, 813f
  thalassemia, 815–816
Hematologic system
  child vs. adult, 805, 805f
  growth and development of, 804–805
Hematoma
  definition of, 427
  hemorrhage from, 427
    clinical manifestations of, 428, 428f,
        430t
    nursing process for, 428–432 (See
        also under Hemorrhage,
        postpartum)
    risk factors in, 427, 427b
    treatment of, 428
Hemoglobin
  glycosylated (HbA$_1$C), in pregnancy, 347
  oxygen saturation of, 509f
  pregnancy, 121

Hemoglobin S (Hgb S), 355
Hemolytic disease of newborn, 469–471
  causes of
    ABO incompatibility, 405, 470
    Rh incompatibility, 404–405, 469–470
  clinical manifestations of, 470
  nursing care for, 471, 471f
  treatment of, 470–471
Hemophilia, 816–819
  causes of, 816
  clinical manifestations of, 817
  clot formation and, 816, 816f
  diagnosis of, 817
  factor IX deficiency, 816–817
  factor VIII deficiency, 816
  nursing process for, 817–819
  treatment of, 817
Hemophilia A, 816–817
Hemophilia B, 817
Hemophilia B$_5$, 816–817
Hemorrhage, early postpartum,
    427–432
  clinical manifestations of
    with hematoma, 428, 428f, 430t
    with lacerations, 428, 430t
    with uterine atony, 427, 430t
  diagnosis of, 428
  nursing process for, 428–432
    assessment, 429, 430t
    evaluation, 432
    implementation, 429–432
      fluid balance, 429–431
      injury prevention, 431
      tissue perfusion, 431–432
    nursing diagnoses, 429
    outcome identification and planning,
        429
  risk factors for, 427, 427b
  treatment of, 428
Hemorrhage, intraventricular, in preterm
    newborn, 457–458
Hemorrhage, late postpartum, 432
Hemorrhage, postpartum
  causes of, 426–427
  definition of, 426
  epidemiology of, 426
Hemorrhage prevention
  after cesarean, 275
  in newborns, 308–309
Hemorrhoids, prenatal care of, 149t,
    150
Hemostasis, early postpartum, 271
Hepadnavirus, 929t
Heparin lock, 692, 692f
Hepatic adaptation, in newborn,
    287–288
Hepatitis, 929t
Hepatitis A, 931t
Hepatitis A virus (HAV), 931t
Hepatitis B virus (HBV), 929t
  newborn infection with, 474t
  in pregnancy, 361
Hepatitis B virus (HBV) immunization,
    neonatal, 316–317
Herbal remedies, prenatal, 154–155
Hernias, 498–499
  definition of, 498
  diaphragmatic, 498
  hiatal, 498
  inguinal, 499, 499f
  omphalocele, 498–499, 499f
  umbilical, 499, 499f

Herpes simplex virus (HSV)
  newborn infection with, 474t
  in pregnancy and neonatal, 363–364,
      364t
Herpes zoster, in pregnancy, 361–362
Heterografts, 915
Heterosexual, 608
Hiatal hernia, 498
Hierarchical arrangement, 593
High birth weigh, problems from, 126
Hind milk, 329
Hip assessment, newborn, 298
Hip dislocation, newborn, 298
Hip dysplasia, 481
Hip dysplasia, congenital, 502–504, 502f,
    503f
Hip subluxation, in newborn, 298
Hirschsprung's disease, 842–845
  clinical manifestations of, 842
  diagnosis of, 842
  nursing process for, 843–845
  pathophysiology of, 842, 842f
  treatment of, 842–843
Hirsutism, 810
Hives, 908
Hodgkin's disease, 701
Holding children, for procedures and
      treatments, 665–666, 666f
Homans' sign, 269–270, 270f
Home apnea monitor, 469, 469f
Home health care. See also Community-
      based nursing
  for child, 34–35, 35f
  prenatal and postpartum, 32, 32f
Homeless family, 522
Homeostasis, 689
Homes, group, children's health care at,
      36
Homografts, 915
Homosexual, 608
Honeymoon period, 856
Hood, oxygen, 670–671, 670t
Hookworms, 848–849
Hordeolum, 749
Horizontal position, for holding child,
      665, 666f
Hormonal changes, in pregnancy, 121
Hormonal implants, contraceptive, 81–82
Hormone replacement therapy (HRT), 92
Hospice care, 730–731
Hospitalism, 6
Hospitalized child care, 643–657
  admission and discharge planning in
    admission interview in, 650
    admission physical examination in,
        650
    discharge planning in, 650–651
    emergency admissions in, 650
    orientation in, 649, 649b
    planned admissions in, 649–650
  in adolescents, 617
  child-life program in, 644
  for child undergoing surgery, 651–655
    postoperative care in, 653–655,
        653f–655f
    preadmission visit in, 649–650, 650f
    preoperative care in, 651–653, 652f
  holding and rocking in, 644, 644f
  in infants, 553–554, 554f
  packing for, 155, 156b
  pediatric hospital setting in, 644–649
    atmosphere in, 644–645

caregiver participation in, 647–649, 647f
early childhood education on, 644, 644f
infection control in, 646–648
intensive care units in, 645
safety in, 646, 646b
play program in, 655–657
hospital play environment in, 655–656, 655f, 656f
play material in, 656–657, 657t
therapeutic play in, 652, 652f, 656, 656f
in preschoolers, 584, 584f
in school-aged children, 598–600, 599t, 600f
in toddlers, 569–570, 569f, 570f
Host, 928b
Hot flashes, 91–92
HPV vaccine, 365, 595
Humalog insulin, 856
Human body, children's concept of, 599t
Human chorionic gonadotropin (hCG), 108
in blastocyst, 103
in fetal well-being assessment, 142
nausea and vomiting from, 123
pregnancy test for, 118
Human Genome Project (HGP), 8–9
Human herpesvirus 6, 932t
Human immunodeficiency virus (HIV)
newborn infection with, 474t
in pregnancy
clinical manifestations of, 366–367, 367b
diagnosis of, 367
epidemiology of, 366
nursing care for, 368
nursing process for, 368–372
assessment, 368–370, 369b–370b
evaluation, 371–372
implementation, 370–371
nursing diagnoses, 370
outcome identification and planning, 370
treatment of, 367–368
Human papilloma virus (HPV), in pregnancy, 365, 368–372. See also Sexually transmitted infections (STIs), nursing process for
Human papilloma virus (HPV) vaccine, 365, 595
Human parvovirus B19, 931t
Human placental lactogen (hPL), 108
Hyaline membrane disease, 457
Hydatidiform mole, 387–389
Hydralazine, on breast-fed infant, 967
Hydrocele, 875
Hydrocephalus, 479f, 482–485
clinical manifestations of, 482–483, 483f
diagnosis of, 483
noncommunicating vs. communicating, 482, 482f
nursing process for, 483–485
pathophysiology of, 482
treatment of, 483, 483f
Hydronephrosis, pregnancy-related, 264
Hydrotherapy, 915
Hydroxyzine, for labor/birth pain, 190, 192t

Hygiene, in pregnancy, 152
Hymen, 49f, 50
Hymen, imperforate, 297
Hymenal tag, 297
Hyperbilirubinemia, 287
Hypercholesterolemia, in children, 16
Hypercoagulability, in pregnancy, 121
Hyperemesis, 381
Hyperemesis gravidarum, 147, 381–383
Hyperglycemia, 347
in children, 860
in pregnancy, 346
Hyperinsulinemia, in pregnancy, 346
Hyperlipidemia, in children, 16, 872
Hyperopia, 744–745
Hypertension
in children, 16
chronic
preeclampsia superimposed on, 403, 403b
pregnancy and, 403
gestational, 394
maternal, 108
pregnancy-related, in diabetic mothers, 350–351
Hypertensive disorders in pregnancy
gestational hypertension, 394
preeclampsia-eclampsia, 394–403 (See also Preeclampsia-eclampsia)
Hyperthermia
definition of, 666
in newborn, 306
Hypertonic dysfunction, uterine, 410–411
Hyperventilation, 222, 691
Hypervolemic, 913
Hypnobirthing, 158b
Hypnosis, for labor/birth pain, 187t, 190
Hypnotics. See also specific hypnotics
on breast-fed infant, 967
in children, 946
Hypochromic, microcytic anemia, 812
Hypochylia, 793
Hypoglycemia, 856
in diabetics in pregnancy, 348
neonatal, 287, 287b, 289
newborn
with diabetic mother, 471–472
preventing, 306, 306f, 307
testing for, 306–307
signs of
in children, 860
in pregnancy, 350, 351b
Hypoglycemic agents, oral, in pregnancy, 349
Hyposensitization, 906
Hypospadias, 297, 500
Hypotension
from epidural anesthesia, 195
postural, in pregnancy, 147
supine hypotensive syndrome in, 122, 122f, 354
Hypothermia
for heart disease, 490
in newborn, 306, 306f
Hypothyroidism
congenital, 507–508, 507f
screen for, in first prenatal visit, 138
Hypotonic dysfunction, uterine, 410–411
Hypovolemic shock, 427
Hypoxemia, 486, 511
Hypoxia, 486, 491–492, 492c
Hyrocodone, on breast-fed infant, 966

Hysterectomy, 63
for uterine fibroids, 68
for uterine prolapse, 69
Hysterosalpingogram, 89
Hysteroscopy, for infertility, 89

I
Ibuprofen
on breast-fed infant, 966
for dysmenorrhea, 64
Identical twins, 113, 113f
Identification, newborn, 309, 313
Identity, 527t, 529
mistaken, of newborn, 309
Idiopathic celiac disease, 832–834, 833f
Idiopathic nephrotic syndrome, 872–875. See also Nephrotic syndrome
Idiopathic thrombocytopenic purpura, 820
Ileostomy, 672
Iliac arteries, 53, 53f
Iliac artery, internal, 53
Ilizarov fixator, 885, 887, 887f
Illness, children's concept of, 599t
Imagery, for labor/birth pain, 186–188, 187t
Imagination, in preschoolers, 577
Immunity
active, 928b
development of, 900
in fetus, 108
natural, 928b
passive, 928b
Immunizations
for infants, 549–550
for newborns, 316–317
for preschoolers, 581–582
recommended childhood and adolescent schedules of, 978
Immunoglobulin, intravenous, for Kawasaki disease, 812
Immunoprophylaxis, 359t
Impending death, child's awareness of, 726–728
Imperforate anus, 498, 498f
Imperforate hymen, 297
Impetigo, 902, 902f
Implanon, 82
Implantation, 102–103, 103f
Implants, contraceptive hormonal, 81–82
Implementation, 21f, 22. See also specific disorders
Impunity, 923
Inborn errors of metabolism, 504–508
congenital hypothyroidism, 507–508, 507f
galactosemia, 507
maple syrup urine disease, 508
overview, 504, 506
phenylketonuria, 506–507
Incest, 714–715
Incompetent cervix, 387
Incomplete abortion, 385t
Incomplete breech presentation, 412
Increment, 172, 174f
Incubation period, 928b
Independence (autonomy)
theories on, 527t, 528, 528f
in toddlers, 558
Independent nursing actions, 22
Independent play, 579
Induced abortion, 72, 86–87, 86t

Induction of labor, 238–241
  cervical ripening in, 240–241
  contraindications for, 239
  elective, 238
  fetal maturity in, 240
  indications for, 239
  labor (cervical) readiness in, 239, 239t
Induration, 692
Industry, 527t, 528, 528f
Inefficiencies, cost, 9–10
Inevitable abortion, 385t
Infant. See also Growth and development,
      28 days to 1 year; Newborn;
      specific topics
  death and dying in, understanding of,
      724
  growth and development of, 538–554
      (See also Growth and
      development, 28 days to
      1 year)
  in health care facility, 553–554, 554f
Infant abduction, 310, 310b, 313
Infant death, 14b
Infantile eczema, 906–908, 906f
Infantile genital stage, 526–527, 526f
Infantile spasms, 757
Infant mortality
  leading causes of, 14b
  rate of, 14–15, 14b, 15f
Infection. See also specific infections
  congenitally acquired newborn, 473,
      474t–475t
  control of, at pediatric hospital,
      646–648
  postoperative, 479t
Infection, postpartum, 432–434
  causes and clinical manifestations of,
      433
  definition of, 432–433
  endometritis, 433–434
  progression of, 433
  risk factors for, 433
Infection prevention
  after cesarean, 276
  after delivery, 233
  with cardiovascular disease in
      pregnancy, 354
  during childbirth, mother to child,
      310–311
  with diabetes in pregnancy, 351
  in labor, first stage, 223
  in newborns, 306–308, 308f, 310–311
      immunization for, 316–317
      parent education on, 318, 320f
  postpartum, early, 272–273
  in preschoolers, 583–584
  in preterm newborn, 461–462
  in umbilical cord stump, 306–308
Infectious diseases, female reproductive
      tract
  pelvic inflammatory disease, 67
  toxic shock syndrome, 66–67
Infectious diseases, in children. See
      Communicable diseases; specific
      diseases
Infectious diseases, in pregnancy,
      359–372
  cytomegalovirus, 363
  hepatitis B, 361
  herpes simplex virus, 363–364, 364t
  overview of, 359
  rubella, 362–363

sexually transmitted infections,
      364–372
  chlamydia, 364
  gonorrhea, 364–365
  HIV/AIDS, 366–368, 367b
  human papilloma virus, 365
  nursing process for, 368–372
  trichomoniasis, 365–366
  syphilis, 361
  terms in, 359t
  TORCH, 360–361, 360b
  Toxoplasmosis, 360–361
  varicella and herpes zoster, 361–362
Inferiority, 528
Infertility, 87–91
  causes and risk factors for, 87, 88b
  comprehensive evaluation and
      diagnostic testing for, 89
  definition of, 87
  initial evaluation of, 87–89
  management of, 89–91
      assisted/advanced reproductive
          therapies in, 90, 90b
      cervical factors in, 89–90
      endometrial and tubal factors in, 90
      gamete intrafallopian transfer in, 90
      intracytoplasmic sperm injection in,
          90–91
      male factors in, 90
      ovarian factors in, 90
      surrogate parenting in, 91
      tubal embryo transfer in, 90
      in vitro fertilization in, 90
      zygote intrafallopian transfer in, 90
  nursing care for, 91
  psychological aspects of, 91
Infiltration, 693
Informed consent
  for cesarean birth, 251, 251f
  for circumcision, 315
Infusion pumps, IV, 692, 693f
Inguinal hernia, 499, 499f
Inhaled deliriants, 597, 597b
Inheritance, of sex, 102, 102f
Inheritance patterns, 813f
Initiative, 527t, 528
Injection, contraceptive, 73f
Injury prevention
  from hypoglycemia, 306, 306f, 307
  in neonates, 317–318, 317b, 318f
  postpartum
      nonimmunity to rubella, 278, 279b
      Rh-negative, 278, 278b
  in pregnancy and delivery
      with diabetes mellitus, 350–351, 351b
      for early postpartum hemorrhage,
          431
      fetal and maternal, 217–219
  in toddlers, 557
Insect bites, 910
Insect stings, 910
Insulin, 828
  administration of, 856–857
  forms of, 856–857, 857t
  injection sites for, in children, 861,
      861f
Insulin-dependent diabetes mellitus
      (IDDM). See Diabetes mellitus
      (DM) type 1
Insulin pump
  in children, 856–857
  in pregnant diabetics, 348–349, 348f

Insulin reaction, 856
Insulin therapy
  in children, 855–856, 856
  in pregnancy, 348–349, 348f
Insurance, private, 12, 12b
Intake measurements, 667
Integumentary changes, in pregnancy, 123
Integumentary disorders, 900–921
  acne vulgaris, 902–903, 903f
  allergic disorders, 905–909
      atopic dermatitis, 906–908, 906f
      diagnosis of, 905
      epidemiology and etiology of, 905
      hyposensitization in, 906
      plant allergies, 908–909, 909f
      skin allergies, 908
  bites
      animal, 909
      insect, 910
      snake, 910
      spider, 909
      tick, 909–910
  burns, 910–920 (See also Burns)
  candidiasis, 901, 902f
  diaper rash, 900–901
  fungal infections
      tinea capitis, 903
      tinea corporis, 903
      tinea cruris, 904
      tinea pedis, 903–904
  impetigo, 902, 902f
  miliaria rubra, 900
  parasitic infections
      pediculosis, 904–905
      scabies, 905
  seborrheic dermatitis, 900
  stings, insect, 910
Integumentary system
  growth and development of, 899–900
  postpartum, 264
Intellectual stimulation, from family, 26
Intensity, of labor contractions, 172–173,
      174f
Intensive care units, pediatric, 645
Intercellular fluid, 690, 690f
Intercurrent infections, 874
Interdependent nursing actions, 22
Intermittent auscultation (IA), of fetal
      heart rate, 211, 218b–219b
Intermittent infusion device, 692, 692f
Internal fixation, 882
Internal iliac artery, 53, 53f
Internal pudendal artery, 53
Internal rotation, in delivery, 176, 177f
Interstitial cell-stimulating hormone
      (ICSH), on male reproduction,
      49t
Interstitial fluid, 690, 690f
Intervention programs, health care at,
      35–36
Intestinal parasites, 848–849
Intimacy, 529
Intimate partner violence (IPV), in
      pregnancy, 372–375
  clinical manifestations of, 372–373,
      373f, 374f
  examples of, 372b
  nursing care for, 374–375
  overview of, 372
  treatment for, 373–374, 374b
Intra-amniotic hyperosmotic fluid
      infusion, 86t

Intracellular fluid, 690, 690f
Intracytoplasmic sperm injection (ICSI), 90–91
Intradermal administration, in children, 687
Intradermal water injections, for labor/birth pain, 187t, 190, 190f
Intramuscular administration, in children, 686–687, 688t–689t
Intrathecal administration, 821
Intrathecal anesthesia, for labor/birth pain, 193, 193t, 194f, 195
Intrauterine device (IUD)
    for contraception, 73f, 82–83, 83b
    for emergency contraception, 84
Intrauterine fetal death, 418–419
Intrauterine growth restriction (IUGR), 108, 108b, 451–455. See also Small-for-gestational-age (SGA) newborn
    cause of, 451
    clinical manifestations of, 453–454
    complications of, 454
    contributing factors to, 451–453, 453t, 454b
    definition of, 451
    nursing care for, 454
Intrauterine pressure catheter, for labor/birth monitoring, 211
Intravascular fluid, 690, 690f
Intravenous immunoglobulin (IVIG) therapy, for Kawasaki disease, 812
Intravenous (IV) therapy, in children, 687, 689–693
    administration of, 691–692
        central IV access in, 692
        infusion control in, 692, 693f
        peripheral IV access in, 691–692, 691f, 692f
    fluid and electrolyte balance in, 689–691 (See also Fluid and electrolyte balance)
        acid-base balance in, 690–691
        electrolytes in, 690
        extracellular fluid in, 690, 690f
        intracellular fluid in, 690, 690f
        regulation of, 691
        water in, 689–690
    total parenteral nutrition in, 692–693
Intraventricular hemorrhage (IVH), in preterm newborn, 457–458
Intrinsic factor, 131
Introitus, 50
Intussusception, 845–846, 845f
Invagination, 845
In vitro fertilization (IVF), 90
Involution
    postpartum, 261
    uterine, 261–262
Iodine
    good sources of, 965
    in pregnancy, 127, 128t, 129
Iron
    foods high in, 813
    good sources of, 965
    in pregnancy, 121
Iron deficiency, 830
Iron-deficiency anemia
    in children, 812–813
    in pregnancy, 355–356

Iron-dextran, 812–813
Iron supplements
    in children, 812
    in pregnancy
        for anemia, 356
        general, 127, 128t, 130
Ischemic phase, 54f, 55
Isoimmunization, 404
Isolation, 529
Isolette, 461, 461f
Isoniazid, 800
Isotretinoin, for acne, 903
Isthmus, uterine, 51, 52f

J
Jacket restraint, 664, 665f
Jaundice, 287–288
    newborn, 292, 321
    physiologic, 287
Jaw thrust-spine stabilization maneuver, 853f
Jock itch, 904
John Tracy Clinic, 751
Joint Commission's "Do Not Use" list, of abbreviations, acronyms, and symbols, 964
Joints, 880. See also Musculoskeletal disorders
Jugular venipuncture, in children, 674, 674f
Jung, Carl, 530–531
Juvenile rheumatoid arthritis (JRA), 891–892, 891t

K
Kangaroo care, 306, 306f, 313
Kawasaki disease, 811–812
Kegel exercises, 69
Kernicterus, 470
Kick counts, fetal, 140
Kidneys. See also Genitourinary disorders
    in children, 867, 868f
    in pregnancy, 123
Kilograms, from pounds, 683
Kissing disease, 927–928, 927f
Klinefelter syndrome, 510
Knot, true, 423t
Kohlberg, Lawrence, 526t, 530
Kussmaul breathing, 855
Kwashiorkor, 829, 829f
Kyphosis, 889

L
Labia, 49–50, 49f
Labia assessment, newborn, 297
Labia majora, 49–50, 49f
Labia minora, 49f, 50
Labor, 167–180. See also Birth
    in asthmatic, 357
    back, 185
    with cardiovascular disease, 354
    communicating expectations about, 155–156
    fetal adaptation to, 180
    fetal scalp pH in, 180, 180t
    food and fluid intake in, 220b
    four components of, 167–174 (See also Labor components)
    maternal adaptation to
        physiologic, 179–180
        psychologic, 180
    nursing care in (See Labor and birth nursing care)

    obstructed, 185
    pain management in (See Pain management, labor and birth)
    postterm, 417–418
    preparing patient for, 155–160
        childbirth education classes, 156, 158b, 159b
        choosing support person, 156
        communicating expectations, 155–156, 157b
        packing for hospital/birthing center, 155, 156b
    preterm, 414–417
    prodromal (false), 120, 175, 176t
    progress of, expected, 409, 410t
    true, 175–176, 176t
Labor, nursing care by stage in, 217–234
    first stage, dilation, 217–225
        active phase, 220–223
            assessment of fetal status, 221
            assessment of labor progress, 220–221
            assessment of maternal status, 221, 221b, 221f
            evaluation, 223
            implementation, 222–223, 223f
            nursing diagnoses, 221–222
            outcome identification and planning, 222
        latent phase, 217–220
            assessment, 217
            evaluation, 220
            implementation, 217, 219–220
            nursing diagnoses, 217
            outcome identification and planning, 217
        overview, 217, 218b–219b
        transition phase, 224–225, 225f
    fourth stage, recovery, 232–234, 233f
    second stage, expulsion of fetus, 225–231
        assessment, 225–226
        definition of, 225
        evaluation, 231
        implementation, 226–230
            effective pushing, 226–227, 228t–229t
            effective pushing despite fatigue, 226
            preparing for delivery, 227, 227f, 229b, 230f
        nursing diagnoses, 226
        outcome identification and planning, 226
    third stage, delivery of placenta, 231–232, 231f
Labor and birth nursing care, 202–234
    in admission, 203–208 (See also Admission, during labor and birth)
    fetal heart rate assessments in, 211–217 (See also Fetal heart rate (FHR) monitoring, labor and birth)
    by labor stage, 217–234 (See also Labor, nursing care by stage in)
    uterine contraction assessments in, 209–211 (See also Uterine contractions, during labor and birth)
Laboratory assessment, in first prenatal visit, 138

Labor at risk, 409–423
  dysfunctional labor, 409–411, 410t
  emergencies
    amniotic fluid embolism, 419–420
    placental and umbilical cord
      abnormalities, 422, 423t
    shoulder dystocia, 420–421, 421f
    umbilical cord prolapse, 421–422, 422f
    uterine rupture, 422
  fetal malpresentation, 411–412, 412f
  intrauterine fetal death, 418–419
  posterm pregnancy and labor, 417–418
  premature rupture of membranes,
    413–414
  preterm labor, 414–417
Labor components, 167–174
  passageway, 167–169
    bony pelvis, 167, 168f
    pelvic dimensions, 169
    pelvic shape, 167–168, 168f
    soft tissues, 169, 169f
  passenger, 170–172
    fetal attitude, 170–171, 171f
    fetal lie, 170, 170f
    fetal position, 171–172, 172b, 172t,
      173f
    fetal presentation, 170, 171f
    fetal skull, 170, 170f
    fetal station, 172, 173f
  powers, 172–174
    frequency, duration, and intensity in,
      172–173, 174f
    phases in, 172, 174f
  psyche, 174, 175b
Labor dystocia, 244, 409–411, 410t
Labor induction, 238–241
  cervical ripening in, 240–241
  contraindications for, 239
  elective induction in, 238
  fetal maturity in, 240
  indications for, 239
  labor (cervical) readiness in, 239, 239t
Labor preferences, on admission for
    labor/birth, 208
Labor process, 174–179
  onset, 174–176
    anticipatory signs of, 174–175
    prodromal vs. true, 175–176, 176t
    theories on causes of, 174
  spontaneous vaginal delivery, 176, 177f
  stages and duration, 176–179, 178t
    factors and variation in, 177
    first: dilation, 177–179, 178t
    fourth: recovery, 179
    second: birth, 178t, 179
    third: delivery of placenta, 178t, 179
Labor readiness, 239, 239t
Labor status
  on admission for labor/birth, 205–208,
    206f
  maternal, 205–208, 206f
Lacerations
  definition of, 427
  hemorrhage from
    clinical manifestations of, 428, 430t
    nursing process for, 428–432 (See
      also under Hemorrhage,
      postpartum)
    risk factors in, 427, 427b
    treatment of, 428
  rimation, 748
  se deficiency, 132

Lactation. See also Breast-feeding
  breast physiology in, 327, 328f
  definition of, 327
  hormonal control of, 327–328, 328f
  physical control of, 327
  sensory stimulation in, 328
Lactational amenorrhea, 74
Lactation consultant, 329, 333
Lactation risk categories (LRC), 966
Lactogen, 328
Lacto-ovovegetarian
  adolescent, 610
  pregnancy in, 130
Lactose, 830
Lactose intolerance
  in children, 830–831, 831t
  in pregnancy, 131–132
Lactovegetarian, adolescent, 610
Lacunae, 102–103
La Leche League, 333
Lamaze method, 158b, 186
Laminaria, 240
Language, in preschoolers, 576–577, 577t
Lanugo, 292, 456
Large-for-gestational age (LGA) newborn,
    455
Laryngitis, spasmodic, 779–780
Laryngopharynx, 488f
Laryngospasm, 779
Laryngotracheobronchitis, acute, 780
Larynx, 488f
Last menstrual period (LMP), 136
Latching on, 330–332, 331f
Latchkey child, 524–525, 524f
Late decelerations, fetal heart rate,
    215–216, 215f, 216f
Latency stage, 527
Latent phase (early labor)
  definition and overview of, 177–178,
    178t
  nursing care in, 217–220
    assessment, 217
    evaluation, 220
    implementation, 217, 219–220
    nursing diagnoses, 217
    outcome identification and planning,
      217
Layette, 159, 159b
Lead poisoning, 16, 850–852
LeBoyer method, 158b
Lecithin/sphingomyelin (L/S) ratio, 285
Leg assessment, newborn, 297
Leg cramps, prenatal care for, 149t, 150
Legg-Calvé-Perthes disease, 890
Leiomyomata, uterine, 67–68
Length. See also Height
  of newborn, 291–292, 292t
Leopold's maneuvers, 205–207, 412
Lesbian family, 28
Leukemia, 820
Leukemia, acute, 820–823
  clinical manifestations of, 820
  diagnosis of, 820
  epidemiology and types of, 820
  nursing process for, 821–823, 822f
  pathophysiology of, 820
  treatment of, 820–821
Leukocytosis
  in children, 809
  postpartum, 263
Leukopenia, 873
Leukorrhea, prenatal care for, 147

Leukotriene inhibitors, for asthma, 784,
    785t
Leuprolide, for endometriosis, 66
Levothyroxine, on breast-fed infant, 967
Lice, 904–905
Lie, fetal, 170, 170f
Life cycle issues, reproductive. See
    Reproductive life cycle issues;
    specific issues
Life support, basic, for infants and
    children, 769t, 770f
Ligaments
  musculoskeletal, 880 (See also
    Musculoskeletal disorders)
  paired, of uterus, 51–52, 52f
Lightening, 174
Lindane, for head lice, 904
Linea nigra, 123, 123f
Linen, 959
Lipoid nephrosis, 872–875. See also
    Nephrotic syndrome
Lispro, 856
Lithium, on breast-fed infant, 967
Lithotomy position, 228t
Liver, newborn, 287–288
Lobes, lung, 489, 489f, 501c
Lochia, 232, 262
  patient teaching on, 278–279
  postpartum, assessment of, 268
  with postpartum hemorrhage, 429
Lochia alba, 262, 279
Lochia rubra, 262, 279
Lochia serosa, 262, 279
Lockjaw, 929t
Long bones, 880. See also
    Musculoskeletal disorders
Longitudinal lie, 170, 170f
Lorazepam, on breast-fed infant, 967
Lordosis
  in children, 888, 890f
  in pregnancy, 122, 122f
Low back pain, prenatal care for,
    148t, 150
Low birth weight (LBW), 451
  causes of, 125
  problems from, 125–126
Lower respiratory tract, 488f, 489f
Low forceps, 243
Low-set ears, in newborn, 296, 296f
LSD, 945
Lumbar puncture, in infants and children,
    675, 675f
Lunelle, 81
Lung capacities, 491t
Lung lobes, 489, 489f, 501c
Lungs, 488f, 489f
  in newborn, 285–286
  in pregnancy, 122
  in preterm newborn, 457
Lung volumes, 491t
Luteal phase, 54f, 55
Luteinizing hormone (LH), in menstrual
    cycle, 54–55, 54f
Lyme disease, 909, 932t
Lymph node biopsy, 514
Lymphoblast, 820
Lymphocytes, 820

M
Macrocytic anemia, 355
Macroglossia, 455
Macrophages, 900

Macrosomia
  in newborn of diabetic mother, 471
  in pregnant diabetic, 347
Macule, 928b
Mafenide acetate, for burns, 915
Magical thinking, 577
Magnesium, for premenstrual syndrome, 65
Magnesium sulfate, for preeclampsia-
      eclampsia, 398–399, 398b
Malathion, for lice, 904
Malattachment, 446–447, 447t
Male sterilization, 73f, 83
Malignant hyperthermia, from general
      anesthesia for labor/childbirth,
      196
Malnutrition
  kwashiorkor, 829, 829f
  marasmus, 829
  nursing process for, 831–832
Malocclusion, dental, 611–612
Malposition, fetal, 410
Malpresentation, fetal, 411–412
Mammography, 60–61, 60f
Managed care, 10
Maple syrup urine disease (MSUD), 508
Marasmus, 829
Marijuana
  child/adolescent use of, 944
  on pregnancy, 155
Mask
  for infection control, 959
  oxygen, 670–671, 670t
Mask of pregnancy, 123
Massage, for labor/birth pain, 187t, 188,
      190f
Mast cell stabilizers, for asthma, 784, 785t
Mastitis, 333, 436–440
  causes and risk factors in, 436
  clinical manifestations of, 436, 436f
  definition of, 436
  diagnosis of, 436
  nursing care for, 436–437
  nursing care plan for, 438–440
  treatment of, 436
Mastoiditis, 752
Maternal–child health care, 3–22
  advance practice nurses in, 18–20
  critical thinking in, 20
  current trends in, 6–11
    bioethical issues in, 8–9
    cost containment in, 9–11 (See also
        Cost containment)
    demographic, 9
    family-centered care in, 6, 8f
    poverty in, 9
    regionalized care in, 6–8
    research advances in, 8
  documentation in, 21
  health status in, 14–18
    child and adolescent, 15–16, 16t
    maternal–infant, 14–15, 14b, 15f
  maternity care in
    anesthesia development on, 5
    germ theory on, 4–5
    history of, 4
  milestones in, 7t
  nurse's changing role in, 19–20
  nursing process in, 21–22, 21f
  payment for services in
    federally funded sources, 12–13, 13f
    private insurance, 12, 12b
    specialized services, 13–14

pediatric care in
    development of, 5–6
    history of, 4
  programs for, 17–18, 17b, 19b
  scientific and technological changes on, 3
  settings for, 20
  sociologic changes on, 3–4
Maternal–fetal medicine, 345. See also
      Pregnancy at risk: complicating
      conditions
Maternal–fetal medicine specialist, 345
Maternal fever, from epidural anesthesia,
      195
Maternal–infant health status, 14–15,
      14b, 15f
Maternal mortality
  causes of, 14b
  rate of, 14–15, 14b, 15f
Maternal–newborn bonding, 270, 270b
Maternal serum alpha-fetoprotein
      (MSAFP)
  in fetal well-being assessment, 142
  prenatal assessment of, 139–140, 139f
Maternal status, on admission for
      labor/birth, 204–205
Maternity blues, 443–444, 444b
Maternity health care
  anesthesia on, 5
  germ theory on, 4–5
  history of, 4
McRoberts maneuver, 420, 421f
Measles, German, 931t
Measles, mumps, and rubella (MMR),
      812, 930t
Measurements. See also specific
      measurements
  of newborn, 291–292, 292f, 292t
Mebendazole
  for hookworms, 849
  for pinworms, 848
Meclofenamate, for dysmenorrhea, 64
Meconium, 107, 298, 468
Meconium aspiration pneumonia, 107
Meconium aspiration syndrome (MAS),
      417–418
  acquired, 468
  in postterm newborn, 467
Meconium ileus, 793. See also Cystic
      fibrosis (CF)
Meconium staining, 417
Mediastinum, 489
Medicaid, 12–13
Medication administration, in children,
      680–689. See also specific
      agents and disorders
  developmental considerations in, 681,
      682t–683t
  dosage calculation in, 681–684
    body surface method, 683–684, 684f
    body weight method, 683
    converting pounds to kilograms in,
        683
  errors in, 681
  intramuscular, 686–687, 688t–689t
  intravenous, 687
  nasal, 686
  ophthalmic, 685, 685f
  oral, 684–685, 684f, 685f, 686b
  otic, 686, 687f
  rectal, 686
  rights of, 680–681
  rules of, 681, 681b

Medication errors, in children, 681
Medications, on pregnancy, 154, 154b
Meiosis, 100–101, 100f
Membranes, fetal, 104, 107, 107f
Menarche, 53, 606, 875
Meningitis, Haemophilus influenzae,
      675f, 759–761
Menopause, 55, 91–93, 92b
Menorrhagia, 63
Menstrual aspiration, 86t
Menstrual cycle, 53–55, 54f
  blood flow in, 54
  length of, 54–55
  menstruation in, 53, 54f
  ovarian cycle in, 54–55, 54f
  uterine cycle in, 54f, 55
Menstrual disorders, 63–66, 875–877
  amenorrhea, 63
  atypical uterine bleeding, 63
  dysmenorrhea, 63–64
  endometriosis, 65–66
  premenstrual dysphoric disorder, 64–65
  premenstrual syndrome, 64–66, 65b
Menstrual periods, postpartum, 262
Menstrual phase, 54f, 55
Menstruation, 53
  absence of, 876
  painful, 876
Mental health. See also Psychosocial
      disorders
  adolescent, 616
Mental retardation, 764–768
  causes of, 764
  clinical manifestations and diagnosis
      of, 764–765
  definition and criteria for, 764
  nursing process for, 765–768
    assessment, 765
    evaluation, 767–768
    implementation, 766–767, 767t
    nursing diagnoses, 765–766
    outcome identification and planning,
        766
  treatment and education for, 765
Meperidine
  on breast-fed infant, 966
  for labor and birth pain, 190, 192t
Mescaline, 945
Mesoderm, embryonic, 104, 104t
Metabolic adaptation, in newborn, 287,
      287b
Metabolism, inborn errors of, 504–508. See
      also Inborn errors of metabolism
Metaphysis, 888
Metaproterenol hydrochloride, for
      asthma, 784, 785t
Metered-dose inhaler (MDI), 784, 785f
Metformin
  for diabetes mellitus type 2 in children,
      863
  in pregnancy, 349
Methamphetamine, 946
Methaqualone abuse, 946
Methicillin-resistant S. aureus (MRSA)
      infection, newborn, 475t
Methyldopa
  on breast-fed infant, 967
  for hypertension in pregnancy, 403
Methylphenidate, for ADHD, 939
Metronidazole
  in children, 849
  for trichomoniasis in pregnancy, 366

Metrorrhagia, 63
Miconazole, for tinea corporis, 903
Microcephaly, 155
Microcytic anemia, 355
Micro drop, 692, 693f
Microsporum audouinii, 903
Microsporum canis, 903
Midforceps, 243
Mifepristone (RU-486)
    for emergency contraception, 84
    for endometriosis, 66
    for induced abortion, 86t
    for uterine fibroids, 68
Milia, 292, 293b
Miliaria rubra, 900
Military presentation, 171, 171f
Milk, breast
    composition of, 328–329
    nutrition in, 324
    for preterm newborn, 463
    pumping of, 334, 334f
    storing of, 334–335, 335t
Milk, witch's, 297
Milk allergy, 830, 831t
Milk ducts, plugged, 333
Milwaukee brace, 893–894, 893f
Mineral insufficiencies, 830
Mineral requirements, in pregnancy,
    127–129, 128t–129t
Minerals. *See also specific minerals*
    good sources of, 965
Mini drop, 692, 693f
Minimal change nephrotic syndrome
    (MCNS), 872–875. *See also*
    Nephrotic syndrome
Mini-pill, 73f, 80–81
Miscarriage, 384–387, 385t. *See also*
    Spontaneous abortion
Misidentification prevention, newborn, 309
Misoprostol, for cervical ripening, 240–241
Missed abortion, 385t
Mistaken identity, of newborn, 309
Mistrust, 528
Mitosis, 100, 100f
Mittelschmerz, 875
Mixed hearing loss, 750
Mode of transmission, 928b
Modified dorsal recumbent position, 228t
Moist heat, 672
Molar pregnancy, 387–389
Molding, 170, 294, 294f
Mongolian spots, 293b
Mono, 927–928, 927f
Monoamniotic-monochorionic twins, 113
Monocytes, 820
Monotherapy, 359t
Monozygotic twins, 113, 113f, 403–404
Mons pubis, 49, 49f
Montelukast, for asthma, 784, 785t
Montgomery's tubercles, 121
Mood stabilizers, on breast-fed infant,
    967
Morbidity, 16
Morning sickness. *See* Nausea
Moro reflex, 299, 300f
    asymmetrical, 297
    exaggerated, 289
Morphine, on breast-fed infant, 966
Mortality, 14, 14b
Morula, 102, 103f
Motor vehicle accidents, toddlers in,
    567–568, 567f

Mottling, of newborn skin, 292
Mouth, of newborn
    assessment of, 295–296
    suctioning of, 305, 305f
Movement, for labor/birth pain, 188,
    189f
Mucocutaneous lymph node syndrome,
    811–812
Mucous plus, passage of, 175
Multifetal pregnancy, 113, 113f, 136b
Multigravida, 136
Multiparity, grand, 262
Multiple gestation, 403–404
Multiple-marker screening, 142
Mummy restraint, 664, 665f
Mumps, 930t
Munchausen syndrome by proxy, 713
Mupirocin, for impetigo, 902
Muscles, 880–881, 882f. *See also*
    Musculoskeletal disorders
Muscular dystrophy, 888–890, 889f, 890f
Musculoskeletal changes, in pregnancy,
    122, 122f
Musculoskeletal disorders, 881–896. *See*
    also specific disorders
    Ewing's sarcoma, 891
    fractures, 882–887
    juvenile rheumatoid arthritis, 891–892,
        891t
    Legg-Calvé-Perthes disease, 890
    muscular dystrophy, 888–890, 889f,
        890f
    osteomyelitis, 888
    osteosarcoma, 890–891
    scoliosis, 892–896
Musculoskeletal system
    anatomy of, 882f
    growth and development of, 880–881
    postpartum, 264
Myelomeningocele, 479f, 480
Myelomeningocele with spina bifida,
    479–480, 479f
Myoclonic seizures, 756
Myomectomy, for uterine fibroids, 68
Myometrium, of uterus, 51, 52f
Myopia, 744
Myotonia, in sexual response cycle, 55–56
MyPyramid
    for Kids, 520, 521f, 562, 580
    for pregnancy, 125, 126f, 151
Myringotomy, 752

N
Nadir, 214, 215f
Nagele's rule, 138
Nail assessment, newborn, 292
Nails, 899
NANDA-approved nursing diagnoses,
    961–963
    activity/rest, 961–962
    comfort, 963
    coping/stress tolerance, 962
    elimination, 961
    growth/development, 963
    health promotion, 961
    life principles, 962–963
    nutrition, 961
    perception/cognition, 962
    role relationships, 962
    safety/protection, 963
    self-perception, 962
    sexuality, 962

Naproxen
    on breast-fed infant, 966
    for dysmenorrhea, 64
    for premenstrual syndrome, 65
Narcotics
    on breast-fed infant, 966
    child abuse of, 945 (*See also* Substance
        abuse)
Nasal administration, in children, 686
Nasal cannula, 670, 670t
Nasal cavity, 487f, 488f
Nasal congestion, in pregnancy, 122
Nasal prongs, 670–671, 670t
Nasal stuffiness, prenatal care for, 147,
    148t
Nasal suctioning, 671, 671f
Nasopharyngitis, 776–777
Nasopharynx, 488f
National Fetal and Infant Mortality
    Review (NFIMR) Program, 18
National Immunization Awareness Month
    (NIAM), 17
National MCHB Center for Child Death
    Review (CDR), 17
Natural immunity, 928b
Nausea and vomiting
    causes of, 117
    prenatal care for, 147, 148t
Nearsightedness, 744
Nebulizer, 784, 785f
Necator americanus, 848–849
Neck assessment, newborn, 296–297,
    296f
Necrotizing enterocolitis (NEC), in
    preterm newborn, 458
Negativism, 558
Neglect, child, 713–714, 716t
Neisseria gonorrhoeae infection
    newborn infection with, 474t
    in pregnancy, 364–365, 368–372 (*See*
        also Sexually transmitted
        infections (STIs), nursing
        process for)
Neonatal Behavioral Assessment Scale,
    288
Neonatal hypoglycemia, 287, 287b, 289
Neonatal mortality rate, 14b
Neonatal substance withdrawal, 473,
    473f
Neonatologist, 4
Nephrotic syndrome, 872–875
    vs. acute glomerulonephritis, 871
    clinical manifestations of, 872, 872f
    diagnosis of, 872
    nursing process for, 873–875
    pathophysiology of, 872
    treatment of, 872–873
Nervous system, 743–744
Neural tube defects, 479. *See also specific*
    defects
Neuromuscular development, in infants,
    540–541
Neuromuscular maturity, 451, 452f,
    453t
Nevus flammeus, 293b
Newborn. *See also* Infant
    gestational and acquired disorders of,
        451–475 (*See also* Acquired
        disorders; Gestational disorders)
    physiology of, *vs.* fetus, 285t
    respiratory distress in, 285b
    toddler sharing with, 561–562, 562f

Newborn care nursing process, general, 309–314
  assessment, 309–310
  evaluation, 313
  implementation
    airway clearance, 310
    first bath, 311–312, 313f
    infection transmission prevention, 310–311
    organized infant behavioral responses, 313
    safety, 313
    skin care, 311–312, 313f
  nursing diagnoses, 310
  outcome identification and planning, 310
Newborn care nursing process, immediate stabilization and transition, 304–309
  assessment, 305
  evaluation, 309
  implementation, 305–309
    cardiovascular and respiratory transition, 305, 305f
    fluid imbalance prevention, 308–309, 308f
    infection prevention, 306–308, 308f
    injury prevention from hypoglycemia, 306, 306f, 307
    misidentification prevention, 309
    thermoregulation, 306, 306f
  nursing diagnoses, 305
  outcome identification and planning, 305
  overview, 304
  standard of care, 304
Newborn circulation, 485, 485f
Newborn discharge preparation nursing process, 314–321
  assessment, 314
  evaluation, 321
  implementation, 315–321
    circumcision assistance, 315–316, 316f
    circumcision family teaching, 317
    infection prevention, immunization, 316–317
    neonatal screening for injury prevention, 317–318, 317b, 318f
    pain prevention and treatment, 315
    parent education, 318–321
      airway clearance, 318, 320f
      crying, 319
      feeding, 319
      handling newborn, 318, 320f
      health maintenance, 319
      infection prevention, 318, 320f
      overview, 318
      safety, 321
      sensory input, 319
      skin care, 321
      sleeping, 319
      stool and urine monitoring, 320–321
      swaddling, 318, 320f
      temperature maintenance, 318–320
  nursing diagnoses, 314
  outcome and identification planning, 314–315
Newborn Hearing Screening program, 17
Newborn nursing care, 304–321
  heel stick in, 307
  IM injection in, 308

Newborn nutrition. See Nutrition, newborn
Newborn rash, 293b
Newborn transition
  fetus vs. newborn physiology in, 285t
  physiologic adaptation in, 284–288
    behavioral and social, 288
    cardiovascular, 285–286
    hepatic, 287–288
    metabolic, 287, 287b
    respiratory, 284–285
    thermoregulatory, 286–287, 286f
  respiratory distress in, 285b
Newborn transition assessment, 288–300
  initial, at birth, 288, 289t
  initial admitting, 289–300
    appearance, body proportions, posture, 290
    Barlow's sign, 298–299
    behavioral, 299–300
    gestational age, 300
    head-to-toe assessment, 292–298
      (See also Head-to-toe assessment, newborn)
    neurologic (reflexes), 298–299, 300f
    Ortolani's maneuver, 298–299
    overview, 289–290
    physical measurements, 291–292, 292f, 292t
    vital signs, 290, 290f, 290t
  throughout transition, 288–289
Newborn weights, pounds to ounces conversion charts for, 977
Niacin. See Vitamin B₃
Niacin insufficiency, 830
Nighttime bending brace, 893–894, 893f
90°–90° traction, 884, 885f
Nipple-feeding, of preterm newborn, 462–463
Nipple sensitivity, 332
Nipple soreness, from breast-feeding, 332
Nissen fundoplication, 834, 834f
Nocturnal emissions, 606
Nonaccidental injury sites, 712, 713f
Noncommunicative language, 577
Non–insulin-dependent diabetes, 862–863
Noninvasive MRI-guided focused ultrasound, for uterine fibroids, 68
Nonorganic failure to thrive (NFTT), 945–948, 946f
Nonsteroidal anti-inflammatory drugs (NSAIDs). See also specific drugs
  on breast-fed infant, 966
  for dysmenorrhea, 64
  for endometriosis, 66
  food with, 892
  for juvenile rheumatoid arthritis, 891–892
  for premenstrual syndrome, 65
Nonstress test (NST), 144–145
North American Nursing Diagnosis Association (NANDA), 21
Nose, 487f, 488f
Nose and throat specimen collection, 672–673
Nose assessment, newborn, 295
Nosebleeds
  in pregnancy, 122
  prenatal care of, 147, 148t
Nose specimen collection, 672–673
Nostril patency, bilateral, in newborns, 295

Nuchal cord
  definition of, 423t
  on fetal heart rate, 214, 215f
Nuchal rigidity, 759
Nuchal translucency, 141
Nuclear family, 27, 27f
Nulli, 136b
Nulligravida, 136, 136b
Nursery school, 580
Nursing diagnoses, NANDA-approved, 961–963. See also NANDA-approved nursing diagnoses
Nursing process, 21–22, 21f
  in community-based nursing, 36
  in cost containment, 11, 11t
  in maternal–child health care, 21–22, 21f
Nutrients. See also specific nutrients
  essential, good sources of, 965
Nutrition
  in adolescents, 609–610, 609t, 610t
  in children, 667–670
    gastrostomy feeding, 667–670, 669f
    gavage feeding, 667–669
    intake and output measurements, 667
  in first year of life, 545–549
    feeding schedule, 547t–548t
    first 4-6 months, 545–546
    solid foods, 546–549
      food preparation, 546, 546f, 548
      infant feeding, 546, 546f
      self-feeding, 548–549, 548f
    weaning, 549
    Women, Infants, and Children Food Program, 549
  gastrostomy feeding, 667–670, 669f
  gavage feeding, 667–669
  on growth and development, 520–522, 521f
  intake and output measurements in, 667
  postpartum, 280
  preconception, 70
  in pregnancy, 125–126, 126f
  in preschoolers, 580–581
    daily nutritional needs, 581, 581t
    eating skills, 581, 582f
    snacks, 581, 581b
  in school-aged children, 593–594, 594t
  Special Supplemental Nutrition Program for Women, Infants, and Children in, 13, 13f
  in toddlers, 562–563, 562t
  total parenteral nutrition, 692–693, 693f
  in utero, 324
Nutrition, newborn, 324–339
  breast-feeding in, 325–335 (See also Breast-feeding)
  breast-feeding vs. formula-feeding in
    culture on, 324–325
    intent to return to work/school on, 325
    nursing considerations in, 325
    past experiences on, 325
    sociodemographics on, 325
  foods in, 338–339, 339t
  formula amounts in, 338–339, 339t
  formula-feeding in, 335–339 (See also Formula-feeding)
  nutritional needs in, 324, 325t

Nutritional intake, in pregnancy, 151
Nutritional needs
    of breast-feeding mother, 329
    of newborn, 324, 325t
    in preterm newborn, 456
Nutritional problems
    food allergies, 830–831, 831t
    iron deficiency, 830
    kwashiorkor, 829, 829f
    marasmus, 829
    mineral insufficiencies, 830
    niacin insufficiency, 830
    nursing process for, 831–832
    riboflavin deficiency, 830
    thiamine deficiency, 830
    vitamin C deficiency, 830
    vitamin D deficiency, 829
Nutritional status assessment, in
        pregnancy, 145–146
Nutrition history, in children, 627
NuvaRing, 73f, 80f, 82
Nystatin
    for candidiasis, 901
    for fetal thrush, 296

O

Obesity, in children, 594, 955
Objective data, 21, 628
Objective data collection in children,
        628–639. See also Data
        collection in children, objective
Obstetric conjugate, 169
Obstetrician, 4
Occupational health, blood-borne
        pathogens and, 959–960
Older adults, respiratory function in, 495t
Oils, skin, 899–900
Oligohydramnios
    on fetal heart rate, 214, 215f
    in postterm pregnancy, 417
Oliguria, 871
Omphalocele, 498–499, 499f
Onlooker play, 579
Oocyte, 100, 100f
Oocyte genesis, 100–101, 100f
Oogenesis, 100–101, 100f
Open adoption, 28
Open fracture, 882f
Open-glottis pushing, 226
Open-heart surgery, for congenital heart
        defects, 490
Operative vaginal delivery. See Assisted
        delivery
Ophthalmia, sympathetic, 748
Ophthalmia neonatorum, 306–308, 308f,
        365
Ophthalmic administration, in children,
        685, 685f
Opioids. See also specific agents and
        substances
    for labor and birth pain, 191, 192t
Opisthotonos, 759
Oral administration, in children,
        684–685, 684f, 685f, 686b
Oral care, in first-stage labor, 222–223
Oral contraceptives. See also specific
        agents
    combination, 73f, 79–80, 80b, 80f,
        81b
    for dysmenorrhea, 64
    for endometriosis, 66
    for uterine cysts, 68

Oral glucose tolerance test (OGTT), 347,
        347b
Oral hypoglycemic agents, in pregnancy,
        349
Oral stage, 525–526
Oral suctioning, 671, 671f
Oral temperatures, in children, 632
Orchiopexy, 875
Orgasm, 56
Oropharynx, 488f
Orthodontia, 612
Orthopedic cast, infant care with,
        505–506
Orthoptics, 748
Ortolani maneuver, 298–299, 502
Osteomyelitis, 888
Osteoporosis
    risk factors for, 92b
    treatment for prevention of, 92
Osteosarcoma, 890–891
Ostomy care, 672
Otic administration, in children, 686, 687f
Otitis media, 745f, 752–753
Otoacoustic emissions, 318
Outcome identification and planning,
        21–22, 21f. See also specific topics
Outcomes, 21–22. See also specific topics
Outlet forceps, 243
Outpatient setting, child health care in, 34
Output measurements, 667
Ova, 45, 52–53
Ovarian artery, 53, 53f
Ovarian cycle, 54–55, 54f
Ovarian cysts, 68
Ovarian vein, 53
Ovaries, 51f, 52–53, 52f
    postpartum, 262
    in pregnancy, 120
Overprotection, 700
Overweight, 954
Oviducts, 51f, 52–53, 52f
Ovulation, 54–55, 54f
Ovulation Predictor Test, 76
Ovum, tubal transport of, 103f
Oximetry, fetal scalp pulse, 210t, 217
Oxygen administration
    in children, 670–671, 670t, 671f
    in preterm newborn, 457
Oxygen croupette, 670, 670t
Oxygen hood, 670, 670t
Oxygen mask, 670t
Oxygen tent, 670–671, 670t, 671f
Oxytocin
    for cervical ripening, 241
    in contraction stress test, 145
    on labor contractions, 185
    in labor onset, 174
    in lactation, 327–328, 328f
    in pregnancy, 121
    for vaginal birth after cesarean, 254–255
    for variables, 215

P

Pain, 184
Pain, labor and birth
    definition of, 184
    factors in, 185
    nursing care plan for, 197–198
    in obstructed labor, 185
    physiology and characteristics of,
        184–185
    uniqueness of, 184

Pain management. See also specific
        disorders
    after cesarean, 276
    in children, postoperative, 653–654, 654f
    postpartum, 271
    postpartum, early, 271–272
Pain management, labor and birth, 185–198
    after delivery, 233–234
    first stage of labor, 222
    nonpharmacologic interventions in,
        186–190
        acupressure and acupuncture, 187t,
            190
        comfort measures, 186
        comparison of, 187t
        continuous labor support, 186, 187t
        intradermal water injections, 187t,
            190, 190f
        relaxation techniques
            attention focusing, 186–188, 187t
            hypnosis, 187t, 190
            movement and positioning, 188,
                189f
            patterned breathing, 186, 187t,
                188t
            touch and massage, 187t, 188, 190f
            water therapy, 187t, 188–189, 190f
    pharmacologic interventions in, 190–196
        analgesia and sedation, 191, 192t
        anesthesia, 191–196, 192t–193t (See
            also Anesthesia, for labor and
            birth pain)
    principles of, 185–186
Pain scales, for children, 654, 654f
Pain threshold, 185
Pain tolerance, 185
Paired ligaments, of uterus, 51–52, 52f
Palmar grasp reflex, 298, 300f
Pancreas
    in children, 828
    in pregnancy, 121
Pandemic, 928b
Papoose boards, 664, 665f
Pap smear
    in first prenatal visit, 137
    in women's health examinatnoi, 61
Pap smear collection, 61–62
Para, 136, 136b
Paracervical block, 192t, 193
Parallel play, 560, 560f
Paramyxovirus, 930t
Parasites, intestinal, 848–849
Parasitic infections
    pediculosis, 904–905
    scabies, 905
Paraurethral glands, 50
Parental behavior, 29–30, 29f
Parenteral nutrition administration, 693,
        693f
Parenthood, preparing patient for, 156,
        157b, 158b
    baby care classes in, 159, 159b
    breast-feeding classes in, 159
    siblings class in, 159–160
Parenting, surrogate, 91
Parent–newborn attachment, early
        postpartum, 274
Parent–newborn bonding, 232–233, 233f,
        270, 270b, 274
Parishes, health care at, 35–36
Parity, 136, 136b
Parotitis, 930t

Parrot speech, 938
Partial seizures, 756
Partial sight, 745
Partograph, 206, 206f
Passageway, 167–169
    bony pelvis, 167, 168f
    pelvic dimensions, 169
    pelvic shape, 167–168, 168f
    soft tissues, 169, 169f
Passenger, 170–172
    fetal attitude, 170–171, 171f
    fetal lie, 170, 170f
    fetal position, 171–172, 172b, 172t, 173f
    fetal presentation, 170, 171f
    fetal skull, 170, 170f
    fetal station, 172, 173f
Passive immunity, 928b
Patch, contraceptive, 73f, 80f, 82
Patellar reflexes, in preeclampsia-
        eclampsia, 396, 397f, 400
Patient-care equipment, 959
Patient-controlled analgesia (PCA) in
        children, postoperative, 654, 654f
Patient placement, 960
Patterned breathing, for labor/birth pain,
        186, 187t, 188t
Pavlik harness, 503, 503f
PCP, 945
Peak flow meter, 782–783, 782f
Pediatric health care
    development of, 5–6, 5f
    history of, 4
Pediculosis, 904–905
Pellagra, 830
Pelvic examination, 61
Pelvic inflammatory disease (PID), 67
    from chlamydia, 364
    from gonorrhea, 365
Pelvic rest, 413
Pelvic support disorders, 68–70, 69f
Pelvis
    android, 168, 168f
    anthropoid, 167–168, 168f
    bony, 167, 168f
    dimensions of, 169
    false, 167, 168f
    gynecoid, 167, 168f
    platypelloid, 168, 168f
    true, 167, 168f
Pemoline, for ADHD, 939
Penicillin
    on breast-fed infant, 967
    for impetigo, 902
    for rheumatic fever, 809
Penis, 45–46, 46f, 47f
Penis assessment, newborn, 297
Pentobarbital, for labor/birth pain, 190, 192t
Perceptive hearing loss, 750
Percutaneous umbilical blood sampling
        (PUBS), 144
Perimenopause, 91
Perinatal transmission, 359t
Perinatologist, 4
Perineal care, postpartum, 278–279
Perineal pain, postpartum, 271–272
Perineum, 49f, 50
    bulging of, 227, 227f
    cleaning of, for delivery, 227, 227f
    postpartum, 262–263
    in pregnancy, 120–121
Periodic changes, in fetal heart rate, 214,
        215f

Period of communicability, 928b
Perioperative period, in cesarean birth, 247
Peripheral intravenous access, 691–692,
        691f, 692f
Personal history, in children, 627
Personality development, in adolescents,
        608, 608f
Perspiration, 899
Pertussis, 929t
Pervasive developmental disorder, 937
Petechiae, 820
Petit mal seizures, 756
Petrolatum gauze dressing, after
        circumcision, 315, 315f
Pfannenstiel's incision, 245, 246f
pH, fetal scalp, 180, 180t
Phallic stage, 526
Phantom pain, 890
Pharynx, in children, 776
Phenobarbital, 758t
Phenothiazines, on breast-fed infant, 967
Phenylketonuria (PKU), 326, 506–507
Phenytoin, 758t
Phimosis, 297
Phobia, school, 940
Phosphorus, in pregnancy, 127, 128t
Photophobia, 748
Phototherapy, for hemolytic disease of
        newborn, 471, 471f
Physical abuse, of children, 712–713,
        713f–715f, 716t
Physical development. See also Growth
        and development
    in adolescents, 606
    in infants, 538–541 (See also Growth
        and development, 28 days to 1
        year)
    in preadolescents, 605–606
    in preschoolers, 575, 576t
    in school-aged children, 589–591, 591t
        (See also Growth and
        development, 6-10 years)
    in toddlers, 558, 558f, 559t
Physical examination. See also specific
        disorders
    in first prenatal visit, 137–138, 138f
    maternal, on admission for labor/birth,
        205, 205b, 206f
Physical examination, in children, 636–639
    abdomen, 637
    back and extremities, 638
    chest and lungs, 637
    ears, 637
    eyes, 636–637
    genitalia and rectum, 637–638
    head and neck, 636
    heart, 637, 638f
    for hospital admission, 650
    neurologic, 638, 639f
    nose, mouth, and throat, 637, 637f
Physical maturity, 451, 452f
Physical neglect, of children, 713–714,
        716t
Physical sustenance, physical, 26
Physiologic adaptation, of newborn,
        284–288
    behavioral and social, 288
    cardiovascular, 285–286
    hepatic, 287–288
    metabolic, 287, 287b
    respiratory, 284–285
    thermoregulatory, 286–287, 286f

Physiologic jaundice, 287
Piaget, Jean, 526t, 529, 529f
Pica
    in children, 850
    in pregnancy, 132
Picornavirus, 931t
Piercings, body, 611
Pike position, 412
Pill, contraceptive, 73f, 79–80, 80b, 80f,
        81b
Pinworm infection, 848
Pitocin. See Oxytocin
Pituitary gland
    anterior
        on menstrual cycle, 54–55, 54f
        on reproductive system, 45, 46f
    in pregnancy, 121
Placenta, 107–108, 107f
    delivery of, 178t, 179, 231–232, 231f
    healthy, 231, 231f
Placenta accreta, 423t
Placental abnormalities, 422, 423t
Placental abruption, 390–392, 391f
Placental circulation, 109
Placenta previa, 244, 389–391, 389f
Plant allergies, 908–909, 909f
Plantar grasp reflex, 298
Plasma, blood, in pregnancy, 121
Plasma thromboplastin component
        deficiency, 816–817
Plateau, sexual, 56
Platform crutches, 887
Platypelloid pelvis, 168, 168f
Play
    childhood, 522
    in preschoolers, 578–579, 578f
    therapeutic
        postoperative, 656, 656f
        preoperative, 652, 652f
    in toddlers, 560–561, 560f
Play program, hospital, 655–657
    hospital play environment in, 655–656,
        655f, 656f
    play material in, 656–657, 657t
    therapeutic play in, 652, 652f, 656, 656f
Plexus, 53
Plugged milk ducts, 333
Plumbism, 850–852
Pneumonia, bacterial, 788–793
    clinical manifestations of, 788
    diagnosis of, 788
    epidemiology and types of, 788
    H. influenzae, 788
    nursing process for
        assessment, 788–789
        evaluation, 792–793
        implementation, 789–792
        nursing care plan, 790–791
        nursing diagnoses, 789
        outcome identification and planning,
            789
    treatment of, 788
Poisoning, 849–850, 850t
    lead, 16
    of toddlers, 568–569
Poison ivy, 908–909, 909f
Poison oak, 908–909
Poison prevention, 849
Poison sumac, 908–909
Polar bodies, 100–101, 100f
Poliomyelitis, 930t
Polyarthritis, 808

Polycythemia, in postterm newborn, 466
Polydipsia, 855
Polyhydramnios, 346
Polyphagia, 855, 955
Polyps, cervical, 67
Polyuria, 855
Port-wine stain, 293b
Position, fetal, 171–172, 172b, 172t, 173f
Positioning
    of infants and small children, 665–666, 666f
    for labor and birth pain, 188, 189f
    for sleep, 666
Positioning, for procedures, 664–666
    holding in, 665, 666f
    restraints in, 664–665, 665f (See also Restraints)
    for sleep, 666
    for transporting, 666
Postcoital test, 89
Postconventional level, 530
Postmature, 451
Postpartum blues, 267, 443–444, 444b
Postpartum care, with cardiovascular disease, 354
Postpartum depression, 443–444, 444b
Postpartum exercise classes, 156, 159
Postpartum home care, 32, 32f
Postpartum infection, 432–434
Postpartum maternal adaptation, 261–267
    physiological, 261–264
        breasts, 263
        cardiovascular system, 263
        cervix, 262, 263f
        gastrointestinal system, 264
        integumentary system, 264
        involution, 261
        musculoskeletal system, 264
        ovaries, 262
        urinary system, 264
        uterus, 261–262, 262f
        vagina and perineum, 262–263
        vital signs, 263–264
        weight loss, 264
    psychological, 265–267
        attachment, 265–266, 266b
        becoming a mother, 265
        bonding, 265–267, 266f, 267f
        postpartum blues, 267
Postpartum nursing process, after cesarean, 274–277
    assessment, 275
    evaluation, 277
    implementation, 275–276
    nursing diagnoses, 275
    outcome identification and planning, 275
Postpartum nursing process, early postpartum
    assessment, 267–270
        complete physical, 268–270, 268f
            bladder and bowel, 269
            breasts, 268
            laboratory studies, 270
            lochia, 268
            lower extremities, 269–270, 270f
            maternal emotional status, 270
            maternal-newborn bonding, 270, 270b
            pain, 270
            perineum, 269, 269f
            uterus, 268–269

data collection, 267–268
initial physical, first hour after delivery, 268
evaluation, 274
implementation, 271–274
    bowel elimination, 273
    fall prevention, 273
    infection prevention, 272–273
    pain management, 271–272
    parent–newborn attachment, 274
    promoting hemostasis, 271
    sleep promotion, 273–274
    thrombus prevention, 273
    urinary elimination, 273
nursing diagnoses, 270–271
outcome identification and planning, 271
Postpartum nursing process, for discharge preparation, 277–280
    assessment, 277
    evaluation, 280
    implementation, 277–280
        danger signs, 278, 279b
        health-seek behavior support, 277–278
        injury prevention, nonimmunity to rubella, 278, 279b
        injury prevention, Rh-negative, 278, 278b
        patient teaching, 278–280, 279b
    nursing diagnoses, 277
    outcome identification and planning, 277
Postpartum period
    changes in, 426
    definition of, 426
Postpartum psychosis, 445
Postpartum woman at risk, 426–447
    grief, 445–446
    hemorrhage, 426–432 (See also Hemorrhage, postpartum)
        early postpartum, 427–432 (See also Hemorrhage, early postpartum)
        late postpartum, 432
    infection (puerperal infection), 432–434
        causes and clinical manifestations of, 433
        definition of, 432–433
        endometritis, 433–435
        progression of, 433
        risk factors for, 433
    malattachment, 446–447
    mastitis, 333, 436–440 (See also Mastitis)
    psychiatric disorders, 443–444
        causes and risk factors for, 443
        definition and overview of, 443
        depression, 443–444, 444b
        psychosis, 445
    urinary tract infection, 437, 440–441 (See also Urinary tract infections (UTIs), postpartum)
    venous thromboembolism, 441–443
    wound infection, 434–436, 435f (See also Wound infection, postpartum)
Postterm, 451
Postterm newborn, 466–467
Postterm pregnancy and labor, 417–418
Postural drainage positions, 796, 796f–797f

Postural hypotension, in pregnancy, 147
Posture, of newborn, 290
Potty chair, 565–567, 565f
Pounds to kilograms conversion, 683, 976
Pounds to ounces conversion, 977
Poverty, 9, 38
Povidone-iodine, for burns, 915
Preadolescent development, 605–606
Precautions, standard and transmission-based, 959–960
Precocious teeth, 296
Preconception care, 70–72, 71b
Preconventional level, 530
Preeclampsia-eclampsia, 394–403
    with chronic hypertension, 403, 403b
    clinical manifestations of, 396–398
    definition and progress of, 394
    epidemiology of, 395
    HELLP syndrome in, 398
    mild vs. severe, 396, 397t
    nursing care for, 399–402
        eclamptic seizures in, 400
        monitoring in, 397f, 400–401
        nursing care plan in, 401–402
        nutrition in, 401
        postpartum care in, 401–402
        psychosocial needs in, 401
    patellar reflexes and clonus in, 396, 397f
    pathophysiology of, 395–396, 396f
    prevention and prediction of, 395, 398, 398b
    risk factors for, 395, 395b
    serious complications of, 395, 395t
    signs and symptoms of, 394–395
    treatment of, 398–399, 398b
Pre-embryonic stage, 101–103, 101f–103f
Preferred provider organizations (PPOs), 12, 12b
Pregestational diabetes mellitus, 346
Pregnancy
    amenorrhea in, 63
    danger signs of, 145b
    ectopic, 112–113, 383–384, 383f
    fetal development in, 99–113 (See also Fetal development)
    multifetal, 113, 113f
    postterm, 417–418
Pregnancy, maternal adaptation in, 117–132
    dietary restrictions in, 130
    dietary supplementation in, 130
    food safety in, 131
    lactose intolerance in, 131–132
    mineral requirements in, 127–129, 128t–129t
    nutritional requirements in, 125–126, 126f
    physiologic, 119–123
        breasts, 121
        cardiovascular changes, 121–122, 122f
        cervix and ovaries, 120, 120f
        endocrine changes, 121
        gastrointestinal changes, 123
        hematologic changes, 121
        integumentary changes, 123
        menstrual cycle, 119–120
        vs. nonpregnant woman, 119t
        respiratory changes, 122
        urinary changes, 123
        uterus, 120, 120f
        vagina and perineum, 120–121

pica in, 132
protein requirements in, 126–127
psychologic, 123–125
  factors in, 123–124
  first-trimester, 124
  second-trimester, 124–125
  third-trimester, 125
signs of pregnancy
  overview, 117, 118b
  positive, 118, 118b
  presumptive (possible), 117–118, 118b
  probable, 118, 118b
vegetarianism in, 130–131
vitamin requirements in, 128t–129t, 129–130
Pregnancy at risk, complicating conditions, 345–378. See also specific conditions
age-related concerns, 375–378
  adolescent pregnancy, 375–377
  pregnancy in later life, 377–378
anemia, 355–356
asthma, 356–358
cardiovascular disease, 352–356 (See also Cardiovascular disease, in pregnancy)
diabetes mellitus, 346–352 (See also Diabetes mellitus (DM), in pregnancy)
epilepsy, 357–359
infectious diseases, 359–372 (See also Infectious diseases, in pregnancy; specific diseases)
intimate partner violence, 372–375 (See also Intimate partner violence (IPV), in pregnancy)
overview, 345
Pregnancy at risk, pregnancy-related complications, 381–405
bleeding disorders, 383–394
  abruptio placentae, 390–392, 391f
  early pregnancy loss, 384–387 (See also Spontaneous abortion)
  ectopic pregnancy, 112–113, 383–384, 383f
  gestational trophoblastic disease, 387–389
  nursing process for, 392–394
  overview of, 383
  placenta previa, 389–391, 389f
blood incompatibilities
  ABO, 405
  Rh, 404–405
chronic hypertension, 403
hyperemesis gravidarum, 381–383
hypertensive disorders in pregnancy
  gestational hypertension, 394
  preeclampsia-eclampsia, 394–403 (See also Preeclampsia-eclampsia)
multiple gestation, 403–404
Pregnancy exercise classes, 156, 159
Pregnancy-related complications. See Pregnancy at risk: pregnancy-related complications; specific complications
Pregnancy-related hypertension, in diabetic mothers, 350–351
Pregnancy Risk Assessment Monitoring System (PRAMS), 18
Pregnancy tests
home, 118
types and use of, 118

Premature, 451
Premature rupture of membranes (PROM), 413–414
Premenstrual dysphoric disorder (PMDD), 64–65
Premenstrual syndrome (PMS), 64–66, 65b, 876
Premoral level, 530
Prenatal care, 135–145
danger signs in, 145b
fetal well-being assessment in, 140–145
  amniocentesis in, 142–143, 142f, 143b
  biophysical profile in, 145
  chorionic villus sampling in, 143–144, 143b
  contraction stress test in, 145
  fetal kick counts in, 140
  maternal serum alpha-fetoprotein screening in, 142
  nonstress test in, 144–145
  percutaneous umbilical blood sampling in, 144
  triple-marker (multiple-marker) screening in, 142
  ultrasonography in, 140–141, 140f, 141b
  vibroacoustic stimulation in, 145
goal of, 135
home, 32, 32f
maternal well-being assessment in, 135–140
  first prenatal visit, 135–139
    due date estimation in, 138–139
    genetic disorder screening in, 137, 137t
    history in, 136–137, 136b
    laboratory assessment in, 138
    length of, 135–136
    physical examination in, 137–138, 138f
    risk assessment in, 139
    STD risk determination in, 137, 137b
    timing of, 135
  subsequent prenatal visits, 139–140, 139f, 140f
statistics on, 135
Prenatal care nursing process, 145–160
assessment, 145–146, 146f
evaluation, 160
implementation, 146–160, 148t–149t
  birth plan, 156, 157b
  offering relief in, 146–151 (See also specific discomforts)
    ankle edema, 149t
    anxiety, 146–147
    backaches, 148t, 150
    breast tenderness, 148t
    constipation and hemorrhoids, 149t, 150
    fatigue, 148t
    feeling faint, 147, 148t
    flatulence, 149t
    gum bleeding, 148t
    heartburn, 148t, 149–150
    leg cramps, 149t, 150
    nasal stuffiness and epistaxis, 147, 148t
    nausea and vomiting, 147, 148t
    round ligament pain, 149t, 150
    safety of woman and fetus, 146b, 155

shortness of breath, 147–149, 148t
    sleep difficulties, 149t, 151
    urination, frequent, 147, 151
    vaginal discharge, 147
    varicose veins, 149t
  preparation for labor, birth, and parenthood, 155–160
    baby care classes, 159, 159b
    breast-feeding classes, 159
    childbirth education classes, 156, 158b, 159b
    choosing support person, 156
    communicating expectations, 155–156, 157b
    packing for hospital/birthing center, 155, 156b
    pregnancy and postpartum exercise classes, 156, 159
    siblings class in, 159–160
  self-care teaching, 151–155
    breast care, 152–153
    clothing, 153
    dental hygiene, 151–152
    employment, 153
    exercise, 152, 152b
    herbal remedies, 154–155
    hygiene, 152
    major components, 151b
    medications, 154, 154b
    nutritional intake, 151
    sexual activity, 153
    travel, 153, 154f
  substance use and abuse teaching, 155
nursing diagnoses, 146
outcome identification and planning, 146
Prenatal screening and testing
antibody, 138
bioethical issues, 9
genetic disorder, 137, 137t
hypothyroidism, 138
maternal serum alpha-fetoprotein, 142
triple-marker (multiple-marker), 142
Preoperational phase, 529
Pre-pregnancy planning, 70–72, 71b
Prepuce, 46, 48f
Preschooler
death and dying in, understanding of, 724
growth and development in, 574–584 (See also Growth and development, 3-6 years)
Presentation, fetal, 170, 171f
Preterm, 451
Preterm labor (PTL), 414–417
clinical manifestations and diagnosis of, 414–415
definition and overview of, 414
epidemiology of, 414
fetal fibronectin test in, 415, 415b
nursing process for, 415–417
risk factors for, 414, 414b
tocolytic agents for, 415, 416t
treatment of, 415
Preterm newborn, 451, 456–466
characteristics of, 456–457, 457f
complication treatment in
  intraventricular hemorrhage, 457–458
  necrotizing enterocolitis, 458
  respiratory distress syndrome, 457
  retinopathy of prematurity, 458

Preterm newborn, (continued)
  muscle weakness in, 457, 458f
  nursing process for, 459–460
    assessment, 459–460
    evaluation, 466
    implementation, 460–465
      body temperature, 461, 461f
      energy conservation, 464
      fluid and electrolyte balance, 462
      growth and development, 464
      infection prevention, 461–462
      neurologic status, 462
      nutrition, 462–463
      parental anxiety, 464–465
      parenting skills and family
        functioning, 465, 465f
      respiratory function, 460–461
      skin integrity, 463–464, 464b
    nursing diagnoses, 460
    outcome identification and planning,
      460
Prevention. See also specific disorders
  in community-based nursing, 39
  primary, 31
  secondary, 31
  tertiary, 31
Prickly heat, 900
Primary germ cells, body structures from,
  103, 103t
Primary prevention, 31
Primi, 136b
Primidone, 758t
Principled level, 530
Private insurance, 12, 12b
Procedures, in children, 662–676.
        See also specific procedures
  for circulation
    cold therapy, 667, 672
    heat therapy, 671–672
  for diagnostic tests and studies,
    675–676
  for elevated body temperature,
    666–667
  for elimination
    enema administration, 672
    ostomy care, 672
  for feeding and nutrition, 667–670
    gastrostomy feeding, 667, 669–670,
      669f
    gavage feeding, 667–669
    intake and output measurements, 667
  follow-up after, 663–664
  holding in, 665–666, 666f
  positioning for, 664–666
    holding in, 665, 666f
    restraints in, 664–665, 665f
      (See also Restraints)
    for sleep, 666
    for transporting, 666
  preparation for, 662–663, 663f
  for respiration, 670–671
    nasal/oral suctioning, 671, 671f
    oxygen administration, 670–671,
      670t, 671f
    tracheostomy care, 671
  for specimen collection, 672–675
    blood, 674, 674f
    lumbar puncture, 675, 675f
    nose and throat, 672–673
    stool, 674
    urine, 673–674, 673f
  transporting in, 666

Prodromal labor, 120, 175, 176t
Progesterone
  on gallbladder in pregnancy, 123
  in menstrual cycle, 54f, 55
  placental, 108
Progesterone intrauterine system, 73f
Progestin-only pills (POPs), 73f, 80–81
Prolactin, in pregnancy, 121
Proliferative phase, 54f, 55
Promethazine, for labor/birth pain, 190,
  192t
Proportions, newborn body, 290
Prospective payment system, 10
Prostaglandin E₁
  for cervical ripening, 240–241
  for vaginal birth after cesarean, 254–255
Prostaglandin E₂
  for cervical ripening, 240
  for vaginal birth after cesarean, 254–255
Prostaglandins
  in dysmenorrhea, 63–64
  in fertilization, 102
  for induced abortion, 86t
  in labor onset, 174
Prostate, 48, 48f
Protein
  good sources of, 965
  pregnancy requirements for, 126–127
Protein malnutrition, 829, 829f
Protest, 647
Protrusion reflex, 546, 546f
Proximodistal, 517, 518f
Pruritus, 830
Pseudohemophilia, 817
Pseudohypertrophic muscular dystrophy,
  888–890, 889f, 890f
Pseudomenstruation, 297
Psilocybin, 945
Psyche, maternal, in labor, 174, 175b
Psychedelic drugs, 945
Psychiatric disorders, postpartum, 443–444
  causes and risk factors for, 443
  definition and overview of, 443
  depression, 443–444, 444b
  psychosis, 445
Psychological status, in children,
  629–630, 629t
Psychomotor seizures, 756
Psychosis, postpartum, 445
Psychosocial development. See under
  Growth and development
Psychosocial disorders, 937–955, 940
  attention deficit hyperactivity disorder
    (ADHD), 939–940
  in adolescents, 616
  autism, 937–938
  children with, 937–958
  eating
    anorexia nervosa, 608–609,
      948–955, 949f (See also
      Anorexia nervosa)
    bulimia nervosa, 949–951
    nursing care plan for, 952–954
    nursing process for, 949–951, 955
  enuresis and encopresis, 940
  nonorganic failure to thrive, 945–948,
    946f
  obesity and overweight, 955
  school phobia, 940
  substance abuse, 941–945 (See also
    Substance abuse)
  suicide, 940–941

Ptyalism, in pregnancy, 123
Puberty, 53
Pubic lice, 904–905
Pudendal artery, internal, 53, 53f
Pudendal block, 191–193
Pudendal veins, 53
Puerperal fever, 4–5
Puerperal infection, 432–434. See also
  Infection, postpartum
Puerperium, 261. See also Postpartum
Pulmonary embolism (PE), 442–443
Pulmonary hypertension, in pregnancy,
  353
Pulmonary tuberculosis, 799–800
Pulse
  in children, 633, 633t, 638f, 975
  sites of, 638f
Pulse count, in infants, 540, 540f
Pulse oximetry
  in children, 634, 634f
  in preterm newborn, 460
Pulse taking
  in children, 633, 633t, 638f
  in newborn, 297, 298f, 305
Pumping, of breast milk, 334, 334f
Punishment, 561
Purpura, 820
Purpuric rash, 759
Pushing
  effective, 226–227, 228t–229t
  open-glottis, 226
  positions for, 226, 228t–229t
  promoting effective, 226
  vigorous, 226
Pustule, 928b
Pyelonephritis, 868
Pyloric stenosis, 839–842
  clinical manifestations of, 839
  diagnosis of, 839
  nursing process for, 839–841
  pathophysiology of, 839, 839f
  treatment of, 839, 839f
Pyloromyotomy, 839, 839f
Pylorus, 839
Pyrantel pamoate
  for hookworms, 849
  for roundworms, 848
Pyrethrin, for lice, 904
Pyridoxine. See Vitamin B₆
Pyrosis
  in pregnancy, 123
  prenatal care for, 148t, 149–150

Q

Quinacrine, 849

R

Rabies vaccination, 909
Radiant warmer, 461, 461f
Radiation, heat loss via, 286–287, 286f
Ranitidine, for gastroesophageal reflux,
  834
Rash
  newborn, 293b
  purpuric, 759
Rationing of health care, 9
Reactive airway disease (RAD). See
  Asthma
Recovery, after delivery, 179
Rectal administration, in children, 686
Rectal temperatures, in children, 632
Rectocele, 68–70, 69f

Rectum assessment, newborn, 298
Recurrent abortion, 385t
Red blood cells (RBCs), in pregnancy, 121
Red reflex, in newborn eyes, 295
Reflex, extrusion (protrusion), 546, 546f
Reflexes, newborn, 298–299, 300f
Refraction, 744
Refractive errors, 744–745
Regional anesthesia, for labor/birth pain, 190–193, 192t
   complications with, 195–196
   epidural, 192t, 193–195, 194f
   intrathecal, 193, 193t, 194f, 195
   overview, 191
   paracervical block, 192t, 193
   pudendal block, 191–193
Regionalized care, 6–8
Rejection, caregiver, 700, 701
Relaxation period, in labor contractions, 173
Relaxation techniques, for labor/birth pain
   attention focusing, 186–188, 187t
   hypnosis, 187t, 190
   movement and positioning, 188, 189f
   patterned breathing, 186, 187t, 188t
   touch and massage, 187t, 188, 190f
   water therapy, 187t, 188–189, 190f
Reproductive life cycle issues, 70–93
   family planning in, 70–86 (See also Family planning)
   induced abortion in, 86–87, 86t
   infertility in, 87–91 (See also Infertility)
   menopause in, 91–93, 92b (See also Menopause)
Reproductive system
   anterior pituitary on, 45, 46f
   complementary male/female structures in, 45
   paired structures in, 45
   purpose of, 45
   regulation of function of
      menopause in, 55
      menstrual cycle in, 53–55, 54f (See also Menstrual cycle)
      in puberty, 53
   sexual response cycle in, 55–56
Reproductive system, female, 49–53
   blood supply, 53, 53f
   clitoris, 49f, 50
   fallopian tubes, 51f, 52, 52f
   labia, 49–50, 49f
   mons pubis, 49, 49f
   ovaries, 51f, 52–53, 52f
   perineum, 49f, 50
   purpose, 49
   uterus, 51–52, 51f, 52f
   vagina, 50–51, 51f
   vestibule, 50
   vulva, 49–50, 49f
Reproductive system, male, 45–49
   accessory glands, 48, 48f
   alkaline fluids, 48
   bulbourethral (Cowper's) glands, 48, 48f
   ejaculatory ducts, 48, 48f
   hormones, 47, 49t
   penis, 45–46, 46f
   prostate, 48, 48f
   role and purpose, 45
   scrotum, 46–47, 46f, 48f

semen (seminal fluid), 48
seminal vesicles, 48, 48f
sperm, 45, 47, 49t
spermatic cord, 47–48, 48f
testes, 47, 48f
testosterone on, 47, 49t
vas deferens, 47–48, 48f
Reproductive tract, in children, 868
Reproductive tract disorders, female, 63–70
   infectious disorders
      pelvic inflammatory disease, 67
      toxic shock syndrome, 66–67
   menstrual, 63–66
      amenorrhea, 63
      atypical uterine bleeding, 63
      dysmenorrhea, 63–64
      endometriosis, 65–66
      premenstrual syndrome, 64–66, 65b
   pelvic support disorders, 68–70, 69f
   of uterus and ovaries
      cervical polyps, 67
      ovarian cysts, 68
      uterine fibroids, 67–68
Residential programs, children's health care at, 36
Resolution, sexual, 56
Respiration, in children
   physiology of, 776, 975
   as vital sign, 633–634, 634f
Respiration procedures, 670–671
   nasal/oral suctioning, 671, 671f
   oxygen administration, 670–671, 670t, 671f
   tracheostomy care, 671
Respiratory adaptation, in newborn, 284–285, 305
Respiratory changes, in pregnancy, 122
Respiratory depression, from spinal/epidural anesthesia, 196
Respiratory disorders, 776–800
   allergic rhinitis (hay fever), 777, 777f
   asthma, 781–788 (See also Asthma)
   bronchiolitis, acute, 781
   croup syndromes
      definition of, 779
      epiglottitis, 780, 780f
      laryngotracheobronchitis, acute, 780
      spasmodic laryngitis, 779–780
   cystic fibrosis, 793–799 (See also Cystic fibrosis (CF))
   nasopharyngitis, acute, 776–777
   pneumonia, bacterial, 788–793 (See also Pneumonia, bacterial)
   respiratory syncytial virus infection, 781
   tonsillectomy, 777–779
   tonsillitis and adenoiditis, 777–778
   tuberculosis, pulmonary, 799–800
Respiratory distress
   in newborn, 285b
   in newborn transition, 288–289, 306
Respiratory distress syndrome (RDS), in preterm newborn, 457
Respiratory hygiene, 960
Respiratory infections. See also specific infections
   family teaching on, 792
Respiratory pattern, monitoring, after cesarean, 275
Respiratory rate
   in infants, 540
   in newborn, 290, 290t

Respiratory rhythm, of newborn, 290, 290t
Respiratory syncytial virus (RSV) infection, 781
Respiratory system
   anatomy of, 776, 776f
   growth and development of, 775–776
Respiratory transition, newborn, 305, 305f
Respite care, 700
Rest, postpartum, 280
Restraints, 664–666, 665f, 666f
   clove hitch, 664, 665f
   crib top, 664, 665f
   elbow, 664, 665f
   for eye surgery, 749
   holding as, 665–666, 666f
   jacket, 664, 665f
   mummy, 664, 665f
   papoose boards, 664, 665f
   use of, 664
Resuscitation, newborn, 305
Retina, detached, 748
Retinopathy of prematurity (ROP), in preterm newborn, 458
Reversibility, 593
Reye syndrome, 753–754, 754t
Rh_0 (D) factor, 404
Rheumatic fever, 807–811
   cause of, 807
   clinical manifestations of, 807–808, 808f
   definition of, 807
   diagnosis of, 808, 808f
   nursing process for, 809–811
      assessment, 809
      evaluation, 811
      implementation, 810–811
      nursing diagnoses, 809
      outcome identification and planning, 810
   prevention of, 809
   treatment of, 808–809
Rheumatoid arthritis, juvenile, 891–892, 891t
Rh factor, 469
Rh incompatibility, 404–405, 469–470
Rhinitis, allergic, 777, 777f
Rh-negative, postpartum care for, 278
RhoGam, 405
Rh_0(D) immune globulin (RhoGAM), postpartum, 278, 278b
Rho(D) positive, 469–470
Rhythm method, 73f, 74–76. See also Fertility awareness methods (FAMs)
Ribavirin, 781
Riboflavin
   deficiency of, 830
   good sources of, 965
   in pregnancy, 128t
Rickets, 829
Rifampin, 800
Rights of medication administration, 680–681
Ring, vaginal contraceptive, 73f, 80f, 82
Ringworm
   of body, 903
   of feet, 903–904
   of inner thighs and inguinal area, 904
   of scalp, 903

Risk assessment. *See also specific disorders*
  on admission for labor/birth, 204
  in first prenatal visit, 139
Risk nursing diagnoses, 21
Ritual, in first-stage labor, 222
Ritualism, 558–560
Rocky Mountain spotted fever, 909
Rohypnol, 615–616
Role confusion, 529
Rooming-in, 647–649, 647f
Rooting reflex, 298, 327
Rotation, in delivery
  external, 176, 177f
  internal, 176, 177f
Round ligament, 52, 52f
Round ligament pain, prenatal care for, 149t, 150
Roundworms, 848
Routine checkups
  for infants, 549
  for preschoolers, 581–582
  for school-aged children, 594–595, 595f
  for toddlers, 563
Rubella, 931t
  development of immunity to, 278, 279b
  newborn infection with, 475t
  nonimmunity to, 278
  in pregnancy, 362–363
Rubella vaccine, in pregnancy, 362
Rubeola, 930t
Rugae
  penile, 46
  scrotal, in newborns, 297
  vaginal, 51
Rumination, 946
Runaway child, 525
Rupture, uterine, 255, 255b, 422
Rupture of membranes
  artificial, 241
  premature, 413–414
Russell traction, 884, 885f

S
Safety
  newborn, educating parents on, 321
  at pediatric hospital, 646, 646b
  in pregnancy, 146b, 155
Salicylates, for rheumatic fever, 809
Saliva production, in pregnancy, 123
Salmeterol, for asthma, 784, 785t
Salpingectomy, 384
Salpingitis, 383
Scabies, 905
Scalp pH, fetal, 180, 180t
Scalp pulse oximetry, fetal, 210t, 217
Scalp sampling, fetal, 210t, 217
Scarf sign, 453t
Scarlet fever, 932t
School-aged child. *See also* Growth and development, 6-10 years; *specific disorders*
  death and dying in, understanding of, 724–725, 724f
  growth and development of, 588–600
School lunch program, 37, 37f
School phobia, 940
Schools, health care at, 35, 35f
Schulze's mechanism, 179, 231
[monito]ring, in cerebral palsy, 762, 762f

Scoliosis, 892–896
  causes of, 892
  checkup for, 595, 595f
  definition and types of, 892
  diagnosis of, 892, 893f
  nursing process for brace for, 894–896
  treatment of, 892–894
    braces, 893–894, 893f
    electrical stimulation, 892–893
    overview, 892
    traction, 894, 894f
Scorpion bites, 909
Screening
  breast cancer, 60–61, 60f
  hearing, newborn, 17, 296, 317–318
  hypothyoidism, prenatal, 138
  multiple-marker, 142
  neonatal, for injury prevention, 317–318, 317b, 318f
  newborn, 317–318, 317b, 318f
  prenatal (*See* Prenatal screening and testing)
  triple-marker, 142
  vision, 745–747, 746f
  women's health, 49–63
    breast cancer, 60–61, 60f
    overview, 59–60
    pelvic examination and Pap smear, 61–62
    vulvar self-examination, 61–63
Scrotum, 46–47, 46f, 48f
Scrotum assessment, newborn, 297
Scurvy, 130, 830
Sebaceous glands, 899–900
Seborrheic dermatitis, 900
Sebum, 902
Secobarbital, for labor/birth pain, 190, 192t
Secondary prevention, 31. *See also specific topics*
Secondary sex characteristics, 53, 606
Secretory phase, 54f, 55
Sedatives. *See also specific sedatives*
  on breast-fed infant, 967
  for labor and birth pain, 190, 192t
Seizure disorders, 756–759
  antiepileptic-anticonvulsant agent for, 758t
  clinical manifestations of, 756–757
  diagnosis of, 757
  generalized seizures, 756–757
  nursing care for, 757–758
  partial seizures, 756
  status epilepticus, 757–759, 758t
  treatment of, 757
Seizures
  in children, acute/nonrecurrent, 754–755
  febrile, 754
Selective estrogen-receptor modifiers (SERMs), for dysmenorrhea, 64
Selective serotonin uptake inhibitors (SSRIs), on breast-fed infant, 967
Self-absorption, 529
Self-care teaching, prenatal, 151–155
  breast care, 152–153
  clothing, 153
  dental hygiene, 151–152
  employment, 153
  exercise, 152, 152b
  herbal remedies, 154–155
  hygiene, 152
  major components, 151b

  medications, 154, 154b
  nutritional intake, 151
  sexual activity, 153
  travel, 153, 154f
Self-examination
  breast, 60, 613f–614f
  on death and dying, in children, 722–724, 723b
  testicular, 47, 615f
  vulvar, 61–63
Self-identity, in adolescents, 605, 605f
Semen, 48
Seminal fluid, 48
Seminal vesicles, 48, 48f
Seminiferous tubules, 47, 48f
Semisitting position, 228t
Semivegetarian, 610
Sensorimotor phase, 529, 529f
Sensorineural hearing loss, 750
Sensory input, newborn, 319
Sensory/neurological disorders, in children, 743–771
  basic life support and CPR for, 769t, 770f
  cerebral palsy, 761–764, 762f
  drowning, 769–771, 769t, 770f
  ears and, 744, 745f
  eye conditions, 747–749
  eyes and, 744, 744f
  foreign bodies, ear or nose, 752–753
  H. influenzae meningitis, 675f, 759–761
  head injuries, 768–769
  hearing impairment, 749–752
  mental retardation, 764–768
  nervous system in, 743–744
  otitis media, 745f, 752–753
  Reye syndrome, 753–754, 754t
  seizure disorders, 756–759, 758t
  seizures, acute/nonrecurrent, 754–755
  vision impairment, 744–747
Separation, of newborns from parents, 6
Separation anxiety, in toddlers, 569, 569f
Seroconversion, 359t
Sex cells, 45, 99
Sex determination, 102, 102f
Sex education, 596
Sex inheritance, 102, 102f
Sexual abuse, of children, 714–715, 716t
Sexual activity, in pregnancy, 153
Sexual assault, 715
Sexual contact, 715
Sexual development, in preschoolers, 578
Sexual excitement, 55–56
Sexual history taking, 369b–370b
Sexuality
  adolescent, 606, 608, 608f, 612–614
  general, 55
Sexually transmitted diseases/infections (STDs/STIs)
  in adolescents, 614–615
  risk of, in first prenatal visit, 137, 137b
  sexual history for, 369b–370b
Sexually transmitted diseases/infections (STDs/STIs), in pregnancy, 364–372
  chlamydia, 364
  gonorrhea, 364–365
  HIV/AIDS, 366–368, 367b
  human papilloma virus, 365
  nursing process for, 368–372 (*See also under* Sexually transmitted infections (STIs), in pregnancy)

assessment, 368–370, 369b–370b
evaluation, 371–372
implementation, 370–371
nursing diagnoses, 370
outcome identification and planning, 370
trichomoniasis, 365–366
Sexual response cycle, 55–56
Sexual responsibility, in adolescents, 614–616
Shaken baby syndrome, 713
Shaking, of infant, 300f
Shame, 528
Shingles, in pregnancy, 361–362
Shivering, 667
Shock, postpartum, 445
Shortness of breath
in pregnancy, 122
prenatal care for, 147–149, 148t
Shoulder dystocia, 420–421, 421f
Shoulder presentation, 170, 411–412
Shriners health care clinics, 35
Shriners Hospital for Children, 13
Sibling order, 29
Siblings class, 159–160
Sickle cell anemia
in children, 813–815, 813f
in pregnancy, 355–356
Sickle cell crisis, 813–814
Sickle cell trait, 355
Side-lying position
for breast-feeding, 330, 331f
for procedures, 228t
Sight, 744, 745f
Sight, partial, 745
Silver nitrate, for burns, 915
Simian crease, 297
Simple fracture, 882f
Simple partial seizures, 756
Sims' position, 269, 269f
Single-parent family, 26, 28
Sitting position, for holding child, 666, 666f
Sitz bath, 271–272
Size variations, 451
Skeletal growth and maturation
in infants, 539
in preschoolers, 575
in school-aged children, 589–590, 590f
Skeletal system defects, congenital, 501–504
definition of, 501
hip dysplasia, 502–504, 502f, 503f
talipes equinovarus, 501–502, 501f, 502f
Skeletal traction, 884, 885f
Skene's glands, 50
Skin. See also Integumentary system
growth and development of, 899–900
newborn, 292, 293b
assessment of, 292–294, 293b
care of, 321
preterm, 463–464, 464b
postpartum, 264
in pregnancy, 123
Skin allergies, 908
Skin disorders. See Integumentary disorders
Skin grafts, 915
Skin tags, newborn, 292
Skin testing
for allergies, 905
tuberculin, 799

Skin traction, 884, 885f
Skull, fetal, 170, 170f
Sleep
Back to Sleep campaign for, 17
early postpartum, 273–274
in infants, 552
in newborns, 273–274, 319
positioning for, 666
postpartum, 280
prenatal care for, 149t, 151
in preschoolers, 583
in toddlers, 567
twilight, 5
Small-for-gestational-age (SGA) newborn, 451–455
cause of, 451
clinical manifestations of, 453–454
complications of, 454
contributing factors to, 451–453, 453t, 454b
definition of, 451
nursing care for, 454
Smegma, newborn, 297
Smokeless tobacco, 944
Smoking
with cardiovascular disease in pregnancy, 354
cessation of, preconception, 70
in children, 944–945
on placental blood flow, 452
on pregnancy, 155
Snacks
for preschoolers, 581b
for school-aged children, 594
Snake bites, 910
Snellen E chart, 746, 746f
Snuff, 944
Social adaptation, newborn, 288
Social history, in children, 627
Socialization, physical, 26–27
Sociologic changes
on child and adolescent health status, 15–16, 16t
on maternal–child health, 3–4
Sodium restriction, for cardiovascular disease in pregnancy, 353
Solid foods, in first year of life, 546–549
food preparation, 546, 546f, 548
infant feeding, 546, 546f
self-feeding, 548–549, 548f
Solitary independent play, 579
Soma cells, 99
Sonogram, in first prenatal visit, 138–139
Spasmodic laryngitis, 779–780
Spasms, infantile, 757
Special Supplemental Nutrition Program for Women, Infants, and Children (WIC), 13, 13f
Specimen collection
nose and throat, 672–673
stool, 674
urine, 673–674, 673f
Specimen collection procedures in children, 672–675
blood, 674, 674f
lumbar puncture, 675, 675f
nose and throat, 672–673
stool, 674
urine, 673–674, 673f
Speed, 946
Sperm (spermatozoa), 45, 47, 49t

Spermatic cord, 47–48, 48f
Spermatid, 100, 100f
Spermatocyte, 100, 100f
Spermatogenesis, 47, 48f, 100–101, 100f
Spermicidal foam, 614
Spermicides, 73f, 76
Spider bites, 909
Spina bifida, 298, 479–482, 479f
clinical manifestations of, 479–480, 479f
degrees and types of, 479, 479f
diagnosis of, 480
nursing process for, 480–482
treatment of, 480
Spina bifida cystica, 480
Spina bifida occulta, 479, 479f
Spina bifida with meningocele, 479, 479f
Spina bifida with myelomeningocele, 479–480, 479f
Spinal block
for labor and birth pain, 193–195, 193t, 194f
total epidural, 195
Spinal headaches, from epidural anesthesia, 195–196
Spine, 881. See also Musculoskeletal disorders
Spine curvature
newborn, assessment of, 298
in pregnancy, 122, 122f
Spinnbarkheit, 55, 75, 75f
Spiral fracture, 882f
Spirituality, family in, 27
Spironolactone, for congestive heart failure, 806
Spongy body, 46, 47f
Spontaneous abortion, 384–387
causes of, 384–385
clinical manifestations and types of, 385–386, 385t
definition and epidemiology of, 384
nursing care for, 386–387
self-care after, 386
treatment of, 385t, 386
Square window, 453t
Squatting position, 228t
Standard days method (SDM), 75–76, 76f
Standard precautions, 959–960
Startle reflex. See Moro reflex
State Child Health Insurance Program (SCHIP, CHIP), 13
Station, fetal, 172, 173f
Status
on admission for labor/birth
fetal, 203–204
maternal, 204–205
labor, maternal, 205–208, 206f
Status asthmaticus, in pregnancy, 357
Status epilepticus, 757–759, 758t
in preeclampsia-eclampsia, 397
in pregnancy, 359
Steatorrhea, 832
Stenotic valves, in pregnancy, 353
Stepfamily, 28
Stepping reflex, 298, 300f
Sterilization, 73f
female, 83
male, 83
transcervical, 73f
Steroids, anabolic, 945
Stethoscope, pediatric, 540, 540f
Stigma, 702

Stings, insect, 910
Stool monitoring, newborn, 320–321, 842
Stool specimen collection, 674
Stork bites, 293b
Strabismus, 295, 747–748, 748f
Streptococcus group B (GBS) infection, newborn, 474t
Stress, cold, 286, 289, 306
Stress ulcer, 915
Stretch marks, breast, in pregnancy, 121
Striae, 873
Striae, breast, in pregnancy, 121
Stridor, 779
Stuttering, in preschoolers, 576
Stye, 749
Subcutaneous administration, in children, 687
Subjective data, 21, 624
Subjective data collection, in children
    client and family caregiver interview in, 623–624, 624f
    client history in, 624–628
        allergies, medications, and substance abuse, 628
        biographic data, 624–627, 625f–626f
        chief complaint, 627
        developmental level, 628
        family health history, 627
        health history, 627
        lifestyle, 628
        review of systems, 627, 627f
Substance abuse, 941–945. See also specific substances
    in adolescents, 616
    alcohol, 943–944
    amphetamines, 945
    anabolic steroids, 945
    analgesics, 945
    in children, 942t
    cocaine, 944–945
    definition of, 155, 941
    dependence, withdrawal, and tolerance in, 941
    depressants/hypnotics, 945
    Ecstasy, 945
    educating school-aged children on, 596–597, 597b
    epidemiology of, 941
    hallucinogens, 945
    marijuana, 944
    miscellaneous abused drugs, 945
    narcotic, 945
    parental, on children, 718–719
    on pregnancy, 155
    prevention of, 942
        in adults, 942
        in children, 597
    resources on, 943
    tobacco, 944
Substance use
    definition of, 155
    on pregnancy, 155
Substance withdrawal
    in children, 941
    neonatal, 473, 473f
Succenturiate placenta, 423t
Sucking
    newborn, 331–332, 331f
    preterm newborn, 462
Sucking calluses, 295
Sucking reflex, 295–296, 298, 300f, 327

Suctioning, nasal/oral, 671, 671f
Sudden infant death syndrome (SIDS), 468–469, 469f
Suffocation, educating parents on, 321
Suicide, 940–941
Sulfadiazine, for burns, 915
Sulfonamide, on breast-fed infant, 967
Supine hypotensive syndrome, 122, 122f, 354
Supplements for mother, 130
    in pregnancy, 130
        iron, 127, 128t, 130
        iron, for anemia, 356
        Special Supplemental Nutrition Program for Women, Infants, and Children in, 13, 13f
Supplements for newborn
    during breast-feeding, 333–334
    during formula-feeding, 338
Support person, for labor and birth, 156
Suppressive therapy, 359t
Suprapubic pressure, 420, 421f
Surfactant
    in fetus, 107
    in newborn, 284–285
Surfactant replacement therapy, 457
Surrogacy, ethical issues in, 9
Surrogate parenting, 91, 569–570, 569f, 570f
Suspensions, 684
Sustenance, physical, family in, 26
Suture lines, 881
Sutures, newborn skull, 294–295
Swaddling, 313, 318, 320f
Swallowing reflex, 298, 828
Sweat glands, 899
Sweats, menopausal, 91–92
Symbols, Joint Commission's "Do Not Use" list of, 964
Sympathetic ophthalmia, 748
Symptothermal method, 75
Syndactyly, 297
Synovitis, 890
Syphilis
    cause and spread of, 921, 922t
    clinical manifestations of, 921–923, 922t
    newborn infection with, 475t
    in pregnancy, 361
    treatment of, 923
Syrups, 684

T
Tachycardia
    fetal, in labor/birth, 213
    in pregnancy, 353
Tailor position, 412
Talipes equinovarus, 481, 501–502, 501f, 502f
Tamoxifen, for dysmenorrhea, 64
Tantrums, temper, 560
Tattoos, 611
Teaching. See Health education; specific topics
Teen pregnancy, 375–377
Teeth, precocious, 296
Telangiectatic nevi, 293b
Temperament, 520
Temperature, body, 666
    in children, 632–633, 633f
    controlling environmental factors for, 667
    elevated, 666–667

high, procedures for, 666–667, 667b
    in infants, 540
    in newborns, axillary, 290, 290f, 290t, 305
    normal, 666
    rectal, 666
Temper tantrums, 560
Temporal temperatures, in children, 632
Tendons, 880. See also Musculoskeletal disorders
Tent, oxygen, 670–671, 670t, 671f
Teratogenicity, 781
Teratogens, 153
    on fetus, 111–112, 111t
    types of, 111–112, 111t
Terbutaline sulfate, for asthma, 784, 785t
Term, 451
Tertiary prevention, 31
Testes, 47, 48f
Testicular self-examination (TSE), 47, 615f
Testosterone
    on male reproduction, 49t
    testes production of, 47
Tetanus, 929t
Tetracycline
    for acne, 903
    on breast-fed infant, 967
    for syphilis, 923
Thalassemia, 815–816
Thalassemia major, 815–816
Thanatologist, 724
Theophylline, for asthma, 784, 785t
Therapeutic abortion, 86, 86t
Therapeutic play
    postoperative, 656, 656f
    preoperative, 652, 652f
Thermoneutral environment, 306
Thermoregulation, newborn, 286
    nursing care for, 306, 306f
    in preterm newborn, 456, 461, 461f
Thermoregulatory adaptation, in newborn, 286–287, 286f
Thiamine. See Vitamin B$_1$ (thiamine)
Thiazide diuretics, for congestive heart failure, 806
Threatened abortion, 385t
Three-month pill, contraceptive, 73f
Threshold, pain, 185
Throat specimen collection, 672–673
Thrombus, 443. See also Pulmonary embolism (PE); Venous thromboembolism (VTE), postpartum
Thrombus prevention
    after cesarean, 276
    early postpartum, 273
Thrush, 296
Thyroid medications, on breast-fed infant, 967
Tick bites, 909–910, 932t
Ticks, wood, 909
Time out, 248
Tinea, 903
Tinea capitis, 903
Tinea corporis, 903
Tinea cruris, 904
Tinea pedis, 903–904
Tissue fluid, 690, 690f
TLSO brace, 893–894, 893f
Tobacco. See also Smoking
    abuse of, 944–945
    on pregnancy, 155

Tocodynamometer, 209, 210t
Tocolytic, 411
Tocolytic agents, 415, 416t
Toddler, growth and development of, 557–570. *See also* Growth and development, 1-3 years
Toe assessment, newborn, 297
Toileting, in preschooler, 582–583
Toilet training, 565–567, 565f
Tolerance
    pain, 185
    substance abuse, 941–945
Tolnaftate
    for tinea corporis, 903
    for tinea pedis, 904
Tongue, in children, 776
Tonic-clonic seizures, 756
Tonic neck reflex, 299, 300f
Tonsillectomy, 777–779
Tonsillitis, 777–778
Tonsils, 776, 777
Tooth eruption, in infants, 539–540, 540f
Total body surface area (TBSA), 913, 914f
Total parenteral nutrition (TPN)
    for burn patients, 913, 920
    for children, 692–693, 693f
Touch, for labor/birth pain, 187t, 188, 190f
Toxic ingestions
    in children, 849–850, 850t
    in toddlers, 568–569
Toxic shock syndrome (TSS), 66–67
Toxin, 928b. *See also specific toxins*
Toxoid, 928b
Toxoplasmosis, on pregnancy, 360–361
Tracheoesophageal fistula, 496–498, 497f
Tracheostomy, 670t, 671
Traction
    for fractures, 884, 885f, 886–887
    for scoliosis, 894, 894f
Transabdominal ultrasound, in prenatal care, 141
Transcervical sterilization, 73f
Transdermal patch, contraceptive, 73f, 80f, 82
Transient tachypnea of the newborn (TTN), 467–468
Transition phase
    in labor, 178–179, 178t, 224–225, 225f
    in newborn (*See* Newborn transition)
Transition stage, of labor, 178–179, 178t
Transmission
    mode of, 928b
    perinatal, 359t
    vertical, 359t
Transmission-based precautions, 646–648, 959–960. *See also* Infection control
Transporting, of infants and small children, 666
Transverse lie, 170, 170f, 411–412
Trauma prevention
    in first stage of labor, 222
    in second stage of labor, 226–227
Travel, in pregnancy, 153, 154f
Treatments. *See* Procedures, in children; *specific treatments*
Treponema pallidum infection
    of children, 921
    of newborn, 475t
    in pregnancy, 361
Tretinoin, for acne, 903
Triamcinolone, for asthma, 784, 785t

Trichomoniasis, in pregnancy, 365–366, 368–372. *See also* Sexually transmitted infections (STIs), nursing process for
Tricyclic antidepressants, on breast-fed infant, 967
Triple-marker screening, 142
Triplets, 113, 403–404
Tripod position, 780, 780f
Trisomy 21, 508–509, 508f, 509f
Trough crutches, 887
True knot, 423t
True labor, 175–176, 176t
True pelvis, 167, 168f
Trust
    in newborns, 313
    theories on, 527t, 528
Tubal embryo transfer (TET), 90
Tubal ligation, 73f, 83
Tubal pregnancy, 383–384, 383f
Tuberculin skin test, 799
Tuberculin testing, of adolescents, 611
Tuberculosis, pulmonary, 799–800
Tunica albuginea, 46, 47f
Turner syndrome, 509–510
Turtle sign, 420
24-hour urine specimen, 674
Twilight sleep, 5
Twin pregnancy, 113, 113f, 122
Twins, 403–404
Twin-to-twin transfusion syndrome, 113
Tympanic temperatures, in children, 622f, 632
Type 1 diabetes mellitus. *See* Diabetes mellitus (DM), in pregnancy; Diabetes mellitus (DM) type 1
Type 2 diabetes mellitus, 862–863

U

Ultrasonography, in prenatal care, 140–141, 140f, 141b
Umbilical arteries, to placenta, 109, 110f
Umbilical cord, 107f, 108–109
    abnormalities of, 422, 423t
    prolapse of, 421–422, 422f
    stump infection of, 306–308
    velamentous insertion of, 423t
Umbilical hernia, 499, 499f
Umbilical vein, 109, 110f
Underwater birth method, 158b
Unfinished business, 726
Unilateral, 491
Unoccupied behavior, 579
Uppers, 946
Upright position, for holding child, 665, 666f
Ureters, in pregnancy, 123
Urethra, male, 46, 47f, 48f
Urethral meatus, 50
Urge-to-push method, 226–227
Urinary changes, in pregnancy, 123
Urinary frequency, in pregnancy, 123
Urinary system, postpartum, 264
Urinary tract, in children, 867, 867f
Urinary tract infections (UTIs)
    in children, 868–870
    postpartum, 437, 440–441
        clinical manifestations of, 437
        definition and causes of, 437
        diagnosis of, 437
        nursing care for, 437, 440–441
        treatment of, 437
    in pregnant diabetics, 351

Urination
    frequent, prenatal care for, 147, 151
    involuntary, 870
Urine, in children, 863. *See also* Genitourinary disorders
Urine monitoring, newborn, 320–321
Urine specimen collection, 673–674, 673f
Urostomy, 672
Urticaria, 830, 908
Urushiol, 909
Uterine artery, 53, 53f
Uterine artery embolization, for uterine fibroids, 68
Uterine atony
    definition of, 426
    hemorrhage from, 426
        clinical manifestations of, 428, 430t
        nursing process for, 428–432 (*See also under* Hemorrhage, postpartum)
        treatment of, 428
Uterine bleeding, atypical, 63
Uterine contractions, during labor and birth
    first stage
        active phase, 221
        transition phase, 224
        monitoring, 209–211
            comparison of techniques for, 209, 210t
            external methods of, 209, 210t
            internal methods of, 210t, 211
            palpation in, 209
    second stage, 225
Uterine contractions, postpartum, 261
Uterine cycle, 54f, 55
Uterine dysfunction, 410
Uterine fibroids, 67–68
Uterine fundus, 107f, 120
Uterine incisions, for cesarean birth, 245–247, 246f
Uterine involution, 261–262
Uterine irritability, 411
Uterine isthmus, 51, 52f
Uterine leiomyomata, 67–68
Uterine prolapse, 68–70, 69f
Uterine rupture, 255, 255b, 422
Uterine subinvolution, 432
Uterine venous plexus, 53
Uteroplacental insufficiency, on fetal heart rate, 215f, 216
Uterosacral ligaments, 52
Uterus, 51–52, 51f, 52f
    boggy, 262
    postpartum, 261–262, 262f
    in pregnancy, 120, 120f
Utilization review, 10

V

Vaccine, 928b
Vacuum-assisted delivery, 242, 243f
Vacuum extractor, 242, 243f
Vagina, 50–51, 51f
    in passageway, 169, 169f
    postpartum, 262–263
    in pregnancy, 120–121
Vaginal artery, 53, 53f
Vaginal birth after cesarean (VBAC), 244, 254–255
    contraindications to, 254
    nursing care in, 255, 255b
    prerequisites for, 254
    risks and benefits of, 254–255

Vaginal care, postpartum, 278–279
Vaginal contraceptive ring, 73f, 80f, 82
Vaginal discharge, prenatal care for, 147
Vaginal examination
    on admission for labor/birth, 206–208, 206f
    in first prenatal visit, 137
Vaginal opening, 50
Vaginal venous plexus, 53
Vaginitis, 876t, 877
Valproic acid
    as anticonvulsant, 758t
    on breast-fed infant, 967
Variability, 213
Variable deceleration, FHR (variables), 214–215, 215f
    first stage, active phase, 221
    in second stage, 225–226
Varicella zoster immunoglobulin (VZIG), in pregnancy, 362
Varicella zoster virus (varicella, VZV), 361–362, 931t
Varicose veins, prenatal care for, 149t
Vascular access port, 692
Vascular hemophilia, 817
Vas deferens, 47–48, 48f
Vasectomy, 73f, 83
Vasocongestion
    in pregnancy, 122
    in sexual response cycle, 55–56
Vasopressin (DDAVP), for hemophilia, 817
Vasospasm, in preeclampsia-eclampsia, 395–396
Vastus lateralis muscle, intramuscular injection via, 688t
Vegan
    adolescent, 610
    pregnancy in, 130–131
Vegetarian
    adolescent, 610
    pregnancy in, 130–131
Velamentous insertion of umbilical cord, 423t
Venipuncture, 692
Venous stasis, in pregnancy, 121
Venous thromboembolism (VTE), postpartum, 441–443
    deep vein thrombosis, 441–442
    definition and incidence of, 441
    pulmonary embolism, 442–443
    risk factors for, 441, 441b
Ventriculoperitoneal shunting (VP shunt), for hydrocephalus, 483, 483f
Ventrogluteal intramuscular injection, 688t
Vernix caseosa (vernix), 292, 312
Version, external, 412, 412f
Vertebral column, 881. See also Musculoskeletal disorders
Vertex presentation, 171, 171f
Vertical transmission, 359t
Very low birth weight (VLBW), 451
Vestibule, 50
Vibroacoustic stimulation, 145
Vigorous pushing, 226
Violence. See also Abuse, in family; Child abuse

cycle of, 372–373, 373f
domestic, 718
in schools, 617
Viral load, 359t
Vision, 744, 744f
Vision impairment, 744–747
    blindness, 745
    clinical manifestations and diagnosis of, 745–747, 746f
    nursing care for, 747
    partial sight, 745
    refractive errors, 744–745
    treatment and education on, 747
Vision screening, 745–747, 746f
Visual development, in preschoolers, 575
Vital signs
    in children, 631–636
        apnea monitor, 634, 635f
        blood pressure, 635–636, 635f, 635t
        pulse, 633, 633t, 638f
        pulse oximetry, 634, 634f
        respirations, 633–634, 634f
        temperature, 632–633, 633f
    in newborn, 290, 290f, 290t
    postpartum, 263–264
Vitamin A
    good sources of, 965
    in pregnancy, 128t, 129
Vitamin B$_1$ (thiamine)
    deficiency of, 830
    good sources of, 965
    in pregnancy, 128t
Vitamin B$_2$
    deficiency of, 830
    in pregnancy, 128t
Vitamin B$_3$ (niacin)
    good sources of, 965
    in pregnancy, 128t
Vitamin B$_6$ (pyridoxine)
    for morning sickness, 147
    in pregnancy, 128t, 130
    for premenstrual syndrome, 65
Vitamin B$_9$ (folic acid)
    for diabetic mothers, 347
    preconception, 70
    in pregnancy, 128t, 129
Vitamin B$_{12}$ (cobalamine), in pregnancy, 130
Vitamin C
    good sources of, 965
    in pregnancy, 129t, 130
Vitamin D
    good sources of, 965
    in pregnancy, 127, 129t
Vitamin D deficiency, 829
Vitamin K, for newborns, 288, 308
Vitamin requirements, in pregnancy, 128t–129t, 129–130
Volunteer service organizations, health care at, 35
Vomiting
    after formula-feeding, 338
    in children, 838
Von Willebrand disease, 817
Vulva, 49–50, 49f
Vulvar self-examination, 61–63

W
Warfarin, in pregnancy, 353
Warmer, radiant, 461, 461f
Warts, genital, 365
Water, 689–690
Water Bugs and Dragonflies, 726, 726f
Water injections, intradermal, for labor/birth pain, 187t, 190, 190f
Water therapy, for labor/birth pain, 187t, 188–189, 190f
Weaning, 549
Weight
    on admission for labor/birth, 205, 206f
    in children, 518, 630–631, 630f, 631f
    in infants, 539, 539f
    in newborn, 291, 292t
    in newborn, daily, 332
    in school-aged children, 589
Weight gain, in pregnancy, 125–126, 151
Weight loss, postpartum, 264
Wellness nursing diagnoses, 21
West nomogram, 683–684, 684f
Wharton's jelly, 108–109, 308
Wheezing, 782
Whiteheads, 902
Whooping cough, 929t
Wilms' tumor, 875
Witch's milk, 297
Withdrawal, 72–74
    substance
        in children, 941
        in neonates, 473, 473f
Withdrawal symptoms, 941
Womb, 51–52, 51f
Women, Infants, and Children (WIC) Food Program, 549
Women's health issues, 59–70
    reproductive tract disorders, 63–70
        (See also Reproductive tract disorders, female)
    screening, 49–63
        breast cancer, 60–61, 60f
        overview, 59–60
        pelvic examination and Pap smear, 61–62
        vulvar self-examination, 61–63
Wood ticks, 909
Working mothers, 29–30
Wound infection, postpartum, 434–436
    clinical manifestations of, 434–435
    diagnosis of, 435
    nursing care for, 436
    risk factors for, 434
    sites of, 434, 435f
    treatment of, 435

X
Xenografts, 915

Z
Zinc, in pregnancy, 127, 129t
Zona pellucida, 102
Zygote, 102, 103f
Zygote intrafallopian transfer (ZIFT), 90